MW01532692

Clinical removable partial prosthodontics

Clinical removable partial prosthodontics

KENNETH L. STEWART, D.D.S., F.A.C.D., F.A.C.P.

Professor, Department of Prosthodontics, The University of Texas Health Science Center at San Antonio, Dental School, San Antonio, Texas

KENNETH D. RUDD, D.D.S., F.A.C.D., F.I.C.D., F.A.C.P.

Associate Dean for Continuing Dental Education, Professor, Department of Prosthodontics, The University of Texas Health Science Center at San Antonio, Dental School, San Antonio, Texas

WILLIAM A. KUEBKER, D.D.S., M.S., F.A.C.P.

Associate Professor, Department of Prosthodontics, The University of Texas Health Science Center at San Antonio, Dental School, San Antonio, Texas

with **1935** illustrations and **3** four-color illustrations

The C. V. Mosby Company

ST. LOUIS • TORONTO • LONDON 1983

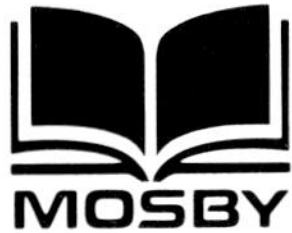

A TRADITION OF PUBLISHING EXCELLENCE

Editor: Darlene A. Warfel
Assistant editor: Melba J. Steube
Manuscript editor: Teri Merchant
Book design: Jeanne Bush
Cover design: Suzanne Oberholtzer
Production: Linda R. Stalnaker, Margaret B. Bridenbaugh, Jeanne A. Gulledge

Printed in the United States of America

The C.V. Mosby Company
11830 Westline Industrial Drive, St. Louis, Missouri 63141

Library of Congress Cataloging in Publication Data

Stewart, Kenneth L.
Clinical removable partial prosthodontics.

Bibliography: p.
Includes index.
1. Partial dentures, Removable. I. Rudd, Kenneth D. II. Kuebker, William A. III. Title.
[DNLM: 1. Denture, Partial, Removable. WU 515 S849c]
RK665.S73 617.6′92 81-22399
ISBN 0-8016-4813-0 AACR2

C/CB/B 9 8 7 6 5 4 3 2 1 01/B/038

Contributors

JAMES S. BRUDVIK, D.D.S.

Associate Professor, Department of Prosthodontics, University of Washington School of Dentistry, Seattle, Washington

MADELINE KURRASCH, B.A., B.S., D.D.S.

Assistant Professor, Department of Removable Prosthodontics, University of California, Los Angeles, School of Dentistry, Los Angeles, California

MERRILL C. MENSOR, Jr., B.A., D.D.S., F.I.C.D.

Consultant in Removable Prosthodontics, Veterans Administration, Wadsworth, Palo Alto, and San Francisco, California; International Circuit Courses Faculty, American Prosthodontic Society; Private Practice, San Mateo, California; Formerly Assistant Clinical Professor, Department of Fixed Prosthodontics, University of the Pacific, School of Dentistry, San Francisco, California

STEPHEN M. PAREL, D.D.S.

Professor and Head, Division of Maxillofacial Prosthodontics, The University of Texas Health Science Center at San Antonio, Dental School, San Antonio, Texas

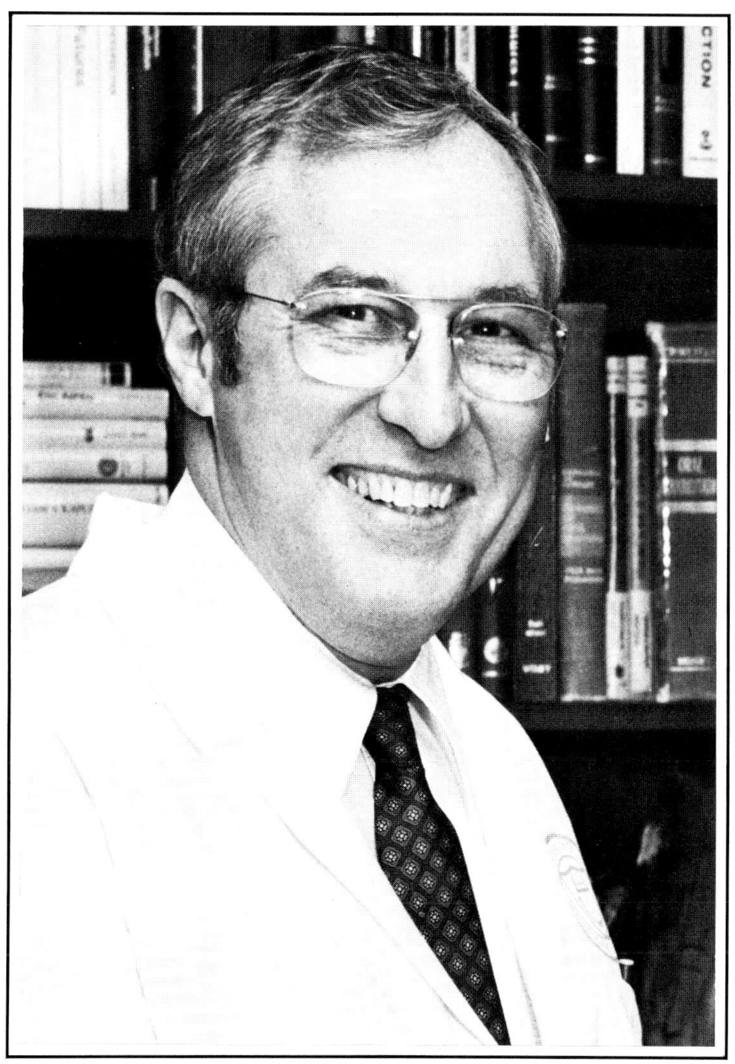

John Joseph Sharry
1925-1981

A dear friend and respected colleague, John Sharry was highly talented in many disciplines of the arts and sciences, well read, an interesting conversationalist and humorist, but most of all deeply and sincerely interested in people. He was an inspirational teacher, a competent clinician, and a firm believer in his country and the concepts upon which it was founded. He shall be sorely missed, but his memory and his beliefs will live forever through his students and the many lives he touched.

Preface

At first thought, a new text in the field of removable partial dentures seemed to us redundant and unnecessary. Several widely accepted books were available and to repeat the information contained in them in a different order did not seem a challenging or a worthwhile project. However, after analyzing the result of years spent teaching dental students, working with recent graduates of dental schools throughout the country, and treating a wide variety of patients in all phases of prosthodontics, we began to realize the possibility of creating a textbook with a new and different concept in its approach to treatment. Before the advent of this book a dental student or general practitioner found it necessary to refer from the front to the back to the center of available texts in order to follow the logical sequence of steps required to treat a partially edentulous patient.

It is the intent of this book that each chapter build upon the preceding chapter in the same order that patient treatment occurs. In this sequence a student or practitioner can develop a basic understanding of removable partial denture components and principles of design and can apply this knowledge in a clinical situation. Relating basic information to clinical practice enables students and practitioners to realize that the two do not exist as separate entities but flow together smoothly and intimately if the relationship can be demonstrated throughout the learning process.

The first chapter prepares the reader to accept and assimilate the material that will follow. A discussion of scientific terminology that is essential to understanding precedes the purposes and indications for removable partial dentures. A knowledge of a system of classifying partially edentulous arches is necessary so that the student, on learning the classification of the partially edentulous arch, can envision the arch and the design factors that must later be considered in carrying out treatment.

The next two chapters describe the component parts of the removable partial denture, knowledge that is essential before the principles and construction of the partial denture can be understood.

The principles concerning the function of the removable partial denture are discussed next, with the emphasis on methods of controlling stresses and forces taking place on the partial denture and the supporting structures. The importance of this chapter is realized when the design of the prosthesis is accomplished.

Chapters 5 and 6 discuss the examination, diagnosis, and treatment planning appointments for the partially edentulous patient. Clinical and laboratory procedures used in gathering data are described. Evaluation of the diagnostic findings, the effect of these findings on the treatment of the patient, and the development of a treatment plan are discussed.

Chapters 7 and 8 are devoted to the survey and design of removable partial dentures. Two philosophies of design are presented: Chapter 7 covers broad stress distribution, and in Chapter 8 Madeline Kurrasch discusses I-bar removable partial denture design. Both philosophies are widely accepted, and either will give excellent clinical results if the complete concepts are followed and attention is given to details in planning, constructing, and delivering the partial dentures. This book intends to favor neither approach but allows the teacher or practitioner to select the one that best serves the interest of the patient.

The preliminary planning for the partial denture is followed by mouth preparation, a frequently overlooked step in treatment, and the making of the master cast. Methods of making preliminary jaw relation records for submitting the casts to the laboratory are described. For patients requiring certain types of anterior tooth replacements, the clinical procedure for trying in the artificial teeth is included.

In Chapter 11 James Brudvik describes the laboratory procedures for constructing the cast framework for a removable partial denture. Most students and practitioners will not construct frameworks, but the knowledge of the procedures involved will enable the dentist to recognize deficiencies or excellence in technique performance.

Following framework construction, discussions of clinical appointments necessary for the completion and delivery of the prosthesis are presented. These appointments include fitting of the framework (an almost totally ignored but vital step in producing a favorable prognosis of the partial denture), making a corrected cast impression to ensure proper distribution of forces to the edentulous ridge, establishing a final jaw relation and setting the artificial teeth, trying in the tooth setup and the laboratory procedures required to complete the partial denture, delivering the prosthesis, and correcting the problems that may be encountered after insertion. These clinical appointments appear in the order in which the patient is treated and should help the student relate one phase of treatment to the others.

The remaining chapters deal with other considerations in removable partial prosthodontics. Chapter 18 discusses the use of temporary and immediate partial dentures, a service important in the general practice of dentistry.

Another clinical situation frequently encountered is the patient who requires a complete denture opposing a removable partial denture. This combination is presented in Chapter 19.

Chapter 20 is devoted to other forms of the removable partial denture: the guide plane removable partial denture to support weakened teeth, the swing-lock partial denture, overdenture abutments in partial denture design, and the unilateral removable partial denture.

In Chapter 21 James Brudvik describes methods of relining and repairing partial dentures, something that dentists in a busy practice must be capable of doing accurately and efficiently.

Internal attachments and other forms of resilient and nonresilient retainers are discussed by Merrill Mensor in Chapter 22. This is a type of removable partial denture that has great appeal to patients conscious of esthetics.

Maxillofacial prosthetic dentistry is able to return severely disfigured or handicapped patients to useful, productive lives. Stephen Parel presents fundamental knowledge necessary to practice this subspecialty of prosthodontics.

For years primary emphasis in dentistry has centered on treating the child and the young adult. Recently, prompted by the added longevity of the population that has resulted in a sizable percentage increase in elderly patients, the study of geriatric dentistry has begun to receive the attention it deserves. James Brudvik discusses important aspects of treating the partially edentulous older adult.

Kenneth L. Stewart
Kenneth D. Rudd
William A. Kuebker

Acknowledgments

It would be improper not to recognize those individuals who have collectively made this book something more than another laborious task. Special thanks of the authors go to the contributors Drs. Kurrasch, Brudvik, Mensor, and Parel. Their dedication and enthusiasm made a difficult sojourn easier.

To Mrs. Wanita Morrow we offer our deepest respect and admiration for her outstanding ability for turning our frenetic henscratching into a readable manuscript—a monumental accomplishment.

To Dr. Rudd's son, Ken E. Rudd, our special thanks for the professionalism and outstanding quality of the photographs that appear in the book.

Dr. William Kuebker is responsible for producing the illustrations and taking the photographs that broaden the scope of the text.

We would be remiss in not making the supreme acknowledgment—to Harriet (Stewart), Helen (Rudd), and Joan (Kuebker) go our undying love for the patience, understanding, and encouragement that we all need so badly and that only a wife can provide.

Removable partial prosthodontics can make a significant contribution to the general health and welfare of the partially edentulous patient. The clinical practice of this phase of dentistry must remain in the hands of the biologically educated dentist. The public must not, for false reasons of economy, allow partially educated lay individuals to practice professional aspects of dentistry.

It is with the hope that this book will contribute to the ability of the dentist to deal with all problems in removable partial prosthodontics that the authors have produced this work.

Contents

Clinical removable partial prosthodontics

1 Introduction and classification

TERMINOLOGY

Several efforts have been made to standardize dental terminology to make communication in the field simpler and more effective, beginning with Dr. Louis Ottofy's compilation of accepted dental terms in 1923.

Undoubtedly the greatest step forward, particularly in prosthodontic terminology, was made by the Academy of Denture Prosthetics, the first and perhaps most sophisticated prosthodontic group. In 1956, it published the *Glossary of Prosthodontic Terms* and has since updated the glossary several times.*

Another significant advance was made in 1963 with the publication of *Current Clinical Dental Terminology*, edited by the late Dr. Carl O. Boucher. A second edition of this book was published in 1974. The glossary includes accepted terms in all disciplines of dentistry.

Because of the existence of these two fine sources of accepted terminology, it is not necessary to repeat definitions. However, to ensure that the terminology used throughout this book will be understood by all readers, some of the most frequently encountered words are defined. In addition, the terms used in this book are limited to those that are recognized as acceptable.

The art or science of replacing absent body parts is termed *prosthetics*, and any artificial part is called a *prosthesis*. As applied to dentistry, the terms *prosthodontics* and *dental prosthesis* are used. Prosthodontics is the branch of dental art and science that pertains to the replacement of missing teeth and oral tissues to restore and maintain oral form, function, appearance, and health. There are three major divisions of prosthodontics: fixed prosthodontics, maxillofacial prosthodontics, and removable prosthodontics (Fig. 1-1).

Fixed prosthodontics is devoted to replacing coronal portions of teeth or one or more missing natural teeth and their associated parts with denture prostheses that are not designed to be removed by the patient. This book discusses fixed prosthodontics only as it relates to removable partial dentures.

*This glossary first appeared in the March, 1956, issue of *The Journal of Prosthetic Dentistry* (published by the C.V. Mosby Co., St. Louis). The latest reprint, published in 1977, can be obtained from the Educational and Research Foundation of Prosthodontics, 211 E. Chicago Ave., Chicago, Ill. 60611.

Maxillofacial prosthodontics, according to Boucher, is "the branch of prosthodontics concerned with the restoration of stomatognathic and associated facial structures that have been affected by disease, injury, surgery, or congenital defect."

Removable prosthodontics is devoted to replacement of missing teeth and contiguous tissues with prostheses designed to be removed by the wearer. It includes two disciplines: removable complete and removable partial prosthodontics. This book deals with the latter. As seen in Fig. 1-1, a removable partial denture prosthesis may be extracoronal (Fig. 1-2) or intracoronal (Fig. 1-3), depending on what type of retention is used to keep it in the mouth.

The terms *prosthesis* and *appliance* are often confused, but they are not interchangeable. *Appliance* is correctly used only to refer to a device worn by a patient in the course of treatment, such as an orthodontic appliance, surgical splint, or space maintainer (Fig. 1-4). A *prosthesis* is an artificial replacement for a missing body part. *Prosthesis, denture, denture prosthesis,* and *restoration* may be used synonymously.

An *abutment* is any tooth that supports a fixed or removable prosthesis. A fixed partial denture (Fig. 1-5) is cemented over the abutment teeth, whereas a removable prosthesis is attached by other methods that are discussed later.

It is regrettable that the term *bridge* continues to be used; it is subprofessional in its connotation and nondescriptive in its scope. Although the word has meaning for the lay person, it does not adequately describe the prosthesis. Many observers believe that *bridge* emphasizes the mechanical aspects of dentistry and that the biologic term *denture* emphasizes the health aspect of the service. In recent years there has been a tendency to avoid the term *bridge*, particularly in teaching centers, and to refer to departments working in this modality as fixed prosthodontic departments rather than crown and bridge departments.

One method used to differentiate types of removable partial dentures is to refer to the form of attachment of the denture to the remaining natural teeth. The fixation device, any form of attachment applied directly to an abutment tooth and used for the fixation of a prosthesis, is called a *retainer*. The most commonly used form of

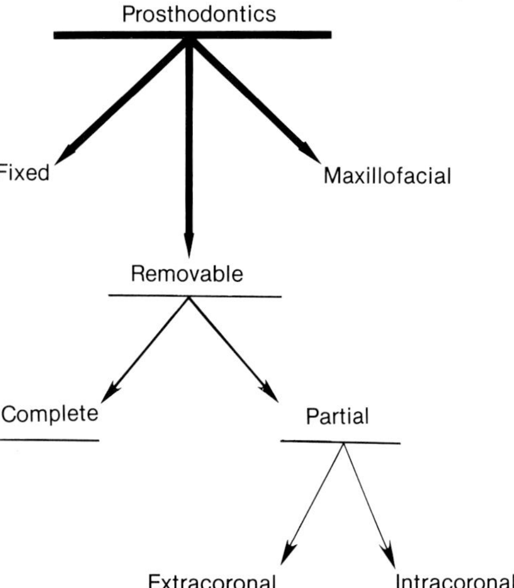

Fig. 1-1. Branches of prosthodontics.

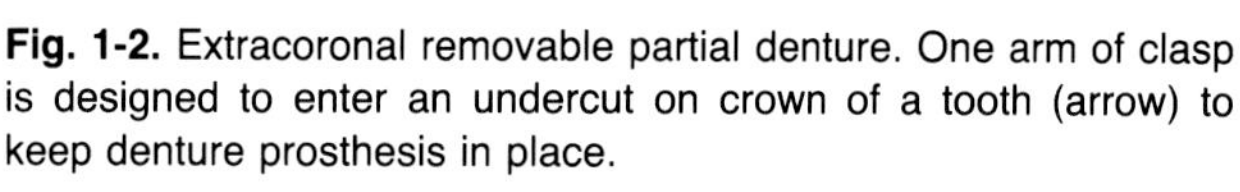

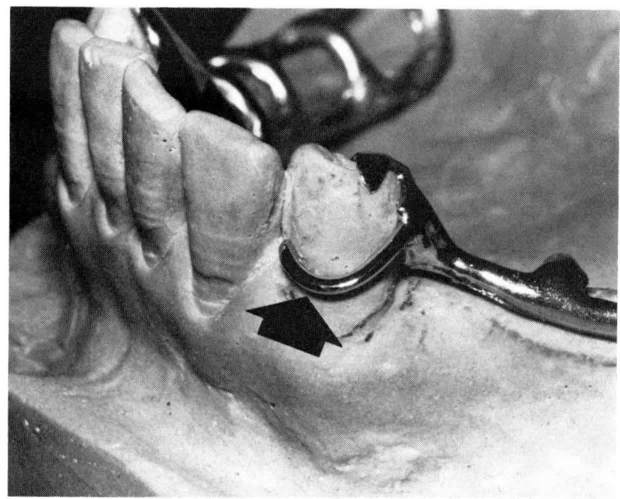

Fig. 1-2. Extracoronal removable partial denture. One arm of clasp is designed to enter an undercut on crown of a tooth (arrow) to keep denture prosthesis in place.

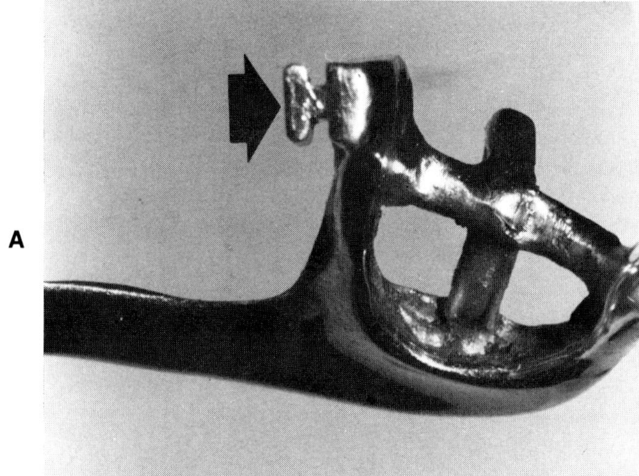

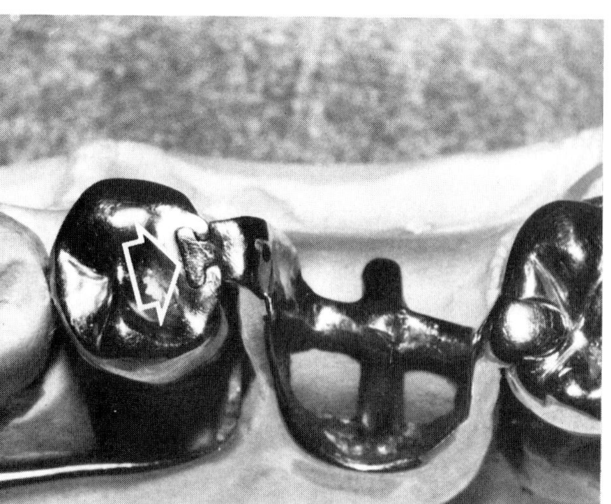

Fig. 1-3. Intracoronal removable partial denture. **A,** Male portion of retaining device (arrow) is designed to fit into female portion, which is part of an artificial tooth crown. **B,** Partial denture is retained in mouth by frictional fit of male and female portions (arrow).

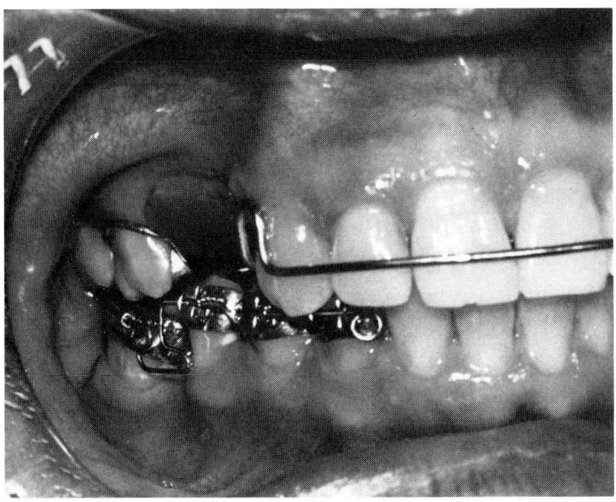

Fig. 1-4. Orthodontic appliance. An appliance is used during treatment to accomplish a specific purpose. Tipped teeth being uprighted before initiation of prosthodontic treatment.

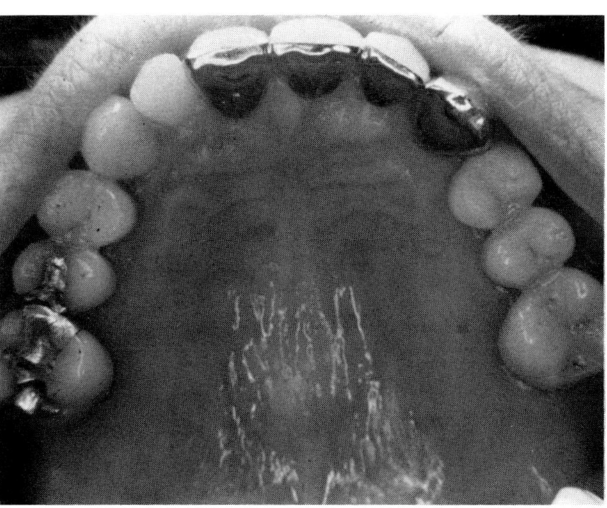

Fig. 1-5. Fixed partial denture. A tooth on each side of an edentulous space is prepared to receive an artificial crown. Artificial tooth, or pontic, is suspended between these two artificial crowns. This unit is then cemented over abutment teeth.

retainer consists of two fingers of metal *(clasps)* that lie on the surface of a tooth crown. One of these clasps, the retentive clasp, is located in an undercut area of the crown, and the other, the reciprocal bracing, or stabilizing clasp, in a nonundercut area. This partial denture is referred to as an *extracoronal partial denture,* because the retentive device lies outside the clinical crown of the natural tooth. In an *intracoronal partial denture,* the retention of the prosthesis depends on the frictional resistance between parallel walls of a male attachment, the key, located on the removable partial denture, and the female receptacle, the keyway, located within an artificial crown on a remaining tooth. The term *internal attachment* refers to this type of retainer. Use of the term *precision attachment* to describe this retentive device should be discouraged because no less precision is required to make an accurate prosthesis with any other form of attachment.

Another method of describing or categorizing removable partial dentures is by the manner of their support. A partial denture that receives support from natural teeth at each end of the edentulous space or spaces is a tooth-supported removable partial denture (Fig. 1-6). Although the artificial teeth are attached to a denture base, the denture base does not receive any significant support from the underlying residual ridge.

A second and larger group of partial dentures categorized by the form of their support are those that have a denture base that extends anteriorly or posteriorly and are supported by teeth at only one end. These are called extension partial dentures, or tooth–tissue–supported partial dentures (Fig. 1-7). The great majority of these are distal extension removable partial dentures in which the denture base extends posteriorly without posterior support from natural teeth. In most cases, the denture receives its support from the teeth anterior to the edentulous space and from the edentulous ridge through the distal extension denture base.

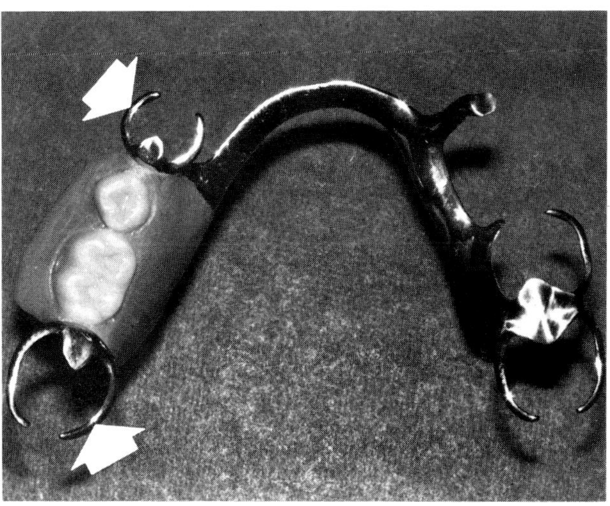

Fig. 1-6. Tooth-supported removable partial denture. Direct retainers, or clasps (arrows), can be seen at each end of artificial teeth, indicating that partial denture is supported entirely by remaining natural teeth.

Temporary removable partial dentures (Fig. 1-8) should never be used as a permanent or prolonged form of treatment because of the danger of destroying the

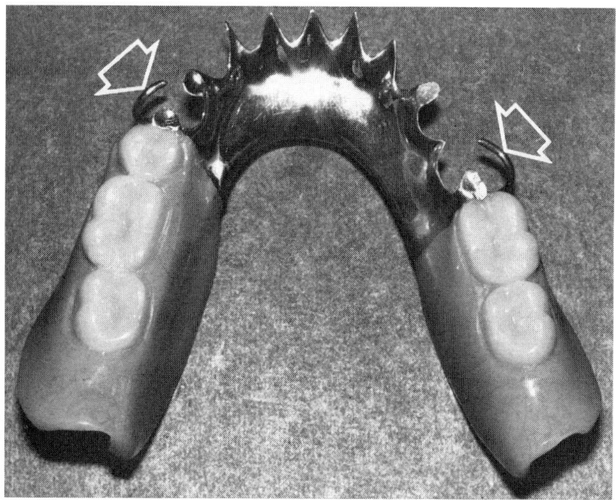

Fig. 1-7. Tooth-tissue–supported removable partial denture. A direct retainer can be seen at anterior end of artificial denture teeth on each side of arch (arrows) indicating that a natural tooth is present at these positions. Posterior end of prosthesis terminates in a denture base, indicating there are no teeth posterior to denture. Artificial teeth are supported partly by underlying edentulous ridge.

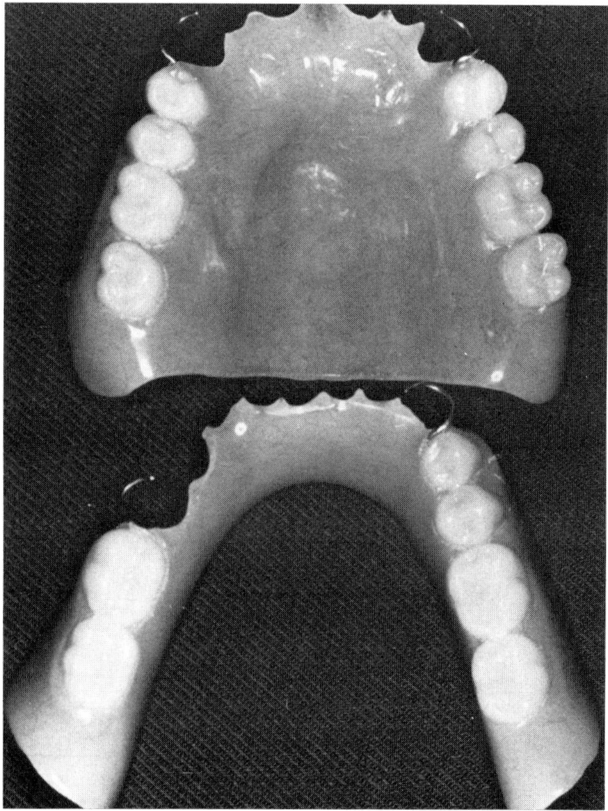

Fig. 1-8. Maxillary and mandibular temporary partial prostheses, constructed of acrylic resin, are supported entirely by underlying soft tissue.

remaining oral tissue. The terms used to describe the various temporary partial dentures denote their purposes.

An *interim denture* is a temporary partial denture used for a short time for reasons of esthetics, masticatory efficiency, or convenience until a more definitive form of treatment can be rendered.

A *transitional denture* may be used when loss of additional teeth is inevitable but immediate extraction is not advisible or desirable. Artificial teeth may be added to the transitional denture when the natural teeth are extracted, either singly or in groups, until all teeth to be extracted have been removed. The denture can then serve as an interim denture until more complete prosthodontic treatment is provided.

A *treatment denture* is used as a carrier for treatment material when the soft tissues have been abused by ill-fitting prosthetic devices, or it may be used after surgery to protect a surgical site or to reposition soft tissue.

Although these three forms of temporary dentures usually derive support solely from soft tissue, it is frequently advisable, when possible, to obtain additional support from the remaining teeth.

Undoubtedly the most defined term in prosthodontics is *centric relation*, closely followed by *centric occlusion*. This book will accept as the basic definition of centric relation, *the most posterior relation of the mandible to the maxilla at an established vertical dimension*. This definition may be embellished in many ways, but if the basic premise of a jaw-to-jaw or bone-to-bone relationship is maintained, acceptance of this simple concept can avoid confusion. Centric occlusion may be defined as *the relation of opposing occlusal surfaces that provides the maximum planned contact or intercuspation, or both* (Fig. 1-9).

The words *model* and *cast* are also frequently misused. *Cast* may be used as a verb (to cast an inlay) or as an adjective (a cast framework). More frequently, it is used as a noun to describe an accurate, positive reproduction of the maxillary or mandibular dental arch, in which case a descriptive adjective gives it a more specific meaning, such as diagnostic cast, master cast, or duplicate cast. A model is a reproduction for demonstration or display purposes; accuracy is in no way implied. It should be a reasonable facsimile of an object, but need not be an accurate reproduction such as that required for construction of a successful prosthesis (Fig. 1-10).

Stability is defined as the quality of a denture to be firm, steady, and constant in position when forces are applied. It refers especially to resistance against horizontal forces, and it implies a stable relationship to the underlying bone. *Retention* is that quality inherent in a prosthesis that resists the force of gravity, the adhesiveness of foods, and the forces associated with opening the jaws. In complete dentures it refers to the maintenance of contact between the denture base and the underlying soft tissue. In removable partial dentures it is the resistance to displacement of the denture from its basal seat; it is spoken of as *direct retention* and is obtained by either internal attachments or by clasps (direct retainers). Retention implies a static relationship to the underlying soft tissue.

Another related series of terms that play a part in the general practice of prosthodontics are *reline*, *rebase*, and *reconstruct*. The words refer to differing extents of correction to improve the fit and/or function of a removable partial denture. When only the tissue surface of the denture base needs to be corrected by adding a layer, or a lining, of new denture base material, a reline is indicated. If the entire denture base needs to be replaced but the artificial teeth are still acceptable, a rebase is the technique of choice. When the denture base and the artificial teeth are no longer usable and only the metal framework is to be retained, a reconstruction must be accomplished.

Those terms that deal directly with the components of a removable partial denture will not be repeated here but will be covered in detail as the components are discussed.

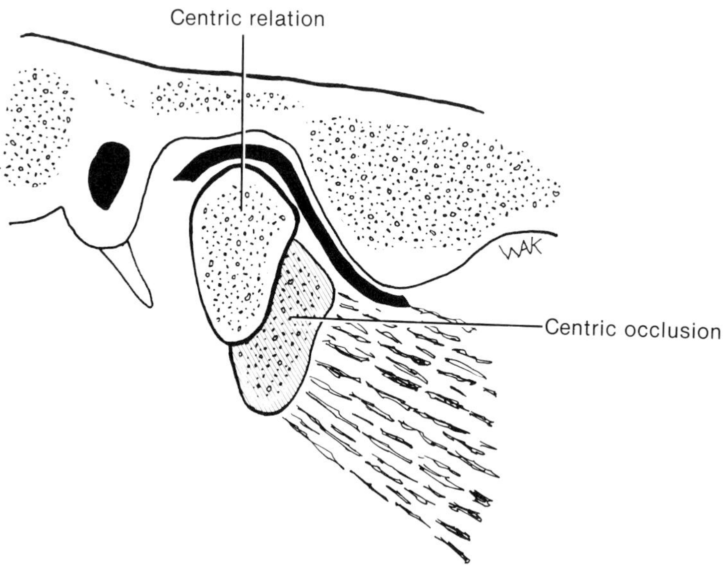

Fig. 1-9. *Centric relation* is bone-to-bone or jaw-to-jaw relationship. At this relation, head of mandibular condyle is seated in its most posterior position in glenoid fossa. *Centric occlusion* is position of mandible at which there is maximum planned intercuspation of teeth. At this position head of mandibular condyle is anterior to its most posterior position in glenoid fossa.

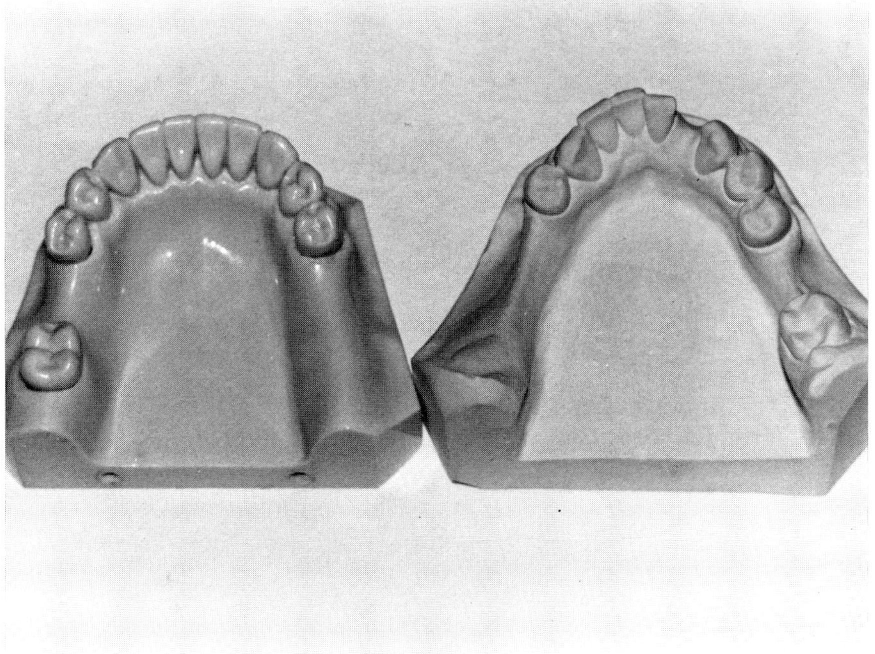

Fig. 1-10. Left, a model, a reasonable facsimile of dental arch, not an accurate reproduction. Right, A dental cast, an accurate reproduction of a patient's dental arch.

TREATING THE PARTIALLY EDENTULOUS PATIENT

The treatment of choice for the partially edentulous patient when all factors are favorable is normally a fixed partial denture. Some factors, however, militate against the use of fixed partial dentures and in favor of removable partial dentures.

Indications against use of fixed partial dentures

Youth or advanced age of patient

Most patients under the age of 17 are poor candidates for fixed partial dentures because of large dental pulps and lack of clinical crown height. Tooth reduction sufficient to reestablish normal coronal anatomy in the cast restoration often compromises the health of the pulpal tissue. An interim partial denture should be considered for patients less than 17 years old. In the aged patient the reduced life expectancy and frequently failing general health contraindicate the expensive and tedious dental procedures required for the fixed partial denture.

Great length of the edentulous span

One of the rules of dentistry that has most successfully passed the judgment of time is that of Dr. Ante. Ante's Law states that the periodontal membrane area of the abutment teeth for a fixed partial denture must be equal to or exceed the periodontal membrane area of the teeth being replaced. Although other conditions may modify this rule to some degree, exceeding the rule by a margin of any significance is almost certain to invite problems.

Excessive loss of bone in the edentulous area

When a large amount of the edentulous ridge has been lost and it is necessary to provide support for the lips or cheek or to obtain proper tooth position for the artificial tooth, the use of a denture base flange is necessary. Several types of composite partial prostheses in which a portion of the restoration is fixed and a superstructure consisting of the artificial teeth and denture base is removable are available. Replacement of all the missing tissues with a fixed partial denture would make the prosthesis cumbersome, and therefore it would be difficult to maintain a healthy oral environment.

Purpose of removable partial denture

The primary purpose of removable partial dentures must always be, as Muller DeVan (1952) stated, "the preservation of that which remains and not the meticulous replacement of that which has been lost." After it has been determined that this primary purpose can be satisfied, one can consider the additional purposes of removable partial dentures: maintaining or improving phonetics, establishing or increasing masticatory efficiency, and developing and restoring esthetics.

If, on the other hand, it is indicated that the health of all or part of the remaining oral structures will be compromised, alternate plans of treatment must be considered. For too many years removable partial dentures were considered by many in the profession to be stepping stones or stumbling blocks on the road to the completely edentulous state. With the materials, equipment, and techniques currently available, thinking of this type must be relegated to the past. Removable partial dentures are and will remain a biologically acceptable form of treatment.

Indications for use of removable partial denture

Length of edentulous span that contraindicates use of fixed partial denture

The teeth adjacent to a long-span edentulous area support a removable partial denture in much the same manner that they would support a fixed partial denture except that the removable denture receives support and stabilization from teeth on the opposite side of the arch as well as from the residual ridge. Without this cross-arch stabilization, the leverage and torque on the abutment teeth would be excessive.

No abutment tooth posterior to edentulous space

Where there is no tooth posterior to the edentulous space to act as an abutment, the choice of suitable methods of replacement is limited. In selected instances when only one tooth need be replaced (either because a complete denture is in opposition or because only a first molar is unopposed, with the two premolars adjacent to the distal extension space having sound periodontal support), a cantilever fixed partial denture may be planned. Other than in this circumstance or in a more controlled environment when a dental implant may be placed, the only practical replacement is a removable partial denture.

Reduced periodontal support of remaining teeth

In many mouths, particularly those of middle-aged or old people and following periodontal therapy, the remaining teeth have lost a considerable amount of bony support and are therefore unable to support a fixed prosthesis. By developing the fit of the denture base to the edentulous ridge, the total support required of the teeth will be diminished.

Need for cross-arch stabilization

When stabilization of the remaining teeth is needed against lateral as well as anteroposterior forces (for example, after treatment of advanced periodontal disease), cross-arch, or bilateral, stabilization is frequently required. The fixed partial denture can provide excellent anteroposterior stabilization but limited lateral, or buccolingual, stabilization.

Excessive bone loss of residual ridge

When a missing tooth is replaced by a fixed partial denture, the artificial tooth (pontic) is so arranged that its base, or neck, lightly contacts the mucosa over the edentulous ridge to simulate the appearance of a natural tooth. This is particularly true of maxillary anterior or premolar teeth. When trauma, surgery, or abnormal resorption patterns have caused excessive bone loss, it is difficult if not impossible to place the artificial tooth in an acceptable buccolingual position. However, if a denture base is used with a removable partial denture to supply the missing portion of the residual ridge, the artificial tooth may be placed in its natural position and the denture base will supply the required support. The denture base will also support the lips and cheeks to reestablish normal facial contours.

Physical or emotional problem of the patient

The lengthy preparation and construction procedures for fixed partial dentures can be trying, especially for patients with a physical or emotional problem. Treatment that will prevent further oral deterioration should be established for such patients, and continued at least until the physical or emotional problem subsides or is controlled. Removable partial dentures are most often indicated. This treatment selection should not compromise the fit and function of the completed prosthesis. Its advantage lies in the reduced patient-dentist contact time.

Esthetics of primary concern in replacement of multiple missing anterior teeth.

It is often possible to attain a more natural tooth position by placing a denture tooth on a denture base than by butting a pontic of a fixed partial denture against the residual ridge. The three-dimentional denture tooth may also have a more lifelike appearance than some pontics that appear flat and dull. In addition, the denture teeth may be arranged more easily to satisfy phonetic and support requirements.

Need to replace teeth immediately after their extraction.

The replacement of teeth immediately following extraction cannot be done successfully with a fixed prosthesis. Many problems are encountered, including future ridge resorption. These teeth are replaced with temporary removable partial dentures that can be relined as resorption occurs. When the edentulous area has stabilized, definitive treatment can be undertaken with either a permanent removable partial denture or a fixed partial denture.

Patient desires

Patients sometimes insist on a removable prosthesis in place of a fixed prosthesis (1) to avoid operative procedures on sound, healthy teeth and (2) for economic reasons. Many patients who have had an unpleasant experience with operative dental procedures object strenously to the tooth preparation necessary for a fixed prosthesis. In addition, it is difficult for the patient to realize it is necessary to cut healthy teeth to replace one or two missing teeth. Patient education in the form of photographs, models, case histories, and so forth can be valuable, and most patients can be convinced of the better service rendered by the fixed replacement.

Some patients, especially those who are retired and living on a fixed income, need and desire replacement of missing teeth but cannot afford a fixed prosthesis. The difference in treatment should be explained, but it should not be implied that they will receive inadequate treatment. Successful treatment with a removable partial prosthesis should be expected if attention is paid to fundamental principles.

Poor prognosis for complete dentures because of size, shape, or relation of residual ridges

This condition is most often encountered in the patient with a retrognathic jaw relation. Retention of some mandibular teeth is of extreme importance. Great effort should be expended to avoid constructing conventional complete dentures for patients with one weak arch opposing a strong arch.

CLASSIFICATION OF PARTIALLY EDENTULOUS ARCHES

For a classification method to be acceptable, it should be able to do the following things:

1. Allow visualization of the type of partially edentulous arch being considered.
2. Permit differentiation between tooth-supported and tooth-tissue–supported partial dentures.
3. Serve as a guide to the type of design to be used.
4. Be universally accepted.

A number of classification systems have been proposed, but few have satisfied these criteria. Some have been overly simplified; others, immensely complex.

One simple system classifies the prostheses according to the type of support they receive from the dental arch (soft tissue–supported, tooth-supported, and tooth-tissue–supported prostheses) (Figs. 1-11 to 1-13). However, there are so many possible variations of the tooth-tissue–supported prostheses that this simplified classification does not adequately describe the design that

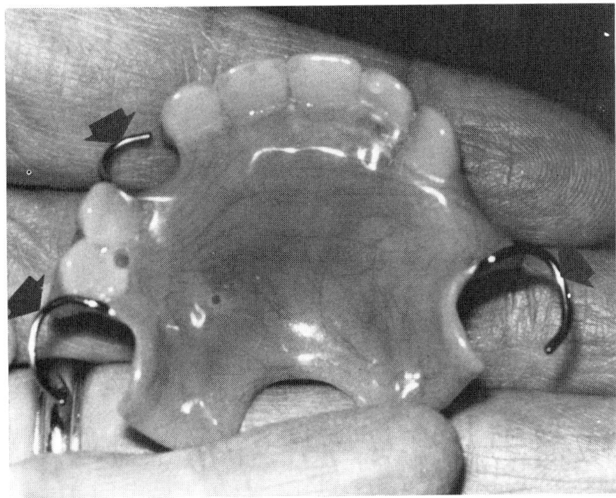

Fig. 1-11. Soft tissue–supported removable partial denture is limited to temporary use. Wire clasps (arrows) retain prosthesis.

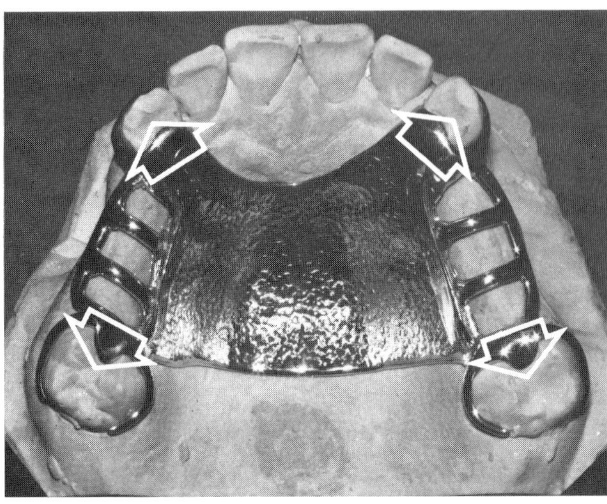

Fig. 1-12. Tooth-supported removable partial denture is supported by abutment teeth (arrows), one at each end of all edentulous spaces.

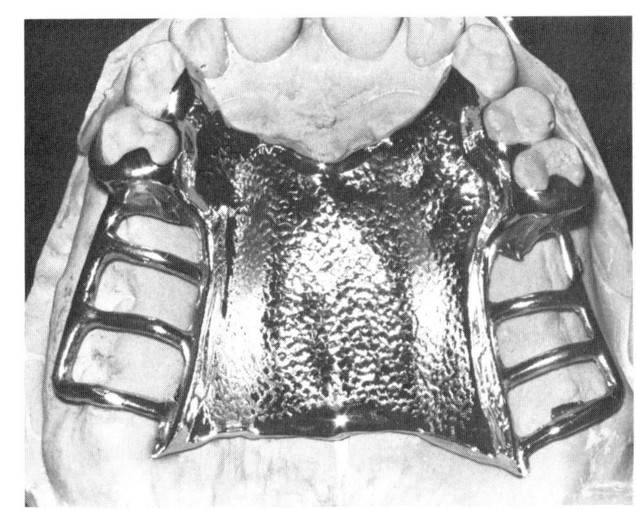

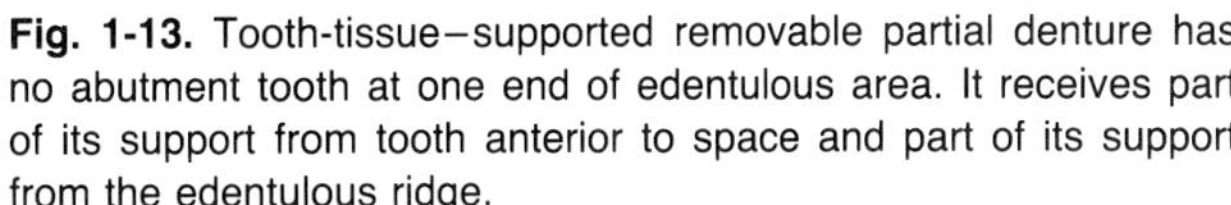

Fig. 1-13. Tooth-tissue–supported removable partial denture has no abutment tooth at one end of edentulous area. It receives part of its support from tooth anterior to space and part of its support from the edentulous ridge.

must be considered. Therefore this system is not suited for general use in discussing, identifying, or planning prostheses.

One of the more complex systems, proposed by Cummer (1942), states that "the classification proposed is that of the finished restoration rather than that of the unrestored condition of the mouth"! Little value can be gained, particularly in discussing design problems, if classification follows the construction of the prosthesis.

Kennedy classification

The most widely used method of classification of the partially edentulous dental arch is the one originally proposed in 1923 by Dr. Edward Kennedy of New York. Although simple, the system can easily be applied to nearly all semiedentulous conditions, and it suggests the main design problems that must be considered.

Kennedy's original classification contains the following four classes, with certain modifications:

Class I. Bilateral edentulous areas located posterior to the remaining natural teeth (Fig. 1-14).

Class II. Unilateral edentulous area located posterior to the remaining natural teeth (Fig. 1-15).

Class III. Unilateral edentulous area with natural teeth both anterior and posterior to it (Fig. 1-16).

Class IV. Single, bilateral edentulous area located anterior to the remaining natural teeth (Fig. 1-17).

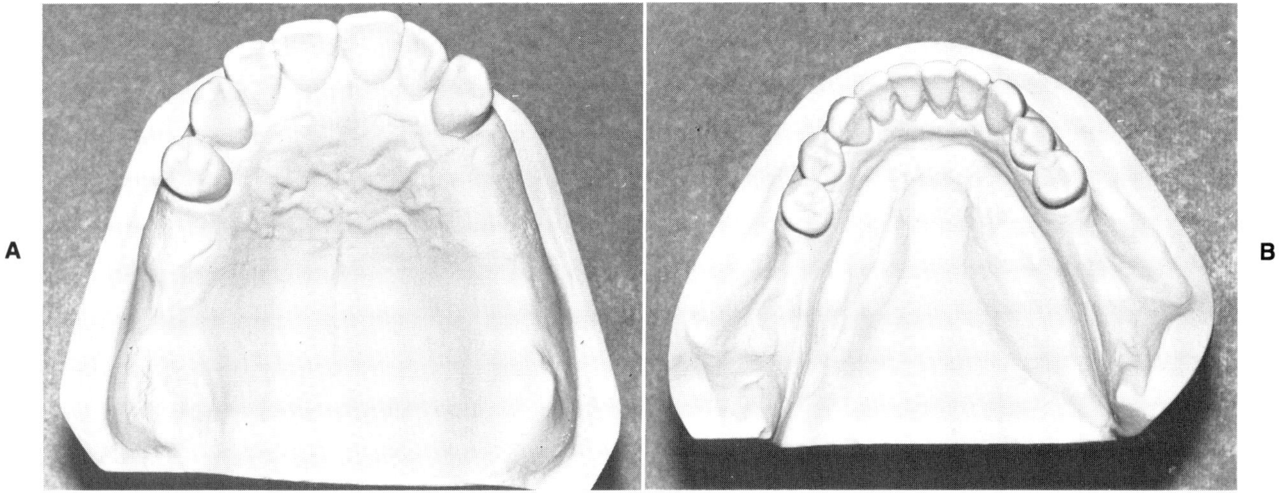

Fig. 1-14. Maxillary cast, **A,** and mandibular cast, **B,** of Kennedy Class I partially edentulous arches.

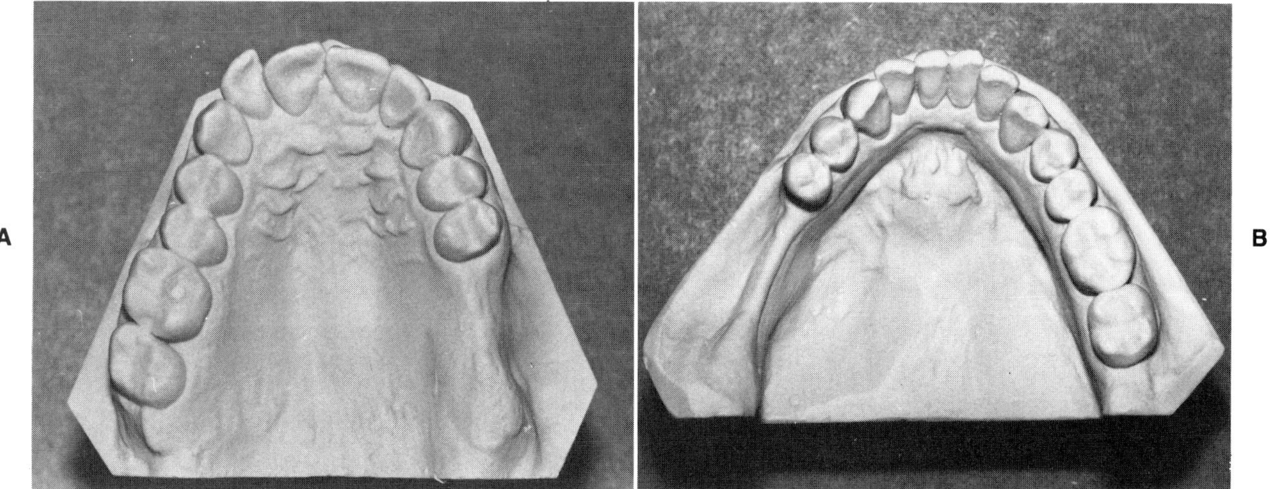

Fig. 1-15. Maxillary cast, **A,** and mandibular cast, **B,** of Kennedy Class II partially edentulous arches.

Each of the classes, except Class I, refers to a single edentulous area in each arch. Since these types of edentulous arches are not in the majority, Kennedy referred to each additional edentulous area, not each additional missing tooth, as a modification area and included them in the classification by the number of such areas (for example, Class I, Modification 1; Class II, Modification 3) (Figs. 1-18 to 1-21).

Dr. O.C. Applegate (1960) later attempted to expand the Kennedy system by adding Classes V and VI. Acceptance has not been universal. Class V is described as an edentulous area bounded anteriorly and posteriorly by natural teeth but in which the anterior abutment (the lateral incisor) is not suitable for support. Class VI is an edentulous situation in which the teeth adjacent to the space are capable of total support of the required prosthesis; it would occur most frequently in a young adult for whom a fixed partial denture is indicated but possible damage to the dental pulp might occur if crown preparation were attempted.

Classes V and VI are not truly indicative of special design considerations and are not included in discussions in this book. Only the four major classes are referred to.

Applegate also provided the following eight rules to govern the application of the Kennedy system:

Rule 1. Classification should follow rather than precede extractions that might alter the original classification.

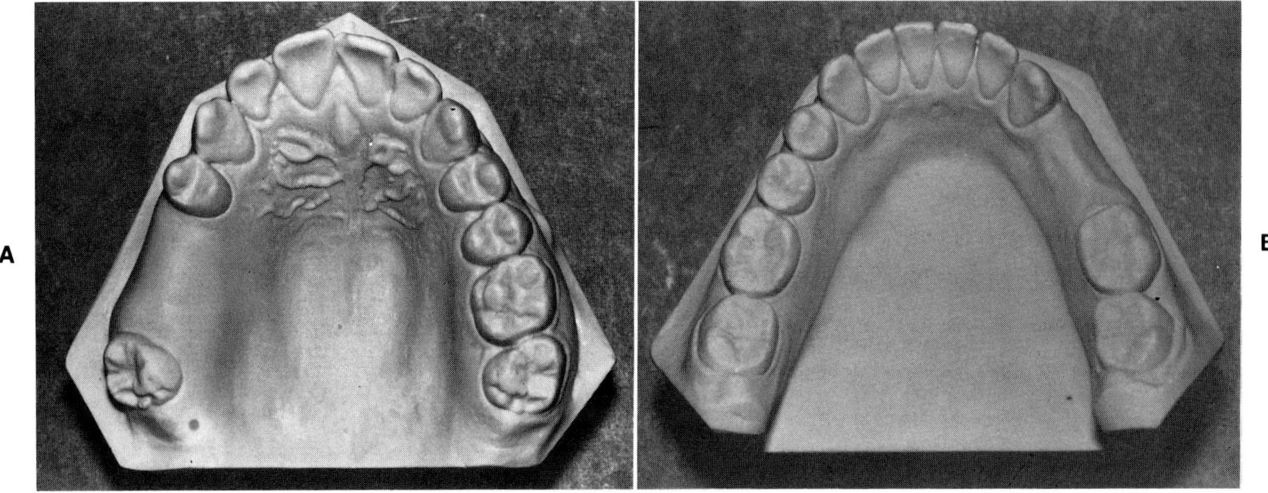

Fig. 1-16. Maxillary cast, **A,** and mandibular cast, **B,** of Kennedy Class III partially edentulous arches.

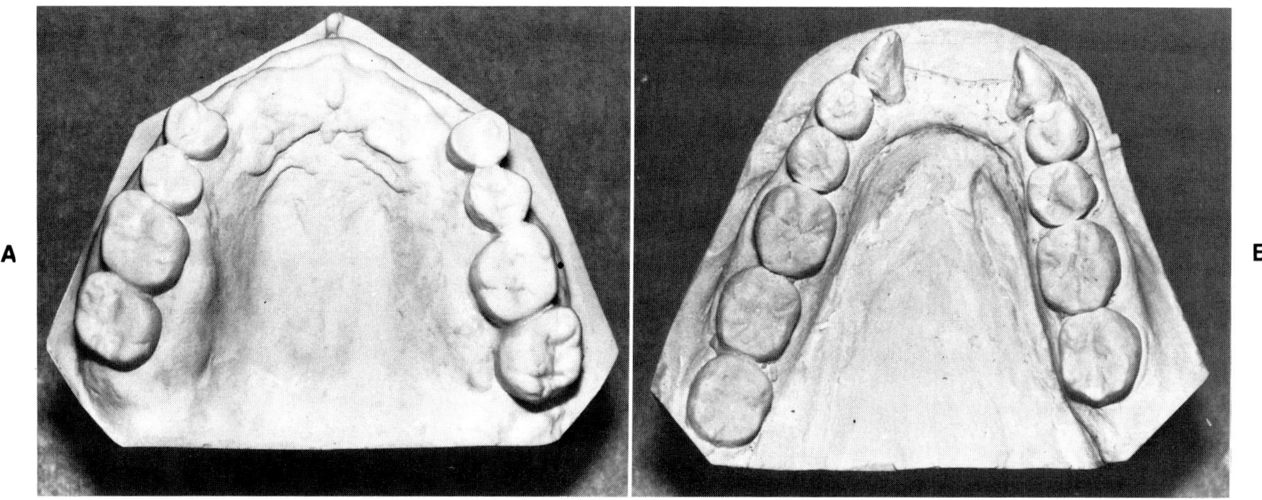

Fig. 1-17. Maxillary cast, **A,** and mandibular cast, **B,** of Kennedy Class IV partially edentulous arches.

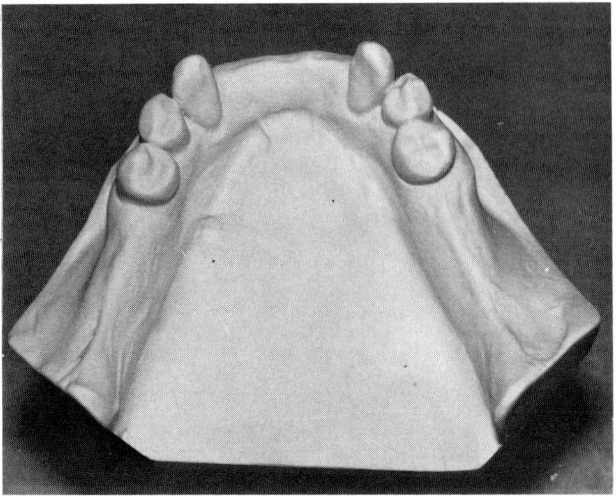

Fig. 1-18. Class I, Modification 1.

A B

C D

Fig. 1-19. **A,** Class II, Modification 1. **B,** Class II, Modification 2. **C,** Class II, Modification 3. **D,** Class II, Modification 4.

A B

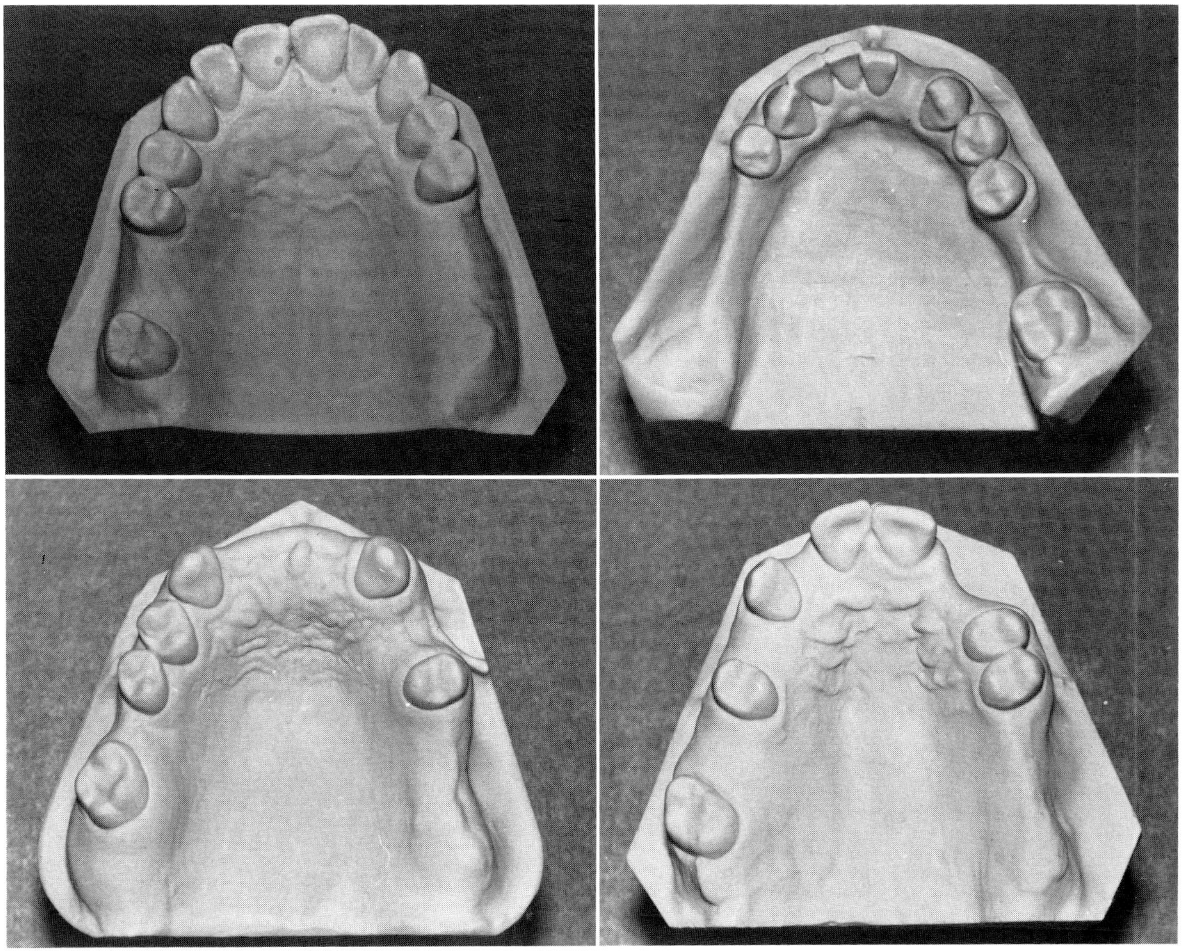

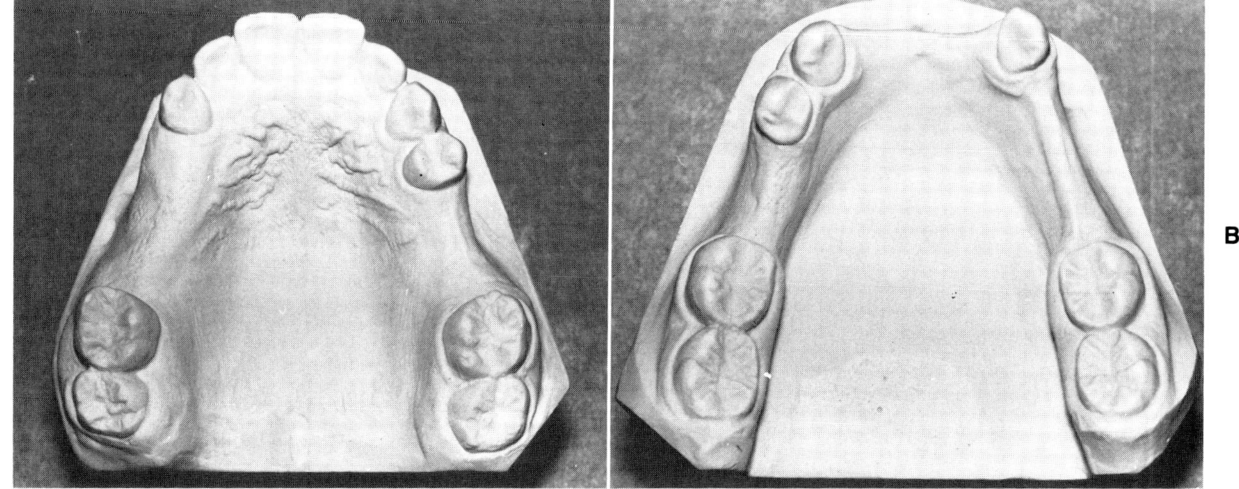

Fig. 1-20. **A,** Class III, Modification 1. **B,** Class III, Modification 2.

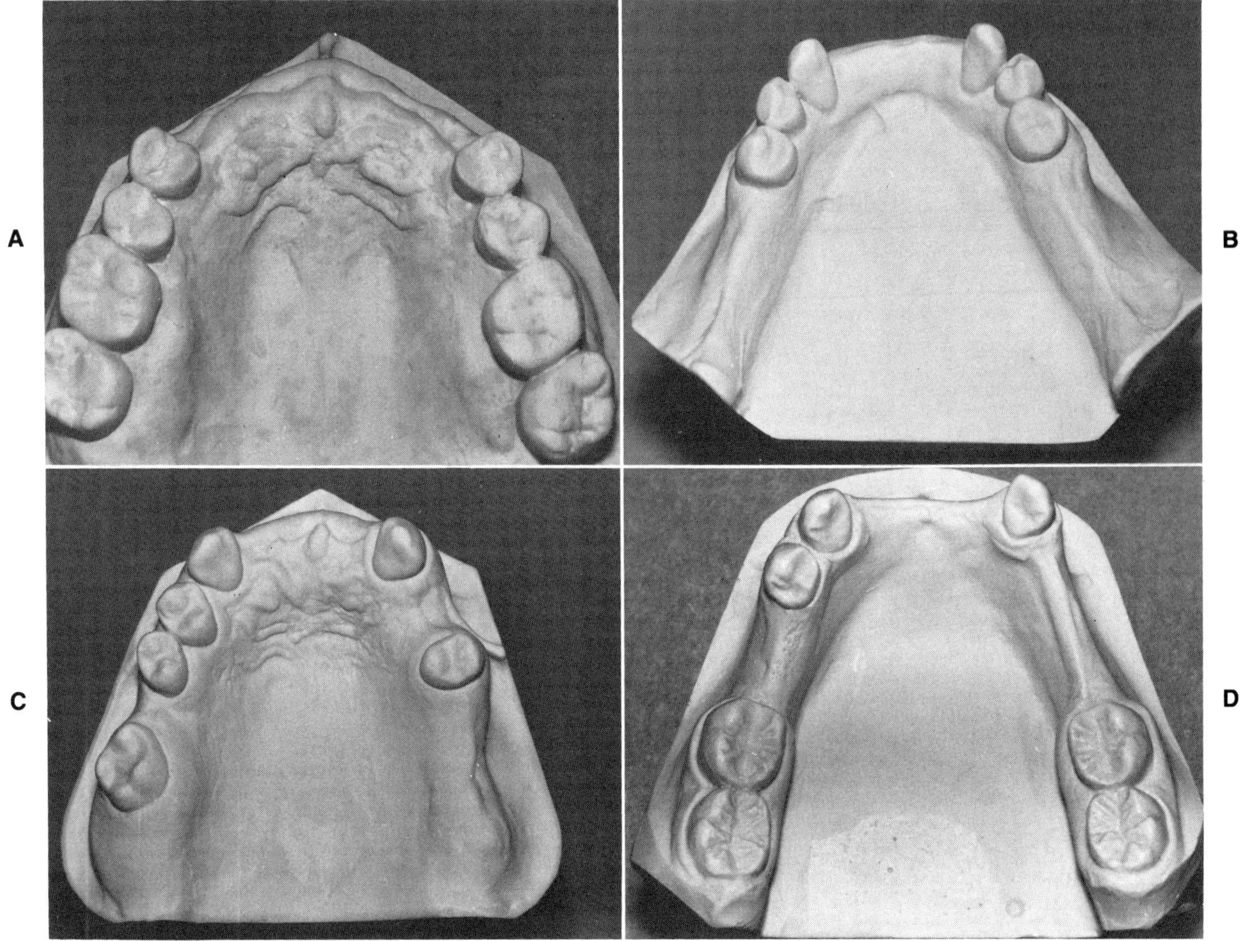

Fig. 1-21. The most posterior space determines the classification. Class IV cannot have modification spaces. **A,** Class IV. **B,** Class I, Modification 1. **C,** Class II, Modification 3. **D,** Class III, Modification 2.

Rule 2. If the third molar is missing and not to be replaced, it is not considered in the classification (Fig. 1-22).

Rule 3. If a third molar is present and is to be used as an abutment, it is considered in the classification (Fig. 1-23).

Rule 4. If a second molar is missing and is not to be replaced (that is, the opposing second molar is also missing and is not to be replaced), it is not considered in the classification (Fig. 1-24).

Rule 5. The most posterior edentulous area or areas always determine the classification (Fig. 1-25).

Rule 6. Edentulous areas other than those determining the classification are referred to as modification spaces and are designated by their number.

Rule 7. The extent of the modification is not considered, only the number of additional edentulous areas (Fig. 1-26).

Rule 8. There can be no modification areas in Class IV arches. Any edentulous area lying posterior to the single bilateral area determines the classification (see Fig. 1-25).

The numeric sequence of the classification system is based partly on the frequency of occurrence, with Class I arches being most common and Class IV arches being least common. The sequence is also based on the principles of design: the Class I partial denture is designed as a tooth-tissue–supported prosthesis, the Class III as a wholly tooth-supported partial denture, and the Class II as a combination of Classes I and III (partly tooth-tissue–supported and partly tooth-supported).

The following three features must be included in the design of a Class I removable partial denture:

1. *Adequate support for the distal extension denture base.* The entire extent of the residual ridge capable of bearing a load must be covered by an

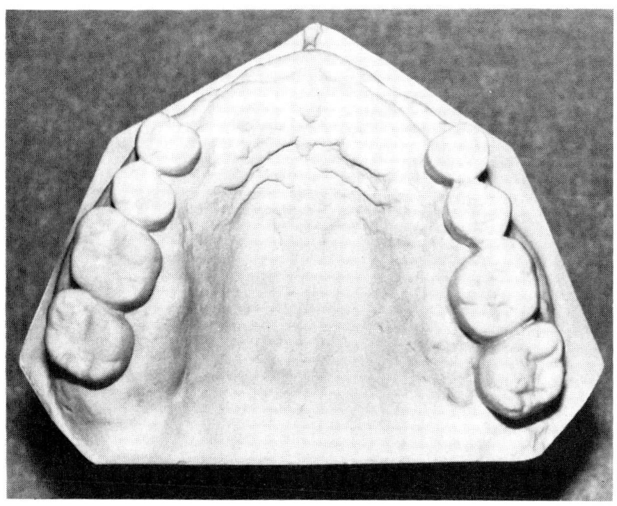

Fig. 1-22. Rule 2. Class IV. If third molar is missing and is not to be replaced, it is not considered in classification.

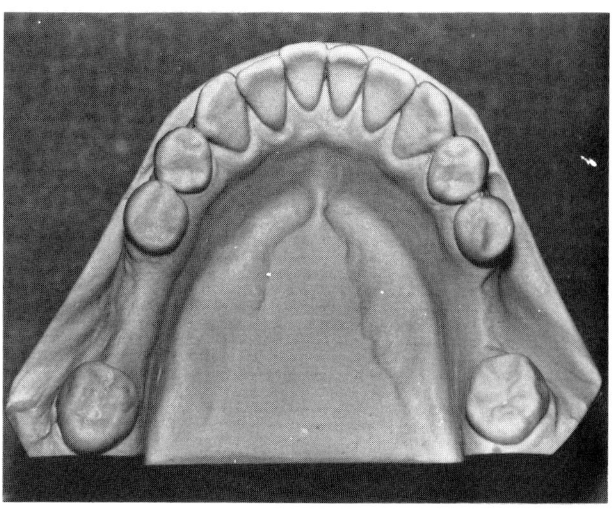

Fig. 1-23. Rule 3. If third molar is present and is to be an abutment, it is considered in classification.

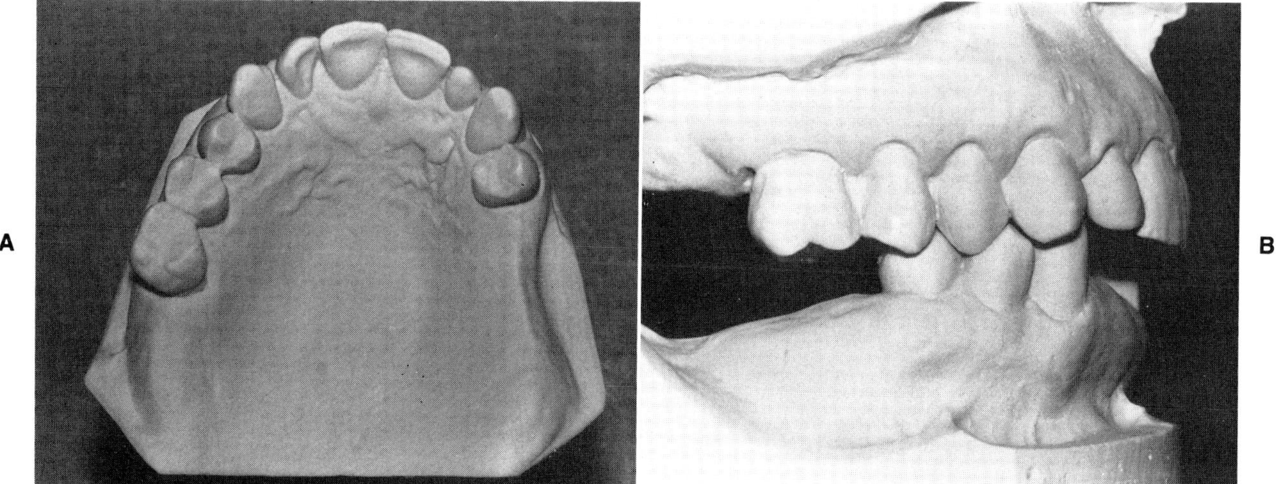

Fig. 1-24. Rule 4. **A,** Because second molar is missing and is not to be replaced, it is not considered in classification. **B,** Opposing second molar is also missing and is not to be replaced.

Fig. 1-25. Rule 5. Class III, Modification 2. The most posterior edentulous area, or areas, always determine classification. Even though posterior edentulous areas have nearly closed as result of mesial drifting of second molars, they still determine classification.

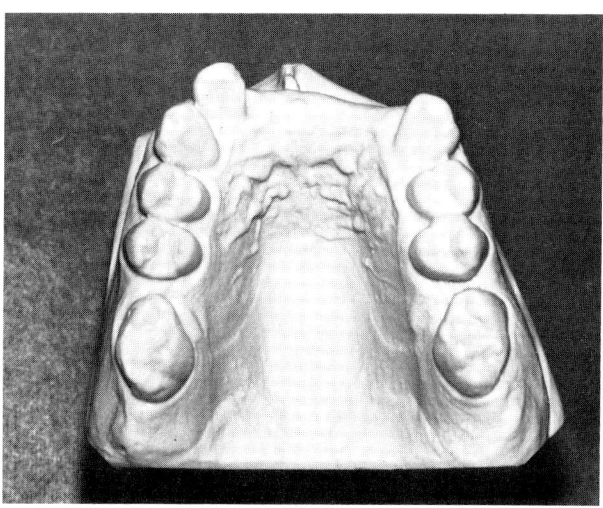

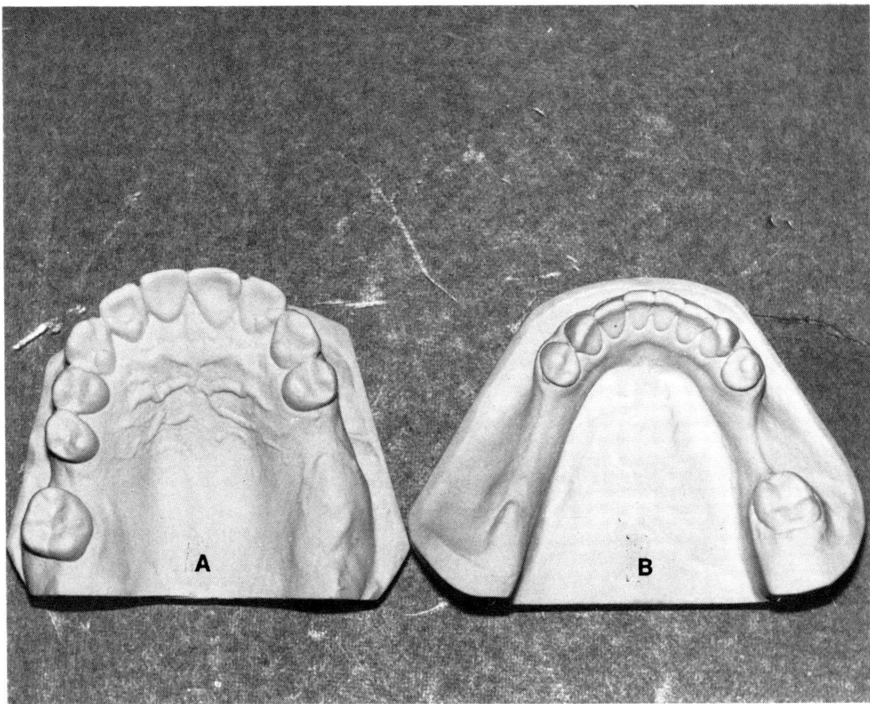

Fig. 1-26. Rule 7. **A,** A single missing tooth representing Modification 1. **B,** A number of missing teeth representing Modification 1.

accurately fitting denture base to minimize the applied stress (Fig. 1-27). Inadequate soft tissue coverage can lead to breakdown of the underlying bone. It is frequently necessary to make a second impression of the edentulous distal extension ridge after the framework has been completed to ensure adequate support for the denture base. The technique for this impression making is covered in Chapter 13.

2. *Flexible direct retention.* The Class I removable partial denture is supported by teeth only at the anterior end of each of the edentulous areas. The posterior end of the denture base is supported by the soft tissue over the edentulous ridge. The soft tissue is compressible, or displaceable, to varying degrees and allows vertical movement of the denture base as occlusal forces occur on the artificial teeth (Fig. 1-28). This vertical movement cannot be completely controlled, and the rocking action results in stress on the terminal abutment teeth. The abutment teeth act as fulcra for these rotational forces. Improperly designed direct retainers on the abutment teeth may magnify the rotational forces by locking the abutment teeth securely, thus forcing them to rock back and forth with eventual damage or destruction of the periodontal attachment. The retentive arm of the direct retainer should be designed so that it will either flex as stresses are applied or move into an area of greater undercut as the denture base moves toward the tissue, thus releasing the abutment tooth from the grasp of the clasp and greatly dissipating the damaging rocking or rotational force. This clasp design is one of the few essentials needed to ensure the success of a removable partial denture.
3. *Indirect retention.* The distal extension denture base is forced toward the tissue during mastication, and it tends to lift away from the tissue after release of the occlusal forces and rebounding of the compressed tissue. The action of sticky food also tends to lift the denture base as the teeth separate. These forces magnify the rotation around the terminal abutment teeth (Fig. 1-29). This lifting force can best be controlled or limited by the placement of an occlusal, lingual, or incisal rest on a tooth or teeth as far anterior to the fulcrum line as practical. This concept of indirect retention is discussed in Chapter 4.

The Class III denture (Fig. 1-30), because it is tooth-borne, does not have the same design requirements. Being supported at both ends of the edentulous spaces, it does not normally tend to rotate or lift, so compen-

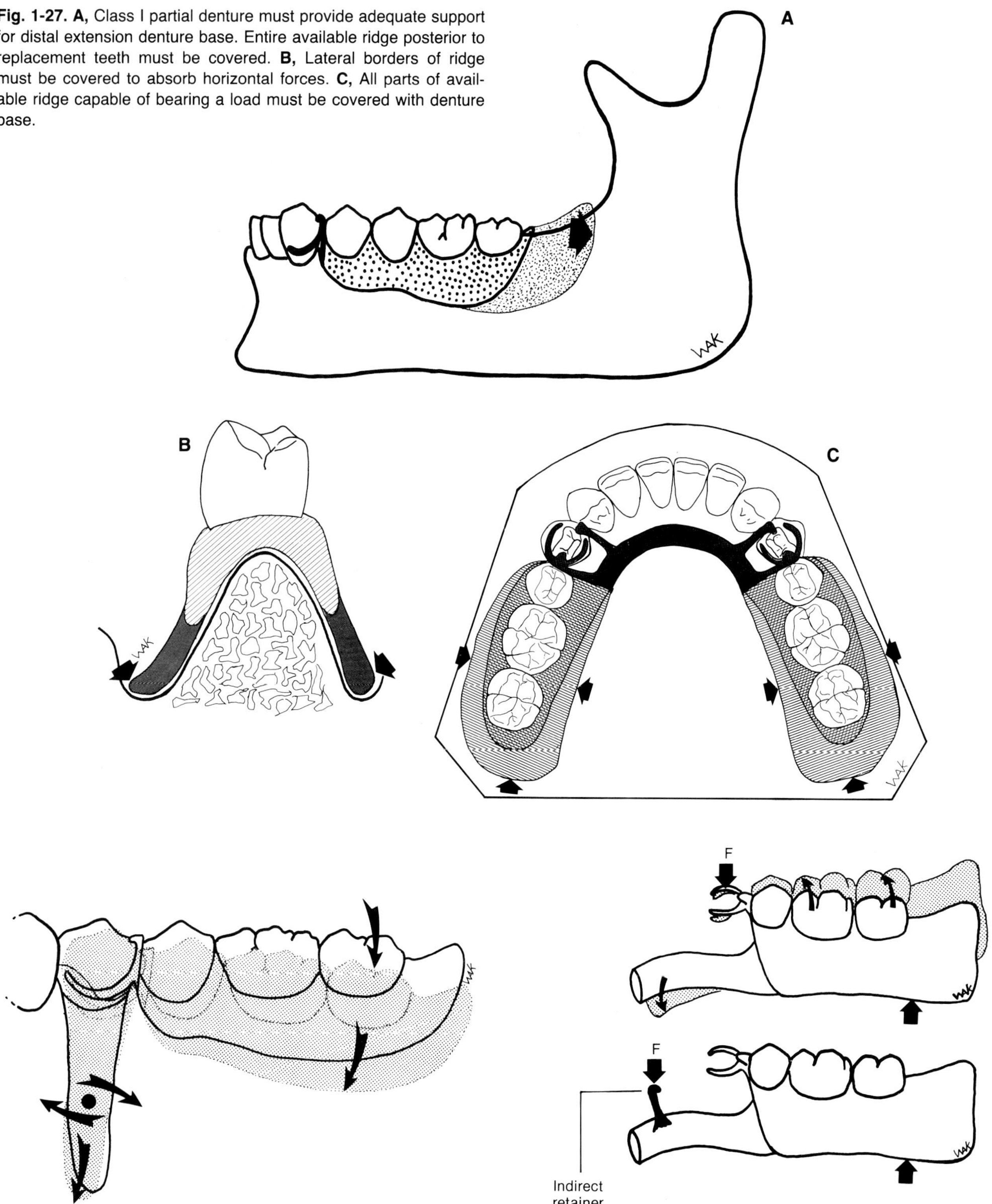

Fig. 1-27. A, Class I partial denture must provide adequate support for distal extension denture base. Entire available ridge posterior to replacement teeth must be covered. **B,** Lateral borders of ridge must be covered to absorb horizontal forces. **C,** All parts of available ridge capable of bearing a load must be covered with denture base.

Fig. 1-28. Class I partial denture must have flexible direct retention. Posterior end of denture base rests on soft compressible tissue. As forces on artificial teeth compress or displace soft tissue, denture base moves vertically. Direct retainers must flex to allow stresses produced by their movement to be dissipated.

Fig. 1-29. Class I removable partial denture base tends to lift away from ridge either because of rebound of soft tissues that were compressed or because of pulling action of sticky foods. Lifting action can be controlled by placing rest on tooth as far anterior to fulcrum line *(F)* as possible. Rest moves fulcrum line anteriorly and provides indirect retention.

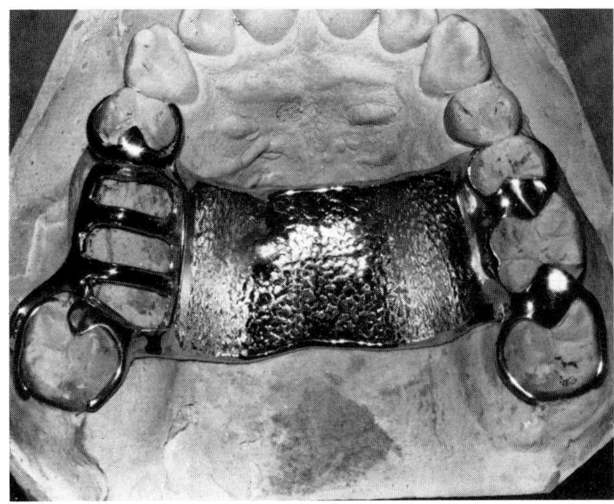

Fig. 1-30. Class III removable partial denture does not tend to rotate or lift in function, so it does not need extensive denture base coverage, flexible direct retainers, or indirect retention.

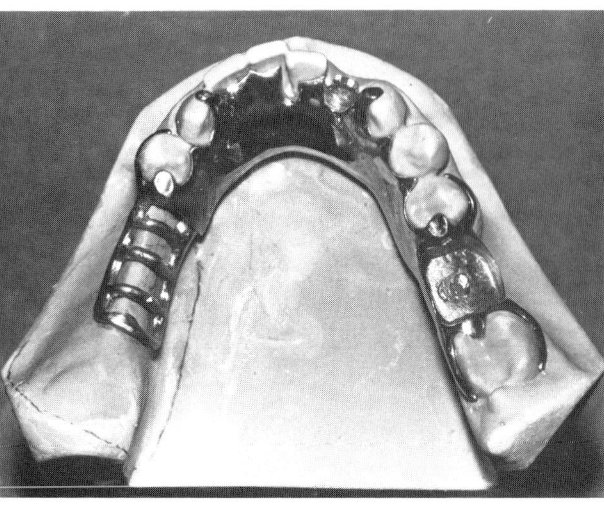

Fig. 1-31. Class II, Modification 2, partial denture must satisfy requirements of Class I partial denture on distal extension side and of Class III partial denture on modification side.

sation for rotational forces is not needed. Generally the Class III denture does not need the following features:

1. *Support from the ridge tissue.* Only when the length of the edentulous span is great or when the abutment teeth are periodontally weak is there a need to use the edentulous ridge for support with a Class III removable partial prosthesis.
2. *Flexible direct retention.* The Class III removable partial denture does not tend to move in function, so the type and position of the retentive arm of the direct retainer are of no significance. Sufficient direct retention is needed only to prevent vertical dislodgment of the prosthesis. However, this requirement may change if direct retention cannot be obtained on one or more of the abutment teeth.
3. *Indirect retention.* Since the Class III denture does not tend to move or rotate in function, there is no need for indirect retention. However, if direct retention is not obtained on one or more abutment teeth, indirect retention may be needed.

The Class II removable partial denture must embody features of both Class I and Class III designs (Fig. 1-31). The dentulous or tooth-supported side, if a modification space exists, must be designed as a Class III denture, and the unilateral distal extension side must be designed as a Class I denture, with adequate support from the denture base, a flexible direct retainer on the terminal abutment tooth, and use of indirect retention.

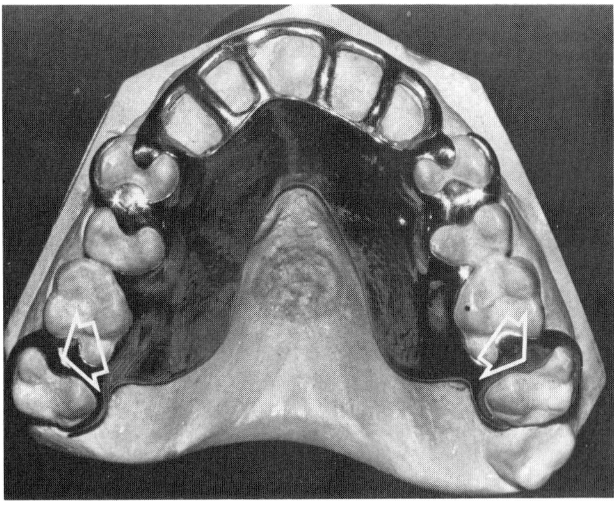

Fig. 1-32. Class IV removable partial denture, particularly for a long space, must be planned as a reverse Class I. Adequate denture base coverage and flexible direct retainers are required, and indirect retention is placed as far posterior as possible (arrows).

The Class IV design, particularly if the edentulous span is lengthy, must be regarded as a Class I denture in reverse (Fig. 1-32). Denture base support and flexible direct retainers must be planned. Forces of rotation will occur around the *anterior* abutment teeth, so indirect retention must be obtained *posterior* to the fulcrum line. If the edentulous span is not lengthy (greater than four teeth), the design may be treated as a tooth-supported, or Class III, partial denture.

REFERENCES

Applegate, O.C.: The rationale of partial denture choice, J. Pros. Dent. **10:** 891-907, 1960.

Boucher, C.O., editor: Current clinical dental terminology, a glossary of accepted terms in all disciplines of dentistry, ed. 2, St. Louis, 1974, The C.V. Mosby Co.

Cummer, W.E.: Partial denture service. In Textbook of prosthetic dentistry, Philadelphia, 1942, Lea & Febiger.

DeVan, M.M.: The nature of the partial denture foundation: suggestions for its preservation, J. Pros. Dent. **2:** 210-218, 1952.

Glossary of Prosthodontic Terms, ed. 4, 1977, The C.V. Mosby Co.

Kennedy, E.: Partial denture construction, Brooklyn, 1928, Dent. Items of Interest Co., pp. 3-8.

Ottofy, L.: Standard dental dictionary, Chicago, 1923, Laird and Lee, Inc., pp. IX.

BIBLIOGRAPHY

Akers, P.E.: A new and simplified method of partial denture prosthesis, J. Amer. Den. Assoc. **12:**711-715, 1925.

Ante, I.H.: The fundamental principles, design and construction of crown and bridge prosthesis, Dent. Items Interest. **1:**215-232, 1928.

Avant, W.E.: A universal classification for removable partial denture situations, J. Pros. Dent. **16:**533-539, 1966.

Friedman, J.: The ABC classification of partial denture segments, J. Pros. Dent. **3:**517-524, 1953.

Godfrey, R.J.: A classification of removable partial dentures, J. Amer. Col. Dent. **18:**5-13, 1951.

Heartwell, C.M., Jr.: Syllabus of complete dentures, ed. 3, Philadelphia, 1980, Lea & Febiger.

Mauk, E.H.: Classifications of mutilated dental arches requiring treatment by removable partial dentures, J. Amer. Dent. Assoc. **29:**2121-2131, 1942.

Miller, E.L.: Systems for classifying partially dentulous arches, J. Pros. Dent. **24:**25-40, 1970.

Skinner, C.N.: A classification of removable partial dentures based upon the principles of anatomy and physiology, J. Pros. Dent. **9:**240-246, 1959.

Terkla, L., and Lacy, W.: Partial dentures, ed. 3, St. Louis, 1963, The C.V. Mosby Co.

2 Components of a removable partial denture

MAJOR CONNECTORS · MINOR CONNECTORS · RESTS AND REST SEATS

Each component of the prosthesis has a name that is most often descriptive of its function. A major connector, for example, does exactly what its name implies: it serves as the major or principal method of connecting the opposing sides of the partial denture. In like manner a clasp clasps or grasps a tooth, and the different varieties of clasps are further named as retentive clasps, because they retain the denture in place, or reciprocal clasps, because they reciprocate or oppose the forces on a tooth caused by a retentive clasp. A minor connector connects smaller components to a larger unit, usually the major connector.

With these definitions in mind, a more in-depth look at the component parts of a removable partial denture will be undertaken along with a description of each part as well as variations that may occur. The structural requirements and function of the components will also be covered.

As can be seen from Figs. 2-1 and 2-2, the names of the components are the same for maxillary and mandibular removable partial dentures. The only variation occurs in the forms of the major connectors.

A removable partial denture will have some of the following components:

Major connector
Minor connectors
Rests
Direct retainers (clasps)
Indirect retainers
One or more denture bases and replacement teeth

The first three components are considered in this chapter; the last three, in Chapter 3.

MAJOR CONNECTORS

The major connector connects the parts of the prosthesis located on one side of the arch with those on the opposite side. All other parts of the partial denture are attached to it either directly or indirectly.

All major connectors must (1) be rigid, (2) provide vertical support and protect the soft tissue, (3) provide a means of obtaining indirect retention where indicated, (4) provide an opportunity of positioning denture bases where needed, and (5) maintain patient comfort.

The first requirement for all major connectors is rigidity. This quality allows stresses that are applied to any portion of the partial denture to be effectively distributed over the entire supporting area, including the abutment teeth, other teeth included in the design of the partial denture, and the underlying bone and soft tissue. Other components of the partial denture such as retentive clasps, occlusal rests, and indirect retainers can be effective only if the major connector is rigid. Perhaps the greatest damage a partial denture can produce is that which results from a flexible major connector. Flexibility allows forces to be concentrated on individual teeth or the edentulous ridge, causing damage to the periodontal support of the teeth, resorption of the bony ridge, and impingement and injury to the soft tissue beneath the major connector.

The second fundamental requirement of a major connector is that it must avoid impingement of the free gingival margin. The major connector must never terminate on gingival tissues because the marginal gingiva is highly vascular and susceptible to injury from pressure. For this reason care should be exercised during the designing procedure to ensure that the gingival margins are not compromised. In the maxillary arch the border of the major connector should be at least 6 mm from the gingival crevice of the teeth (Fig. 2-3), and in the mandibular arch it should be at least 3 mm from the gingival margin (Fig. 2-4). If it is impossible to obtain this clearance, it will be necessary to extend the major connector onto the lingual surfaces of the teeth in the form of lingual plating. This form of major connector is discussed in greater detail when various types of major connectors are considered.

The border of the major connector should run parallel to the gingival margin of the teeth (Fig. 2-5). If the gingival margin must be crossed, the crossing should be at right angles to the margin to produce the least pos-

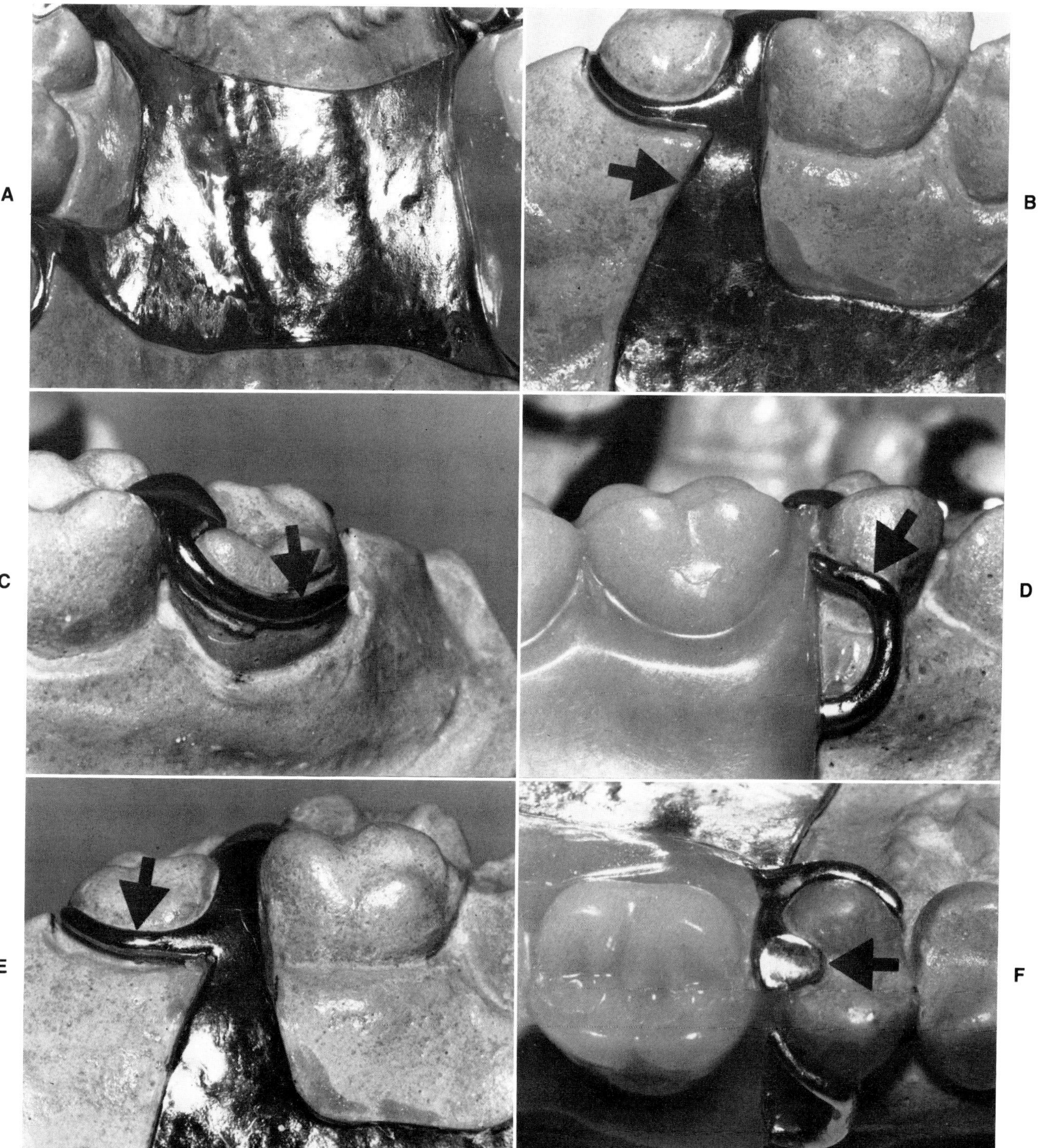

Fig. 2-1. Components of a maxillary removable partial denture. **A,** Maxillary major connector. **B,** Minor connector. **C,** Circumferential retentive clasp. **D,** Vertical projection retentive clasp. **E,** Reciprocal clasp. **F,** Occlusal rest.

Continued

G

H

I

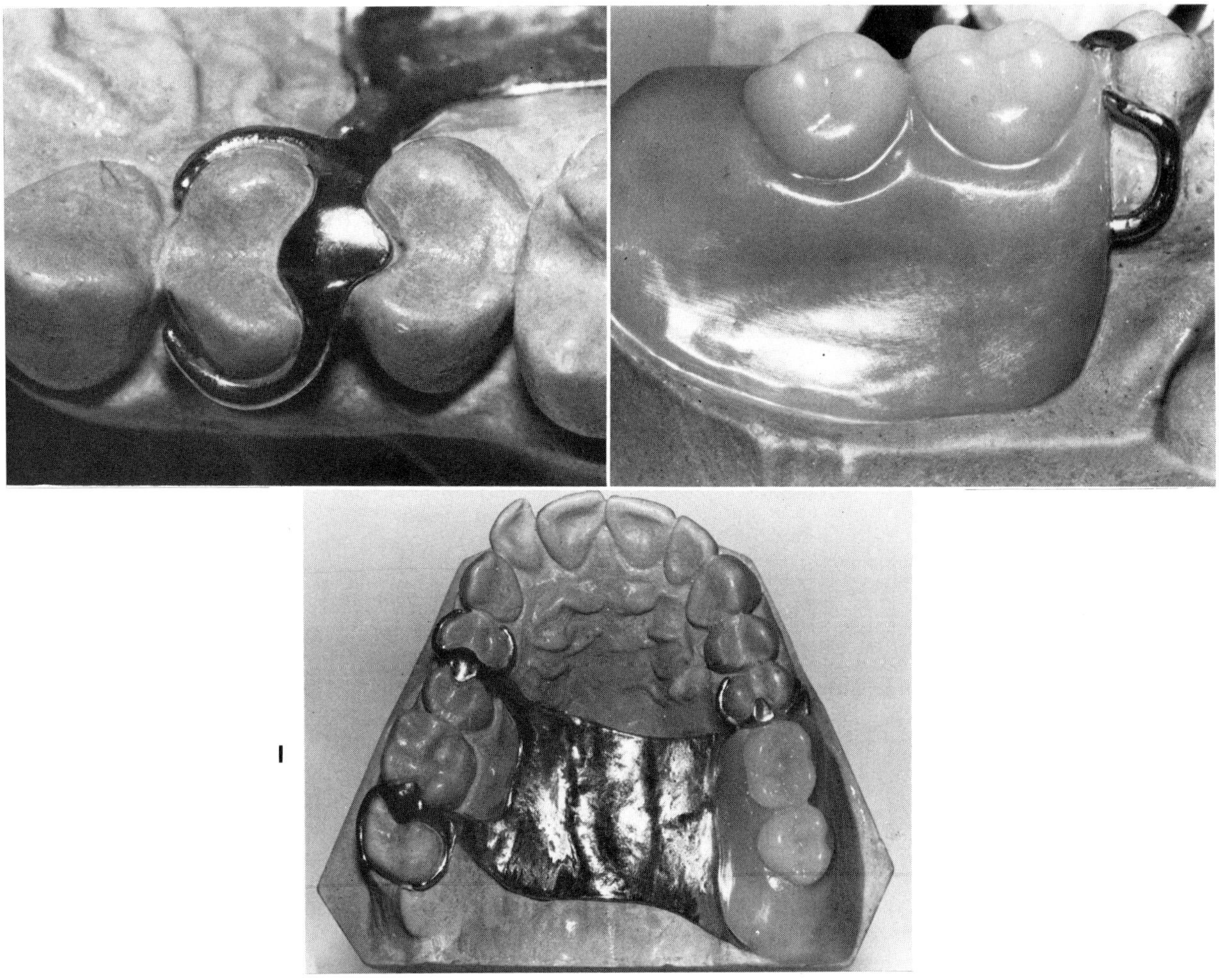

Fig. 2-1, cont'd. G, Clasp assembly: retentive and reciprocal clasps, occlusal rest, and minor connector. **H,** Denture base and artificial teeth. Entire prosthesis is shown in **I.**

A

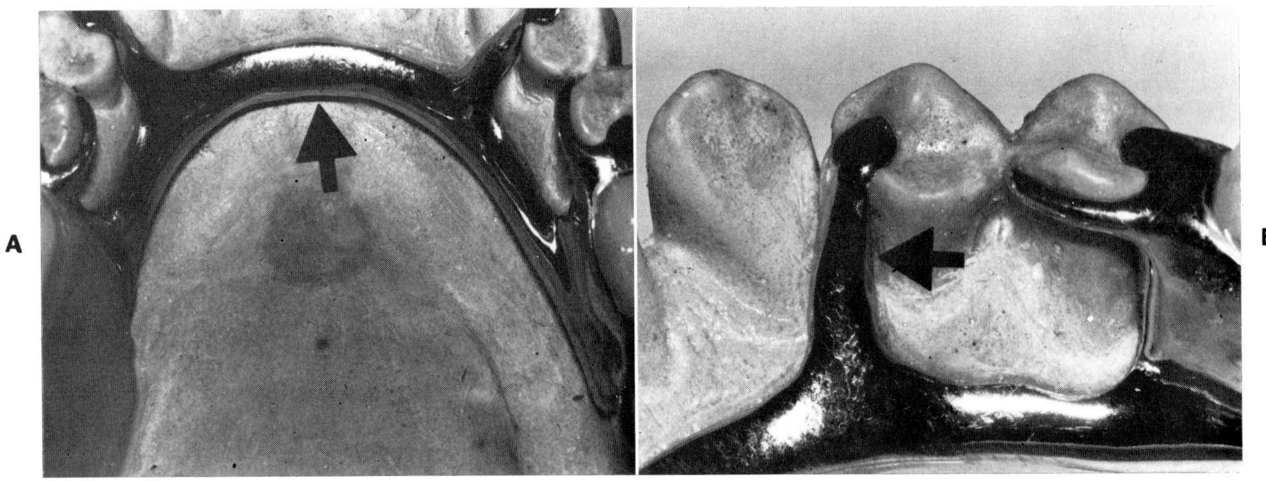

B

Fig. 2-2. Components of a mandibular removable partial denture. **A,** Mandibular major connector. **B,** Minor connector.

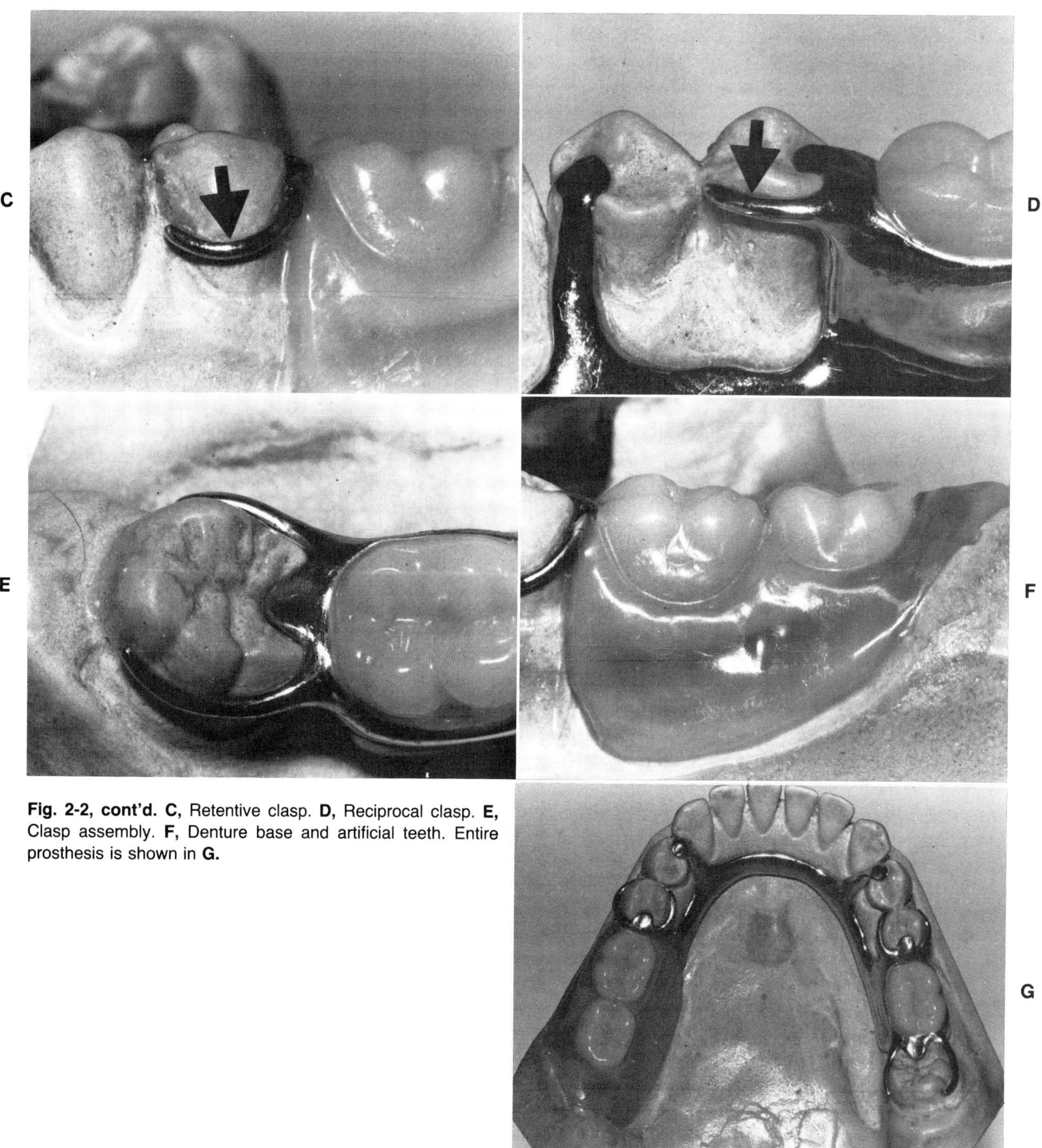

Fig. 2-2, cont'd. C, Retentive clasp. **D,** Reciprocal clasp. **E,** Clasp assembly. **F,** Denture base and artificial teeth. Entire prosthesis is shown in **G.**

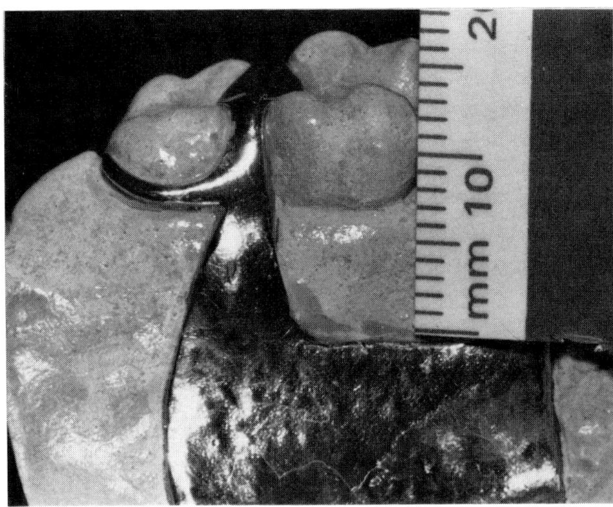

Fig. 2-3. In maxillary arch, border of major connector must be no closer than 6 mm to gingival crevices of teeth.

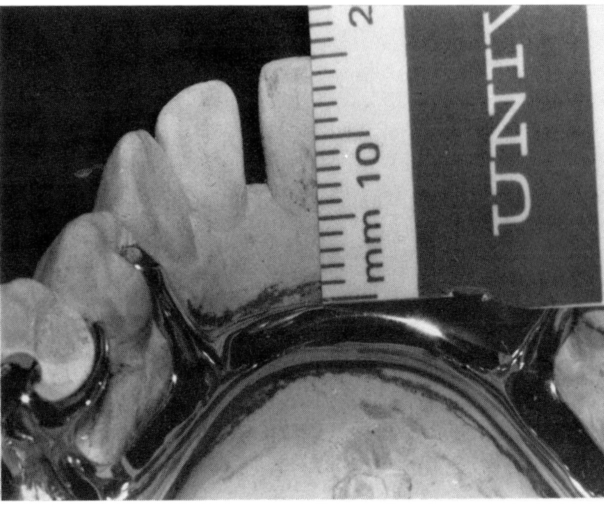

Fig. 2-4. In mandibular arch, border of major connector must not be closer than 3 mm to gingival margin.

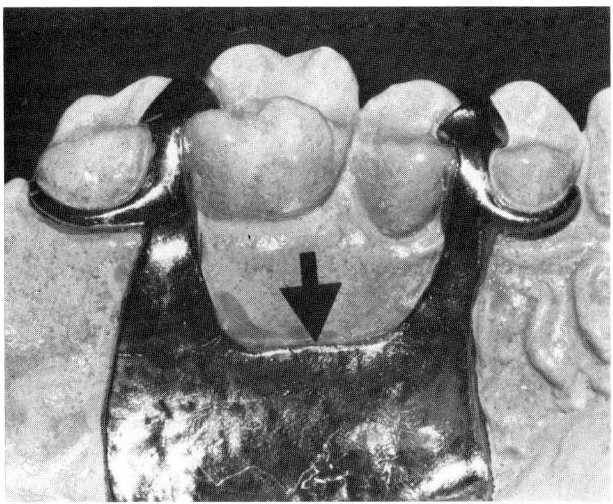

Fig. 2-5. Border of any major connector must be parallel to gingival margin (arrow).

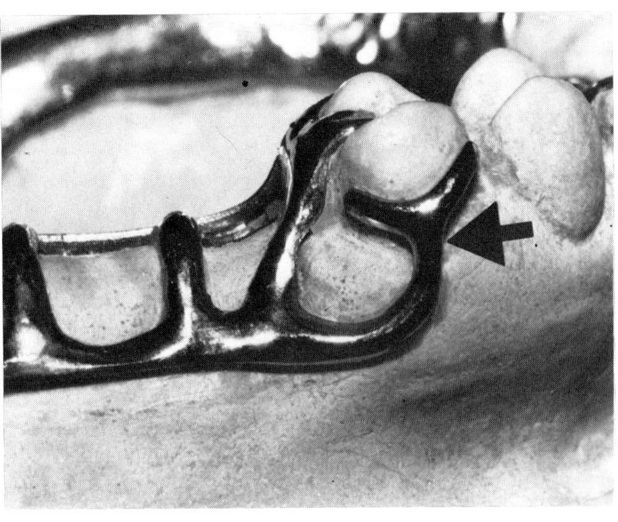

Fig. 2-6. If gingival margin is crossed by metal, crossing should be made at right angles to margin (arrow).

sible contact with the soft tissue (Fig. 2-6). Whenever the major connector does cross the gingival margin, relief, or a space, must be provided between the metal and the soft tissue. Methods of providing this relief are presented in Chapter 10. If relief is inadequate, edema and inflammation of the soft tissue will result.

When the free gingival margin is covered by metal, the patient must be thoroughly schooled in oral physiotherapy procedures to provide the soft tissues with the stimulation needed to maintain oral health. These tissues, when covered by a denture, lose the stimulation otherwise provided by food, the tongue, and surrounding musculature.

To prevent the major connector from being forced in a gingival direction or from transmitting horizontal or lateral forces to teeth that it contacts, adequate rests must be provided. Otherwise settling or movement of the major connector will cause damage to the underlying bone and soft tissue or orthodontic movement of the supporting teeth, or both.

A removable partial denture that is not supported at each end of an edentulous space tends to rotate around a fulcrum line. This concept of partial dentures undergoing rotational displacement is discussed in Chapter 3. One method of preventing or controlling this movement is by the use of an indirect retainer. The major

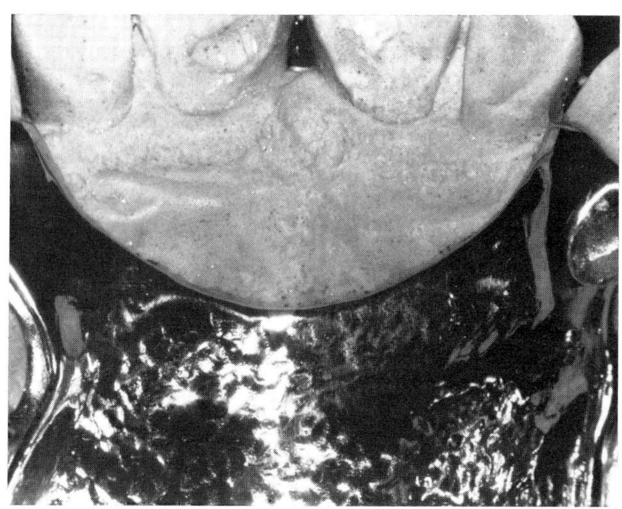

Fig. 2-7. Anterior border of a maxillary major connector should end in valley between rugae.

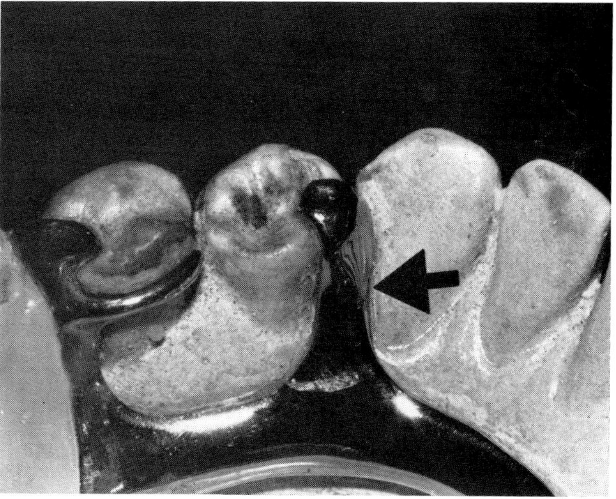

Fig. 2-8. Metal components extending onto teeth (arrow) should be placed in tooth embrasures to disguise their thickness.

connector in the form of lingual plating may be used to assist in indirect retention. The contact of the major connector with the teeth helps control the rotational movement.

The selection of the type of major connector will at times be dictated by the location of the denture bases that replace the missing teeth. Certain major connectors can be used to replace anterior teeth; others cannot. Some major connectors may be selected for a tooth-supported partial denture but not to replace distal extension edentulous areas. The location and number of denture bases influence the type of major connector that must be used.

A major connector must not create food entrapment areas. A partial denture must always be designed to be as self-cleansing as possible. As a general rule it is best to avoid covering the lingual surfaces of teeth with the metal of the major connector. However, when freeing the gingival margin will result in a design that may cause the entrapment of food or other debris, the area may be covered with a thin layer of metal. Food entrapment is most frequently encountered when an attempt is made to free the gingival margin around a single tooth. The inferior border of a mandibular major connector may cause food entrapment if it is not positioned as far inferiorly as function will permit.

Finally, the major connector should be selected and designed with consideration of the comfort of the patient. The edges of the connector should be rounded and tapered toward the tissues. Adding a portion of the connector to a tooth surface that is already convex can produce discomfort. This is particularly true of the anterior or leading edge of a maxillary major connector that crosses the rugae area. The anterior border of the major connector should not end on the crest of a prominent ruga. Rather, it should end in the valleys between the rugae crests (Fig. 2-7). If it is necessary to cross a ruga, the crossing should be as abrupt as possible.

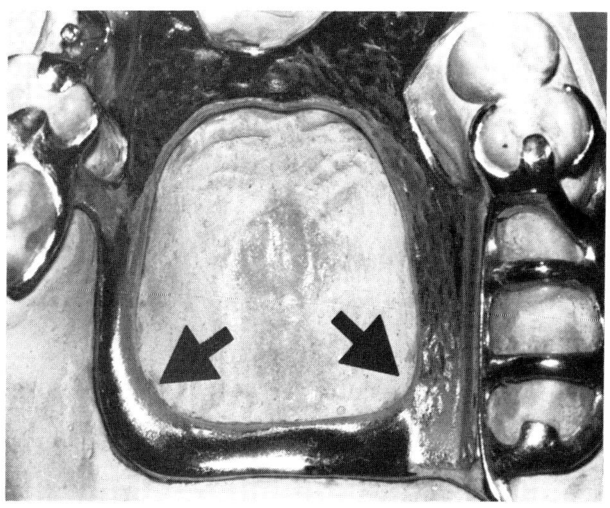

Fig. 2-9. Border outlines of a major connector should be curved (arrows) to prevent annoying tongue.

When it is necessary to extend components of the partial denture in the form of extensions of metal onto the teeth, tooth embrasures should be used to hide the presence of the metal (Fig. 2-8).

The borders of the major connector should be as inconspicous to the tongue as possible. Sharp angles or corners should be avoided and the border outline should have gentle curves (Fig. 2-9).

It is good design policy to make the major connector

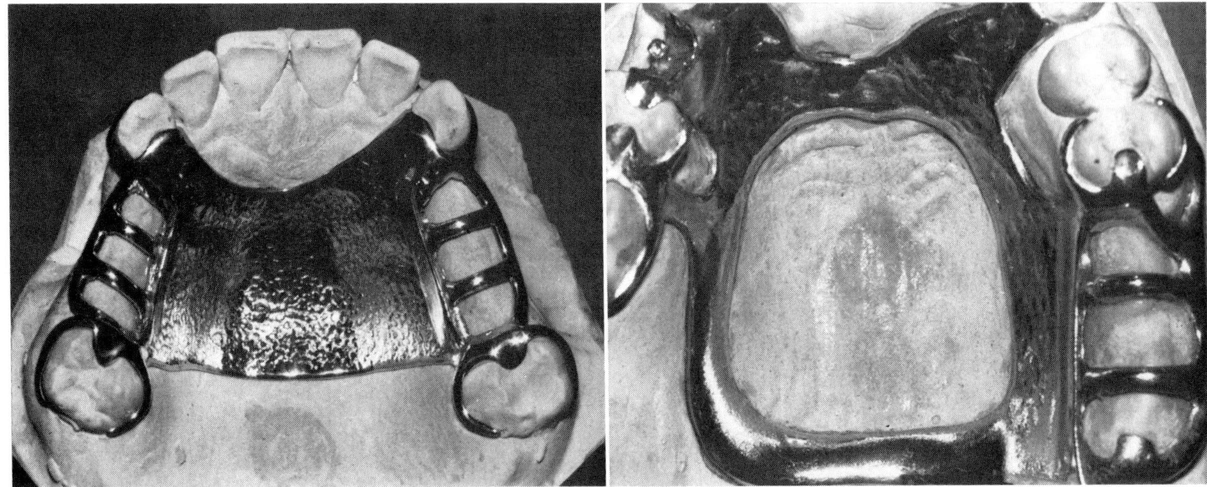

Fig. 2-10. The major connector should be as symmetric as possible and should cross the palate in a straight line.

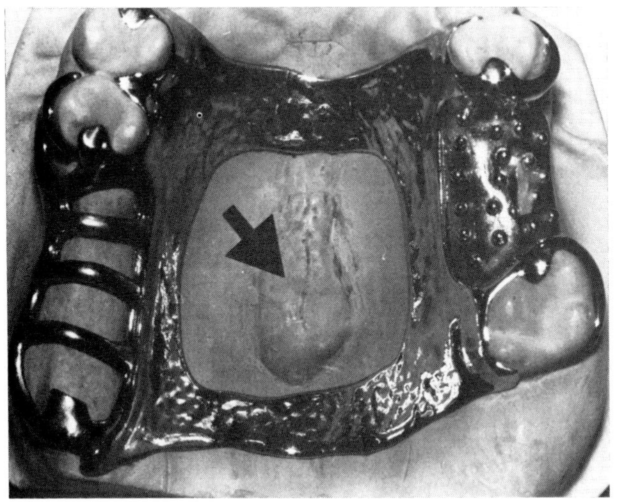

Fig. 2-11. The major connector should avoid crossing bony prominences such as this small torus palatinus (arrow).

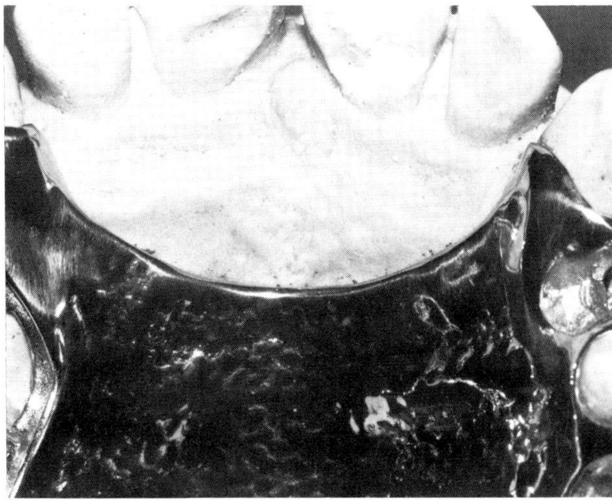

Fig. 2-12. Anterior portion of palate or rugae area should not be covered by metal, if possible, to avoid problems with speech.

symmetric and to have it cross the palate in a straight line (Fig. 2-10).

It is best to design the major connector so that its margins do not cross bony or soft tissue prominences (Fig. 2-11). In the palate a small torus may be completely covered by a major connector if its surgical removal is impossible and the torus cannot be avoided by changing the design of the major connector. One of the few instances in which relief is used in the maxillary arch is when a torus is to be covered. Avoiding mandibular tori is much more complicated, and as a general rule these tori should be surgically removed.

It is important that the major connector not interfere with speech or phonetics. An attempt should be made not to cover the anterior portion of the palate or the rugae area, because of possible problems with phonetics (Fig. 2-12).

These design details are fundamental to all major connectors. The importance of each requirement depends on the type of partially edentulous arch that is being treated. Therefore the type of major connector is selected on the basis of the individual patient's needs. Specific design concerns and types of major connectors will be considered for each arch.

Maxillary major connectors

Special structural requirements

All maxillary major connectors should have a specially prepared seal along all borders that contact soft tissue (Fig. 2-13). This seal forms a beading that will slightly displace the soft tissue. The beading is scribed on the surface of the master cast before duplication in investment material. It is best prepared with a small spoon excavator. It should have a depth and width of approximately 0.5 to 1.0 mm and should fade out approximately 6 mm from the gingival margin if the metal is to continue up on the teeth. The depth of the beading should also be reduced in areas of thin tissue coverage such as a torus or the midpalatine raphae. When the partial denture is not in the mouth, the outline of the beading should be evident in the palatal tissue, but there should be no evidence of irritation or inflammation (Fig. 2-14).

Beading prevents food debris from collecting under the major connector and provides an excellent visual finish line for the technician who finishes and polishes the metal framework. The extra thickness of metal provided by the beading also makes it possible to thin the metal on the polished surface side while maintaining the necessary strength. This helps make the junction of the metal and soft tissue less noticeable to the tongue.

Except in the presence of a palatal torus or a prominent median suture line, relief is not used under a maxillary major connector. The intimate contact between the palatal soft tissue and the metal connector enhances the retention and stability of the denture. To maintain this intimate metal–soft tissue contact, the tissue side of the major connector is not brought to a high finish during the polishing procedure. Electrolytic polishing is sufficient to produce a smooth, well-finished surface without disturbing the accuracy of the casting.

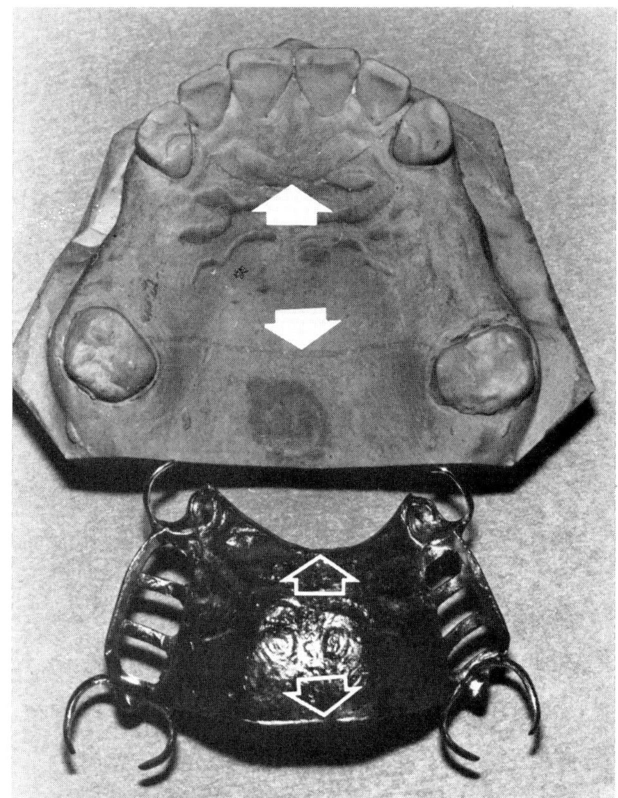

Fig. 2-13. Borders of a maxillary major connector that contact soft tissue should have a specially prepared seal, or beading (arrows).

Types of maxillary major connectors

The following six types of maxillary major connectors are used: (1) single posterior palatal bar, (2) palatal strap, (3) anteroposterior, or double, palatal bar, (4) horseshoe, or U-shaped connector, (5) closed horseshoe, or anteroposterior palatal strap, and (6) complete palate.

Single posterior palatal bar. The single posterior palatal bar is a narrow half-oval with its thickest point at the center. The bar is gently curved and should not form a sharp angle at the juncture with the denture base (Figs. 2-15 and 2-16).

Advantages. Although for many years it was one of the most widely used maxillary major connectors, at present the main and perhaps only indication for the single posterior palatal bar is as an interim partial denture until more definitive treatment can be rendered.

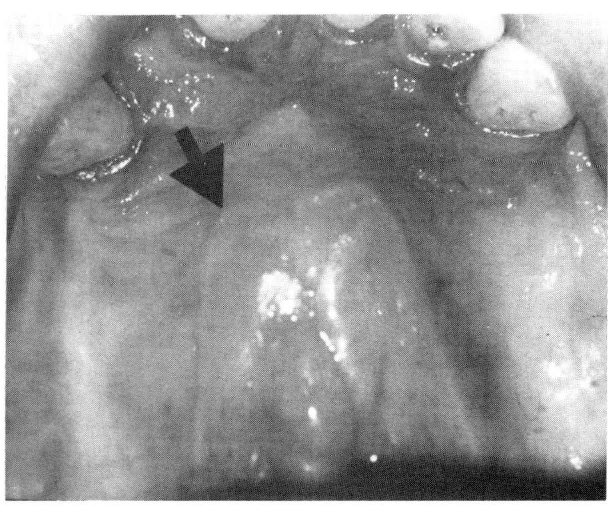

Fig. 2-14. When maxillary partial denture is removed from mouth, beading should be seen in soft tissue of palate (arrow). There should be no evidence of inflammation or irritation as seen in anterior palate.

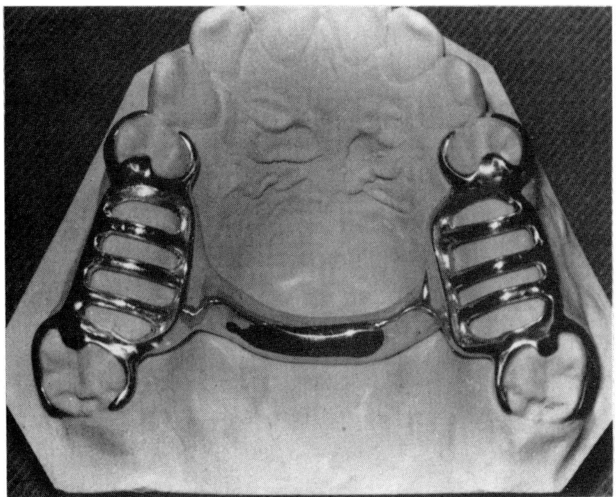

Fig. 2-15. Single posterior palatal bar has limited indication for use.

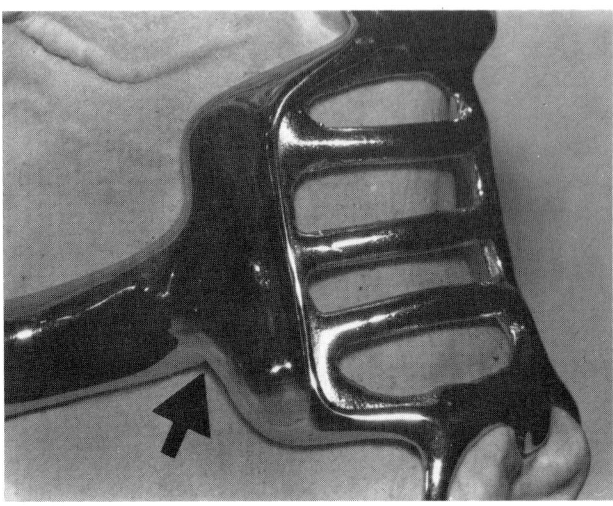

Fig. 2-16. Sharp angles should be avoided at junction of palatal bar and denture base (arrow).

Disadvantages. The single posterior palatal bar is one of the most difficult maxillary major connectors for a patient to adjust to, because to maintain any degree of rigidity it has to be bulky. Because of its narrow anteroposterior width it derives little vertical support from the bony palate and must therefore be supported positively by rests on remaining teeth. If used at all, it should be limited to replacing one or two teeth on each side of the arch and should be placed no further anteriorly than the second premolar position. There must be teeth capable of bearing an additional load both anterior and posterior to the edentulous space.

If the bar is placed any farther forward than the center of the dental arch, severe interference with tongue action will be encountered.

The single palatal bar should never be used in a distal extension edentulous situation, nor should it be used when anterior teeth require replacement.

Palatal strap. The palatal strap is the most versatile maxillary major connector. It consists of a wide, thin band of metal that crosses the palate in an unobtrusive manner. It can be made fairly narrow anteroposteriorly for a tooth-supported denture when the edentulous spaces are small, but should not be less than 8 mm wide or its rigidity may be compromised (Fig. 2-17).

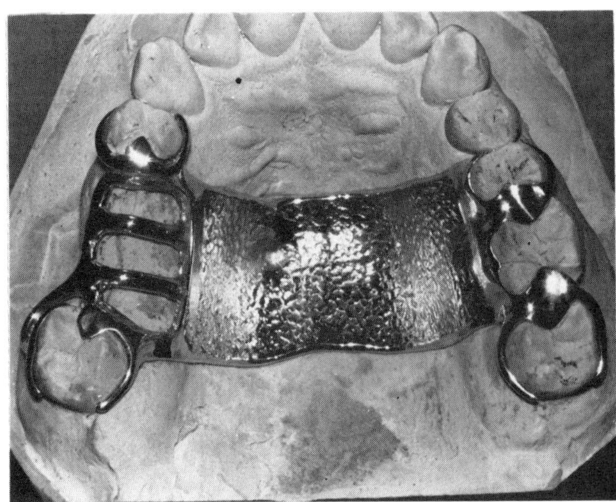

Fig. 2-17. Palatal strap is the most widely used maxillary major connector. Width of strap can vary but should not be less than 8 mm.

The width should be increased as the edentulous space increases in length. This increase in width not only ensures rigidity, but also provides greater support from the hard bony palate. The wider the palatal strap, the vaguer the difference between it and a modified complete palate. (If the edentulous areas are extensive, bilateral, and not supported posteriorly with natural teeth and if the major connector extends posteriorly to the junction of the hard and soft palates, the connector is a modified complete palate.) The wide palatal strap may be used for a unilateral distal extension edentulous partial denture, but rarely in a bilateral situation.

Advantages. Because the palatal strap is located in three planes (the horizontal, or vault of the palate; the vertical, or lateral slopes of the palate; and the sagittal, or anterior slope of the palate), it offers great resistance to bending and twisting forces. Thus greater rigidity with less bulk of metal is produced. This theory is similar to the L-bar principle used in building construction. Forces transmitted on different planes are counteracted more easily.

Because the palatal strap is inherently strong, it can

be kept thin, thus increasing patient comfort. It offers little interference to tongue action and as a result is accepted well. In addition, by covering a relatively large area of palatal tissue it helps distribute stress over a broad area.

Retention of the partial denture through the forces of adhesion and cohesion is enhanced by the intimate contact between the metal and soft tissue.

The strap also contributes some indirect retention, preventing the partial denture from rocking anteriorly when the pull of sticky foods or the force of gravity tends to unseat the posterior end of the denture. This is accomplished because the relatively firm palatal tissues are intimately contacted on several planes. However, there is a limit to the amount of force or pressure to which the palatal tissue can be submitted without an adverse reaction, such as inflammation or ulceration.

Disadvantages. The patient may complain of excessive palatal coverage. This complaint frequently can be traced to improper positioning of the strap borders. The anterior border should be posterior to the rugae area; if this is not possible, the border should be terminated in the valley of the rugae. The posterior border should terminate short of the junction of the hard and soft palates and must avoid crossing a torus or a prominent median suture.

Another possible disadvantage is an adverse soft tissue reaction in the form of papillary hyperplasia. (See Chapter 6 for further discussion.) This condition is seen when the partial denture is worn 24 hours a day and is normally accompanied by poor oral hygiene and poor care of the prosthesis. The cause can be traced to a lack of patient instruction or faulty communication between the dentist and the patient. Complete instruction on wearing and caring for any removable prosthesis must be given and repeated to every patient.

Anteroposterior, or double, palatal bar. The greatest asset of the anteroposterior palatal bar is excellent rigidity. At the same time, because of its narrow bars, or straps, it offers little in the way of support to the partial denture, which must rely almost exclusively on support from the remaining teeth (Fig. 2-18). Therefore this connector should not be used unless the remaining teeth have good periodontal support.

The flat anterior bar is narrower than the palatal strap. It's borders are positioned in the valleys between the rugae, never on the rugae crests. The posterior bar is half-oval, similar to the single posterior palatal bar connector but less bulky. The two bars are joined by flat longitudinal elements on each side of the lateral slopes of the palate. This configuration gives the effect of a circle and is considerably more rigid than any of the individual elements. The two bars, lying in different planes, produce a structurally strong L-beam effect.

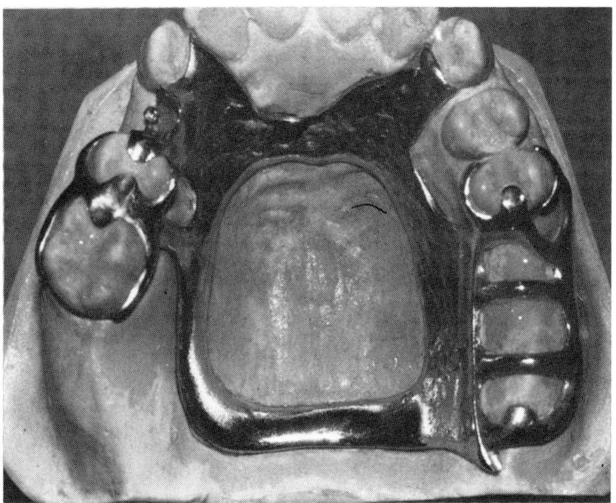

Fig. 2-18. Anteroposterior palatal bar is a rigid major connector that receives little vertical support from hard palate.

Advantages. The only advantage of the anteroposterior palatal bar is its rigidity. In comparison to the amount of soft tissue coverage, it is by far the most rigid maxillary major connector.

The anteroposterior palatal bar may be used when support is not a major consideration and when the anterior and posterior abutments are widely separated.

Occasionally this major connector may be considered when a patient objects to a large amount of palatal coverage, but the lack of vertical support must be weighed against the possible advantage of patient comfort.

In patients with a large palatal torus for whom surgery has been ruled out, the anteroposterior palatal bar may be the major connector of choice.

Disadvantages. Because of the limited palatal tissue contact, little support is derived from the bony palate. In many instances the extra rigidity offered by the anteroposterior palatal bar would be desirable, but its use is contraindicated because of reduced periodontal support of the remaining teeth that necessitates additional support from the palate.

As a general rule the anteroposterior palatal bar should not be considered as a first choice for a maxillary major connector. It should be selected only after other choices have been considered and eliminated. It is definitely not indicated when a high narrow vault is present because the anterior bar will interfere with phonetics.

The anteroposterior palatal bar is frequently uncomfortable. In addition to the extra bulk of metal needed because of the narrow bars, the many borders of the bars are a nuisance because the tongue tends to want to investigate them.

Horseshoe, or U-shaped, connector. The horseshoe connector consists of a thin band of metal running along the lingual surface of the posterior teeth and extending onto the palatal tissue for 6 to 8 mm (Fig. 2-19). Anteriorly the metal normally covers the cingula of the present teeth and extends on to the palate to cover the entire rugae area. Some variation of this outline form may occur.

The borders of the horseshoe connector must either be 6 mm from the gingival margin or extend onto the lingual surfaces of the teeth. The borders should also be placed in the valleys of the rugae. The lateral palatal borders should be at the junction of the horizontal and vertical slopes of the palate. The rigidity can be increased by extending the borders slightly onto the horizontal palate surface. The connector should be symmetric, with the palatal borders extending to the same height on both sides.

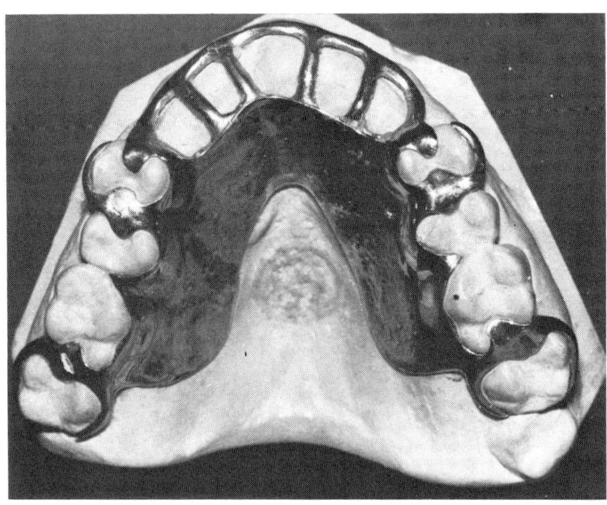

Fig. 2-19. Horseshoe, or U-shaped, connector is useful for replacement of anterior teeth. It is not indicated for Class I partially edentulous arches.

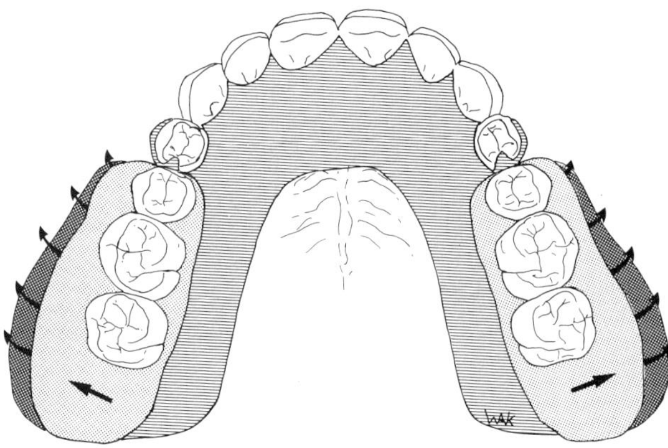

Fig. 2-20. One weakness of horseshoe major connector is its tendency to spread apart as force is applied to artificial teeth. This spreading can damage abutment teeth.

All borders or angles of the connector should be gently curved and smooth.

Advantages. This major connector is used primarily when several anterior teeth are being replaced. It is a reasonably strong connector that can derive some vertical support and some indirect retention from the palate. In patients with considerable vertical overlap of the anterior teeth, the horseshoe is thin yet strong enough to support the replacement teeth.

In the presence of a hard median suture line or an inoperable torus, this major connector may offer some definite advantages. The torus can be avoided without sacrificing strength or loss of vertical support.

Disadvantages. When vertical force is applied to either or both ends of the horseshoe major connector, there is a tendency for the connector to spread or straighten (Fig. 2-20). Therefore it is a poor choice for a distal extension partial denture. For the same reason this is not a good connector when cross-arch stabilization is required. It has less resistance to flexing, and movement can occur at the open end.

To avoid the tendency to flex, the metal crossing the rugae area must be thicker than that used in most other major connectors. This places the greatest bulk of metal in the area where the tongue needs the most space. Interferences with phonetics and patient comfort can result.

Closed horseshoe, or anteroposterior palatal strap. The closed horseshoe (Fig. 2-21) is a structurally strong and rigid major connector that may be used in most maxillary partial denture designs and is particularly indicated when numerous teeth are to be replaced and when a torus palatinus is present.

The thickness of metal in the straps should be uniform, and the borders of the connector should be kept 6 mm from the free gingival margin or should extend onto the lingual surfaces of the teeth.

In instances in which anterior teeth are not being replaced, the anterior strap should be as far back in the rugal area as possible to minimize interference with speech. The posterior strap should also be as posterior as possible but should not contact the soft palate.

All the borders should be finished in smooth, gentle curves.

Advantages. The closed horseshoe is a rigid connector that derives good support from the palate even though an opening is provided in the palate.

The corrugated contour of the metal over the rugae adds strength to the connector and allows the metal to be made thinner. The circle effect of the anterior and posterior straps contributes to the rigidity of the connector. The shape of this connector also provides a definite L-beam effect (that is, the metal lying in two planes increases the resistance to flexing).

Disadvantages. Even though the metal over the rugae area may be thinner than in some other major connectors, interference with phonetics may occur in some patients. In addition, the extensive length of borders for the tongue to contact may cause annoyance or discomfort.

Complete palate. The complete palate (Fig. 2-22) provides the ultimate in rigidity and support. It also provides the most tissue coverage, so the need for maximum support and rigidity should be determined before this connector is selected.

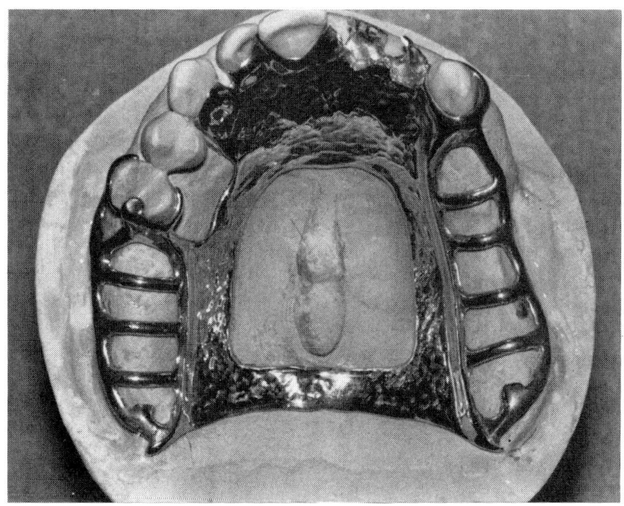

Fig. 2-21. Closed horseshoe, anteroposterior palatal strap, is rigid major connector that is indicated for Class I or II arches when anterior teeth are also to be replaced.

The posterior border of the complete palate normally extends to the juncture of the soft and hard palate. The anterior border must be kept 6 mm from the marginal gingiva or must cover the cingula of the anterior teeth. The connector can be made in the following three forms:

1. *All acrylic resin* (Fig. 2-23). The entire connector is made of acrylic resin. It covers the entire palate and usually extends to two or more edentulous areas and to the juncture of the hard and soft palates.
2. *Combination metal and acrylic resin* (Fig. 2-24). The anterior portion of the connector, covering the rugal area, is constructed of metal cast to conform to the convolutions of the rugae. Extending posteriorly from the metal are projections of metal around which can be processed the acrylic resin that will cover the remainder of the palate. This resin extends posteriorly to the junction of the hard and soft palates.
3. *All cast metal.* The entire palate is covered with a thin metal casting, which also extends posteriorly to the junction of the hard and soft palates.

The posterior palatal seal that is used with complete dentures should not be employed with a removable partial denture. It is not possible to produce a peripheral seal in a removable partial denture such as is produced by border molding a complete denture.

Attempts to use a posterior palatal seal not only fail

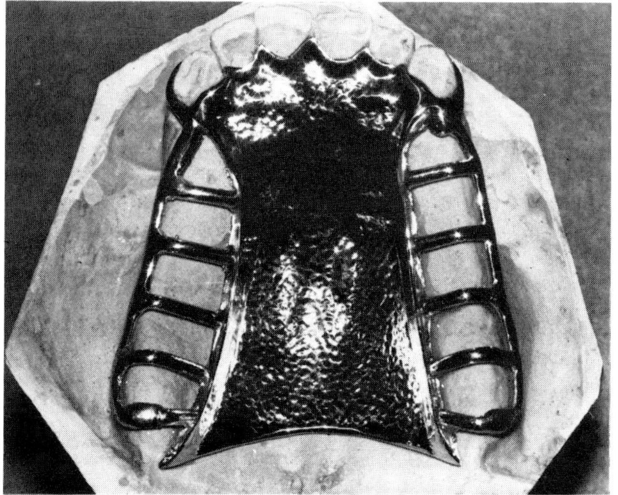

Fig. 2-22. Complete palate, the most rigid major connector, is indicated when maximum support from hard palate is needed.

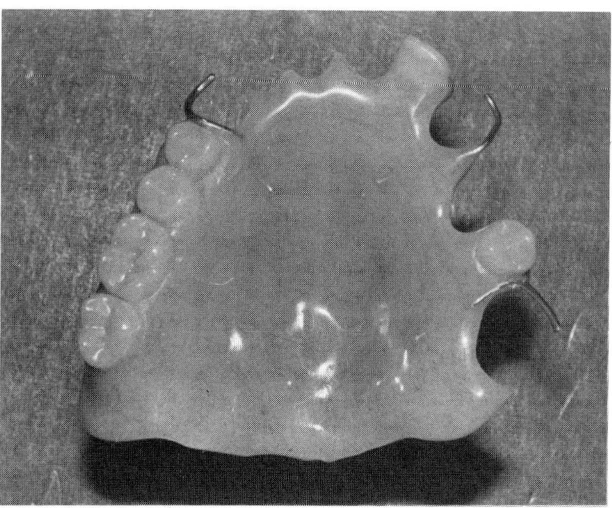

Fig. 2-23. All-acrylic resin palate must cover entire palate and is usually indicated for a temporary removable partial denture.

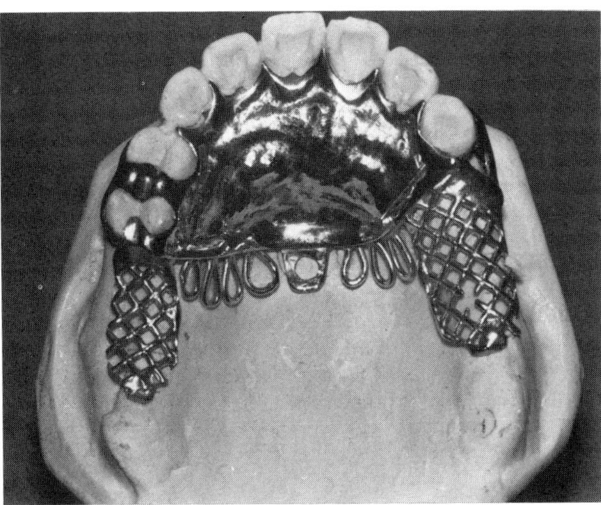

Fig. 2-24. Combination cast metal and acrylic resin palate is indicated when obtaining an accurate *casting* of the palate is difficult or when major connector may need to be relined after palatal surgery.

to accomplish the desired purpose, but also, because of the rebound of the tissues under compression, place unnecessary extra forces on the abutment teeth.

A slight border seal, or bead is needed along the posterior border of the connector to prevent debris from collecting beneath the complete palate. The intimate contact of the cast metal palate aids retention through adhesive and cohesive forces.

Many practitioners resort to complete or partial coverage of the palate with acrylic resin in preference to cast metal because of the mistaken belief that it is difficult if not impossible to obtain an accurate casting of the size needed to cover the palate. Inaccurate castings can most frequently be traced to inaccurate impressions of the palatal vault area. Impression materials of the type generally used for removable partial dentures tend to slump away from the palatal tissues during their gelation period if the material is not supported adequately. This slumping will produce an impression that appears accurate but in reality is distorted. This problem is discussed in greater detail in Chapter 9.

Advantages. Complete palatal coverage is indicated when all posterior teeth are to be replaced bilaterally. It is also indicated when anterior teeth require replacement along with bilateral distal extension replacements.

In individuals with well-developed muscles of mastication and a full complement of mandibular teeth, heavy occlusal forces can be anticipated, and the extra support against vertical displacement offered by the complete palate major connector may be beneficial.

When flat or flabby ridges or a shallow vault is present, the complete palate can provide the best stabilization for the prosthesis. Undesirable lateral or horizontal forces are dissipated well by the intimate contact between this connector and the soft tissue.

Occasionally, patients are treated with a transitional partial denture in preparation for treatment with a complete denture. Allowing the patient to feel the sensation of complete palatal coverage at this point makes the accommodation to complete dentures less frustrating. Transitional partial dentures with a complete palate major connector, like complete dentures, are usually constructed of all-acrylic resin.

In the maxillary arch any acrylic resin partial denture that replaces posterior teeth should have full palatal coverage for strength.

Cleft palate patients frequently require treatment with a maxillary removable partial denture. Many of these patients have a narrow, steep palatal vault. To gain intimate tissue contact and to close any patent air passage between the nasal and oral cavities a cast-complete palate is most often the connector of choice. This problem will be expanded on in Chapter 23.

The cast metal palate can be produced as a uniformly thin plate that reproduces the anatomic contour of the palate. The surface irregularities feel natural to the patient, and the major connector serves as a secondary masticatory surface.

The corrugations resulting from the rugal contours and the coverage of different palatal planes provides an L-beam effect, making this a rigid major connector.

The all-metal connector also enhances the transfer of temperature changes to produce a more natural sensation during eating and drinking. This advantage is lost when acrylic resin is used.

Disadvantages. Because of the extensive tissue coverage, adverse soft tissue reaction in the form of inflammation or hyperplasia may occur if adequate oral hygiene is not practiced. Problems with phonetics may occasionally be encountered.

Review of structural requirements for maxillary major connectors

1. The borders are placed a minimum of 6 mm from gingival margins or are positioned on the lingual surfaces of the teeth (Fig. 2-25). The location is determined by the need for support, stabilization, and/or oral hygiene.
2. Relief is normally not required under the major connector.
3. Anterior borders of major connectors that extend onto the rugae area should follow the valleys between the crests of the rugae (Fig. 2-26).
4. The posterior component of an anteroposterior palatal bar or a closed horseshoe should be either half-oval or straplike with a minimal width of 8

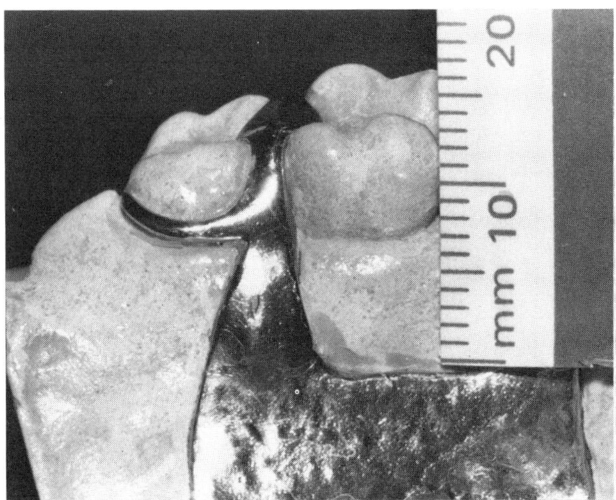

Fig. 2-25. Borders of maxillary major connectors must be positioned 6 mm from gingival margins of teeth or must extend onto lingual surfaces of teeth.

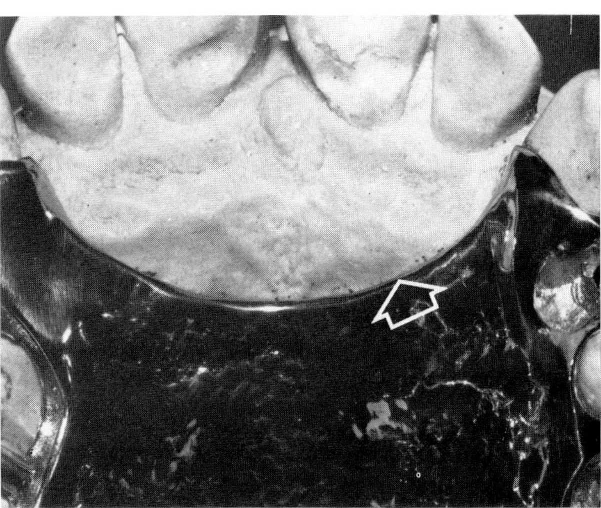

Fig. 2-26. Anterior border of major connector should be located in valleys between major rugae to help disguise thickness of metal (arrow).

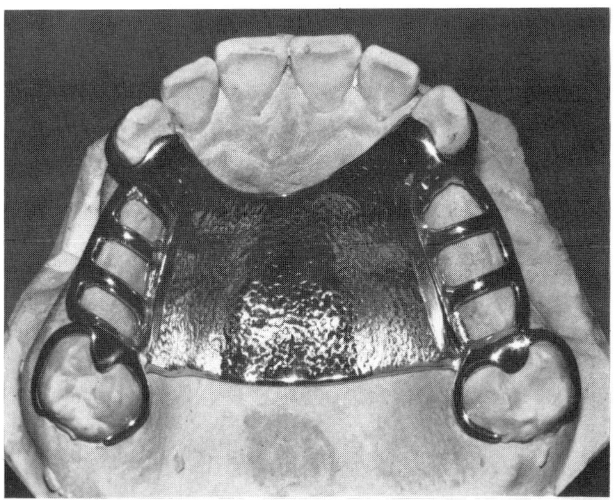

Fig. 2-27. Anterior and posterior border of major connector should cross midline at right angle to it.

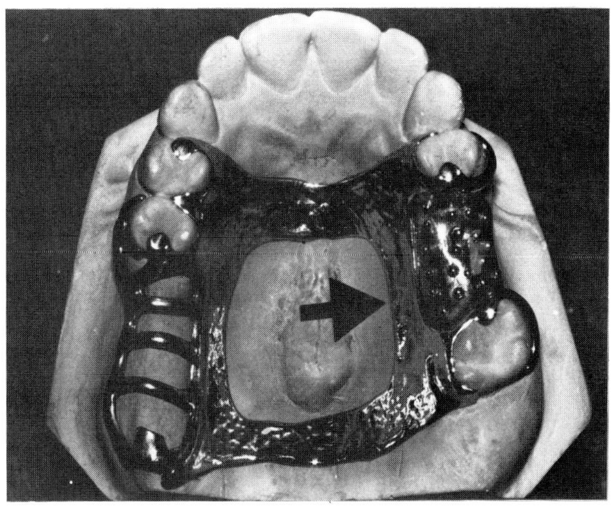

Fig. 2-28. Lateral borders of major connector are positioned at junction of horizontal and vertical surfaces of palate (arrow).

mm, and should be located as far posteriorly as possible without contacting the movable soft palate.

5. All borders should taper slightly toward the soft tissue.
6. Both anterior and posterior borders should cross the midline at right angles, never diagonally (Fig. 2-27).
7. The lateral borders of the connectors are positioned at the junction of the vertical and horizontal surfaces of the palate. In a flat or gently curved palate this location is approximated. These borders should be symmetric to prevent tongue awareness and patient discomfort (Fig. 2-28).
8. Thickness of the metal should be uniform throughout the palate.
9. The finished borders of the metal should be gently curved, never angular.
10. The metal should be smooth but not highly polished on the tissue side.
11. All borders on soft tissue should be beaded with the bead fading out near the gingival margins of the teeth.

Review of indications for maxillary major connectors

1. If the periodontal support of the remaining teeth is weak, more of the palate should be covered; thus a wide palatal strap or a complete palate is indicated.
2. If the remaining teeth have adequate periodontal support and little additional support is needed, a palatal strap or double palatal bar can be used.
3. For long-span distal extension bases where rigidity is critical, a closed horseshoe or complete palate is indicated.
4. When anterior teeth must be replaced, a horseshoe, closed horseshoe, or complete palate may be used. The final selection must be based on modifying factors such as number and location of posterior teeth missing, support of remaining teeth, and type of opposing occlusion.
5. If a torus is present and is not to be removed, a horseshoe, closed horseshoe, or anteroposterior palatal bar may be used; which one to use depends on other factors.
6. A single palatal bar is rarely indicated.

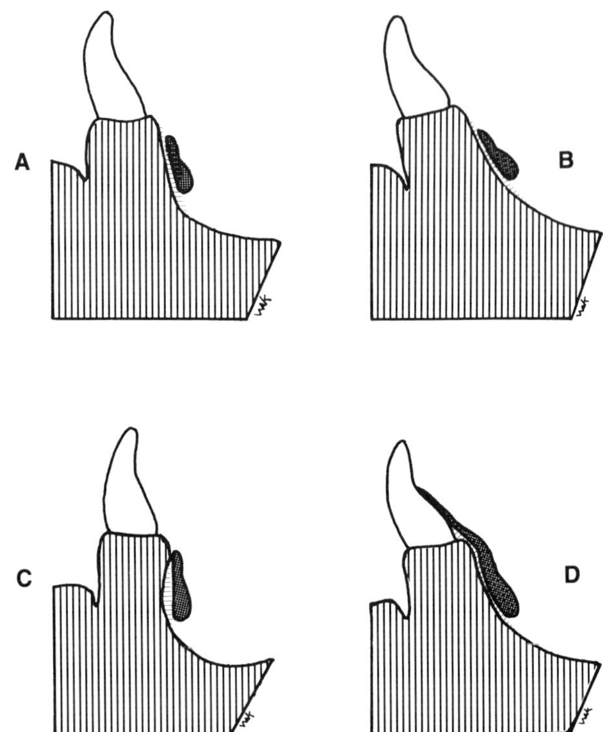

Fig. 2-29. Relief is required beneath mandibular major connector. Amount of relief required depends partially on anatomy of tissue lingual to anterior teeth. **A,** Slope of tissue is nearly vertical; minimal relief is necessary. **B,** Tissues slope toward tongue; maximum relief is needed to prevent major connector from compressing soft tissue during function. **C,** Lingual ridge is undercut; no additional relief is required. Undercut must be blocked out by laboratory technician, and this process automatically furnishes relief. **D,** In addition to relief under a lingual plate major connector, relief is required between gingival crevice and metal. This is essential to prevent damage to gingival tissue.

Mandibular major connectors

Special structural requirements

Many mandibular major connectors are long and relatively narrow because of space limitations caused by the height of the floor of the mouth, the position of the lingual frenum, or the presence of mandibular tori. This is especially true when compared with the space available for maxillary major connectors. For this reason consideration must be given to maintaining rigidity of the connector without making it so bulky that it is unacceptable to the patient. Structural considerations to maintain rigidity for each mandibular connector are offered as each is discussed.

In contrast to the maxillary major connectors, for which relief is infrequently required, relief must be routinely provided between the mandibular major connector and the soft tissue. The amount of relief depends on the type of removable partial denture. For an all-tooth-supported prosthesis a minimum of relief is needed because the denture does not tend to move, whereas a distal extension partial denture needs more relief because it tends to rotate during function. Relief prevents the margins of the connector from lacerating the friable and sensitive lingual mucosa as a result of this movement.

The slope of the lingual tissue also influences the amount of relief needed (Fig. 2-29). Tissue that slopes toward the tongue requires the greatest amount of relief because any movement of the connector will bring it into contact with the mucosa.

If the lingual soft tissues are vertical or nearly so, minimal relief need be used. (For the actual amount of relief as measured by the gauge of relief wax, see Chapter 11.) If the lingual ridge as viewed from above is undercut, sufficient space may be created when the technician blocks out the undercut area.

Because of the need for relief under all mandibular major connectors, beading is never indicated.

Types of mandibular major connectors

The following four types of mandibular major connectors are used: (1) lingual bar, (2) lingual plate, (3) double lingual bar, or Kennedy bar, and (4) labial bar.

Lingual bar. The lingual bar (Fig. 2-30) is by far the most frequently used mandibular major connector, and because of its basic simplicity it should be used if no contraindications are evident.

The basic form of the lingual bar is that of a half-pear-shaped bar with the broadest portion at the inferior border of the bar (Fig. 2-31). The thickness of the bar

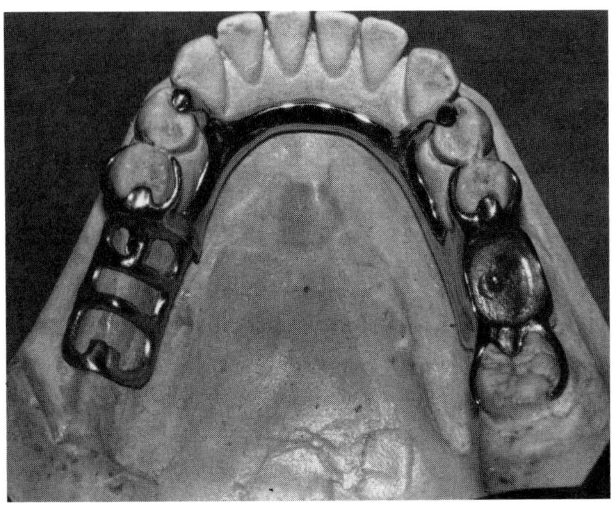

Fig. 2-30. Lingual bar, the most frequently used mandibular major connector, should be selected if no contraindications are present.

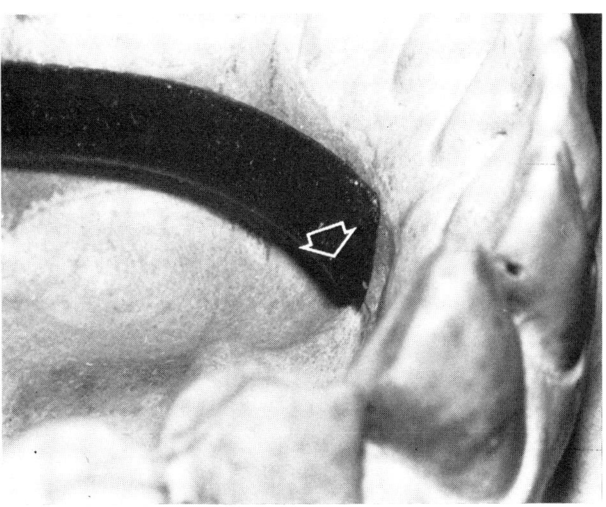

Fig. 2-31. The cross section of a lingual bar has a half-pear shape, with broadest portion at inferior border of bar (arrow).

may be altered to some degree during the waxing procedure if additional rigidity is needed, but care must be taken to avoid making the bar so bulky that tongue interference during speech or mastication will result. The normal thickness of the bar is that of a 6-gauge half-pear-shaped wax or plastic pattern. This will usually result in a rigid major connector unless the span or length is excessive. If there is concern that the bar will not be rigid, wax may be added to the half-pear shape to increase the thickness and, if space is available, to increase the width or height of the bar slightly.

Availability of space is one determining factor as to whether the lingual bar can be used. At least 8 mm of vertical space between the active tissues of the floor of the mouth and the gingival margins of the teeth is required (Fig. 2-32). This permits the major connector to have a minimum width or height of 5 mm and an essential space of 3 mm between the gingival margin and the superior border of the bar. Any closer encroachment of the bar to the marginal gingiva can produce an adverse soft tissue response in the form of hypertrophy or hyperplasia.

The simplest and most accurate way to determine the amount of space available for the lingual bar is by measuring with a periodontal probe. The patient is instructed to elevate and protrude the tongue so that the tip touches the vermilion border of the upper lip. This activates the floor of the mouth and raises the tissues to the height that occurs during normal functions such as speech, mastication, and deglutition. While the patient maintains this position, the periodontal probe can be inserted and measurements taken lingual to each of the canines and between the central incisors. The tip of the probe should rest at the junction of the soft tissues, and

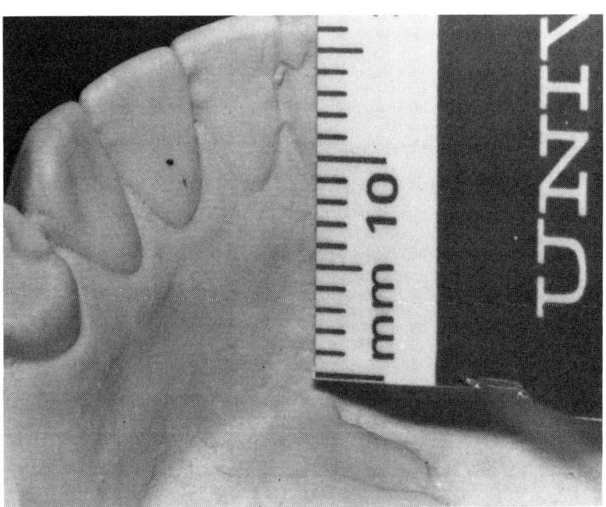

Fig. 2-32. Lingual bar major connector requires a minimum vertical space of 8 mm between active tissues of floor of mouth and gingival margins of teeth.

the readings should be taken at the most inferior point of the gingival margins. These readings may then be transferred to the diagnostic or master cast.

The lingual bar should be located as inferior as the patient can tolerate not only to permit more freedom of movement for the tongue, but also to permit more space between the marginal gingiva and the superior border of the bar.

Because of its simplicity in design and construction, the lingual bar should be used unless one of the other connectors offers a definite advantage. It is indicated for all tooth-supported removable partial dentures unless there is insufficient space lingual to the remaining teeth.

Although many patients with a maxillary torus may be treated successfully, the reverse is true of patients with mandibular tori. Surgical removal of the tori is usually required for a successful prognosis. If mandibular tori cannot be surgically removed, the lingual bar can rarely be used successfully. The soft tissue over lingual tori is thin and responds to minimal pressure or irritation with ulceration and pain. Attempting to construct a partial denture by avoiding the tori or by trying to gain adequate relief for the tori usually renders the partial denture unacceptable as far as patient comfort is concerned. It may also jeopardize the rigidity of the major connector.

Positioning the bar over an undercut area of the lingual surface of the ridge should be avoided. Otherwise gross food entrapment with accompanying patient discomfort will occur.

Advantages. In addition to the previously mentioned advantage of simplicity, the lingual bar has minimal contact with the oral tissues. It does not contact the teeth, so decalcification of tooth surfaces because of food or plaque collecting around the major connector does not occur.

Disadvantages. The greatest disadvantage is a potential one. If care is not taken by the laboratory or if proper instructions are not given to the technician, the lingual bar may not be rigid. This usually occurs when one attempts to use the lingual bar as a major connector when there is not enough space to place it correctly. The resulting bar is almost inevitably too thin and therefore flexible.

Lingual plate. The structure of the lingual plate is basically that of a pear-shaped lingual bar with a thin, solid piece of metal extending upward from the superior border of the bar onto the lingual surfaces of the teeth (Fig. 2-33). The lingual bar, which constitutes the lower portion of the lingual plate, is positioned as low in the mouth as possible without interfering with the functional activity of the floor of the mouth. This lower portion of the lingual plate may be slightly less bulky than the lingual bar major mandibular connector, but no compromise in rigidity can be made. The use of chrome metal is advocated because it allows the connector to be thin and finished to a fine edge and yet still retain the needed strength.

There must be adequate blockout and relief for both soft tissue undercuts and undercuts in the proximal areas of the teeth that are included under the plate (Fig. 2-34). The free gingival margin and the sulcus area must be relieved. Special consideration must be given to providing relief for the gingival crevicular tissue because damage can occur rapidly to this vital area if metal is allowed to compress or project into the gingival crevice. Minimal relief is required under the pear-shaped inferior portion of the connector as well as other soft tissue coverage areas.

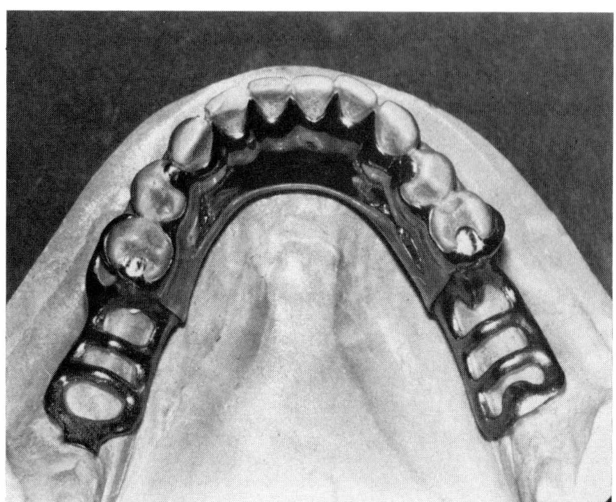

Fig. 2-33. Lingual plate has same basic configuration as lingual bar with an added extension of metal superiorly on lingual surface of teeth. This extension provides added rigidity and support.

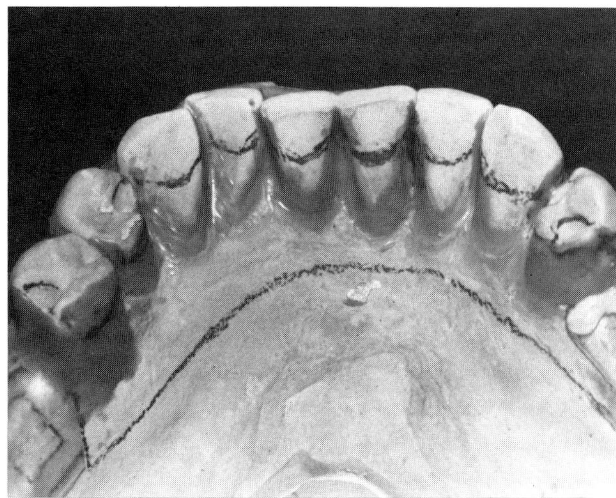

Fig. 2-34. Blockout and relief of master cast is required before construction of lingual plate major connector to eliminate undercuts and to provide space between soft tissue and metal of connector. Relief, in form of wax, is described in detail in Chapter 11.

The superior border of the plate must be contoured to intimately contact the lingual surfaces of the teeth above the cingula and to completely close off the spaces between the teeth up to the contact points. Sealing of the teeth embrasures from the lingual aspect prevents food from being packed into this area. As a result of this

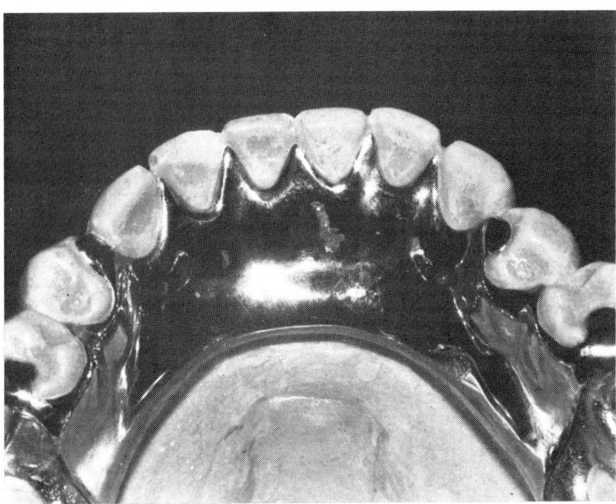

Fig. 2-35. A properly designed and constructed lingual plate major connector has a scalloped appearance on superior margin. This is necessary to adequately close interproximal spaces between teeth.

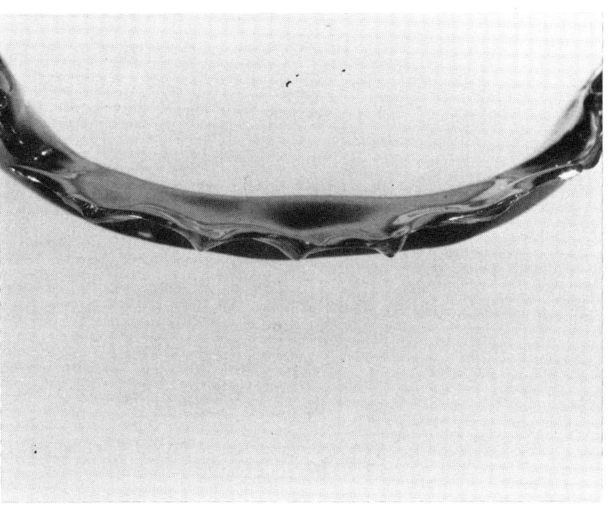

Fig. 2-36. With use of chrome metal, lingual plate major connector can be made thinner and can be finished to a fine edge.

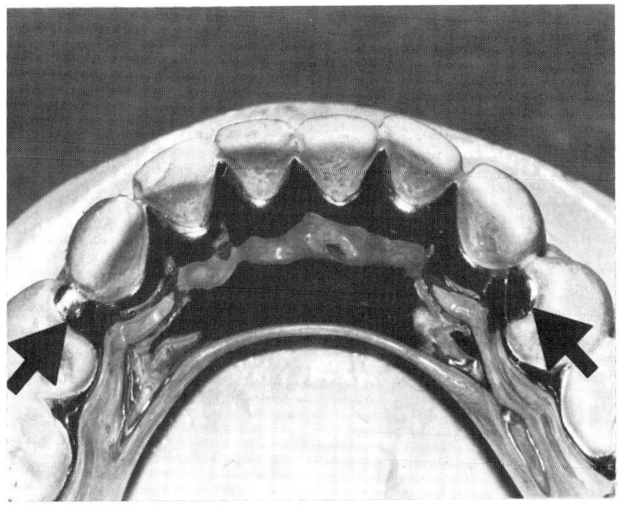

Fig. 2-37. Anterior lingual plate must always be supported by rests at each end of anterior span. In this case occlusal rests have been positioned on mesial fossae of first premolar teeth (arrows). Incisal rests on canines are an optional choice.

contouring, the lingual plate has a scalloped appearance (Fig. 2-35). The margins of the metal should be knife-edged to avoid a ledging effect on the lingual surfaces of the teeth. Consequently the points on the scalloping are sharp enough to puncture the finger if handled carelessly; however, fitted correctly, they will not damage the oral tissue. Chrome is an excellent material for this type of major connector (Fig. 2-36).

Patient discomfort may be produced if the superior margin of the plate is designed as a straight line running across the lingual surfaces of the teeth because the tongue will not adapt to this unnatural configuration.

The anterior lingual plate, whether acting as part of the indirect retention or not, must always be supported at each end of the anterior span by a rest located no further posteriorly than the mesial fossae of the first premolars (Fig. 2-37).

When loss of tissue height interproximally has occurred as a result of recession or periodontal surgery or when mandibular anterior teeth are widely spaced, special design considerations can be made to avoid having the metal show between the teeth or through the embrasures. Cut-backs or step-backs of the plating can be designed to completely hide the metal without compromising the strength or rigidity of the connector (Fig. 2-38). The superior border of the plate should normally be designed with the metal covering the cingula, rising upward to the contact point, or approximately where the teeth are spaced, and then dropping gingivally along the marginal ridges of the teeth to the gingiva. The metal crosses the gingiva to the next tooth and then rises up the marginal ridge to the contact point. The potential danger in using this approach is to make the cut-back so severe that the connector may not be rigid. The pear-shaped portion of the lingual plate should be increased slightly in thickness to compensate for this danger.

Advantages. There are a number of indications for the choice of the lingual plate as the major connector. The first is when most posterior teeth have been lost and there is a need for additional indirect retention.

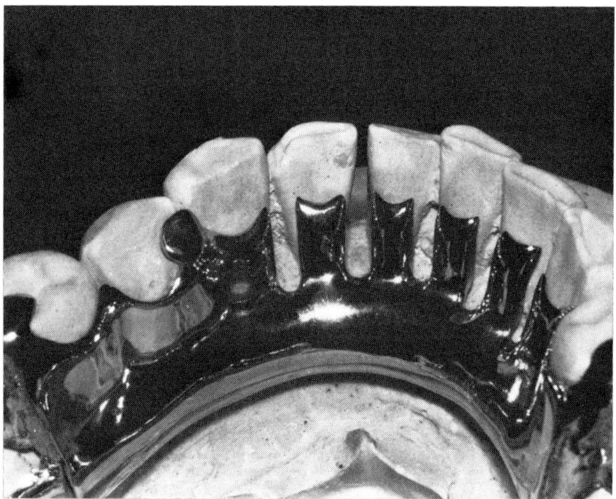

Fig. 2-38. For patients with wide spacing of anterior teeth or large interproximal embrasures, a series of step-backs of lingual plate can be designed to effectively prevent an unnecessary display of metal.

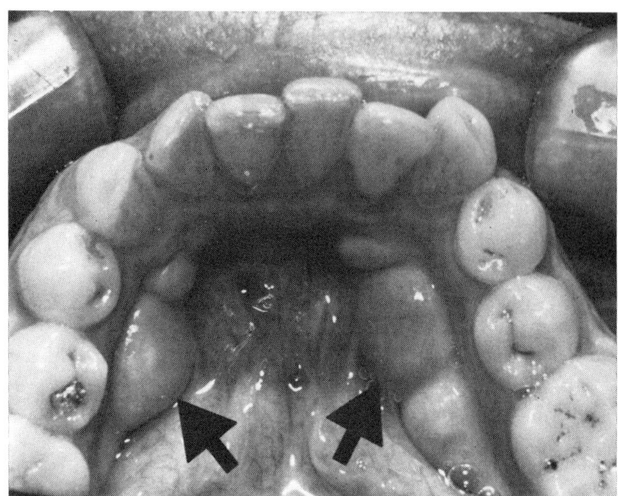

Fig. 2-39. Lingual plate major connector may be used at times to provide additional strength if mandibular tori are present (arrows) and cannot be surgically removed. The treatment of choice would be to remove tori before construction of partial denture.

The lingual plate by itself is not an indirect retainer, but when it is supported at each end of the anterior teeth by a rest it contributes to the action of indirect retention. This point will be discussed further in Chapter 3.

The second principal indication is remaining teeth that have lost much of their periodontal support and require splinting.

In addition, when there is insufficient space for the lingual bar, the lingual plate must be used. Insufficient space may arise as a result of the tissues of the floor of the mouth rising so high that they leave too little space between the movable tissues and the lingual marginal gingiva of the teeth to accommodate a lingual bar. Inadequate space may also be caused by the high attachment of the lingual frenum on the lingual surface of the ridge, or excessive recession of the lingual marginal gingiva.

The presence of mandibular tori in a patient who is unable to tolerate surgery is another indication for the lingual plate (Fig. 2-39).

In a patient who has bilateral distal extension edentulous areas and has lost much of the residual ridges because of resorption, the lingual plate can be used on the remaining teeth to provide resistance against horizontal or lateral movement of the partial denture.

When one or more remaining teeth, usually the incisor teeth, have lost much of their bony support yet may still provide service for a time, these teeth may be supported by a lingual plate until their extraction is necessary. As the teeth are lost, a retentive loop of metal may be soldered to the lingual plate and an artificial tooth attached to the loop. This permits the patient to replace the tooth without the expense required of remaking the partial denture.

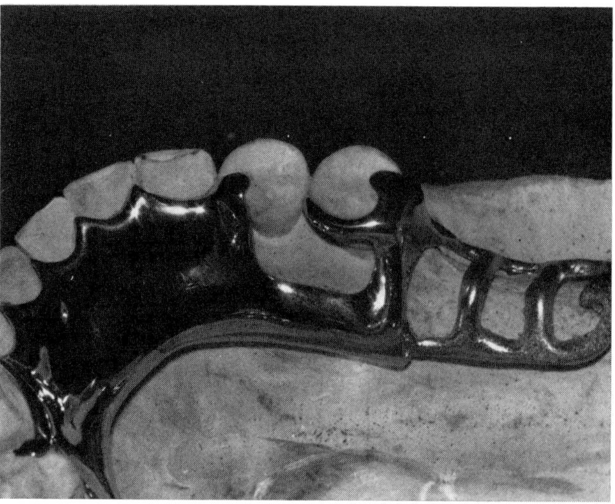

Fig. 2-40. A step-back of lingual plating away from posterior teeth is acceptable, provided space left is large enough to be self-cleansing. Space should be greater than a single tooth.

At times a lingual plate is used for some of the teeth, the anterior teeth usually, and the lingual surfaces of one or more premolars are left uncovered for a variety of reasons. This is an acceptable approach provided the space left by avoiding the lingual surfaces of these teeth is large enough to be self-cleansing (Fig. 2-40). Too often not only is the space so small that it acts as a food trap, but the margins of the metal, not being in inti-

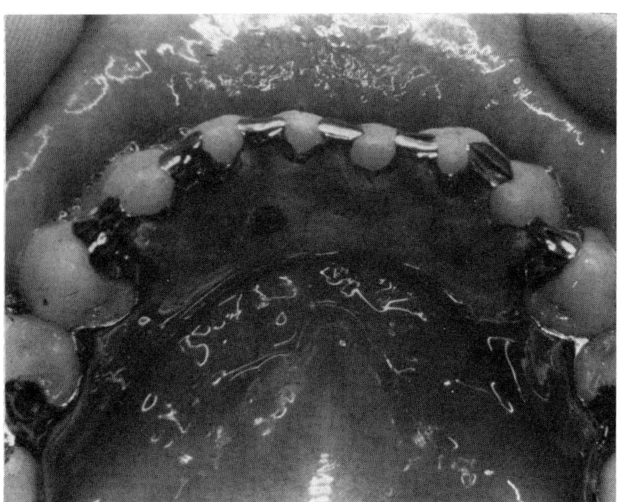

Fig. 2-41. Lingual plate major connector can be modified by adding incisal rests to mandibular anterior teeth to prevent overeruption of these teeth.

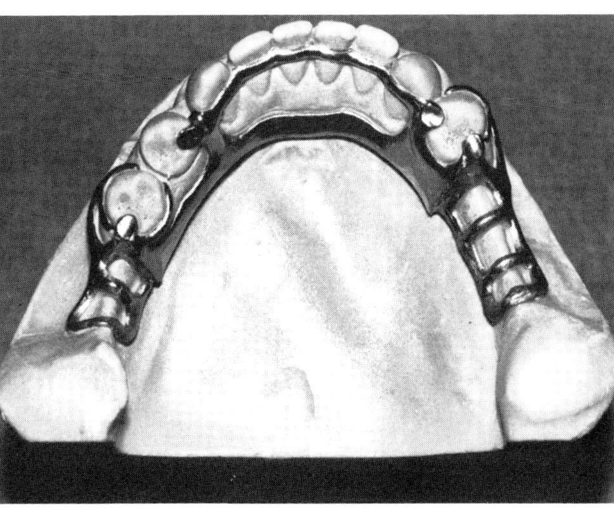

Fig. 2-42. Double lingual bar is same major connector as lingual plate with metal removed from below superior margin of plate down to half-pear-shaped bar.

mate contact with the soft tissue or teeth, act as an irritant to the tongue.

The lingual plate may also be used with slight modification to help prevent mandibular anterior teeth from overerupting. This condition is seen most frequently when a retrognathic jaw relation is accompanied by a deep vertical overlap of the anterior teeth (Fig. 2-41). The lingual plate will usually need to be assisted by rests placed on the incisal edges of the teeth.

The lingual plate is the most rigid mandibular connector, and it provides more support and stabilization than do the other connectors. It is particularly useful in stabilizing periodontally weakened teeth. Patients frequently consider the lingual plate to be more comfortable and more acceptable for tongue comfort and ease in phonetics than the lingual bar.

Disadvantages. The lingual plate's extensive coverage of teeth and soft tissue may contribute to decalcification of enamel surfaces or irritation of the soft tissue if the patient's oral hygiene habits are poor. A thorough examination and diagnosis are essential to recognize those patients for whom this major connector should not be selected.

Double lingual bar, or Kennedy bar. The double lingual bar (Fig. 2-42) differs from the lingual plate in that it has no sheet of metal extending from below the superior border of the plate to the pear-shaped lingual bar. This leaves the major part of the lingual surfaces of the teeth and the interproximal soft tissues exposed.

The lower bar should have the same design as a single lingual bar, pear-shaped in cross section with the greatest diameter at the inferior margin. The upper bar should be half-oval in cross section and approximately 2 to 3 mm high and 1 mm thick at its greatest diameter. The bar should not run straight across the lingual surfaces of the teeth but should dip from the contact points of the teeth downward to the upper limit of the cingula. If there is diastema between the anterior teeth, a step-back design such as that used with the lingual plate can hide the metal (Fig. 2-43). Because this step-back design can reduce the strength of the major connector, additional thickness should be added to the lower bar in the areas of step-back to retain rigidity.

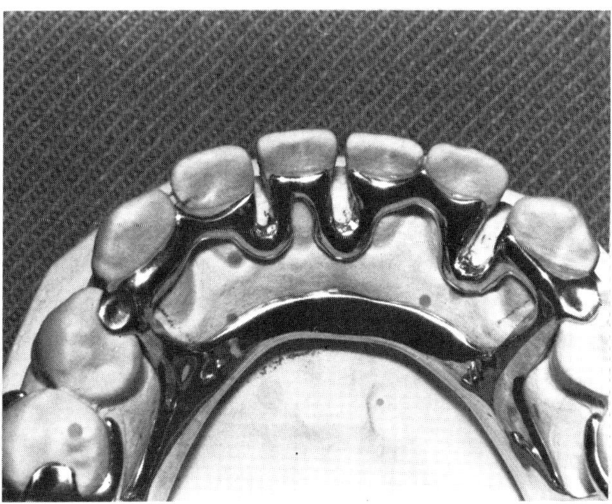

Fig. 2-43. A step-back can be designed for upper bar of double lingual bar if anterior teeth are spaced and display of metal between teeth would be unsightly.

The two bars are joined by rigid minor connectors at each end of the upper bar (Fig. 2-44). The minor connectors should be located in the interproximal spaces, usually between the canines and first premolars, to disguise the thickness of the metal and to be less noticeable to the tongue.

Rests must be placed at each end of the upper bar, usually attached to the rigid minor connector and no farther posterior than the mesial fossae of the first premolar, to prevent the bar from settling and causing orthodontic movement of the anterior teeth (Fig. 2-45).

Advantages. The double lingual bar effectively extends indirect retention in an anterior direction provided it is supported by adequate rests at each end. It also contributes to horizontal stabilization of the prosthesis because stress on the partial denture is distributed to all the teeth that it contacts. Thus the total stress on each tooth is reduced.

Because the gingival tissues and the interproximal embrasures are not covered by the double lingual bar, a free flow of saliva is permitted and the marginal gingiva receives natural stimulation.

The double lingual bar is indicated primarily when some degree of indirect retention is required and when periodontal disease and its treatment have resulted in large interproximal embrasures. The upper bar should be positioned at the contact points of the teeth; therefore it is well hidden from view.

Disadvantages. Patients frequently feel more tongue annoyance with the double lingual bar than is usually encountered with the lingual plate.

The major disadvantage of this connector, the entrapment of gross portions of food debris, arises from the marked crowding that mandibular anterior teeth frequently exhibit. The numerous undercuts created by the overlapping teeth make it difficult to fit the upper bar accurately to the lingual surface of each tooth. If the bar does not maintain intimate contact with tooth surface, food entrapment with resultant patient discomfort will ensue. For this reason the selection of the double lingual bar in preference to the lingual plate for other than esthetic reasons is questionable in most cases.

Labial bar. The labial bar, as its name suggests, runs across the mucosa labial to the mandibular anterior teeth (Fig. 2-46) or, in some instances, facial to the posterior teeth.

It has a half-pear shape similar to that of the lingual bar. For the same degree of rigidity, however, the height and thickness of the labial bar must be correspondingly greater than those of a lingual bar designed to act as a connector for the same clinical situation. The arc or length of the labial bar must also be greater than that of a lingual bar. Relief is required beneath the bar, as it is for all mandibular major connectors.

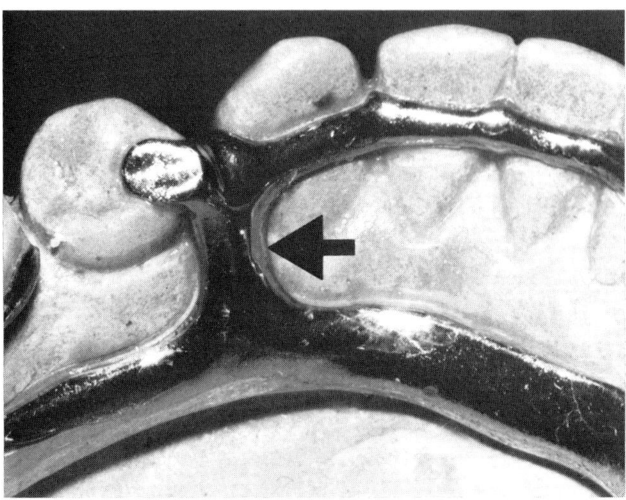

Fig. 2-44. Minor connector joining upper bar to lower bar (arrow) must be rigid and must be positioned in interproximal spaces, usually between first premolar and canine.

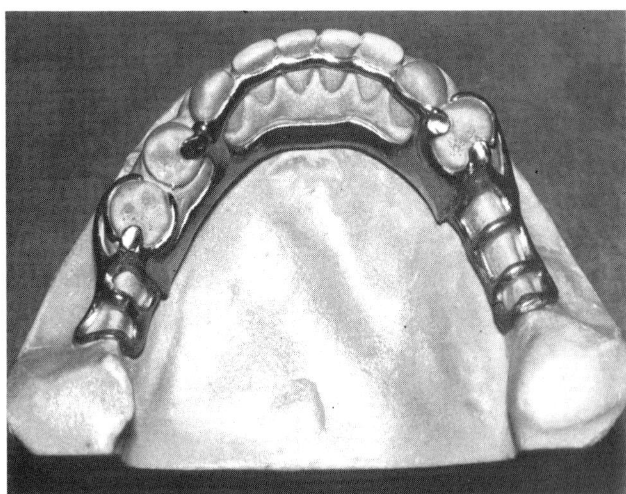

Fig. 2-45. Rests must be placed at each end of upper bar, no farther posterior than mesial fossae of first premolar, to prevent orthodontic movement of anterior teeth.

The only justification for its use is a gross noncorrectable interference that makes the placement of a lingual major connector impossible (Fig. 2-47). Indications for the use of the labial bar are rare. It is difficult, if not impossible, for a patient to adjust to the bulk of metal between the lip and the labial gingival tissue.

The interferences that usually lead to the selection of the labial bar as the major connector are malposed or

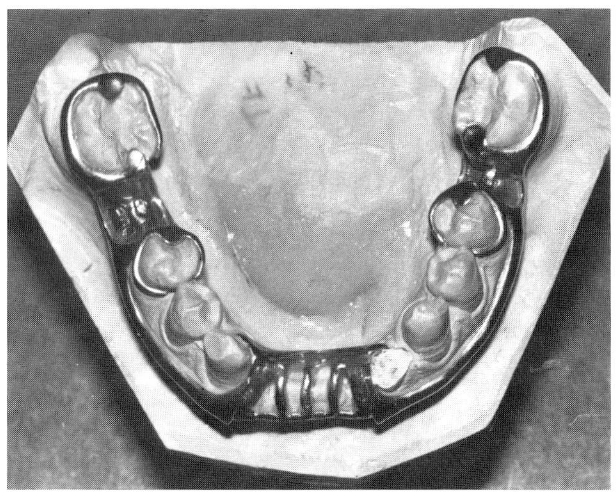

Fig. 2-46. Labial bar runs across mucosa labial to mandibular anterior teeth. Length of bar is greater than that of a lingual bar for same edentulous situation; therefore labial bar must be thicker than corresponding lingual bar, resulting in more patient discomfort.

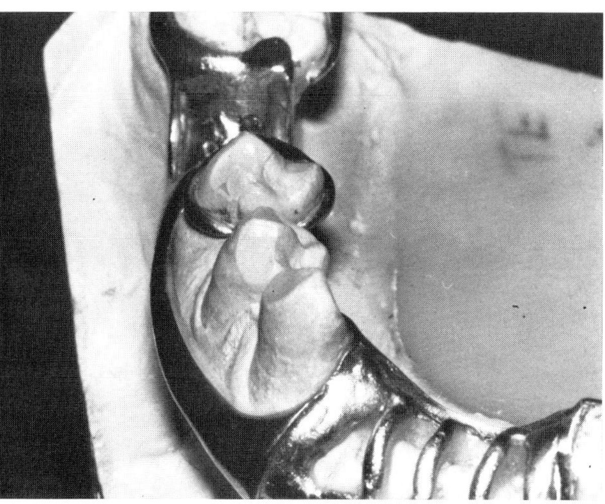

Fig. 2-47. Mandibular teeth that are lingually tipped to an excessive degree and cannot be corrected orthodontically or by placement of crowns can be treated by use of labial bar major connector.

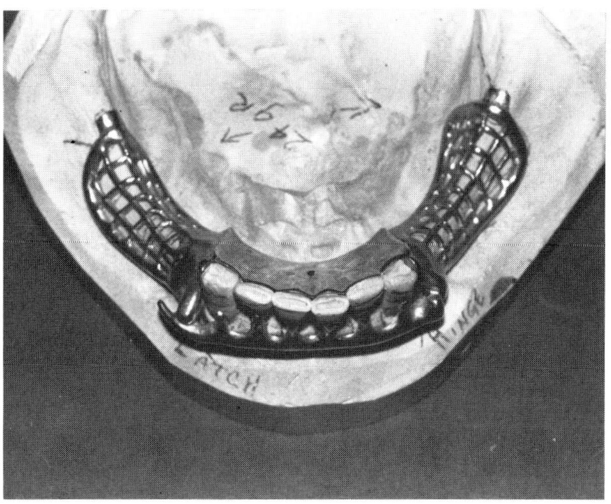

Fig. 2-48. The swing-lock partial denture is a variation of labial bar major connector. Hinged labial arm of swing lock is less bulky than a labial bar major connector.

lingually inclined teeth and/or large mandibular tori that preclude the use of a lingual plate. Every attempt should be made to correct the condition by extraction of severely malposed teeth, by orthodontic correction of lingually inclined teeth, by placement of crowns, or by surgical intervention to remove tori. The chance of successful treatment with a labial bar is limited.

A modification of the labial bar, the swing-lock labial bar, is currently undergoing limited but successful use. The swing-lock partial denture has as one of its components a bar labial to the anterior teeth. This bar, however, is not the major connector and does not require the bulk of the conventional labial bar for rigidity (Fig. 2-48). The swing-lock labial bar has a hinge device at one end and a locking device at the opposite end. Its hinging action permits it to be positioned more intimately against the gingival tissue; at times it is even positioned in undercuts on the labial surface of the ridge. This helps disguise the thickness of the bar and is more acceptable as far as patient comfort is concerned. The use of the swing-lock removable partial denture is discussed at length in Chapter 20.

Advantages. When the lower anterior teeth and the premolars are so severely lingually inclined that a conventional lingual major connector cannot be used, the labial bar can be considered. However, every possible means of avoiding use of the labial bar should be entertained before it is incorporated into the design of the partial denture. Recontouring the teeth by enameloplasty, by placement of restorations, or by orthodontic treatment should be considered.

Disadvantages. The results of a labial bar are generally poor. The bulk of the connector distorts the lower lip unless the lip is relatively immobile, and the mere presence of the metal between the gingival tissue and the lip causes patient discomfort. In addition, the labial vestibule is usually not deep enough to permit a connector of sufficient rigidity without encroaching on the free gingival margin.

Review of indications for mandibular major connectors

1. For a tooth-supported removable partial denture, the lingual bar is normally the mandibular major connector of choice.
2. For long-span edentulous ridges in which there is no posterior abutment tooth and indirect retention is needed, the lingual plate is generally indicated.
3. When the anterior teeth have reduced periodontal support and need stabilization, the lingual plate or, occasionally, the double lingual bar may be used.
4. When the tissues of the floor of the mouth are active and less than 8 mm is available between the tissues and the marginal gingiva, when inoperable tori are present, or when a high lingual frenum is present, a lingual plate must be used.
5. For patients who have had periodontal surgery and who have large interproximal spaces that could cause esthetic problems by the display of the metal of a lingual plate, a double lingual bar may be indicated.
6. The labial bar is rarely indicated.

MINOR CONNECTORS

The primary function of a minor connector is to join other units of the prosthesis such as clasps, rests, indirect retainers, and denture bases to the major connector. The minor connector is also responsible for distributing the stresses that occur against certain components of the partial denture to other components, thus preventing any buildup of force at a single point. The need for rigidity is emphasized by this function. If the minor or major connector were to flex, stresses could not be distributed evenly throughout the prosthesis.

The minor connector also distributes forces on the edentulous ridge to the ridge and the remaining teeth. Occlusal force on the minor connector that attaches the denture base to the major connector is passed to several other minor connectors that serve as attachments for clasps, rests, or indirect retainers. This broad distribution of force prevents any one tooth or one portion of the edentulous ridge from bearing a destructive amount of stress.

Types of minor connectors

There are four types of minor connectors: those that (1) join the clasp assembly to the major connector, (2) join indirect retainers or auxiliary rests to the major connector, (3) join the denture base to the major connector, and (4) serve as an approach arm for a vertical projection or bar-type clasp (Fig. 2-49).

Minor connectors that join clasp assembly to the major connector

Minor connectors that join the clasp assembly to the major connector must be rigid, because they support the active component of the partial denture, the retentive clasp. They also support the component of the prosthesis that prevents vertical movement toward the tissue, the rest. They must have sufficient bulk to ensure rigidity, but the bulk must be concealed or it will irritate the tongue. Most minor connectors that support clasp assemblies are located on proximal surfaces of teeth adjacent to edentulous areas. In this location the correct configuration of the minor connector should be broad buccolingually but thin mesiodistally (Fig. 2-50). The thickest portion buccolingually should be at the lingual line angle of the tooth and it should taper evenly to its thinnest point at the buccal line angle of the tooth. This shape will make it easier to arrange the artificial tooth in a natural position.

If the clasp assembly is not being placed on a tooth adjacent to an edentulous space, the minor connector must be positioned in the embrasure between two teeth (Fig. 2-51). Using this triangular space for the metal results in sufficient bulk without encroaching on tongue space. The minor connector should never be positioned on the convex lingual surface of a tooth.

Minor connectors that join indirect retainers or auxiliary rests to major connector

Minor connectors that join indirect retainers or auxiliary rests to the major connector generally arise from the latter. They should form a right angle with the major connector, but the junction should be a gentle curve rather than a sharp angular connection (Fig. 2-52). The minor connector should be designed to lie in the embrasure between teeth to disguise its bulk as much as possible (Fig. 2-53).

Minor connectors that join denture base to major connector

Minor connectors that join the denture base to the major connector may be (1) of latticework construction, (2) of mesh construction, or (3) bead, wire, or nailhead minor connectors (used with a metal base) (Fig. 2-54). They must be strong enough to anchor the denture base securely, they must be rigid enough to resist breakage or flexing, and they must interfere as little as possible with arrangement of the artificial teeth.

In the maxillary arch if the denture base is a distal extension base (no tooth posterior to the edentulous space), the minor connector must extend the entire length of the residual ridge to cover the tuberosity. When a distal extension ridge in the mandibular arch is

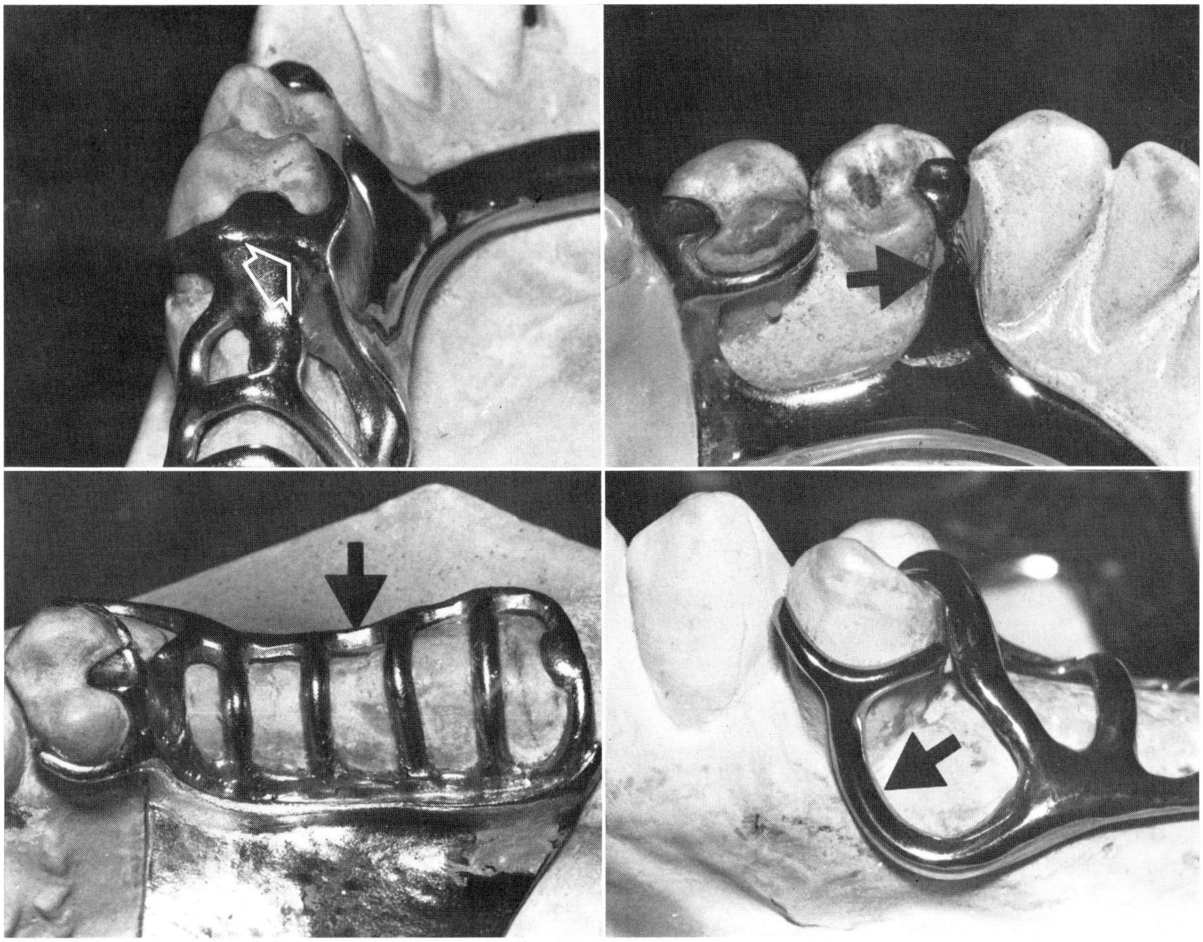

Fig. 2-49. Minor connectors serve one of four functions. **A,** Primary function is to join components of partial denture to major connector. Minor connector shown is connecting clasp assembly to major connector (arrow). **B,** Minor connector is used to join indirect retainer or other auxillary rests to major connector (arrow). This minor connector must be positioned in interdental embrasure to prevent irritating tongue. **C,** Acrylic resin retention minor connector (arrow) joins denture base to major connector. Acrylic resin denture base containing artificial denture teeth will be molded around struts of minor connector. **D,** Minor connector that serves as approach arm (arrow) is the only minor connector that is not rigid; it must have a limited amount of flexibility.

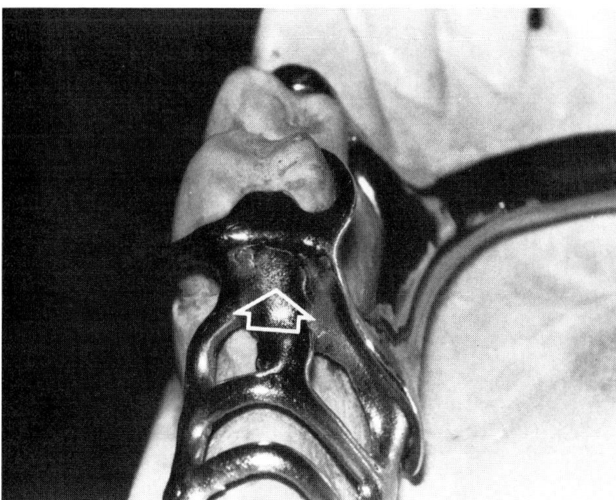

Fig. 2-50. Minor connector that joins clasp assembly to major connector (arrow) must be broad buccolingually but thin mesiodistally to help arrange artificial teeth in a more natural position.

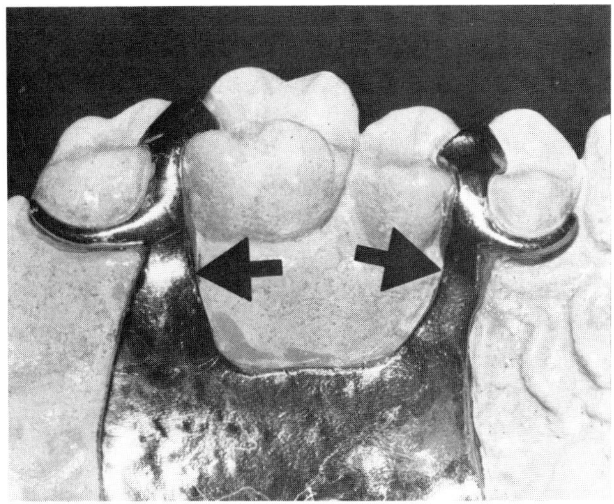

Fig. 2-51. If a clasp assembly is not placed adjacent to an edentulous space, minor connector must be positioned in embrasure between two teeth (arrow).

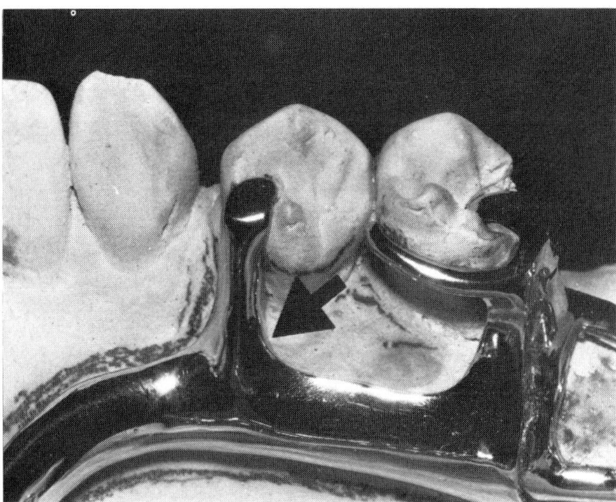

Fig. 2-52. Minor connectors should exit from major connector at right angles, with junction being gentle curves, not sharp angulations (arrow).

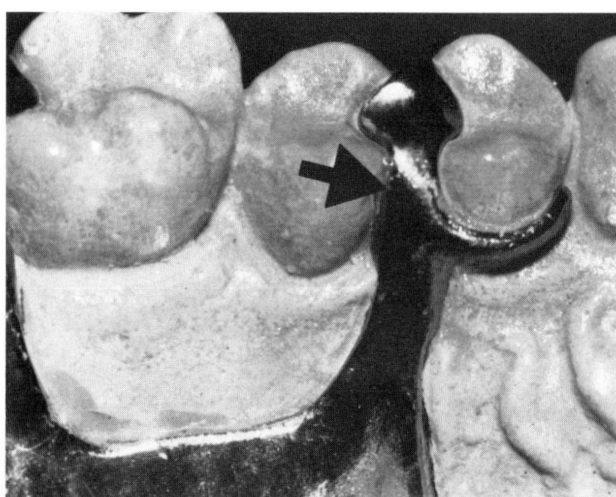

Fig. 2-53. Minor connector positioned in embrasure to prevent feeling of bulk (arrow).

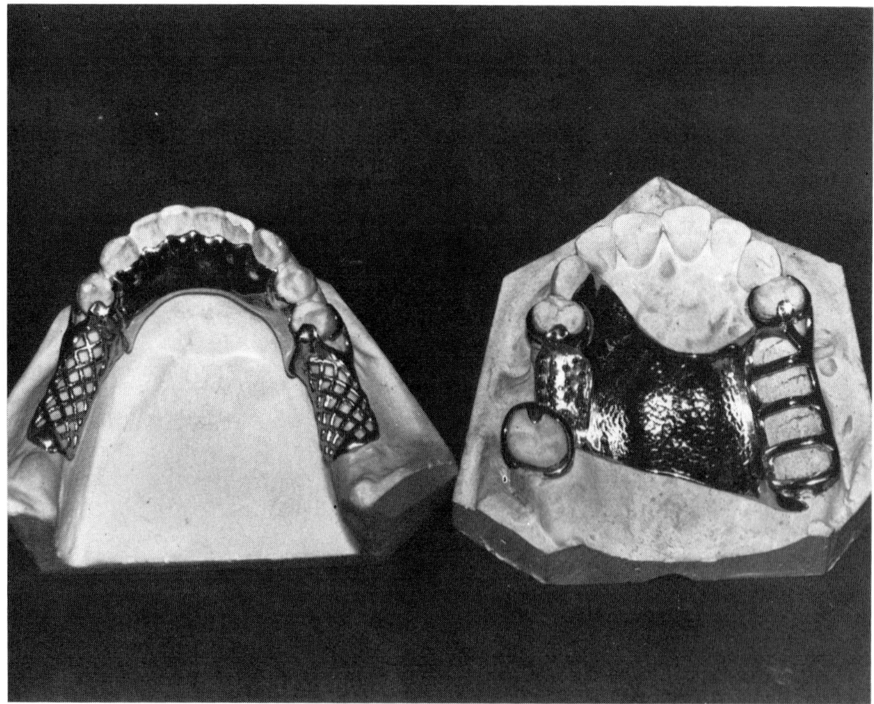

Fig. 2-54. Minor connectors that join denture base to major connector are in three forms. Left, mesh type minor connectors are illustrated on mandibular partial denture. Openings through mesh are fine but are capable of supporting denture base. Right, maxillary partial denture has an open latticework minor connector on right side (patient's left) and a metal base with bead retention, on left side.

being treated, the minor connector should extend two-thirds the length of the edentulous ridge.

Open latticework construction. The latticework (Fig. 2-55) consists of two struts of metal, usually 12 to 16 gauge thick, extending longitudinally along the edentulous ridge. In the mandibular arch one strut should be positioned buccal to the crest of the ridge and the other lingual to the ridge crest.

In the maxillary arch one strut is positioned buccal to the ridge crest, and the border of the major connector acts as the second strut. Smaller struts, usually 16 gauge thick, connect the two struts and form the latticework (Fig. 2-56). These connecting struts run over the crest of the ridge and should be positioned to interfere as little as possible with arrangement of the artificial teeth. The number of cross struts is not critical; however, too many of them make it more difficult to form the denture base. Generally, one cross strut between each of the teeth to be replaced should be satisfactory.

Positioning of a longitudinal strut down the crest of the ridge must be avoided. This not only interferes with the placement of artificial teeth, but also sets up a cleavage action on the denture base. Longitudinal fracture of the denture base in such situations is not unusual.

Wax forms of the struts are positioned on the refractory, or investment, cast, which is duplicated from the master cast after the latter has been relieved. It is necessary to provide a relief space over the edentulous ridges for both the latticework and the mesh minor connectors so that there will be a space between the struts or mesh and the underlying ridge. It is in this space and around the struts or mesh that the acrylic resin denture base will be formed. The locking of the acrylic resin around and through the latticework or the mesh provides the retention of the denture base.

The latticework minor connector can be used whenever multiple teeth are to be replaced. Studies have shown that it provides the strongest attachment of the acrylic resin denture base to the removable partial denture. It is also the easiest of the denture base retainers to reline if this becomes necessary because of ridge resorption.

Mesh construction. The mesh type of minor connector consists of a thin sheet of metal with multiple small holes that extends over the crest of the residual ridge to the same buccal, lingual, and posterior limits as does the latticework minor connector (Fig 2-57). It can be used whenever multiple teeth are to be replaced. The main drawback in using mesh is that it makes it more difficult to pack the acrylic resin dough because more pressure is needed against the resin to force it through the small holes. It also does not provide as strong an attachment for the denture base. Studies have shown that the smaller the openings in this minor connector, the weaker the attachment.

Tissue stop. On all distal extension partial dentures using latticework or mesh retention a provision must be made to stabilize the framework during the acrylic resin packing and processing procedure.

As mentioned previously, latticework and mesh mi-

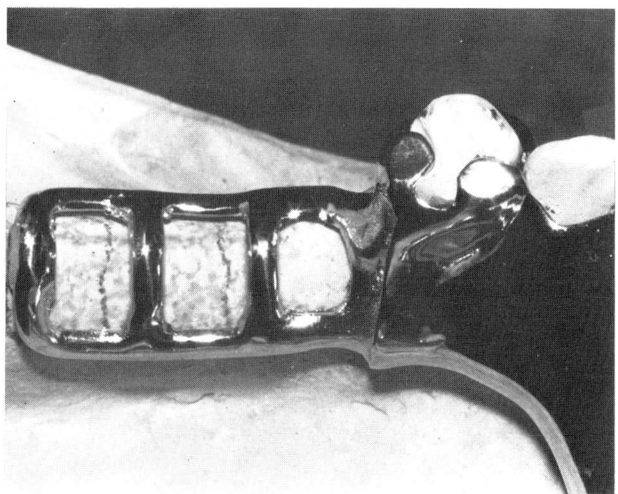

Fig. 2-55. Open latticework acrylic resin retention provides strongest retention of denture base to major connector. Two longitudinal struts are positioned, one buccal and one lingual, to crest of ridge. In mandibular arch, as shown, retentive latticework should extend posteriorly two-thirds the length of edentulous ridge from terminal abutment tooth to pear-shaped pad.

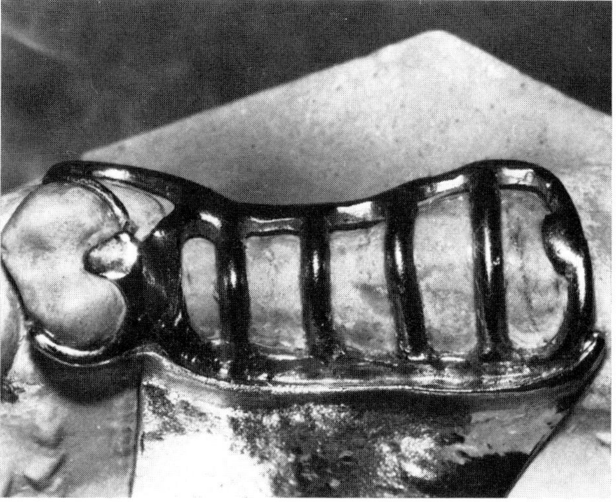

Fig. 2-56. Open latticework in maxillary arch for distal extension ridge differs to the extent that one longitudinal strut is positioned buccal to edentulous ridge and lingual strut is replaced by palatal extent of major connector. Horizontal struts attach directly to major connector. Minor connector must cover tuberosity.

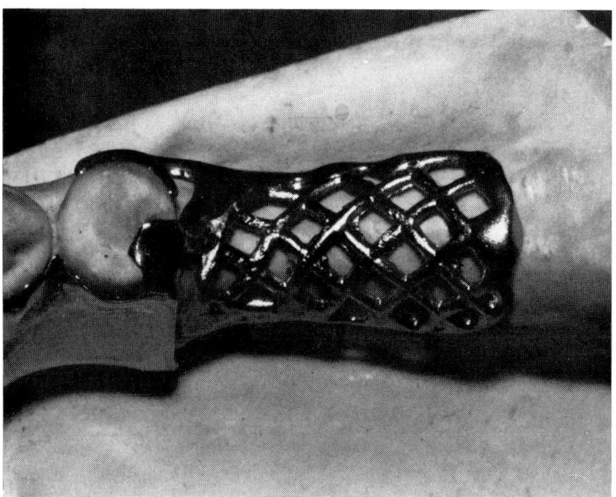

Fig. 2-57. Mesh retention for acrylic resin denture base may be of type shown or may have holes with even smaller diameters. This is an effective denture base retainer but does not possess strength of latticework type.

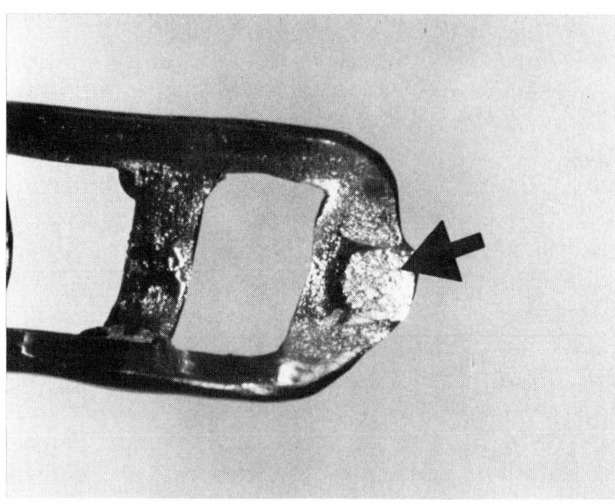

Fig. 2-58. Tissue stop is a small square of metal in contact with ridge that prevents framework from being displaced when acrylic resin is packed under pressure.

nor connectors are constructed with a space between them and the underlying ridge. Considerable force must be used in packing the acrylic resin so that the resin will flow completely around the latticework or mesh. This force could displace or distort the framework if the terminal portion of the minor connector is not supported. The tissue stop is used to provide this support (Fig. 2-58). The tissue stop is made by removing approximately 2 square mm of the relief wax used to create the space beneath the latticework or mesh (Fig. 2-59) from the point where the posterior end of the minor connector crosses the center of the ridge. During waxing of the framework, this little depression is waxed as a projection of the latticework or mesh. After the framework has been cast and returned to the master cast, this projection will contact the edentulous ridge of the cast and will prevent the framework from being distorted during the acrylic resin packing procedure.

Bead, wire, or nailhead retention minor connectors. The bead, wire, or nailhead minor connector (Fig. 2-60) is used with a metal denture base, which is cast so that it fits directly against the edentulous ridge; no relief is provided beneath the minor connector. The denture base is attached to the outer or superior surface of the metal base, and retention is gained by projections of metal on this surface. These projections may be beads made by placing beads of acrylic resin polymer on the waxed denture base and investing, burning out, and casting these beads; they may be wires that project from the metal base, or they may be in the form of nailheads.

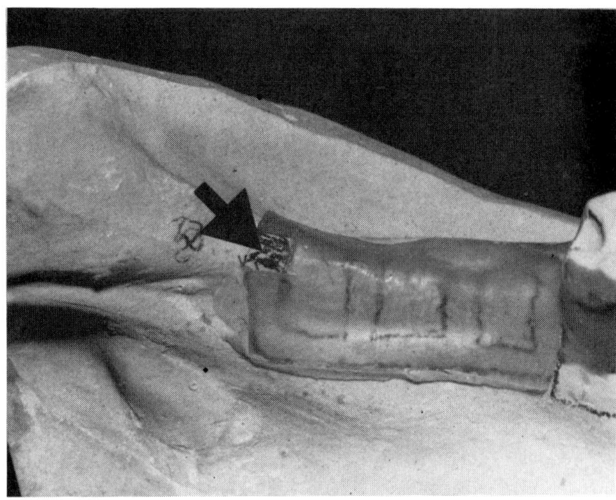

Fig. 2-59. Approximately 2 square mm of relief wax is removed at posterior extent of relief wax to create tissue stop.

This form of denture base is hygienic because of better soft tissue response to metal than to acrylic resin. There are shortcomings however. It is difficult to adjust the metal base. It cannot be relined adequately in the event that ridge resorption takes place. This attachment is the weakest of the three types. Clinically, it will function successfully if used properly. It should be used on tooth-supported, well-healed ridges when the interarch space is limited and acrylic resin by itself would not have sufficient strength to withstand the forces of occlusion.

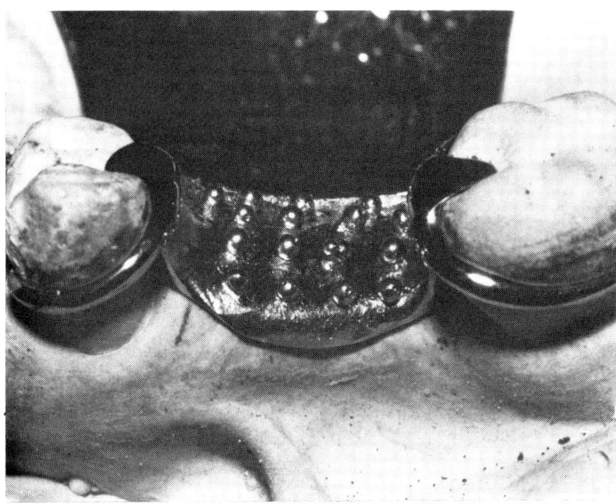

Fig. 2-60. Metal base with bead, or wire, or nailhead minor connector. Metal is cast directly onto ridge, and extrusions of beads or wire on superior surface of metal are used to retain acrylic resin denture base and artificial teeth. This minor connector is used principally on tooth-supported segments because of difficulty in relining if need should arise.

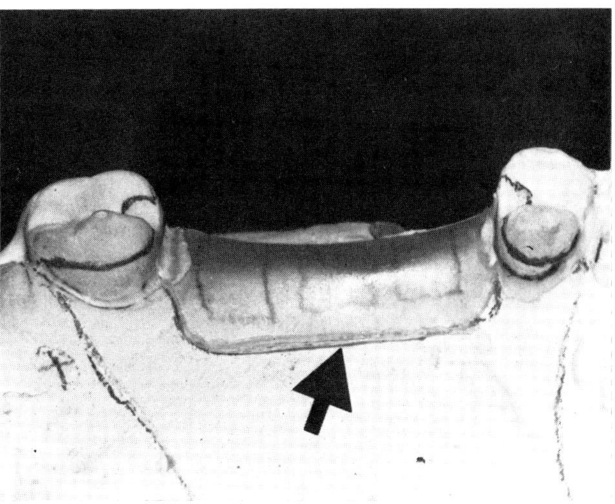

Fig. 2-61. Internal finish line is developed as master cast is relieved before duplication. Relief wax is placed over edentulous ridge (arrow) to provide space for acrylic resin denture base to lock around retention struts of minor connector.

Attachment to major connector

The acrylic resin minor connector must be joined to the major connector with sufficient bulk to avoid fracture. The denture base and artificial teeth that will be supported by the minor connector will be subjected to considerable occlusal forces, and breakage at the junction of the connectors is a possibility.

The acrylic resin that will eventually be processed around the latticework and mesh minor connector must join the major connector in a smooth, even joint. Any irregularity between the two surfaces will irritate either the tongue or the mucosa of the ridge. Acrylic resin cannot be finished to a thin edge. If this is attempted, chips and fractures of the material will occur, creating an unhygienic and potentially irritating situation.

To prevent the acrylic resin from being thinned excessively in order to produce a smooth joint, the design and construction of the joining of the major and minor connectors must provide space for a butt joint so that the acrylic resin can blend evenly with the major connector.

Because the acrylic resin is processed completely around the latticework and mesh minor connectors, space for these butt joints must be made on both internal and external surfaces of the major connector. In the case of the metal base minor connector, the acrylic resin is processed only on the external surface, so only a single butt joint is required. These butt joints are referred to as *finish lines*. If they occur on the outer aspect of the major connector, they are called *external* finish lines; if they are on the internal or tissue side of the major connector, they are *internal* finish lines.

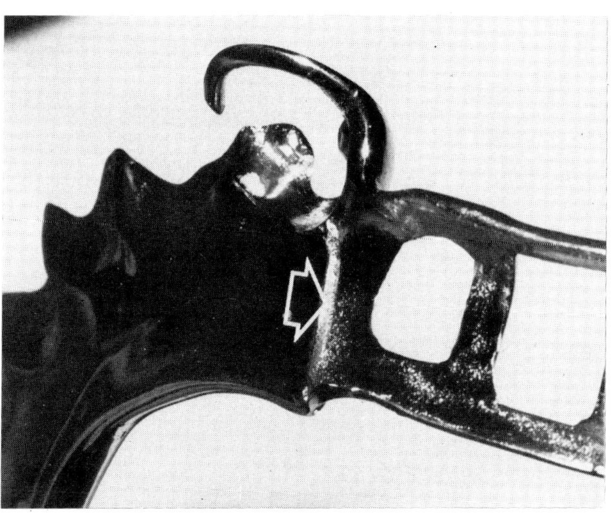

Fig. 2-62. Edge of relief wax establishes a sharp wall in metal against which acrylic resin may be finished (arrow). Wall is necessary because acrylic resin cannot be finished to a thin or feather edge.

Internal finish lines. Internal finish lines are formed from the relief wax used over the edentulous ridges on the master cast before duplication of the cast in investment material on which the framework will be waxed (Fig. 2-61). The relief wax, usually 24 to 26 gauge, creates the space that is needed for the acrylic resin denture base under latticework or mesh minor connectors (Fig. 2-62). The margins of the relief wax become the

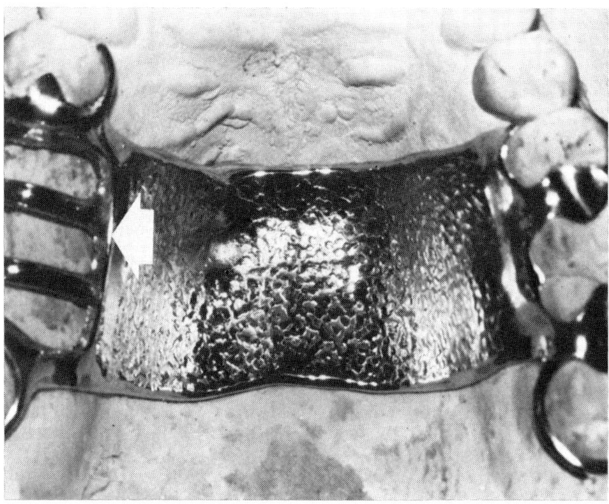

Fig. 2-63. External finish line as viewed from above must be undercut (arrow). This undercut, an angle of less than 90 degrees to major connector, is necessary to mechanically lock acrylic resin denture base in position.

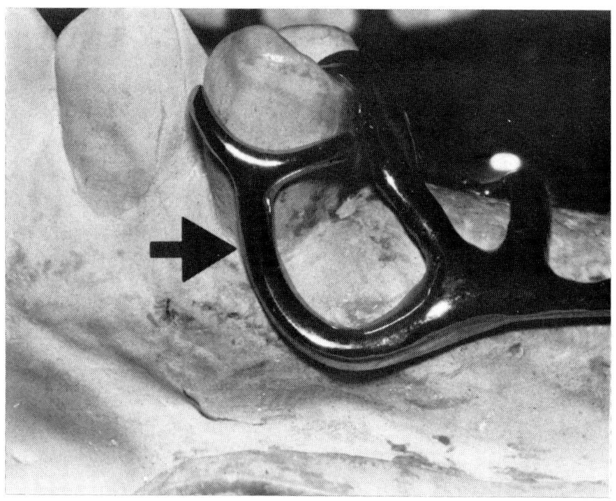

Fig. 2-64. Approach arm of a vertical projection or bar-type clasp is the only minor connector not required to be rigid (arrow). It must have a smooth, even taper from its origin to its terminus, the retentive clasp, and it must not cross a soft tissue undercut.

internal finish line. The ledge created by the margin of the wax must be sharp and definite.

External finish lines. The external finish line must also be sharp and definite and should be slightly undercut to help lock the acrylic resin securely to the major connector. The angle the finish lines form with the major connector should be less than 90 degrees (Fig. 2-63).

The external finish line is formed by placement of the wax during the waxing procedure and by carving the wax. It should extend onto the proximal surfaces of the teeth adjacent to the edentulous space. The finish line begins at the lingual extent of the rest seat and continues down the lingual aspect of the minor connector on the proximal surface of the tooth.

Minor connectors that serve as approach arm for vertical projection or bar-type clasp

The approach arm for a vertical projection or bar-type clasp is the only minor connector that is not required to be rigid. It supports a direct retainer (clasp) that engages an undercut on a tooth from below rather than above (Fig. 2-64). It approaches the tooth from the gingival margin. It should have a smooth, even taper from its origin to its terminus. It must not cross a soft tissue undercut, and for this reason its use is contraindicated in some instances. This minor connector is considered in greater depth when direct retainers are discussed (Chapter 3).

RESTS AND REST SEATS

The components of a removable partial denture that serve primarily to transfer forces occurring against the prosthesis down the long axis of the abutment teeth are called rests, and a rest seat is the prepared surface of a tooth or fixed restoration into which a rest fits.

The relationship between the rest and the surface of a tooth must be such that forces transmitted from the prosthesis to the rest are directed apically down the long axis of the tooth (Fig. 2-65). In this fashion stress can be absorbed by the fibers of the periodontal ligament without damaging the ligament or the supporting bone.

In the case of the tooth-supported denture, all the stresses are transferred to the abutment teeth. In the combination partial denture, only a portion of the stress is transferred to the teeth, and the edentulous ridge must absorb the remainder.

In addition to transferring forces, the rest must act as a vertical stop, preventing injury and overdisplacement of the soft tissues under the partial denture bases or major connectors (Fig. 2-66). It is unfortunate that many temporary partial dentures do not possess this function, with resulting damage to underlying soft tissue and supporting structures of abutment teeth.

The rest must also maintain the retentive clasp in its proper position. If the clasp is not supported, it will lose the ability to retain as it was designed to do (Fig. 2-67).

The rest that is a component part of a direct retainer unit is referred to as a primary rest, whereas additional rests that may be used for indirect retention or extra support are called auxiliary, or secondary rests.

Auxiliary, or secondary, rests are used as indirect re-

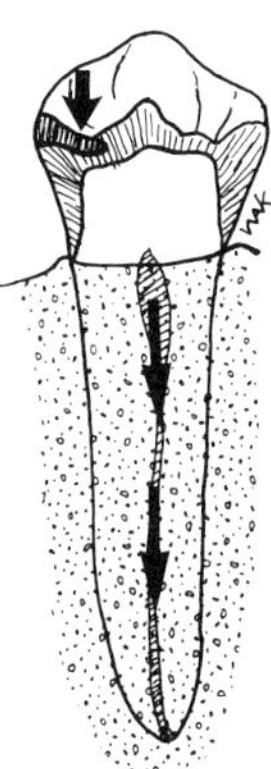

Fig. 2-65. Force on a partial denture is transmitted to occlusal rest, and because of design of rest seat, force is further transmitted down long axis of abutment tooth. Fibers of periodontal ligament withstand vertical forces better than lateral or horizontal forces.

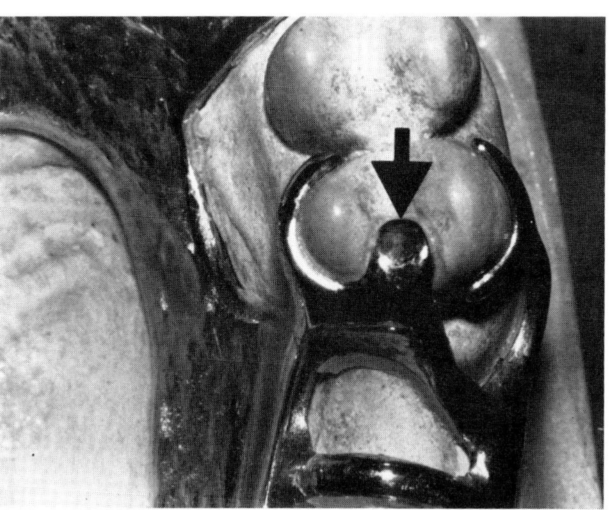

Fig. 2-66. In addition to transferring forces against partial denture, rest (arrow) also acts as a vertical stop to prevent prosthesis from displacing and damaging underlying soft tissue.

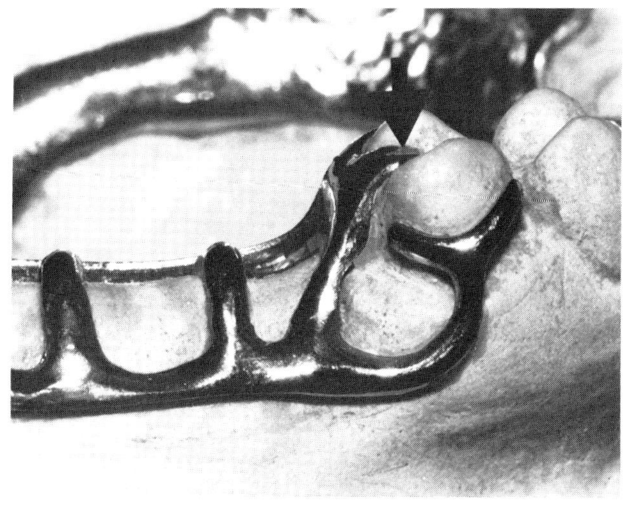

Fig. 2-67. Rest (arrow) also maintains retentive clasp in proper position. Without rest, clasp would not remain in amount of undercut designed.

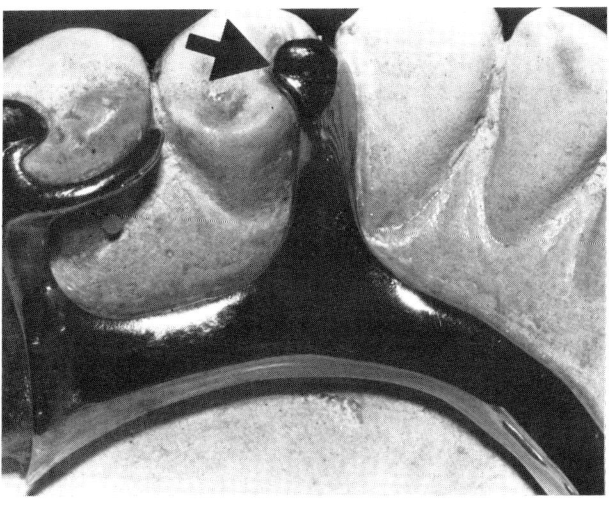

Fig. 2-68. Auxillary or secondary rests shown in mesial fossa of first premolar (arrow) are placed anterior to axis of rotation of distal extension partial denture to prevent denture base from lifting away from edentulous ridge.

tainers in distal extension partial dentures. These rests are placed anterior or posterior to the axis of rotation to prevent the unsupported distal extension denture base from lifting away from the edentulous ridge (Fig. 2-68).

Primary rests prevent vertical movement of the prosthesis toward the tissue and also help transmit lateral or horizontal forces applied to the partial denture during function to the supporting teeth. This action of transmitting lateral forces may be increased by deepening the rest seat, but this should be done only for an all-tooth–supported prosthesis. For a distal extension partial denture, the rest seat should be shallow and saucer-shaped so that the rest can move slightly, like a ball and socket joint, allowing the horizontal forces to be dissipated (Fig. 2-69). Supporting teeth are capable of withstanding vertical forces, but lateral or horizontal forces of much less magnitude can be destructive.

On the proximal surface of an abutment tooth adjacent to an edentulous space food may be impacted between the minor connector and the tooth if a rest is not

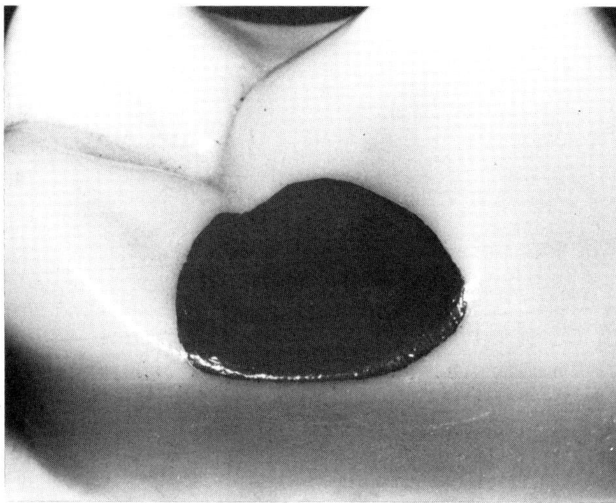

Fig. 2-69. Occlusal rest seat should be saucer-shaped so that rest may move slightly in function, like a ball-and-socket joint, to dissipate horizontal forces.

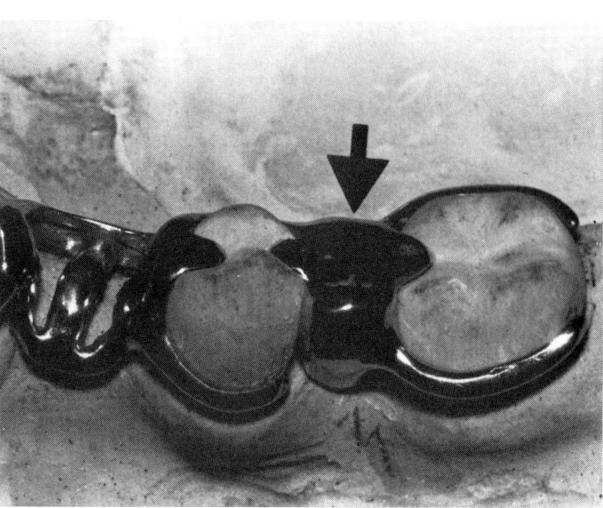

Fig. 2-70. Occlusal rests may be designed between spaced teeth (arrow) to reestablish continuity of arch and prevent further drifting or tipping of teeth.

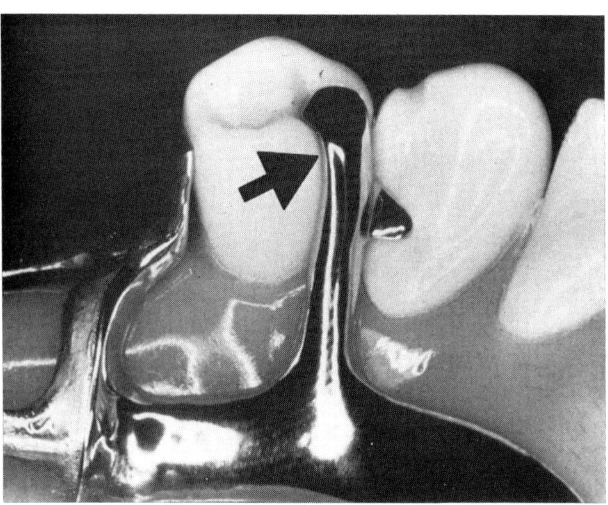

Fig. 2-71. Occlusal rest may be positioned on side of a tooth opposite retentive clasp to act as a reciprocal clasp. Minor connector in combination with rest performs reciprocation (arrow).

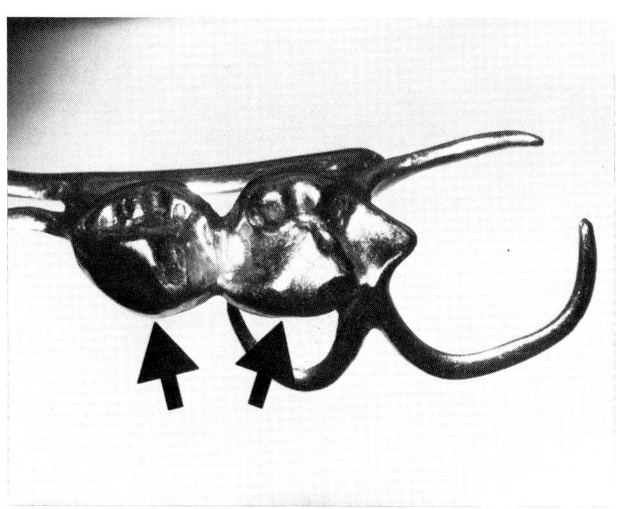

Fig. 2-72. It is possible to use occlusal rests in form of onlay rests (arrows) to reestablish acceptable plane of occlusion. This is usually done on tipped molars. This type of rest has limitations and should be used judiciously.

used on the proximal-occlusal or incisal surface. It is our philosophy of removable partial denture design that rests should be placed on the proximal surfaces of all teeth adjacent to edentulous spaces. (This principle, however, may be altered in the case of anterior edentulous spaces.)

Many patients requiring a removable partial denture have a small space or spaces between remaining posterior teeth as a result of tooth drift or migration. The space may be too small to receive a normal-sized replacement. It may be tempting to ignore this space in the design of the prosthesis, but this lack of continuity in the arch will prolong the problem of drifting teeth. If esthetics is not a concern, occlusal rests can be placed on the adjacent teeth with a metal pontic between to close these spaces and reestablish a continuous arch, preventing further drifting or tipping of posterior teeth and improving periodontal health (Fig. 2-70).

Some practitioners use a strategically positioned minor connector and rest to reciprocate the forces gener-

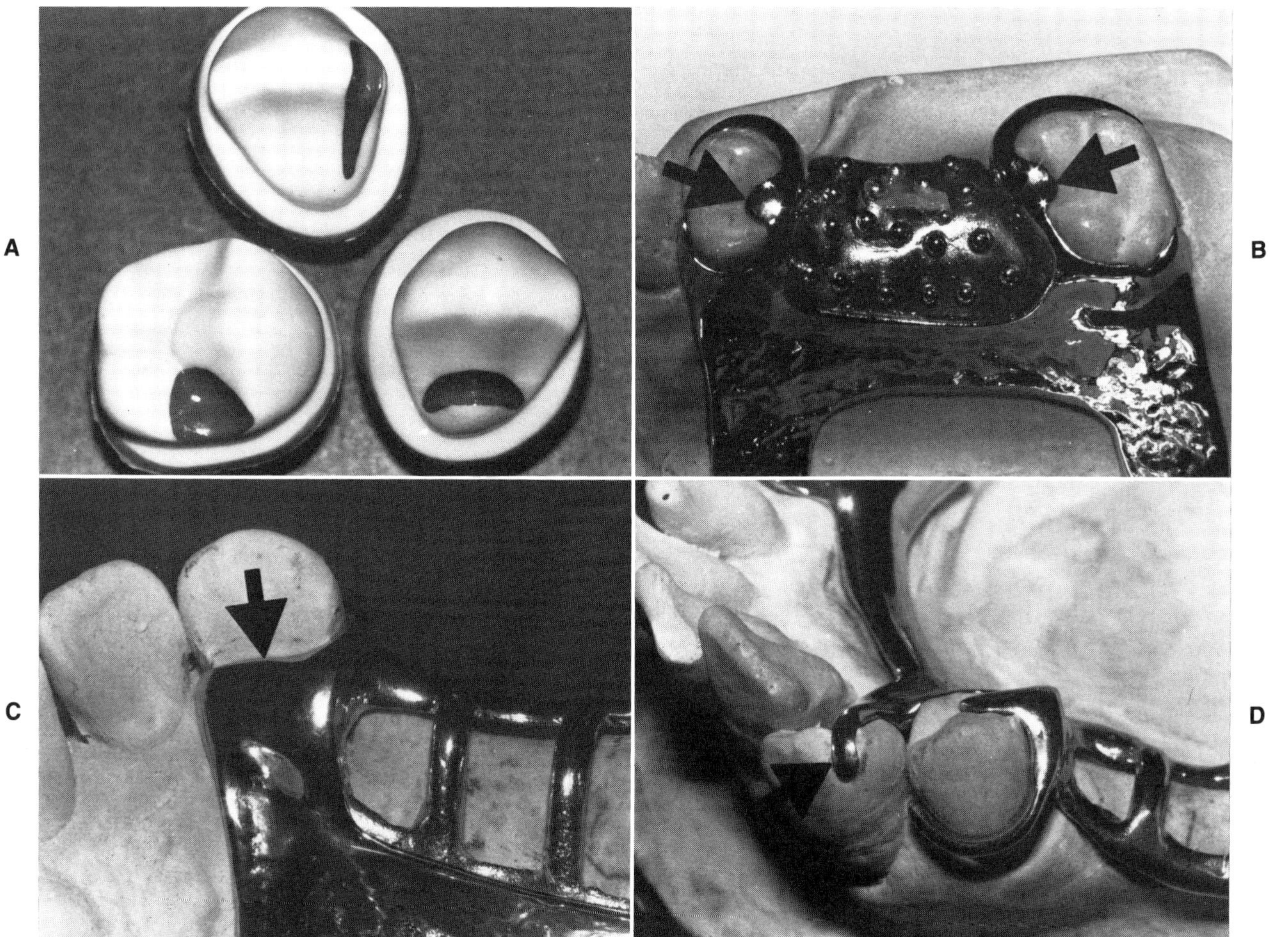

Fig. 2-73. A, Three forms of rests. Lower left, occlusal rest in a fossae of a premolar. Lower right, lingual or cingulum rest in lingual surface of a maxillary canine. Top, mesial rest on incisal surface of a mandibular canine. **B,** Occlusal rests are seated in a depression on occlusal surface of posterior teeth (arrows). Rests serve to transmit forces occurring against partial denture down long axis of abutment teeth. **C,** Cingulum rest (arrow) forms a positive rest seat for lingual plate to grasp to direct forces apically and to support the prosthesis. **D,** Incisal rest (arrow) extends slightly to labial surface of canine to prevent tooth from being orthodontically moved in that direction.

ated against an abutment tooth by the retentive clasp arm (Fig. 2-71). The rest must be designed so that it and another minor connector act as the reciprocal clasp arm. This procedure does not alter the normal contour of at least half of the crown of the abutment. This concept is discussed in greater detail in Chapter 8.

Rests may also help establish a more acceptable occlusal plane. Occasionally a large occlusal onlay rest may be used on a tipped molar to produce an acceptable plane of occlusion (Fig. 2-72). Obviously, this type of rest has limited applications. Restoration of the plane by a crown or onlay must be ruled out before this is attempted. If the onlay rest must occlude with opposing natural dentition, the occlusal surface of the onlay rest should be changed to tooth-colored acrylic resin. The technique for accomplishing this change is covered in Chapter 11.

There are three forms of rests: (1) the occlusal rest, so named because it is seated on the occlusal surface of a posterior tooth, (2) the lingual, or cingulum, rest, seated on the lingual surface of a tooth, usually a maxillary canine, and (3) the incisal rest, seated on the incisal edge of a tooth, usually a mandibular canine (Fig. 2-73). Lingual and incisal rests may under certain circumstances be used on any or all incisor teeth, but the indications are limited and are covered in the following discussion. Characteristics of each of the rests and their seats are covered. The technique and instrumentation to accomplish each of the rest seat preparations are included in Chapter 9.

Occlusal rests and rest seats

It is essential that a rest seat be prepared in the occlusal surface of a tooth for each occlusal rest. A rest should never be placed on a tooth that has not been adequately prepared.

The outline form of an occlusal rest should be triangular, with the base of the triangle resting on the marginal ridge and the rounded apex directed toward the center of the tooth (Fig. 2-74).

If there is one descriptive phrase that can be applied to occlusal rest seats, it is "smooth gentle curves." All angles, walls, and ledges must be avoided. Any portion of the rest seat that restricts movement of the rest may transmit undesirable horizontal forces to the tooth.

The shape of the rest should follow as closely as possible the outline of the mesial or distal fossa of the occlusal surface of the tooth in which the rest seat is prepared (Fig. 2-75). The size of the rest varies from one-third to one-half the mesiodistal diameter and approximately half the buccolingual width of the tooth measured from cusp tip to cusp tip (Fig. 2-76).

The floor of the occlusal rest seat must be inclined slightly toward the center of the tooth. The enclosed angle formed from a line dropped down the proximal surface of the tooth parallel to the long axis of the tooth and the floor of the rest seat must be less than 90 degrees so that the transmitted occlusal forces can be directed along the vertical axis of the tooth (Fig. 2-77). An angle greater than 90 degrees not only will not transmit the forces vertically, but will create an inclined

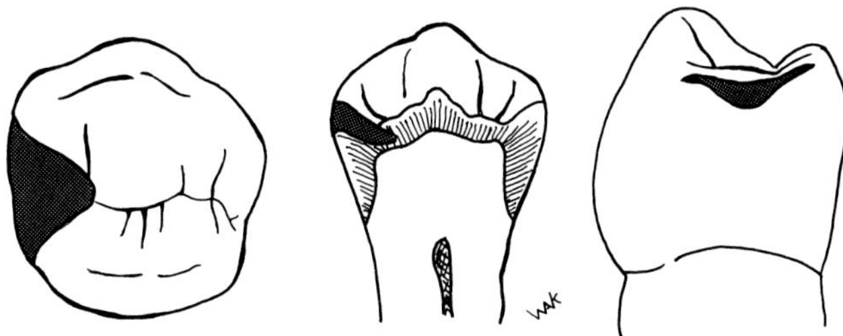

Fig. 2-74. Left, outline form of an occlusal rest is triangular, with base of triangle resting on marginal ridge. Center, floor of rest seat must incline toward center of tooth to transmit forces down long axis of tooth. Right, rest seat must be saucer-shaped with no angles. If otherwise horizontal forces cannot be dissipated by rotation of rest in rest seat.

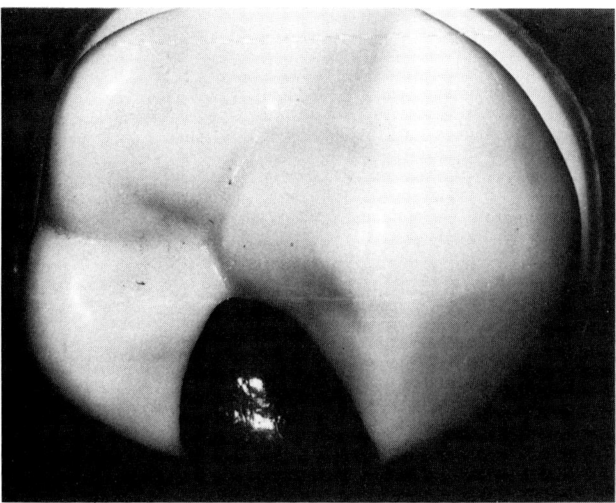

Fig. 2-75. Outline form of rest should follow that of mesial or distal fossa of occlusal surface.

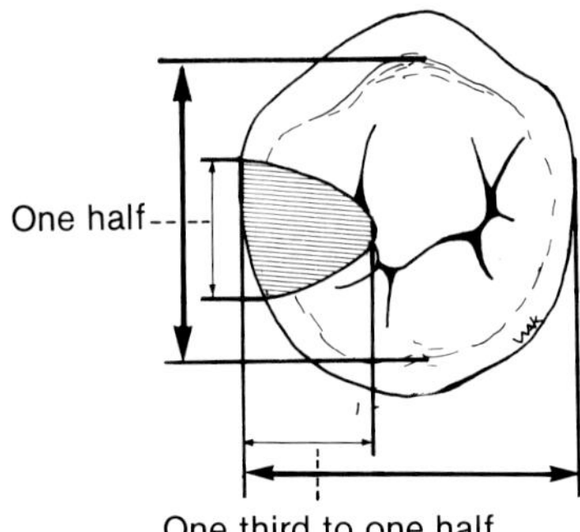

Fig. 2-76. Size of occlusal rest should be one-half the buccolingual width of tooth from cusp tip to cusp tip and one-third to one-half the mesiodistal width.

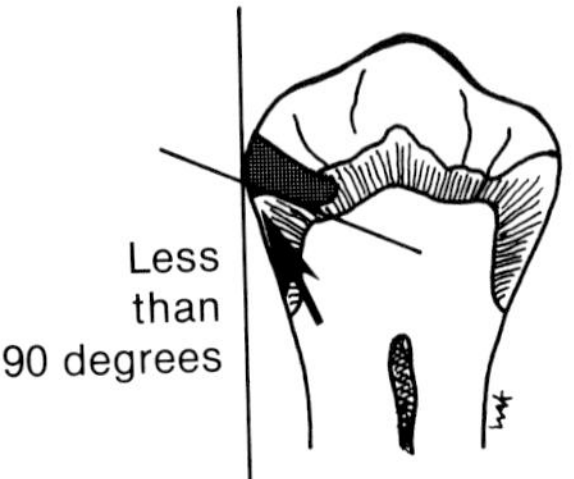

Fig. 2-77. Enclosed angle formed by floor of rest seat and a line dropped down the proximal surface of tooth parallel to long axis of tooth must be less than 90 degrees if rest is to be effective in transmitting forces on partial denture vertically down the tooth.

plane effect (Fig. 2-78). This inclined plane could produce slippage of the prosthesis away from the abutment tooth, which would place unnecessary strain on other supporting teeth. The inclined plane could also, and frequently does, cause orthodontic movement of the abutment tooth with concurrent pain and eventual bone loss.

The deepest part of the occlusal rest seat should be in the center of the preparation, with the base of the preparation rising gradually to join the enamel of the occlusal surface in a smooth, curving junction.

The greatest cause of failure of an occlusal rest is insufficient reduction of the marginal ridge. This leads to construction of a rest that is too thin and will eventually break in function. The occlusal rest must be at least 0.5 mm thick at its thinnest point and should be between 1.0 and 1.5 mm thick where it crosses the marginal ridge (Fig. 2-79). Techniques of determining the available space for the rest are covered in Chapter 9.

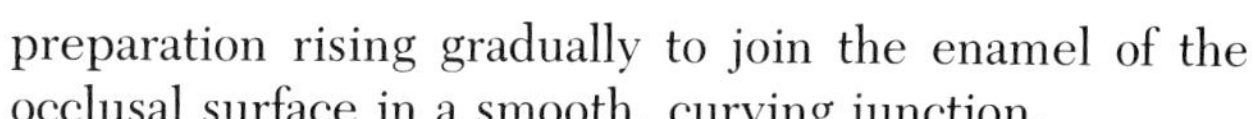

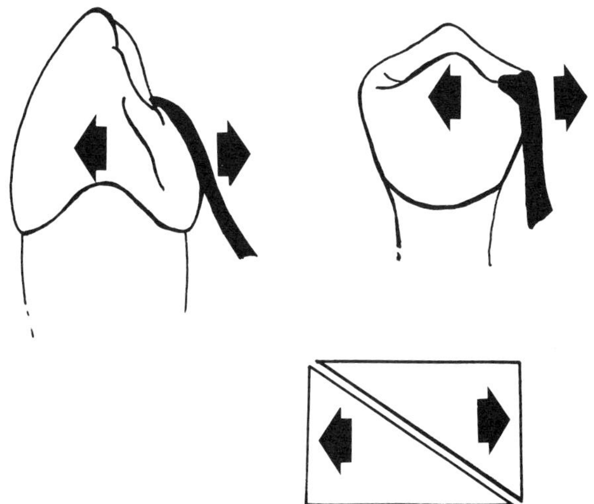

Fig. 2-78. Bottom, improperly prepared rest seats have the effect of inclined planes between tooth and prosthesis. Left, improperly prepared lingual rest seat results in forces against partial denture shunting abutment tooth facially. Right, same result occurs when enclosed angle of floor of rest seat and long axis of tooth is greater than 90 degrees.

Occlusal rests in amalgam restorations

Placing occlusal rests on amalgam alloy restorations is hazardous at best. The primary reason given for attempting this is economics (an amalgam restoration costs less than a comparable cast gold restoration). This justification is hardly logical. The flow characteristics and the lower yield strength of amalgam make the possibility of fracturing the restoration high. Replacing a defective restoration under an existing removable partial denture is difficult, and the result is usually less than completely successful. A technique for placing a cast restoration under an existing prosthesis is discussed in Chapter 21.

Perhaps the only indication for using amalgam alloy to support the partial denture is if the remaining teeth have a guarded prognosis and the denture is considered interim or temporary until the completely edentulous state is reached.

Occlusal rests in gold restorations

When a gold restoration (inlay, onlay, or crown) is planned for an abutment tooth, the wax pattern for the

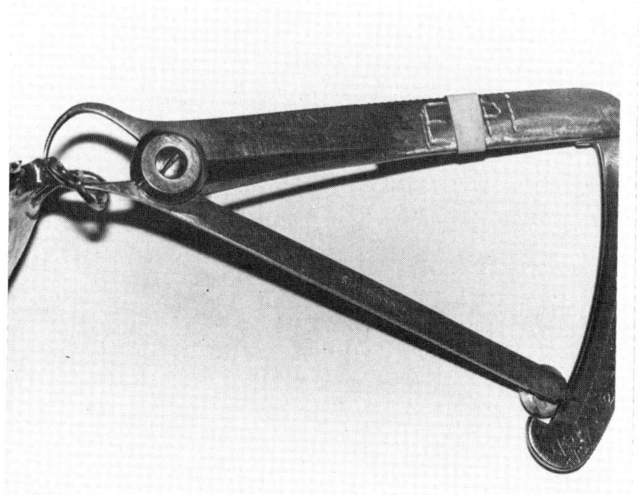

Fig. 2-79. A crown gauge, calibrated in 0.1 mm is used to measure occlusal rests.

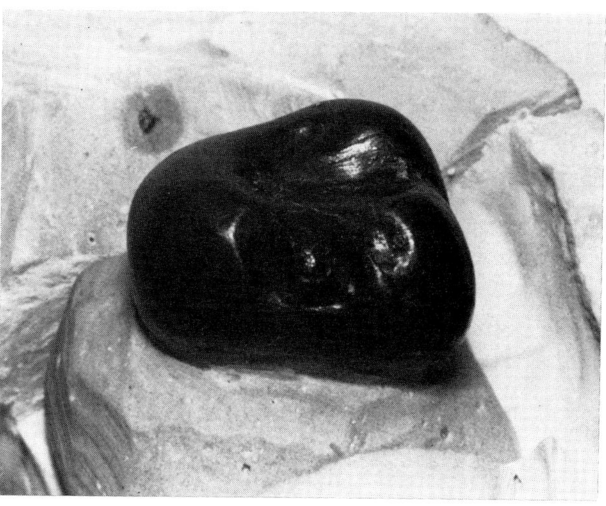

Fig. 2-80. If a gold crown has been planned for an abutment tooth, rest seat must be carved in wax pattern.

restoration must be shaped to properly receive the removable partial denture. The rest seat must be carved in the wax and refined in the cast gold before the restoration is seated in the mouth (Fig. 2-80). The entire technique for this procedure is discussed in Chapter 7.

Lingual, or cingulum, rests

The lingual, or cingulum, rest is used primarily on maxillary canines. The normal morphology of the tooth is such that a satisfactory rest seat can be formed with a minimum of tooth preparation (Fig. 2-81). The thickness of enamel on the lingual surface of mandibular canines rarely allows a lingual rest to be used (Fig. 2-82). Lingual rests on incisor teeth are also rarely used. The main indication for their use is missing canines. In this instance multiple incisor teeth must receive lingual rests to distribute the stresses over a number of teeth, because a single incisor tooth seldom offers adequate support.

Although a lingual rest may be used successfully, an occlusal rest in the mesial fossa of the first premolar is preferred, if occlusion permits, because of its mechanical advantage and because it is easier to prepare than a lingual rest.

A lingual rest, however, is preferred to an incisal rest. The lingual rest is nearer the center of rotation of the supporting tooth, so it does not tend to tip the tooth (Fig. 2-83). (The longer minor connector required for an incisal rest magnifies the forces being transferred to the abutment tooth.) In addition, since the lingual rest is confined to the lingual surface of the anterior tooth, it is more acceptable esthetically. Because of the configuration of the lingual rest, it is also less subject to breakage and distortion.

Form of lingual rests

The rest seat for a lingual rest is V shaped. The labial incline of the lingual surface of the tooth makes up one wall of the V-shaped notch, and the other wall begins at the top of the cingulum and inclines labiogingivally toward the center of the tooth to meet the other wall of the preparation (Fig. 2-84).

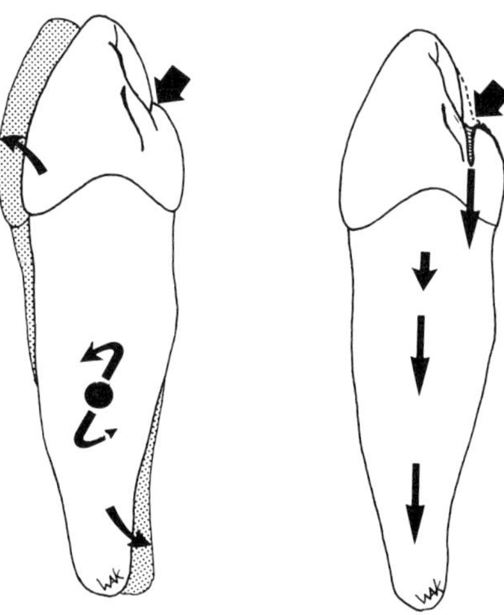

Fig. 2-81. Maxillary canine is naturally suited to receive a lingual rest because of morphology of crown. Left, a failure to prepare rest seat. Right, adequate tooth preparation directs forces down long axis of tooth.

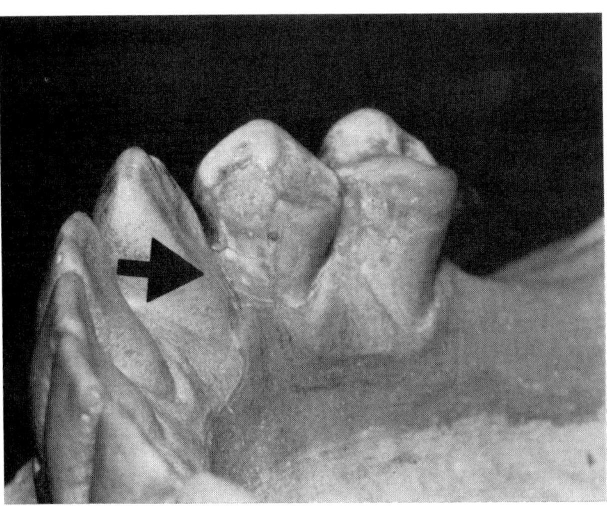

Fig. 2-82. Mandibular canines are poor candidates for lingual rest because of slope of lingual surface of tooth (arrow). Preparation of an adequate rest seat would require penetration through enamel surface of tooth.

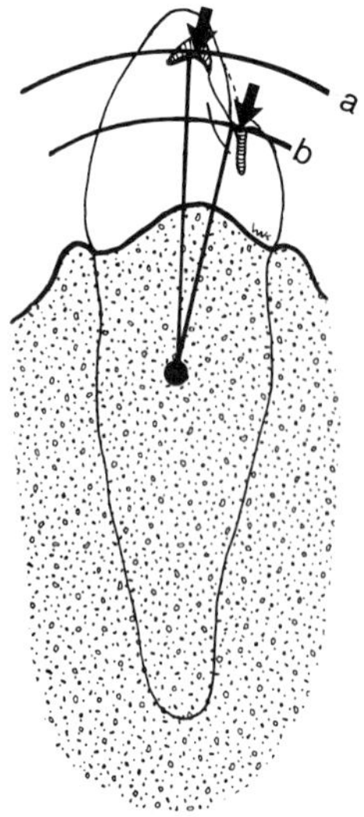

Fig. 2-83. Lingual rest is always preferred over an incisal rest on an anterior tooth because lingual rest is closer to center or rotation of tooth (b) and resultant forces on partial denture passing through a lingual rest are of less magnitude than those taking place against an incisal rest (a).

Sharp line angles and corners must be avoided because they complicate the fit of the cast framework of the partial denture.

Placement of lingual rest seats in enamel surfaces is a sound practice provided (1) the cingulum is prominent enough to present a gradual slope to the lingual surface rather than a vertical slope as is usually the case with mandibular canines, (2) the patient practices good oral hygiene, and (3) the caries index is low.

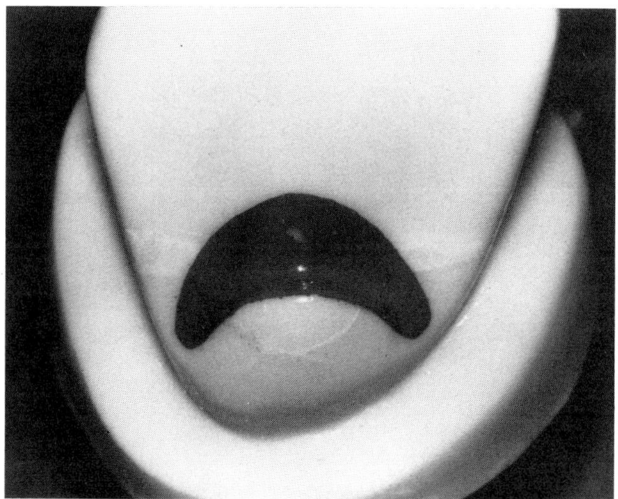

Fig. 2-84. Outline form of a lingual rest is half-moon shaped. Sharp angles must be avoided and slope of outer lip of rest seat must be labiogingival, forming an angle of less than 90 degrees to long axis of tooth.

Lingual rest seats in crowns

When crowns are to be placed on anterior teeth and rest seats are required, the rest seat should be placed in the wax pattern. The cingulum of the tooth should be accentuated in the restoration to allow development of a rest preparation that will direct the forces of occlusion through the long axis of the tooth (Fig. 2-85). The lingual form of the tooth should be restored by the metal of the partial denture framework.

Incisal rests and rest seats

Incisal rests are less desirable for anterior teeth than lingual rests. They may be used successfully, however, if the abutment tooth is sound and a cast restoration is not indicated (Fig. 2-86). If a cast restoration such as a crown is planned for an anterior tooth that is to function as an abutment tooth for a partial denture, an incisal rest is never indicated. A lingual rest incorporated in the wax pattern is the method of choice.

Incisal rests are most frequently used on mandibular canines but may be used on maxillary canines. They are not generally indicated on incisor teeth except under unusual circumstances. If stabilization of incisor teeth is indicated and fixed stabilization is not warranted because of a poor prognosis, incisal rests may be incorporated into a lingual plate to support these teeth (Fig. 2-87).

Incisal rests are positioned near the incisal angles of abutment teeth. Whether they are designed for the mesioincisal or distoincisal angle depends on the type of clasp planned for that tooth. If the tooth is not to be clasped, the rest is placed on the distoincisal surface for esthetic reasons (Fig. 2-88).

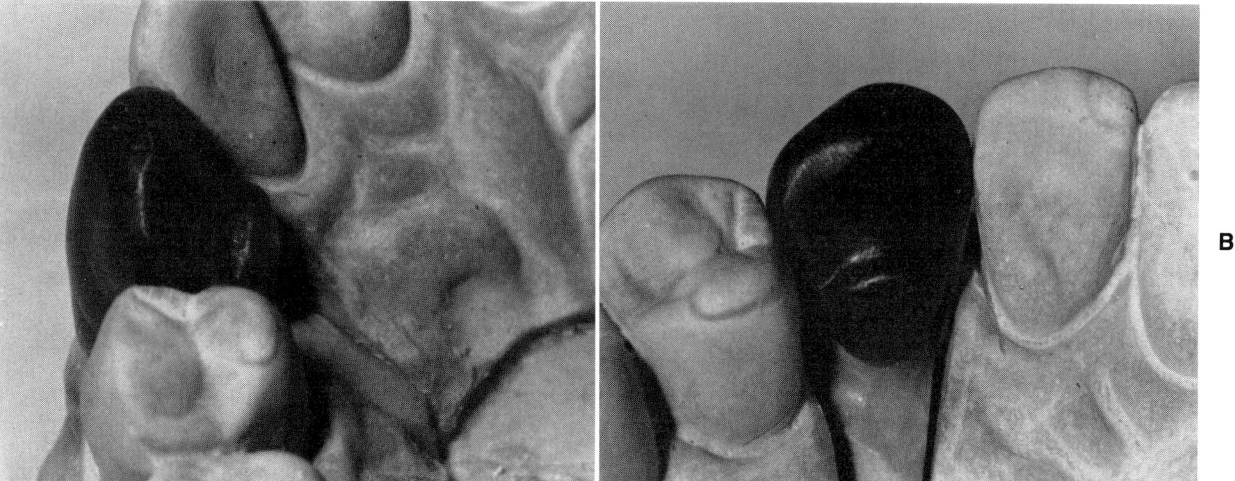

Fig. 2-85. Lingual rest must be prepared in wax pattern when a crown is planned for an abutment tooth. Same form of rest seat must be carved in wax as would be prepared in an enamel surface. **A,** Proximal view. **B,** Lingual view.

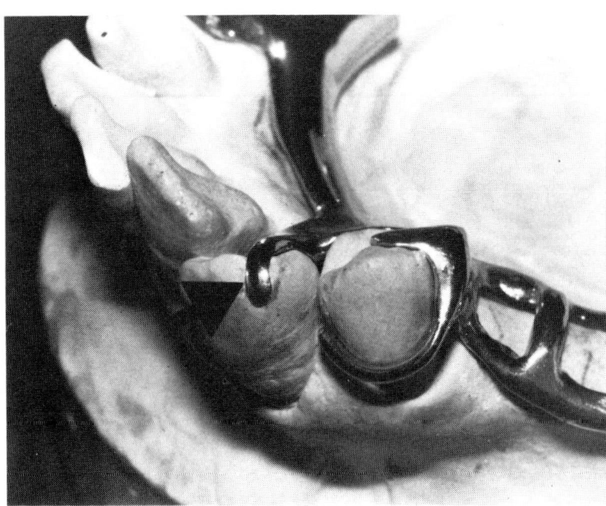

Fig. 2-86. Incisal rests are indicated most often on mandibular canines (arrow). Incisal rest is considered to be the least desirable of rests for anterior teeth because of tipping forces generated against abutment tooth.

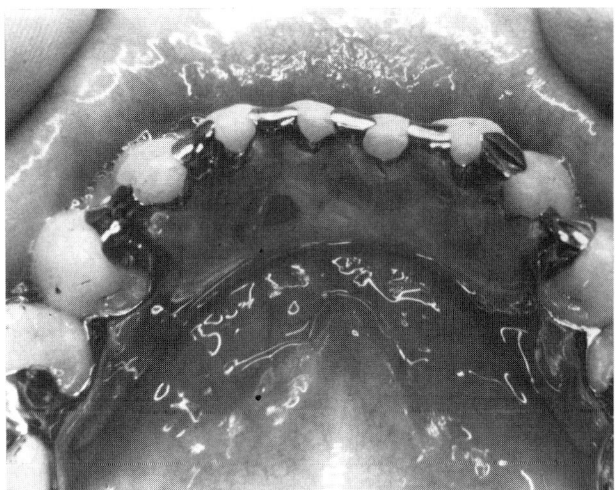

Fig. 2-87. Incisal rests may be used on incisor teeth for stabilization if other forms of stabilization with fixed prosthodontics are not warranted.

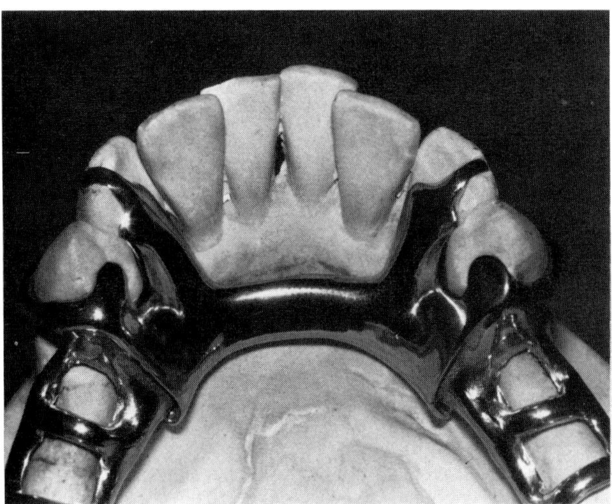

Fig. 2-88. Incisal rest is positioned near incisal angle of abutment teeth. For esthetic reasons the distoincisal angle is more acceptable.

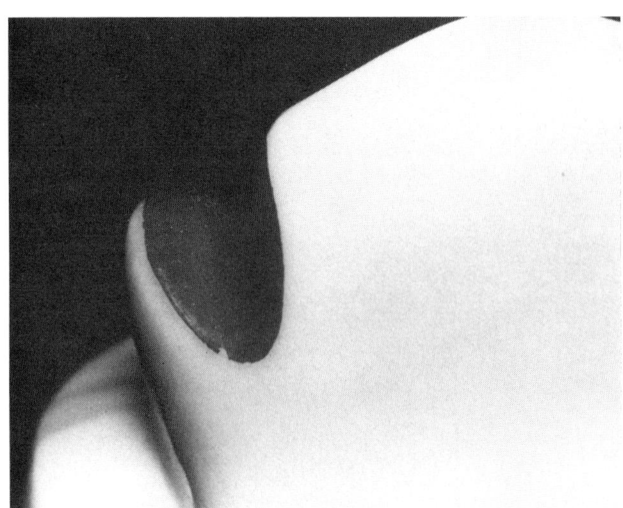

Fig. 2-89. Incisal rest seat is a V-shaped notch 1.5 to 2 mm from proximal-incisal angle of tooth (arrow). Rest seat must extend onto labial surface to prevent tooth from being forced to move in that direction.

Form of incisal rests

The incisal rest is a small, V-shaped notch located approximately 1.5 to 2.0 mm from the proximal-incisal angle of the tooth (Fig. 2-89). The deepest part of the preparation should be toward the center of the tooth mesiodistally. The notch must be rounded and should extend slightly onto the facial surface to provide a positive seat for the rest.

The enamel on the lingual surface should be prepared as a shallow depression to accommodate the minor connector and avoid annoying the tongue. Because of the greater length of this minor connector, care must be taken to maintain rigidity.

BIBLIOGRAPHY

Anderson, J.N.: Dimensions of cast palatal and lingual bars. Dent. Pract. Dent. Rec. **8**:270-274, 1958.

Applegate, O.C.: The partial denture base, J. Prosthet. Dent. **5**:636-648, 1955.

Askinas, S.W.: Facings in removable partial dentures, J. Prosthet. Dent. **33**:633-636, 1975.

Beck, H.O.: Alloys for removable partial dentures, Dent. Clin. North Am. **4**:591-596, 1960.

Berg, T., and Caputo, A.A.: Anterior rests for maxillary removable partial dentures, J. Prosthet. Dent. **39**:139-146, 1978.

Buckner, H., and La Velle, W.E.: Metal backings for denture teeth, J. Prosthet. Dent. **32**:579-581, 1974.

Campbell, L.D.: Subjective reactions to major connector designs for removable partial dentures, J. Prosthet. Dent. **37**:506-517, 1977.

Cecconi, B.T.: Lingual bar design, J. Prosthet. Dent. **29**:635-639, 1973.

Cecconi, B.T.: Effect of rest design on transmission of forces to abutment teeth, J. Prosthet. Dent. **32**:141-151, 1974.

Dirksen, L.C., and Compagna, S.J.: Mat surface and rugae reproduction for upper partial denture castings, J. Prosthet. Dent. **4**:67-72, 1954.

Dunny, J.A., and King, G.E.: Minor connector design for anterior acrylic resin bases, a preliminary study, J. Prosthet. Dent. **34**:496-502, 1975.

Fisher, R.L., and Jaslow, C.: The efficiency of an indirect retainer, J. Prosthet. Dent. **33**:24-30, 1975.

Henderson, D.: Major connectors for mandibular removable partial dentures, J. Prosthet. Dent. **30**:532-548, 1973.

Henderson, D.: Major connectors—united it stands, Dent. Clin. North Am. **17**:661-668, 1973.

Laney, W.R., and Desjardins, R.P.: Comparison of base metal alloys and Type IV gold alloys for removable partial denture framework, Dent. Clin. North Am. **17**:611-630, 1973.

LaVere, A.M., and Krol, A.J.: Selection of a major connector for the extension base removable partial denture, J. Prosthet. Dent. **30**:102-105, 1973.

MacKinnon, K.P.: Indirect retention in partial denture construction, Dent. J. Aust. **27**:221-225, 1955.

Seidin, A.: Occlusal rests and rest seats, J. Prosthet. Dent. **8**:431-440, 1958.

Skinner, F.W., and Chung, P.: The effect of surface contact in the retention of a denture, J. Prosthet. Dent. **1**:229-235, 1951.

Wallace, D.H.: The use of gold occlusal surfaces in complete and partial dentures, J. Prosthet. Dent. **14**:326-333, 1964.

3 Components of a removable partial denture

DIRECT RETAINERS · INDIRECT RETAINERS · TOOTH REPLACEMENTS

DIRECT RETAINERS

The component that engages an abutment tooth and in so doing resists dislodging forces applied to a removable partial denture is called the direct retainer. The amount and location of this retention on an abutment tooth must be carefully controlled to prevent damage to the supporting structures of the tooth.

There are two types of direct retainers currently in use, intracoronal and extracoronal.

Intracoronal retainers

The intracoronal retainer, or internal attachment, was developed by Dr. Herman E.S. Chayes in 1906. It consists of two units (Figs. 3-1 and 3-2), one of which is a receptacle that is built into a crown or inlay constructed for an abutment tooth. The second unit is an insert that is attached to the removable partial denture. The insert is machined to fit precisely into the receptacle. When two or more of these units are used to retain a prosthesis, the exact parallelism of these retainers results in a binding action when a dislodging force is applied to the partial denture. The retention does not result from friction between the insert and receptacle but from the binding, or wedging, that occurs when a dislodging force attempts to alter the parallel relationship. The patient can remove the prosthesis by applying finger pressure equally on each side parallel to the long axis of the receptacles.

This aspect of direct retention, the intracoronal attachment, is considered in greater detail in Chapter 22.

Extracoronal retainers

The extracoronal direct retainer or clasp, operates on the principle of the resistance of metal to deformation. It is designed so that one terminal of each clasp is located on an external surface of a tooth that converges apically to produce an undercut (Fig. 3-3). When two or more of these clasp terminals engage undercuts, the partial denture will resist dislodging forces. The amount of retention can be varied by the depth of the undercut and the flexibility of the clasp arm positioned in the undercut.

It must be understood that a removable partial denture is designed so that it has a definite path of insertion into and removal from the mouth. The areas used for extracoronal retention must be undercut in relation to this path or there will be no retention (Fig. 3-4). Dislodging forces such as sticky foods or the force of gravity that tend to unseat the partial denture in function act at right angles to the plane of occlusion; to resist them, the undercut areas must be present when the cast is viewed with the occlusal surfaces of the teeth parallel to the floor (Fig. 3-5). A complete understanding of this principle will resolve many of the problems involved in the design of areas of retention for a removable partial denture. If there are no undercuts related to a line dropped perpendicularly from the occlusal plane, another means must be used to retain the prosthesis. Alternate methods are considered in Chapter 7.

To further the understanding of how an extracoronal direct retainer resists dislodging forces, the shape of premolar and molar teeth should be considered. In 1916 Prothero advanced a cone theory as the basis for clasp retention. He described the shape of crowns of premolar and molar teeth as that of two cones sharing a common base (Fig. 3-6). A clasp arm or tip that ends on a cervical cone would resist movement in the occlusal direction because to release from the tooth it would be forced to undergo deformation. The metal used for clasp construction is resilient and will deform, but will resist deformation when stressed not to exceed its proportional limit. The degree of resistance to deformation determines the amount of the clasp's retention.

The line at which the two converging cones meet (or more practically, the line at which occlusally sloping surfaces meet cervically sloping surfaces) is called the *height of contour*, a term first used by Kennedy (Fig. 3-7). It represents the greatest bulge or diameter of a crown when viewed from a specific angle. The height of contour of a tooth will change as the vertical position

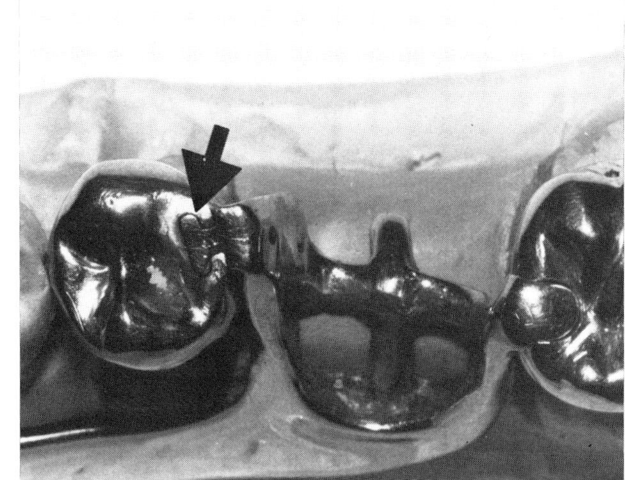

Fig. 3-1. An internal attachment in place (arrow). Female receptacle in artificial crown on abutment tooth. Male unit is attached to removable partial denture. Prosthesis is retained by relative parallelism of two or more of these units.

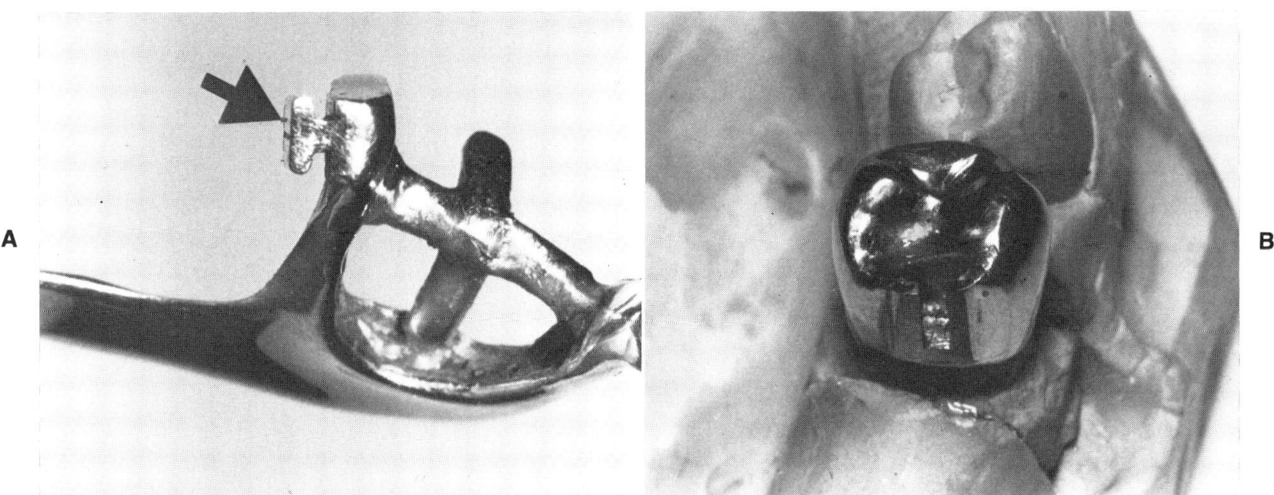

Fig. 3-2. A, Male portion of intracoronal retainer attached to minor connector of partial denture (arrow). **B,** Female unit in crown of abutment tooth.

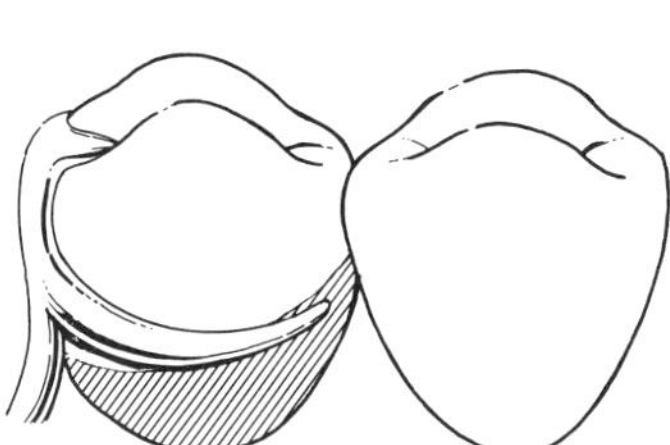

Fig. 3-3. Extracoronal retainer (clasp) is designed so that one terminal of each clasp assembly will be in an undercut (shaded area). This retainer will prevent partial denture from being dislodged during function.

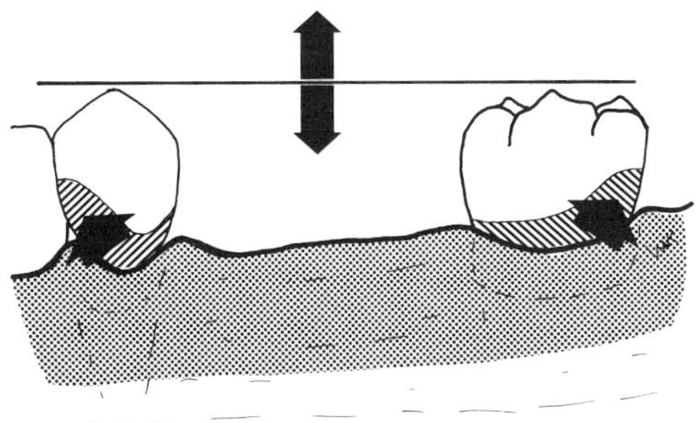

Fig. 3-4. The areas selected to retain the prosthesis must be undercut in relation to partial denture's path of insertion and withdrawal.

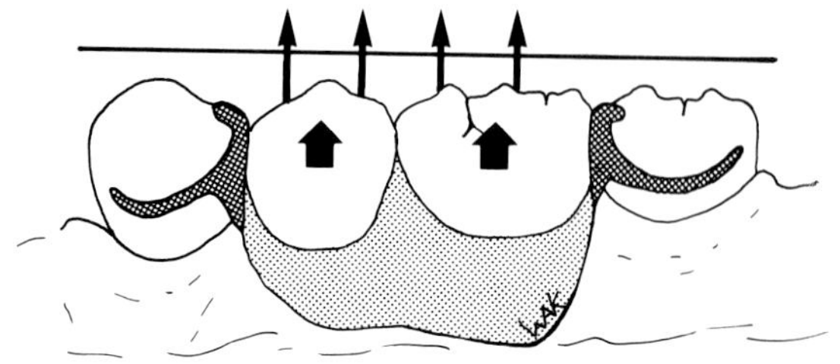

Fig. 3-5. Dislodging forces that tend to unseat partial denture, such as pull of sticky food or force of gravity, always act perpendicular to plane of occlusion.

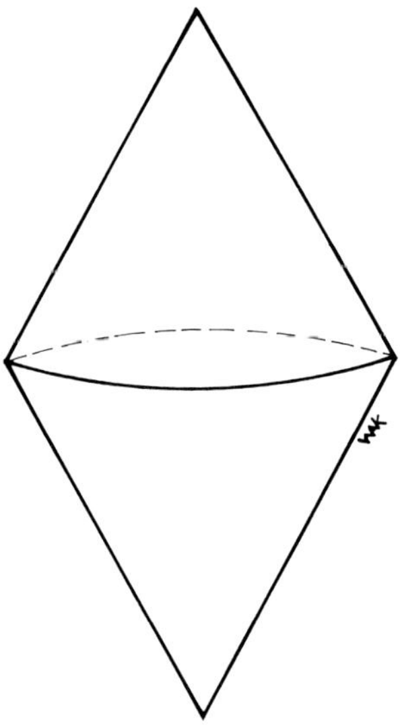

Fig. 3-6. Shape of crown of molar and premolar teeth is similar to that of two cones placed so that they share a common base. One cone approximates the cervical portion of the tooth, and one the occlusal portion. A clasp arm on cervical cone would have to undergo deformation to move in occlusal direction; therefore such movement is resisted.

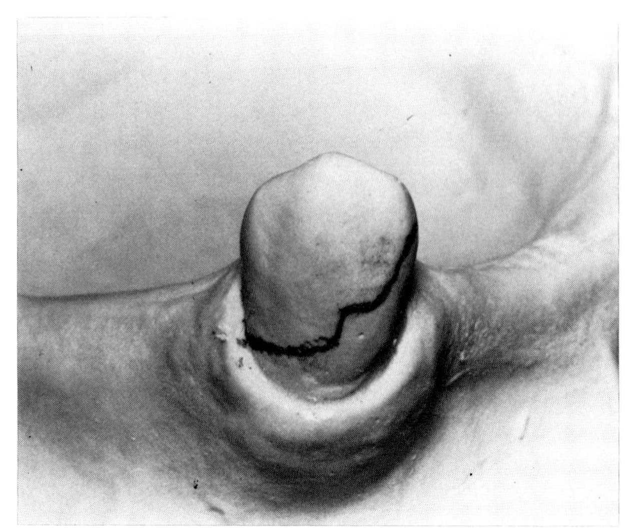

Fig. 3-7. The line at which occlusally or incisally sloping surface of crown meets cervically sloping surface is called height of contour.

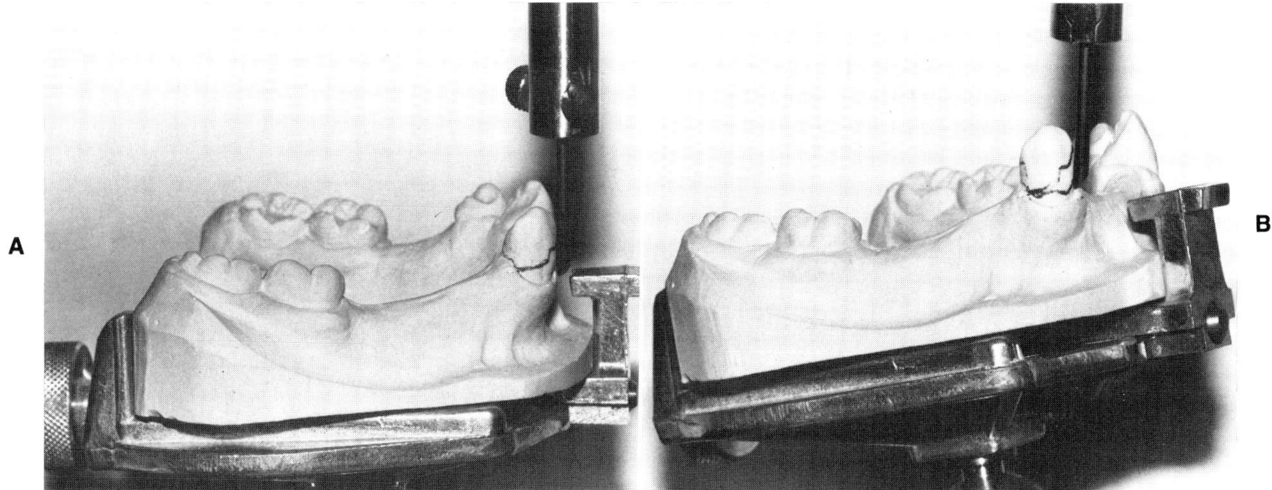

Fig. 3-8. Changing tilt of cast in relation to vertical plane moves height of contour. Line drawn to indicate height of contour in **A** was no longer correct when cast was tilted, **B.** Note new (lower) line drawn on tooth in **B.**

of the tooth is changed. Tipping or tilting a cast will cause the height of contour to move accordingly (Fig. 3-8).

DeVan (1955) used some clarifying terms to describe retention. He referred to the surface of a tooth that is occlusal to the height of contour as *suprabulge*, and the surface inclining cervically as *infrabulge*. A tooth surface may be said to be retentive if it is cervical to its height of contour, or infrabulge.

There are two basic categories of clasps: (1) circumferential, or Akers, clasps and (2) vertical projection, or bar or Roach, clasps. This book follows the currently favored practice of using the descriptive terms rather than the eponyms.

A circumferential clasp has two clasp arms that partially encircle the abutment tooth. The clasp, with the exception of the retentive clasp terminal, is always located occlusal to the height of contour (Fig. 3-9). Thus, the retentive tip approaches the undercut from above the greatest bulge of the tooth. This is the principal difference between the two basic categories of clasps: circumferential clasps approach the undercut from above the height of contour, whereas vertical projection clasps approach it from below the height of contour.

The *combination clasp* is a type of circumferential clasp. Its retentive arm is of wrought metal, which makes it more flexible than a similar arm constructed of cast alloy (Fig. 3-10). The reciprocal arm must be rigid to counteract the forces generated by the flexible wrought metal; therefore it is made of cast metal. The retentive terminal reaches the undercut from above the height of contour, as do those of all the circumferential clasps. The wrought metal or wrought wire clasp arm is

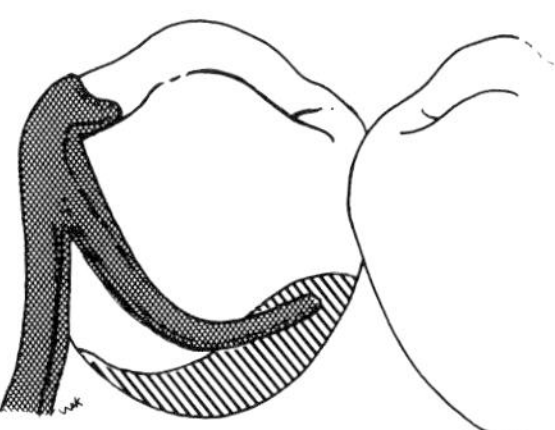

Fig. 3-9. Circumferential clasp approaches retentive undercut from above greatest bulge of tooth.

usually attached to the metal framework of the partial denture during the framework wax-up procedure. The wax framework with the wrought wire clasp is invested, and the metal for the framework is cast directly to the wrought wire clasp arm. This results in mechanical union between the cast framework and the wrought wire.

The vertical projection, or bar, clasp is an extension of the metal framework of the partial denture that projects along the mucosa, crosses the gingival margin of the abutment tooth, and approaches the infrabulge of the tooth in a cervico-occlusal direction (Fig. 3-11).

The clasp, or more properly the clasp assembly, has the following component parts (Fig. 3-12):

rest (Fig. 3-12, *1*) Part of the clasp that lies on the occlusal, lingual, or incisal edge or surfaces of a tooth and resists tissueward movement of the clasp by ensuring that the retentive terminal of the clasp remains fixed in the desired, or planned depth, of undercut.

body (Fig. 3-12, *2*) Part of the clasp that connects the rest and shoulders of the clasp to the minor connectors. It,

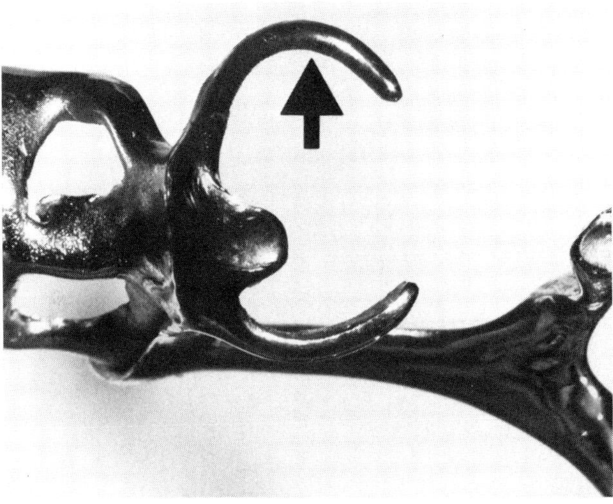

Fig. 3-10. Combination clasp is a clasp that has a retentive arm made of wrought metal (arrow). Consequently, it is more flexible than a comparable cast arm would be. Reciprocal arm is of cast metal and is nonflexible.

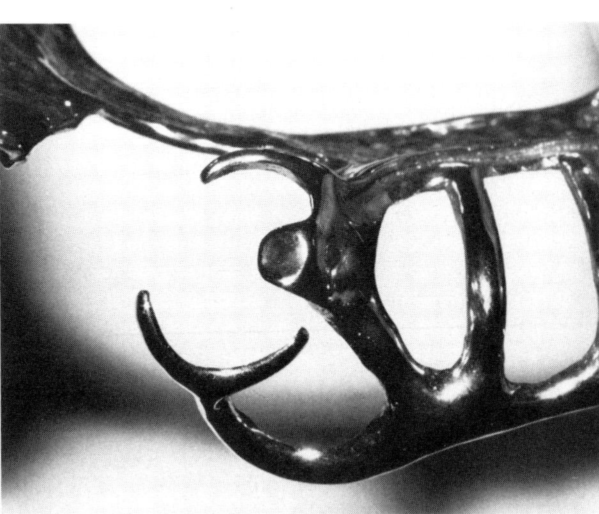

Fig. 3-11. The vertical projection, or bar, clasp approaches retentive undercut from below height of contour.

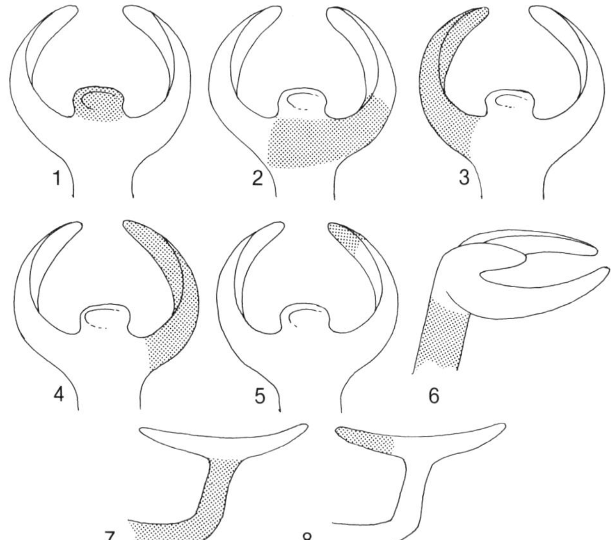

Fig. 3-12. Components of clasp assembly: *1,* Rest provides support for prosthesis. *2,* Body connects rest and clasp arms to minor connector. *3,* Reciprocal clasp arm must be rigid and lie above height of contour. *4,* Retentive clasp arm includes shoulder and retentive terminal. *5,* Retentive terminal, distal third of retentive clasp arm, is positioned below height of contour and provides direct retention for prosthesis. *6,* Minor connector joins body of clasp assembly to remainder of framework. *7,* Approach arm is a component of vertical projection clasps. It is a minor connector that joins body and retentive terminal of clasp to framework. It is the only minor connector that is not rigid. *8,* Retentive terminal is portion of vertical projection clasp positioned below survey line.

like all components, except the retentive terminal, must be rigid and must lie above the height of contour.

shoulder Part of the clasp that connects the body to the clasp terminals. The shoulder must lie above the height of contour and provide some stabilization against horizontal displacement of the prosthesis.

reciprocal arm (Fig. 3-12, *3*) A rigid clasp arm placed above the height of contour on the side of the tooth opposing the retentive clasp arm. One of its purposes is to resist the tipping force generated by the retentive terminal as it passes over the height of contour when the partial denture is inserted into or withdrawn from the mouth. As the retentive terminal passes over the greatest bulge of the tooth, the metal must deform. This deformation generates a positive lateral force against the tooth. If the tooth were not supported against this destructive lateral force, damage to the supporting periodontal ligament and bone could occur. The position of the reciprocal arm in relation to the retentive arm is critical. It must be designed to contact the tooth before the retentive clasp does, and to *remain in contact* while the retentive terminal passes the height of contour (Fig. 3-13). This requires that the surface of the abutment tooth on which the reciprocal arm is placed be as parallel as

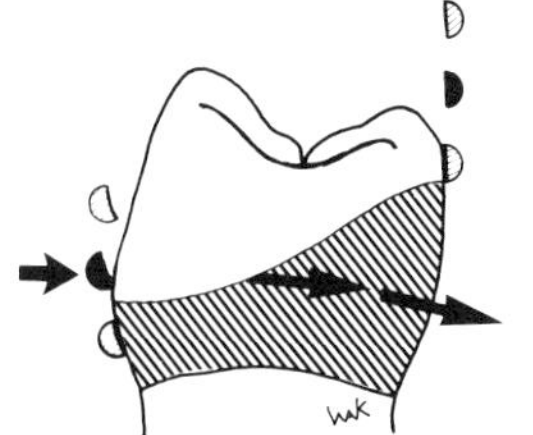
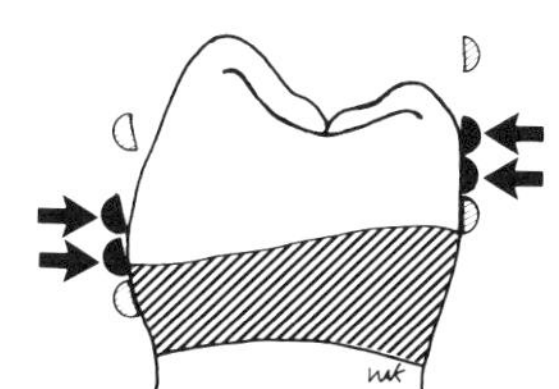

Fig. 3-13. Reciprocal clasp arm must contact tooth before retentive clasp arm passes over height of contour. By bracing tooth, it reciprocates force exerted against tooth by retentive clasp.

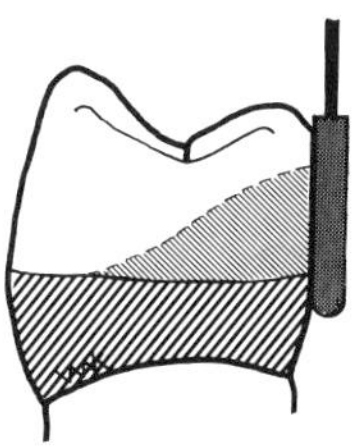

Fig. 3-14. Recontouring of enamel surfaces can effectively change height of contour. In this case height of contour is being lowered to allow placement of a reciprocal clasp arm in a more favorable position.

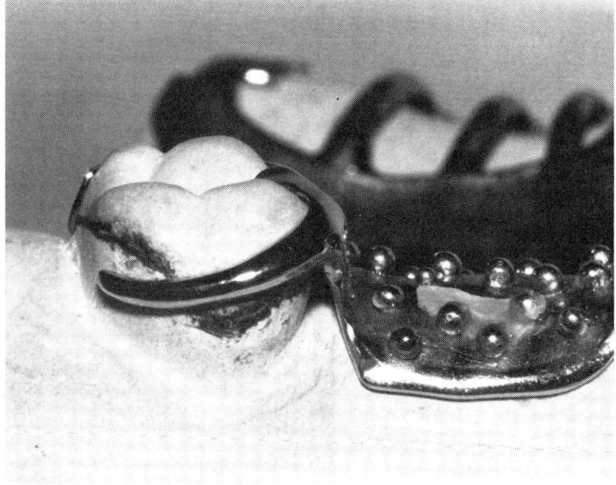

Fig. 3-15. Shoulder of circumferential clasp is rigid and must remain above height of contour, represented by line drawn on this tooth. Terminal third of clasp (retentive terminal) must be positioned below height of contour.

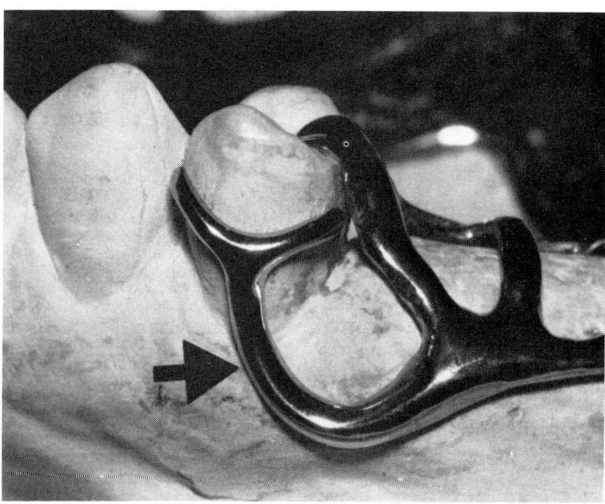

Fig. 3-16. Approach arm (arrow) of vertical projection clasp joins body and retentive terminal of clasp to framework. It is in intimate contact with underlying mucosa and may be slightly flexible.

possible to the path the prosthesis takes as it is inserted into or withdrawn from the mouth. The enamel surface can usually be contoured to produce this desired result (Fig. 3-14).

As an additional function the reciprocal arm helps stabilize the partial denture against lateral movement. Also, because it lies on the suprabulge, it contributes somewhat to vertical support of the prosthesis.

retentive clasp arm (Fig. 3-12, *4*) Part of the clasp comprising the shoulder, which is not flexible and is located above the height of contour, and the retentive terminal (Fig. 3-15).

retentive terminal (Fig. 3-12, *5* and *8*) The distal third of the clasp arm. It is the only component of the removable partial denture to lie on the tooth surface cervical to the height of contour. It is this position of the flexible terminal in the undercut that provides the direct retention.

minor connector (Fig. 3-12, *6*) Part of the clasp that joins the body of the clasp to the remainder of the framework. It must always be rigid.

approach arm (Fig. 3-12, *7*) Component of bar, or vertical projection, clasps (those that engage the undercut from below the height of contour). The approach arm is a minor connector that projects from the framework, runs along the mucosa, and turns to cross the gingival margin of the abutment tooth. The body and retentive terminal are attached to it. The approach arm may be slightly flexible (Fig. 3-16).

Requirements of clasp design

All clasps must be designed so that they satisfy the following six basic requirements: (1) retention, (2) support, (3) stability, (4) reciprocation, (5) encirclement, and (6) passivity.

Retention. The function of the retentive clasp arm is to provide retention for the prosthesis against dislodging forces. The retentive clasp is divided into three parts, each with its own functional requirements. The terminal third is flexible and engages the undercut

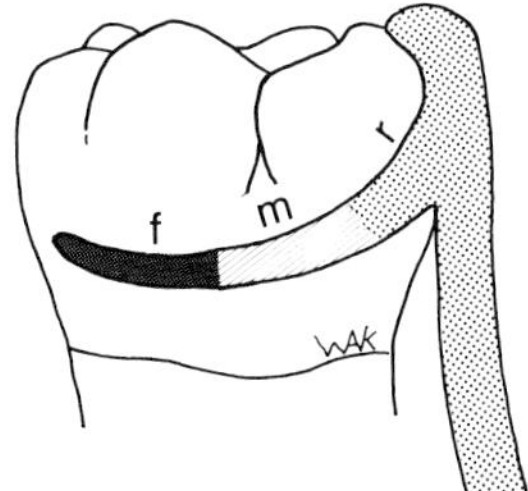

Fig. 3-17. Retentive clasp is divided into three parts. Terminal third *(f)* is flexible and is placed below the height of contour. Middle third *(m)* has a limited degree of flexibility. Proximal third *(r)* is rigid and must be positioned above height of contour.

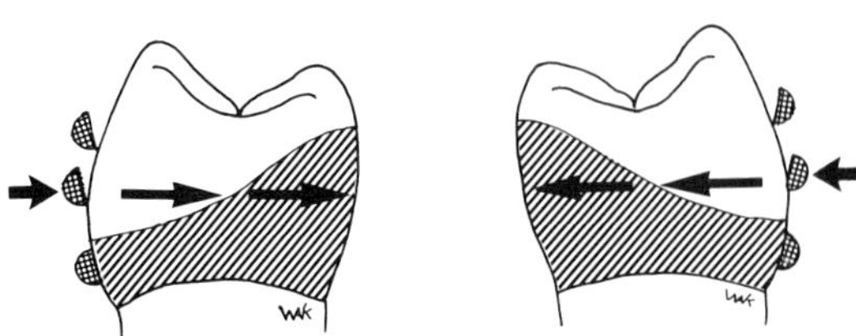

Fig. 3-18. A retentive clasp passing over the greatest bulge of a tooth to enter a retentive undercut exerts lateral forces against tooth. These lateral forces can damage abutment tooth.

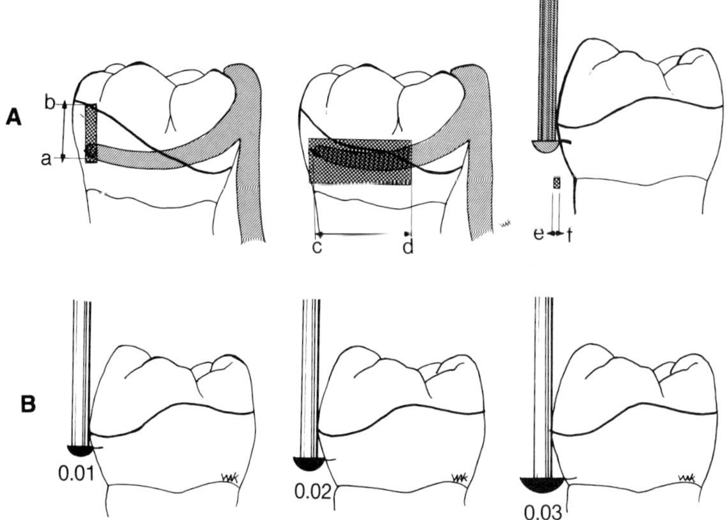

Fig. 3-19. A, Three dimensions of a retentive undercut. Distance between tip of clasp and height of contour *(a-b)* is not significant. Mesiodistal length of clasp arm that is positioned below height of contour *(c-d)* is significant only to extent that the longer the distance, the greater will be the flexibility of the clasp. This would influence amount of retention required. Actual measured amount of undercut in a bucco lingual dimension *(e-f)* is the critical dimension of the three. **B,** Buccolingual depth of retentive undercut can be measured with an undercut gauge. A retentive clasp constructed of cast chrome metal is normally placed in a 0.010-inch undercut. Clasps made of wrought metal are normally positioned in an undercut of 0.020 inch. A 0.030-inch undercut would rarely be used in a conventional partial denture.

area, the middle third has a limited degree of flexibility and may engage a minimal amount of undercut, and the proximal third, or shoulder, is rigid and must be positioned above the height of contour (Fig. 3-17).

The amount of retention that a clasp arm provides depends on the flexibility of the clasp arm, the depth that the retentive terminal extends into the undercut, and the amount of clasp arm that extends below the height of contour.

The amount of retention used should always be the minimum necessary to resist reasonable dislodging forces. A rigid clasp flexing over the greatest bulge of a tooth to enter a deep undercut will apply harmful stresses to the abutment teeth (Fig. 3-18).

The retentive undercut has three dimensions (Fig. 3-19, *A*). The buccolingual depth of the undercut (*e-f* in Fig. 3-19, *A*) may be measured by an undercut gauge and expressed in thousandths of an inch (Fig. 3-19, *B*). It is measured on a line *dropped* cervically from the height of contour. The distance between the height of contour and a given buccolingual measurement depends on the angle formed by the infrabulge and this vertical line. The less sharp this angle, the greater distance needed between the height of contour and the retentive terminal to achieve the same amount of retention.

The clasp's flexibility also affects its placement. Most clasps made of cast chrome metal are placed in under-

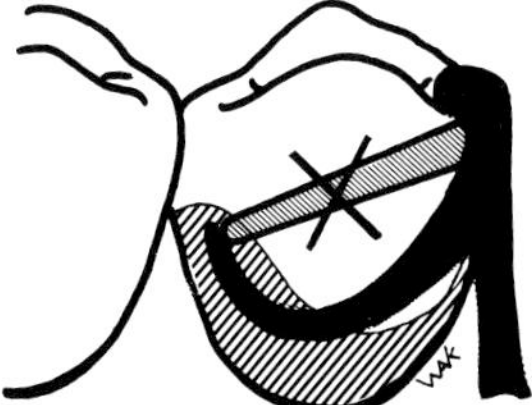

Fig. 3-20. Flexibility of a clasp arm increases as length of clasp increases. A clasp arm should not cover surface of a tooth in a straight line but should be curved as much as possible. This clasp tip should be pointed occlusally.

cuts of 0.010 inch. Cast clasps of gold are generally designed for 0.015-inch undercuts, and casts of wrought alloy are designed for a maximum 0.020-inch undercut. These statements are generalizations; the specific clinical situation must be considered when the required amount of retention is determined. (See Chapter 7.)

Another dimension of the retentive undercut, the distance between the survey line and the tip of the retentive clasp (a-b in Fig. 3-19, *A*), affects the clasp arm length, which in turn influences the flexibility of the clasp. In actual clasp placement this dimension is not seriously considered.

The third dimension of the undercut is the mesodistal length of the clasp arm below the height of contour (*c-d* in Fig. 3-19, *A*). The longer this measurement, the more flexible the clasp will be and the more important is the buccolingual dimension of the retentive undercut.

The most variable factor in determining retention for a removable partial denture is clasp flexibility. Flexibility is determined by the length of the clasp, the diameter of the clasp arm, its taper, the cross-sectional form, and the material from which the clasp is made.

The greater the *length* of the clasp arm, the greater will be its flexibility, because flexure is directly proportional to the cube of the length (Fig. 3-20). By doubling the length of a clasp arm, its flexibility is increased five times. By increasing the clasp's flexibility, the magnitude of horizontal stresses against an abutment tooth can be reduced. However, flexibility should not be so great that the clasp's ability to provide retention is lost.

Flexibility is inversely proportional to the *diameter* of the clasp arm (Fig. 3-21).

A uniform *taper* in both thickness and width is essential for both the approach arm of a bar clasp and the retentive arm of a cast clasp. A clasp should be half as thick at the tip as at the origin (Fig. 3-22).

The *cross-sectional form* also affects flexibility. A round clasp has greater flexibility than a half-round clasp with the same diameter. It also has the ability to flex in all spatial plans, whereas a half-round clasp normally flexes in only a single plane.

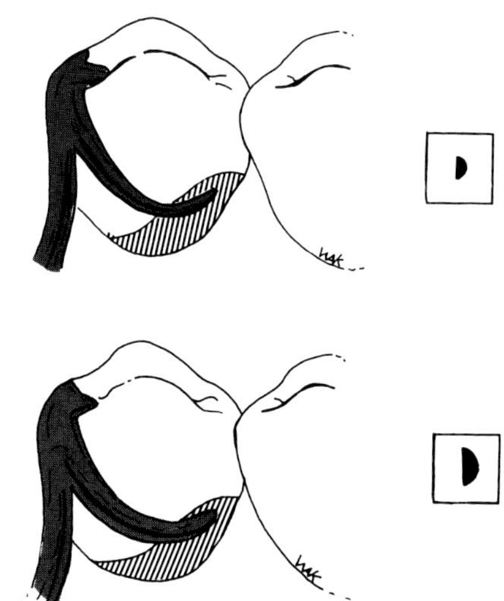

Fig. 3-21. Flexibility of a clasp is inversely proportional to its diameter. Clasp above will be twice as flexible as one below.

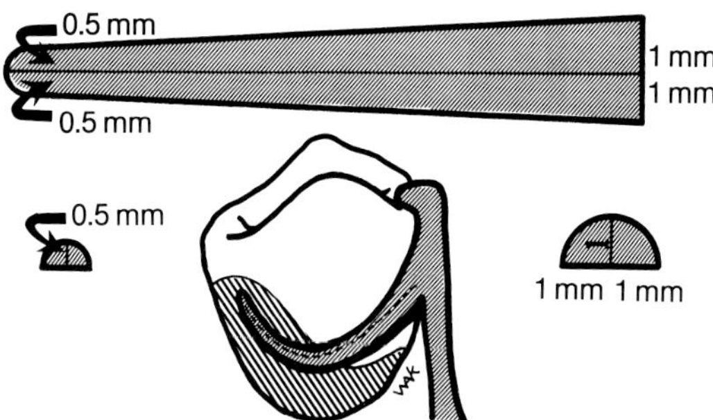

Fig. 3-22. A uniform taper in both thickness and width is necessary for proper function of a clasp. Clasp terminal should be half as thick as origin.

The *material* of which the clasp is made is also important (Figs. 3-23 and 3-24). Chrome alloys have a higher modular of elasticity than do gold alloys and are therefore less flexible. Therefore a smaller cross-sectional form of the clasp and less depth of retentive undercut must be used when chrome alloy is the metal selected for the framework of the partial denture. Because of the internal structure of wrought wire, it has greater ability to flex than is permitted by the crystalline structure of cast alloy. To obtain equal retention, therefore, a greater depth of undercut is required for a wrought wire clasp than for a cast clasp.

Support. Support is the property of a clasp that resists displacement of the clasp in a gingival direction. The prime support units of a clasp are occlusal, lingual, or incisal rests. The manner in which rests provide support has been discussed previously, but it will be repeated that rests should provide only vertical support.

Other elements of the partial denture must resist horizontal displacement (provide stability).

Stability. Stability is resistance to horizontal displacement of a prosthesis. All clasp components except the retentive clasp terminals contribute to this property in varying degrees. The cast circumferential clasp offers the greatest amount of stability because its shoulder is rigid and aids in stabilization. The wrought wire clasp has a flexible shoulder, and the bar clasp does not have a shoulder, so both provide less stability.

All three clasp types have rigid reciprocal, or bracing, arm which provides equal amounts of stability.

Reciprocation. Each retentive clasp terminal must be opposed by a reciprocal clasp arm or another element of the partial denture capable of resisting horizontal forces exerted on the tooth by the retentive arm.

The reciprocal arm of the clasp is positioned on the opposite side of the tooth from the retentive arm. In addition to reciprocating stress generated against the tooth by the retentive clasp, it also plays an important role in stabilizing the denture against horizontal movement.

A lingual plate may at times by used to provide reciprocation (Fig. 3-25). In certain removable partial denture designs an additional occlusal rest is positioned on the opposite side of the tooth and it, with its minor connector, will provide reciprocation. (See Chapter 8).

The reciprocal clasp arm must be rigid. It is not tapered as is the retentive clasp. The reciprocal arm should be positioned on a surface of a tooth that is reasonably parallel to the denture's path of insertion and withdrawal. If the arm is positioned on a surface that is tapered occlusally, a slight movement of the denture will cause the clasp to lose contact with the tooth, and as a result reciprocation and retention will be lost.

Because the reciprocal clasp must be rigid, it must be positioned above the height of contour. It should, however, be placed as close to the height of contour as possible, no higher than the middle third of the tooth and preferably at the junction of the gingival and middle thirds (Fig. 3-26). To reciprocate forces properly, it should contact the tooth at the same time or before the retentive arm does. In this way the tipping forces generated by the retentive clasp terminal as it flexes over

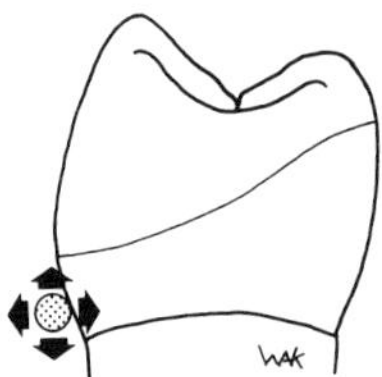

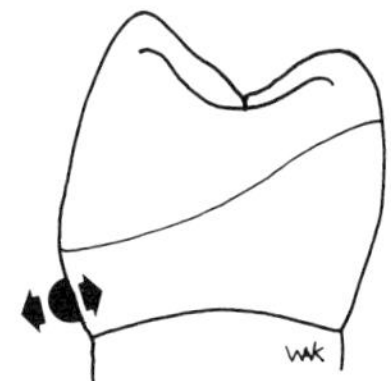

Fig. 3-23. A wrought wire clasp, left, is capable of flexing in all spatial planes. This allows clasp to be adjusted in all directions to improve retention. Cast clasp, right, will flex in only a single plane, either inward or outward perpendicular to its flat surface. This makes clasp more difficult to adjust.

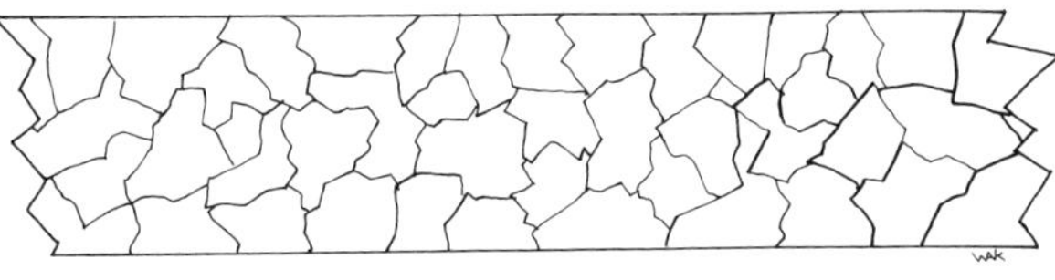

Cast grain structure

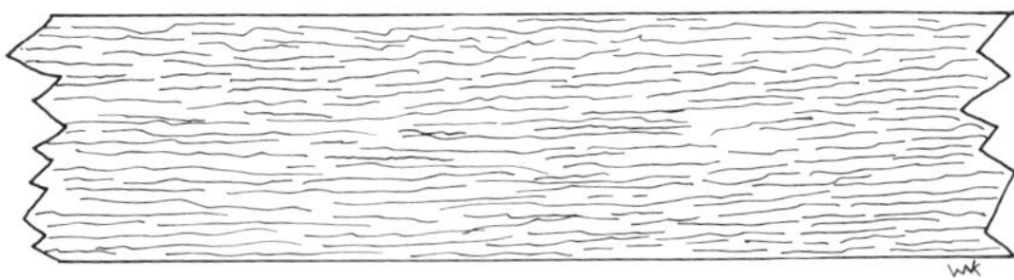

Wrought wire

Fig. 3-24. Longitudinal structure of wrought wire clasp permits a greater degree of flexing than does grain structure of cast alloy clasp. For this reason wrought wire clasps are placed in slightly greater undercuts than are cast clasps.

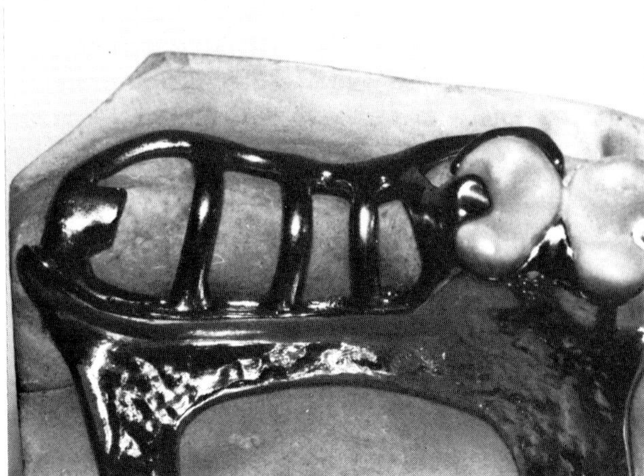

Fig. 3-25. A lingual plate may be used in place of a reciprocal clasp to provide reciprocation.

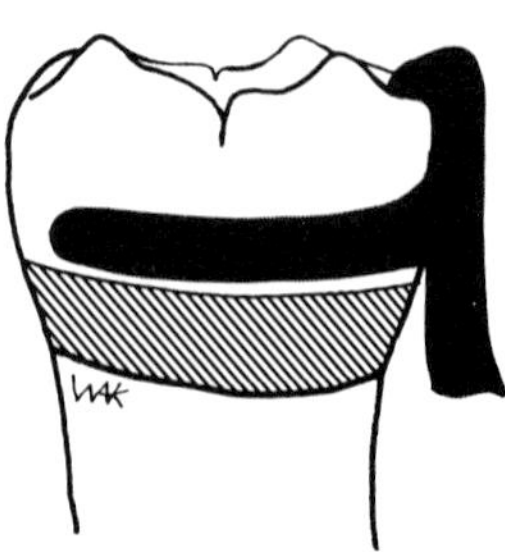

Fig. 3-26. The rigid, nontapered, reciprocal clasp arm must be positioned above height of contour. Its ideal position is at junction of gingival and middle thirds of abutment tooth.

the greatest bulge of the tooth are neutralized.

If the height of contour lies in the occlusal third of the tooth and cannot be changed by reshaping the enamel surface, a lingual plate is more effective in providing reciprocation.

Encirclement. Each clasp must be designed to encircle more than 180 degrees (more than half the circumference) of the abutment tooth. Encirclement may be in the form of continuous contact, as is the case with circumferential clasp arms, or broken contact, as with bar clasps. If broken encirclement is planned, the clasp assembly must contact at least three different tooth areas (normally the occlusal rest, the retentive terminal, and the reciprocal terminal) that embrace more than half the tooth's circumference (Fig. 3-27). This prevents the tooth from moving out of the confines of the clasp assembly as stresses or orthodontic forces are applied to the prosthesis (Fig. 3-28).

Passivity. A clasp in place should be completely passive. The retentive function is activated only when dislodging forces are applied to the partial denture. One of the main causes of pain or tenderness in an abutment tooth following insertion of a partial denture is incomplete seating of the clasp. If the clasp is not seated, the retentive terminal cannot reach the depth of undercut it was planned to reach and therefore always applies force to the tooth, producing pain. (Fig. 3-29).

Location of retentive terminals

In circumferential and bar retentive clasps the retentive terminal is located at the mesial or distal line angle of the tooth (Fig. 3-30). There is another category of clasps, used in a special design concept, that locates the retentive terminal near the center of the facial, or infrequently the lingual, surface of the tooth. This concept is discussed in Chapter 8.

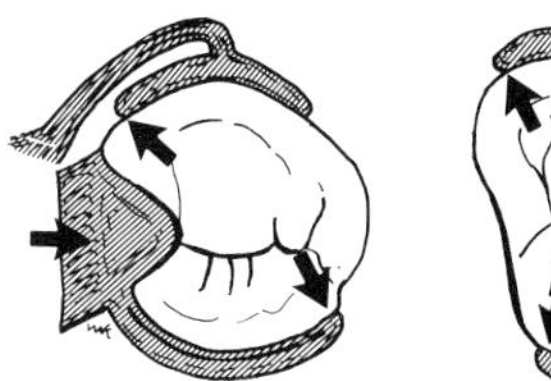

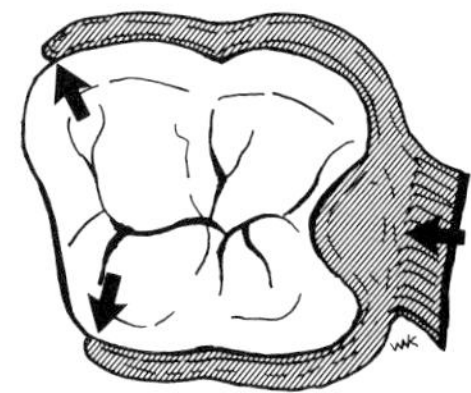

Fig. 3-27. Each clasp assembly, whether it be of vertical projection group, left, or circumferential group, right, must encircle more than 180 degrees of abutment tooth. The encirclement is continuous with circumferential clasps but broken with vertical projection clasps. If broken contact is used, contact must be provided between clasp and tooth in at least three places. The three points of contact are normally at occlusal rest and at retentive and reciprocal terminals.

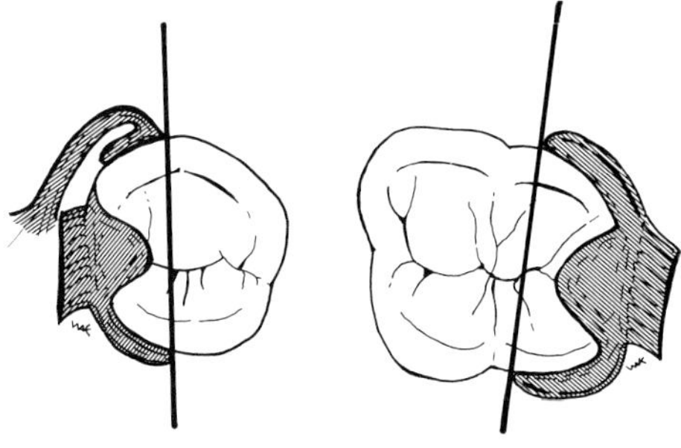

Fig. 3-28. A clasp that fails to provide encirclement will act as an orthodontic appliance, forcing abutment tooth to move out of contact with clasp.

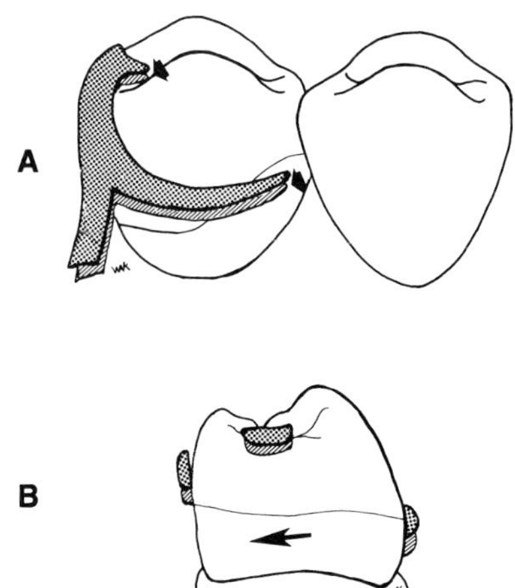

Fig. 3-29. A, A clasp must be completely seated on a tooth to be completely passive (arrow). If a clasp designed to reach a retentive undercut of 0.010 inch cannot reach that depth, it will exert a constant force on tooth. **B,** Over time this can produce pain or tooth movement (arrow).

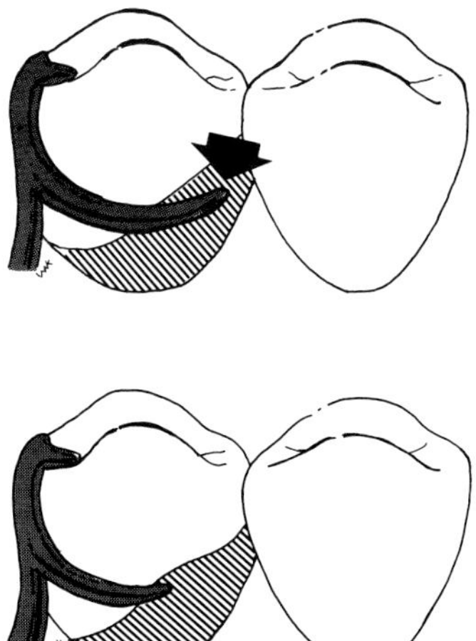

Fig. 3-30. In conventional circumferential or vertical projection clasps, area of tooth selected for retentive undercut should be mesial or distal line angle. If center of facial or lingual surface were used, clasp would be shortened, thus reducing its flexibility and compromising encirclement.

The retentive terminal is normally positioned at the mesiofacial or distofacial line angle. The facial or buccal positioning is preferred over the use of the lingual surface. In most mouths the mandibular premolars have a decided lingual axial inclination, and as a result the height of contour is located near the occlusal surface. Therefore if a lingual retentive area were selected, the clasp would have insufficient length to provide the flexibility needed.

Maxillary premolars rarely demonstrate a lingual undercut because of the normal buccal inclination of these teeth, so lingual retention cannot be considered.

Molar teeth, on the other hand, often exhibit undercuts on either or both the facial or lingual surfaces. The mesiodistal dimension of these teeth is also great enough to permit a clasp of sufficient length to provide the required flexibility to engage a retentive undercut. Therefore on molar teeth either buccal or lingual retention may be used, depending on the most desirable or available undercut.

As a general rule, if buccal retention is selected for use on one side of the arch, it should be opposed by buccal retention on the opposite side of the arch. In the same manner if lingual retention is used on one side of the arch, it also should be opposed by lingual retention on the opposite side.

If two retentive clasps are to be used on each side of the arch, it is possible to have one clasp on each side engage a buccal undercut and the other clasp on each side engage a lingual undercut. When a unilateral distal extension ridge is being treated, one clasp on the dentulous side, usually on a molar, may engage a lingual retentive area. The other two clasps, usually on premolars or canines on opposite sides of the arch, will engage buccal undercuts.

An important rule, with two exceptions, is that only one retentive clasp arm is used on a tooth and that each clasp arm must be opposed by a reciprocal arm or its equivalent on the opposite side of the tooth. The first exception, a unilateral partial denture (Fig. 3-31), and the potential hazards involved are discussed in Chapter 20. The other exception is a maxillofacial prosthesis designed for a patient with teeth on only one side of the arch (that is, a patient who has had a hemimaxillectomy or hemimandiblectomy). This design will be discussed in Chapter 23.

Comparison of retentive qualities of circumferential and bar clasps

The bar clasp approaches the undercut from below the greatest bulge of the tooth, and to resist dislodgment the clasp pushes toward the occlusal surface of the abutment tooth. The circumferential clasp, on the other hand, engages the retentive undercut from above the height of contour. It pulls toward the occlusal surface from the undercut to resist displacement. The bar clasp is easier to seat on the tooth and more difficult to remove than the circumferential clasp. Therefore if all factors (for example, length of clasp arm, flexibility of clasp arm, depth of undercut) are the same, the bar clasp is more retentive than the circumferential clasp. This may be an important consideration when a partial denture is being designed.

A
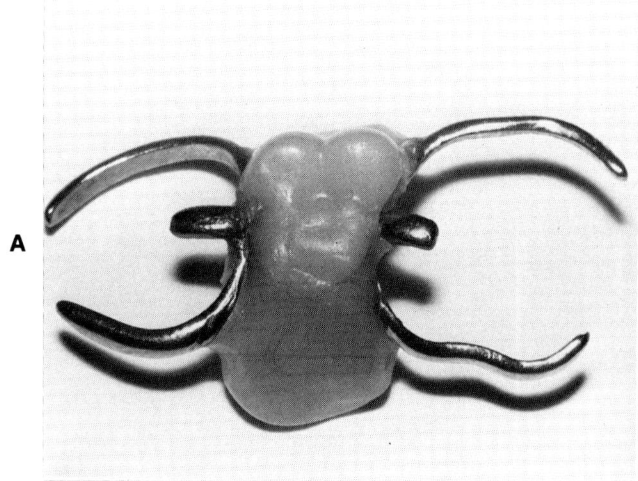
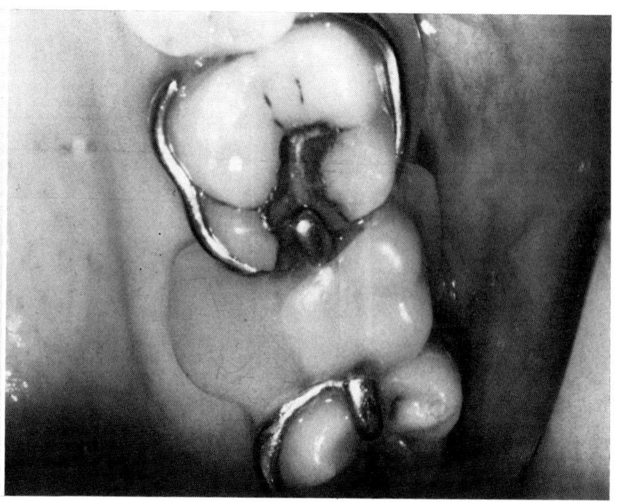
B

Fig. 3-31. A unilateral partial denture (**A,** alone; **B,** in place) must be designed with retentive terminal on both the buccal and facial surfaces. This is an exception to rule that usually only one retentive terminal is used for each clasp assembly. Potential hazards of unilateral removable partial denture are discussed in Chapter 20.

Cast circumferential clasps

The cast circumferential clasp is the easiest clasp to design and construct. It is the most logical clasp choice for tooth-supported partial dentures because of its excellent support, bracing, and retentive qualities. In addition, this clasp is the easiest to repair, and it causes fewer problems of food retention than does the bar clasp. The many varieties of the cast circumferential clasp allow them to be used in practically all cases, although they may not be the clasp of choice in some instances.

Certain disadvantages, however, are inherent in the design of the cast circumferential clasp. More tooth surface is covered than with the bar clasp, which may lead to decalcification of the enamel surface or caries. The circumferential clasp also changes the morphology of the abutment crown. The normal buccolingual contour of the tooth is altered, which may interfere with the normal food flow pattern. This could lead to damage of the gingival tissue because of a lack of physiologic stimulation of this tissue. If these clasps are positioned high on the tooth, they can increase the width of the food table, which in turn causes greater occlusal force to be exerted on the tooth (Fig. 3-32).

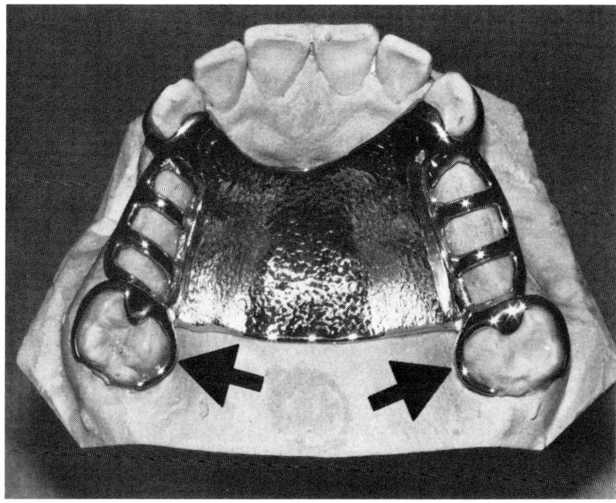

Fig. 3-32. Clasps positioned near occlusal surfaces of abutment teeth widen food table (occlusal surface) (arrows). This interferes with stimulating normal food flow pattern and may damage supporting tissues.

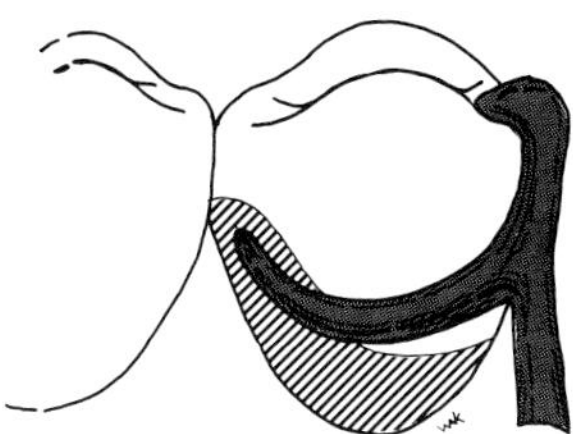

Fig. 3-33. Retentive tip of all clasps should point toward occlusal surface of abutment tooth. This produces a curved clasp of greater length and greater flexibility.

Because of the half-round configuration of the cast circumferential clasp, it is not possible to truly adjust the clasp with pliers. The clasp can be adjusted only in a plane perpendicular to its flat inner surface. Adjusting the clasp inward or outward against the tooth surface may increase or decrease its frictional resistance but does not change its retentive capability.

Rules for use. The retentive clasp arm should originate above (occlusal to), and its terminal third should be positioned below (gingival to) the height of contour.

The retentive terminal should always point toward the occlusal surface, never toward the gingiva. This helps produce a curved clasp and results in greater flexibility (Fig. 3-33).

The retentive tip should terminate at the mesial or distal line angle of the abutment tooth, never in the center of the facial or lingual surface.

The clasp arm should be kept as low on the tooth as possible without violating its relation with the height of contour. In this position it will have greater mechanical advantage against a lever action on the tooth than if it were positioned near the occlusal surface. In addition, the lower the clasp is placed on the tooth, the less the clasp arms will compromise the esthetic result.

Simple circlet clasp. The simple circlet is the most versatile and widely used clasp (Fig. 3-34). It is most

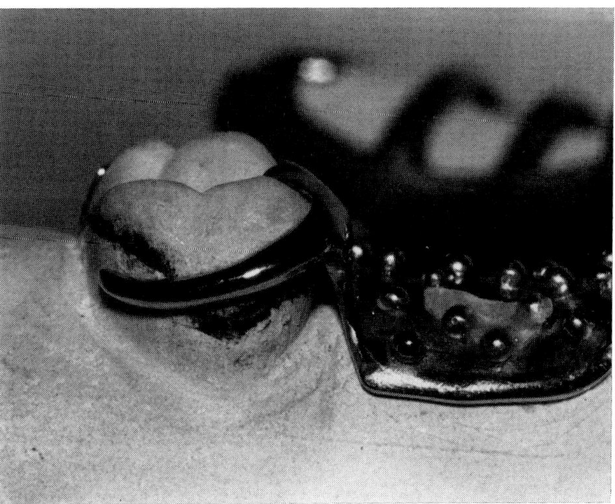

Fig. 3-34. Simple circlet clasp is the most versatile of all clasps. It fulfills requirements of support, stabilization, reciprocation, encirclement, and passivity better than any other type, and it is the easiest clasp to construct and maintain.

often the clasp of choice on tooth-supported removable partial dentures where the available retention undercut permits its use. This clasp usually approaches the undercut on the abutment tooth from the edentulous area and engages the undercut remote from the edentulous space.

When there is a choice to be made between the simple circlet clasp and another of apparently equal capability, the simple circlet should be the clasp of choice.

The clasp fulfills the requirements of support, stability, reciprocation, encirclement, and passivity better than any other type of clasp.

It is easy to construct because the design is not complicated, and it is relatively simple to repair.

The limitations to the use of the simple circlet clasp are the same as for all cast circumferential clasps. The clasp tends to increase the circumference of the crown, which interferes with the normal food flow pattern and deprives the gingival tissue of needed physiologic stimulation. In the anterior part of the mouth it is not always acceptable from an esthetic standpoint. The simple circlet clasp also covers more tooth surface than the bar clasps and can be conducive to caries. The clasp can be adjusted in a buccolingual direction but not in an occlusogingival direction (the more frequently needed adjustment).

Reverse, or reverse approach, circlet clasp. The reverse circlet clasp is used when the retentive undercut is located on the surface of the abutment tooth adjacent to the edentulous space (Fig. 3-35). A more expedient approach to this type of undercut is normally through the use of a bar clasp that approaches the abutment tooth across the mucosa and turns upward to engage the undercut adjacent to the edentulous area. If, however, the mucosa is in an undercut area caused by buccoversion of the abutment tooth or in an undercut area in the ridge itself, then the bar clasp is contraindicated and the reverse circlet is the clasp of choice.

In a distal extension edentulous ridge partial denture the reverse approach circlet clasp helps control stresses transmitted to the terminal abutment tooth on the edentulous side. As the denture base is depressed under function, the retentive clasp tip rotates gingivally to enter a greater amount of undercut and reduce the torsional stresses transmitted to the abutment tooth. When dislodging forces in the form of sticking food or gravity tend to unseat the prosthesis, the retentive tip engages the undercut and the denture is retained.

The greatest problem encountered with this clasp is obtaining sufficient occlusal clearance so that the clasp has the necessary thickness to maintain strength. The clasp must travel on the marginal ridges, in prepared rest seats, of two adjacent teeth to reach the retentive undercut on the buccal surface of the abutment tooth. If the opposing occlusion is tight, it is often difficult to obtain adequate clearance to place the rests and clasp without removing a prohibitive amount of tooth structure on the abutment tooth and its antagonist (Fig. 3-36).

An occlusal rest on the surface of the tooth away from the edentulous space does not protect the marginal gingiva adjacent to the abutment tooth. This marginal gingiva may be traumatized if food packs between the denture and the proximal surface of the tooth. It is frequently advisable to place an additional occlusal rest next to the edentulous space to eliminate this problem.

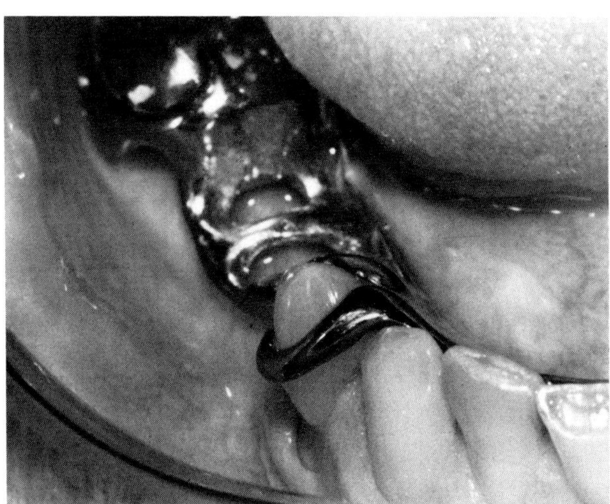

Fig. 3-35. Reverse circlet clasp is exact opposite of simple circlet clasp. Whereas simple circlet clasp normally engages a mesial undercut on an abutment tooth, reverse circlet usually engages a distal undercut.

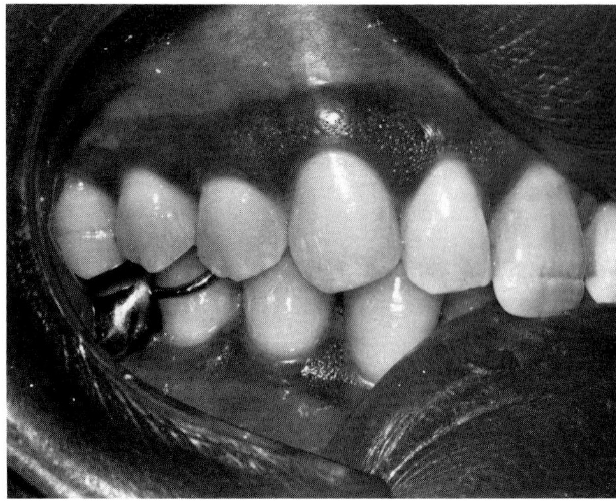

Fig. 3-36. One problem encountered with reverse circlet clasp is obtaining sufficient clearance with opposing occlusion so that clasp can have enough thickness to maintain strength.

This additional rest will, however, decrease or eliminate the releasing action of the clasp tip as the denture base is depressed on the distal extension side.

Because this clasp is positioned most frequently on the mesial occlusal side of the abutment tooth and crosses the facial surface from mesial to distal, it is a poor clasp from an esthetic viewpoint and is not often the clasp of choice on premolars (Fig. 3-37).

Unless the occlusal rests are well prepared on the abutment and its adjacent tooth, wedging may occur between the teeth when the distal extension denture base is subjected to occlusal loading.

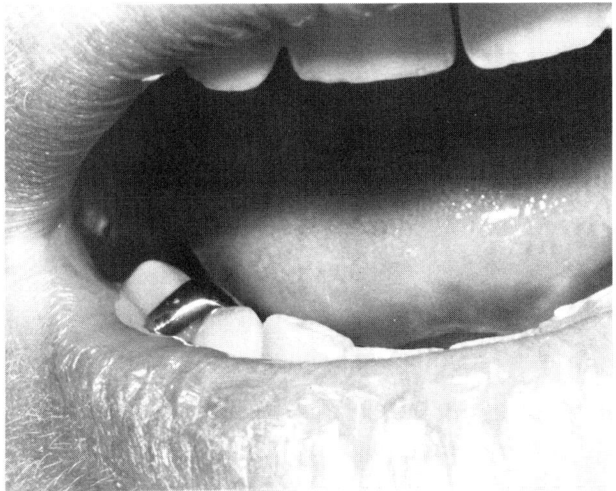

Fig. 3-37. Reverse circlet clasp often gives a poor esthetic result with excessive display of metal, particularly on premolar.

Multiple circlet clasp. The multiple circlet clasp is essentially two opposing simple circlet clasps joined at the terminal end of the two reciprocal arms (Fig. 3-38). Its use is primarily in sharing the retention responsibilities among several abutment teeth on one side of the arch when a principal abutment tooth has lost some of its periodontal support. This may be considered a form of splinting weakened teeth by a removable partial denture. This concept is discussed in Chapter 20.

The disadvantages of the multiple circlet clasp are the same as those of simple circlet and reverse circlet clasps.

Embrasure clasp, or modified crib clasp. The embrasure clasp is essentially two simple circlet clasps joined at the body (Fig. 3-39). It is most frequently used on the side of the arch where there is no edentulous space. The clasp must cross the marginal ridges of two teeth, emerge to cross the facial surfaces of both teeth, and engage undercuts on the opposing line angles of these teeth. Occlusal rest preparations must be made on both teeth, and tooth structure must be removed from the buccal inclines of both teeth to provide space for adequate thickness of metal. Breakage of these clasps in function is not uncommon because of insufficient tooth preparation. It is best to avoid using this clasp unless the opposing occlusion is such that gaining necessary space is not a problem.

Ring clasp. The ring clasp is most often indicated on tipped molars (Fig. 3-40). Most unsupported mandibular molars tend to drift and tip in a mesiolingual direction, whereas maxillary molars tip in a mesiobuccal direction. This means the available retentive undercut will be located on the mesiolingual line angle of a man-

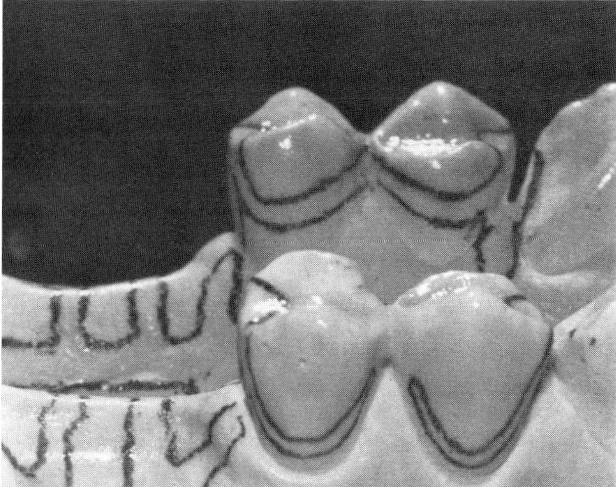

Fig. 3-38. Multiple circlet clasp is two opposing simple circlet clasps joined together at terminals of reciprocal arms. It is used to share retention among several teeth.

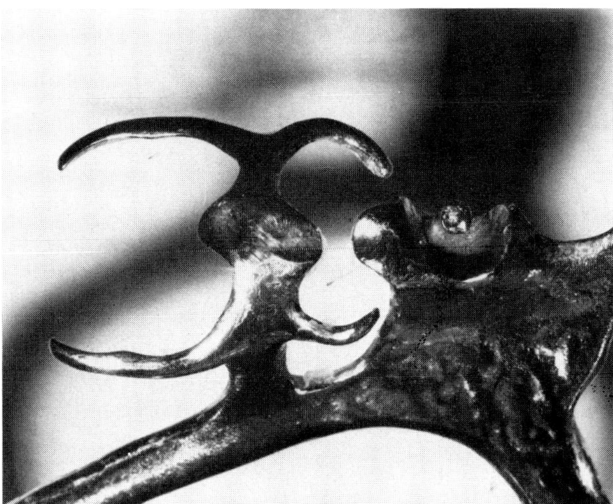

Fig. 3-39. Embrasure clasp is two simple circlet clasps joined at body. It is indicated most frequently on side of arch where there is no edentulous space. The greatest problem with this clasp is providing sufficient space for adequate thickness of metal.

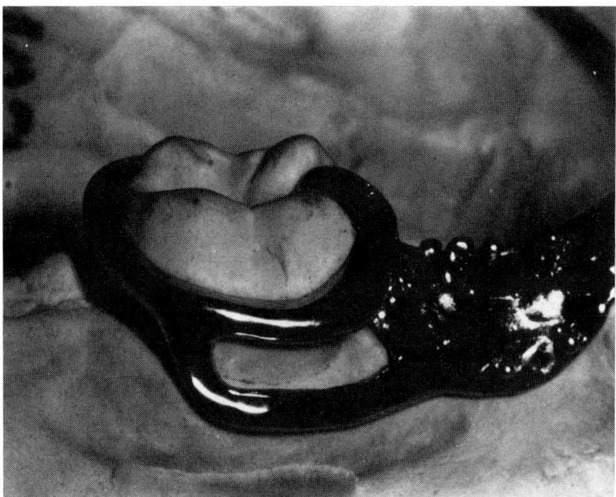

Fig. 3-40. Ring clasp may be used on tipped molars. Clasp requires additional support because of its greater length. An auxiliary bracing arm is needed to prevent excessive flexing. Clasp has limited indication.

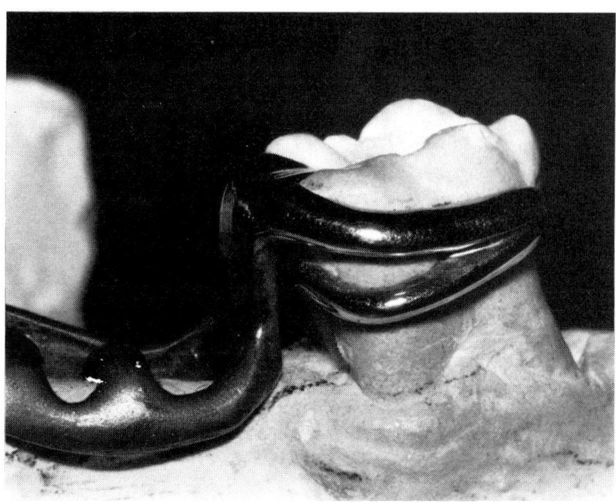

Fig. 3-41. The C clasp is basically a simple circlet clasp in which retentive clasp arm reverses direction after crossing tooth surface and loops back to engage an undercut below its point of origin. Clasp must be designed for an abutment tooth with a long clinical crown because clasp requires adequate occlusogingival height to accommodate this double width of metal.

dibular molar and the mesiobuccal line angle of a maxillary molar.

The ring clasp permits engagement of this undercut by encircling almost the entire tooth from its point of origin. On a mandibular molar the clasp encircles the tooth beginning on the mesiobuccal surface and terminating in an infrabulge area on the mesiolingual surface. On a maxillary molar the direction of the clasp is reversed; it begins at the mesiolingual surface and terminates in an undercut on the mesiobuccal surface.

Because of the great length of the clasp, it must be designed with additional support, usually in the form of an auxiliary bracing arm. In the mandible the bracing arm usually projects from the acrylic resin retention metal, runs across the mucosa, and turns upward to engage the buccal arm of the ring clasp near the center of the buccal surface. Without the rigid bracing element the clasp would not possess reciprocity and would contribute little to stability of the denture. The entire clasp with the exception of the retentive tip must be placed above the height of contour. This means that a large amount of the tooth surface is covered with metal. In addition, the contour of the crown is drastically altered, and interference with normal stimulation of the surrounding mucosa may occur. With or without the auxiliary bracing arm, the clasp is prone to get out of adjustment, and it is difficult to adjust or repair.

An additional occlusal rest on the opposite side of the tooth from the clasp origin may provide additional support and prevent further movement of the mesially inclined tooth. However, problems may be encountered in obtaining the occlusal space needed for this additional rest seat.

The ring clasp should not be considered on a mandibular molar where the attachment of the buccinator muscle is so close to the tooth that the auxiliary bracing arm encroaches on it. It is also contraindicated when the bracing arm must cross a soft tissue undercut.

In general, the ring clasp should not be considered if another form of clasp can be used.

C, fishhook, or hairpin clasp. The C clasp is essentially a simple circlet clasp in which the retentive arm, after crossing the facial surface of the tooth from its point of origin, loops back in a hairpin turn to engage a proximal undercut below its point of origin (Fig. 3-41).

The upper part of the retentive arm must be considered to be a minor connector and should be rigid. The lower part of the clasp arm should be tapered; it is the only flexible part of the clasp arm.

The crown of the abutment tooth must have sufficient occlusogingival height to accommodate this double width of the clasp arm. The upper and lower arms of the retentive clasp must also be shaped such that food debris will not be retained between them. In addition, there must be sufficient space between the arms so that the metal may be adequately finished and polished.

If the C clasp is designed on mandibular posterior teeth, the upper arm must be positioned so as not to interfere with the opposing occlusion (Fig. 3-42). The C clasp is indicated for use when the retentive clasp must engage an undercut adjacent to the occlusal rest

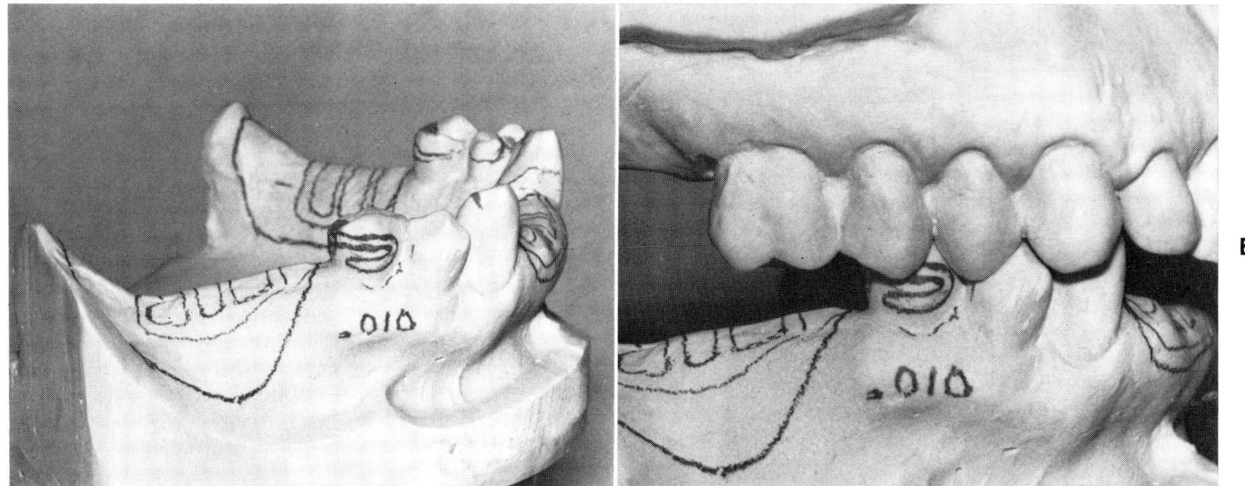

Fig. 3-42. A, C clasp drawn on mandibular abutment tooth. **B,** Clasp causes occlusal interference with maxillary buccal cusp.

or edentulous space and a soft tissue undercut precludes the use of a bar clasp. (The approach arm of a bar clasp must never cross a soft tissue undercut.) The C clasp is also indicated when the reverse circlet clasp cannot be used because of lack of occlusal space.

The clasp covers a considerable amount of tooth structure, which may trap food debris. It is not a good choice for a young patient or one who is prone to caries, and it is often unacceptable esthetically, particularly on premolar teeth.

Onlay clasp. The onlay clasp is an extended occlusal rest with buccal and lingual clasp arms (Fig. 3-43). The clasp may originate from any point on the onlay that will not create occlusal interferences. This clasp is generally indicated when the occlusal surface of the abutment tooth is below the occlusal plane, usually as a result of the tooth being tipped or rotated. The onlay is used to restore the normal occlusal plane (Fig. 3-44). The onlay clasp should be employed only in caries-resistant mouths unless the tooth is covered by a gold crown. If a gold crown is to be used, the need for the onlay clasp would be questionable. It would be better to restore the occlusal plane with the crown and plan a different, more conventional, clasping system.

If the onlay clasp is constructed of chrome alloy and is opposed by a natural tooth, the occlusal surface should be constructed of acrylic resin or gold (Fig. 3-45). Chrome alloy, because of its extreme hardness, will cause rapid wear of enamel surfaces.

Combination clasp. The combination clasp consists of a wrought round wire retentive clasp arm and a cast reciprocal clasp arm (Fig. 3-46). The cast reciprocal arm is normally a circumferential clasp, but a bar clasp may

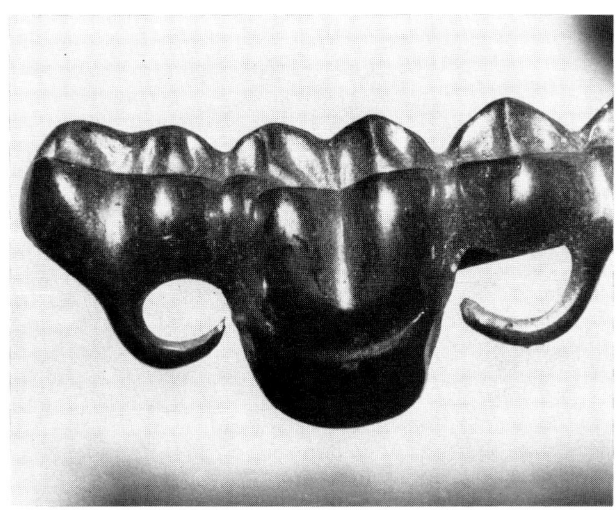

Fig. 3-43. Onlay clasp is an extended occlusal rest with buccal and lingual clasp arms.

be used. The wrought wire retentive arm is a circumferential clasp arm.

If the partial denture framework is to be constructed of gold or low-heat chrome alloy, the wrought wire clasp can be incorporated into the framework during the waxing step and the alloy can be cast directly to the wrought wire clasp. If a high-heat chrome alloy is used, the wrought wire must be soldered to the completed framework.

The combination clasp is most often indicated on an abutment tooth adjacent to a distal extension space when the usable undercut on the tooth is on the me-

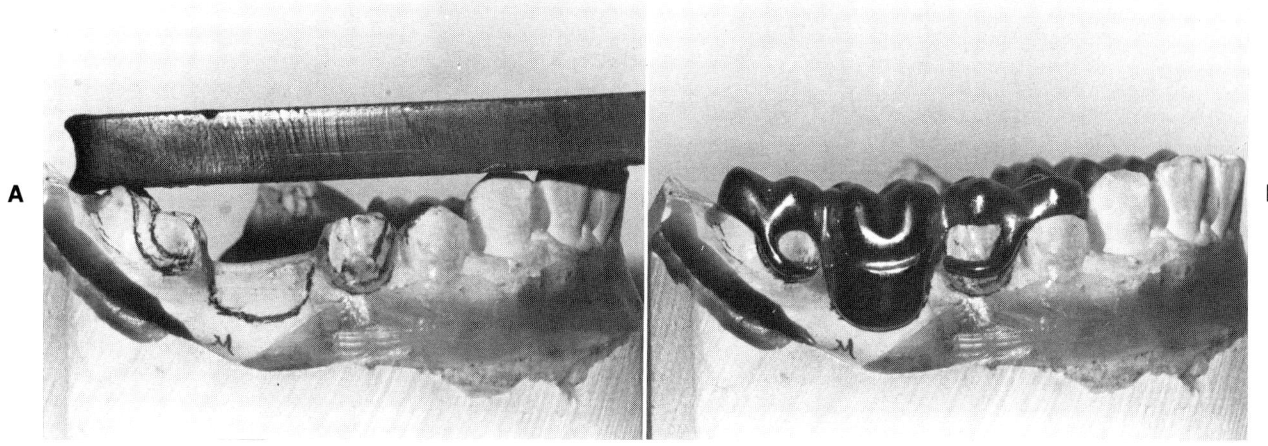

Fig. 3-44. A, Onlay clasp may be indicated where occlusal surface of one or more teeth is below occlusal plane. However, there are frequently better treatment plans than the use of onlay clasps. **B,** Onlay clasp covers a large amount of tooth structure and may lead to breakdown of enamel surfaces. Opposing enamel occlusal surfaces may also be subjected to rapid wear.

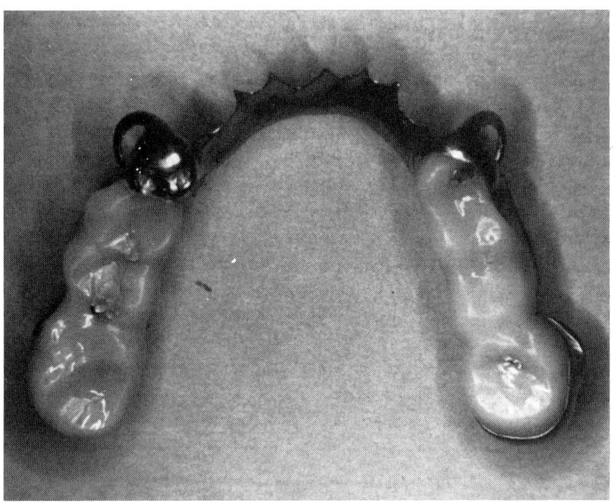

Fig. 3-45. If onlay clasps must oppose natural tooth surfaces, metallic onlay should be overlaid with tooth-colored acrylic resin to prevent excessive wear of opposing tooth structure. Acrylic resin may require frequent replacement as wear takes place.

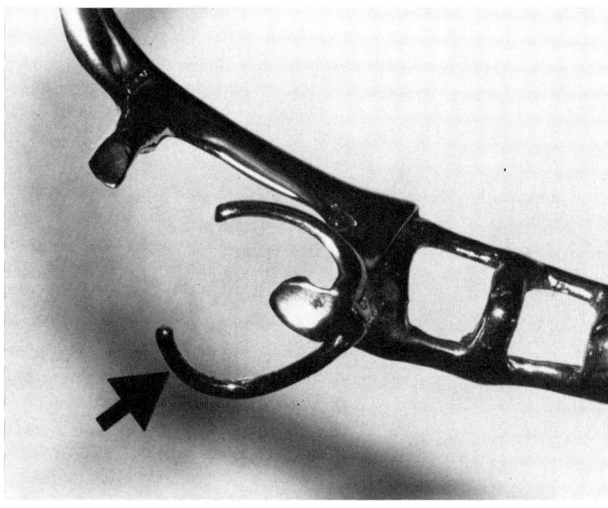

Fig. 3-46. Combination clasp has a wrought wire retentive arm (arrow) and a cast reciprocal arm. It is indicated when greater flexibility of retentive arm is desired. It may be used when a vertical projection clasp is contraindicated because of a soft tissue undercut below tooth.

siobuccal surface. The greater flexibility of the wrought wire acts as a stress equalizer, preventing the undesirable forces created by the lever action of the retentive clasp tip from lifting or torquing the abutment tooth as downward forces occur on the denture base. The partial denture tends to rotate around a fulcrum, the occlusal rest, producing potentially damaging stresses to the abutment tooth. For this reason *a cast circumferential clasp must never be used to engage a mesiobuccal undercut on an abutment tooth adjacent to a distal extension space.*

The greater flexibility of the combination clasp allows it to be placed in a greater, or deeper, undercut area. It can frequently be placed in the gingival third of the clinical crown of the abutment tooth, resulting in a more acceptable esthetic appearance. It is often used

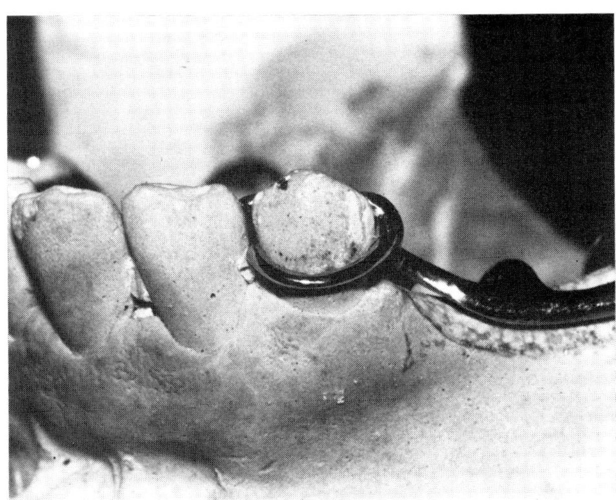

Fig. 3-47. Because of greater flexibility of wrought wire, a combination clasp can be placed in a deeper undercut area. Usually clasp can be positioned lower on crown of a tooth, in gingival third, resulting in a more esthetic appearance.

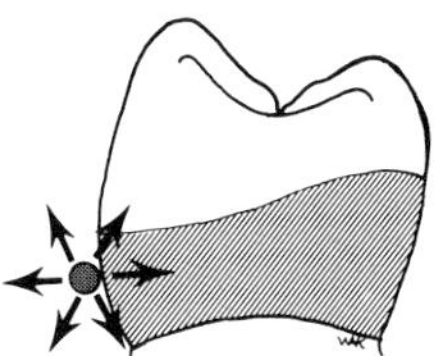

Fig. 3-48. Round wrought wire clasp makes only a line contact with tooth surface, right. Therefore its use is indicated in caries-prone individuals.

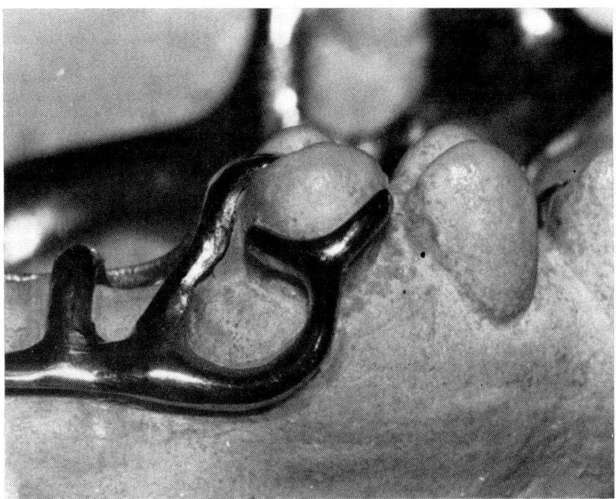

Fig. 3-49. Vertical projection clasps approach retentive undercut from a gingival direction. Entire approach arm must contact mucosa.

on maxillary canines or premolars for this reason (Fig. 3-47).

The round wrought wire clasp can flex in all spatial planes, which allows it to dissipate torquing forces exerted on the abutment tooth and to be adjusted in all planes.

The round wire makes only a line contact with the surface of the abutment tooth rather than the surface contact of a cast clasp. This minimal surface contact makes its use in caries-prone mouths somewhat more beneficial (Fig.3-48).

The main disadvantage of the combination clasp is that it does require extra steps in laboratory fabrication. It is also more prone to breakage or damage than a cast clasp. It can be easily distorted by careless handling by patients, who tend to remove the partial denture from the mouth by lifting on the retentive portion of the wrought wire clasp. This leads to the clasp's coming out of adjustment. The patient should be taught the correct technique of removing the partial denture—either grasping the denture base with the fingers or lifting the clasp at its point of origin in the metal framework.

Because of the increased flexibility of the retentive arm, it does not possess the bracing or stabilizing qualities of most circumferential clasps. If stabilization of the teeth or of the partial denture against horizontal forces is needed, the combination clasp would not be a good choice.

Bar, or vertical projection, clasps

The bar clasps (Fig. 3-49) approach the undercut or retentive area on the tooth from a gingival direction, resulting in a "push" type of retention (Fig. 3-50). This push retention of bar clasps is more effective than the "pull" retention characteristic of circumferential clasps. A patient encounters less difficulty inserting and more difficulty removing a removable partial denture with bar clasps than one with circumferential clasps.

The flexibility of the bar clasp can be controlled by the taper and length of the approach arm. The greater the length and the more marked the taper, the more flexible the clasp will be.

Because of the gingival approach of the bar clasp, it is usually more esthetic than a circumferential clasp. There are a variety of bar clasps, giving it a wide range of adaptability.

Among the disadvantages of bar clasps is the greater tendency to collect and hold food debris. Also, because of the increased flexibility of the retentive arm, it does not contribute as much to bracing and stabilization as most circumferential clasps do. Additional stabilizing units should be employed in the design of a partial denture when bar type clasps are used.

Rules for use. The approach arm of the bar clasp must not impinge on the soft tissue it crosses. It is not

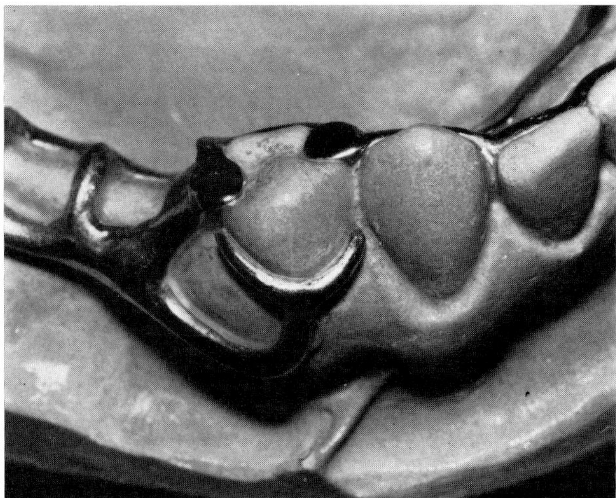

Fig. 3-50. Because of gingival approach to the retentive undercut, bar clasp is said to have "push" type retention.

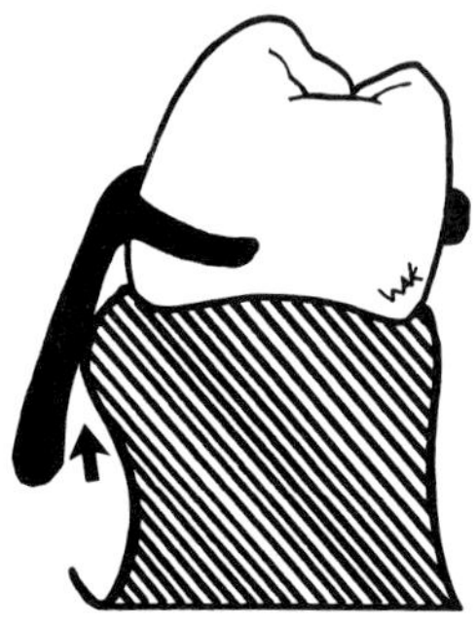

Fig. 3-51. Approach arm positioned over a soft tissue undercut will collect food and irritate lips or cheeks.

desirable to provide an area of relief under the arm, but the tissue side of the approach arm should be smoothed and polished.

The minor connector that attaches the occlusal rest to the framework should be strong and rigid to provide some bracing.

The approach arm must always be tapered uniformly from its attachment at the framework to the clasp terminal.

The approach arm must never be designed to bridge a soft tissue undercut. Otherwise, food will be trapped, and the cheeks or lips will be irritated (Fig. 3-51).

The approach arm should cross the gingival margin at a 90-degree angle (Fig. 3-52). This sensitive and critical area must be protected from irritation by as little interference with normal function as possible.

The bar retentive clasp is used only when the retentive undercut is adjacent to the edentulous area from which the approach arm originates. The approach arm must extend on the abutment tooth to the height of contour. The retentive terminal leaves the approach arm at that point and extends into the undercut area. The other terminal, the one away from the edentulous area, is positioned above the height of contour. As is the case with the circumferential clasp, the retentive terminal tip must point toward the occlusal surface, never toward the gingiva (Fig. 3-53).

The bar clasp should also be placed as low on the tooth as possible while honoring the height of contour to reduce the leverage-induced stress to the abutment tooth.

The bar clasps are designated by the shape formed by the terminals as they join the approach arm. Although a variety of clasps are included in this classifi-

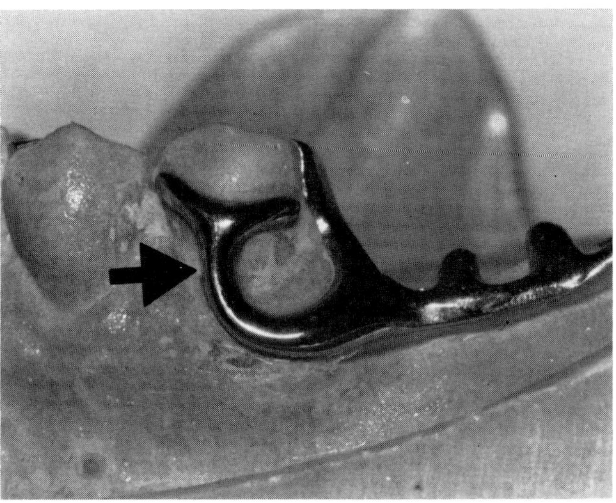

Fig. 3-52. Approach arm must cross sensitive gingival margin at a 90-degree angle (arrow).

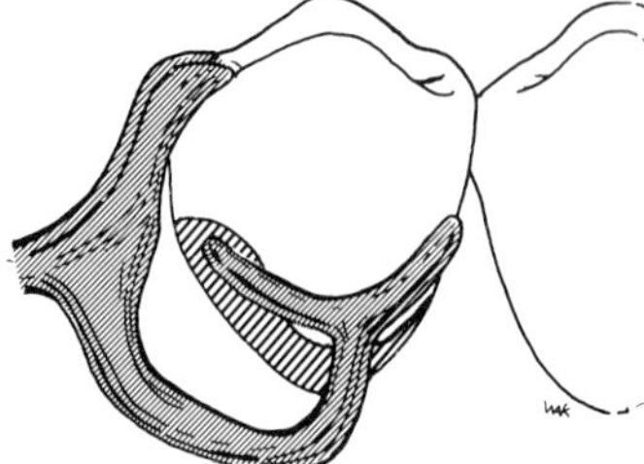

Fig. 3-53. Retentive terminal of bar clasp, as tip of circumferential clasp, should point toward occlusal surface. Clasp must be kept as low on tooth as possible.

cation, this book primarily deals with four. Most functions intended to be performed by bar clasps can be accomplished by these four.

Types of bar clasps

T *clasp*. The T clasp is used most often in combination with a cast circumferential reciprocal arm. The retentive terminal and its opposing encircling finger project laterally from the approach arm to form a T (Fig. 3-54). Both projections should point toward the occlusal surface of the abutment tooth. The retentive terminal must cross under the height of contour to engage the retentive undercut, while the other finger of the T stays on the suprabulge of the tooth. The approach arm should taper gradually and uniformly from its origin to the retentive terminal. The approach arm contacts the tooth only at the height of contour.

The T clasp is used most frequently on a distal extension ridge where the usuable undercut is on the distobuccal surface of the terminal abutment tooth. In this position, as tissueward forces occur on the denture base, the terminal clasp tip rotates cervically into a greater undercut, which reduces the torquing stresses to the abutment tooth. For any removable partial denture with one or two distal extension denture bases, the clasp retention most desired is distobuccal retention on the terminal abutment. This retention can best be secured by T clasps projecting from the metal acrylic resin retention.

The T clasp can also be used for a tooth-supported partial denture when the retentive undercut is located on the abutment tooth adjacent to the edentulous space. In this all-tooth–supported type of removable partial denture, the retentive clasping can be accomplished by using the natural retentive undercuts on the abutment teeth. This concept of retentive clasping can be called "clasping for convenience," because rotationary forces that occur with any distal extension denture base partial dentures do not occur. For this reason, instead of changing the contour of the abutment tooth to meet the prerequisites for "ideal" clasping, the dentist uses the retentive undercuts present with any available *acceptable* clasp types.

The T clasp should not be used on a terminal abutment adjacent to a distal extension base if the usable undercut is located on the side of the tooth away from the edentulous space. This is an often misunderstood concept of clasping.

The T clasp can never be used if the approach arm must bridge a soft tissue undercut. This produces a food retention area as well as potential irritation to the lips and cheeks.

There are also instances when the height of contour is close to the occlusal or incisal surface of an abutment tooth. If a T clasp is used under these conditions, a large space will be created between the approach arm of the clasp and the tooth, which could result in irritation to the lips or cheeks and in trapping food debris (Fig. 3-55).

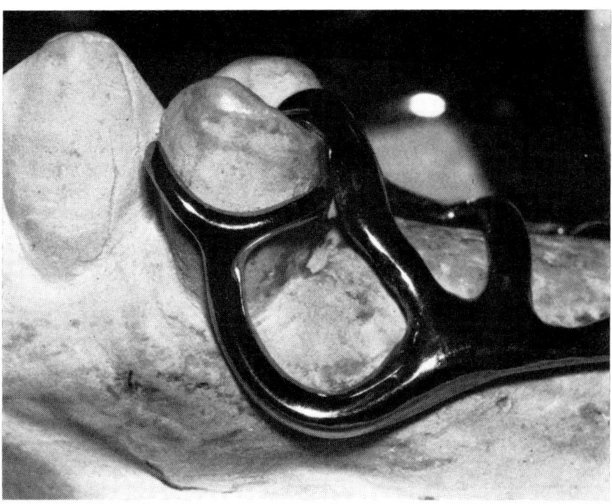

Fig. 3-54. T clasp, the most frequently used vertical projection group clasp is most often used on terminal abutment tooth on distal extension edentulous ridge.

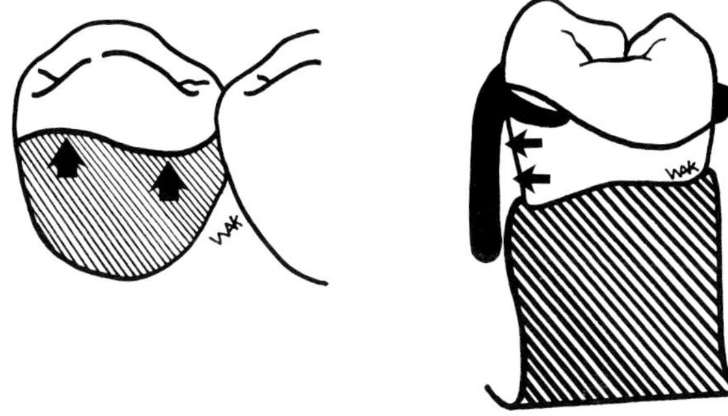

Fig. 3-55. T clasp should be avoided if height of contour of abutment tooth lies close to occlusal surface, right. If a T clasp is used under these circumstances, a large space would be created between approach arm of clasp and tooth. Space would trap food. High position would also be unesthetic.

The T clasp for the most part is esthetically superior to the circumferential clasp group. However, because of the flexibility of the approach arm, it does not possess the bracing qualities of most circumferential clasps.

Modified T *clasp*. The modified T clasp is essentially a T clasp with the nonretentive (usually mesial) finger of the crossbar of the T terminal omitted (Fig. 3-56).

This clasp is most often used on canines or premolars for esthetic reasons. The potential danger in its use is that encirclement, or 180-degree coverage, of the abut-

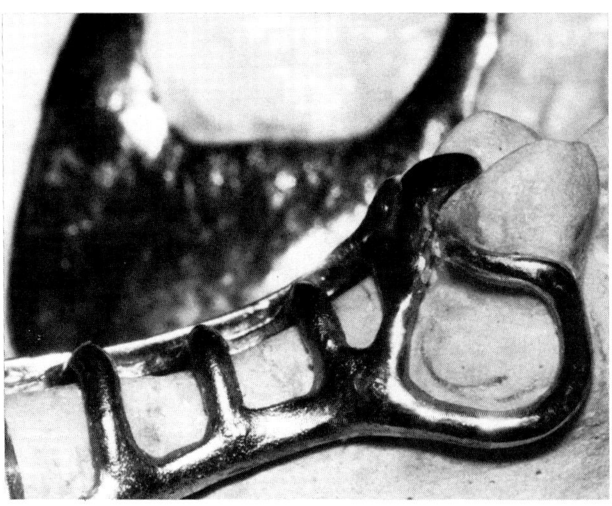

Fig. 3-56. Modified T clasp is basically a T clasp with no nonretentive finger. Clasp is indicated for premolars and canines for esthetic reasons. Care must be taken to ensure 180-degree encirclement of abutment.

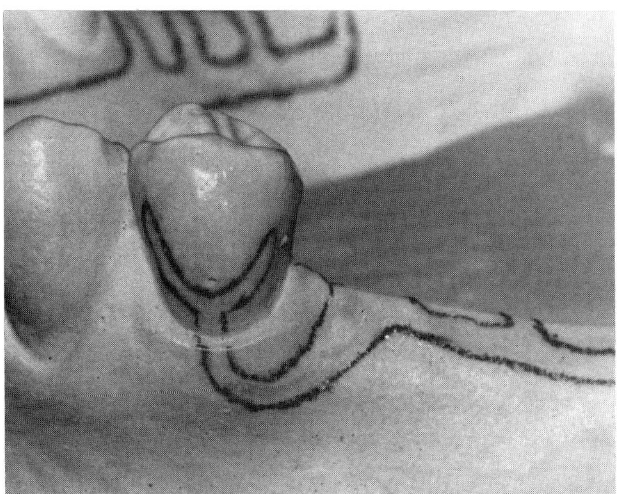

Fig. 3-57. The T clasp acquires a Y configuration when height of contour on abutment tooth is high on mesial and distal line angles and low on center of facial surface. Body or center of the Y clasp should be kept as low on tooth as possible, and fingers should be permitted to rise as dictated by height of contour.

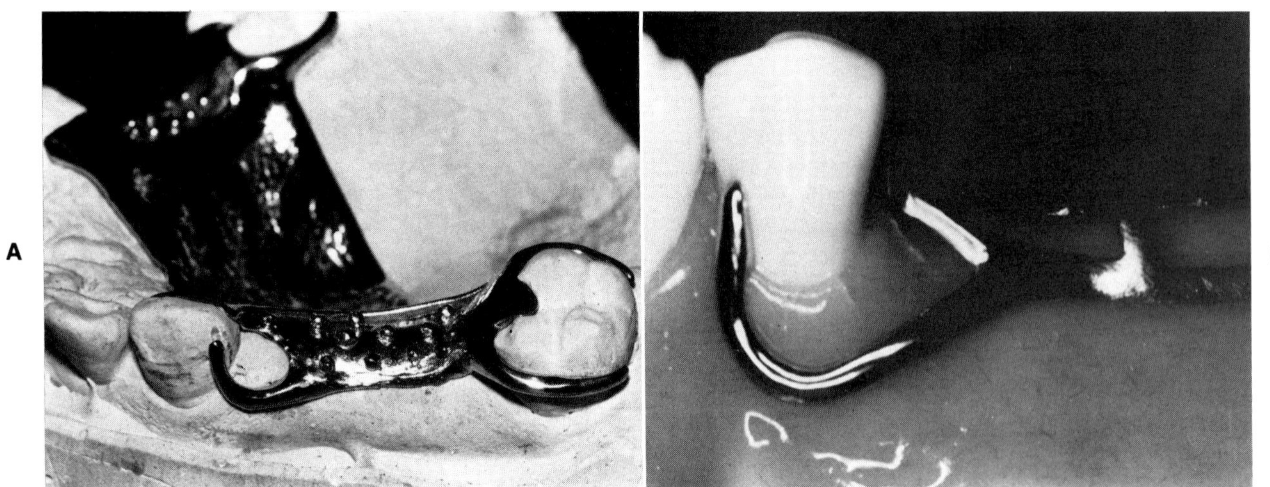

Fig. 3-58. A, The I clasp may be used on the distobuccal surface of maxillary canines for esthetic reasons. There must be a posterior abutment tooth for this clasp to be successful. Encirclement may be a problem. **B,** I bar is a component part of a partial denture design philosophy, the rest, proximal plate, I bar retentive clasp (RPI) concept. It differs from I clasp in position on abutment tooth that retentive undercut is selected. I bar retention is normally near center of facial surface of tooth. RPI philosophy is detailed in Chapter 8.

ment tooth may be sacrificed to esthetics. Esthetics should always be considered when the partial denture is being designed, but its consideration must not supersede the necessity of making the prosthesis mechanically acceptable. An esthetically superior denture that leads to ultimate destruction of the remaining oral tissues is not in the best interests of the patient.

All other aspects of the modified T clasp are the same as for the T clasp.

Y *Clasp*. The Y clasp is basically a T clasp; its configuration occurs when the height of contour on the facial surface of the abutment tooth is high on the mesial and distal line angles but low on the center of the facial surface (Fig. 3-57).

The use and other considerations of the Y clasp are the same as for the T clasp. On occasion, careful recontouring of the enamel surface of the abutment tooth will permit the Y clasp to be converted to the standard T clasp.

I *clasp and* I *bar*. The I-clasp may occasionally be used on the distobuccal surface of maxillary canines for esthetic reasons (Fig. 3-58). There is a definite danger involved in using this clasp. Because the only contact of the retentive clasp with the abutment tooth is the tip of the clasp, an area of 2 to 3 mm, encirclement and horizontal stabilization may be compromised.

The I bar is a component part of a partial denture design philosophy referred to as the RPI concept. The concept advocates the use of a retentive I bar, an occlusal or lingual rest positioned on the opposite side of the tooth from the proximal plate, which is located on the proximal surface of the tooth adjacent to the edentulous area. This concept is discussed in Chapter 8.

Summary of extracoronal direct retainers

The clasp, or extracoronal direct retainer, selected for use on an abutment tooth should conform to the shape of the existing retentive undercut. The clasp should not be preselected and then made to fit the usable undercut.

The selection of the direct retainer should not be the first or primary consideration when removable partial denture design is undertaken. For the most part, the tendency is to overretain the denture.

Clasp selection is critical only when the abutment tooth is adjacent to a distal extension ridge. In this instance stresses resulting from movement of the partial denture during function build up or concentrate on that abutment tooth. If a mesiobuccal undercut is available on the terminal abutment tooth, a combination clasp with the wrought wire retentive clasp should be used to dissipate the stresses. If the retentive undercut is located on the distobuccal surface, a bar clasp should be selected. This mode of retention also releases stress on the abutment tooth by allowing the retentive tip to move into a greater undercut. If there are contraindications to the use of the bar clasp (such as soft tissue undercut, high height of contour), a reverse circlet clasp or a C clasp should be used.

The clasp designs should be kept as simple as the situation permits. The less desirable clasp designs should be avoided by changing the form of the abutment teeth by means of full crown restorations to create contours that will be compatible with a simpler direct retainer design.

INDIRECT RETAINERS

A removable partial denture that is supported entirely by remaining natural teeth usually does not require additional support other than that furnished by the primary abutment teeth. If positive direct retainers are located on the abutment teeth, forces will not tend to rotate or dislodge the prosthesis.

If the partial denture is not supported by natural teeth at each end of the edentulous space or spaces (that is, it covers a unilateral or bilateral distal extension ridge or a long-span anterior edentulous space), some provision must be made for the denture to resist rotational forces to which it will be subjected. In the case of a bilateral distal extension partial denture, the occlusal rests on the terminal abutment teeth act as fulcra, and an imaginary line drawn between the occlusal rests will be the fulcrum line (Fig. 3-59). Rotational movement around this fulcrum line, either toward the tissue or away from the tissue or ridge, may occur as forces are applied to the artificial teeth on the denture base. Movement toward the supporting ridge will be limited

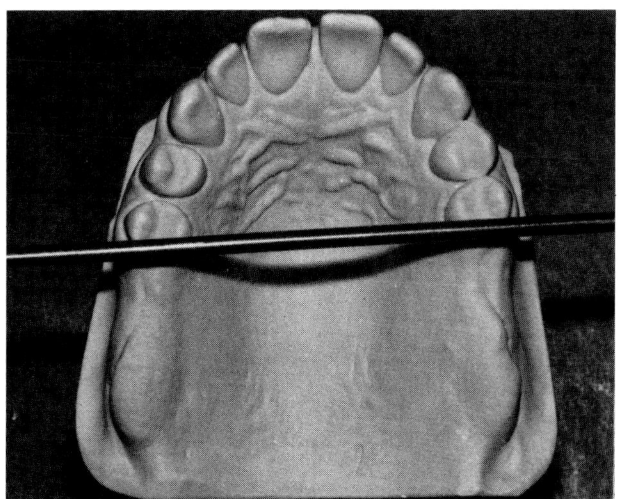

Fig. 3-59. Rotational forces occur on a Class I partial denture. Rotation will take place around a fulcrum line, an imaginary line between occlusal rests on terminal abutment teeth.

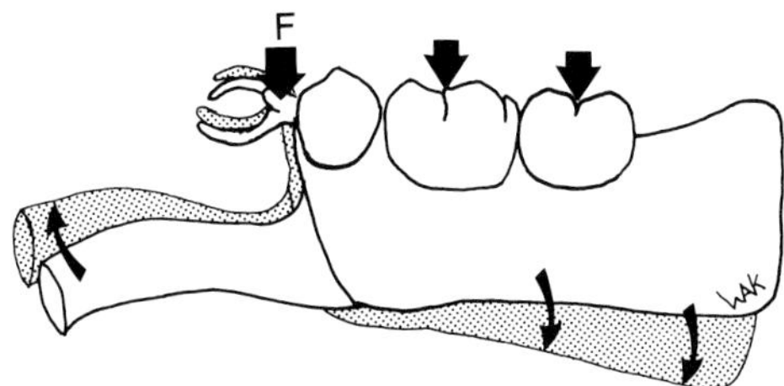

Fig. 3-60. Tissueward movement of partial denture is controlled or limited by denture base in contact with mucosa covering edentulous bony ridge. An indirect retainer cannot control this movement. (*F*, fulcrum.)

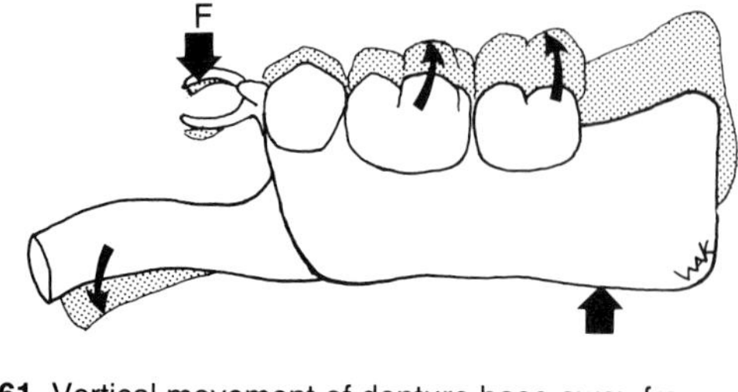

Fig. 3-61. Vertical movement of denture base away from supporting ridge occurs as a result of sticky foods or rebound of soft tissues compressed by force of occlusion. (*F*, fulcrum.)

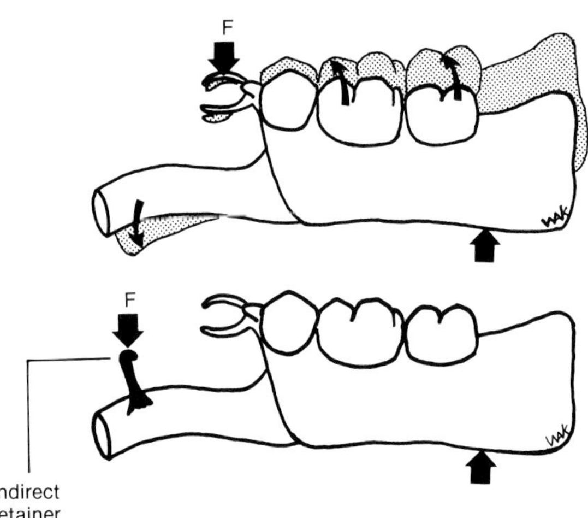

Fig. 3-62. Top, as lifting forces take place on partial denture, fulcrum line moves from posterior occlusal rests to retentive tips of clasps *(F)*. Bottom, indirect retainer *(F)* positioned anterior to fulcrum line counteracts lifting force and stabilizes denture base.

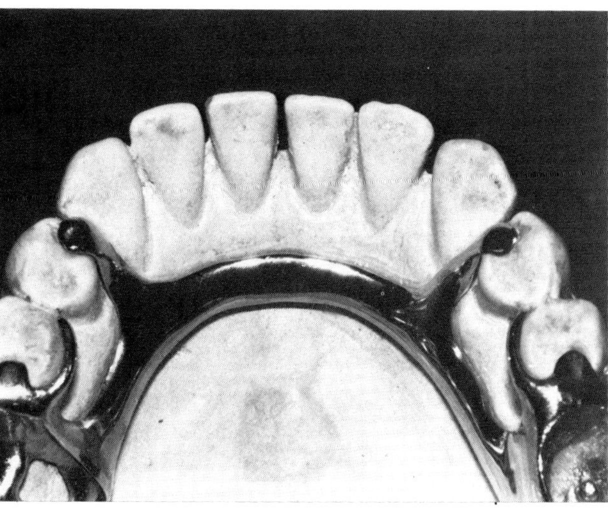

Fig. 3-63. Indirect retainers, shown here as occlusal rests in mesial fossae of first premolars, contribute to support and stability of partial denture.

by the supporting ridge and will be equal to the amount of compressible mucosa or the amount of bone resorption that has taken place since the partial denture was constructed. This vertical component of the rotating motion toward the ridge can be controlled only by stable denture base support. An indirect retainer does not control this movement (Fig. 3-60).

Vertical movement also occurs in the direction away from the supporting ridge. Sticky foods or other substances may exert a pull on the artificial teeth that tends to lift the denture base away from the ridge (Fig. 3-61). Tissues adjacent to the borders of the denture base, such as the tongue or buccinator muscle, may also lift the denture base from the underlying ridge when they are activated by speech, chewing, or swallowing. In addition, gravity exerts an unseating force on maxillary prosthesis. The principal reason for using the indirect retainer is to counteract the movement produced by these forces.

When the bilateral or unilateral distal extension partial denture is under occlusal loading, the fulcrum line runs between the most posterior rests. When the denture is subjected to dislodging forces such as sticky food, the fulcrum line runs through the retentive tip of the direct retainer (clasps). The indirect retainer in the distal extension partial denture uses the mechanical advantage of leverage by moving the fulcrum line farther from the force (Fig. 3-62).

The indirect retainer has several additional functions. It contributes to the support and stability of the partial denture, particularly in counteracting horizontal forces applied to the denture (Fig. 3-63). When a long-span mandibular lingual bar major connector is used, even if tooth-supported, an indirect retainer provides additional support and rigidity for the lingual bar. It also prevents impingement of the lingual bar on the mucosa during function.

The indirect retainer also acts as a third point of con-

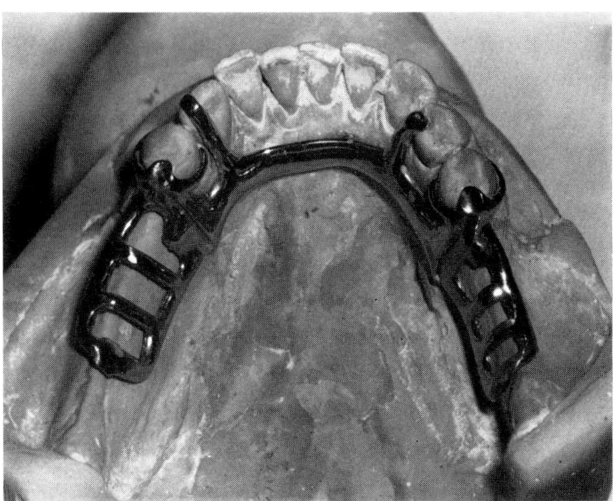

Fig. 3-64. To ensure that framework is positioned accurately on teeth, there must be at least three points of contact between metal of framework and teeth. On this framework there are four points of contact: two distal occlusal rests on terminal abutment teeth, distal incisal rest on left canine, and occlusal rest in mesial fossae of right first premolar.

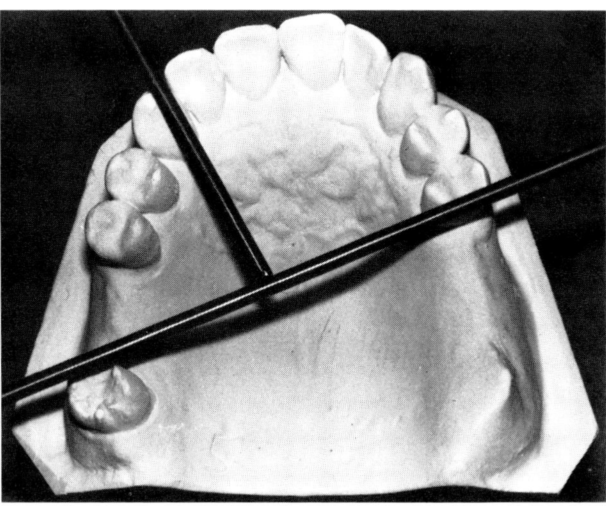

Fig. 3-65. Fulcrum line in this maxillary arch runs between rests of the most posterior teeth. A perpendicular line projected anteriorly from this fulcrum line indicates the most effective location of an indirect retainer. A lingual rest on right canine would be ideal.

tacting tooth structure to ensure accurate repositioning of the framework on the teeth during relining or rebasing. Occlusal rests on the terminal abutment teeth act as the other two of the three points of the tripod (Fig. 3-64). If final impressions are to be made with the framework as a support for the impression tray, this accurate repositioning is absolutely essential.

Factors determining effectiveness of indirect retainers

Indirect retainers must be placed in rest seats that transmit applied forces through the long axis of the abutment tooth. Several factors influence the effectiveness of the indirect retainer. The greater the distance between the fulcrum line and the indirect retainer, the more effective will be the indirect retainer. A line projected at right angles from the fulcrum line and ending in a tooth that is capable of supporting a suitable rest preparation will indicate the most effective location for the indirect retainer (Fig. 3-65). The longer this line, the more favorable will be the result.

The direct retainer must prevent the denture base and rests from being lifted from the tissues and abutment tooth in order for the indirect retainer to function. If the denture base and rests lift from their support, the action is one of displacement and not of rotation. The indirect retainer does not resist displacement.

The indirect retainer must be rigid. If the arm of the indirect retainer were to flex, forces would be multiplied instead of dissipated.

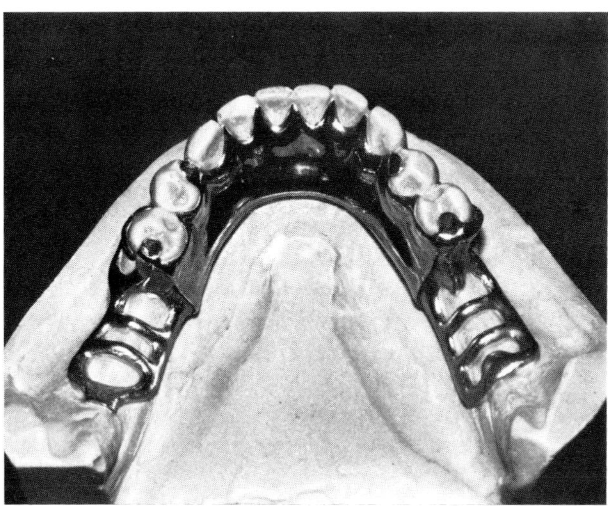

Fig. 3-66. Lingual plating of anterior teeth does not by itself act as an indirect retainer. Because plate contacts inclined surfaces of incisor teeth, lingual plate can force teeth in a labial direction unless plate is supported. Support is best provided by rests. In this case occlusal rests on first premolars are primary indirect retainer.

Confusion exists as to the part that lingual plating plays in indirect retention. A lingual plate by itself cannot act as an indirect retainer. However, if it is adequately supported at each end, normally by an incisal or lingual rest on the canines or by an occlusal rest in the mesial fossae of the first premolar, it can greatly increase the efficiency of the primary indirect retainer. The anterior teeth as a group can counter lifting forces on the denture base. The occlusal or lingual rest will prevent the lingual plate from displacing the incisor teeth (Fig. 3-66).

Form of indirect retainer

The indirect retainer is most often an auxiliary rest—usually an occlusal rest but on occasion, where an occlusal rest cannot be used, an incisal or lingual rest on a canine tooth. An occlusal rest seat can best be prepared on an occlusal surface so that forces transmitted to it can be directed apically through the long axis of the tooth.

An incisal rest must be used if there are no other possible sources of indirect retention, normally on mandibular canines where a lingual or cingulum rest cannot be used (Fig. 3-67). The length of the approach arm of the incisal rest and the concentration of stresses on the incisal edge of the crown can produce detrimental tipping forces to the tooth. In situations like this, consideration should be given to preparing the mandibular canine to receive a crown and carving the lingual rest in the wax pattern of the crown. This type of approach greatly decreases the length of the lever arm and helps direct the forces down the long axis of the abutment tooth.

Cingulum rests acting as indirect retainers can be used to great advantage on maxillary canines. The normal morphology of the canine lends itself to rest seat preparations with minimal tooth structure removal. In addition, opposing mandibular teeth most often occlude into the mesial fossae of the first premolar, making occlusal rest seat preparations difficult, if not impossible.

Incisor teeth are not good candidates to serve as support for indirect retainers. If they must be used, it must be as a group and not individually. Rest seats may be placed in enamel surfaces, but more effective seats may be placed on crowns prepared for these teeth. The prognosis of these teeth should be carefully considered before they are selected (Fig. 3-68).

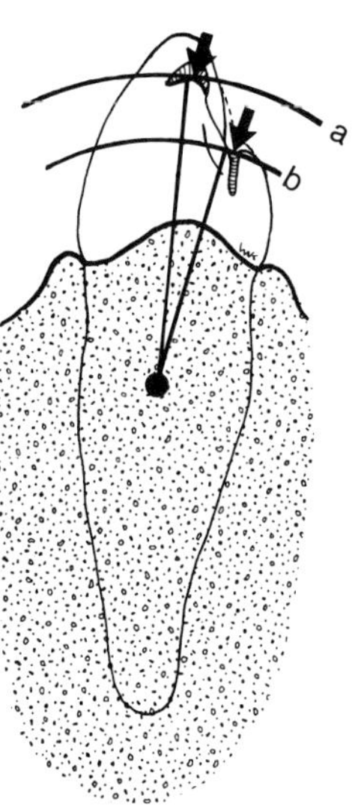

Fig. 3-67. Lingual, or cingulum, rest is preferred over incisal rest because of its mechanical advantage. Incisal rest represents a long lever arm *a* that concentrates stresses transmitted to partial denture on incisal edge of abutment teeth. This magnifies forces beyond those that would take place if lingual rest were used *b*.

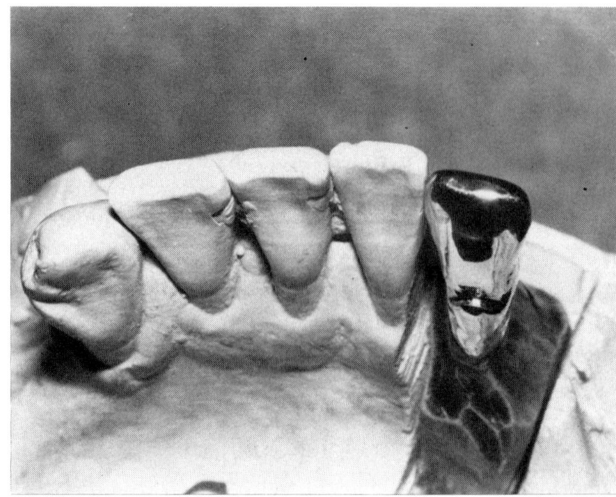

Fig. 3-68. Incisor teeth are not normally selected to support indirect retainers. If an incisor tooth must be used, it should be prepared to receive a crown and a lingual rest seat should be prepared in crown.

As mentioned earlier, incisor teeth can be used to assist the action of the indirect retainer when lingual plating or a double or split lingual bar is selected as the major connector. Rest seats are not necessary on the incisor teeth under these circumstances. However, when weakened, periodontally involved incisor teeth need additional stabilization, incisal or lingual rests can be incorporated into the design of the major connector. This permits the weakened teeth to be supported rigidly and also provides additional horizontal stabilization for the prosthesis.

Treatment of bilateral distal extension edentulous ridges in the maxillary arch with only the six anterior teeth remaining constitutes a special problem. Not only are the usual rotationary forces present, but in the maxilla the force of gravity is a constant factor. Frequently the lower anterior teeth strike the lingual surface of the upper anterior teeth in the area where rest seats should be prepared. Rest seats must be provided, so recontouring the enamel surfaces of the opposing teeth to gain sufficient occlusal clearance must be attempted. If recontouring cannot provide the needed space, a crown must be prepared and the rest seat must be incorporated in the wax pattern. Compromise in the selection of teeth as indirect retainer abutments in the maxillary arch is sometimes required. Broad coverage of the major connector over relatively firm palatal tissues will contribute some indirect retention, but should not be relied on to provide all of it.

Movement of tissue adjacent to the borders of the partial denture is another cause for denture displacement, with resulting rotational force along the fulcrum line. Normal movement of the lips and cheeks (for example, during speaking and mastication) will tend to unseat the prosthesis, particularly if the borders of the denture base have been overextended. Movement of the tongue and floor of the mouth will constantly apply lifting forces to the partial denture. Proper placement of the components of the partial denture will minimize these displacing forces, but the indirect retainer is the prime source for controlling rotational forces on the prosthesis.

TOOTH REPLACEMENTS

The majority of artificial teeth on a removable partial denture are positioned on a denture base (Fig. 3-69). However, there are instances (for example, single missing tooth, confined space, small interocclusal distance) in which facings, tube teeth, reinforced acrylic pontics (RAP), or metal pontics have a more favorable prognosis (Fig. 3-70). The characteristics of the various tooth replacements are considered following this discussion of denture bases.

Denture bases

Plastic (acrylic resin) and metal denture bases are available. The acrylic resin denture base may be used when denture teeth are indicated as replacement teeth except when the edentulous span is too great for other forms of replacement teeth and the interarch space is restricted. In the latter situation extra strength to prevent breakage is required, and a metallic denture base must be used (Fig. 3-71). The main drawback to a metal denture base, particularly on a distal extension edentulous ridge, is the inability to reline it in the event of ridge resorption. The metal base is more indicated for tooth-supported edentulous areas. The metal is somewhat easier for the patient to clean and is not subject to breakage as acrylic resin is. Because the denture base is metal, thermal changes are more quickly transferred

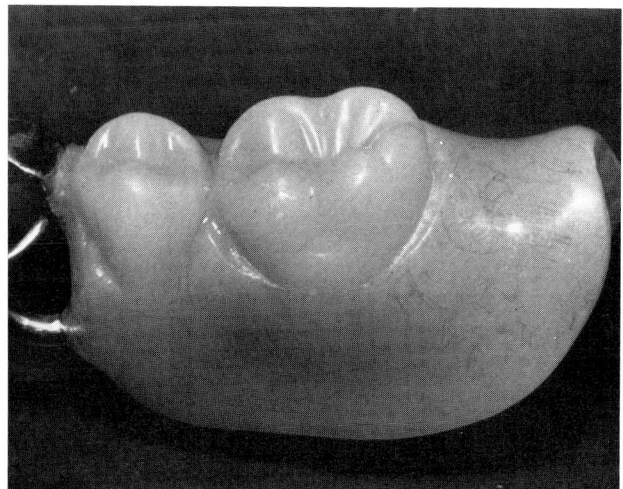

Fig. 3-69. Artificial denture teeth are most often attached to partial denture by denture bases made of acrylic resin. This is most versatile form of tooth replacement. It is most often indicated when multiple teeth are being replaced, but may be used for single tooth replacement.

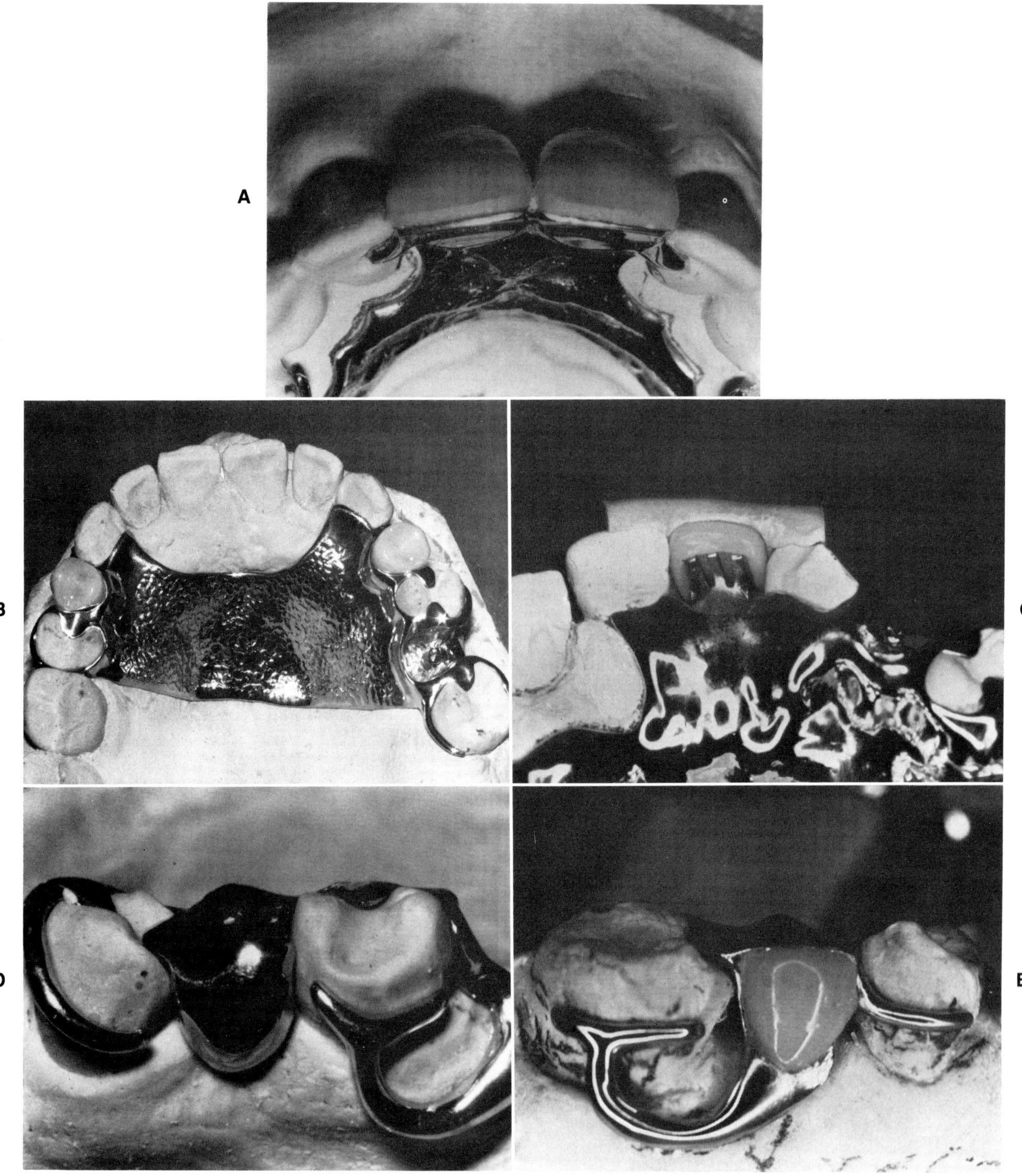

Fig. 3-70. Other types of tooth replacements. **A,** A facing, a thin veneer of tooth-colored porcelain or acrylic resin attached to a metal backing, is a strong tooth replacement. **B,** Tube teeth are porcelain or plastic teeth cemented over a post or tube. Tube teeth shown are attached to a framework. **C,** Reinforced acrylic pontic (RAP) consists of an acrylic resin denture tooth hollowed out and attached to metal projection of framework. This is an excellent replacement for single missing anterior teeth. **D,** Metal pontics are used as replacement teeth when edentulous space is restricted and strength is required. **E,** Metal pontic can be made more esthetic by preparing a cavity, or window, in facial surface of pontic and adding tooth-colored acrylic resin to window.

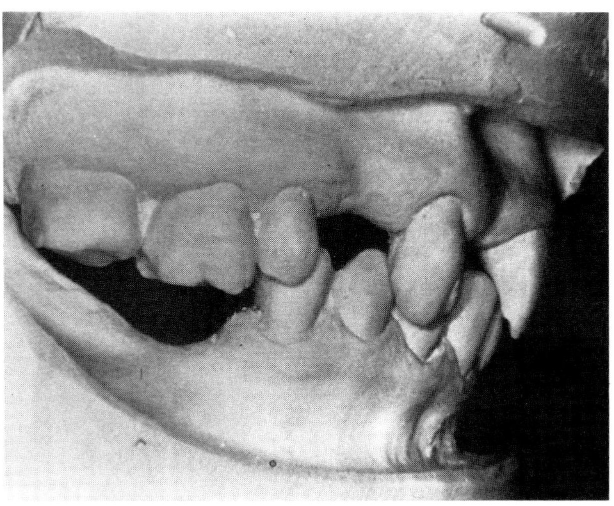

Fig. 3-71. Where the interarch spaces are restricted, such as in the maxillary premolar and mandibular molar areas, forms of tooth replacement other than denture teeth on an acrylic resin denture base may be indicated for additional strength. Metal denture bases and tube teeth may be indicated in this instance.

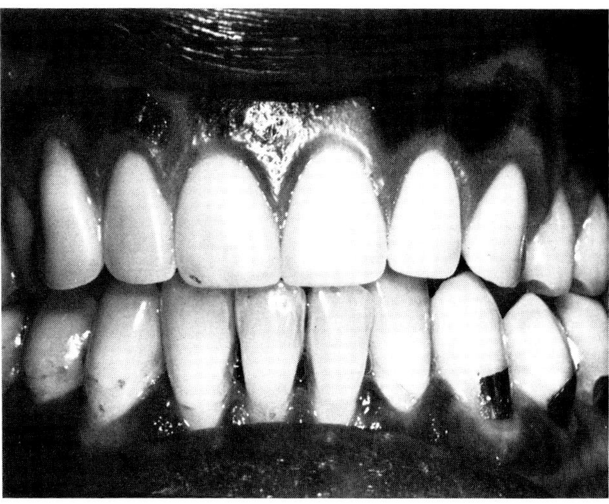

Fig. 3-72. Acrylic resin of denture base may be characterized to duplicate soft tissue tones of patient.

to the underlying mucosa, stimulating the soft tissue in a manner not possible with a plastic base.

If a metal denture base is planned for the partial denture, extreme care must be used in the impression-making procedure. Overextension of the denture base borders must be avoided because adjusting the metallic borders is not an easy office procedure. Underextension of the denture must also be avoided because the forces generated by function of the partial denture must be distributed over as large an area as possible to prevent the edentulous ridge from being overstressed, which could lead to ridge resorption. In addition, esthetics restricts use of the metal denture base to the placement of posterior teeth.

The use of characterized acrylic resin to duplicate the soft tissue tones of each individual patient can permit the placement of esthetically acceptable denture bases in the anterior part of the mouth (Fig. 3-72). One of the great advantages of an acrylic resin denture base is that the artificial teeth may be positioned exactly where the original teeth were, regardless of the loss of ridge that may have occurred, thus restoring the normal contour of the edentulous ridge. This cannot be done with other forms of tooth replacement. In selected cases the resin of the denture base may be used as a "plumper" to fill out or reestablish the normal contours of the lips or cheeks. Care must be taken in this instance not to overstress the abutment teeth.

Anterior tooth replacements

Replacement of anterior teeth, particularly single tooth replacement, should normally be accomplished with a fixed partial denture. In the following instances, however, an anterior replacement may be part of a removable partial denture:

1. In a young patient in whom tooth preparation might compromise a healthy pulp, this treatment may be used as an interim prosthesis.
2. Poor general health of the patient may contraindicate the more prolonged treatment with a fixed prosthesis.
3. The periodontal support of the abutment teeth may not be sufficient for a fixed partial denture.
4. The edentulous span may be too long or the curve of the arch too great to permit the use of a fixed replacement (Fig. 3-73).
5. Excessive loss of the edentulous ridge would make positioning the artificial teeth with a fixed partial denture difficult, if not impossible (Fig. 3-74).

Methods

There are basically four methods of replacing anterior teeth with removable partial dentures. Other replacement forms exist but can be considered to be modifications of these four.

1. Porcelain or plastic denture teeth on denture base
2. Facings
3. Tube teeth
4. Reinforced acrylic pontics (RAPS)

Each of these replacements is discussed and described, and its indications and limitations presented.

Porcelain or plastic denture teeth on denture base. If there is any doubt as to the type of tooth replacement

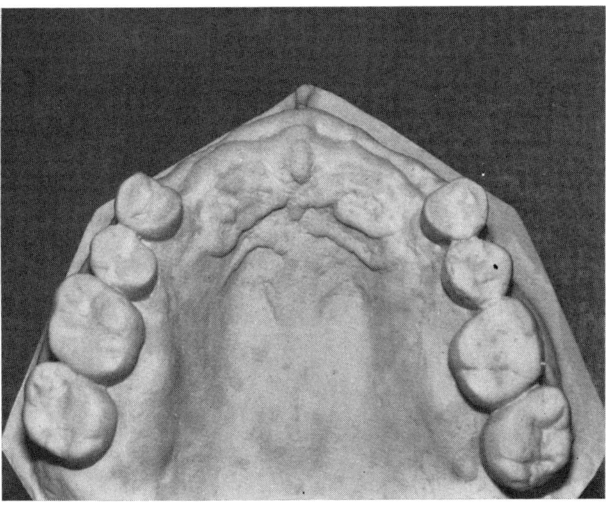

Fig. 3-73. Length of edentulous space is too long and curve of arch is too great to restore missing teeth with a fixed partial denture. A removable partial denture is indicated.

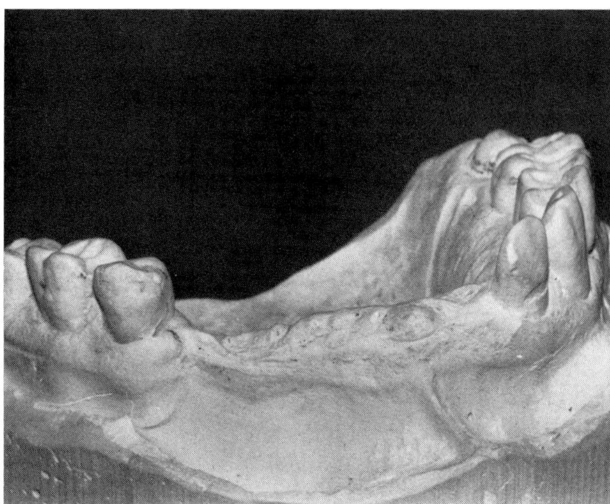

Fig. 3-74. An excessive amount of edentulous ridge has been lost. Replacing these teeth other than by a removable partial denture would be difficult if not impossible.

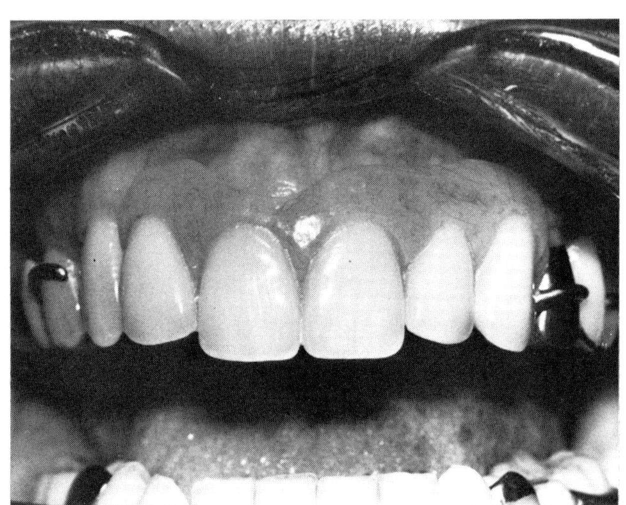

Fig. 3-75. Denture teeth on a denture base is most widely used form of tooth replacement. It can be used anywhere sufficient space is available. It is perhaps most esthetic type of replacement, because position of denture teeth can be varied to produce a natural result. Varying position of other forms of tooth replacement is more difficult.

to use, it will seldom be wrong to use denture teeth on a denture base (Fig. 3-75).

Porcelain teeth. Porcelain (and plastic) denture teeth can be produced in such a variety of shades that any remaining natural teeth can be matched nearly perfectly.

The hardness and resistance to abrasion of porcelain teeth may be considered favorable, because the teeth wear very minimally in function. The proper vertical dimension of occlusion is therefore accurately maintained. Their durability, however, is a potential hazard when the porcelain teeth oppose natural teeth. The porcelain, particularly glazed porcelain, can wear the porcelain, particularly unglazed porcelain, can wear the enamel surfaces of natural teeth rapidly.

One major disadvantage of porcelain teeth on a removable partial denture is that porcelain is fractured easily by impact stresses (Fig. 3-76). Artificial teeth for a partial denture must be ground and reshaped in order to fit the space between remaining natural teeth in the same arch, between and around components of the metal framework of the denture, and to occlude properly with opposing teeth. This grinding and reshaping further weakens the porcelain tooth, and fracture frequently occurs.

As a general rule the use of porcelain teeth should be limited to those removable partial dentures that oppose a complete denture and where adequate interarch space is present so that the teeth will not need to be

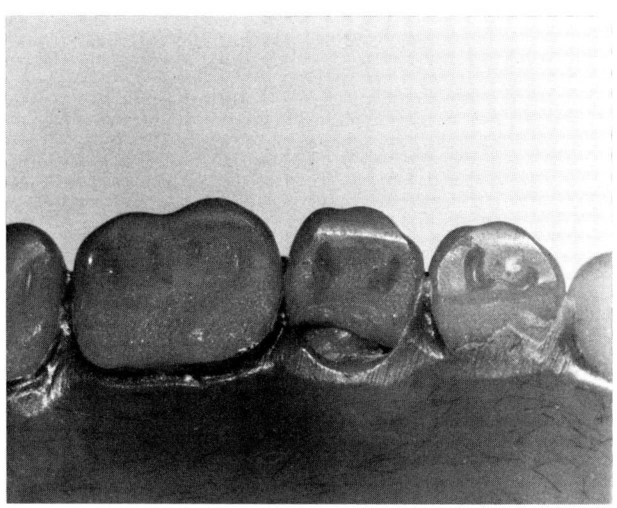

Fig. 3-76. Inherent weakness of porcelain to impact contraindicates use of porcelain teeth in removable partial dentures.

ground excessively. Other than this indication, the use of porcelain teeth in removable partial dentures should be discouraged.

Plastic teeth. The plastic denture tooth has very high impact strength, and fracture or breakage is rarely a problem (Fig. 3-77). The plastic tooth can also be ground and reshaped to fit available space without sacrificing strength. The esthetic quality of present-day plastic teeth is comparable to that of porcelain teeth.

The main weakness of plastic teeth is their relative lack of resistance to wear and abrasion. New forms of plastic teeth are being produced that have improved abrasive resistance, but plastic still wears more rapidly than porcelain.

Summary of denture teeth on denture base.

ADVANTAGES

1. Most esthetic form of replacement.
2. Permits wider distribution of vertical forces.
3. Restores lost portion of edentulous ridge.
4. May be easily relined if needed.
5. In case of plastic teeth, opposing occlusion is against acrylic resin.

LIMITATIONS

1. Difficult to use for single tooth replacement.
2. Requires bulk for adequate strength.

Facings. Facings used to be popular replacements for anterior teeth, possibly because of their strength (Fig. 3-78). They can be placed in very restricted spaces and require only a minimum of interocclusal space. They are also convenient, because the laboratory prefabricates the restorations; the dentist only has to cement the facing on at the time of insertion. In addition, because the facings are interchangeable, they can easily be replaced if the need arises. Without question facings are one of the strongest, most durable replacements available, and they serve as a last resort if less than 1 mm of interocclusal space is available for an anterior pontic.

However, the virtues of facings are overshadowed by their shortcomings. Their biggest drawback is in their poor esthetic quality, particularly for multiple anterior replacements. The lingual half of the facings, the backing, consists of cast gold or chrome and is part of the framework. The metal tends to influence the shade of the plastic or porcelain facing, and it is difficult to select a shade that will blend with adjacent natural teeth. Also, thin plastic or porcelain veneer offers no sense of depth, resulting in a lifeless appearance.

Another major drawback of facings, particularly in the case of a deep vertical overbite, is that the opposing teeth will be striking against metal. This can result in rapid wear to these teeth.

The facing must be butted against the edentulous ridge to give a natural appearance, so a broad well-healed ridge is a requirement. No freedom of position is allowed.

Summary of facings

ADVANTAGES

1. May be used as a single tooth replacement when interocclusal space is limited and strength is required.
2. May be used when a broad, well-healed ridge is present with little resorption having taken place.

LIMITATIONS

1. Difficult to obtain a good esthetic result.
2. Opposing occlusion is against metal.
3. Cannot be relined.
4. Little or no support is derived from the underlying ridge.
5. Cannot be used on resorbed ridge.

Tube teeth. The tube tooth consists of a plastic or porcelain denture tooth prepared by drilling a channel, or tube, from the base of the tooth upward (Fig. 3-79). As the framework is being waxed, the tooth is positioned and connected to the framework by waxing the prepared tube to the rest of the denture. Before investing, the artificial tooth is removed, leaving the wax post that is subsequently cast.

After the framework has been finished and polished, the tooth is cemented back on the post.

Because the entire thickness of the tooth is either plastic or porcelain, esthetics is generally good. It is easy to produce the correct shade, and because of the thickness of the tooth it has a lifelike quality.

The tube tooth must be butted against the ridge to have a natural appearance; for this reason it must be used on a broad nonresorbed ridge. It is not an especially strong replacement and should not be used where mesiodistal or occlusogingival space is restricted.

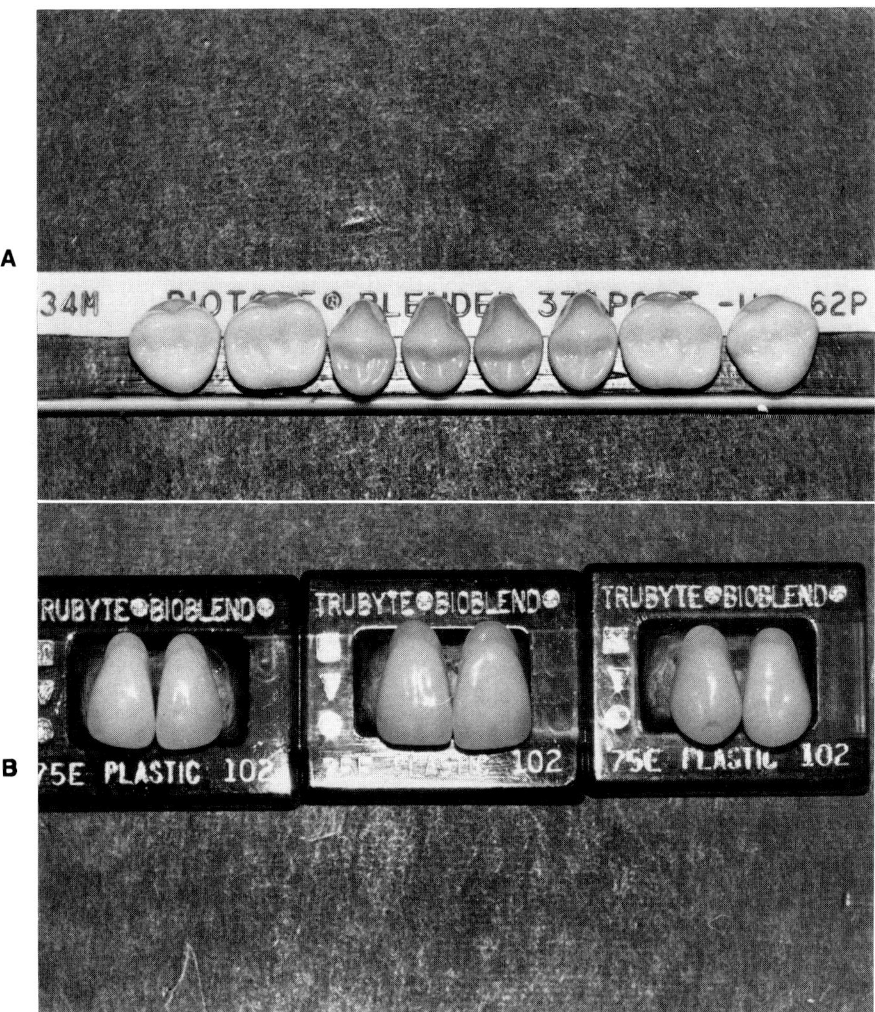

Fig. 3-77. A, Plastic, or acrylic resin, teeth are supplied in same molds and shades as are porcelain teeth. Their advantages and disadvantages are reverse of those of porcelain teeth. Plastic teeth will wear or abrade when opposing natural teeth. However, they can be cut and recontoured to fit edentulous spaces without noticeably weakening teeth. **B,** Plastic anterior teeth are available in same molds and shades as are porcelain anterior teeth.

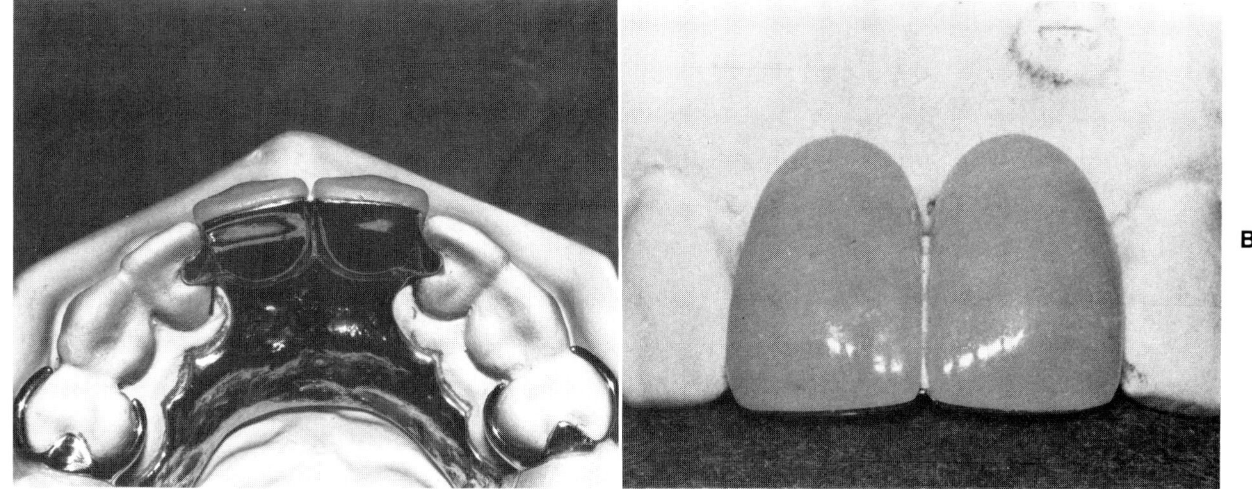

Fig. 3-78. The only redeeming features of facings as a form of tooth replacement are strength and ease of replacement. **A,** Facing is a thin veneer of resin backed by metal. **B,** Natural tooth's three dimensions of depth cannot be matched.

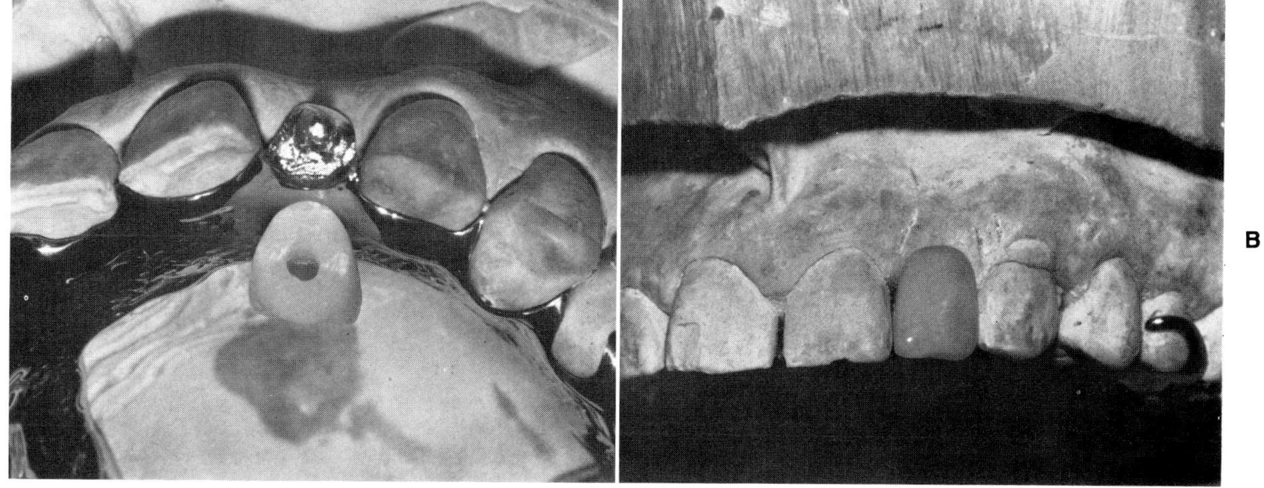

Fig. 3-79. Tube tooth is an acrylic resin or porcelain tooth that has been prepared by drilling a channel from base of tooth upward. Tooth is waxed into framework and removed, leaving wax post or tube. After framework is complete, **A,** tooth is cemented to post, **B.**

Laboratory time may be saved by its use, because investing or processing resin is not necessary. The tube tooth can be a good single tooth replacement but is not good for multiple adjacent teeth replacements. Little or no support can be gained from the underlying ridge.

Summary of tube teeth.

ADVANTAGES

1. Provides good esthetic replacement for a single tooth where space is available (Fig. 3-80).
2. Opposing teeth will occlude against the acrylic resin tooth.
3. Not necessary to invest and process the denture after the framework has been finished.

LIMITATIONS

1. Must have ample space mesiodistally and occlusogingivally.
2. Requires a well-healed, nonresorbed ridge; even moderate resorption of the ridge contraindicates its use.
3. Derives no support from the soft tissue and cannot be relined.

The tube tooth also makes an excellent single tooth *posterior* replacement, particularly in the premolar area.

Reinforced acrylic pontics (RAPs). The RAP is a fairly new tooth replacement, and some commercial

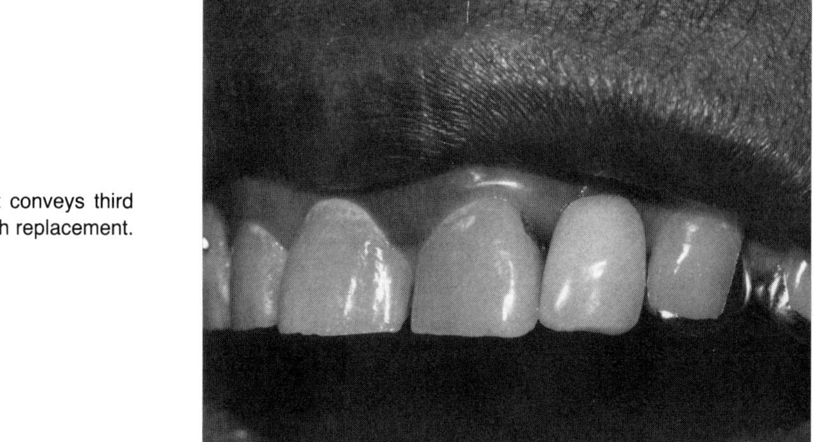

Fig. 3-80. Because tube tooth has full thickness, it conveys third dimension of depth. It makes an excellent single tooth replacement.

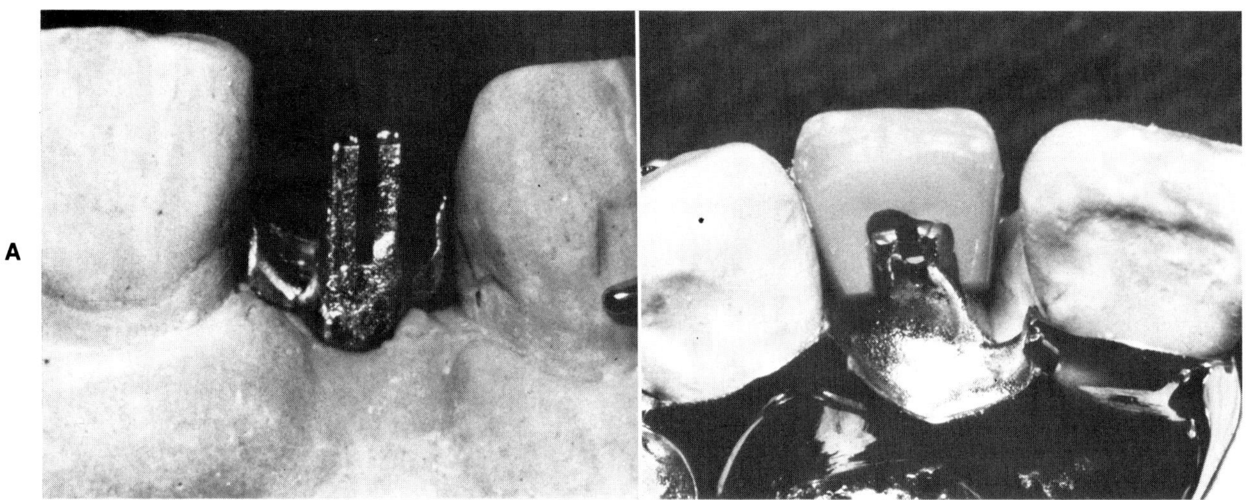

Fig. 3-81. A, Gingival half of lingual surface of RAP consists of projections of metal around which artificial tooth is processed. **B,** Lingual projection of metal adds to strength of the replacement tooth without detracting from esthetic value. RAP is an excellent single tooth replacement.

laboratories may not be equipped to make it. It combines most of the good features of facings and tube teeth and eliminates many of their shortcomings.

The gingival half of the lingual surface of the RAP consists of projections, or loops of metal, around which the artificial tooth is processed (Fig. 3-81). The metal ensures that the replacement has strength, thus allowing its use in areas in which space is restricted. The incisal half is solid plastic, which provides easy shade control and generally good esthetics.

As for the facing or tube tooth, a well-healed broad ridge is necessary. The RAP is used only for anterior teeth and maxillary first premolars.

Summary of RAPs.

ADVANTAGES

1. Excellent strength and esthetics.
2. Can be designed so that occlusion is confined to the plastic.
3. Can be used in a restricted space.

LIMITATIONS

1. Unhealed ridge or resorbed ridge contraindicates use.
2. Little support can be gained from the ridge.
3. Cannot be relined.

Posterior tooth replacements

Plastic teeth

The vast majority of missing posterior teeth will be replaced by acrylic resin denture teeth supported on a denture base. However, the wear and abrasion of plastic teeth may be dangerous when most of the posterior teeth have been replaced by plastic teeth. Over time the occlusal surfaces of the teeth tend to flatten, not only producing inefficient masticating surfaces, but also causing a gradual decrease in the vertical dimension of occlusion and a change in the occlusal relationship (Fig. 3-82). Patients wearing this type of prosthesis must be maintained on a strict recall program to prevent this occlusal change.

After plastic or resin teeth have been adjusted to function against opposing natural teeth, the occlusal surfaces of the substitute teeth will flatten and become devoid of nearly all occlusal anatomy. Teeth with flat surfaces generate stress against the oral structures during mastication because of the lack of cutting efficiency. The use of flat, inefficient teeth in removable partial dentures is probably the single greatest cause of overloading or stressing the remaining teeth and soft tissues. Fortunately, it is relatively easy to recarve the occlusal surfaces of plastic teeth to produce spillways, cusps, and accessory grooves that will restore cutting efficiency (Fig. 3-83). This process is much more difficult with porcelain teeth.

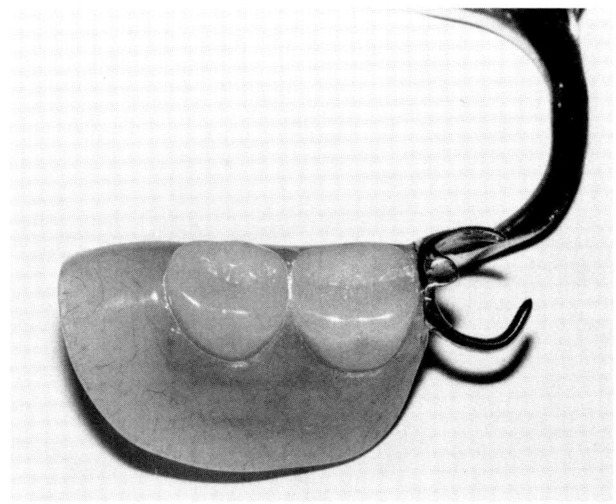

Fig. 3-82. Occlusal surfaces of plastic teeth opposed to natural teeth will eventually show evidence of wear. This can change occlusal relationship of teeth. Plastic teeth require periodic examination by dentist and replacement when necessary.

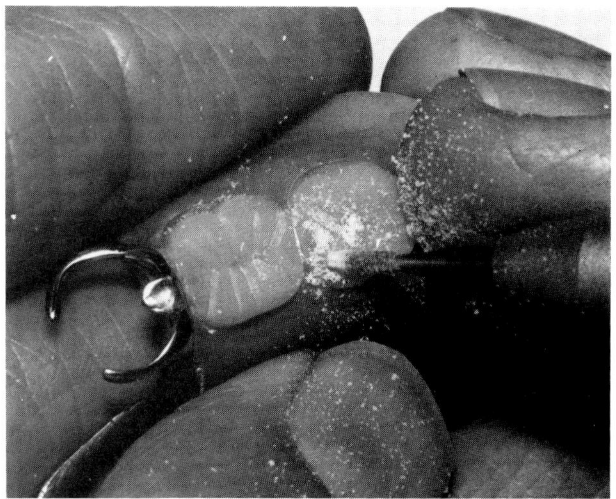

Fig. 3-83. Surfaces of plastic posterior teeth that have been worn should be redeveloped. A straight fissure burr can be used to define spillways, cusps, and accessory grooves to restore masticatory efficiency.

Porcelain teeth

Porcelain teeth should be used only when artificial teeth are opposed by artificial teeth (Figs. 3-84 and 3-85).

Metal pontics

The use of the metal tooth, or pontics, is obviously restricted to the replacement of posterior teeth (Figs. 3-86 and 3-87). A veneer of tooth-colored resin can be processed on the facial surface of the metal pontic to produce an acceptable esthetic result.

The metal tooth is indicated where the interarch space is severely restricted or where drifting of the remaining teeth has resulted in a space too small for a plastic or porcelain tooth.

Normally the tooth is made of the same metal from which the rest of the framework is constructed, either gold or chrome alloy. If chrome alloy teeth contact opposing natural teeth, the very hard metal will wear enamel surfaces rapidly. Therefore occlusal surfaces should be processed in tooth-colored resin and attached to the metal tooth (Fig. 3-88). The technique for constructing the occlusal surfaces is covered in Chapter 14.

The ideal material for the occlusal surfaces of substitute teeth on a removable partial denture that opposes natural teeth or other artificial teeth is gold (Fig. 3-89). Gold has adequate strength to be used in restricted areas and can be produced in forms necessary to restore complete functional and efficient occlusion. It is the material of choice whenever long-term maintenance is required. The occlusal surfaces may be produced originally in wax or resin, invested, and then cast in gold. The technique for producing gold occlusal surfaces is described in Chapter 14.

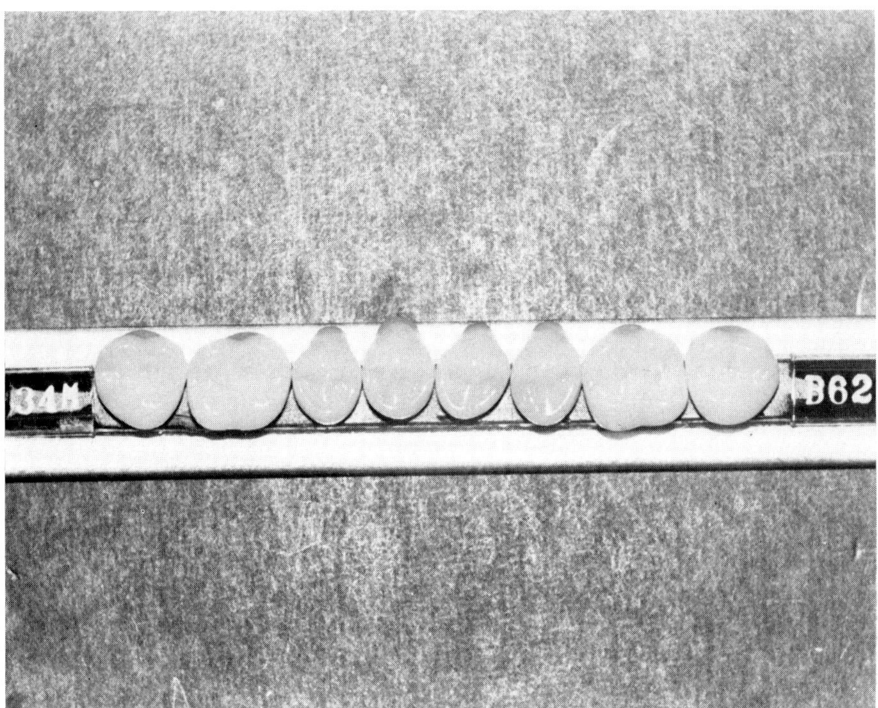

Fig. 3-84. Porcelain posterior denture teeth are supplied in groups of eight on a card showing mold of teeth, 34M, and shade of teeth, B62. One main advantage of porcelain teeth is hardness. Teeth will wear or abrade minimally in function.

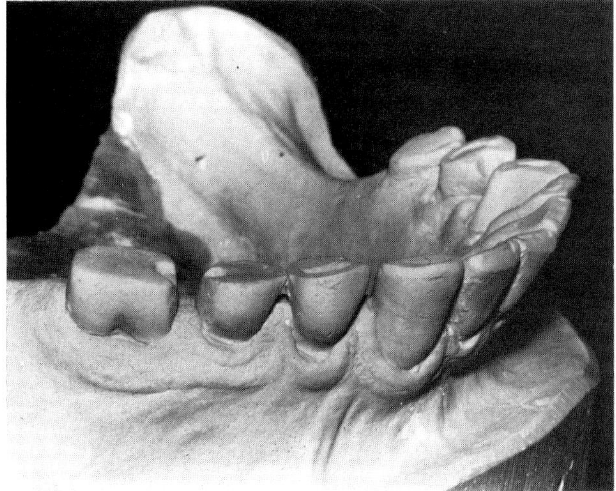

Fig. 3-85. Advantage of porcelain teeth, hardness, is a major disadvantage when porcelain denture teeth oppose natural teeth. Occlusal surfaces of molar and premolars depicted have been completely destroyed by occlusion with porcelain teeth.

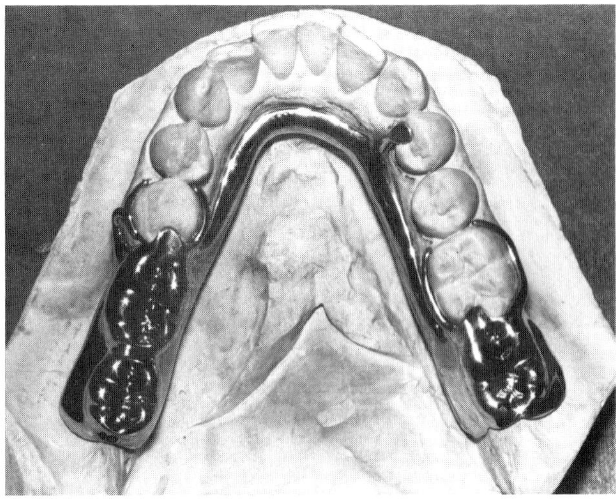

Fig. 3-86. Use of metal teeth as illustrated is limited. Impact of occlusion against metal teeth is magnified and can be damaging not only to opposing teeth but also to supporting ridge. Restricted interarch space is the only indication for use of metal teeth.

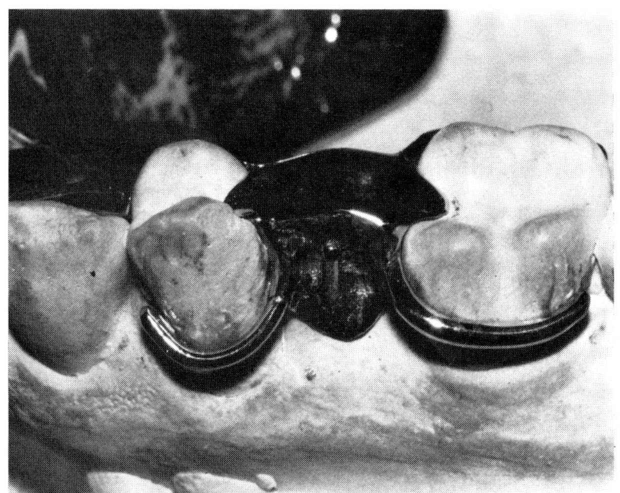

Fig. 3-87. Metal pontic is used only in areas where space is restricted and strength of replacement teeth is required. If esthetics is a factor, pontic can be prepared to receive a tooth-colored plastic facing.

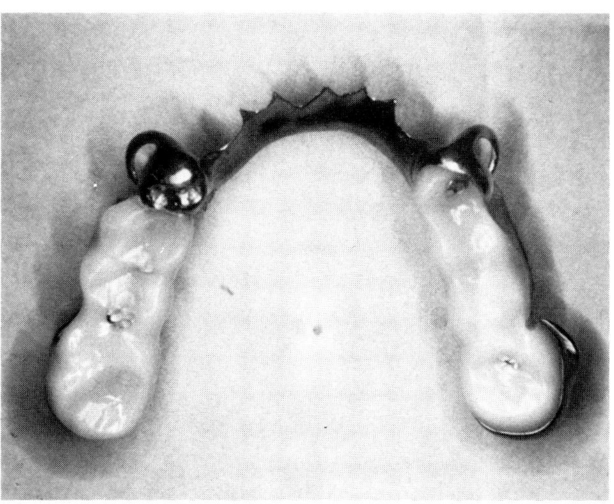

Fig. 3-88. Tooth-colored acrylic resin can be processed on occlusal surfaces of metal teeth to reduce occlusal force on ridge and prevent wear of opposing teeth.

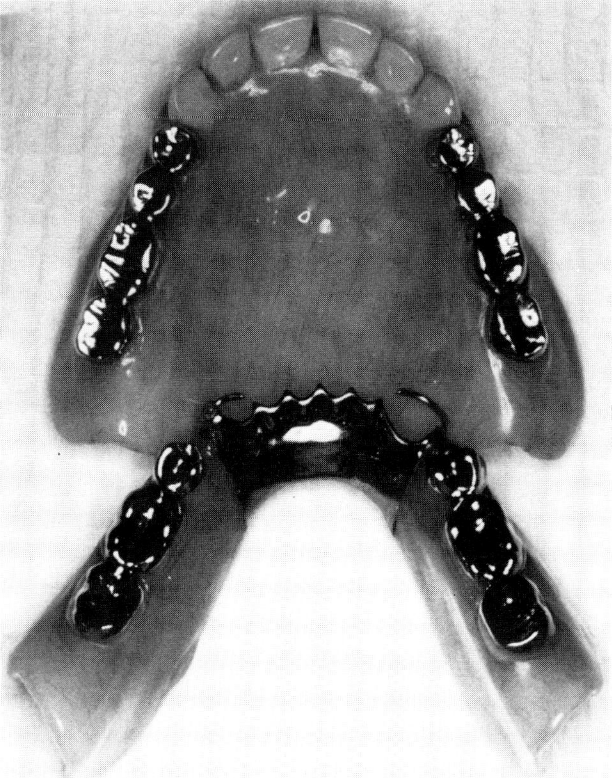

Fig. 3-89. Gold occlusal surfaces of posterior teeth are most efficient and least damaging form of occlusion that can be restored to partially edentulous patient.

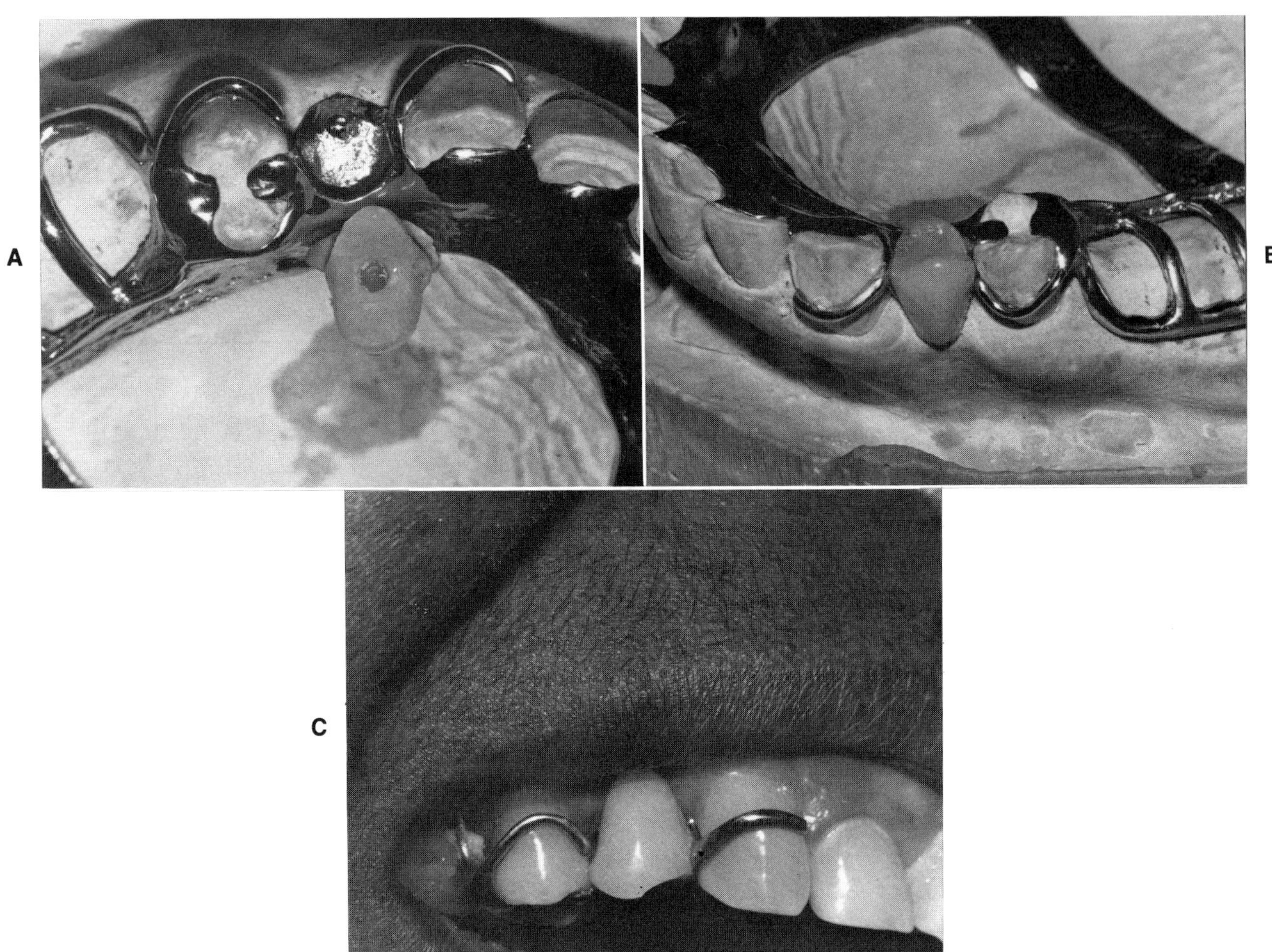

Fig. 3-90. Posterior tube tooth is an excellent replacement for single teeth. It is a particularly esthetic replacement for maxillary first premolars. **A,** Framework and prepared tooth. **B,** Tooth placed on framework. **C,** In mouth.

Metal pontics with acrylic window. In the event that esthetics are of concern and the edentulous space is restricted, the buccal surface of the pontic may be cut away during framework wax-up, and tooth colored resin processed in the recess.

Tube teeth

Tube teeth are the most used form of posterior tooth replacement next to denture teeth on a denture base (Fig. 3-90). They should be limited to one, two, or three teeth and should usually be tooth supported.

A tube tooth makes an excellent esthetic replacement for maxillary first premolars. In this position it should be butted to the edentulous ridge.

Tube teeth are seldom indicated for a distal extension ridge. The ridge should be well healed, because there is no possibility of relining this type of replacement.

REFERENCE

DeVan, M.M.: Preserving natural teeth through the use of clasps, J. Prosthet. Dent. **5**:208-214, 1955.

BIBLOGRAPHY

Anthony, E.P.: American textbook of prosthetic dentistry, ed 7, Philadelphia, 1949, Lea & Febiger.

Avant, W.E.: Indirect retention in partial denture design, J. Prosthet. Dent. **16**:1103-1110, 1966.

Bates, J.F.: Cast clasps for partial dentures, Int. Dent. J. **13**:610-613, 1963.

Blatterfein, L.: Study of partial denture clasping, J. Am. Dent. Assoc. **43**:169-185, 1951.

Blatterfein, L.: Design and positional arrangement of clasps for partial dentures, N.Y. J. Dent. **22**:305-306, 1952.

Breisach, L.: Esthetic attachments for removable partial dentures, J. Prosthet. Dent. **17**:261-267, 1967.

Brudvik, J.S., and Wormley, J. H.: Construction techniques for wrought wire retention clasp arms as related to clasp flexibility, J. Prosthet. Dent. **30**:769-774, 1973.

Cecconi, B.T., Asgar, K., and Dootz, E.: The effect of partial denture clasp design on abutment tooth movement, J. Prosthet. Dent. **25**:44;56, 1971.

Cecconi, B.T., Asgar, K., and Dootz, E.: Clasp assembly modifications and their effect on abutment tooth movement, J. Prosthet. Dent. **27**:160-167, 1972.

Chayes, H.E.S.: Movable-removable bridgework, New York, 1922, Chayes System Laboratories, Inc.

Chick, A.O.: Correct location of clasps and rests on dentures without stress-breakers, Br. Dent. J. **95**:303-309, 1955.

Clayton, J.A., and Jaslow, C.: A measurement of clasp forces on teeth, J. Prosthet. Dent. **25**:21-43, 1971.

Craddock, F.W., and Bottomleys, G.A.: Second thoughts on clasping, Br. Dent. J. **46**:134-137, 1954.

Firtell, D.N.: Effect of clasp design upon retention of removable partial dentures, J. Prosthet. Dent. **20**:43-52, 1968.

Frank, R.P., and Nicholis, J.I.: An investigation of the indirect retainer, J. Prosthet. Dent. **38**:494-506, 1977.

Garver, D.G.: A new clasping system for unilateral distal-extension removable partial dentures, J. Prosthet. Dent. **39**:268-273, 1978.

Gindea, A.E.: A retentive device for removable dentures, J. Prosthet. Dent. **27**:501-508, 1972.

Grasso, J.E.: A new removable partial denture clasp concept J. Prosthet. Dent. **43**:618-621, 1980.

Kabcenell, J.L.: Effective clasping of removable partial dentures, J. Prosthet. Dent. **12**:104-110, 1962.

Kennedy, E.: Removable partial dentures, Brooklyn, 1928, Dental Items of Interest Pub. Co.

Kotowicz, W.E.: Fisher, R.L., Reed, R.A., and Jaslow, C.: The combination clasp and the distal extension removable partial denture, Dent. Clin. North Am. **17**:651-660, October, 1973.

Kratochvil, F.: Influence of occlusal rest position and clasp design on movement of abutment teeth, J. Prosthet. Dent. **13**:114, 1963.

Krol, A.J.: Clasp design for extension base removable partial dentures, J. Prosthet. Dent. **29**:408-415, 1973.

Langer, A.: Combinations of diverse retainers in removable partial dentures, J. Prosthet. Dent. **40**:378-384, 1978.

McCall, J.O.: The periodontist looks at the clasp partial denture, J. Am. Dent. Assoc. **43**:439-443, 1951.

McKinnon, K.P.: Indirect retention in partial denture construction, Dent. J. Aust. **27**:221-225, 1955.

Morrison, M.L.: Internal precision attachment retainers for partial dentures, J. Am. Dent. Assoc. **64**:209-215, 1962.

Prothero, J.H.: Prosthetic dentistry, ed. 3, Chicago, 1923, Medico-Dental Publishing Co.

Rad, M.N., and Yarmand, M.A.: Design of a direct retainer for removable partial dentures, J. Prosthet. Dent. **31**:457-459, 1974.

Roach, F.E.: Principles and essentials of bar clasp construction, J. Am. Dent. Assoc. **17**:124-138, 1930.

Shohet, H.: Relative magnitudes of stress on abutment teeth with different retainers, J. Prosthet. Dent. **21**:267-282, 1969.

Smith, G.P.: Cast clasps: their uses, advantages, and disadvantages, Am. J. Orthodont. Oral Surg. **33**:479-483, 1947.

Steffel, V.L.: Simplified clasp partial denture designed for maximum function, J. Am. Dent. Assoc. **32**:1093-1100, 1945.

Stone, E.R.: Tipping action of bar clasps, J. Am. Dent. Assoc. **23**:596-617, 1936.

Warr, J.A.: An analysis of clasp design in partial dentures, Phys. Med. Biol. **3**:212-232, 1959.

Weinberg, L.A.: Lateral force in relation to the denture base and clasp design, J. Prosthet. Dent. **6**:785-800, 1956.

4 Principles of removable partial dentures

It is axiomatic in prosthodontics that a properly constructed fixed partial denture is superior to a removable partial denture. The reason for this is that the fixed partial denture does not move in function, and forces against it from any direction are directed down the long axis of the abutment teeth (Fig. 4-1). The last statement is somewhat oversimplified, but basically it is true. This is in direct contrast to what happens to forces directed against a removable partial denture.

Of all partial dentures, an all-tooth–supported, or Class III, partial denture can best resist forces because it, like the fixed partial denture, is supported by abutment teeth (Fig. 4-2). Limited movement is possible, however, and the prosthesis may lift in function. These movements create stresses that need to be countered or controlled by additional teeth, soft tissue, or components of the denture.

Classes I, II, and IV removable partial dentures are subjected to greater stresses because their support is a combination of tooth and soft tissue (Fig. 4-3). Forces must be controlled by maximum coverage of soft tissue, by proper use of direct retainers, and by placement of the components in the most advantageous position.

A better understanding of the methods of controlling forces on removable partial dentures may be achieved by a brief review of the development of forces. A removable partial denture in the mouth can perform the action of two simple machines, the lever and the inclined plane (Fig. 4-4). It may also act like a wedge but not in the normal course of events.

The lever is a rigid bar supported at some point along its length. If the lever rests against its support and a weight is applied at another point, rotation or movement will occur around the support (Fig. 4-5). The support is known as the fulcrum, and movement takes place around the fulcrum.

There are three types of levers, first-, second-, and third-class, and each magnifies or disguises the force to a different degree (Fig. 4-6).

The inclined plane is the other simple machine to be concerned with. Forces against the inclined plane may result in deflection of that which is applying the force or may result in movement to the inclined plane. Neither of these results is desirable.

It is in distal extention removable partial dentures that the type of prosthesis controlling stress is important. The all-tooth–supported partial denture is rarely subjected to induced stresses, because leverage-type forces are not involved and there are no fulcrums around which the partial denture may rotate. Inclined planes are also not a factor when the partial denture is tooth supported.

The distal extension partial denture, on the other hand, is subjected to rotation around three principal fulcrums (see Figs. 4-7, 4-10, and 4-11). Movement usually takes place around all three fulcrums simultaneously. During the formulation of a design for a partial denture, these three fulcrums and the movement that may take place around them must be kept in mind. Components of the denture may then be positioned to counteract or prevent as much of the rotation as possible. Components should not be added to the partial denture indiscreetly or because of design habit. A technician, who does not understand the biologic or physiologic requirement of a prosthesis, will design all partial dentures of a class the same. This is one main reason that removable partial dentures have not enjoyed overwhelming acceptance in years past. Only the dentist, who knows the health and condition of the oral tissues, is qualified to design a removable prosthesis. Components of a partial denture must be selected and positioned to perform a specific function. To omit a component because of a patient's objection to it or to make the prosthesis lighter or smaller renders a disservice to the patient and compromises the basic philosophy of prosthodontics—preserving that which remains rather than merely attempting to replace that which has been lost.

FORCES ACTING ON PARTIAL DENTURE

The forces acting on a partial denture are a result of a composite of forces arising from three principal fulcrums.

One fulcrum is on the horizontal plane that extends

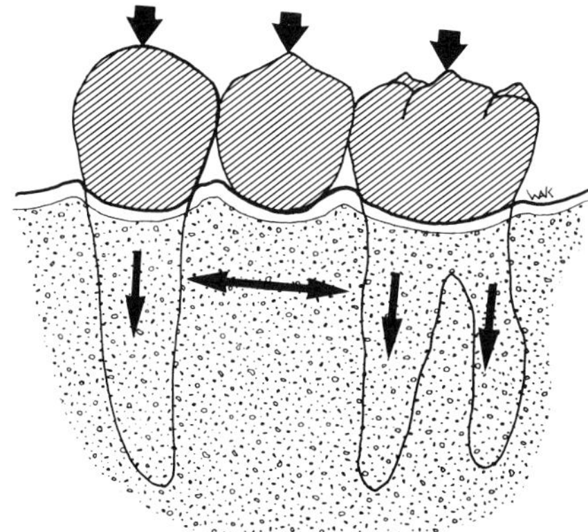

Fig. 4-1. All forces against fixed partial denture are directed down long axis of abutment teeth (arrows).

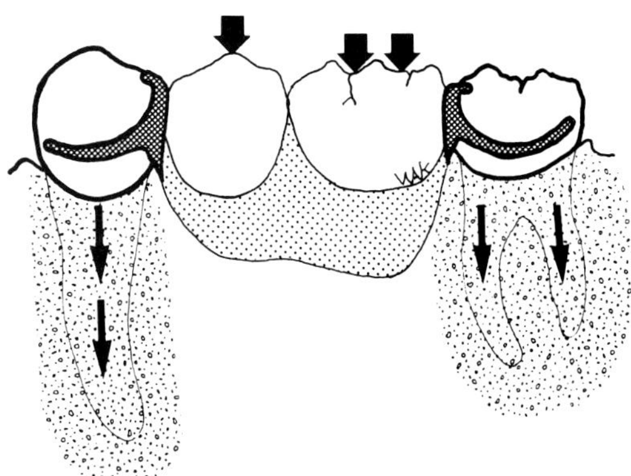

Fig. 4-2. Tooth-supported, or Class III, removable partial denture, like fixed partial denture, is supported by abutments. Most forces against it are transmitted down long axis of abutment teeth (arrows). However, limited movement, including a tendency to lift in function, is possible.

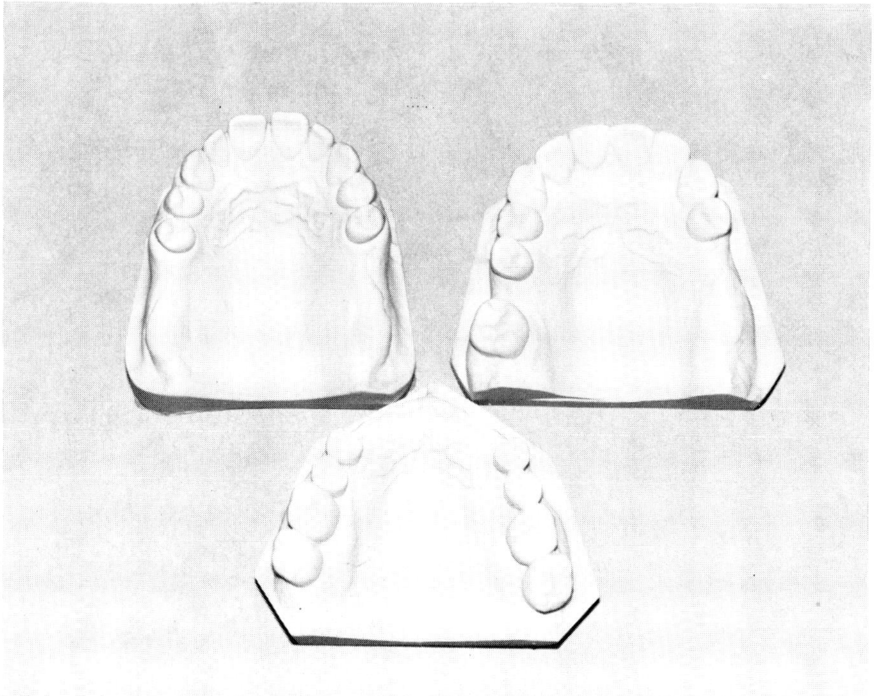

Fig. 4-3. Class I, upper left, Class II, upper right, and Class IV, lower, partially edentulous arches are subjected to greater stresses than Class III arch because support for a prosthesis must be derived from both teeth and soft tissue. Soft tissue, being compressible, permits vertical and rotational movement.

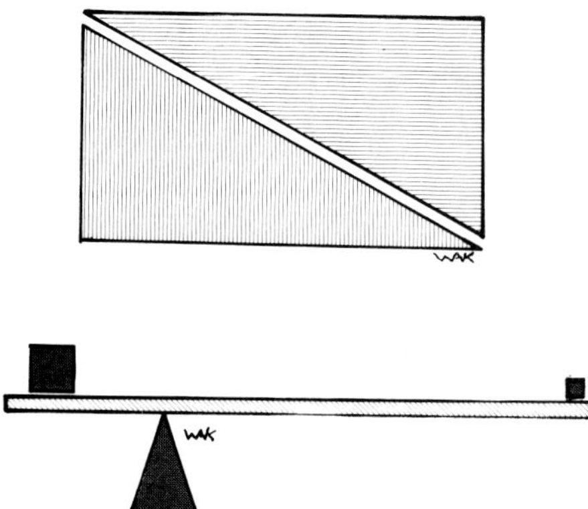

Fig. 4-4. Removable partial denture can perform action of two simple machines: lever, bottom, and inclined plane, top.

Fig. 4-5. Distal extension denture base of partial denture is a lever arm. As downward forces occur against denture base, downward movement results because underlying soft tissue is compressed. As downward force is removed, denture base moves in opposite direction because of rebound of soft tissue. This downward and upward movement is rotational. Center of rotation is occlusal rest of denture in rest seat of tooth, referred to as a fulcrum.

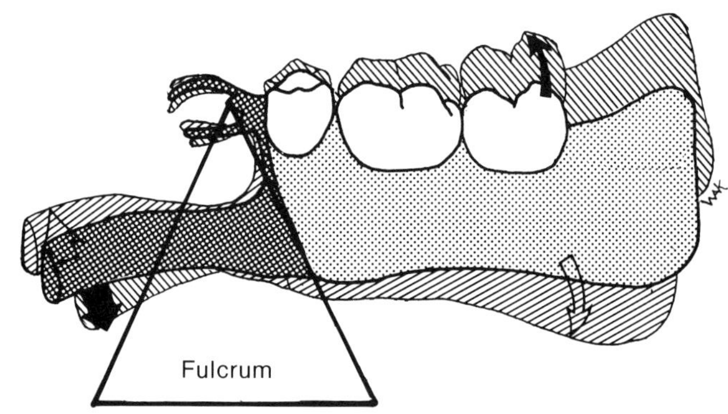

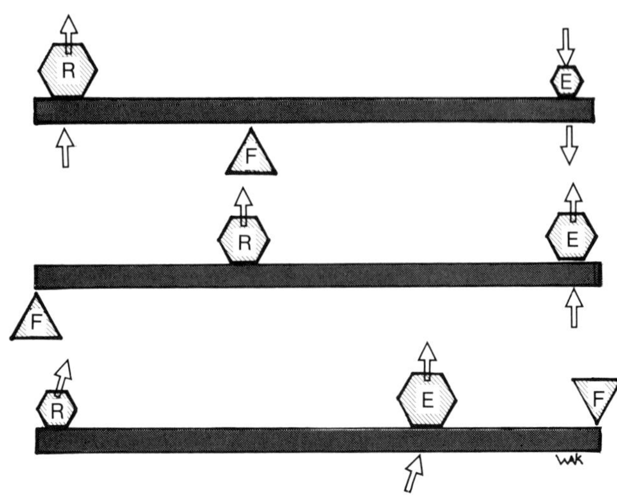

Fig. 4-6. Top, first-class lever. Fulcrum is in center, resistance is at one end, and effort, or force, is at opposite end. This is most efficient and easily controlled lever. Center, second-class lever with fulcrum at one end, effort at opposite end, and resistance in center. This type is seen as indirect retention in removable partial dentures. Bottom, third-class lever with fulcrum at one end, resistance at opposite, and effort in center. This class is not encountered in partial dentures.

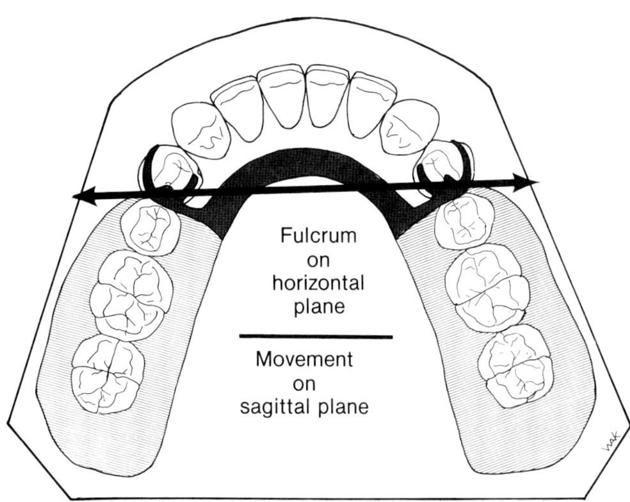

Fig. 4-7. Horizontal fulcrum line passing between two principal abutment teeth controls rotational motion of denture toward or away from supporting ridge.

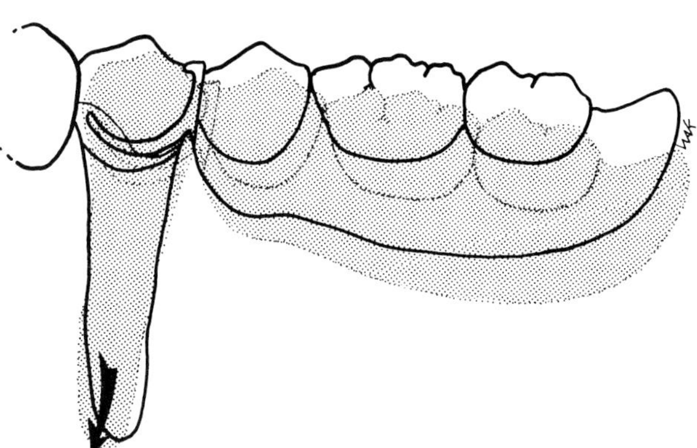

Fig. 4-8. Resulting force on abutment tooth from rotation in sagittal plane is usually in a mesioapical or distoapical direction (arrow) with greatest magnitude in apical direction.

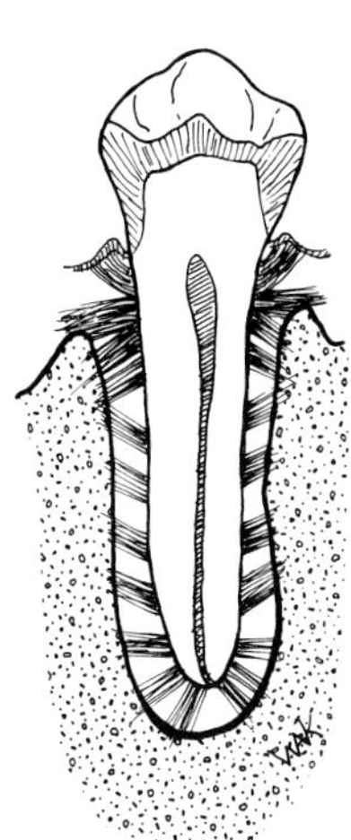

Fig. 4-9. Fibers of periodontal ligament are basically arranged such that resistance to vertical forces is much greater than that to horizontal or torsional forces. The fibers act as a sling to counter vertical displacement.

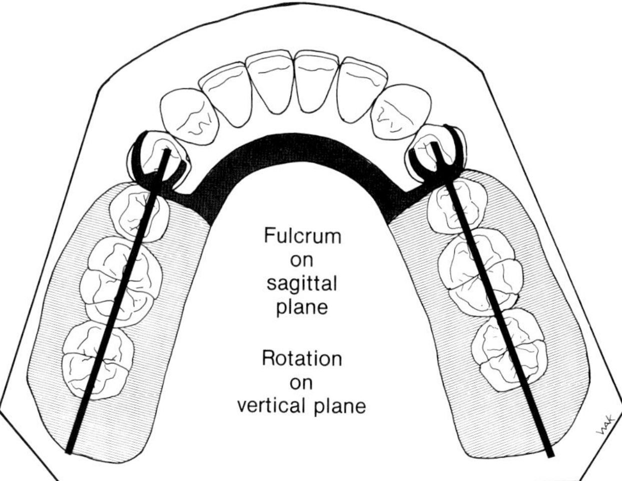

Fig. 4-10. Second rotational fulcrum extends from occlusal rest on terminal abutment posteriorly along crest of residual ridge. This fulcrum controls rocking, or side-to-side, movement that takes place over crest of ridge. In a Class I arch there are two such fulcrums.

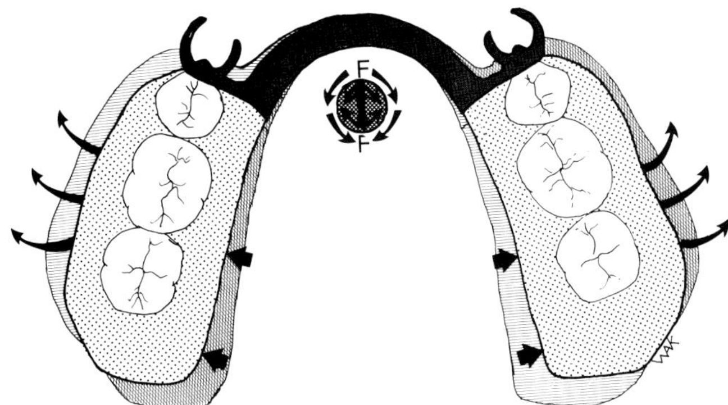

Fig. 4-11. Third fulcrum is vertical and is located in midline lingual to anterior teeth. It controls movement of denture in horizontal plane.

through two principal abutments, one on each side of the dental arch, and is termed the *fulcrum line* (Fig. 4-7). This fulcrum controls the rotational movement of the denture in the sagittal plane (denture movement toward or away from the supporting ridge). Rotational movement around this horizontal fulcrum line or axis is of the greatest magnitude of that around the three fulcrums but not necessarily the most damaging. The resulting force on the abutment teeth is usually mesial-apical or distal-apical, with the greatest vector in the apical direction (Fig. 4-8). Fibers of the periodontal ligments are so arranged that vertical forces are resisted to a much greater degree than are horizontal or torsional forces (Fig. 4-9). Horizontal or lateral forces of much less magnitude can be destructive to the supporting structures of the teeth as well as to the alveolar ridge.

A second fulcrum (Fig. 4-10) is on the sagittal plane and extends through the occlusal rest on the terminal abutment and along the crest of the residual ridge on one side of the arch. In a Class I situation there would be two of these fulcrums, one on each side of the arch. This fulcrum controls the rotational movements of the denture in the vertical plane (rocking, or side-to-side, movements over the crest of the ridge). This movement, although easier to control than the first and usually not of great magnitude, can be damaging. The main direction of the resulting force is more nearly horizontal and not well resisted by the tissues.

The third fulcrum (Fig. 4-11) is located in the vicinity of the midline just lingual to the anterior teeth. This fulcrum line is vertical, and it controls the rotational movement of the denture in the horizontal plane or the flat circular movements of the denture.

Every effort must be made in the design of a removable partial denture to control or minimize the rotational movements related to these three principal fulcrums.

FACTORS INFLUENCING MAGNITUDE OF STRESSES TRANSMITTED TO ABUTMENT TEETH

Length of span

The longer the edentulous span, the longer will be the denture base and the greater will be the force transmitted to the abutment teeth. The fulcrum is located at or near the occlusal rest on the terminal abutment tooth. The load is applied to the artificial teeth, and the length of the lever arm, the denture base, determines how much force the abutment tooth must withstand. As Archimedes wrote "Give me a lever long enough and a support strong enough and I can move the world" (Fig. 4-12). Other factors such as thickness of the mucosa over the ridge and total area of ridge covered by the denture base mitigate the amount of force resulting, but the length of the edentulous span is a factor to be aware of. When treatment is being planned, every effort should be made to retain a posterior abutment tooth to avoid a Class I or Class II situation. Preserving a posterior tooth to serve as vertical support or even as an overdenture partial denture abutment is rendering the patient an outstanding service.

Quality of support of ridge

The form of the residual ridge can play a large part in dissipating forces created by function of the partial denture. Large, well-formed ridges (Fig. 4-13) are capable of absorbing greater amounts of stress than are small, thin, or knife-edged ridges. Broad ridges with parallel sides permit the use of longer flanges on the denture base, which helps stabilize the denture against lateral forces.

The type of mucoperiosteum influences the magnitude of stresses transmitted to abutment teeth. A healthy mucoperiosteum approximately 1 mm thick is capable of bearing a greater functional load than is a thin atrophic mucosa. Soft, flabby, displaceable tissue

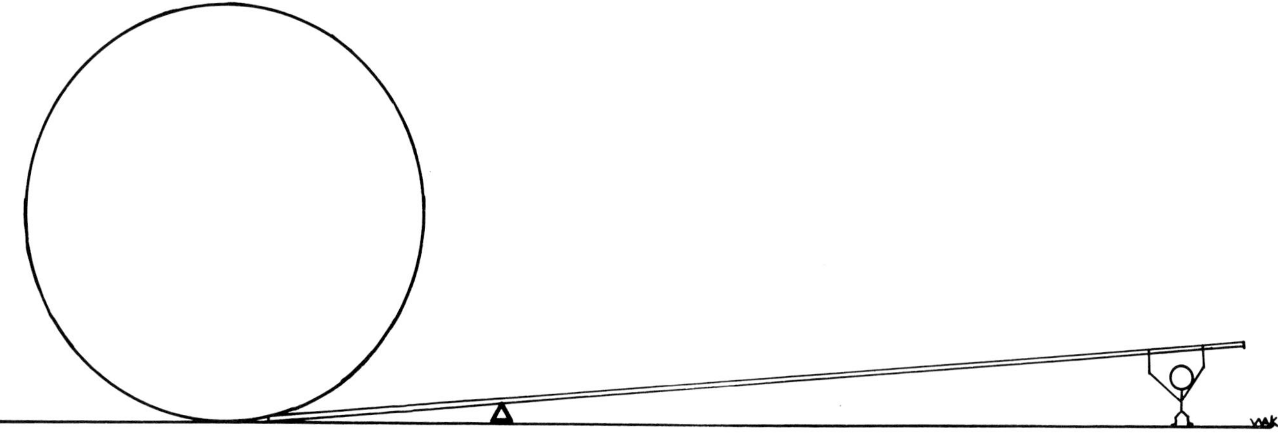

Fig. 4-12. Given a lever long enough and support strong enough, a person can move the world.

contributes little to the vertical support of the denture and nothing to the lateral stability of the denture base. This type of tissue allows excessive movement of the denture, with resultant transmission of stress to the adjacent abutment tooth.

Qualities of clasp

In the discussion of the components of the partial denture it was noted that the more flexible the retentive arm of the clasp, the less stress is transmitted to the abutment tooth. This is the reason the combination or wrought wire retentive clasp was suggested for the terminal abutments for Class I or II partial dentures in certain cases. It was also noted, however, that a flexible clasp arm contributes less resistance to the more destructive horizontal stresses (Fig. 4-14). Therefore, as the flexibility of the clasp increases, both the lateral and vertical stresses transmitted to the residual ridge increase. On the basis of findings made during the examination phase of the treatment, a decision has to be made as to whether the ridge or the abutment tooth requires the most protection. If the periodontal support of the abutment tooth is good, a less flexible clasp such as a T bar vertical projection clasp would be indicated because the tooth would more likely be able to withstand a greater amount of stress. If, on the other hand, the periodontal support has been weakened, a more flexible clasp such as the combination clasp with a wrought wire retentive arm should be used so that the residual ridge would share more of the resistance to horizontal forces acting on the partial denture.

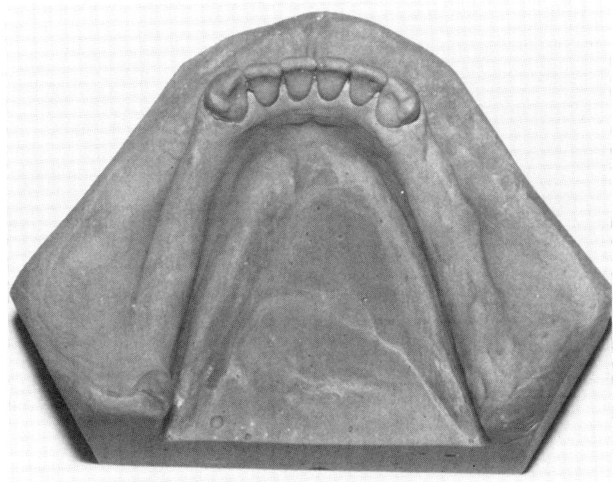

Fig. 4-13. Large, broad, well-formed ridges can absorb more stress than can knife-edged ridges.

Clasp design

A clasp that is designed so that it is passive when it is completely seated on the abutment tooth will exert less stress on the tooth than one that is not passive. Removable partial denture frameworks need to be fitted to the natural teeth to ensure that the prosthesis is completely seated. Only when the framework is completely seated will the retentive clasp arms be passive. If a retentive tip is designed and constructed to lie in a 0.010-inch undercut and the framework does not go

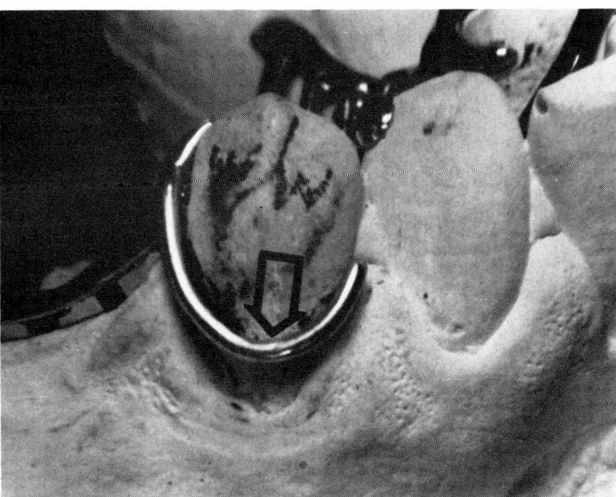

Fig. 4-14. A wrought wire clasp (arrow), which is more flexible than a cast clasp, tends to dissipate forces transmitted to abutment tooth and increase forces transferred to edentulous ridge. It also provides less horizontal stability.

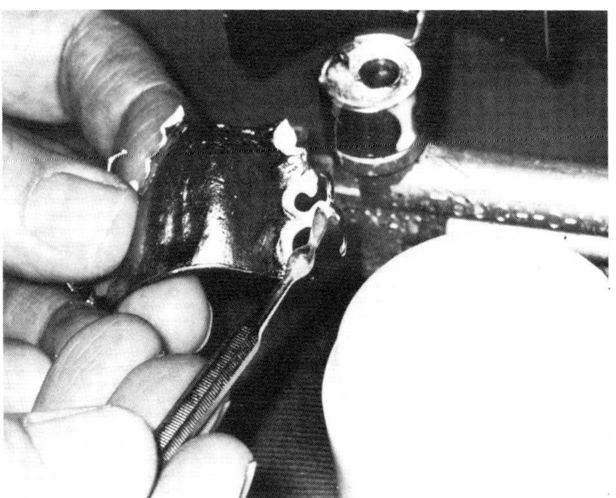

Fig. 4-15. Refining fit of cast framework to teeth is an integral part of controlling undesirable forces transmitted by framework. The more accurate the adaptation of metal to teeth, the less the tendency for teeth to be pushed or twisted. Disclosing wax is being used as refining agent.

completely to place, that retentive tip will not be passive but will exert a continuous force to the abutment tooth. Fitting of the framework is best accomplished by using a disclosing wax on the framework surfaces that contact the teeth. (Fig. 4-15). As the wax is displaced, areas of showthrough of the metal framework are adjusted until the framework is completely seated and the clasp arms become passive. The technique for fitting the framework is covered in detail in Chapter 12.

A clasp should be designed so that during insertion or removal of the prosthesis the reciprocal arm contacts the tooth before the retentive tip passes over the greatest bulge of the abutment tooth. This will stabilize or neutralize the stress to which the abutment tooth is subjected as the retentive terminal passes over the greatest bulge of the tooth.

Length of clasp

As previously mentioned, the more flexible a clasp, the less stress it will exert on the abutment tooth. Flexibility can be increased by lengthening the clasp. Doubling the length of a clasp will increase its flexibility five times. Clasp length may be increased by using a curved rather than a straight course on an abutment tooth (Fig. 4-16).

Material used in clasp construction

A clasp constructed of chrome alloy will normally exert greater stress on the abutment tooth than a gold clasp, all other factors being equal, because of the greater rigidity of the chrome alloy. To compensate for this property, clasp arms of chrome alloys are constructed with a smaller diameter than a gold clasp would be to accomplish the same purpose (Fig. 4-17).

Abutment tooth surface

The surface of a gold crown or restoration offers more frictional resistance to clasp arm movement than does the enamel surface of a tooth. Therefore, greater stress is exerted on a tooth restored with gold than on a tooth with intact enamel.

Occlusal harmony

A disharmonious occlusion, one in which deflective occlusal contacts between opposing teeth are present, generates horizontal forces that, when magnified by the factor of leverage, can transmit destructive forces to both the abutment teeth and residual ridges.

The type of opposing occlusion can play a role in determining the amount of stress generated by occlusion. Some individuals with natural teeth can exert a closing force of 300 pounds per square inch, whereas the closing force of a person wearing complete dentures may not exceed 30 pounds per square inch. Therefore a par-

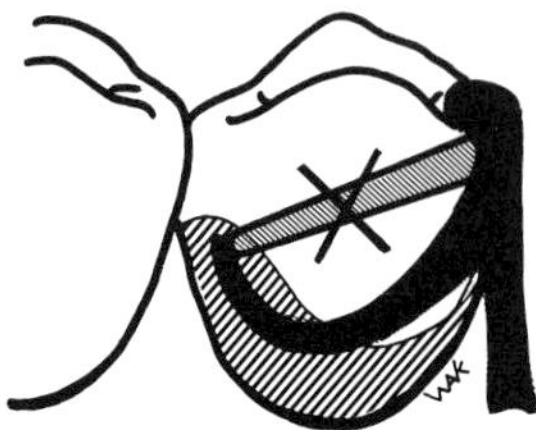

Fig. 4-16. Stress transmitted to an abutment tooth by a retentive clasp can be decreased by increasing flexibility of clasp. Because clasp flexibility is related directly to length of clasp, it can be increased by curving clasp into retentive undercut. A clasp should not cross a tooth surface in a straight line.

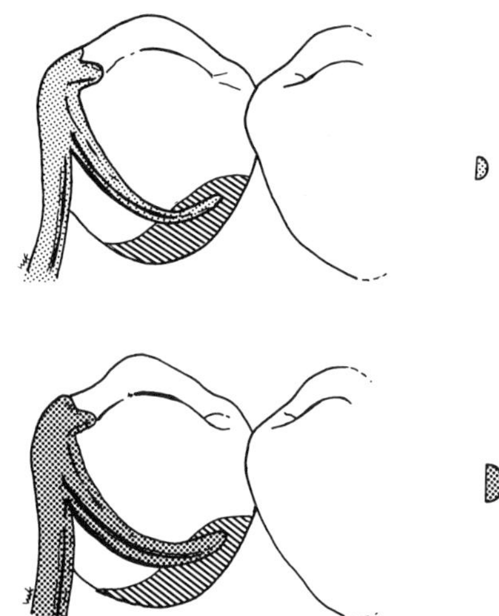

Fig. 4-17. Comparative diameter of retentive clasps designed to accomplish same purpose, one constructed of chrome alloy, top, and other constructed of gold alloy, bottom. Because of greater rigidity, chrome alloy clasp must be smaller in diameter.

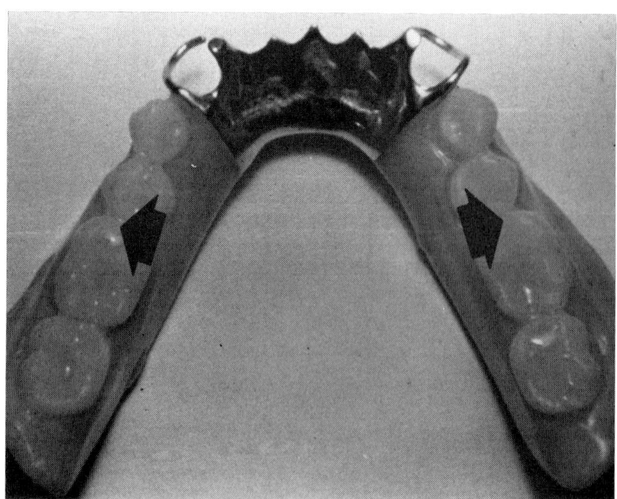

Fig. 4-18. Greatest concentration of occlusal load should be in center of denture-bearing area—usually second premolar and first molar area (arrows).

tial denture constructed to oppose a complete denture will be subjected to much less occlusal stress than one opposed by natural dentition.

The area of the denture base against which the occlusal load is applied significantly influences the amount of stress transmitted to the abutment teeth and ridge. If the occlusal load is applied to the base adjacent to the abutment tooth, there will be less movement of the denture base and less stress transmission than if the load is applied at the distal end of the denture base.

Ideally the occlusal load should be applied in the center of the denture-bearing area, both anteroposteriorly and buccolingually. In most mouths the second premolar and first molar represent the best areas for the application of the masticating load. Artificial teeth should be arranged so that the bulk of the masticating force is applied in that area (Fig. 4-18).

CONTROLLING STRESS BY DESIGN CONSIDERATIONS

It is often argued that the theoretical aspects of partial denture design are of primary importance. However, clinical observation and experience must be used to balance what should happen with what will happen. The statement "no removable partial denture can be designed or constructed that will not be destructive in the mouth" can be thoroughly justified if all rotational forces and other stresses are considered. At present there is no way that all forces can be totally countered or negated. However, long-term clinical observation has proved that a design philosophy that strives to control these forces within the physiologic tolerance of the teeth and supporting structures can be successful. Therefore the design philosophy of this book is a combination of theoretical and clinical knowledge, which a student can learn and use with predictably successful clinical results. Much too often in the past the unending arguments concerning whether a clasp exerts a destructive or a beneficial force has resulted only in the student being confused and rejecting any attempt to design a removable partial denture. If the book tends to oversimplify the design process, it is done with the ultimate desire that the student or the dentist will accomplish the design and not allow the technician to do a clinically oriented procedure.

Direct retention

The retentive clasp arm is the element of the partial denture that is responsible for transmitting most of the destructive forces to the abutment teeth. A removable partial denture should always be designed to keep clasp retention to a minimum yet provide adequate retention to prevent dislodgement of the denture by unseating forces.

Other components of a denture, considered in the following discussion, used to contribute to the retention of the prosthesis so that the amount of retention provided by clasps can be reduced. Exploiting this retentive potential in widely separated areas of the mouth can result in stress on the abutment teeth being effectively reduced; the support and stability of the prosthesis may be enhanced as well.

Forces of adhesion and cohesion

To secure the maximum possible retention through the use of the forces of adhesion and cohesion, the denture base should cover the maximum area of available support and must be accurately adapted to the underlying mucosa (Fig. 4-19). Adhesion is the attraction of saliva to the denture and the tissues, and cohesion is the internal attraction of the molecules of saliva for each other. Although it is not possible to develop a complete peripheral seal around the borders of a partial denture because of the presence of the teeth, atmospheric pressure may still contribute a slight amount of retention. This may be noted in particular on a maxillary complete palate major connector when an accurate metal casting is used and the margins of the connector are beaded. A partial vacuum can occur beneath the major connector or denture base, or both.

Frictional control

The partial denture should be designed so that *guide planes* are created on as many teeth as possible (Fig. 4-20). Guide planes are areas on teeth that are created so that they are parallel to each other and parallel to the

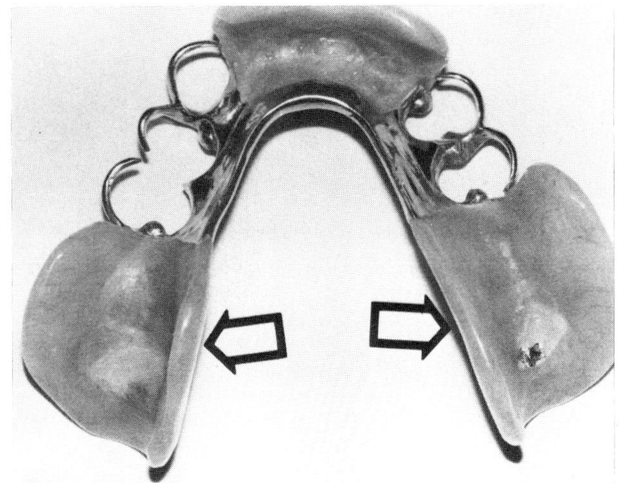

Fig. 4-19. To enhance quality of retention through adhesion and cohesion, denture base (arrows) must fit edentulous ridge accurately and must cover maximum area of available support.

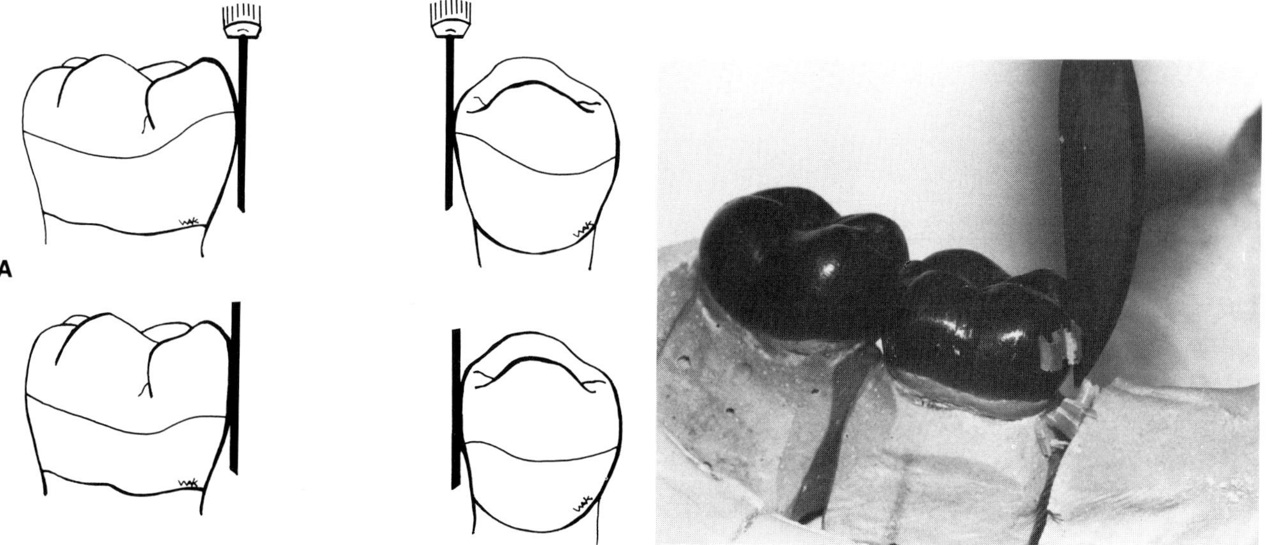

Fig. 4-20. Development of guide planes on proximal surfaces of teeth adjacent to edentulous spaces will increase retention of partial denture by frictional contact. These guide planes may be created in enamel surfaces, A, Or in restorations placed on the teeth, B.

path the denture takes as it is inserted and withdrawn from the mouth. The planes may be created on the enamel surfaces of the teeth or in restorations placed on the teeth. The frictional contact of the prosthesis against these parallel surfaces can contribute significantly to the retention of the denture.

Neuromuscular control

The innate ability of the patient to control the action of the lips, cheeks, and tongue can be a major factor in the retention of a denture. A patient who lacks the ability or coordination to control the movement of these tissues may not be able to retain a prosthesis. The design and contour of the denture base can greatly affect the patient's ability to retain the prosthesis. Any overextension of the denture base either facially, lingually in the mandible, or posteriorly onto the soft palate will contribute to the loss of retention, and the abutment teeth bearing the direct retainers will be overly stressed because of the denture's being constantly dislodged. A properly contoured denture base, however, can aid the patient's neuro-muscular control of the prosthesis (Fig. 4-21).

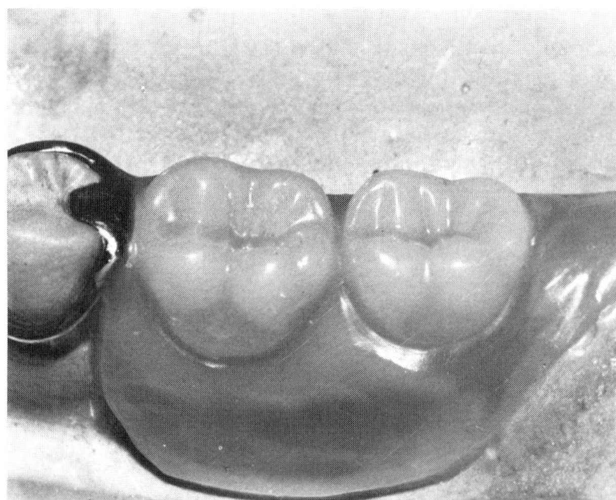

Fig. 4-21. Properly contoured borders of a denture base can aid in retention by permitting patient to use neuromuscular skills to avoid dislodging base. Overextended denture bases will constantly be unseated by action of border tissues.

Clasp position

Most people who design removable partial dentures use too many retentive clasps. Usually the position or the relation of the retentive clasp to the height of contour is more important in retention and in controlling stress than is the number of clasps. The number of clasps that should be used in the design is most often dictated by the classification.

Quadrilateral configuration. The quadrilateral configuration (Fig. 4-22) is indicated most often for Class III arches, particularly when there is a modification space on the opposite side of the arch. A retentive clasp should be positioned on each abutment tooth adjacent to the edentulous spaces. This results in the denture being confined within the outline of the four clasps, and

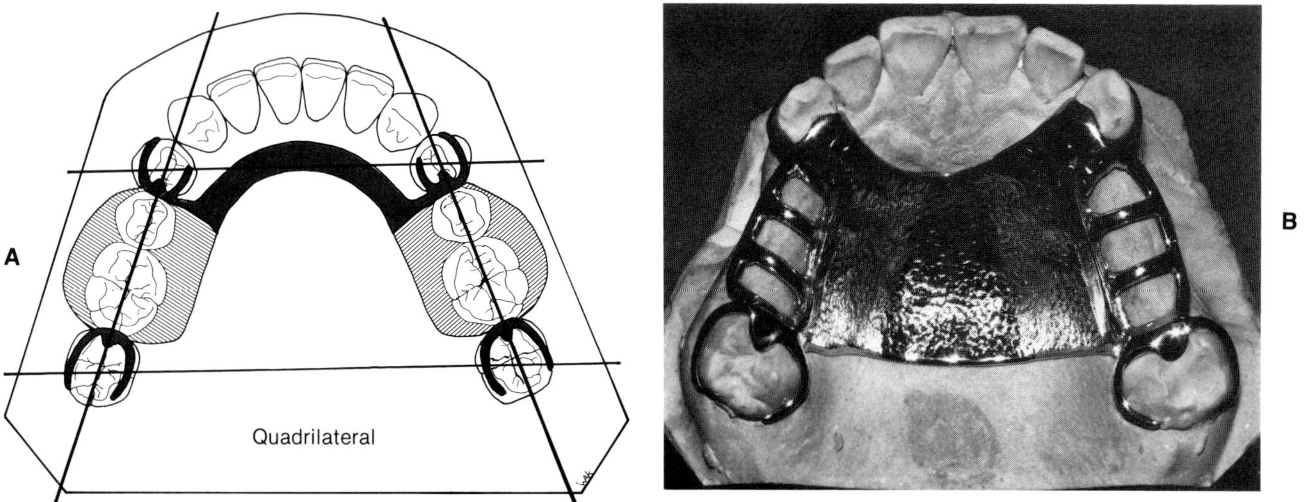

Fig. 4-22. Quadrilateral clasping consists of a retentive clasp at each end of edentulous space. This provides maximum in retention and stability.

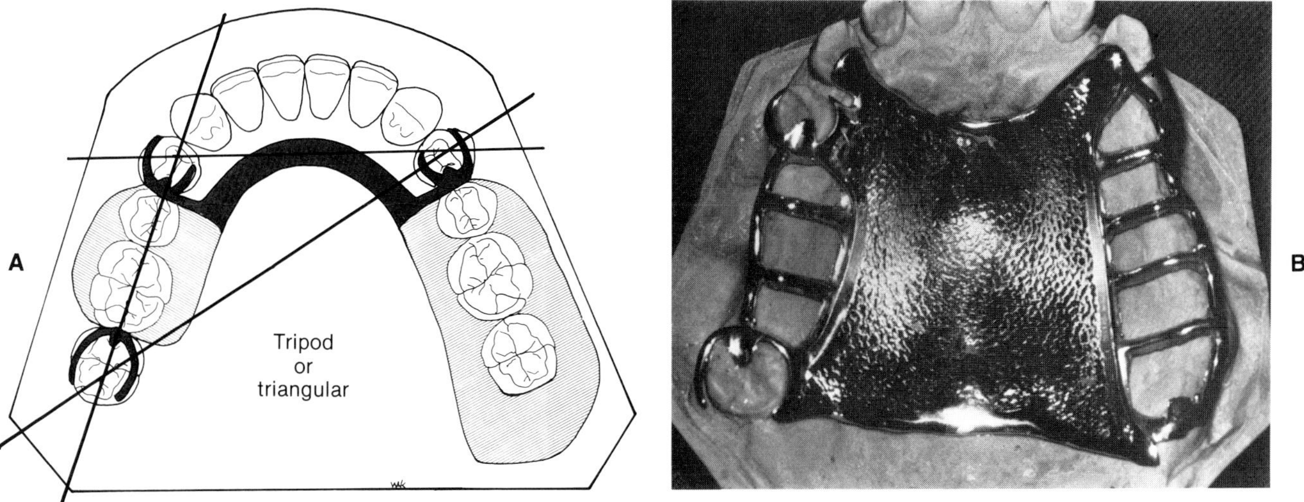

Fig. 4-23. A, Triangular, or tripod, configuration is ideal for a Class II arch. **B,** If a modification space is present, teeth adjacent to that space are clasped. If no modification space exists, clasps of dentulous side should be separated as much as possible, one as far anteriorly as esthetics and occlusion permit, and one as far posteriorly as possible.

leverage on the denture is effectively neutralized. For a Class III arch where no modification space exists, the goal should be to place one clasp as far posterior on the dentulous side as possible and one as far anterior as space and esthetics permit. This retains the quadrilateral concept and is the most effective way to control stress.

Tripod configuration. Tripod clasping (Fig. 4-23) is used primarily for Class II arches. If there is a modification space on the dentulous side, the teeth anterior and posterior to the space are clasped and the terminal abutment on the distal extension side is clasped to bring about the tripod configuration. If a modification space is not present, one clasp on the dentulous side of the arch should be positioned as far posterior as possible, and the other, as far anterior as factors such as interocclusal space, retentive undercut, and esthetic considerations will permit. By separating the two

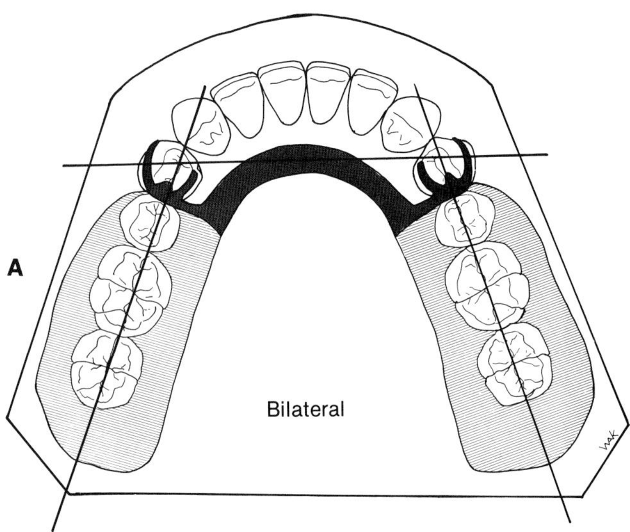

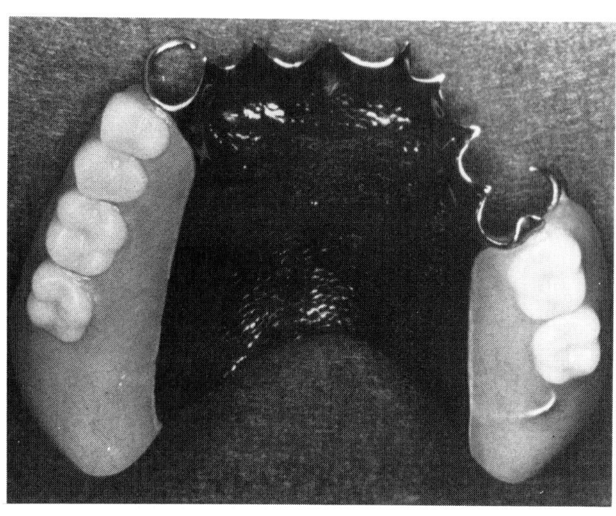

Fig. 4-24. A, For a Class I partially edentulous arch, a bilateral clasping configuration is required. Although this configuration cannot be considered ideal, it is best for problem at hand. **B,** Bilateral clasping for maxillary Class I removable partial denture.

abutments on the tooth-supported side as far as possible, the largest possible area of the denture will be enclosed in the triangle formed by the retentive clasps. This design is not as effective as the quadrilateral configuration, but is most effective in neutralizing leverage in the class II situation.

Bilateral configuration. Unfortunately most removable partial dentures fall into the bilateral distal extension group, or Class I (Fig 4-24). Ideally, the single retentive clasp on each side of the arch should be located near the center of the dental arch or denture-bearing area. For practical purposes, however, the terminal abutment tooth on each side of the arch must be clasped regardless of where it is positioned. In the bilateral configuration the clasps exert little neutralizing effect on the leverage-induced stresses generated by the denture base. These stresses must be controlled by other means.

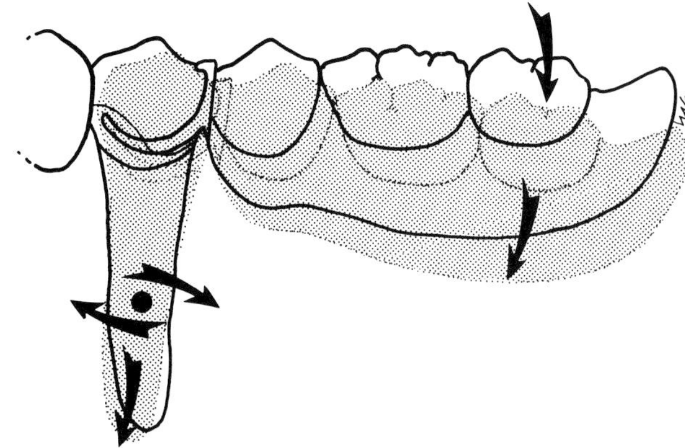

Fig. 4-25. As force directed toward tissue occurs on distal extension denture base, rotational forces take place around distal occlusal rest. Cast circumferential clasp places an extremely destructive distal tipping or torquing force on abutment tooth (arrows).

Clasp design

Circumferential cast clasp. The conventional circumferential cast clasp originating from a distal occlusal rest on the terminal abutment tooth and engaging a mesiobuccal retentive undercut should *not* be used on a distal extension removable partial denture. The terminal of this clasp reacts to movement of the denture base toward the tissue by placing a distal tipping, or torquing, force on the abutment tooth (Fig. 4-25). This particular force is the most destructive force a retentive clasp can exert. This clasping concept must be avoided at all costs.

The reverse circlet, a cast circumferential clasp that approaches a distobuccal undercut from the mesial surface of a terminal abutment tooth, is acceptable (Fig. 4-26). The effect on the abutment tooth is reversed from that of the conventional circumferential clasp. As an occlusal load is applied to the denture base, the retentive terminal moves further gingivally into the undercut area and loses contact with the abutment tooth. In this manner torque is not transmitted to the abutment tooth. The reverse circlet clasp, because it normally projects between two teeth, may produce some wedging force. This can usually be countered by occlusal rests on the approximating surfaces of both teeth.

Vertical projection, or bar, clasp. The vertical projection, or bar, clasp is used on the terminal abutment tooth on a distal extension partial denture when the re-

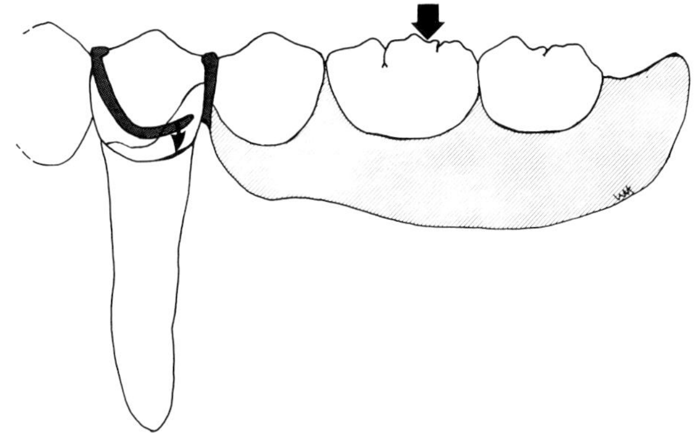

Fig. 4-26. A reverse circlet clasp, approaching a distobuccal undercut from mesial occlusal surface, may be acceptable for a distal extension partial denture. As denture base moves toward the tissue, retentive clasp tip will tend to move into an area of greater undercut (arrow). This action releases torquing forces that can damage an abutment tooth.

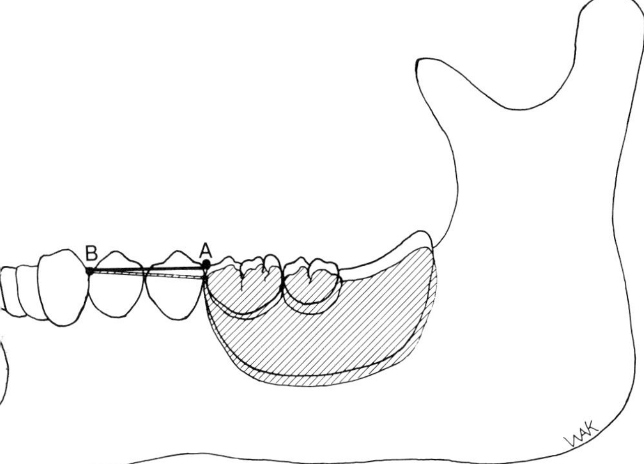

Fig. 4-28. One advantage claimed for eliminating distal occlusal rest *(A)* and placing a mesial rest more anteriorly *(B)* is that lever arm, represented by distance from rest to denture base, is increased. This increase in length makes rotational action caused by up-and-down movement of denture base in function more vertical. A vertical force is better tolerated by ridge than is a horizontal oblique force.

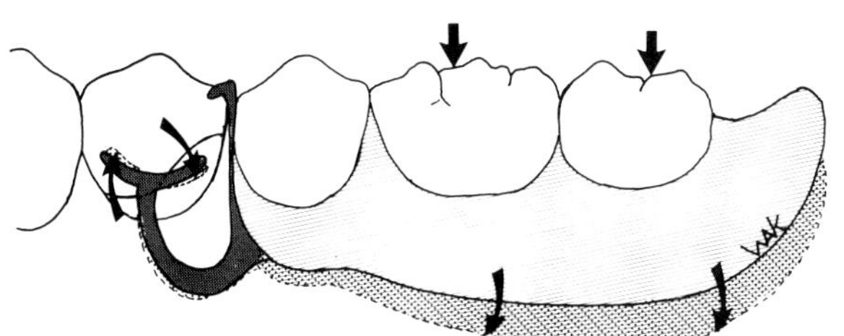

Fig. 4-27. The vertical projection T clasp releases torsional stress on terminal abutment tooth. This releasing action is accomplished when retentive clasp tip rotates gingivally into a greater undercut as tissueward forces are applied to denture base (arrows). Rotation takes place around distal occlusal rest.

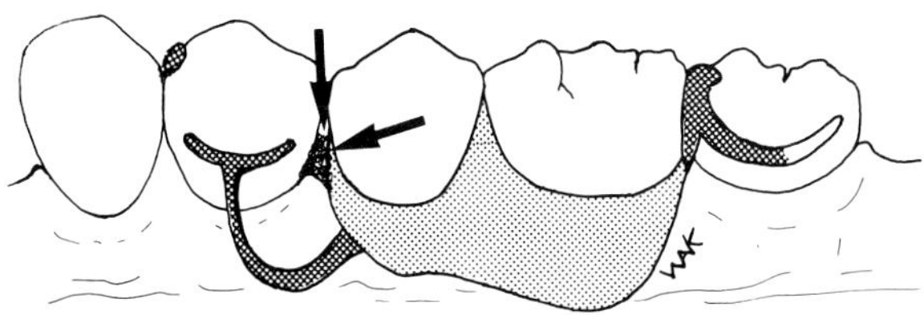

Fig. 4-29. Omitting a rest adjacent to an edentulous space permits packing of food between minor connector of partial denture and tooth (arrows). This area is susceptible to injury.

tentive undercut is located on the distobuccal surface. It is never indicated when the tooth has a mesiobuccal undercut.

The bar clasp functions in a manner similar to the reverse circumferential clasp. As the denture base is loaded toward the tissue, the retentive tip of the T clasp rotates gingivally to release the stress being transmitted to the abutment tooth (Fig. 4-27). The bar clasp does not produce the wedging force sometimes produced by the reverse circumferential clasp.

One school of thought on the philosophy of removable partial denture design has advocated omitting the distal occlusal rest from the terminal abutment in favor of a mesial rest when a bar clasp is used. The belief is that a distal rest would cause the fulcrum line around which the denture tends to rotate to be distal to the retentive clasp terminal. Theoretically the retentive tip could not release if the denture base were to move toward the tissue. Another advantage claimed for moving the occlusal rest more anteriorly is that the lever arm (the distance from the rest to the denture base) is increased, which causes the force directed toward the residual ridge to be more vertical and thus better tolerated by the ridge (Fig. 4-28).

These advantages must be weighted very carefully against certain disadvantages. If the distal rest, or a rest adjacent to any endentulous space, is omitted, a space is left between the framework and tooth surface in which food debris will collect and be trapped against the most critical and sensitive area of the tooth, the gingival crevice (Fig 4-29). It may be argued that a properly prepared guiding plane will prevent this food impaction, but as long as there is space enough to provide for the vertical movement of the minor connector, a space will exist. If vertical movement does not or cannot take place, then the advantage in repositioning the rest is lost.

A number of research reports on the effect of various clasping schemes for terminal abutments have been written. The consensus of these reports is that the clasp that subjects the abutment tooth to the least unfavorable torque is the T clasp with a distal-occlusal rest and a rigid circumferential reciprocating clasp.

Combination clasp. When a mesiobuccal undercut exists on an abutment tooth adjacent to a distal extension edentulous ridge, the combination clasp can be employed to reduce the stress transmitted to the abutment tooth. Wrought alloy wire, by virtue of its internal structure, is more flexible than a cast clasp. It can flex in any spatial plane, whereas a cast clasp flexes in the horizontal plane only. The wrought wire retentive arm has a stress-breaking action that can absorb torsional stress in both the vertical and horizontal planes. A cast circumferential clasp under the same circumstance would transmit most of the leverage-induced stress to the abutment tooth.

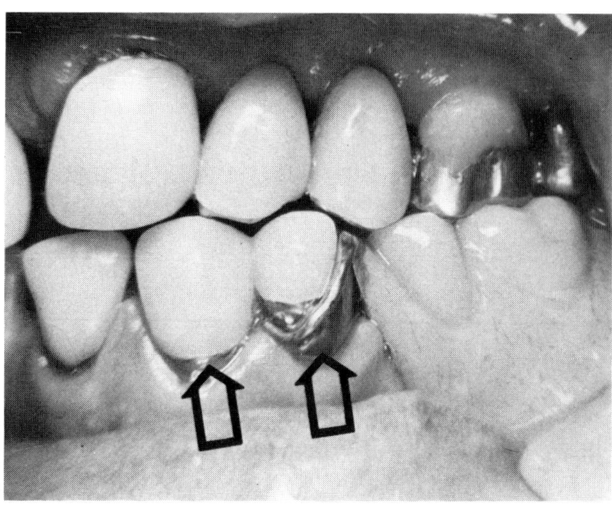

Fig. 4-30. Canine and first premolar have been splinted by acrylic resin veneer crowns (arrows) to increase periodontal membrane area and distribute applied stress over a greater area.

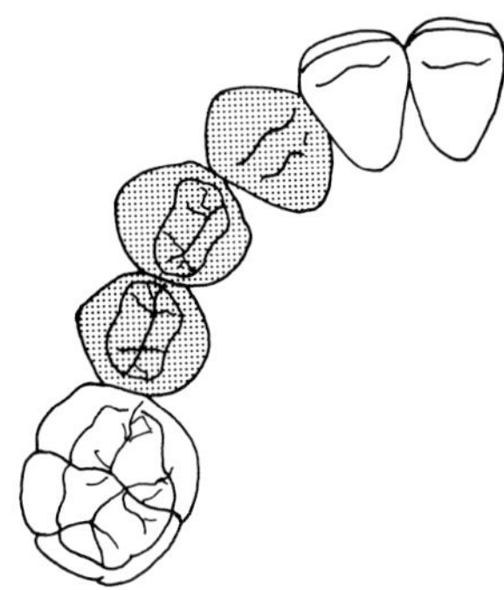

Fig. 4-31. For a splint to stablize teeth in a buccolingual direction, splint must extend around curve of arch. Canine would have to be included in splint.

Splinting of abutment teeth

Adjacent teeth may be splinted by means of crowns to control stress transmitted to a weak abutment tooth (Fig. 4-30). Splinting two or more teeth actually increases the periodontal ligament attachment area and distributes the stress over a larger area of support.

Splinting by means of crowns also has the effect of stabilizing the abutment teeth in a mesiodistal or anteroposterior direction. If one of the included abutment teeth in the fixed splint is a canine or if the splint extends anteriorly around the curve of the arch, the abutment teeth will be stabilized in the buccolingual direction as well (Fig. 4-31). Two posterior teeth, molar or premolar, splinted together will not improve the buccolingual resistance to stress. The removable partial denture will provide the needed cross-arch stabilization and will help resist lateral or horizontal forces.

Fixed splinting may be indicated when some loss of periodontal attachment has occurred after periodontal disease and therapy. It is seldom beneficial to splint an extremely weak abutment tooth to a strong tooth; the result is to weaken the strong abutment rather than to strengthen the weak one.

Splinting is also indicated when the proposed abutment tooth has either a tapered root or short roots such that there is not an acceptable amount of periodontal ligament attachment present. The tying together of two such teeth by crowns will in effect produce an acceptable multirooted abutment tooth (Fig. 4-32).

One of the most important and frequently indicated needs for splinting is when the terminal abutment tooth on the distal extension side of the arch stands alone, that is, an edentulous space exists both anterior and posterior to it. This situation is most often seen in second premolars, both maxillary and mandibular. Such a premolar is potentially a weak abutment because of the rotational forces it must withstand. Splinting of this tooth to the tooth anterior to it, usually the canine, should be accomplished with a fixed partial denture (Fig. 4-33).

Splinting by means of clasps (Fig. 4-34) on the removable partial denture is possible under some condi-

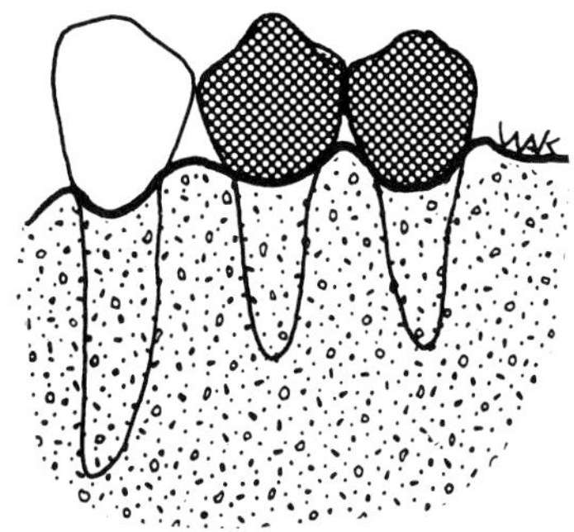

Fig. 4-32. When roots of a proposed abutment tooth are short or conical, splinting to an adjacent tooth may in effect produce a multirooted abutment tooth.

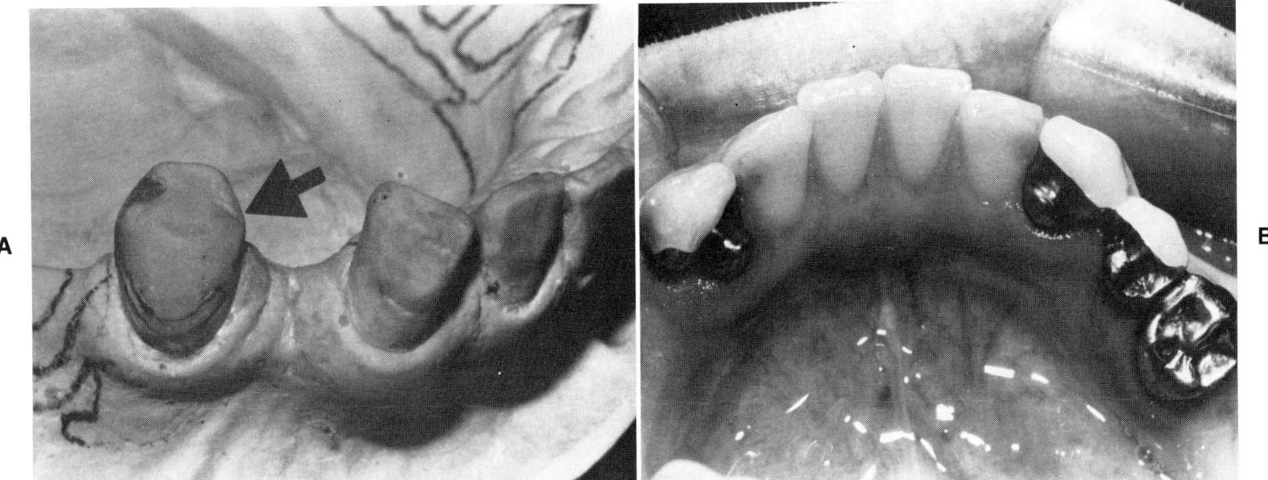

Fig. 4-33. A, An isolated premolar (arrow) is a weak abutment tooth. B, Normally this tooth should be splinted to canine with a three-unit fixed partial denture.

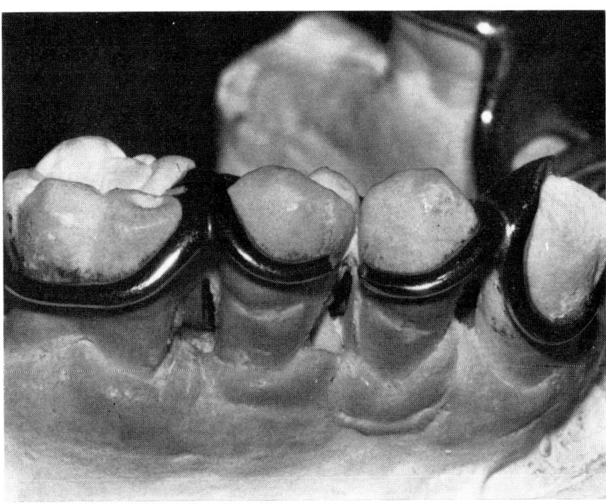

Fig. 4-34. Periodontally weakened teeth can be stabilized against horizontal forces by a removable partial denture. Multiple rests and clasps are used to contribute this horizontal stabilization. Not all clasps should be retentive. Some are positioned above height of contour and are used for stabilization only.

tions. This should not be attempted if fixed splinting is possible because it is considered a compromise form of treatment. It is indicated when no other approach is feasible. The splinting consists of clasping more than one tooth on each side of the arch, using a number of rests for additional support and stabilization, and preparing guiding planes on as many teeth as possible to contribute to horizontal stabilization of the teeth and the prosthesis. The multiple clasps should not all be retentive. Research has shown that if periodontally weakened teeth are supported rigidly, their mobility will either decrease or remain the same. Most of the clasp arms, both buccal and lingual, will not pass over the greatest bulge of the tooth and enter undercuts.

A principal advantage of splinting with a removable prosthesis is cross-arch stabilization. The teeth on both sides of the arch, supported by lingual plating, can be held together rigidly to prevent damage from horizontal forces.

Other forms of removable prostheses such as the swing-lock partial denture can be used to splint teeth effectively. These special partial dentures are discussed in detail in Chapter 20.

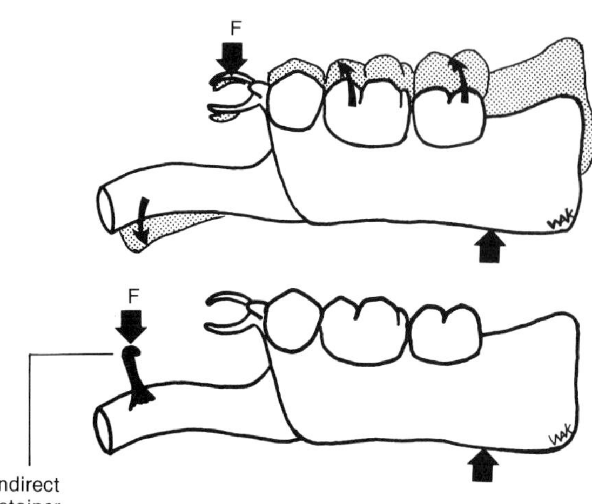

Fig. 4-35. Top, forces attempting to move denture base away from the residual ridge cause rotational movement around a fulcrum line *(F)* located near retentive clasps. Bottom, placement of a rest anterior to fulcrum line provides indirect retention. Fulcrum line *(F)* is moved to rest, which is farther from force attempting to unseat denture base. This changes lever from Class I to Class II, which reduces potential for movement of denture base.

Indirect retention

An indirect retainer is a part of the removable partial denture that helps the direct retainer prevent displacement of the distal extension denture by resisting the rotational movement of the denture around the fulcrum line established by the occlusal rests. The indirect retainer is located on the opposite side of the fulcrum line from the denture base. The action of the indirect retainer is discussed in Chapter 3.

The indirect retainer is essential in the design of Classes I and II partial dentures. By using the mechanical advantage of leverage (Fig. 4-35), it counteracts the forces attempting to move the denture base away from the residual ridge by moving the fulcrum farther from the force. In a Class I prosthesis the fulcrum line would be moved from the tips of the retentive clasp to the most anteriorly located component, the indirect retainer.

Because the indirect retainer resists lifting forces at the end of a long lever arm, it must be positioned in a definite rest seat so that the transmitted forces are diverted apically through the long axis of the abutment tooth.

The indirect retainer also contributes, to a lesser degree, to the support and stability of the denture.

The need for indirect retainers varies with the type of removable partial denture.

In a Class I arch indirect retention must always be used. The indirect retainer or retainers must be positioned as far anterior to the fulcrum line as possible. (Fig. 4-36).

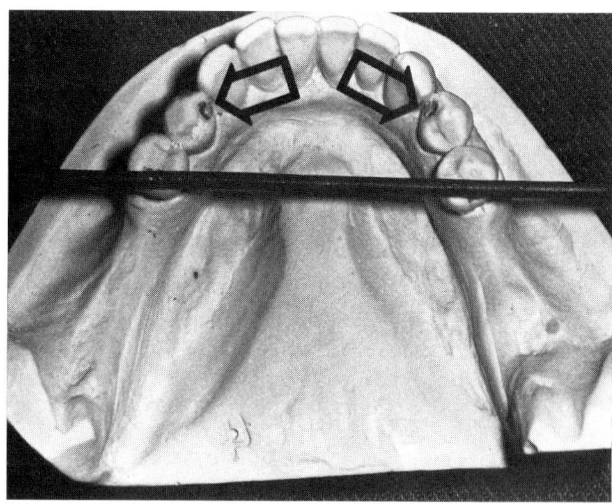

Fig. 4-36. Fulcrum line of a Class I partially edentulous arch runs through distal occlusal rests of terminal abutment teeth. Two indirect retainers should be used, one on each side of arch. Indirect retainer should be positioned as far anterior to fulcrum line as strength of remaining teeth will permit. In instance shown, mesial fossa of first premolar has been selected (arrows). Incisal rests on canines might also have been considered.

Although indirect retention is not as critical in a Class II arch as in a Class I arch, it is still required. If a modification space exists on the tooth-supported side, abutment teeth on both sides of the space should be selected. The fulcrum line will run through the most posterior abutment on the tooth-supported side and the terminal abutment on the distal extension side (Fig. 4-

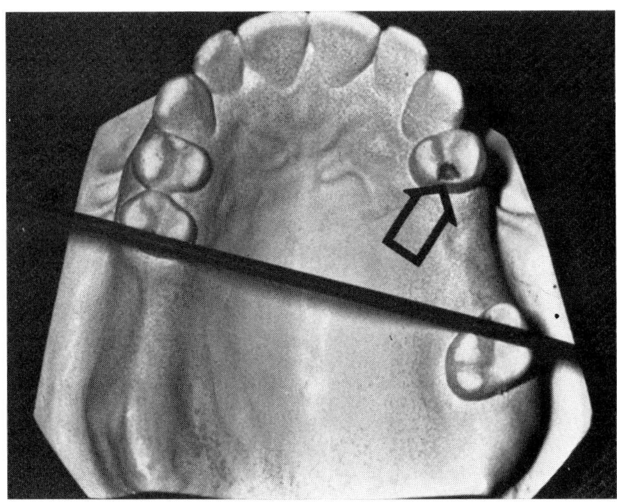

Fig. 4-37. In a Class II partially edentulous arch with a modification space, fulcrum line runs through the most posterior occlusal rests. It is around this line that rotational movement in sagittal plane takes place. A single indirect retainer is needed on side of arch opposite distal extension edentulous ridge. In this case distal occlusal rest on first premolar can act as indirect retainer (arrow).

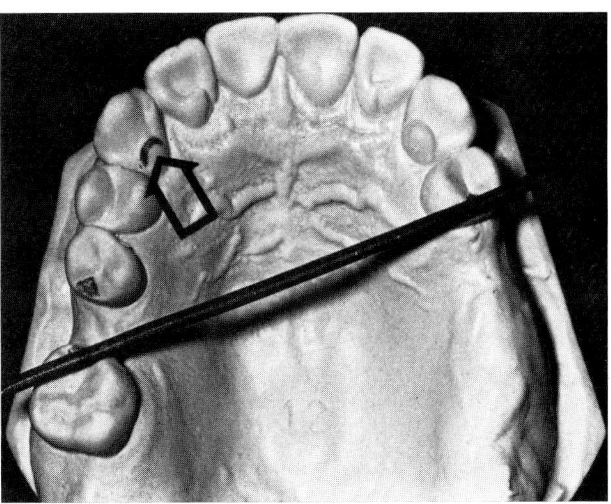

Fig. 4-38. If modification space is not sufficiently long for occlusal rest on abutment tooth anterior to edentulous space to act as an indirect retainer, another rest should be placed to provide indirect retention. In this case a lingual rest was placed on canine (arrow). This rest is as far anterior to fulcrum line as can be properly used.

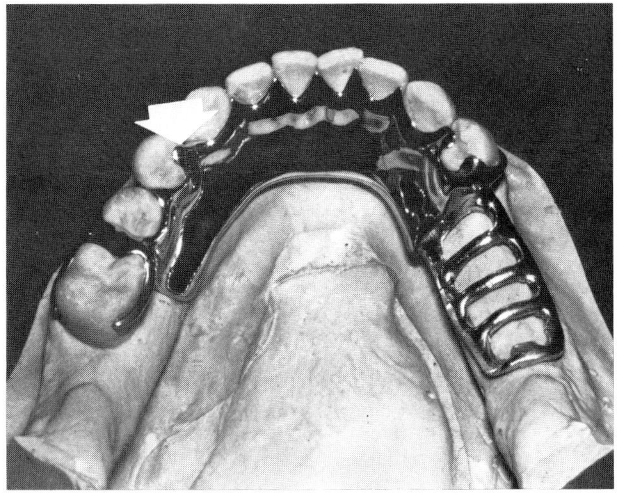

Fig. 4-39. For Class II partially edentulous arch with no modification space, one clasp on dentulous side should be positioned as far posterior as possible, in this case on left first molar. An indirect retainer must be selected as far anterior as practical. In case shown an occlusal rest in mesial fossa of first premolar was used (arrow). Second premolar was also clasped (not shown) to complete triangular clasp configuration.

37). The most anterior abutment on the tooth-supported side, with its rest and clasp assembly, may be located far enough anterior to the fulcrum line to serve as the indirect retainer. However, a definite rest seat positioned even farther anterior, if possible, may increase the effectiveness of the indirect retention, (Fig. 4-38).

If there is no modification space in the tooth-supported side of the arch, the most posterior tooth on that side with favorable contours for clasping should be used as one abutment (Fig. 4-39). This design places the fulcrum line in a posterior position, allowing the indirect retainer to be placed farther from the fulcrum line. To develop a good triangular configuration of clasping, an additional abutment tooth with suitable contours for clasping should be selected as far anterior on the tooth-supported side as possible. This abutment tooth, with its rest and clasp assembly, may serve as the indirect retainer if it is located far enough anterior to the fulcrum line.

For the Class III arch, indirect retention is not ordinarly required because there is no distal extension denture base to create a lever arm. However, auxiliary rests may be needed to provide additional vertical support for a long lingual bar major connector or an extensive palatal major connector. Auxiliary rests are always indicated for support of a lingual plate major connector (Fig. 4-40).

There are times when the contours of the posterior abutment teeth of a Class II or III partial denture are not suitable for retention and the prognosis for the teeth may be such as not to warrant construction of cast gold restorations. These teeth, even with reduced periodontal support, can usually provide support and stability for the prosthesis. An occlusal rest and nonretentive stablizing clasp should be designed for them. Under these circumstances the clasp design for the an-

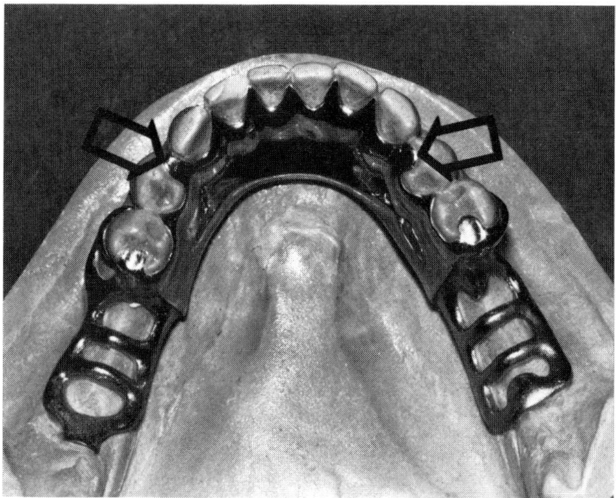

Fig. 4-40. A lingual plate major connector must always be supported at each end of anterior teeth by rests. Vertical support supplied by rests prevents lingual plate from shunting incisor teeth anteriorly because of an inclined plane action. Mesial fossae of both first premolars (arrows) are used to provide vertical support for lingual plate and to act as indirect retainers.

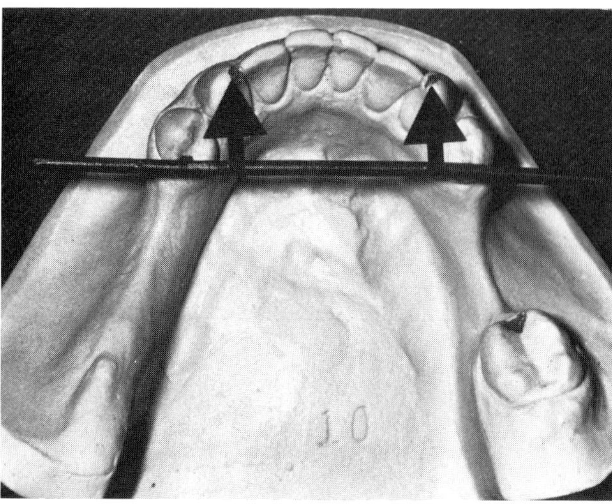

Fig. 4-41. If contours of posterior teeth for a Class II (shown here) or III partially edentulous arch do not permit use of retentive clasps, design of partial denture must provide for indirect retainers. Without posterior retention, rotation will take place around fulcrum line, posterior rests of anterior abutment teeth. In case shown, mesial incisal rests on canine have been selected for indirect retention.

terior abutment teeth need not be the same as for the terminal abutments on a Class I or II partial denture, but indirect retention is required. (Fig. 4-41).

The consideration for the Class IV arch is the reverse of that for Class I and Class II arches, and the design of the partial denture, in order to resist the rotational forces in the opposite direction, must also be reversed. The lever arm is anterior to the fulcrum line, so the indirect retainer must be located as far posterior as possible. Occlusal rests and clasp assemblies are placed on the most posterior teeth with favorable contours for both direct retention and support. (Fig. 4-42).

Occlusion

A smoothly functioning occlusion that is in harmony with the movements of both the temperomandibular joints and the neuromusculature will minimize the stress transferred to the abutment teeth and residual ridge.

Neither the metal of the framework nor the artificial teeth of the partial denture should receive the initial occlusal contact as the jaws come together. They should not guide the movement of the mandible in protrusive or lateral movements. They must be coordinated with mandibular movements and the guiding influence of the remaining natural teeth. The contacts of the remaining natural teeth must be the same when the removable partial denture is in the mouth as when the prosthesis is not in place.

The occlusal surfaces, or food table, of the artificial

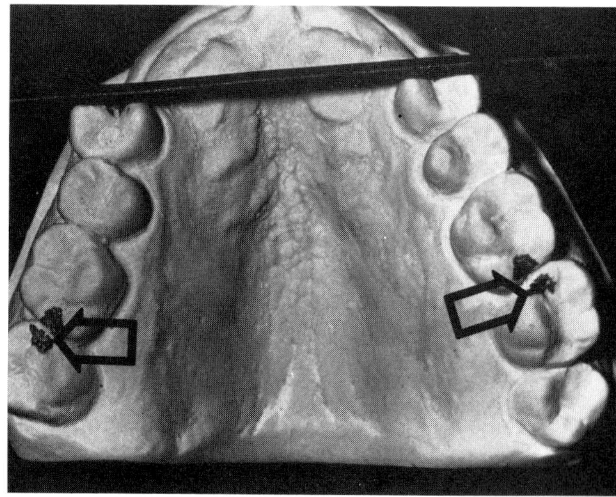

Fig. 4-42. For Class IV arch, lever arm is anterior to fulcrum line, mesial occlusal rest of anterior teeth. Rotational forces will occur around fulcrum line in a direction opposite to that in Class I or II arch. Therefore indirect retainer is positioned posterior to fulcrum line. For this patient, indirect retainers are shown as distal occlusal rests on first molars and mesial occlusal rests on second molars (arrows).

teeth can transmit various amounts of stress to the supporting structures. A large or broad occlusal surface delivers more stress than does one that has been reduced in buccolingual width. The number of teeth being replaced may also be reduced to decrease the stress.

Artificial posterior teeth should possess sharp cutting

surfaces and sluiceways for the escape of food between the teeth to be as efficient as possible and to relieve some of the unnecessary force in mastication. Steep cuspal inclines on the artifical teeth should be avoided because they tend to introduce horizontal forces that can produce torsional stresses on the abutment teeth.

Denture base

The denture base should be designed to cover as extensive an area of supporting tissue as possible. The stress created by the partial denture in function will thus be distributed over a large area, so no single area will be subjected to stress beyond its physiologic limit.

The denture base flanges should be made as long as possible to help stabilize the denture against horizontal movements.

The distal extension denture bases must always extend onto the retromolar pad area of the mandible and cover the entire tuberosity in the maxilla. Both structures are capable of absorbing more stress than is the alveolar ridge anterior to them.

Equal care must be taken not to overextend the borders of the denture base. Interference with the functional movements of the surrounding tissues by an overextension will produce and transmit significant stresses to the remaining teeth.

The more accurate the adaptation of the denture base to the residual ridge, the better will be the retention, in part because of the forces of adhesion and cohesion. There will be less tendency for the denture base to move in function, and as a result less stress will be transmitted to the abutment teeth.

The type of impressions used to record the mucoperiosteum of the residual ridge will influence the amount of stress the residual ridge can effectively absorb. The mucosa of the ridge is displaceable to varying degrees and can be recorded with a free-flowing impression material. An impression is made of the supporting or functional form of the residual ridge while the soft tissues are subjected to an occlusal load. This is accomplished by using a slowly flowing or slightly resistant impression material or by using a selectively relieved impression tray. This special tray permits more occlusal pressure to be applied to portions of the ridge that are capable of bearing greater stress.

Several techniques are used to make this functional impression of the residual ridge. Each technique is based on the theory that if the ridge were recorded in its functional state rather than in its resting form, when the denture base is actually subjected to occlusal loading, the tissue would not be displaced to any great extent. The magnitude of the stress transmitted to the abutment teeth, therefore, would be minimal. The clinical technique used to develop this functional or selected pressure form of the residual ridge is discussed in Chapter 13.

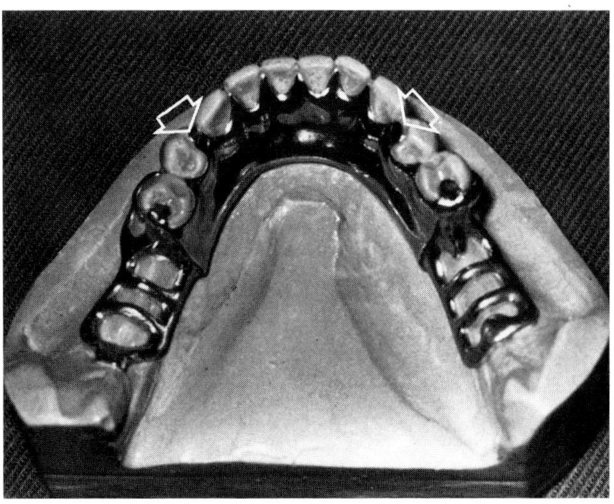

Fig. 4-43. Major connector, in this case anterior lingual plate, can help control functional stresses on remaining teeth. By contacting a number of teeth, major connector reduces amount of force transmitted to each tooth. Major connector must be supported by rests at each end of anterior span (arrows).

The contours of the polished surface of the denture base need to be developed in order to assist in retention of the denture. If done properly, this will reduce movement of the partial denture and thereby decrease the stress transferred to the abutment teeth and supporting tissues.

Major connector

In the mandibular arch the lingual plate major connector that is properly supported by rests can aid in the distribution of functional stresses to the remaining teeth (Fig. 4-43). It is particularly effective in supporting periodontally weakened anterior teeth.

The lingual plate also adds rigidity to the major connector. The added rigidity contributes to the effectiveness of cross-arch stabilization. Stresses created on one side of the arch are transmitted through the major connector to the teeth on the opposite side, thus reducing the stress applied to any single portion of the arch.

In the maxillary arch the use of a broad palatal major connector that contacts several of the remaining natural teeth through lingual plating can distribute stress over a large area. (Fig. 4-44). The major connector must be rigid and must receive vertical support through rests from several teeth.

The hard palate often provides a valuable area for support. A maxillary major connector that uses maximum coverage of this area can contribute greatly to the support, stability, and retention of the prosthesis. This

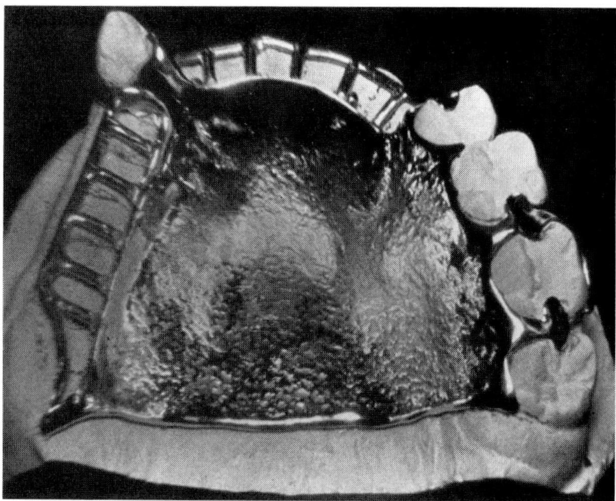

Fig. 4-44. In maxillary arch, major connector should cover a broad area of bony palate to distribute functional forces and prevent excessive forces on individual teeth. In this case few natural teeth remain, so a complete palate major connector that contacts lingual surfaces of all remaining teeth was used. Functional forces will be distributed as widely as possible.

in turn substantially reduces the stress that ordinarily would be transferred to the abutment teeth.

Minor connector

The most intimate tooth-to–partial denture contact takes place between the minor connector joining the clasp assembly to the major connector and the guiding planes on the abutment tooth surface. This close metal-to-enamel contact serves two purposes. First, it offers horizontal stability to the partial denture against lateral forces on the prosthesis. The tooth with its supporting bone helps dissipate these displacing stresses. Second, through the contact of the minor connector and the abutment tooth, the tooth receives stabilization against lateral stresses.

Because lateral forces are the most destructive, their control is essential. If guiding planes on additional abutment teeth are incorporated, the force resisted by each tooth can be minimized. In this way the physiologic limit of any single tooth will not be surpassed.

Rests

Properly prepared rest seats, as discussed in Chapter 9, help control stress by directing forces transmitted to abutment teeth down the long axis of those teeth. The periodontal ligament is capable of withstanding vertical forces of far greater magnitude than horizontal or torsional forces.

One of the most critical points of the rest seat is that the floor of the preparation must form an angle of less than 90 degrees with a perpendicular line dropped down the long axis of the tooth. This permits the rest, whether occlusal, incisal, or lingual, to grasp the tooth securely and prevent its migration. If the enclosed angle formed by the base of the rest seat and the long axis of the tooth is greater than 90 degrees, an inclined plane action is set up and the stress against the abutment tooth is magnified.

In all Class I and II partial dentures the rest seat preparation must be saucer-shaped, completely devoid of any sharp angles or ledges. As forces are applied to the partial denture, the rest must be free to move within the rest seat to release stresses that would otherwise be transferred to the tooth. This movement of the rest within the rest seat is similar to the action of a ball-and-socket joint. If ledges or walls are developed in the rest seat, the releasing action cannot take place and undesirable forces are concentrated on the abutment tooth.

The number of abutment teeth influences the amount of force each tooth must absorb. The more teeth that bear rest seats, the less will be the stress placed on each individual tooth.

BIBLOGRAPHY

Applegate, O.C.: Keeping the partial denture in harmony with biologic limitations, J. Am. Dent. Assoc. **43**:409-419, 1951.

Applegate, O.C.: Stresses induced by a partial denture upon its supporting structures and partical methods of control, Proc. D. Centenary pp. 308-319, 1940.

Angsberger, R.H.: Abutment stabilization through endosseous and cross-arch splinting, J. Prosthet. Dent. **26**:406-413, 1971.

Avant, W.E.: Factors that influence retention of removable partial dentures, J. Prosthet. Dent. **25**:265-269, 1971.

Craig, R.G., and Farah, J.W.: Stresses from loading distal-extension removable partial dentures, J. Prosthet. Dent. **39**:274-277, 1978.

Frechette, A.R.: Partial denture planning with special reference to stress distribution, J. Ontario Dent. Assoc. **30**:318-329, 1953.

Friedman, J.: Abutment sites and spaces in partial denture case analysis, J. Prosthet. Dent. **4**:803-812, 1954.

Granger, E.R.: Mechanical principles applied to partial denture construction, J. Am. Dent. Assoc. **28**:1943-1951, 1941.

Herkneby, M.: Model experiments on the transmission of forces from a lower free-end partial denture to the supporting teeth, Tandlaegebladet, 1067, 1967.

Henderson, D., and Steward, T.E.: Design and force distribution with removable partial dentures, J. Prosthet. Dent. **17**:350-364, 1976.

Hughes, G.A.: Review of the basic principles of removable partial denture prosthesis, Fort. Rev. Chicago, Dent. Soc. **13**:9-13, 1947.

Mahler, D.B., and Terkla, I.G.: Analysis of stress in dental structures, Dent. Clin. North Am. **2**:789-798, 1958.

McLean, D.W.: Fundamental principles of partial denture construction, J. Tenn. Dent. Assoc. **19**:108-118, 1939.

Schuyler, C.H.: The partial denture as a means of stabilizing abutment teeth, J. Am. Dent. Assoc. **28**:1121-1125, 1941.

Weinberg, L.A.: Lateral force in relation to the denture base and clasp design, J. Prosthet. Dent. **6**:785-800, 1956.

White, J.T.: Visualization of stress and strain related to removable partial denture abutments, J. Prosthet. Dent. **40**:143-151, 1978.

5 Examination and evaluation of diagnostic data

THE FIRST DIAGNOSTIC APPOINTMENT

IMPORTANCE OF DIAGNOSTIC PHASE OF TREATMENT

The treatment of the partially edentulous patient requires the knowledge and the skill of the dentist in almost every phase of dental practice. The actual construction of the removable partial denture is usually the last of many complex procedures.

Many failures in removable partial denture treatment can be traced to an inadequate diagnosis and an inappropriate or incomplete treatment plan. A logical, properly sequenced treatment plan is essential to the successful treatment of this type of patient.

The formulation of an appropriate treatment plan requires the careful evaluation of all pertinent diagnostic data. Essential diagnostic data are obtained from a patient interview; radiographs; mounted and surveyed diagnostic casts; a definitive oral examination, including periodontal probing, percussion, and vitality tests; and consultations with medical and dental specialists when appropriate.

All too often the design of the prosthesis is determined after all the other phases of definitive patient treatment have been completed. This approach is as ludicrous as designing a building after the foundation has been constructed. Decisions relative to teeth to be retained, surgical procedures to be employed, and types of restorations to be placed must be made with the ultimate design of the prosthesis in mind. Therefore the making of accurate casts that can be analyzed with a dental surveyor is an integral part of the diagnostic procedure.

It is usually advisable to have a separate fee for the diagnostic service. The patient should be informed of the fee and the importance of the diagnostic service. The patient should understand the value and necessity of this service and how it relates to the ultimate prognosis of treatment.

ORGANIZING THE EXAMINATION

The examination can be completed most effectively and expeditiously if two appointments are used. During the first appointment, which will be described in detail in this chapter, the patient fills out a health questionnaire and is interviewed; a cursory examination of the oral cavity is made to identify any condition that requires immediate attention; an oral prophylaxis is accomplished; a radiographic survey is completed; and accurate diagnostic impressions and casts are made. In addition, a face-bow transfer and centric jaw relation records may be made for mounting the diagnostic casts on an adjustable articulator if a sufficient number of occlusal contacts remain. Usually it is more convenient to defer the mounting procedures until the second appointment, because a baseplate is frequently needed to provide the necessary occlusal contacts for accurate mounting of the casts.

During the second appointment the diagnostic casts are mounted (if this procedure was not accomplished at the first appointment), a definitive examination of the oral cavity is completed, the radiographs are interpreted and correlated with the clinical findings, arrangements are made for any needed consultation with a medical or dental specialist, the diagnostic data are analyzed, and a definitive treatment plan is formulated when possible. These procedures are detailed in Chapter 6.

HEALTH QUESTIONNAIRE

The objective of the health questionnaire (Fig. 5-1) is to assess the patient's general health. It should be inclusive enough to provide information concerning any systemic condition that may affect the prognosis of the patient's treatment. Any positive responses or questionable answers should be explored during the patient interview. The importance of the health questionnaire is emphasized by the fact that two thirds of the patients completing the questionnaire will have at least one positive response.

An important part of any health evaluation should be an entry for blood pressure measurements (Fig. 5-2). It has been estimated that 23 million Americans have hypertension, of which only half have been diagnosed and

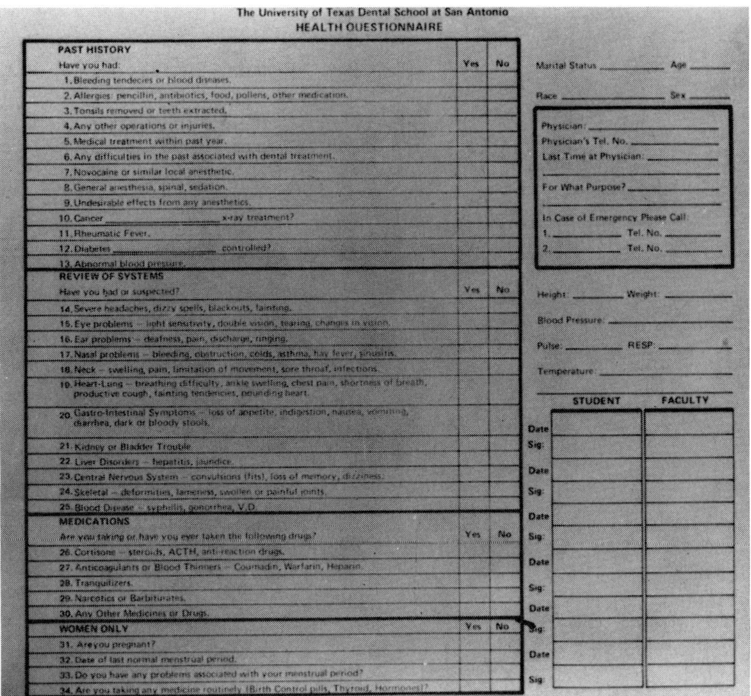

The University of Texas Dental School at San Antonio
HEALTH QUESTIONNAIRE

PAST HISTORY Have you had:	Yes	No
1. Bleeding tendecies or blood diseases.		
2. Allergies: pencillin, antibiotics, food, pollens, other medication.		
3. Tonsils removed or teeth extracted.		
4. Any other operations or injuries.		
5. Medical treatment within past year.		
6. Any difficulties in the past associated with dental treatment.		
7. Novocaine or similar local anesthetic.		
8. General anesthesia, spinal, sedation.		
9. Undesirable effects from any anesthetics.		
10. Cancer ______ x-ray treatment?		
11. Rheumatic Fever.		
12. Diabetes ______ controlled?		
13. Abnormal blood pressure.		
REVIEW OF SYSTEMS Have you had or suspected?	Yes	No
14. Severe headaches, dizzy spells, blackouts, fainting.		
15. Eye problems – light sensitivity, double vision, tearing, changes in vision.		
16. Ear problems – deafness, pain, discharge, ringing.		
17. Nasal problems – bleeding, obstruction, colds, asthma, hay fever, sinusitis.		
18. Neck – swelling, pain, limitation of movement, sore throat, infections.		
19. Heart-Lung – breathing difficulty, ankle swelling, chest pain, shortness of breath, productive cough, fainting tendencies, pounding heart.		
20. Gastro-Intestinal Symptoms – loss of appetite, indigestion, nausea, vomiting, diarrhea, dark or bloody stools.		
21. Kidney or Bladder Trouble		
22. Liver Disorders – hepatitis, jaundice.		
23. Central Nervous System – convulsions (fits), loss of memory, dizziness.		
24. Skeletal – deformities, lameness, swollen or painful joints.		
25. Blood Disease – syphilis, gonorrhea, V.D.		
MEDICATIONS Are you taking or have you ever taken the following drugs?	Yes	No
26. Cortisone – steroids, ACTH, anti-reaction drugs.		
27. Anticoagulants or Blood Thinners – Coumadin, Warfarin, Heparin.		
28. Tranquilizers.		
29. Narcotics or Barbiturates.		
30. Any Other Medicines or Drugs.		
WOMEN ONLY	Yes	No
31. Are you pregnant?		
32. Date of last normal menstrual period.		
33. Do you have any problems associated with your menstrual period?		
34. Are you taking any medicine routinely (Birth Control pills, Thyroid, Hormones)?		

Marital Status ______ Age ______

Race ______ Sex ______

Physician: ______
Physician's Tel. No. ______
Last Time at Physician: ______
For What Purpose? ______
In Case of Emergency Please Call:
1. ______ Tel. No. ______
2. ______ Tel. No. ______

Height: ______ Weight: ______

Blood Pressure: ______

Pulse: ______ RESP: ______

Temperature: ______

	STUDENT	FACULTY
Date		
Sig:		
Date		
Sig:		
Date		
Sig:		
Date		
Sig:		
Date		
Sig:		
Date		
Sig:		

Fig. 5-1. Health questionnaire used by students at University of Texas Dental School at San Antonio. Exact wording of questionnaire is not as important as follow-up of all leads by dentist.

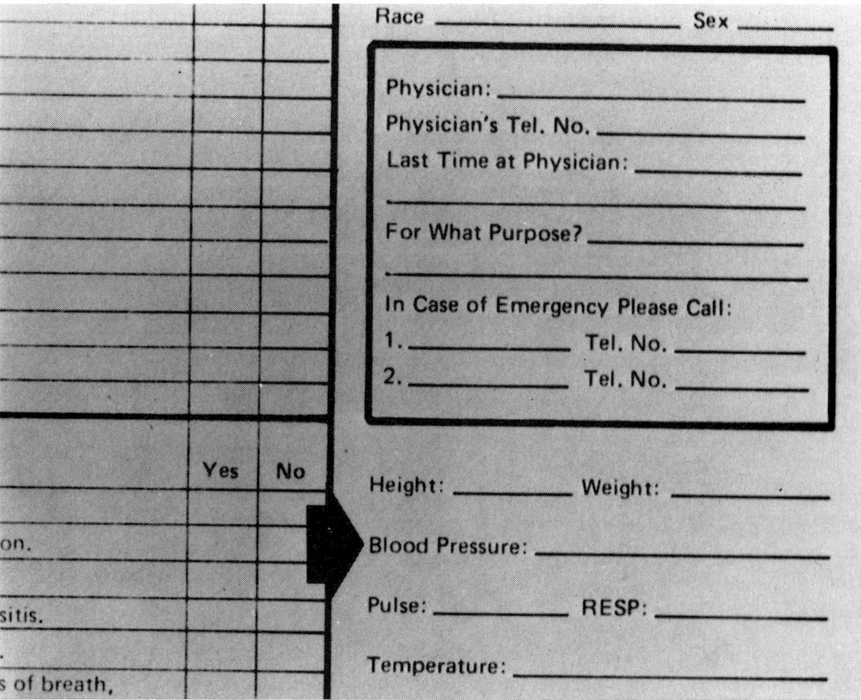

Race ______ Sex ______

Physician: ______
Physician's Tel. No. ______
Last Time at Physician: ______
For What Purpose? ______
In Case of Emergency Please Call:
1. ______ Tel. No. ______
2. ______ Tel. No. ______

Yes No

on.

sitis.

s of breath,

Height: ______ Weight: ______

Blood Pressure: ______

Pulse: ______ RESP: ______

Temperature: ______

Fig. 5-2. Questionnaire with area for entry of blood pressure recordings (arrow).

only a fourth are receiving adequate therapy. These facts should motivate all health professionals to routinely screen patients for hypertensive disease. Any patient with diastolic pressure of 130 mm Hg or above should be considered to have a medical emergency problem and medical consultation is indicated. In addition, most geographic areas have specified blood pressure levels at which medical consultation is advised. If repeated blood pressure measurements equal or surpass these levels, the patient should be referred to a physician.

PATIENT INTERVIEW

The next step in the examination procedure is the patient interview, during which the dentist should establish rapport with the patient, gain insight into the psychologic makeup of the patient, explore any physical problems that may affect the treatment, and ascertain the patient's expectations of treatment.

Establishing a rapport

Devan (1961) stated it well when he said we should meet the mind of the patient before we meet the mouth of the patient. The patient's attitudes and opinions relative to the dentist and dentistry can greatly influence the success or failure of the treatment. Many clinically acceptable prostheses are not worn because the patients were not mentally prepared to receive them. Boucher (1970) put the initial contact with the patient in its proper perspective when he said the first 5 minutes spent with the patient are the most important period the dentist spends with the patient. Patients should be made to feel that the dentist is genuinely interested in them and in helping to solve their dental problems.

Gaining insight into psychologic makeup of patient

The patient's attitudes and psychologic makeup have considerable influence on the success of the treatment and on the degree of difficulty the dentist will have in treating the patient.

In 1950 Dr. M.M. House classified patients into the following four psychologic types: the philosophical, the exacting, the hysterical, and the indifferent patient.

Philosophical patients are the easiest to treat. They are well adjusted and easygoing. They can accept their share of the responsibility for having lost their teeth, they can recognize the need for replacement of the missing teeth, and they can understand that they have a role in maintaining their dental health. These individuals adjust to any prosthesis that is reasonably well designed and constructed, and usually do not present problems for the dentist.

Exacting patients are precise in everything they do. Usually they are immaculate in dress and appearance. Their nature is to be satisfied only by perfection. They may demand that the dentist explain every step of treatment in detail. These patients should not be promised or led to believe that they will be able to wear a prosthesis without any inconvenience or discomfort, because they will expect the dentist to live up to this promise. Potential problems and inconveniences should be explained in detail *before* treatment is initiated; a logical explanation may be construed to be an excuse if given after a problem has arisen. Additional appointment time should be scheduled for exacting patients because they need the dentist's extreme care, effort, and patience. These patients have high expectations and are difficult to treat. However, they can be satisfied, and then they become enthusiastic supporters and valuable assets to a dental practice.

The hysterical patient must be recognized before treatment is initiated to avoid an extremely unpleasant experience for both patient and dentist. Hysterical patients are emotionally unstable and may be excessively apprehensive about having dental treatment. Whereas exacting patients have complaints with valid reasons, hysterical patients tend to complain without justification. Many are convinced that they will never be able to wear a prosthesis. They cannot accept the responsibility for any of their dental problems. Patients who have chronic or debilitating systemic disorders and who have subsequently become depressed are included in this category. They must be made aware that their dental problems are primarily related to their systemic or emotional problems. Psychiatric and medical treatment may be useful. Unless the mental attitude of these patients is changed, the possibility for success in treatment is poor.

Indifferent patients also present problems to the dentist. They are characterized by lack of motivation or concern about their oral health. These patients tend to ignore instructions and to be uncooperative in treatment. Frequently they exhibit little concern even though several missing anterior and posterior teeth detract from their appearance. They may believe that they function sufficiently well with their remaining teeth. Unless the patient can be educated to appreciate the importance of replacing missing teeth and maintaining oral health, the prognosis for treatment with a removable partial denture is poor.

Evaluating effect of physical problems on treatment

Another objective of the patient interview is to evaluate physical problems that may affect the patient's treatment. Any positive responses in the health questionnaire must be explored in detail and evaluated.

There are so many systemic disturbances that one should not rely on memory alone, but should consult appropriate, current reference material. The symptoms, manifestations, and prognosis of the disease should be reviewed and then carefully evaluated to determine what effect it will have on the treatment of the patient. When any doubt exists, the most prudent action is to seek a medical consultation before dental treatment is initiated. Knowing that the patient has a systemic disturbance is not enough; the dentist must understand how the disease may affect the treatment of the patient.

Systemic disturbances that can have a significant effect on the treatment of the patient include the following.

Diabetes

Uncontrolled diabetes is frequently accompanied by multiple small oral abscesses and poor tissue tone. The disease should be brought under control before prosthodontic treatment is accomplished. The lessened resistance to infection exhibited by diabetic patients necessitates special care during treatment and follow-up. The diabetic patient often has a reduced salivary output, which significantly reduces the ability of a patient to wear a prosthesis with comfort and increases the possibility that caries will occur.

Arthritis

If arthritic changes occur in the temporomandibular joint, the making of jaw relation records can be difficult, and changes in the occlusion may occur.

Paget's disease

Patients with Paget's disease may have enlargement of the maxillary tuberosities, which can cause changes in the fit and the occlusion of a prosthesis. A frequent recall program should be instituted for such patients.

Acromegaly

Patients with acromegaly may have enlargement of the mandible. They should be observed frequently to evaluate the fit and occlusion of the prosthesis.

Parkinson's disease

Parkinson's disease is characterized by rhythmic contractions of the musculature, including the muscles of mastication. The symptoms are sometimes so severe that it is impossible for the patient to insert and remove a removable partial denture, let alone practice the oral hygiene procedures necessary for the maintenance of oral health. Impression procedures are also compromised by the presence of an excessive quantity of saliva.

Pemphigus vulgaris

Pemphigus vulgaris is a disease that usually begins by formation of bullae in the oral cavity with gradual spreading to the skin. Before 1959 the disease was usually fatal, but with current treatment the prognosis is good. In the acute phase a painful oral cavity and dryness of the mouth are common symptoms. These symptoms may be interpreted as being caused by a prosthesis the patient is wearing, and patients have been known to go from dentist to dentist for the relief of pain or the remake of a prosthesis because the true problem had not been diagnosed. When the disease is controlled with medication, these patients can wear a prosthesis successfully. However, care must be taken to establish smooth and well-polished contours and borders of the prosthesis. Greater than normal postinsertion care can be anticipated.

Epilepsy

The epileptic patient presents special problems in treatment planning and in treatment. A grand mal seizure may result in fracture and aspiration of the prosthesis, and possibly the loss of additional teeth. Consultation with the patient's physician is essential before treatment is initiated. Complete information concerning the patient's condition is indispensable. The construction of removable partial dentures is usually contraindicated if the patient has frequent, severe seizures with little or no warning. However, if the seizures are controlled by medication or if the patient has adequate premonition of a seizure so that the prosthesis can be removed, a removable partial denture can be used. All materials used in the construction of a prosthesis for an epileptic patient must be radiopaque so that any part of the prosthesis that is accidentally aspirated or swallowed during a seizure can be located radiographically. If the patient's medication includes diphenylhydantoin (Dilantin), one must take particular care to ensure that the removable partial denture does not irritate the gingival tissues, or hypertrophy of these tissues may result.

Cardiovascular disease

Patients with the following require medical consultation before any dental procedures.

Acute or recent myocardial infarction
Unstable or recent onset of angina pectoris
Congestive heart failure
Uncontrolled arrhythmia
Uncontrolled hypertension

The patient's physician should be consulted and written approval should be obtained before any dental treatment is initiated.

Several other cardiovascular conditions may warrant

medical consultation. Prophylatic antibiotic therapy is always recommended if surgical procedures are to be accomplished for patients with a history of congenital or rheumatic valvular heart disease, cardiac murmurs, or repaired coarctation of the aorta. However, there is conflicting evidence as to the need for prophylactic medication when lesser degrees of tissue trauma are antitipated, such as the placement of restorations and the making of impressions, and many physicians do not recommend antibiotic prophylaxis for patients with a history of rheumatic fever if there has not been cardiac involvement. Because the patient's knowledge of his condition may not be completely accurate, the most prudent procedure for the dentist is to request a medical consultation with the patient's physician.

Cancer

Cancer is a common disease. Modern treatment modalities enable many patients to be treated as outpatients. Therefore the dental care of cancer patients is no longer the exclusive responsibility of the hospital dentist. Many oral complications result from radiation treatment for cancer of the head and neck. Radiation caries is common if the patient does not practice meticulous oral hygiene and apply fluoride to the teeth daily. Certainly the wearing of a removable partial denture will compound the patient's problems in maintaining adequate oral hygiene. Radiation treatment can cause a greatly diminished blood supply to the jaws, particularly the mandible. Osteoradionecrosis may result from even minor irritation caused by a prosthesis or dental procedure. The selection of teeth to be retained and those to be removed before the initiation of radiation treatment is critical. Teeth that are likely to create problems because of peridontal disease or a periapical pathologic condition should be removed provided there is adequate time for healing before the initiation of radiation treatment. Timing is critical because a common cause of osteoradionecrosis is the initiation of radiation treatment before adequate healing has occurred. Obviously the physician is anxious to initiate radiation therapy as soon as possible. The radiologist and the dentist must work closely together to formulate a plan that benefits the patient to the greatest degree. If the patient will die if the radiation treatment is not initiated immediately, the danger of osteoradionecrosis in the future is of small concern. However, if treatment can be deferred until selected teeth have been removed and adequate healing has occurred, the quality of the patient's life after treatment of the malignancy may be better.

Oral complications are also a common side effect of radiation and chemotherapy for malignancies in areas other than the head and neck. The most common oral complications are mucosal irritations, xerostomia, and bacterial and fungal infections. These symptoms will complicate the construction and wear of a removable partial denture. A recent study (Sonis and others, 1978) indicated that 40% of all patients treated with chemotherapy and radiotherapy for malignancies remote from the oral cavity developed some form of oral complication. The incidence varied with the type of malignancy: Hodgkin's disease, 100%; leukemia, 66.7%; mesenchymal cancer, 37.5%; gynecologic cancer, 33.3%; non-Hodgkin's lymphoma, 33.3%; adenocarcinoma of bowel, 20%; and breast cancer, 11.5%.

Transmissible diseases

Hepatitis, tuberculosis, influenza, and other transmissible diseases pose a particular hazard for the dentist, patients, and dental auxiliaries. These diseases may be transmitted by contact with the patient's blood or saliva, contaminated dental instruments, and aerosal from the handpiece. In addition, several other potential hazards exist in the prosthodontic phases of treatment. Impression trays and materials may be contaminated when impressions are made. The handling of the impression and the cast made from it, as well as the grinding of the cast, may cause contamination or transmission of the disease. Contaminated polishing wheels, pumice, and pumice pans, as well as grindings from the patient's prosthesis may cause aerosal contamination of both the laboratory and the dental office (Fig. 5-3). It is imperative that the dentist know of any infectious disease that the patient may have and take precautions to prevent contamination and transmission of the disease. The regular use of fresh sterilized pumice and sterilized

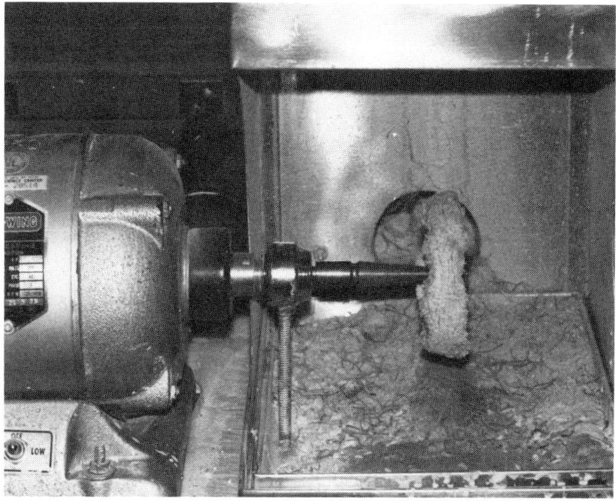

Fig. 5-3. Contaminated polishing and finishing equipment can be a health hazard for everyone in dental office and laboratory.

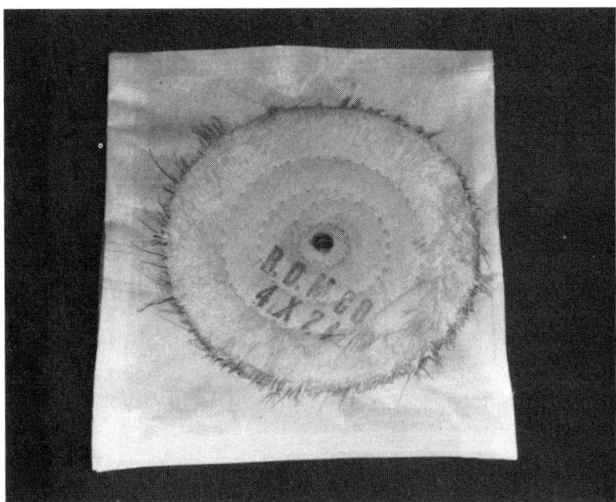

Fig. 5-4. Sterilization of polishing wheels and use of fresh pumice will contribute to a healthier environment in dental office and laboratory.

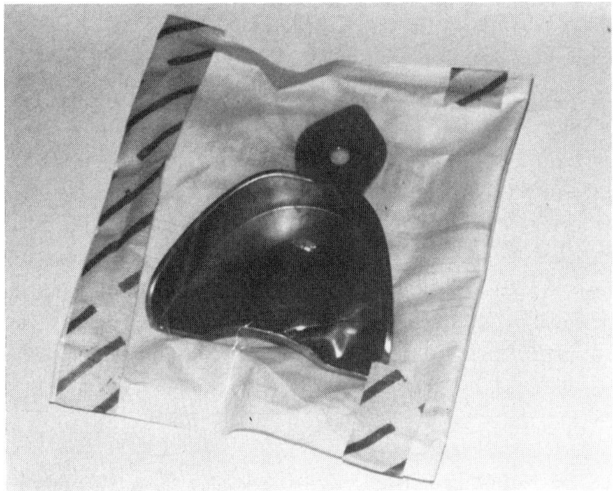

Fig. 5-5. Impression trays should be sterilized after use and stored in a sterile manner.

rag wheels will help maintain a healthy environment (Fig. 5-4). Impression trays should be cleaned, sterilized, and stored in an aseptic manner (Fig. 5-5). Rubber gloves, face masks, protective eye wear, and acceptable sterilization and decontamination techniques are essential in the treatment of patients with transmissible diseases.

High risk for hepatitis. An increasing number of individuals must be considered at high risk for the transmission of hepatitis. Included in this group are patients with a history of hepatitis, drug abuse, dialysis treatment, cancer therapy, frequent whole blood or blood product transfusions, living in an institutional environment such as a nursing home, or having been refused as a blood donor, and those with recent jaundice. Patients from this group may be carriers of hepatitis even though they have a negative history of the disease. They should be treated with all the precautions mentioned for patients with transmissible diseases. Exposure to the patient's blood or saliva through puncture by a contaminated needle or instrument or contamination of an open wound or the mucous membrane by the patient's saliva, blood, or aerosal spray should be immediately and thoroughly cleansed with soap and water, and the patient should be tested to determine whether the dentist or assistant should receive treatment.

Evaluating effect of drugs on treatment

No dentist or physician can be expected to remember the effects, side effects, and drug interactions of every available drug. However, the dentist is responsible for determining what medication the patient is taking and then using current reference information to determine what, if any, effect the medication will have on the treatment of the patient.

Increasing age usually means an increase in (1) the need for some type of prosthodontic treatment and (2) the use of prescribed and over-the-counter drugs. The proportion of persons on some type of medication is 1 in 4 for teenagers, 1 in 3 for young adults, 1 in 2 for persons in their forties, and 2 in 3 for persons age 50 and older. Therefore at least half the patients requiring prosthodontic treatment are likely to be taking a drug that could affect their treatment.

Some of the frequently prescribed drugs that can affect prosthodontic treatment are discussed.

Anticoagulants

Postsurgical bleeding could be a problem for patients receiving anticoagulants who undergo extractions or soft tissue or osseous surgery. These patients should be referred to an oral surgeon for management of the surgical phases of treatment.

Antihypertensive agents

The most significant side effect of the antihypertensive drugs is orthostatic, or postural, hypotension, which may result in syncope when the patient suddenly assumes the upright position. Therefore care must be taken when the patient gets up from the dental chair. The patient should be questioned about feeling dizzy or weak. If symptoms persist, the patient should not be allowed to leave the office unaccompanied. Another fact to consider is that treatment for hypertension usually includes prescription of a diuretic agent, which can contribute to a decrease in saliva and an associated dry mouth.

Endocrine therapy

Patients receiving endocrine therapy may develop an extremely sore mouth. If the patient is wearing a prosthesis, it could incorrectly be blamed for causing the discomfort.

Saliva-inhibiting drugs

Methantheline bromide (Banthine), atropine, and their derivatives are sometimes used to control excessive salivary secretion, particularly when it is necessary to make accurate impressions. They are generally contraindicated for use by patients with cardiac disease because of their vagolytic effect. Other contraindications for these drugs include prostatic hypertrophy and glaucoma. Saliva should be controlled by mechanical means in these patients.

Ascertaining patient's expectations of treatment

The fourth objective of the interview is to ascertain the patient's expectations of treatment and determine whether they are realistic in the light of the oral and physical conditions. Any removable partial denture will complicate oral hygiene procedures, occupy space in the oral cavity, and necessitate a learning and adaptation period. If the patient's expectations are such that these inconveniences are not acceptable, chances for successful treatment are extremely limited. Termination of the treatment would be in the best interest of both the patient and the dentist if the patient's expectations cannot be changed through explanation and education.

Obstacles to successful interview

Several obstacles must be overcome in interviewing the patient if the dentist is to meet the goals just described.

The first obstacle is the dentist. Too often the dentist is lecturing when he should be listening to the patient. Information cannot be gained from the patient if the dentist is doing all the talking. Certainly patient education is an extremely important part of the treatment of the partially edentulous patient, but the patient interview is not the appropriate time for this phase of treatment. Valuable information may be gained from many patients by simply allowing them to talk. Their opinion of dentists, past dental treatment, the importance they attach to their teeth, their fears, their health, and their expectations of treatment may be learned by asking a few general questions.

Other patients may require the dentist's best efforts at phrasing leading and specific questions. However, many dentists are reluctant to ask questions because they are uncomfortable "prying" into the personal life of the patient. Although many patients are reluctant to answer questions about anything other than their teeth, the dentist should not use this resistance as an excuse to terminate the interview, thereby missing information critical to the success of the treatment.

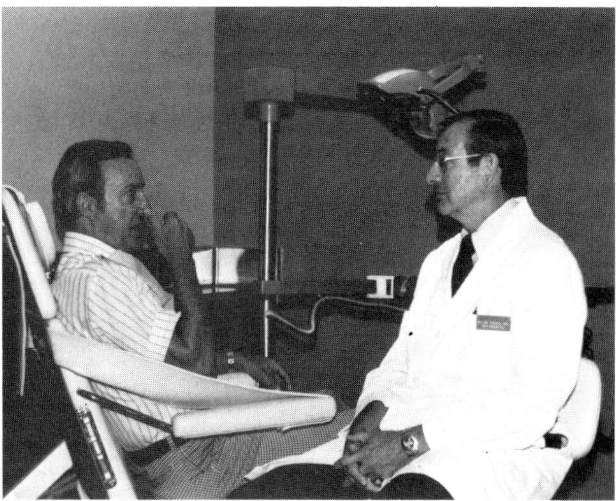

Fig. 5-6. Hand placed in front of mouth during speech may indicate patient's embarrassment over appearance of teeth.

Too often the dentist is nonattentive or merely hearing words when complete attention and interpretation of the patient's communication is called for. The patient's body language and things that are left unsaid may be more indicative of what the patient means than the words that are used. Simple actions such as holding the lips over the teeth when speaking or smiling, smiling with a closed mouth, or placing the hand in front of the mouth when speaking may indicate patients' true feelings about the appearance of their teeth or their prosthesis or about their oral health (Fig. 5-6). Patients who describe obscure pain or functional problems may really be communicating that they are uncomfortable with their teeth or prosthesis. Middle-aged patients may say that obtaining good function and comfort is all they expect from a partial denture, whereas their immaculate or youthful dress, excessive use of cosmetics, or youthful speech or mannerisms may communicate that appearance is of critical importance and that they may be expecting the treatment to restore their youth.

Another obstacle to a successful interview may be the dentist's choice of words. Professional terms such as *esthetics, centric jaw relation, vertical dimension, stability, hypertrophy,* and *edema* may be misinterpreted or completely misunderstood by the patient. Special care must be taken in interviewing the elderly because their educational level may limit their vocabulary, organic brain damage may impair their memory of recent events, and loss of auditory acuity may increase their anxiety. Patience, clarity of speech, and the use of understandable terms are essential in interviewing any patient.

Probably the greatest obstacle to the successful use of the patient interview is failure to consider or use the elicited information in the treatment of the patient. This error is likely to result in inferior treatment, as well as loss of confidence in the dentist if the patient is aware of this oversight.

Patients may also present obstacles to the fulfillment of the objectives of the patient interview. Patients may be fearful of their condition or of the possible treatment. They may be nervous or feel inferior to the denitst. Patients who feel vulnerable may give responses that are evasive or difficult to interpret. The dentist must attempt to relax patients, to alleviate their fears, and to make them feel they are equals if the communication process is to succeed.

Patients may be reluctant to provide information that they believe is irrelevant to their condition or treatment. Information relative to systemic problems or drug usage may be particularly difficult to obtain. The dentist must explain the importance of this information and be relentless in obtaining all relevant information. A patient's failure to provide appropriate information after adequate explanation of its importance should result in termination of treatment by mutual consent. Treatment based on inadequate information may be more harmful to the patient than no treatment at all.

A patient's lack of response to questions may be the result of inability to verbalize thoughts and feelings or a lack of understanding of the question rather than unwillingness to cooperate. The dentist must determine the actual cause of the lack of response, patiently and persistently ask understandable questions, and carefully interpret what the patient says and does.

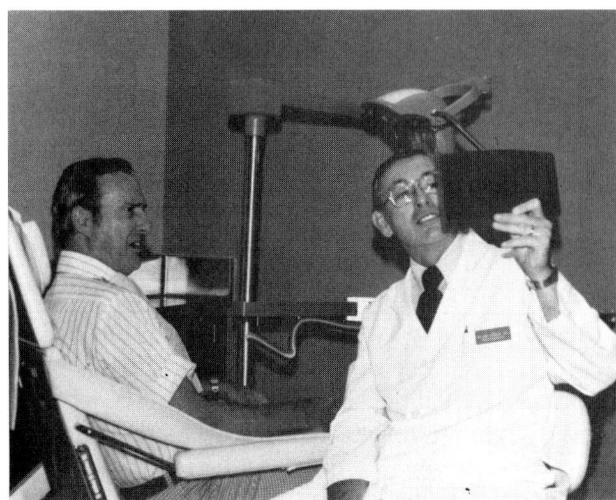

Fig. 5-7. This dentist's actions might be interpreted by patient as lack of interest.

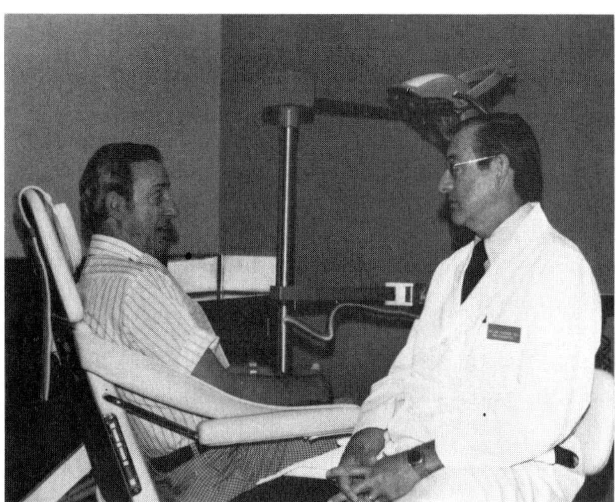

Fig. 5-8. Dentist should face patient at same level and should appear relaxed and unhurried.

Aids for successful interview

Dentist's attitude and behavior

The dentist's attitude and behavior during the interview have a great impact on its ultimate success or failure. A patient who perceives the dentist as caring, understanding, and respectful is more likely to be honest and cooperative. The dentist can communicate concern for the patient by employing the following behaviors:

1. The dentist should make eye contact with the patient, looking directly at the patient and displaying complete attention rather than studying radiographs or writing (Fig. 5-7).
2. The dentist should maintain a relaxed and attentive physical posture. The dentist should face the patient, preferably at the same level, and should appear relaxed and unhurried (Fig. 5-8). Impatient activity such as frequently glancing at a watch may cause the patient to feel anxious or rushed and is likely to be counterproductive to a successful interview (Fig. 5-9).
3. The dentist should employ appropriate head nodding, verbal following, and verbal reflection. In verbal following the dentist makes a short comment such as "I see," "I understand," or "that is unusual" to indicate attention to what is being said and to encourage the patient to continue to provide information. A nod of the head can perform the same function. In verbal reflection the dentist

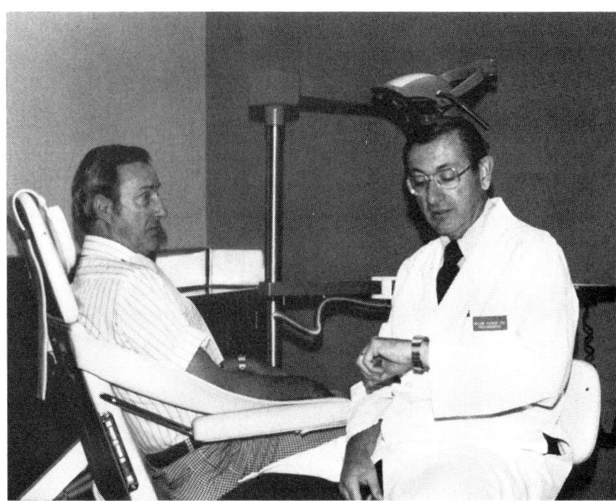

Fig. 5-9. Impatient activity such as looking at watch may cause patient to feel anxious or rushed.

restates the essential content of what the patient has expressed. This helps reassure patients that what they have said is understood and that it is important to the dentist.

Phrasing of questions

The phrasing of questions is very important to the success of the patient interview. When general information such as attitudes and experiences is sought, the question should be phrased so that a simple "yes" or "no" will not suffice as an answer. For example, if the patient is asked, "Are you frightened or nervous when you have to go to the dentist?" "yes" or "no" may be the only response. By using a *open-ended question* such as "Tell me about your feelings when you have to go to the dentist," a much greater insight into the patient's feelings about dentists and dental treatment is likely to be gained. As the interview progresses, more *specific questions* are usually necessary to gather information about a particular subject or to focus on a particular problem.

The dentist can control the direction of the interview by the content of the questions that are asked. *Leading questions* can be used to shift the conversation from one subject area to another.

Structure of interview

Breaking the ice

Although the interview should seem informal and relaxed to the patient, it must have some structure, or sequence pattern. Otherwise considerable time can be wasted. The interview should be opened with questions to break the ice so the patient will feel relaxed. Questions about the patient's family or job such as "Where do your children go to school?" or "What kind of work do you do?" help reduce the tension that may be present at the beginning of the interview.

Chief complaint

It is imperative that the patient's chief complaint be obtained early in the interview. Far too often patients never get the chance to explain why they are consulting the dentist. A question such as "Why did you seek dental treatment at this time?" or "Tell me about the problems that brought you in today" should obtain the critical information.

General health

A leading question such as "What do you think of your general health?" will direct the conversation to that subject and may gain information not included in the health questionnaire. Then specific questions are usually needed to clarify positive responses to the questionnaire relative to health problems or the use of drugs.

Dental history

A considerable amount of valuable information can be obtained from the review of the patient's dental history. It is important to find out why teeth have been lost. A question such as "Have you had any of your permanent teeth removed?" followed by "Why were these teeth removed?" will provide valuable information for treatment planning. If the teeth were lost because of *caries*, special emphasis will have to be placed on improving the patient's dietary intake and oral hygiene procedures. The presence of a removable partial denture in the mouth will increase the possibility of further carious activity and will complicate the maintenance of good oral hygiene. If the teeth were lost because of *periodontal disease*, every effort must be made to discover and eliminate its cause. Since a removable partial denture will undoubtably increase the stress placed on the remaining teeth, it will likely hasten the loss of the remaining teeth unless the etiologic factors of the disease are controlled.

The response to a question such as "How do you feel about the loss of your natural teeth?" will indicate whether the patient has a strong motivation or an indifferent attitude toward retaining the remaining natural teeth.

Asking "How do you feel about the dental treatment you have had in the past?" may help determine the psychologic type of the patient. Favorable responses may indicate that the patient is of the philosophic type, whereas unfavorable responses may indicate an exacting or hysterical patient. It should be remembered, however, that the patient may have had an unpleasant experience that justifies a negative response. Obviously an unfavorable reply should be thoroughly explored to determine whether the response is justified.

If a removable partial denture has been constructed previously for the patient, it is important to learn as much as possible about the patient's experience during and following treatment. A question such as "How many partial dentures have you had made?" is important. If several prostheses have been constructed over a relatively short time, the patient may be of the exacting type. The patient's response to a question such as "Why were you dissatisfied with the partial dentures?" should help the dentist avoid repeating the same errors that caused the patient's previous discontent. Or further questioning may indicate whether the patient's expectations are too great to be met.

If the patient has had only one removable partial denture and it has simply worn out, the patient's experience has probably been favorable and a similar experience may be anticipated from future treatment. The patient should be asked "What did you like best about your present partial denture?" and these features should be incorporated in the new design, provided, of course, there was no adverse tissue response to the previous design.

If a prosthesis needs to be remade because of loss of abutment teeth as a result of recurrent caries or other factors, patient education and changes in patient habits must be effected.

If the patient does not wear or is unhappy with a prosthesis that has been constructed, the reasons for patient dissatisfaction must be found. An indifferent patient may not understand the need for wearing the prosthesis or may understand the importance of wearing the prosthesis but simply not be motivated to do so. A hysterical patient may be dissatisfied with the prosthesis because it does not fulfill his unrealistically high expectations. For the exacting or philosophic patient the simple removal or change in position of an unsightly clasp may be all that is needed to change an unfavorable to a favorable response.

Answers to questions such as "How do you clean your partial denture and your teeth?" "Do you wear your partial denture while sleeping?" and "Do you ever keep your partial dentures out of your mouth to rest the tissues?" indicate whether patient education is needed in these areas.

Diet

The patient's diet should be evaluated. If cough drops, breath mints, soft drinks, hard candy, coffee with sugar, or other sugar containing products are used continually throughout the day, a change must be effected. The problems caused by sugar are compounded by the wear of a removable partial denture because the prosthesis shields the microorganisms from the cleansing and buffering action of the patient's saliva.

Habits

Patient habits should also be evaluated to determine whether they will affect the prognosis of treatment.

Pipe smoking and gum and tobacco chewing. If a patient smokes a pipe, it is important to know how the pipe is held in the mouth. If a prospective abutment tooth is involved, the added stress may cause loss of the tooth.

The chewing of gum or tobacco produces additional and unnecessary stress on the abutment teeth and these habits should be discouraged.

Bruxism and clenching. Bruxism and clenching have a significant adverse effect on the prognosis (Fig. 5-10). If either habit persists following treatment with removable partial dentures, it will probably cause early loss of the abutment teeth.

Bruxism is often initiated by interceptive occlusal contacts. The occlusion should be analyzed to determine whether correction is indicated. If efforts to eliminate the bruxism are unsuccessful, the patient should wear an occlusal splint at night to help protect the remaining teeth.

Clenching is used by some patients to help relieve tension. Some patients have such an ingrained clenching habit that they do not realize that an interocclusal space is normal. Patient education as to the need for an interocclusal space and special isometric and isotonic jaw exercises help make the patient aware of the habit and help the patient reduce the clenching and its damaging effects.

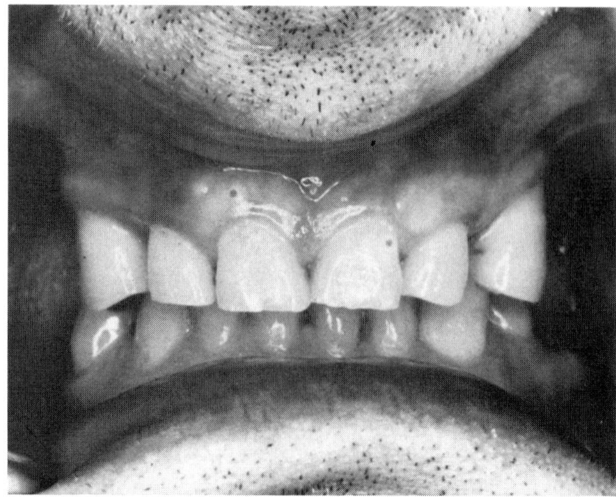

Fig. 5-10. Bruxism has caused extensive loss of occlusal and incisal tooth structure.

Tongue thrusting. If a tongue thrust habit has been a contributing factor in the loss of the patient's teeth, continuation of the habit could cause extensive stress on the teeth retaining and supporting a removable partial denture. The habit should be eliminated before a prosthesis is constructed. If the habit persists, the removable partial denture should be designed to distribute the resultant forces to as many teeth and supporting structures as possible.

Expectations of treatment

Some indication of the patient's expectations may have been gained when the dental history was reviewed. However, further questions may provide more insight. "What do you expect from having a partial denture made?" or "What things would you like to have changed if a new partial denture is made?" will help the dentist find out whether the patient's expectations are realistic. If the patient has unrealistic expectations (for example, a removable partial denture without a major connector crossing the palate or without clasps; one that will not feel bulky; or one that will feel, look, and work just like the natural teeth), the treatment plan should be altered or patient expectations should be changed through education. If neither can be accomplished, it would be inappropriate to treat the patient.

Questions from patient

Asking whether the patient has any questions is a good way to terminate the interview, and it allows the patient to open any new subject areas or to add to any previous areas that have been discussed.

Patient's physical characteristics

Additional important information can be gained by simply observing the patient's physical characteristics. For instance, clenching and tongue thrust problems should be apparent.

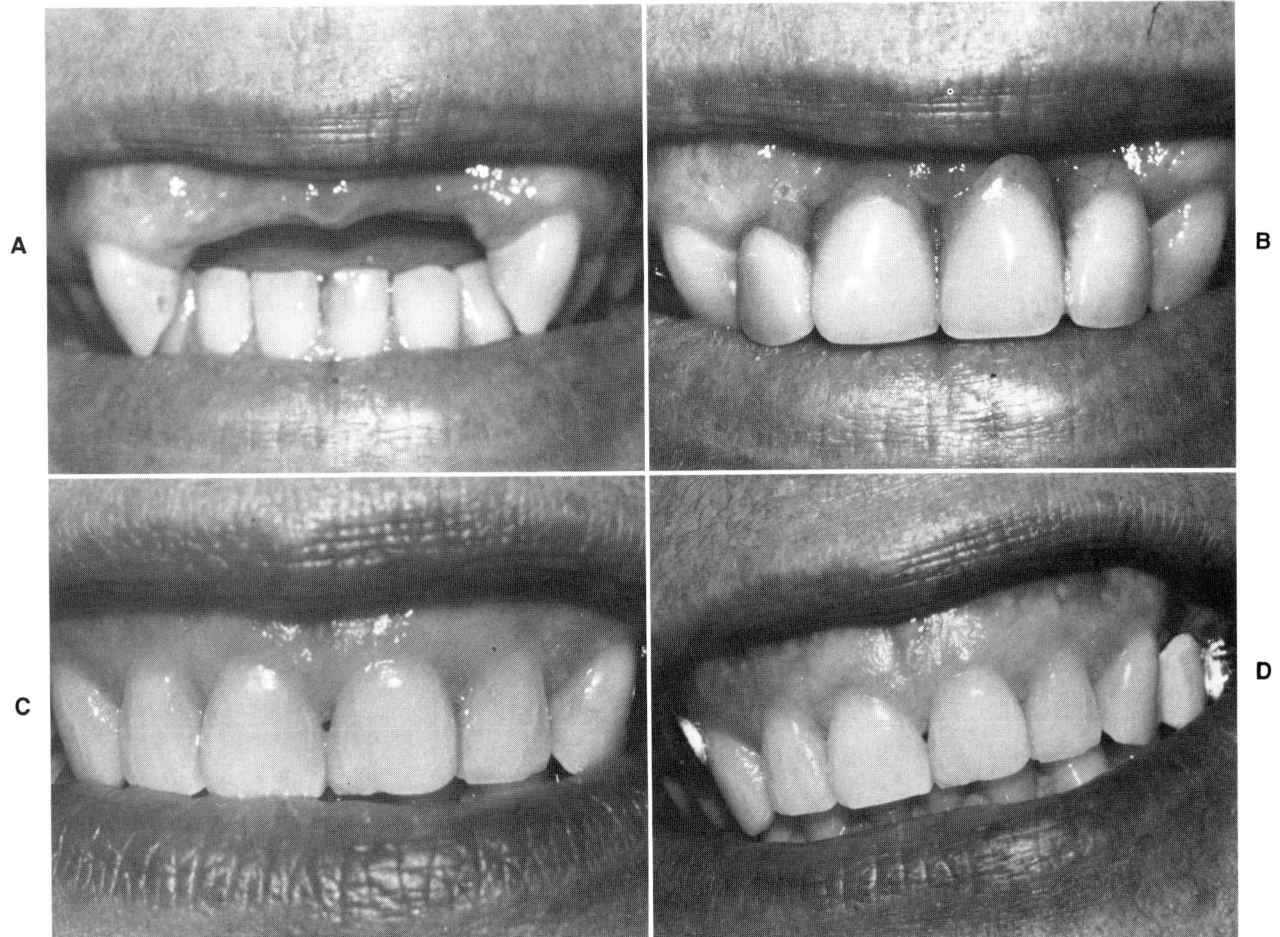

Fig. 5-11. A, Patient shows ridge when smiling, indicating potential problems in developing good esthetics. **B,** Attempt made to butt teeth to ridge, but resorption made it necessary to use some tissue-colored acrylic resin. **C,** Patient with very mobile upper lip. **D,** Clasps show when patient smiles.

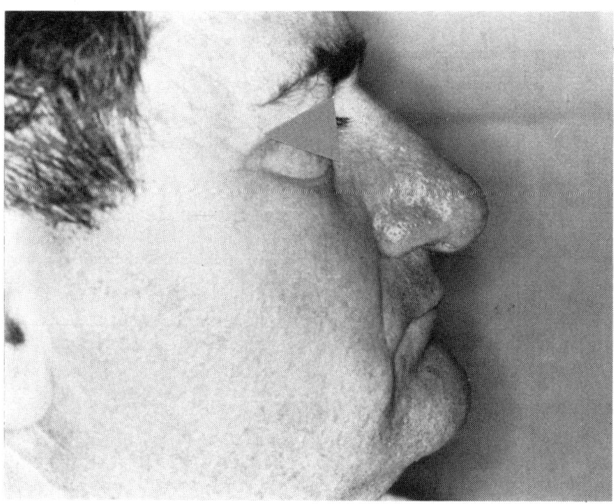

Fig. 5-12. Patient with extensive wear of teeth and apparent closure of vertical dimension of occlusion. Patient requires careful diagnostic workup.

If the patient has a speech problem, it is important that the problem be recognized before the construction of the removable partial dentures. Otherwise the patient or the dentist may blame the prosthesis for the problem. Patients with a history of corrected speech problems generally require a longer period to learn good speech with a new prosthesis.

An observation that the patient exhibits poor coordination indicates a good possibility that the patient will require longer than normal to adapt to wearing a removable partial denture. An elderly patient or one who has suffered a stroke or other neuromotor damage is likely to have difficulty placing and removing a removable partial denture. Patients with poor coordination may have difficulty maintaining an adequate level of hygiene of the oral cavity and the prosthesis.

The length and the mobility of the patient's lips are important characteristics that should be observed. Patients with short or highly mobile lips present problems in the construction of any type of prosthesis (Fig. 5-11). Esthetics are compromised because most or all of the clasp arms, denture borders, and other components will show when the patient smiles or speaks.

Facial changes suggesting an apparent loss of vertical dimension of occlusion indicate the need for great caution and care (Fig. 5-12). If loss and migration of teeth have allowed an overclosure of the vertical dimension of occlusion, special considerations are required in treatment planning. Opening or restoring an apparent overclosure with removable partial dentures alone is usually contraindicated because intrusion and migration of the remaining teeth frequently result. Instead, a diagnostic occlusal splint should be constructed at the new vertical dimension of occlusion and should be worn by the patient for several months. The splint can be adjusted during that period to determine the most acceptable vertical dimension of occlusion. Definitive treatment procedures should be deferred until it has been demonstrated that the new position is well tolerated and does not cause problems in speech or other functions. When comfort is ensured, crowns and fixed partial dentures should be constructed to maintain the new vertical dimension of occlusion. The splint should be modified at the time of insertion of the crowns and fixed units so that it can be worn until the removable partial denture is completed. An alternative procedure is the final insertion of the crowns, fixed partial dentures, and removable partial dentures at the same appointment. Altering the vertical dimension of occlusion is discussed in detail in Chapter 14.

The patient's cosmetic index also can provide valuable information. If the patient has used great care with makeup or is very meticulous in dress and appearance, there is a good chance that the patient will be equally concerned with the appearance and the feel of the prosthesis.

CURSORY EXAMINATION

Detection of problems requiring immediate attention

It is essential that a superficial examination be performed at the first appointment to detect problems that need immediate attention. Large carious lesions may have to be excavated to determine whether there is pulpal involvement (Fig. 5-13). Temporary restorations should be placed to relieve discomfort and to restore tooth contours so that accurate diagnostic casts can be made.

Oral conditions caused by ill-fitting removable partial dentures may also require immediate attention. Adjustment or temporary reline of the prosthesis should be accomplished to eliminate patient discomfort and allow recovery of the damaged tissues.

Evaluation of oral hygiene

Evaluation of the patient's oral hygiene is critical to the prognosis of the patient's treatment. Inadequate oral hygiene must be recognized early in the diagnostic procedure so that a preventive dentistry program can be initiated (Fig. 5-14). When one has experienced the disappointment of seeing a beautifully restored mouth destroyed by dental disease in a relatively short time because of the patient's poor oral hygiene, one realizes that education in preventive dentistry is perhaps the most valuable service that can be provided for the patient. The ultimate success of the treatment depends on the home care of the patient no less than on the quality

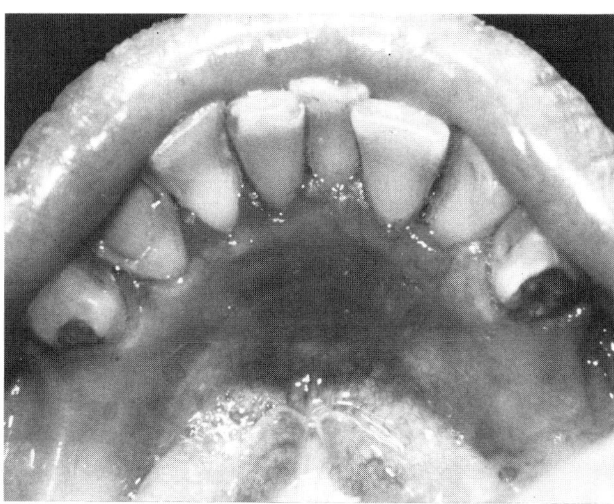

Fig. 5-13. Teeth with large carious lesions require immediate care.

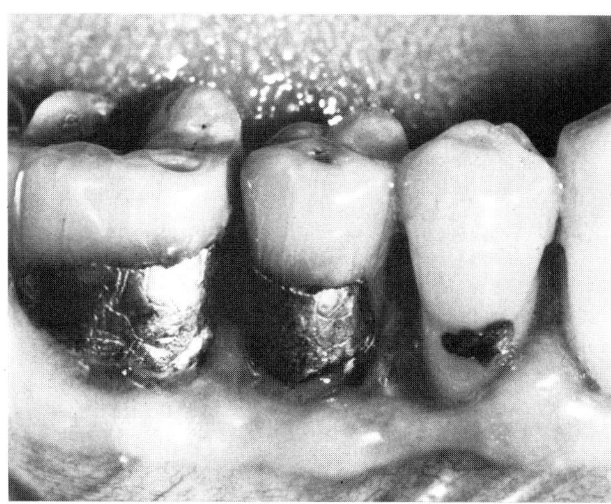

Fig. 5-15. Presence of large numbers of restored teeth and signs of recurrent caries indicate that this patient is susceptible to caries.

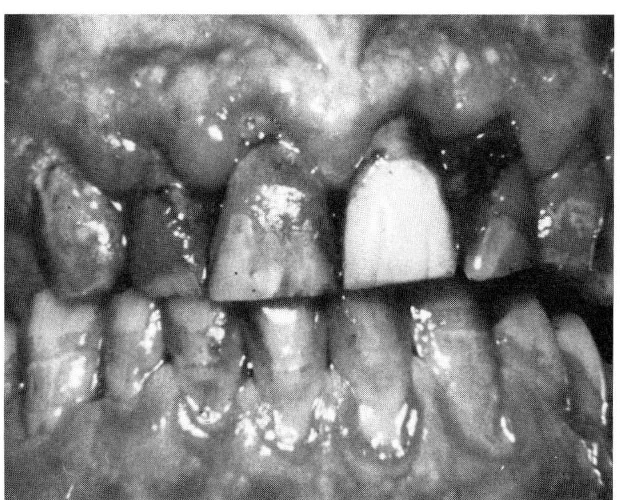

Fig. 5-14. Patient with totally inadequate oral hygiene.

of the technical procedures provided by the dentist.

A patient requiring extensive restorative and prosthodontic treatment should demonstrate the motivation and ability necessary to maintain an adequate level of oral hygiene. At times a preventive dentistry program may require several weeks of patient education and motivation. Some patients may never reach the desired level of oral hygiene performance, and a compromise or interim treatment plan may have to be initiated.

It is the dentist's responsibility to explain to the patient (1) the signs and symptoms of dental disease, (2) the equipment and techniques for proper home care, and (3) the patient's responsibilities in preventing further dental disease and their importance for the long-term success of treatment.

Only after patients have acknowledged their responsibilities and demonstrated their motivation and ability to maintain good oral hygiene should extensive fixed and removable partial denture treatment be initiated.

Evaluation of caries susceptibility

The presence of a large number of restored teeth, signs of recurrent caries, and evidence of decalcification indicate that the patient is susceptible to caries (Fig. 5-15). Unless an exceptional level of plaque control can be achieved, the prognosis for treatment will be poor. The placement of crowns on the abutment teeth may be indicated for a patient with a high degree of caries susceptibility; however, crowning of the teeth without exceptional plaque control will not necessarily prevent the recurrence of dental disease and subsequent failure of the dental treatment.

Detection of oral-antral and oral-nasal communications

A routine part of the cursory examination should be the inspection of the palate and posterior ridge areas for communication between the oral cavity and the maxillary sinus or nasal cavity (Fig. 5-16). These areas should be dried with a light flow of compressed air, and any dimples or craters should be carefully inspected. Paper or gutta percha points can be used to probe the area. Before diagnostic impressions are made, any communication should be closed with gauze tied to dental floss or any other material that can close the opening without danger of being forced into the antrum or nasal cavity (Fig. 5-17). Impression materials confined in an impression tray can flow through the smallest communication in great quantity. All impression materials

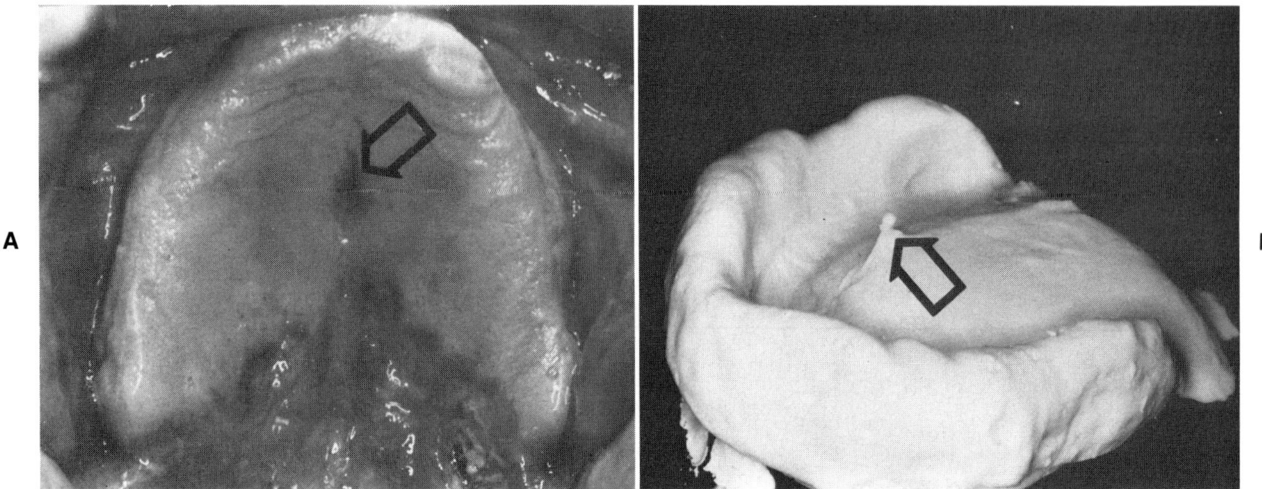

Fig. 5-16. A, Dimpled area in center of palate (arrow). **B,** Raised area in impression (arrow). A large amount of irreversible hydrocolloid had been forced into nasal cavity and broke off during removal of impression. Assistance from an otolaryngologist was needed for removal of impression material. (Courtesy Dr. Steven Parel, University of Texas Dental School at San Antonio.)

A B

C

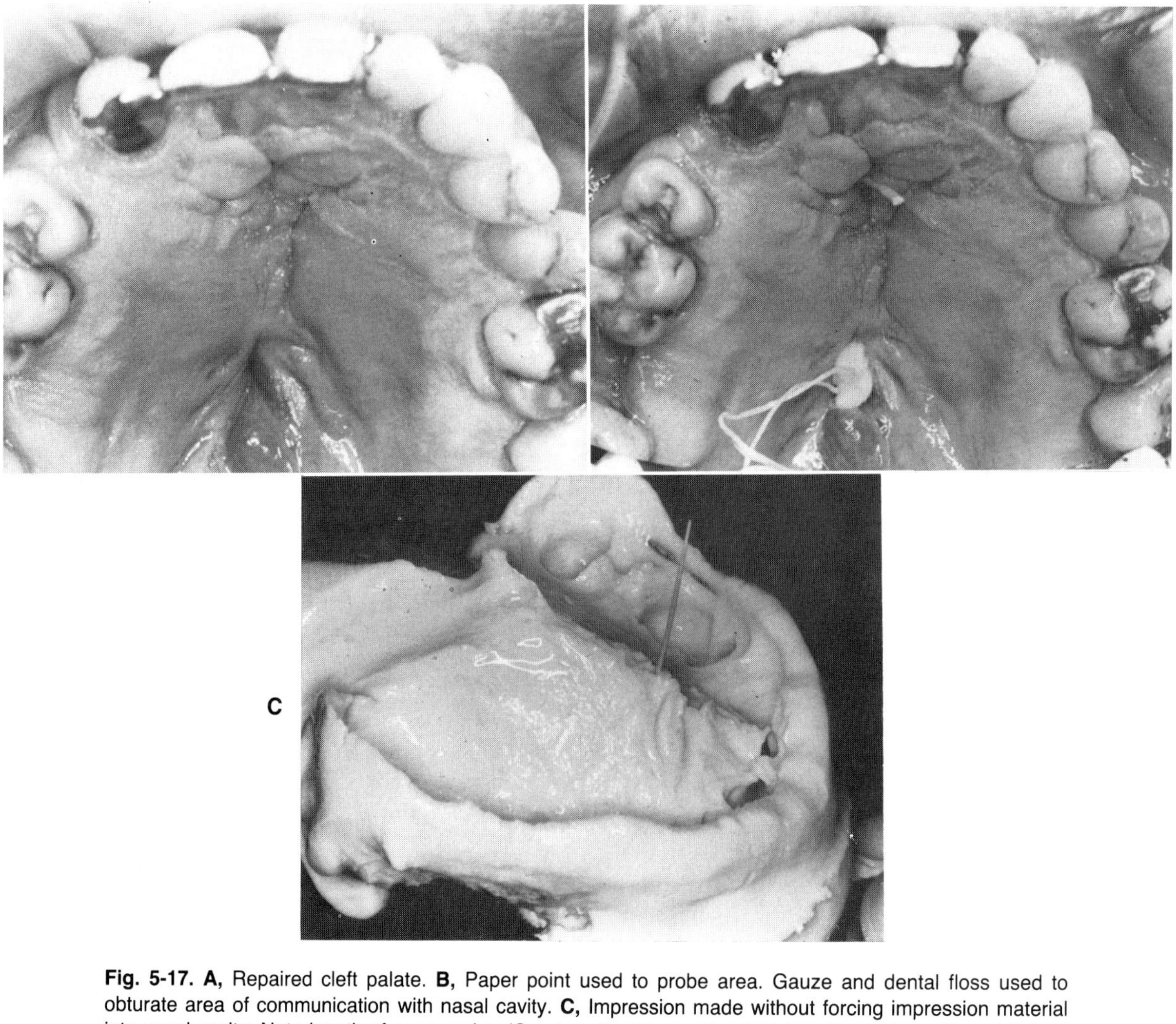

Fig. 5-17. A, Repaired cleft palate. **B,** Paper point used to probe area. Gauze and dental floss used to obturate area of communication with nasal cavity. **C,** Impression made without forcing impression material into nasal cavity. Note length of paper point. (Courtesy Dr. Steven Parel, University of Texas Dental School at San Antonio.)

cause inflammation when present in either the sinus or nasal cavity; they must be removed if accidently forced into these areas. Therefore it is far more prudent to take the time to examine the patient for the possible presence of a communication than to have to refer the patient to a specialist for the removal of impression material from one of these cavities.

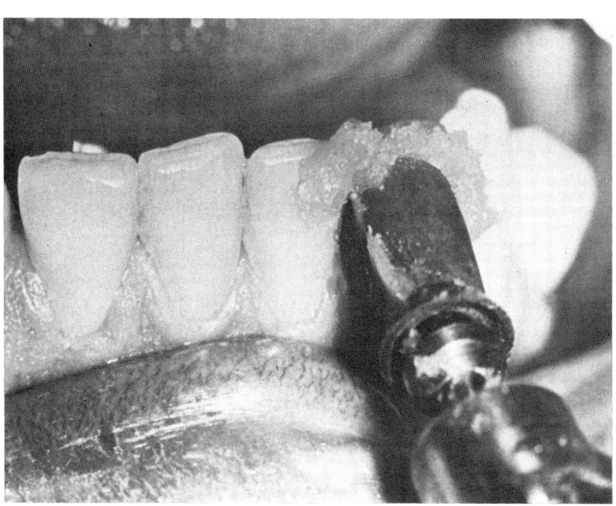

Fig. 5-18. Oral prophylaxis accomplished before making diagnostic impressions and performing definitive oral examination.

ORAL PROPHYLAXIS

Supragingival calculus should be removed and oral prophylaxis should be performed if these procedures have not been accomplished recently (Fig. 5-18). The diagnostic casts and the definitive intraoral examination will be more accurate if the teeth are clean.

RADIOGRAPHS

A complete series of periapical and bite-wing radiographs is an essential part of the complete examination of the prospective removable partial denture patient. The panoramic radiograph (Fig. 5-19) is ideal for screening for pathologic conditions but is not adequate for the definitive examination of this type of patient. Excellent periapical radiographs, preferably made using the long cone technique, are essential for determining the crown/root ratio of the remaining teeth, the status

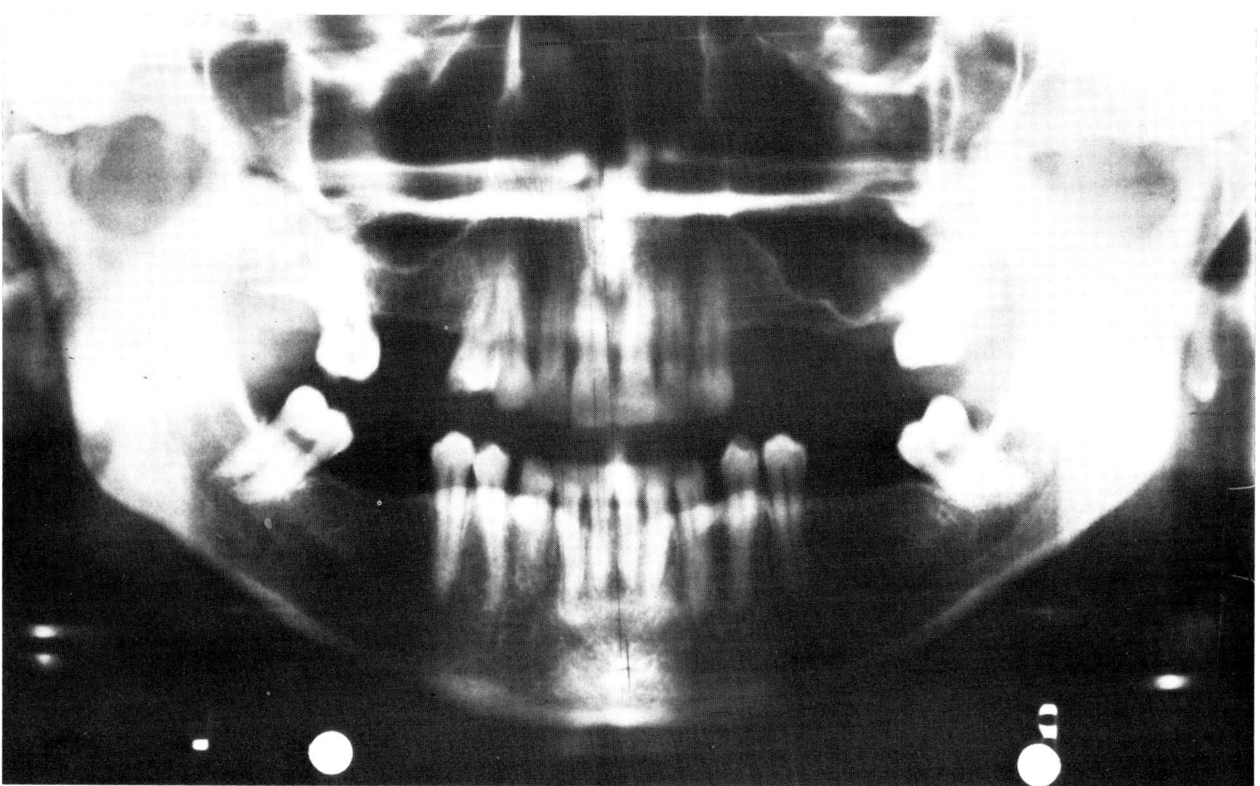

Fig. 5-19. Panoramic radiograph ideal as a screening tool.

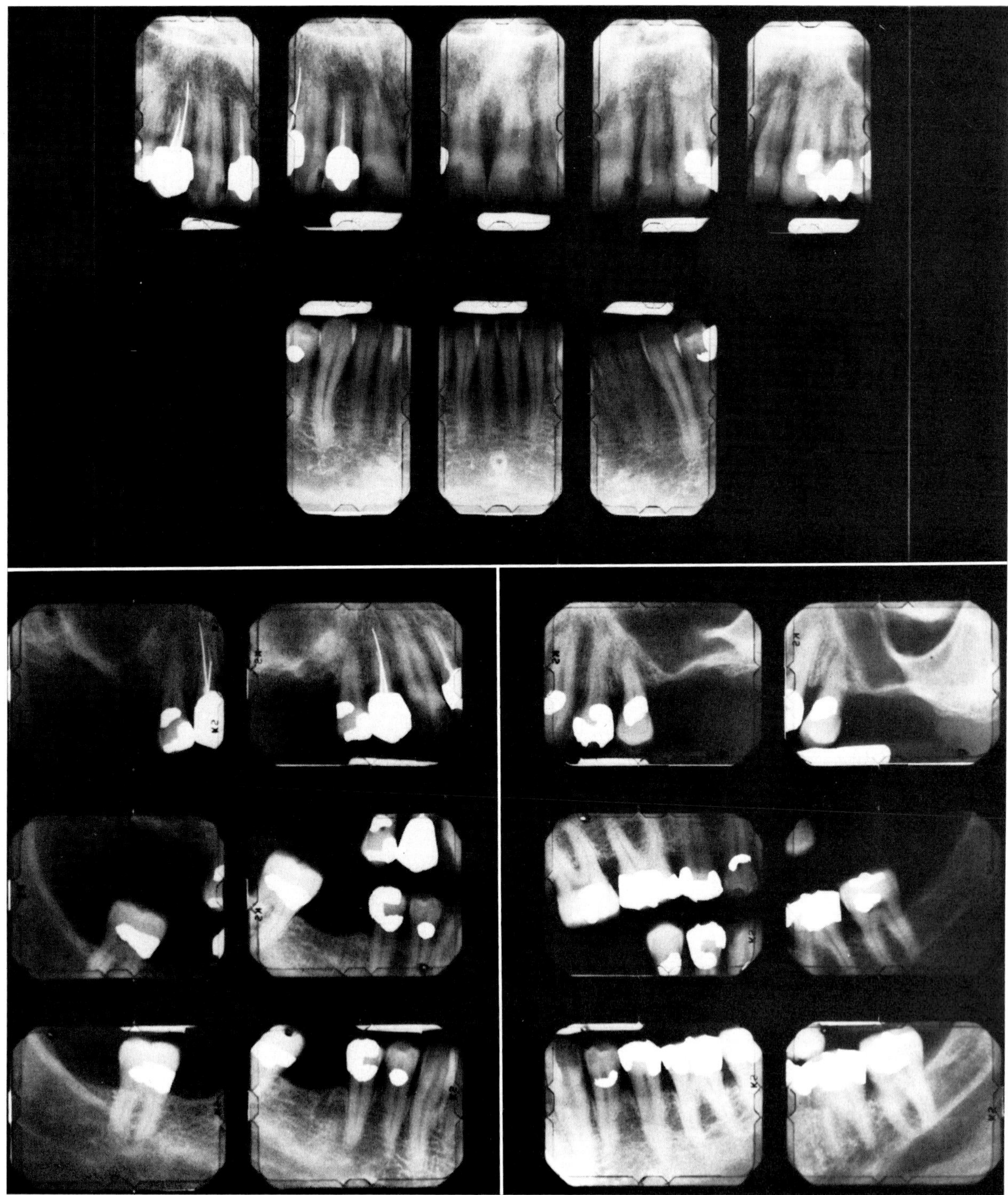

Fig. 5-20. Periapical radiographs essential for definitive examination of partially edentulous patient.

of the periodontal ligament space and lamina dura of the prospective abutment teeth, and the quality of the bone of the residual ridge in the edentulous areas of the mouth (Fig. 5-20). Evaluation of the radiographs is discussed in detail in Chapter 6.

DIAGNOSTIC IMPRESSIONS AND CASTS

A diagnostic procedure for a partially edentulous patient must be considered incomplete unless it includes the evaluation of accurate diagnostic casts (Fig. 5-21). Diagnostic casts permit analysis of the contour of both the hard and soft tissues of the mouth; determination of the types of restorations to be placed on the abutment teeth; and determination of the need for surgical correction of exostoses, frena, tuberosities, and undercuts. The diagnostic casts are surveyed, and the proposed design is drawn on the casts (Fig. 5-22). The casts then serve as a blueprint for the placement of restorations, the recontouring of teeth, and the preparation of rest seats. The designed casts aid in the presentation of the proposed treatment plan to the patient. Patients are more likely to approve the treatment plan if they can "see" the problem rather than just hear it described.

Diagnostic casts that are accurately mounted on a suitable articulator permit analysis of the patient's occlusion, of the adequacy of interarch space, and of the presence of overerupted or malposed teeth and tuberosity interferences (Fig. 5-23).

Because the casts are normally mounted and evaluated during the second diagnostic appointment, these procedures are discussed in Chapter 6. The procedure for making diagnostic impressions and casts is discussed here.

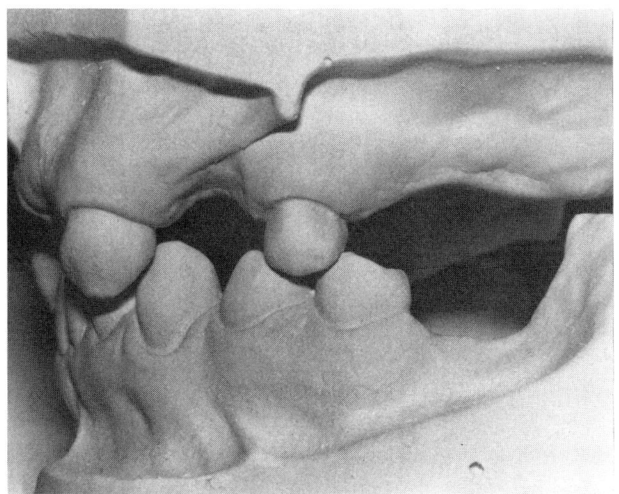

Fig. 5-21. Accurate diagnostic casts are essential.

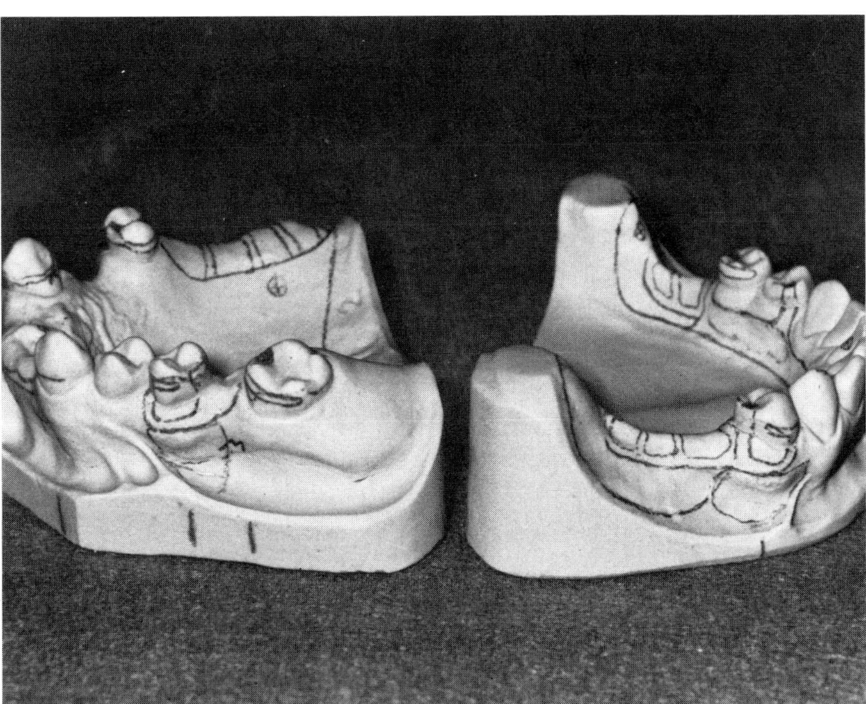

Fig. 5-22. Design drawn on diagnostic casts.

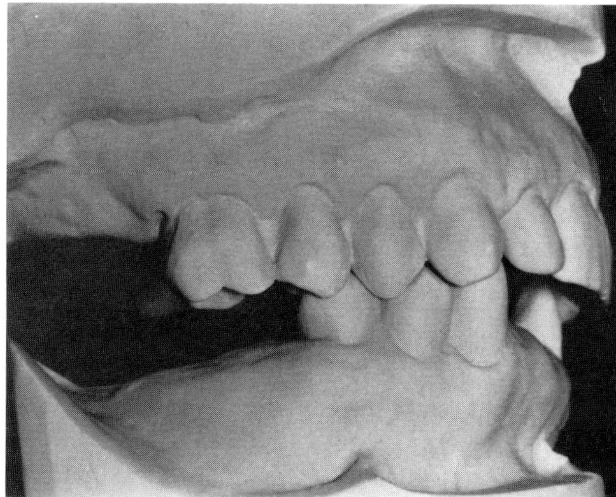

Fig. 5-23. Diagnostic casts mounted on articulator for analysis.

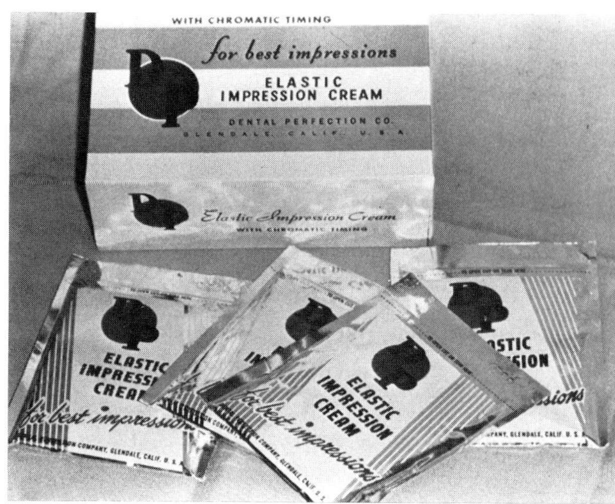

Fig. 5-24. Preweighed packaged alginate is convenient but expensive.

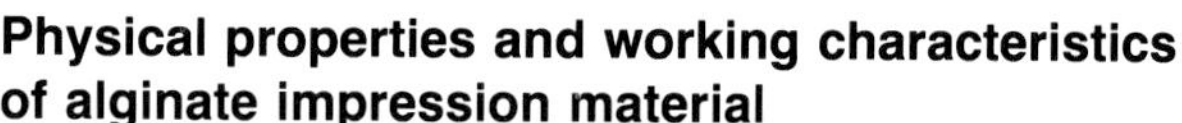

Physical properties and working characteristics of alginate impression material

Irreversible hydrocolloid impression material, commonly known as alginate, is the material of choice for diagnostic impressions.

Although alginate does not record the same degree of surface detail as some other impression materials, it is accurate and it is suitable for making diagnostic and final impressions for removable partial dentures. Alginate is easy to use and is relatively inexpensive. However, it is one of the most abused impression materials used by dentists. Knowledge of the physical properties and working characteristics of irreversible hydrocolloid is essential if the material is to be used successfully.

Alginate impression material is supplied in powdered form. Water is mixed with the powder to form a viscous sol, which forms an elastic gel through a series of chemical reactions after it is placed in the mouth.

The alginate powder is available in preweighed pouches containing sufficient material for most impressions and in bulk containers (Figs. 5-24 and 5-25). The individual packages are considerably more expensive than the bulk alginate.

Although irreversible hydrocolloid is not usually considered to have a shelf life, the method of storage is very important. Alginate deteriorates rapidly in elevated temperatures and high humidity. Alginate stored at 65° C for 1 month has been shown to be unsuitable for use. Evidence of deterioration has even been shown after storage at 54° C. This deterioration is thought to be caused by depolymerization of the alginate constituent. Once a can of alginate is opened, it can show measurable deterioration within 3 days. Repeated opening of the can and exposure of its contents to humidity contribute to rapid deterioration of the powder that remains. Alginate that has deteriorated because of heat or moisture will become thin during mixing, exhibit erratic setting times, have reduced strength, and produce high degrees of permanent deformation of the impression. Alginate can also be contaminated by gypsum. Small amounts of dental stone left in the mixing bowl or on the spatula can contaminate the alginate and accelerate its set (Fig. 5-26).

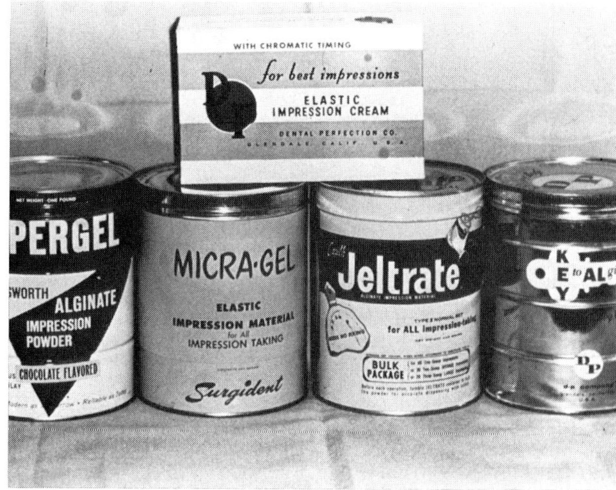

Fig. 5-25. Alginate impression material in bulk containers.

The accuracy of irreversible hydrocolloid is not affected by changes in the water/powder ratio. Extremely thin mixes of alginate may be used for duplicating casts with no loss of accuracy, but with loss of strength. However, the water/powder ratio does have a signifi-

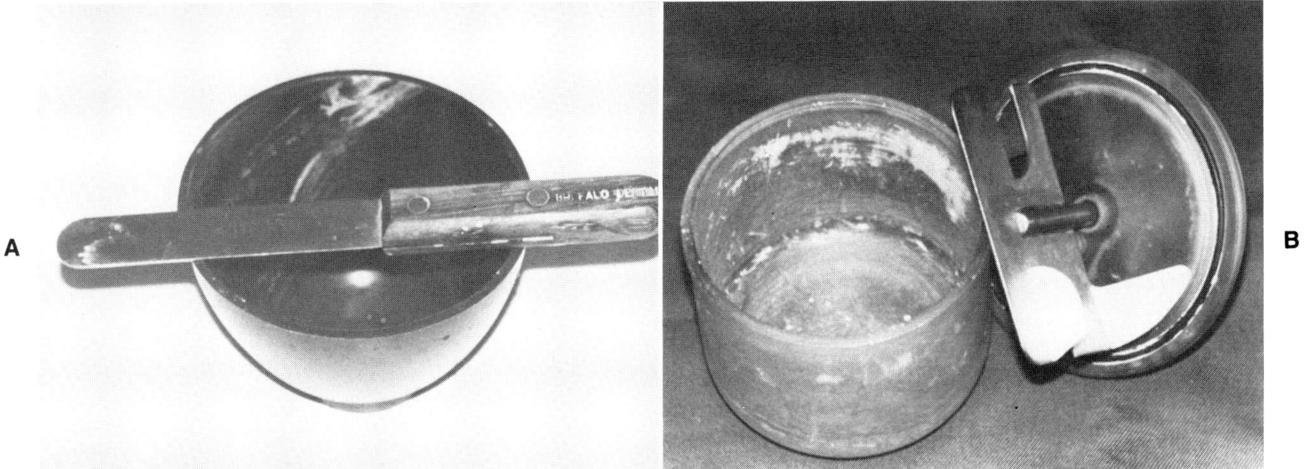

Fig. 5-26. A, Remnants of dental stone on spatula or rubber bowl can contaminate alginate. **B,** Contaminated mechanical mixer.

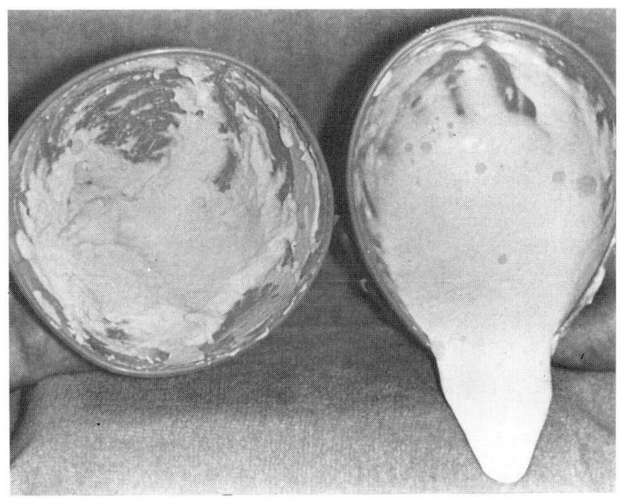

Fig. 5-27. Uncontrolled water/powder ratio can result in too thick or too thin a mix for clinical use.

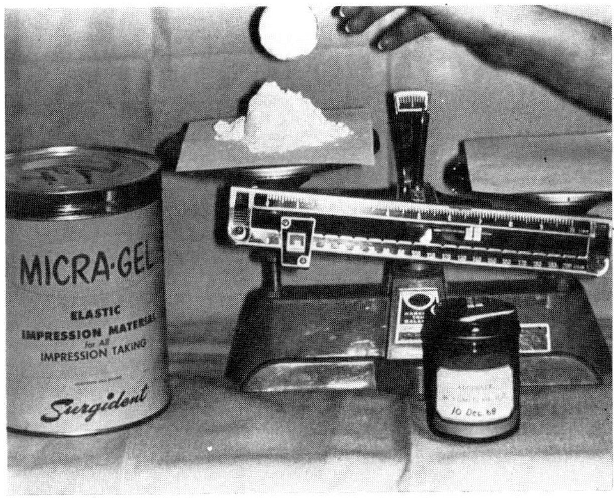

Fig. 5-28. Accurate scale used to weigh bulk alginate.

cant effect on the working characteristics of the alginate when it is used for making impressions of the mouth. Changes in the water/powder ratio will affect the consistency and setting time of the mixed material and the strength and quality of the impression. Too heavy or thick a mix will not flow sufficiently to record all detail. Too thin a mix will tend to flow out of the tray and away from the tissue being recorded, will tear too easily on removal from the mouth, and will result in an unacceptable impression (Fig. 5-27). Ideally, the dentist should work with a predetermined amount of powder for every impression, varying the amount of water slightly to obtain subtle changes in consistency to meet specific clinical requirements. The consistency of the mix can vary considerably if the powder is measured by the scoop provided by the manufacturer. The amount of powder in one scoop depends on whether the powder in the can had been fluffed or was left compacted and on whether the scoop handle was tapped to compress the material or the excess was simply scraped off the top of the scoop. Considerable variation is also present in the preweighed packages of alginate; the equipment used for weighing the material apparently has a low degree of accuracy.

Bulk alginate is the most economical means of using alginate. Once the can is opened, its entire contents should be accurately weighed into three scoop equivalent amounts (Fig. 5-28) and then tightly sealed in oint-

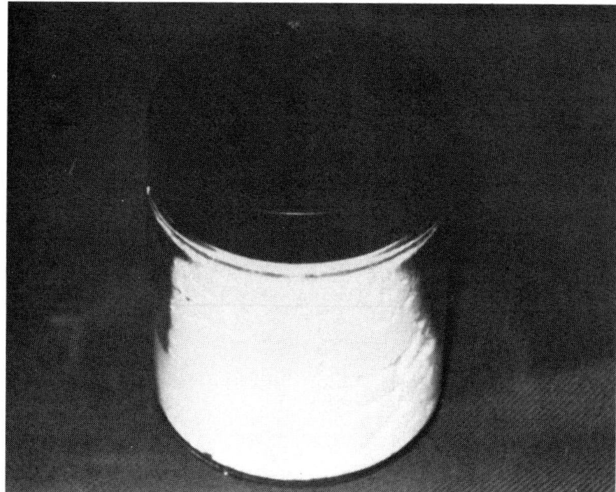

Fig. 5-29. Alginate stored in an airtight container.

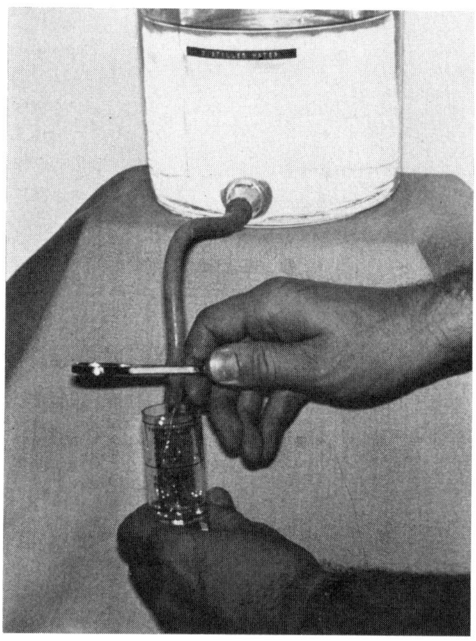

Fig. 5-30. Measuring distilled water for a mix of alginate.

ment jars or plastic bags (Fig. 5-29). This quantity is adequate for most impressions. With this method the only variable will be the amount of water used, which can be varied to satisfy the requirements of the patient being treated.

Some water supplies contain large amounts of minerals. These impurities can adversely affect the accuracy and the setting time of the alginate. The routine use of distilled or demineralized water can preclude these problems (Fig. 5-30).

The setting time of alginate is determined by the formulation used by the manufacturer. Both fast- and regular-set alginate are available. The dentist can control the setting time somewhat by varying the temperature of the water used. Most manufacturers recommend the use of 22° C (72° F) water. Cooler water will provide more working time, whereas slightly warmer water will hasten the set of the impression material. Some brands of alginate exhibit greater sensitivity to temperature change than others. Some products have shown as much as a 20-second change in gelation time for each 1° C change in the temperature of the water. Refrigeration of the mixing bowl and water can greatly increase the working time. Prepackaged and preweighed alginate can also be refrigerated, but a can of bulk alginate should not because when the cooled can of alginate is opened, the water that has condensed on the inside of the lid will fall on the powder, making it unfit for use.

Storage of alginate impressions

A definite disadvantage of the alginate impression material is that it cannot be stored for any appreciable length of time. Measurable distortion occurs if the cast is not poured within 12 minutes. No method of storage for longer periods is safe if accuracy is to be achieved.

The alginate expands if it comes in contact with liquids because the alginate will imbibe water. Therefore wrapping the impression in wet paper towels or soaking the impression in water or other solution is contraindicated. Evaporation and shrinkage of the alginate occur if it is exposed to the atmosphere. In addition, dimensional change will result from the release of strains within the material as the moisture content changes. Even in a completely humid environment the alginate shrinks through a process called syneresis, in which a fluid exudate forms on the surface of the impression.

Alginate should not be used for diagnostic impressions unless the time and facilities are available for pouring the impression within 12 minutes from the time the impression is removed from the mouth. An important point is that anything that will cause the alginate to gain or lose water will allow the release of strains that invariably develop during the making and removal of the impression.

Sticking of alginate

A potential problem in using irreversible hydrocolloid is the tendency for this material to stick to the teeth (Fig. 5-31). The sticking usually occurs on the flat labial and buccal teeth surfaces and occasionally on the tips of the cusps. Rarely will there be sticking on the lingual surfaces of the teeth. The sticking is caused by a chemical bond between the alginate radical and the

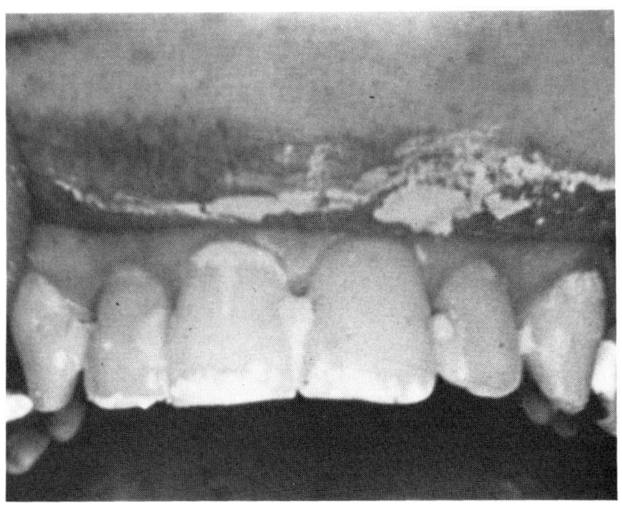

Fig. 5-31. Alginate tends to stick to teeth.

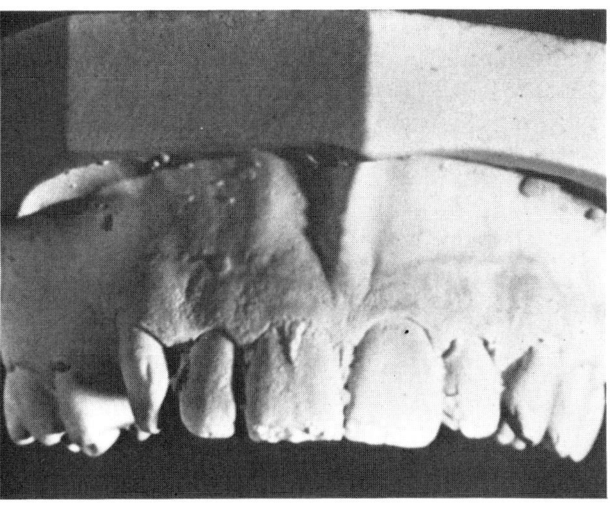

Fig. 5-32. Inaccurate cast resulting from alginate sticking to teeth.

hydroxyapatite crystal of the surface enamel. If the alginate sticks to the teeth, the impression and the cast will be inaccurate (Fig. 5-32). The inaccuracy will range from a small degree of surface roughness in the area of sticking to gross distortion if the sticking is severe enough to pull the alginate away from the tray. The dentist must know that the problem exists, how to determine whether sticking has occurred, what factors contribute to sticking, how to prevent sticking, and how to proceed once sticking has occurred.

The dentist should make a habit of examining the labial and buccal surfaces of the teeth immediately after removing an alginate impression. If sticking occurs, the alginate will have to be scraped off the teeth because it adheres tightly. The impression itself presents a characteristic appearance if sticking has occurred: the buccal or facial surfaces will have a roughened or scaly appearance. Therefore the impression should be thoroughly examined immediately after its removal.

Three factors contribute to the sticking. First, sticking occurs more frequently when the teeth are very clean. Most dentists polish the teeth following mouth preparation for removable partial dentures or early in the diagnosis and treatment planning phase of treatment. If impressions are made after thorough or vigorous polishing of the teeth, sticking is more likely to occur. Therefore only light cleaning of the teeth should be accomplished immediately before impressions are made. If thorough cleaning is necessary, the impression making should be deferred until a later appointment. Second, there is a greater tendency for the alginate to stick if the teeth are dry. Saliva must be controlled or it will displace the alginate. Adequate control of the saliva can be accomplished by packing the mouth with gauze pads before making the impression. Drying with compressed air, however, is contraindicated because the degree of dryness achieved in this manner contributes to the sticking of the alginate. Third, there is a greater tendency for sticking to occur if repeated impressions are made of an arch. The film that protects the enamel from the sticking of alginate is apparently lost during repeated attempts to make a satisfactory impression. Invariably, once sticking begins, it becomes increasingly more severe with every attempt to make an impression. Good technique should be followed in making the impressions so that several attempts are not necessary. And once sticking has occurred, it is foolish to make further attempts during that appointment unless other measures are taken to prevent the alginate from sticking.

A good preventive measure is to use a prophylactic paste to which silicone ointment has been added. The thin film of silicone will usually prevent sticking. An alternative method of applying the silicone is to wipe a small amount of silicone ointment onto the vulnerable areas of the teeth. Excess silicone must be removed or it will make the impression inaccurate.

Once the dentist recognizes that alginate has stuck to the patient's teeth, one of two courses of action should be followed. (1) The dentist may choose to clean the alginate from the teeth and make another appointment for the patient. Usually sticking will not be a problem the next day if the teeth are not recleaned at that time. (2) The dentist may try to prevent the sticking from recurring and repeat the impression procedure. After the adhering alginate has been scraped away, silicone can be applied to the teeth using one of the two methods just described. (Petrolatum is not a satisfactory substitute for the silicone.) Or the patient may suck on sour candy, chew sour gum of one of the citrus flavors, or swish whole milk in the oral cavity to accelerate the production of a protective film over the enamel of the teeth. However, for some patients none of these measures is effective, and the only solution is to defer the making of the impression.

Technique for making diagnostic impressions

Position of patient and dentist

The position of the patient and the dentist can facilitate or complicate the making of impressions. This procedure can be accomplished most conveniently and with greatest comfort for the patient if the dentist is standing and the patient is seated upright. The occlusal plane of the arch for which the impression is being made should be parallel to the floor when the patient's mouth is open (Fig. 5-33). Therefore some adjustment of the chair is necessary between impressions. The height of the chair should be adjusted so that the patient's mouth is at the same level as the dentist's elbow.

When making the maxillary impression, the dentist should stand at the right rear of the patient.* This permits the dentist's left arm and hand to encircle the patient's head and manipulate the left corner of the mouth and lips (Fig. 5-34). For the mandibular impression the dentist stands at the right front of the patient. With the impression tray held in the right hand, the dentist can manipulate the right corner of the patient's mouth with the left thumb and index finger (Fig. 5-35).

*Instructions as to the dentist's position are for a right-handed dentist. The left-handed practitioner should substitute *left* for *right* and vice versa in following these instructions.

Impression trays

Stock impression trays for dentulous and partially edentulous dental arches are of three basic types: rim lock trays, perforated metal trays, and plastic disposable trays. The tray of choice is the rim lock tray because it is rigid and it confines the impression material, helping to force it into all the areas to be included in the impression. Although perforated trays are rigid, they do not confine the material as well as the rim lock tray (Fig. 5-36). Many of the disposable plastic trays are too flexible to ensure the accuracy of impression and cast that is needed for removable partial dentures (Fig. 5-37).

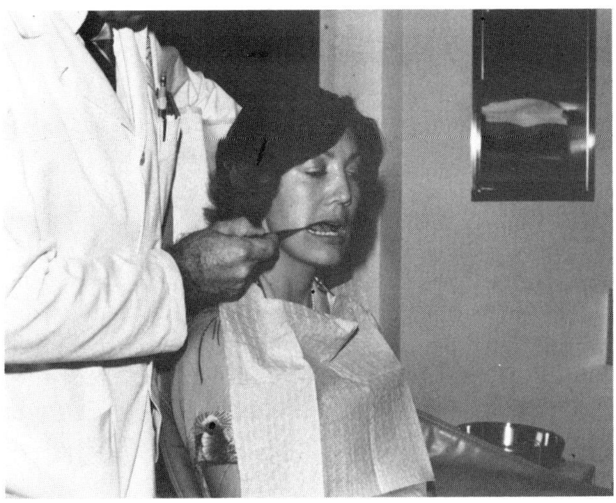

Fig. 5-33. Occlusal plane should be parallel to floor when impressions are made.

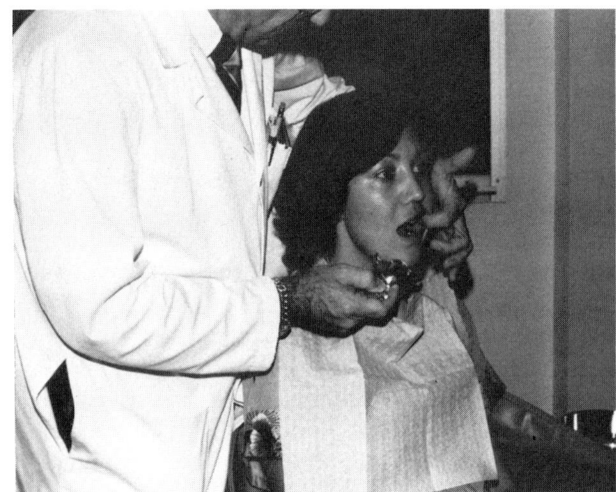

Fig. 5-34. Dentist's position at right rear allows manipulation of left corner of mouth and lips when maxillary impression is made.

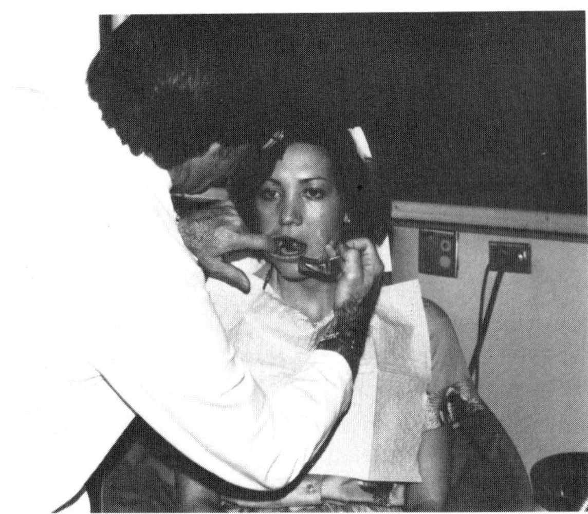

Fig. 5-35. Dentist's position at right front allows manipulation of right corner of mouth when mandibular impression is made.

Checking maxillary tray for correct size. The width of the tray is the determining factor in the selection of the size of the tray. There should be a buccal clearance of 5 to 7 mm between the inner flanges of the tray and the facial surfaces of the remaining teeth and the edentulous ridge (Fig. 5-38). The operator should stand at the right rear of the patient in checking the maxillary tray. The impression tray is held in the right hand with the thumb on top of the tray and the index and middle fingers under the handle. The left arm is behind the patient's head and the chair, and the left hand is used to manipulate the patient's left cheek and upper lip to allow easier insertion of the tray and better vision for the operator. The right posterior flange of the tray is used to stretch the right corner of the mouth, and the tray is rotated into the mouth while the dentist stretches the patient's left cheek and lifts the upper lip with his left hand. By standing behind and being above the patient, the operator can see the relation of the flanges of the tray to the facial surfaces of the teeth. The 5- to 7-mm space is necessary so that the impression material will be thick enough to spring over the undercuts. Too large a tray may be difficult to insert, and interference with the coronoid processes of the mandible may be encountered in seating the tray. Frequently a tray that has the proper width is not long enough to cover the entire desired impression area, or a considerably greater space is present between the tray and the palatal tissues than the desired 5 to 7 mm. If an impression is attempted with such a tray, a great bulk of alginate tends to sag before gelation is complete, and an inaccurate impression of the palatal vault results. Unfortunately, this inaccuracy is not readily apparent. As the bulk of the alginate sags, the surface that has developed sufficient gelation to record anatomic contours also sags away from the tissues, resulting in an impression that looks accurate but is not. The length of the tray and excessive palatal space can be easily corrected by the use of modeling plastic. It is not always necessary to modify the tray when diagnostic impressions are made, but is always necessary for the maxillary final impression.

Checking mandibular tray for correct size. A mandibular tray should provide 5 to 7 mm of space both buccal and lingual to the remaining teeth and the residual ridge. If the tray extends too far from the teeth in a

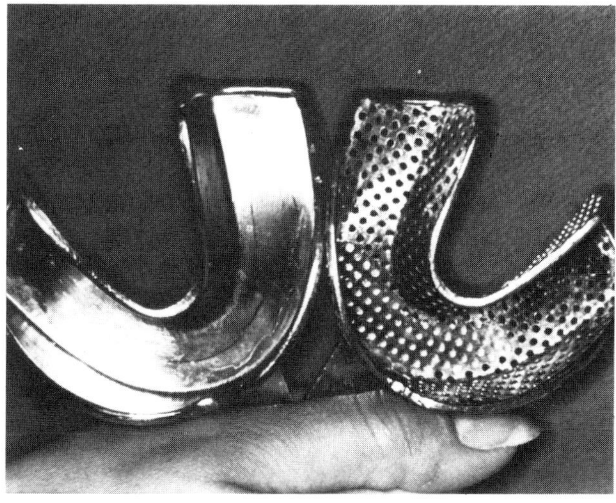

Fig. 5-36. Left, rim lock tray. Right, perforated impression tray.

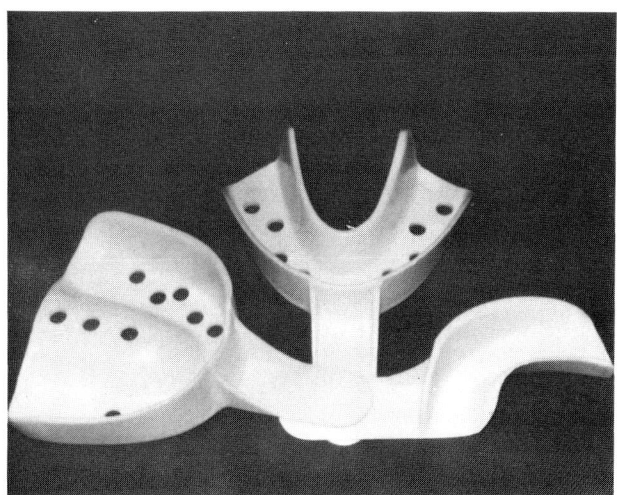

Fig. 5-37. Most disposable plastic trays are too flexible to ensure accuracy.

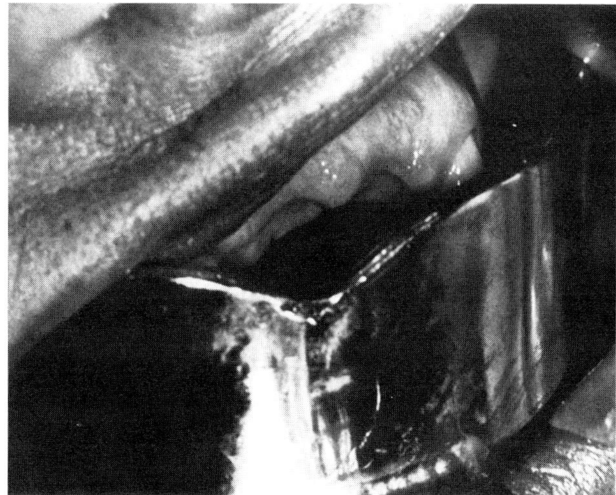

Fig. 5-38. Tray should have buccal clearance of 5 to 7 mm.

lingual direction, there is a tendency to trap the tongue or the floor of the mouth. The problem should be corrected by selecting a tray of a different size or by bending the lingual flanges of the tray to provide the 5 to 7 mm of clearance.

A right-handed dentist should be positioned at the right front of the patient. The patient's mandibular occlusal plane should be at the level of the dentist's elbow. The impression tray is held in the right hand, and the left thumb and index fingers are used to manipulate the right corner of the patient's mouth. The impression tray is rotated into the mouth by contacting the left corner of the mouth with the left posterior flange of the tray. As the right flange of the tray is rotated toward the mouth, the left thumb and index finger are used to stretch the right corner of the mouth and depress the lower lip. The patient is asked to raise the tongue gently out of the mouth. This will ensure that the tongue is out from under the tray. The patient should hold the tongue in a relaxed forward position while the tray is seated. Once the tray has passed the corner of the mouth, it is straightened and positioned over the teeth. With the lower lip depressed, the dentist can easily see the buccal and lingual clearance between the teeth and the tray.

Extending an impression tray. Frequently an impression tray that has a correct width is too short to cover the entire desired impression area. The impression tray can be lengthened by the use of modeling plastic (Figs. 5-39 and 5-40). The modeling plastic is softened in a 60° C (140° F) water bath, kneaded, and adapted to the tray to form the general contours of the impression area. The modeling plastic is flamed, tempered in the water bath, and seated in the mouth. If undercuts are present, the tray should be seated and partially removed several times to prevent the locking of the tray into the undercuts. After the modeling plastic has been chilled, it is relieved with a sharp knife to provide approxi-

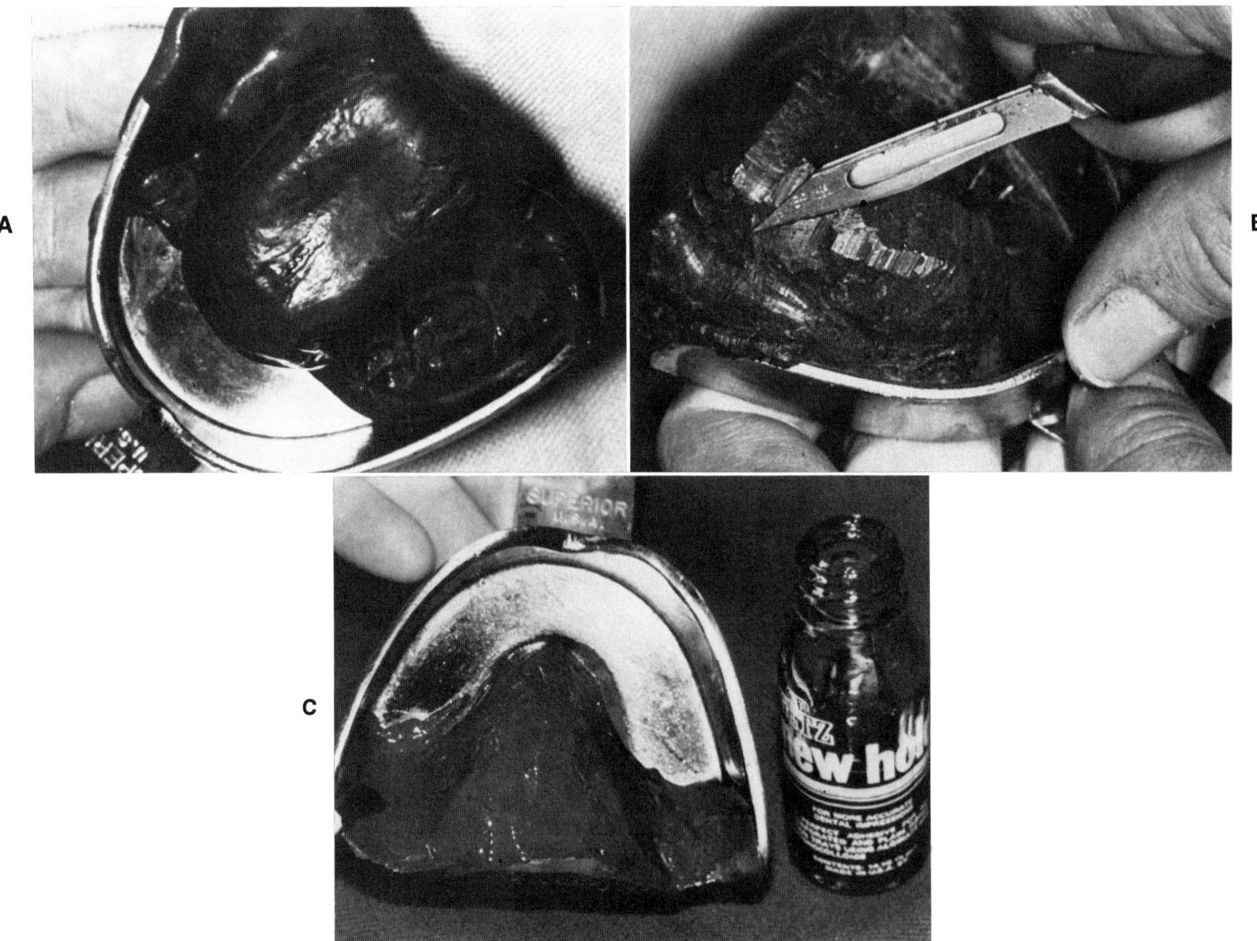

Fig. 5-39. A, Maxillary tray modified with softened modeling plastic. **B,** Modeling plastic relieved to make room for impression material. **C,** Tray and modeling plastic painted with alginate adhesive.

mately 5 to 7 mm of clearance. Alginate adhesive should be painted on the modeling plastic and the inner surface of the tray.

Control of gagging

It is usually a mistake to make too big an issue over the making of impressions. The dentist definitely should not bring up the subject of gagging. The dentist should ask whether the patient has had impressions made previously. If this is to be the patient's first experience, a brief description of the procedure should be given. That the material to be used has the consistency of thick whipped cream and that it sets up to a rubbery consistency in several minutes is usually all the explanation that is necessary. The dentist should proceed in a confident, efficient manner. Dentists usually encounter more problems with gagging when they are in initial stages of dental practice and approach the making of impressions with an unsure and nervous demeanor.

Procedures that will help to prevent gagging include

1. Seating the patient in an upright position with the occlusal plane parallel with the floor.
2. Correcting the maxillary tray with modeling plastic and leaving sufficient unrelieved modeling plastic at the posterior border so that positive contact can be maintained against the posterior palate during the setting of the alginate.
3. Not overfilling the tray with alginate.
4. Seating the posterior part of the tray first and then rotating the tray into position, thereby forcing excess alginate in an anterior direction rather than out the posterior border of the tray.
5. Asking the patient to keep the eyes open during the impression procedure (this usually reduces the patient's tension).
6. Asking the patient to breathe through the nose.
7. Asking the patient to keep the eyes focused on some small object.

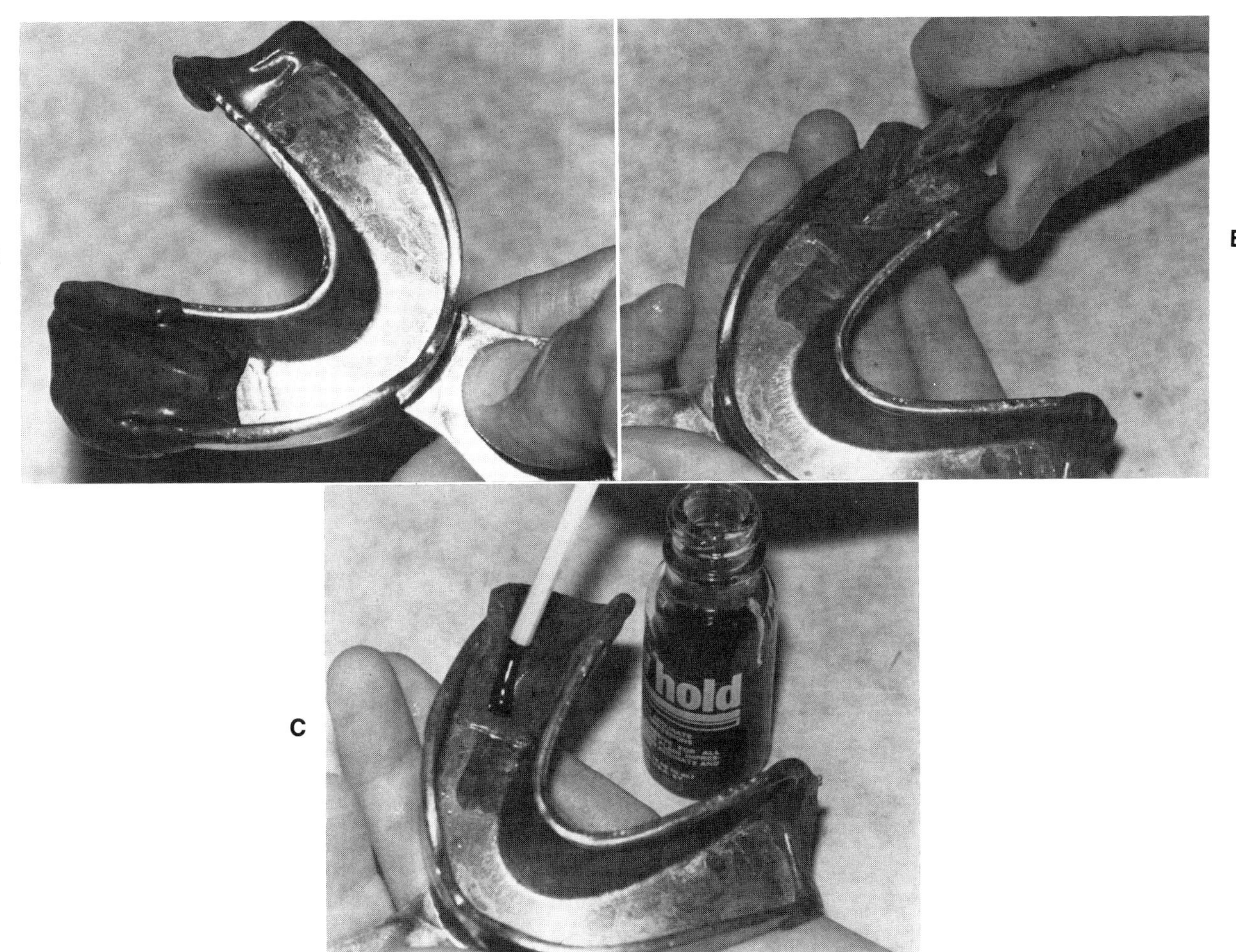

Fig. 5-40. A, Mandibular tray modified with softened modeling plastic. **B,** Scraping relief. **C,** Tray painted with alginate adhesive.

8. Giving all instructions to the patient in a firm, controlled manner.
9. Having the patient use astringent mouth rinse and cold water rinses before the impression is made. The use of an anesthetic spray is usually contraindicated because it will cause numbness of the tongue and palate and may contribute to the urge to gag.

Most gagging problems are psychologic rather than physical, and confidence in the dentist will help eliminate many of them.

A very small percentage of patients has a true, uncontrollable gag reflex. The simple procedure of attempting to introduce an empty tray into the mouth may initiate severe gagging. Obviously, other measures in addition to those previously described are necessary if impressions are to be successfully made for these patients. The following procedures will allow the dentist to make impressions for almost any patient who is physically and psychologically able to follow the instructions that are given.

1. The patient is asked to take a deep breath and hold the breath while the dentist quickly checks the size and fit of the tray. Most patients will not gag while holding the breath so the dentist can complete simple, short procedures such as fitting the tray, correcting the tray with modeling plastic, and drying the palate without the danger of the patient gagging.
2. The patient is asked to rinse the mouth with astringent mouthwash and then hold cold water in the mouth, provided the teeth are not sensitive.
3. A fast-setting alginate or slightly warmer than normal (approximately 24° C [75° F]) water is used to hasten the set of the alginate.
4. The "leg lift" procedure is used before and during the making of the impression. The patient is asked to lift one leg off the dental chair and to keep it raised at all times (Fig. 5-41). As fatigue sets in, it will usually be necessary to firmly command the patient to keep the leg lifted. The mixing of the alginate is not begun until the patient appears to be in some distress at efforts to keep the leg raised. When fatigue is noticeable, the alginate is mixed, the palate or floor of the mouth is quickly dried with gauze, the alginate is placed in critical areas, and the tray is seated in the mouth. The dentist should be giving commands to keep the leg raised throughout these procedures to distract the patient. Once the patient has been shown that an impression can be made successfully, all further procedures can be accomplished with a greatly reduced tendency toward gagging. The success of the leg lift procedure is probably based on a combination of some disorientation of the patient caused by fatigue, focusing the patient's attention on the difficult task of keeping the leg raised, and anger at the dentist. However, the success of making impressions is almost always accompanied by an exhibition of appreciation and relief by these patients.

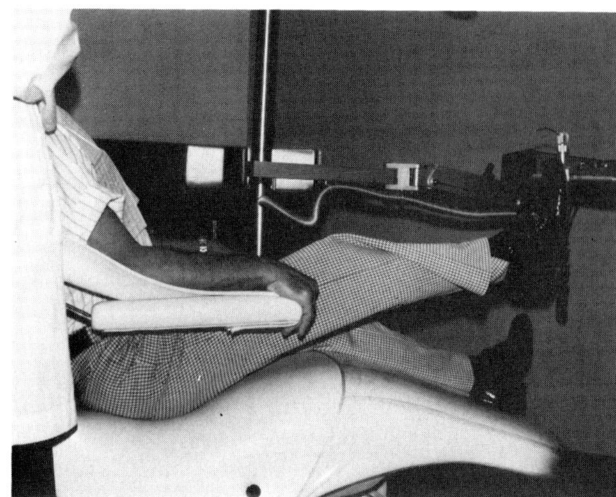

Fig. 5-41. Patient elevating leg to combat gagging during impression making.

Control of saliva

Alginate has a tendency to stick to teeth if the teeth are too dry. Therefore the teeth should not be air dried before making an impression. However, excessive amounts of saliva, particularly of the thick mucous type, will displace the alginate impression material and will contribute to an inaccurate impression. The saliva can be controlled for most patients by having the patient rinse the mouth with an astringent mouthwash followed by a rinse of cold water (Fig. 5-42) and then packing the mouth with 2 × 2 inch gauze that has been unfolded to form a strip of 2-inch gauze (Fig. 5-43). In the maxillary arch one gauze strip is placed in the right buccal vestibule and another in the left vestibule. The patient can be asked to lightly hold a third piece of gauze in the palate. Because too much force by the patient may displace the tissue to be recorded in the impression, the dentist may prefer to wipe the palatal area just before making the impression. In the mandibular arch one gauze strip is placed in each of the buccal vestibules and another is placed in the linguoalveolar sulcus by having the patient raise the tongue, placing the gauze in the sulcus, and then having the patient relax the tongue to hold the gauze in position.

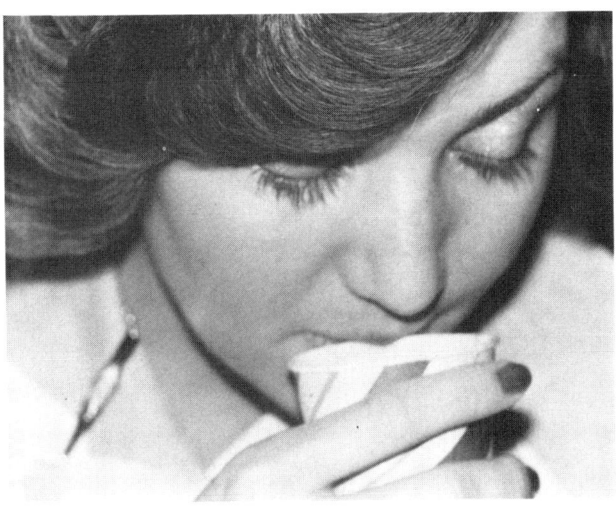

Fig. 5-42. Patient rinsing with astringent mouthwash before impression is made.

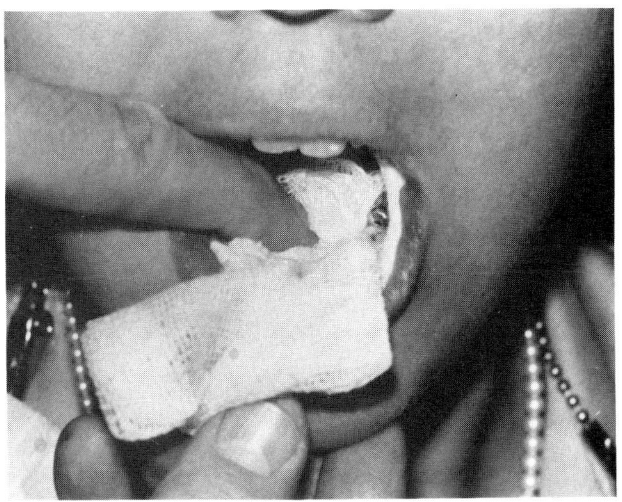

Fig. 5-43. Mouth packed with gauze to control saliva.

The gauze is removed immediately before the impression is made.

A few patients secrete an excessive amount of thick mucinous saliva from the palatal salivary glands. This heavy saliva displaces the alginate and results in an inaccurate and rough surface to the impression. These patients should be instructed to rinse with an astringent mouth rinse. Then 2 × 2-inch sponges dampened in warm water should be used to place pressure over the posterior palate in an attempt to milk the glands. This is followed by an ice water rinse immediately before the impression is made.

In rare instances the patient will secrete such copious amounts of saliva that impression making becomes extremely difficult if not impossible. The use of an antisialagogue in combination with mouth rinses and gauze packs effectively controls this salivation. A 15-mg propantheline bromide (Pro-Banthine) tablet taken 30 minutes before the impression appointment will also help control the excessive salivation. These drugs should never be prescribed in the presence of medical contraindications such as glaucoma, prostatic hypertrophy, and cardiac conditions in which any increase in the heart rate is to be avoided.

Mixing impression material

Alginate may be mixed by hand spatulation, mechanical spatulation, or mechanical spatulation under vacuum. The objective is a smooth, bubble-free mix of alginate. In hand spatulation a measured amount of distilled water at approximately 22° C (72° F) is placed in a rubber mixing bowl. The preweighed alginate powder is sifted from its container into the water. The mixing should begin slowly using a stiff, broad-bladed spatula. When the powder is thoroughly wet, the speed of the spatulation should be increased. The spatula should crush the material against the sides of the bowl to ensure that the material is completely mixed. The spatulation should continue for a minimum of 45 seconds. The strength of the gel can be reduced 50% if the mixing is not complete. Insufficient spatulation can result in failure of the ingredients to dissolve sufficiently. Then the chemical reaction of changing from a sol to a gel will not proceed uniformly throughout the mass of alginate. An incompletely spatulated mix will appear lumpy and granular and will have numerous areas of trapped air. Complete spatulation will result in a smooth, creamy mixture. The mixing should be completed by wiping the alginate against the side of the bowl with the spatula to remove any trapped air (Fig. 5-44). The most consistent method of making a smooth, bubble-free mix is mechanical spatulation under vacuum (Fig. 5-45). The preweighed powder is added to the premeasured water in the mechanical mixing bowl. The powder is thoroughly incorporated into the water by hand spatulation. The mix is then mechanically spatulated under 20 pounds of vacuum for 15 seconds. Longer spatulation will result in a greatly reduced setting time of the alginate and could affect the strength of the gel.

Loading impression tray

Small increments of the impression material should be placed in the tray and forced under the rim lock (Fig. 5-46). Placing too large a portion of alginate at one time increases the possibility of trapping air. The tray should be filled level with the flanges of the tray. Overfilling should be avoided.

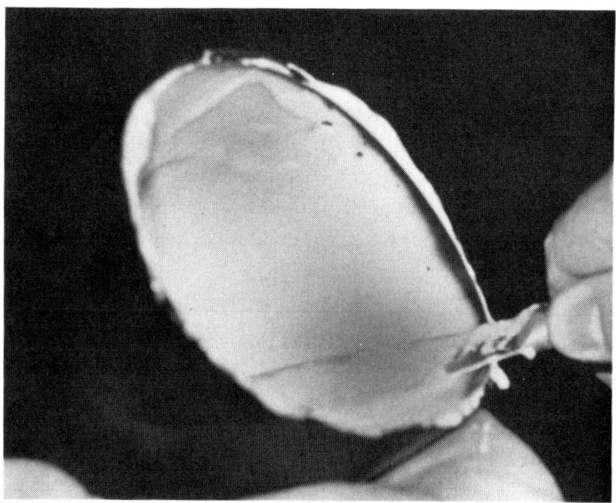

Fig. 5-44. Alginate wiped against side of bowl with spatula to remove trapped air.

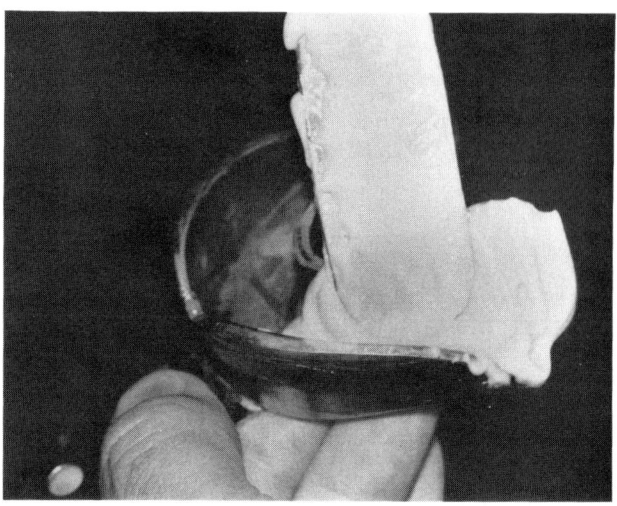

Fig. 5-46. Small increments of alginate are forced under rim lock when tray is loaded.

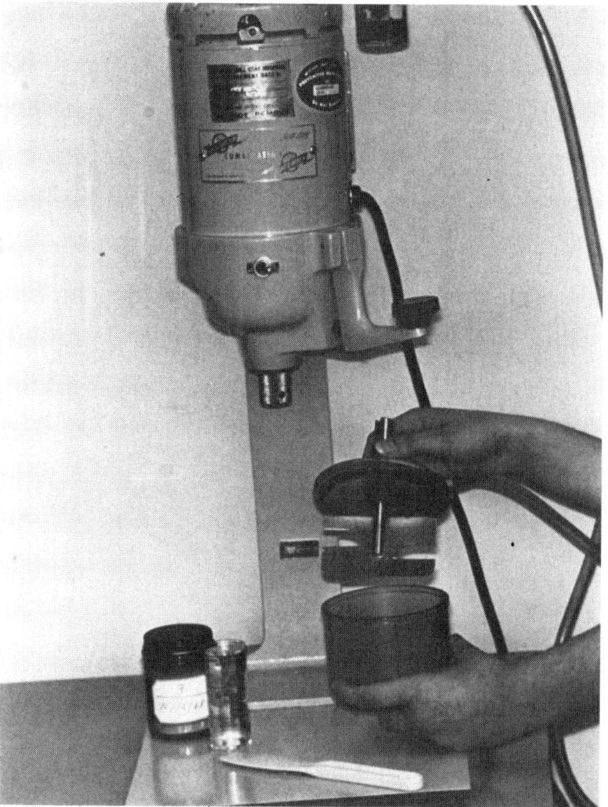

Fig. 5-45. Most consistent mix of alginate is made with mechanical spatulation under vacuum.

Making impressions

The mandibular impression is made first because it usually entails less patient discomfort. Patient confidence is increased when an impression has been successfully completed.

While holding the tray with the left hand, the dentist uses the right hand to remove the gauze pads from the patient's mouth. Impression material remaining in the bowl is picked up with fingers of the right hand and painted over the occlusal surface of the teeth and into the vestibular and alveololingual sulcus areas (Fig. 5-47). The impression material will remain in place if the tissues are fairly dry. A tendency for the alginate to form a ball and not remain where placed indicates that the tissues are too moist and that voids are likely to be present in the impression. There is not enough time to repack the mouth before gelation begins, so the impression procedure should be completed. The impression should be carefully inspected and if voids are present in critical areas, the impression procedure should be repeated. Packing the mouth with more or larger gauze pads and avoiding removal of the gauze until ready to apply the alginate will usually prevent this problem. The layer of alginate applied with the fingers should be 3 to 4 mm thick; if it is too thin, the heat of the tissues of the oral cavity may cause the material to set before the tray is seated, resulting in a layered impression. The tray is then rotated into the mouth in the manner described for checking the fit of the tray. The fingers of the left hand that are retracting the right cheek should depress the lower lip to provide good visibility (Fig. 5-48). When the tray is correctly lined up over the teeth, the patient is asked to protrude the tongue. The tray is carefully seated

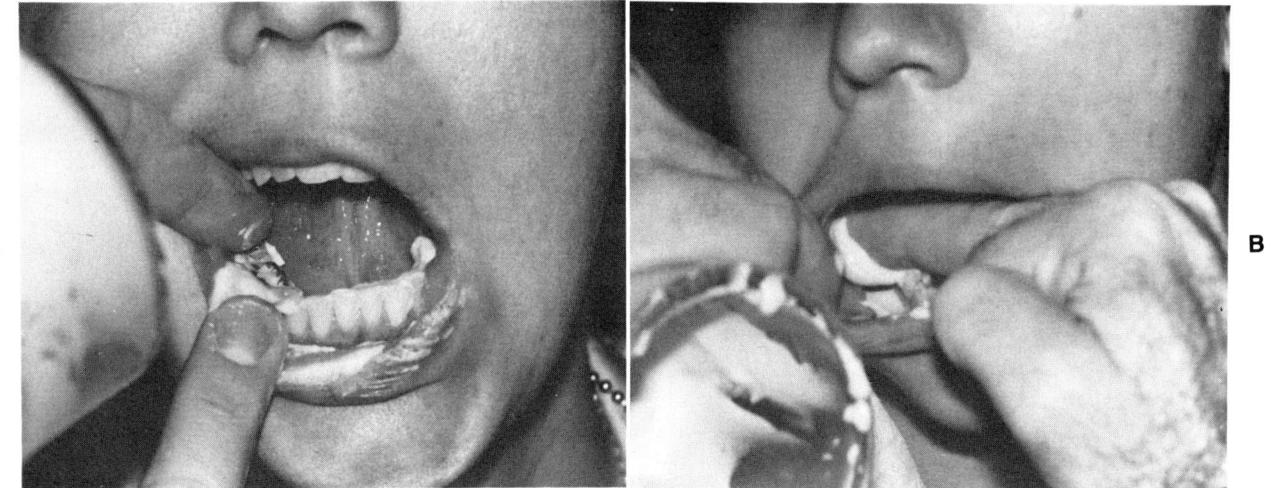

Fig. 5-47. Alginate wiped onto teeth, **A,** and into vestibular areas, **B.**

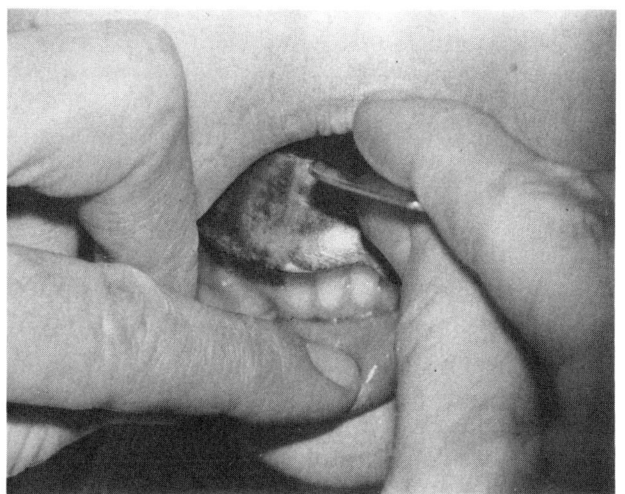

Fig. 5-48. Lower lip depressed to provide visibility when tray is seated.

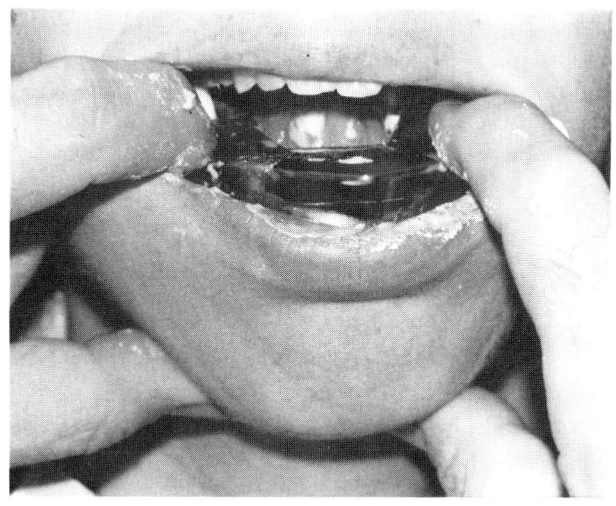

Fig. 5-49. Mandibular tray held in position by forefingers in premolar areas and thumbs under patient's chin.

so that its flanges are below the gingival margins of the teeth. The tray should not be overseated because this could result in the cusps of the teeth contacting the tray, causing an inaccurate impression. Great care must be exercised in seating the tray if the patient has mandibular tori or other exostoses, or the making of this impression can be a very painful experience for the patient. As the tray is being seated, the cheeks are pulled out to prevent the trapping of buccal tissues under the tray. The patient is asked to keep the tip of the tongue in contact with the upper surface of the tray during the gelation of the impression material. The dentist must maintain the position of the tray during the entire gelation period. This can be accomplished most conveniently and effectively by placing the forefinger of each hand on the top of the tray in the premolar area and by placing the thumbs under the patient's chin (Fig. 5-49). The dentist through tactile sense can maintain an even amount of pressure on the tray even if the patient swallows or opens or closes the mouth. Any movement of the tray during the gelation period will result in an inaccurate impression. Allowing the patient or the assistant to hold the tray or leaving the patient unattended must be avoided. Within 3 to 4 minutes the alginate should be set.

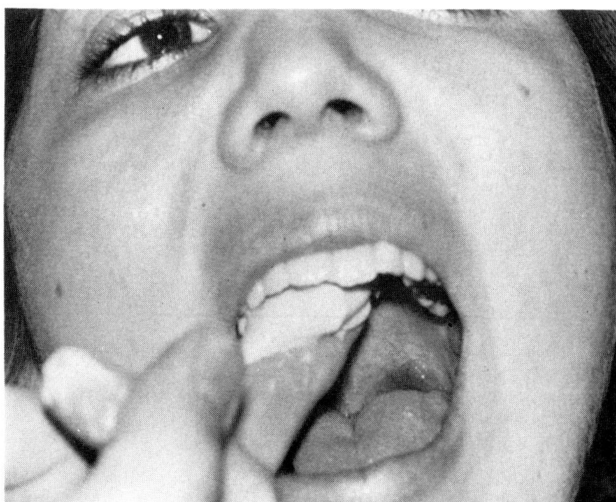

Fig. 5-50. Impression material wiped into palate to avoid trapping air.

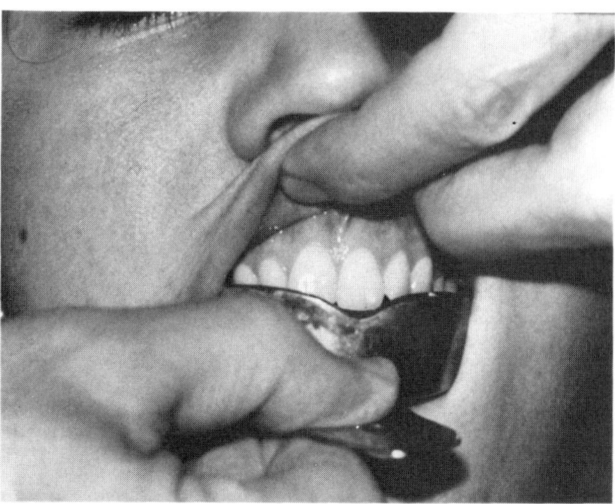

Fig. 5-51. Upper lip raised to provide visibility when maxillary tray is being seated.

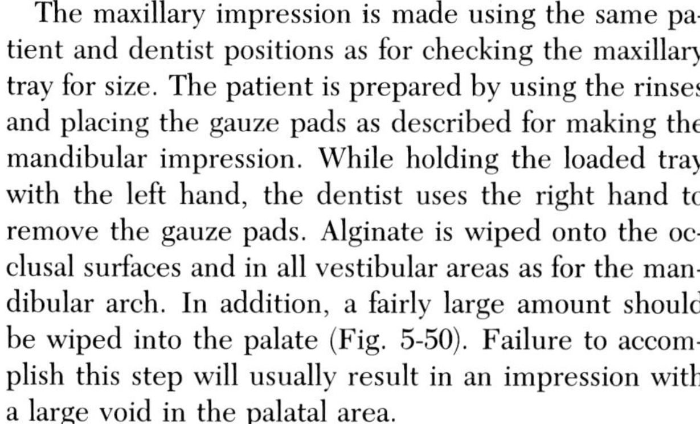

The maxillary impression is made using the same patient and dentist positions as for checking the maxillary tray for size. The patient is prepared by using the rinses and placing the gauze pads as described for making the mandibular impression. While holding the loaded tray with the left hand, the dentist uses the right hand to remove the gauze pads. Alginate is wiped onto the occlusal surfaces and in all vestibular areas as for the mandibular arch. In addition, a fairly large amount should be wiped into the palate (Fig. 5-50). Failure to accomplish this step will usually result in an impression with a large void in the palatal area.

The loaded maxillary tray is grasped by the thumb and forefinger of the right hand. As the right posterior flange of the impression tray stretches the right corner of the mouth, the dentist's left arm should be behind the patient's head and headrest so that the thumb and index finger may grasp the left corner of the mouth and distend it slightly to allow the impression tray to enter the mouth in a straight line. No attempt should be made to seat the tray until the tray is in its correct anteroposterior position. Once the tray is in the mouth, the thumb and forefinger of the left hand should raise the upper lip to allow the dentist to see the relationship between the labial flange of the tray and the anterior teeth or the residual ridge (Fig. 5-51). The tray must be centered and properly aligned. This position can best be verified by looking at the patient's face from above and observing the position of the handle of the tray. It should protrude straight from the center of the mouth (Fig. 5-52). After the proper position has been verified, the tray is seated by using the fingers of both hands over the premolar areas. As the tray is being seated, the cheeks must be lifted outward and upward

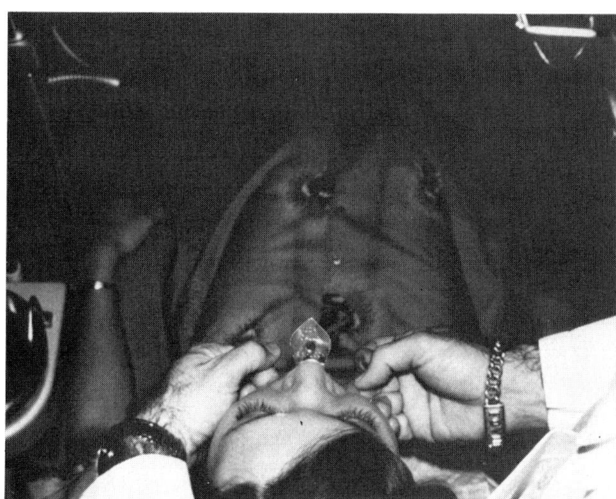

Fig. 5-52. Position of tray verified by observing handle of tray protruding from center of mouth.

to prevent the buccal tissues from being trapped under the flanges of the tray. The lip must also be lifted up and out to allow good visibility and to avoid trapping the lip between the flange of the tray and the anterior teeth. Care must be taken not to overseat the tray to avoid contact between the tray and the cusp tips or incisal edges of the teeth. The tray should be stabilized throughout the set of the impression material by keeping light pressure over the premolar areas on both sides of the arch. The alginate should set in 3 to 4 minutes.

Effect of movement of tray

Gelation of alginate occurs by a chemical reaction. When mixed with water, the sodium alginate and calcium sulphate in the powder react to form a latticework of fibrils of insoluble calcium alginate. The heat of the oral tissues accelerates the chemical reaction, causing the alginate next to the tissues to gel first. If the dentist exerts pressure or allows the tray to move during gelation of the remainder of the alginate, internal stresses are created that can distort the impression as it is removed from the mouth.

Removal of impression from mouth

Clinically, the initial set of alginate is determined by a loss of surface tackiness. The impression should be left in the mouth for an additional 2 to 3 minutes to allow the development of additional strength. Early removal of the weak alginate may lead to unnecessary tearing of the impression. The gel strength doubles during the first 4 minutes after initial gelation. No further strengthening was found after that time. In fact, impressions left in the mouth for 5 minutes rather than the recommended 2 to 3 minutes after initial gelation exhibited definite distortion. Most alginates improve their elasticity with time, providing a better opportunity for accurate reproduction of undercuts. Impressions removed too early after initial gelation produce a rough surface of the poured cast. These data indicate that alginate impressions should not be removed from the mouth for at least 2 to 3 minutes after initial gelation. There are two reliable methods of determining the correct time for removal of the impression: (1) a timer can be used to measure the 2 to 3 minute period after initial gelation or (2) a small mound of the original mix of alginate can be placed on a glass or metal surface; when this alginate will fracture cleanly with finger pressure, the impression is ready to be removed from the mouth (Fig. 5-53).

The physical strength of the alginate gel is such that a sudden force is more successfully resisted than a slowly applied force. The gel recovers from distortion better when the compression is of a shorter time interval. The following technique makes it possible to remove the impression without fracture or distortion of the alginate. After the lips and cheeks are retracted to release some of the seal, the impression should be removed with a sudden jerk, with the force directed as closely as possible along the long axes of the teeth. Rocking the tray or teasing out the impression will result in unacceptable distortion and tearing of the impression.

Inspecting the impression

The impression should be inspected under a good light source and magnification (Fig. 5-54). The surface should not be dried with compressed air because this will contribute to loss of moisture and release of strains in the impression. An impression should be repeated if there is any doubt as to its accuracy. The following are some reasons for rejecting an impression:

1. Alginate sticking to the teeth.
2. Alginate pulling away from any area of the tray (Although it appears that the alginate can be pushed back into contact with the tray, the overwhelming odds are that the cast will be inaccurate.)
3. Voids in critical areas.
4. Layered impression (indicating that the material wiped on the teeth and tissue had set before the tray was seated).

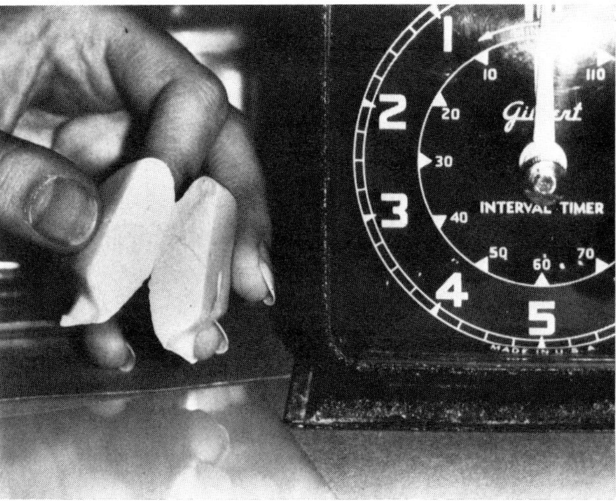

Fig. 5-53. Setting time of alginate may be determined by timer or when it fractures cleanly with finger pressure.

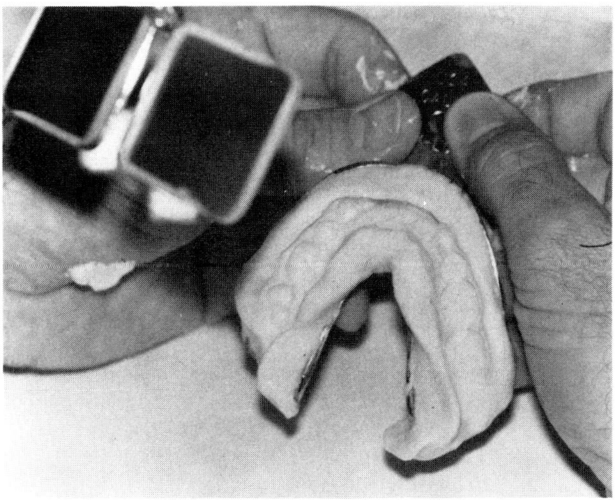

Fig. 5-54. Impression inspected under good light and magnification.

5. Granular impression with poor tissue detail (indicating inadequate spatulation or premature removal).
6. Trapping of the lip, cheeks, tongue, or floor of the mouth.
7. Inadequate extension to the soft tissue areas.
8. Tearing of important areas of the impression.
9. Contact between cusps of teeth and the impression tray.

The causes of and solutions for common problems encountered in alginate diagnostic impressions are presented in Table 1 at the end of this chapter.

Cleaning the impression

Failure to remove the saliva from the impression will result in a rough cast. A saliva-free alginate surface will feel grainy or coarse to the finger, whereas a surface covered with saliva will feel slick or greasy. Most patients have thin, serous saliva. This type of saliva can be easily removed by holding the impression under gently running cool tap water. If running tap water is not effective, the saliva can be removed by a soft camel's hair brush and soap suds. Thick ropy salva is tenacious and difficult to remove. A thin layer of artificial dental stone powder can be sprinkled on the surface of the impression (Fig. 5-55). The stone adheres to the saliva and acts as a disclosing agent. When the impression is placed under running tap water, the saliva will be easily seen and can be physically removed by light brushing with a wet camel's hair brush (Fig. 5-56). All traces of saliva must be removed before the cast is poured.

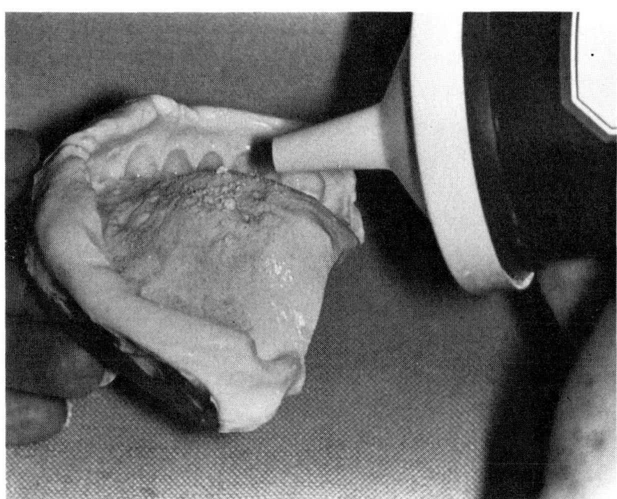

Fig. 5-55. Dental stone sprinkled on impression to act as disclosing agent for saliva.

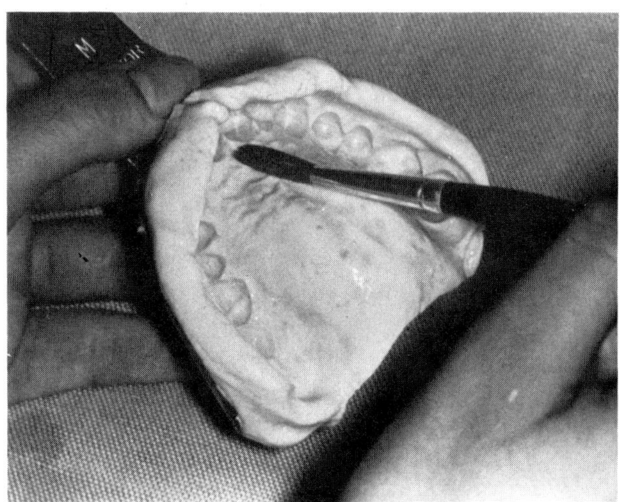

Fig. 5-56. Saliva can be removed with camel's hair brush and running water.

Pouring the cast

A poor impression cannot be improved, but an acceptable impression can be ruined during the procedures of pouring and trimming the casts. The technique for the pouring and trimming of diagnostic casts should be as exacting as that used for making final impressions for master casts. The only difference between the pouring of diagnostic and master casts is that the master cast is usually poured in a minimal expansion improved stone, whereas diagnostic casts are poured in less expensive dental stone. Dental plaster of paris is unacceptable for either type of cast.

Two-stage pour technique

Alginate and other elastic impressions of partially edentulous arches are not easily boxed as are impressions for complete dentures. Therefore a two-stage, or double pour, technique should be used for all casts used in the construction of removable partial dentures. The two-stage pour technique produces a cast in which the teeth and soft tissue areas are the densest and hardest parts.

When a fresh mix of stone is tapped or vibrated, water immediately rises to the surface. A frequently used pouring technique calls for the impression to be filled with stone, a patty or mound of stone to be placed on the bench top, and the filled impression to be inverted and placed into the mound of stone. When the stone is shaped with an instrument or any other movement or vibration occurs in the laboratory, the water in the mix of stone rises to the surface. Therefore the stone that makes up the teeth and anatomic portions of the cast will be the weakest or least dense areas of the cast.

The two-stage pour technique avoids this problem. After the impression is filled with a mix of stone, the tray is suspended by its handle until it reaches its initial set in 10 to 12 minutes. If any movement or vibration

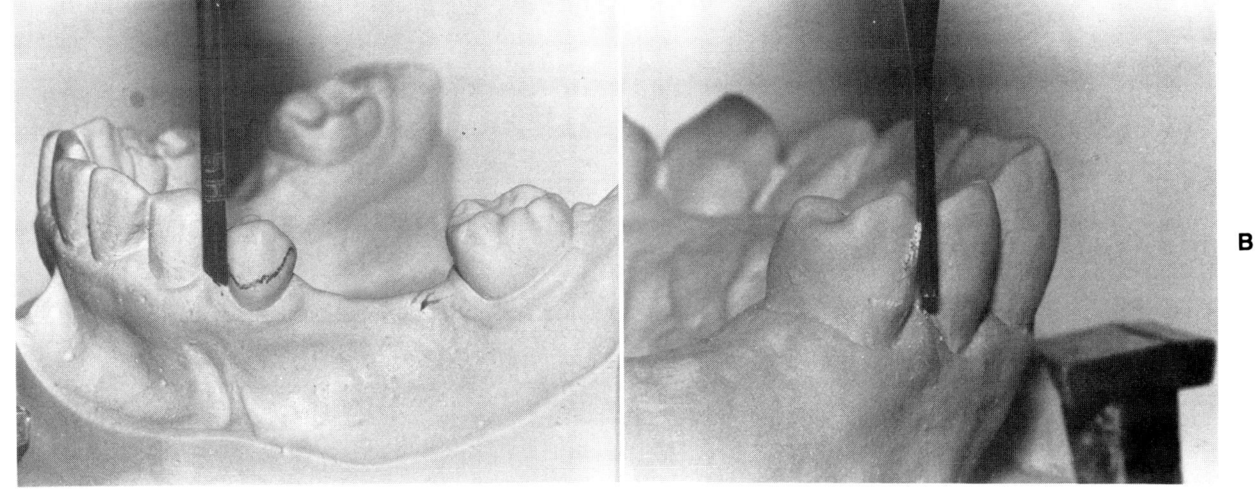

Fig. 5-57. A, Cast with a hard surface is essential because of procedures used in construction of the prosthesis. **B,** Cast with soft surface will be abraded during survey with analyzing rod.

occurs during this period, the water that rises will not affect the anatomic areas of the cast. In fact, the stone in the tooth and other anatomic areas will become denser as the excess water rises away from these areas. When the first pour of stone has reached its initial set, the impression and cast are placed in clear slurry water (a supersaturated solution of calcium sulfate made by placing chips of stone in water for 48 hours). After the first pour has soaked for 5 minutes, the impression is inverted into a patty of a second mix of stone without endangering the density of the cast surface.

Importance of water/powder ratio

A cast with a hard surface is essential in all phases of designing and constructing a removable partial denture (Fig. 5-57). The surface hardness of a stone cast is directly related to its compressive strength, and the compressive strength of a stone cast is directly affected by the water/powder ratio used in making the cast. All gypsum products, whether dental plaster, dental stone, or improved stone, require only 18.61 ml of water to react with 100 g of powder to form calcium sulfate dihydrate. All the remaining water used in making the mix occupies space in the cast, thereby reducing the compressive strength. The main reason that improved stone yields a harder and stronger cast than dental plaster is that it has been refined so that it will mix into a workable consistency with much less water. (Dental plaster requires approximately 50 ml of water to mix with 100 g of powder to produce a workable consistency. The compressive strength is only 1600 pounds per square inch. The same amount of dental stone can be mixed with 27 ml of water to produce a cast with compressive strength of 4500 pounds per square inch; and 100 g of improved stone may be mixed with 24 ml of water,

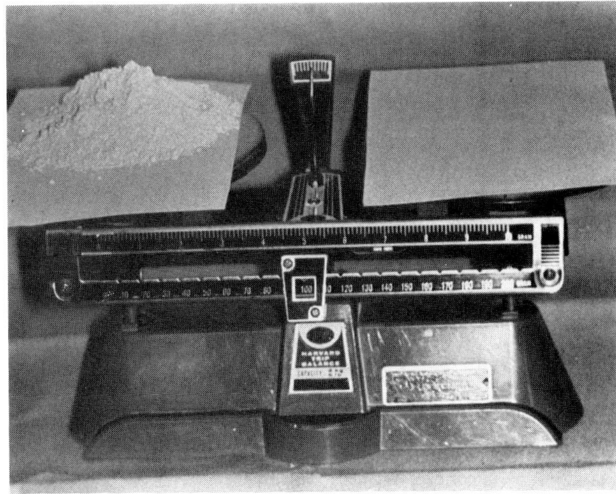

Fig. 5-58. Measuring dental stone on a Harvard trip balance.

with a resultant compressive strength of approximately 5500 pounds per square inch.) Compressive strength is lost even when only a few extra milliliters of water is used. For example, if 30 rather than 27 ml of water is mixed with 100 g dental stone, the compressive strength is reduced from 4500 to 3000 pounds per square inch. No more water should be used than is actually necessary to produce a mix that will flow into the impression.

The powder of all gypsum products must be measured by weight rather than by volume because of the packing effect (Fig. 5-58). The most economical, efficient, and accurate method of handling gypsum products is to weigh out amounts suitable for pouring a single impression and to store the weighed material in an

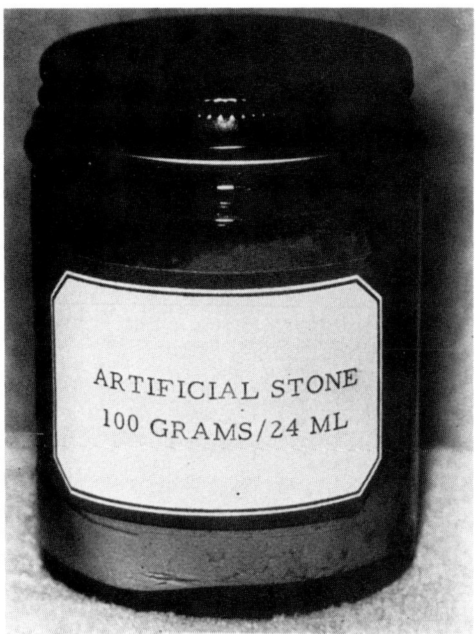

Fig. 5-59. Gypsum products should be stored in an airtight container.

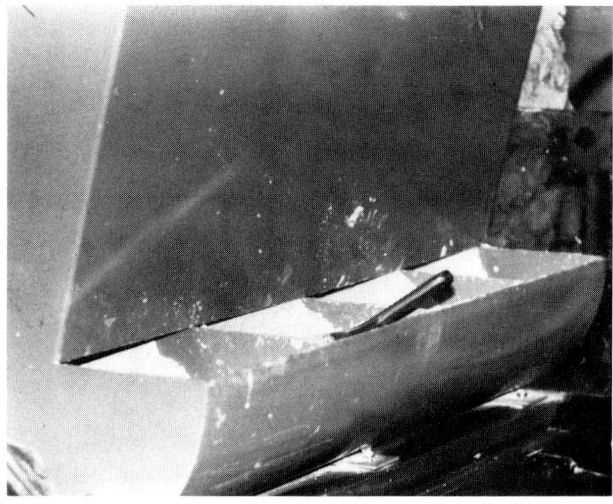

Fig. 5-60. Storage of artificial stone in open bins causes rapid deterioration of physical properties.

airtight container such as an ointment jar (Fig. 5-59). Usually 150 g is adequate for a single pour. This procedure will reduce waste, ensure a correct water/powder ratio, and prevent deterioration. If gypsum products are exposed to the air in an open container, the hemihydrate of gypsum products takes up moisture from the air (Fig. 5-60). Moisture contamination will cause a reaction with the hemihydrate, forming calcium sulfate dihydrate and resulting in a film of gypsum on the hemihydrate particles. With slight moisture contamination, the gypsum crystals will act as a nuclei of crystallization and will accelerate the set. More prolonged contamination may result in a film of gypsum covering the entire particle, preventing the water in a mix from contacting the powder particle. This will greatly prolong the setting time. In addition, moisture contamination reduces both the compressive strength and the surface hardness of the cast.

Mixing dental stone

The objective in mixing dental stone is to make a smooth, homogenous, bubble-free mix that will produce an accurate, strong, hard, dense cast. The water that has been accurately measured should be placed in the mixing bowl first. The preweighed powder should be slowly sifted into the water to avoid air entrapment. Care should be taken to avoid a whipping action, which would incorporate air when mixing by hand. The mixing should continue until a smooth consistency is achieved. Usually 1 to 2 minutes is adequate. Prolonged spatulation can break up the crystals of gypsum that have formed and weaken the final cast. After the mixing is complete, light vibration should be used until no more air bubbles rise to the surface. Mechanical spatulation will produce a mix with smaller air bubbles and result in a stronger, denser cast with less chance of voids. Mechanical spatulation under vacuum will produce an even better cast with reduced porosity. Mixing time should be reduced to 20 to 30 seconds when mechanical spatulation is used.

Danger of soaking casts in water

Dental stone is soluble in tap and distilled water. If a stone cast is immersed in running water, its linear dimensions may decrease approximately 0.1% for every 20 minutes of exposure. Therefore casts should never be cleaned or soaked in tap or distilled water. Clear slurry water should be used when it is necessary to clean or soak a cast (Fig. 5-61).

Causes of rough surface of casts

There are several potential causes of roughness on the surface of the casts. If this is a consistent problem, one should suspect incompatibility between the alginate and the stone used for pouring the cast. Changing the brand of either the alginate or stone may correct the problem.

A rough surface can also be caused by saliva or excess water on the surface of the impression. Excess water should be blotted with a dry tissue. Compressed air should not be used because it may dehydrate the impression, causing increased evaporation, syneresis, and release of strains.

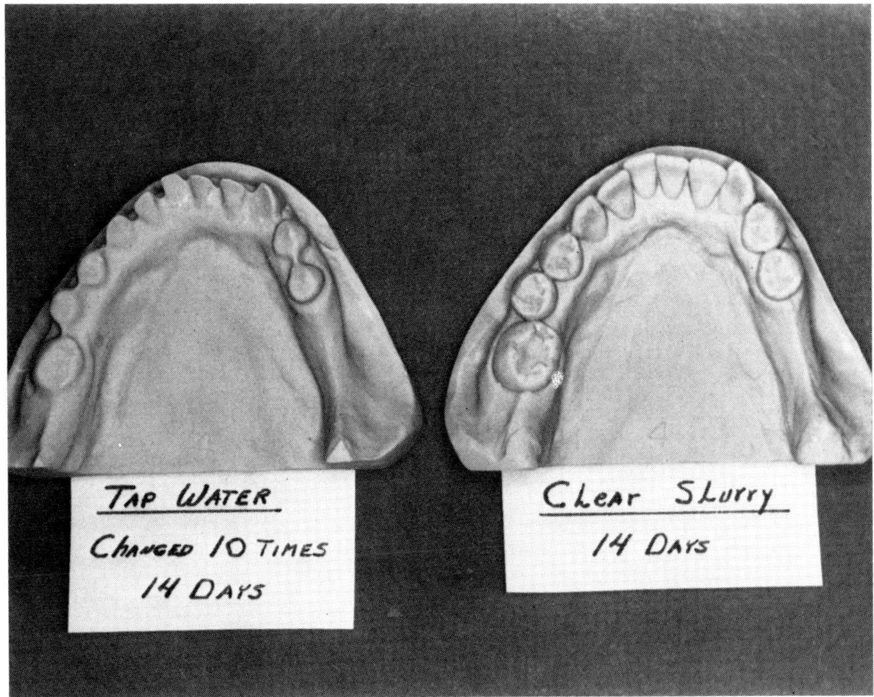

Fig. 5-61. Cast on left stored in tap water for 14 days. Cast on right stored in clear slurry water for 14 days.

Insufficient spatulation of the alginate or premature removal of the impression from the mouth can also cause a rough surface. The sticking of alginate to the teeth will cause roughness in the area of sticking.

Insufficient spatulation of stone, the use of contaminated stone, and the use of the single-pour technique can cause a rough and soft surface on the cast.

An alginate impression should be removed from the cast 45 to 60 minutes after the first pour. Leaving the impression on the cast for several hours or overnight can produce a chalky surface. There is also danger that the cast will be scraped or broken as the alginate shrinks and hardens.

The causes of and solutions for common problems in diagnostic casts are presented in Table 2 at the end of this chapter.

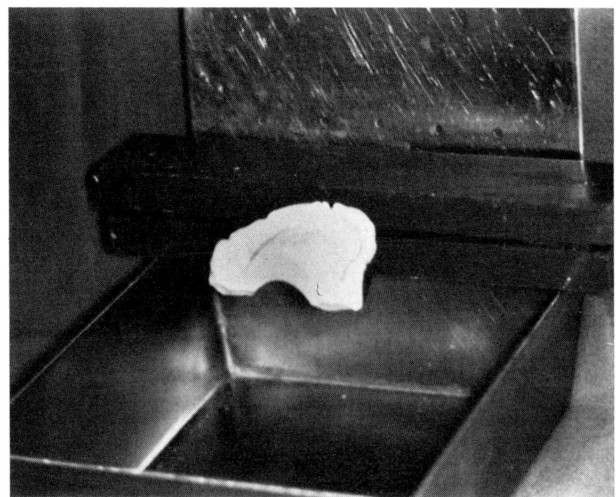

Fig. 5-62. Impression suspended by tray handle to avoid distortion that could be caused by setting impression on bench top.

Steps in pouring diagnostic cast

1. The impression is cleaned to remove all saliva. Excess water remaining on the surface, particularly the tooth areas of the impression, is blotted.
2. The tray is suspended by its handle in a tray holder or a slightly open drawer (Fig. 5-62). Laying the tray on the table may displace the alginate from the tray or cause distortion of the alginate.
3. Dental stone, 150 g, is gently sifted into a mixing bowl containing 42 ml of water, then, hand mixed for 1 to 2 minutes or mechanically spatulated under vacuum for 20 to 30 seconds. The mixture is vibrated on a vibrator until no air bubbles rise to the surface. *The pour must be begun within 12 minutes after the impression is removed from the mouth.*

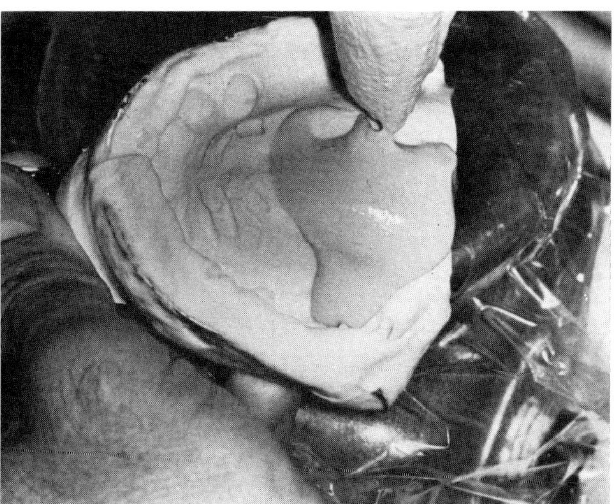

Fig. 5-63. Small amounts of stone added to one posterior side of impression, stone allowed to flow slowly over surface of impression.

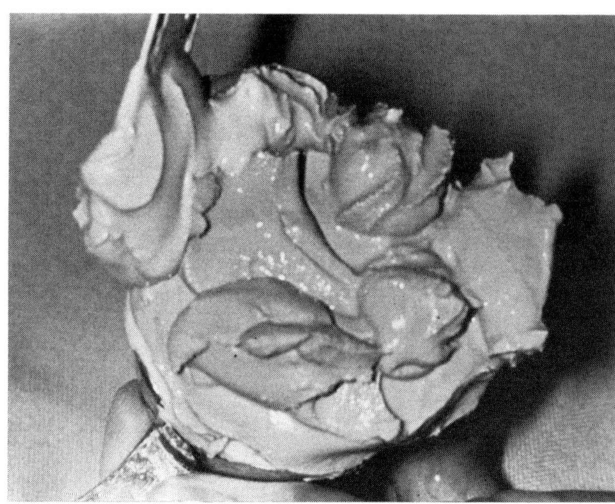

Fig. 5-64. Stone added to cover all borders with 6 to 8 mm of stone, and small mounds of stone added for retention of second pour.

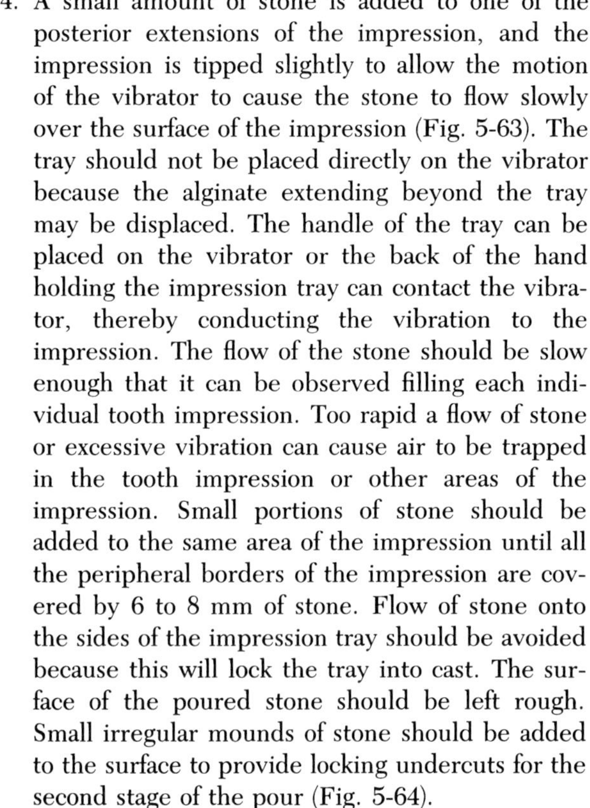

4. A small amount of stone is added to one of the posterior extensions of the impression, and the impression is tipped slightly to allow the motion of the vibrator to cause the stone to flow slowly over the surface of the impression (Fig. 5-63). The tray should not be placed directly on the vibrator because the alginate extending beyond the tray may be displaced. The handle of the tray can be placed on the vibrator or the back of the hand holding the impression tray can contact the vibrator, thereby conducting the vibration to the impression. The flow of the stone should be slow enough that it can be observed filling each individual tooth impression. Too rapid a flow of stone or excessive vibration can cause air to be trapped in the tooth impression or other areas of the impression. Small portions of stone should be added to the same area of the impression until all the peripheral borders of the impression are covered by 6 to 8 mm of stone. Flow of stone onto the sides of the impression tray should be avoided because this will lock the tray into cast. The surface of the poured stone should be left rough. Small irregular mounds of stone should be added to the surface to provide locking undercuts for the second stage of the pour (Fig. 5-64).
5. The tray should be suspended by the tray handle for 10 to 12 minutes, until the stone has reached its initial set (Fig. 5-65).
6. After the intial set, the impression is placed in a bowl of clear slurry water for 4 to 5 minutes to thoroughly wet the first pour of stone (Fig. 5-66).
7. A second mix of stone with the same water/powder ratio is mixed. A patty of the stone is placed on a glass slab and formed into the approximate shape of the impression. Some of the remaining stone is vibrated onto the roughened surface of the first mix of stone (Fig. 5-67). The impression is then inverted and placed into the patty of stone. An instrument is used to shape the base (Fig. 5-68). Care should be taken to avoid locking the impression tray into the stone. Special care should be taken to smooth the tongue space of the mandibular impression.

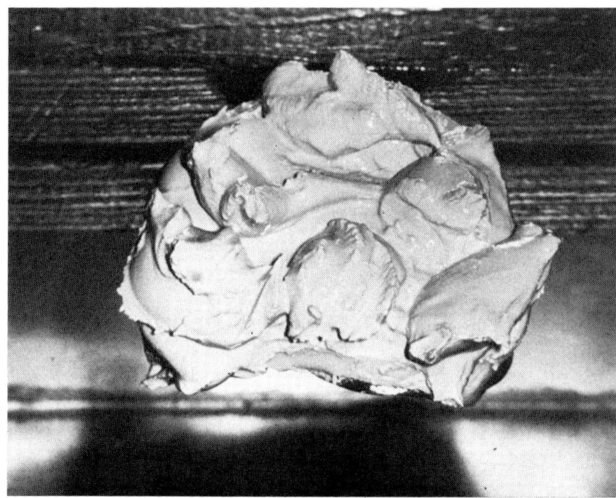

Fig. 5-65. Tray suspended by handle until stone reaches its initial set.

8. Between 45 and 60 minutes after the first pour, the impression is separated from the cast. The impression must not be allowed to remain on the cast for a prolonged period or damage to the cast will result.

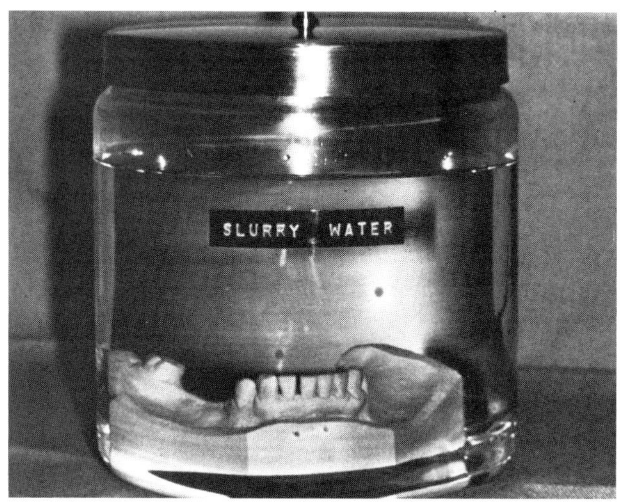

Fig. 5-66. Clear slurry water is made by soaking of old casts for 48 hours to supersaturate the water with calcium sulfate. A cast placed into this solution will not dissolve.

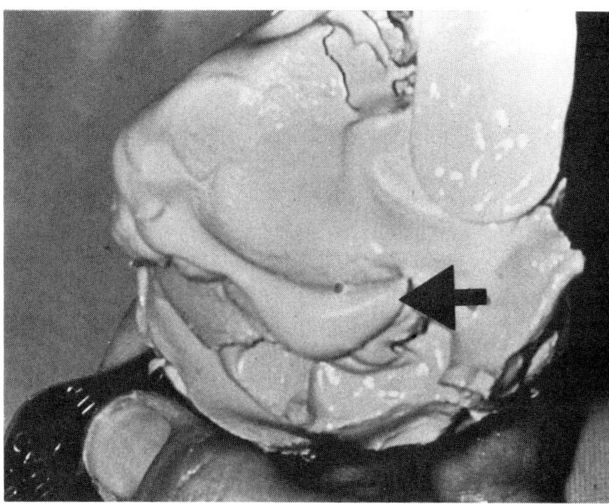

Fig. 5-67. New mix of stone is vibrated onto rough surface of first pour (arrow).

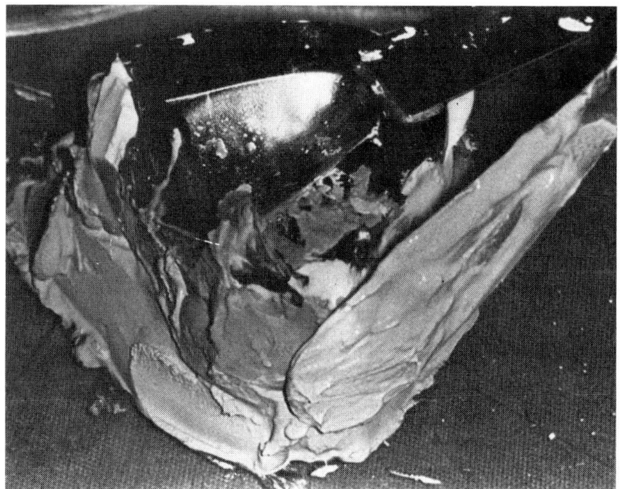

Fig. 5-68. Impression is inverted into patty of stone, and base is shaped with spatula.

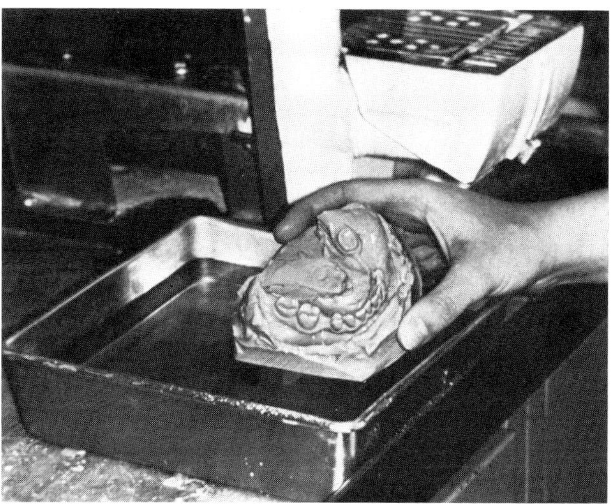

Fig. 5-69. Cast is soaked in clear slurry water before being trimmed on model trimmer.

Trimming the cast

1. The cast is thoroughly soaked in clear slurry water (Fig. 5-69) to prevent the slurry of stone and water from the model trimmer from adhering to the surface of the cast. A dry cast placed on a model trimmer acts like a blotter or a sponge. The stone slurry from the model trimmer is absorbed onto the surface and is impossible to remove (Figs. 5-70 and 5-71). Attempts to wash or brush off the attached slurry will further ruin the surface of the cast. The only way to avoid this problem is to wet the cast thoroughly before shaping it on the model trimmer. It is advisable to have a pan of clear slurry water next to the model trimmer so that the stone slurry that accumulates on the surface of the cast during trimming can be rinsed off periodically.
2. The base of the cast is trimmed so that the occlusal surfaces of the teeth are parallel to the base. A stream of water should be flowing through the model trimmer throughout the shaping procedure. The base should be trimmed until it is 10 mm thick at its thinnest point, usually the center of the hard palate for the maxillary cast and the depth of the lingual sulcus for the mandibular cast (Fig. 5-72).

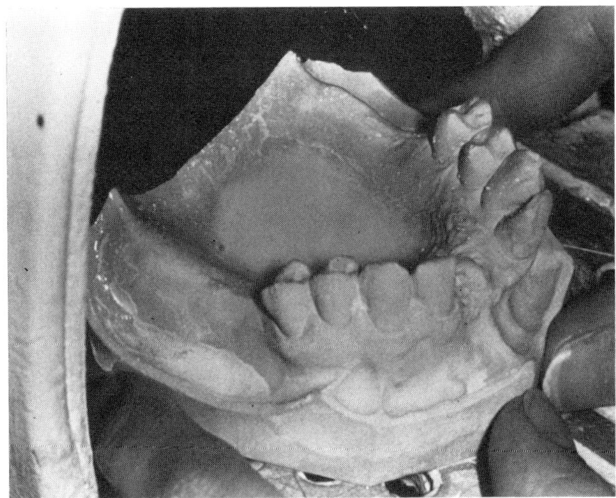

Fig. 5-70. Dry cast absorbs stone slurry from model trimmer like a sponge.

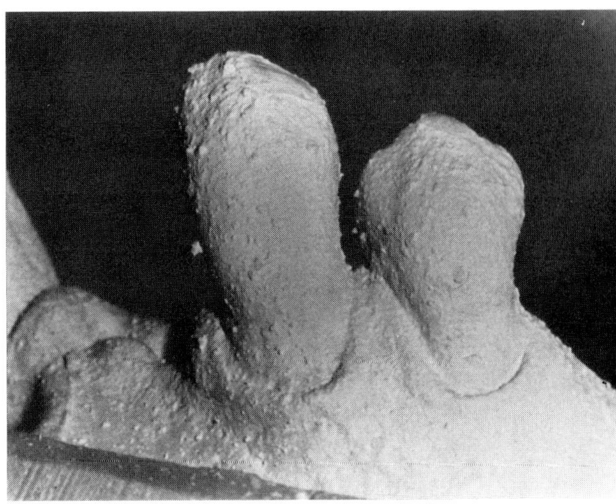

Fig. 5-71. Stone slurry from model trimmer cannot be removed; therefore cast is ruined.

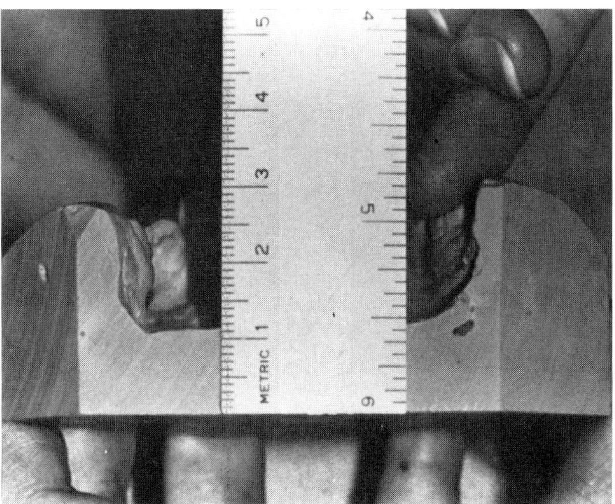

Fig. 5-72. Trimmed casts should be at least 10 mm thick at thinnest point.

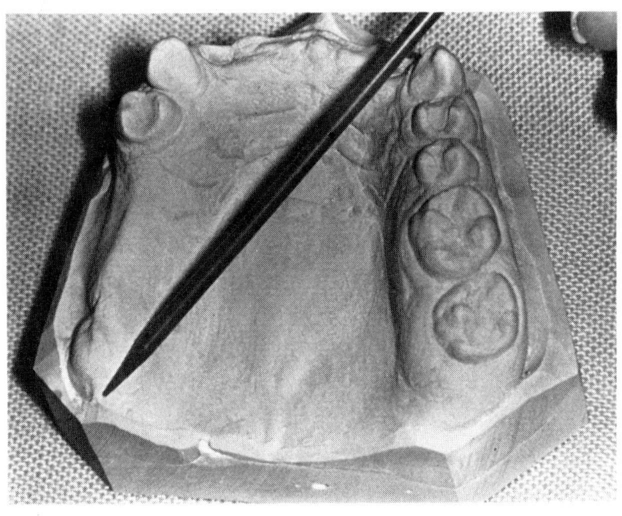

Fig. 5-73. Hamular notch area must be preserved.

3. The posterior border of the cast is trimmed so that it forms an angle of 90 degrees with the base and is perpendicular to a line passing between the central incisors. Care must be taken to avoid trimming the hamular notch and tuberosity areas of the maxillary cast and the retromolar pad areas of the mandibular cast(Fig. 5-73).
4. The sides of the casts are trimmed so that they form an angle of 90 degrees with the base of the cast and so that they are parallel to the buccal surfaces of the posterior teeth or the crest of the edentulous ridge (Fig. 5-74). Care must be taken to avoid overtrimming, which could obliterate the vestibular and buccal shelf areas. A land area of 2 to 3 mm should be maintained around the entire cast.
5. The sides and the posterior borders are joined by trimming just posterior to the hamular notch or retromolar pad. Overtrimming these areas and thereby removing the hamular notch or the retromolar pad is a frequent error. These are essential landmarks and must be preserved.
6. The anterior borders of the maxillary cast are trimmed differently from those of the mandibular cast, although both must form an angle of 90 degrees to the base. The anterior borders of the

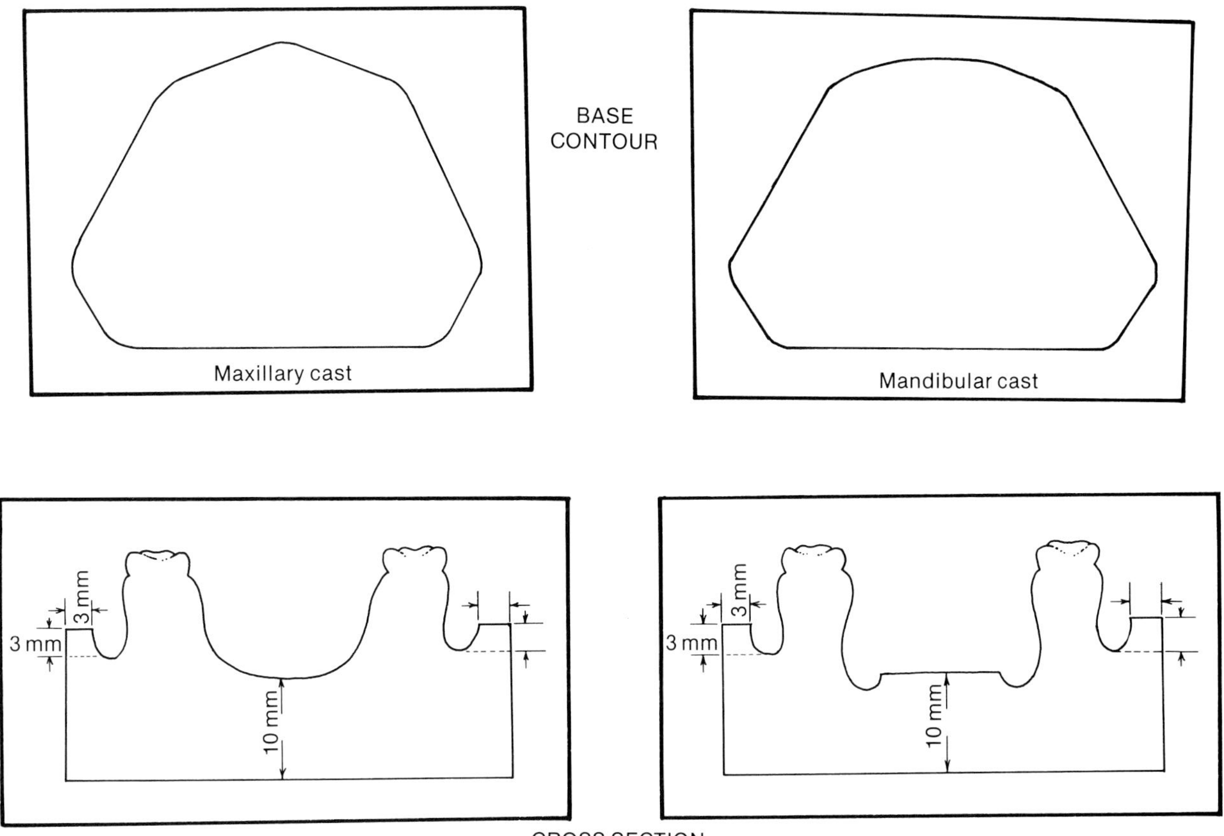

Fig. 5-74. Base contour and cross-sectional form of correctly trimmed diagnostic casts.

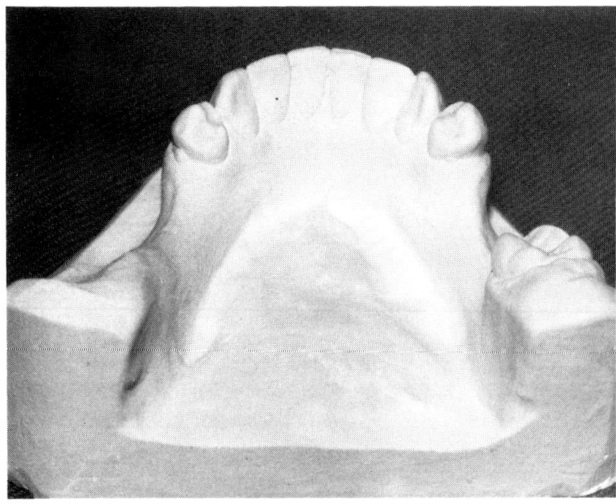

Fig. 5-75. Tongue space of mandibular cast is trimmed flat.

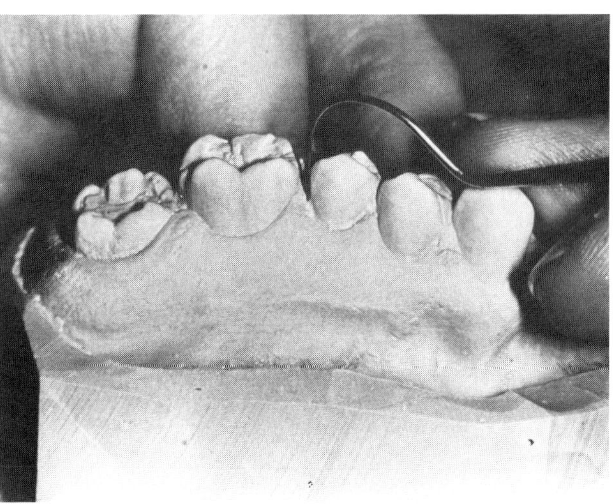

Fig. 5-76. Stone nodules are scraped from noncritical areas to improve appearance of cast.

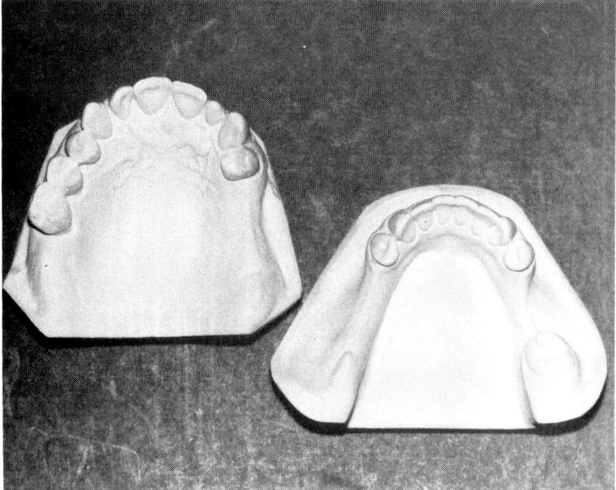

Fig. 5-77. Completed diagnostic casts.

maxillary cast are formed by trimming from the canine area on each side to a point anterior to the interproximal area of the central incisors. The anterior border of the mandibular cast is formed by creating a curving wall from the canine on one side to the canine on the other. The curve should follow the form of the arch. On both casts care must be taken to avoid removal of the vestibular area or damage to the anterior teeth.

7. The tongue space should be trimmed flat while the integrity of the lingual frenum and the entire alveololingual sulcus is maintained (Fig. 5-75).
8. Nodules of stone caused by voids in the impression can be scraped from noncritical areas (Fig. 5-76). Voids in the base and other noncritical areas of the cast can be filled with a thin mix of stone to improve the appearance of the cast. The cast must be thoroughly soaked in clear slurry water before the new mix of stone is added to the deficient areas.
9. The casts are now ready for the second diagnostic appointment (Fig. 5-77). The casts should never be placed under running water, brushed or soaked in anything except clear slurry water.

LENGTH OF APPOINTMENT

Most practicing dentists will use auxiliary personnel to help the patient complete the health questionnaire, to record the blood pressure, to perform the prophylaxis, and to make and develop the radiographs. The patient interview, the cursory examination, and the making of diagnostic impressions can easily be completed in a 1-hour appointment if the procedures are efficiently organized.

Dental students, who will likely be completing all the steps will probably require 3 to 4 hours to complete the first diagnostic appointment.

TABLE 1 COMMON PROBLEMS IN MAKING ALGINATE DIAGNOSTIC IMPRESSIONS

Problem	Probable cause	Solution for problem
1. Alginate sticks to teeth	Teeth too clean from too vigorous pumicing	Pumice lightly; delay impression making after thorough prophylaxis; use silicone as protective coating for teeth.
	Teeth too dry	Avoid air drying of teeth; isolate arch with gauze packs.
	Loss of protective film from teeth because of repeated impressions	Use good technique so repeated impressions not necessary; delay impression to another day.
	Any of the above	Use silicone as protective film; have patient suck on sour candy (citrus); have patient swish with whole milk.
2. Voids in impression	Poor mix of alginate	Spatulate for 45 to 60 seconds by hand or 15 seconds mechanically; wipe alginate along side of bowl duiing spatulation; use mechanical spatulation under vacuum.
	Alginate did not flow to all areas	Wipe alginate on teeth, in palate, and into vestibular areas after mouth has been isolated with gauze packs; avoid mix that is too thick or too thin by using correct water/powder ratio; measure alginate by weight, not by volume; avoid deterioration of alginate by heat or by moisture contamination.
3. Peripheral underextension	Alginate did not flow into peripheral areas or poor mix of alginate	See No. 2.
	Tray too small, so material not carried into vestibule	Use tray with 5 to 7-mm. clearance
	Tray incorrectly seated	Center tray with handle pointing straight out of mouth; retract lips with fingers so correct position of tray can be seen; seat tray so borders go below gingival marginal areas; avoid too large a tray, which will interfere with coronoid processes of mandible.
	Cheeks, lips, or floor of mouth trapped under tray	Pull out cheeks, retract lips, have patient protrude tongue before final seating of tray.
4. Alginate tears when impression removed	Too thin or too thick a mix of alginate	Use water/powder ratio recommended by manufacturer; measure alginate by weight not by volume; avoid deterioration of alginate by heat or moisture.
	Impression removed from mouth too soon	Keep impression in mouth 2 to 3 minutes after it loses its tackiness.
	Inadequate bulk of alginate	Select tray with 5- to 7-mm clearance; center tray properly; relieve modeling plastic used to modify tray for 5- to 7-mm clearance.
	Use of deteriorated alginate	Store bulk alginate in airtight containers at room temperature.
	Prolonged or insufficient spatulation	Hand spatulate 45 to 60 seconds, or mechanically spatulate 15 seconds.
	Improper removal from mouth	Avoid rocking or teasing out of impression; remove with snap with force along long axis of tooth.

Continued.

TABLE 1 COMMON PROBLEMS IN MAKING ALGINATE DIAGNOSTIC IMPRESSIONS—cont'd

Problem	Probable cause	Solution for problem
5. Lack of detail or grainy appearance	Prolonged or insufficient spatulation	Hand spatulate 45 to 60 seconds; or mechanically spatulate 15 seconds.
	Insufficient flow of material	Use tray that confines alginate; avoid too thick or too thin a mix by using correct water/powder ratio, measuring by weight, and avoiding deterioration of alginate by heat or moisture.
	Impression removed from mouth too soon	Hold steady in mouth for 2 to 3 minutes after tackiness is gone from alginate surface.
6. Alginate sets before tray completely seated	Mixing water too warm	Use water temperature of 22°C (72° F), or lower if more working time required.
	Particles of dental stone (calcium sulfate) in mixing bowl	Use different mixing bowls and spatulas for alginate and stone.
	Prolonged spatulation of alginate	Hand spatulate 45 to 60 seconds, or mechanical spatulate 15 seconds.
	Use of deteriorated alginate	Store at room temperature; avoid moisture contamination by measuring and sealing all contents of bulk containers of alginate.
	Layer of material painted in mouth too thin	Wipe larger amounts onto teeth and into vestibules; introduce tray immediately by having tray filled before painting in mouth.
	Fast-set alginate used	Use regular-set alginate.
7. Patient gags when tray is fit or impression made	Patient is fearful and lacks confidence in dentist	Proceed with confident, well-organized manner; use simple explanation; avoid talk about gagging.
	Alginate flowing out of tray and into patient's throat	Seat patient upright with occlusal plane parallel with floor; correct maxillary tray with modeling plastic; avoid overfilling of tray.
	Patient tense	Instruct patient to keep eyes open and focused on some small object; instruct patient to breathe through nose at normal rate.
	Palate numb because of use of topical anesthetics	Avoid topical anesthetics; use astringent mouth rinses and cold water rinses instead.
	Patient has severe gag reflex	Ask patient to hold breath while tray is fit or corrected; use the "leg lift" procedure; use fast-set alginate or accelerate the set of alginate by using warmer water.
8. Alginate displaced by saliva in palate	Mucous saliva not removed from palate	Have patient use astringent mouth rinse and cold water rinse; wipe and isolate palate with 2 × 2 inch gauze.
	Excessive secretion by palatal mucous glands	Use warm gauze pads to milk palatal glands followed by cold pads to constrict gland openings.
	Patient produces copious amounts of saliva	Premedicate with 15 mg of propantheline bromide (Pro-Banthine) 30 minutes before procedure if no contraindications.
9. Alginate pulled away from the tray	Alginate not forced under rim lock	Use small increments and force alginate into rim lock areas
	Alginate does not stick to modeling plastic	Use alginate adhesive to coat entire inner surfaces of tray and modeling plastic.
	Alginate stuck to teeth	See No. 1.

TABLE 2 **COMMON PROBLEMS OF CASTS MADE FROM ALGINATE IMPRESSIONS**

Problem	Probable cause	Solution for problem
1. Cast has rough surface	Incompatibility between alginate and dental stone	Change brand of alginate or stone to obtain compatible combination.
	Insufficient spatulation of stone	Spatulate until smooth homogenous mix is attained—1 to 2 minutes by hand or 20 to 30 seconds by mechanical spatulation under vacuum.
	Sticking of alginate to teeth	See No. 1 in Table 1.
	Saliva retained on impression	Rinse in running water until alginate has rough feel; use soapsuds/and camel's hair brush to remove saliva; use dry dental stone as a disclosing agent and remove saliva with camel's hair brush and running water.
	Water left on impression	Blot water with dry tissue paper; avoid use of compressed air.
	Poor mix of alginate; insufficient spatulation	Hand spatulate 45 to 60 seconds, or mechanically spatulate 15 seconds.
	Use of single-stage pour technique; water rose to tissue/tooth surface of impression	Use two-stage pour technique.
2. Surface of cast has chalky appearance	Incompatible alginate/stone combination	Change brand of alginate or stone to find compatible combination.
	Film of stone slurry on cast after dry cast trimmed on model trimmer	Thoroughly soak cast in clear slurry water before trimming; rinse periodically in clear slurry water while trimming.
	Impression left in contact with cast for prolonged period	Separate impression from cast 45 to 60 minutes after first pour.
3. Cast has a soft surface	Too much water in mix of stone	Use acceptable water/powder ratio; measure stone by weight, not volume.
	Use of inverted single-stage pour technique; water rose to tissue/tooth surface of impression	Use two-stage pour technique.
	Use of stone that has been contaminated by moisture	Premeasure stone and store in airtight container; avoid use of open bins for stone storage.
	Water or stone powder added to improper water/powder ratio mix after mixing has been started	Measure correct amount of water, and weigh correct amount of stone for acceptable water/powder ratio.
	Stone spatulated too long	Hand spatulate 1 to 2 minutes, or mechanically spatulate 20 to 30 seconds.
4. Cast breaks when impression separated from cast	Premature removal of impression from cast	Separate cast from impression 45 to 60 minutes after first pour.
	Too much water in mix of stone	Measure water and weigh powder for correct water/powder ratio.
	Use of single-stage pour technique	Use two-stage pour technique.
	Water left in tooth impression	Blot all water with dry tissue paper.
	Low compressive strength of dental stone because of moisture contaminated stone, adding powder or water while mixing stone, or prolonged spatulation	Store stone correctly; measure water and weigh powder before mixing; spatulate 1 to 2 minutes by hand or 20 to 30 seconds mechanically.
	Alginate impression left in contact with cast overnight	Separate impression from cast 45 to 60 after first pour.

Continued.

TABLE 2 COMMON PROBLEMS OF CASTS MADE FROM ALGINATE IMPRESSIONS—cont'd

Problem	Probable cause	Solution for problem
5. Separation of cast between first and second pours of stone	Failure to leave surface of first pour with mechanical retention for second pour	Leave surface of first pour rough; add small irregular mounds of stone to soft surface of first pour.
	Failure to thoroughly wet first pour before adding second pour	After initial set of first pour, soak cast and impression in clear slurry water for 5 minutes.
6. Voids in surface of cast	Air trapped in mix of stone because of inadequate or improper mixing	Sift powder into water to avoid air entrapment; hand spatulate 1 to 2 minutes, avoiding any whipping action; lightly vibrate mix until no more air bubbles come to surface; mechanically mix stone under vacuum for 20 to 30 seconds.
	Cast poured too rapidly and air trapped on surface of impression	Add small increments of stone to the same posterior extension of impression with light vibration and allow stone to flow slowly to fill all areas of impression.
	Overvibration during pouring	Use light vibration only; flowing stone should not bounce.
7. Underextension of cast	Cast overtrimmed; hamular notch, retromolar pad, or vestibular areas obliterated	Take care in trimming of casts on model trimmer to avoid removal of critical areas.
	First pour of alginate did not cover all peripheral areas of impression	Fill impression completely and cover all peripheral border areas with 5 to 6 mm of stone when making first stage of pour.
	Peripheral underextension of alginate impression	See No. 3 in Table 1.
8. Erratic setting time of stone	Contamination of stone by heat or moisture	Preweigh and store stone in airtight containers.
9. Cast is inaccurate; not a true reproduction of the anatomy of the mouth	Loss of moisture content of impression because of syneresis, resulting in release of strains	Pour cast within 12 minutes after removal of impression from mouth; avoid excessive drying of impression.
	Release of strains and swelling because of water	Do not store impression in water or other solutions; do not wrap impression in wet paper towel.
	Strains or distortion in impression caused by its movement during gelation	Maintain impression in position until it is ready for removal; do not have assistant or patient hold impression.
	Impression removed before gelation complete	Maintain impression in position for 2 to 3 minutes after alginate has lost its tackiness.
	Strains induced in impression during its removal from mouth	Remove impression with a snap, with force directly along long axes of teeth.
	Use of nonrigid impression tray	Avoid use of tray that lacks rigidity.
	Use of inaccurate impression	See Table 1.
	Surface of cast lost by washing or soaking cast in tap water	Use clear slurry water whenever cast needs to be soaked or washed.
	Teeth contacted tray during making of impression, allowing stone to flow between impression and tray	Retract lips for good visibility when seating tray; use gingival margins as landmark when seating tray; seat tray slightly beyond this landmark.
	Alginate displaced or strains induced by setting tray on bench top	Suspend tray by its handle in a tray holder or a slightly opened drawer.
	Distortion in palate because of failure to correct tray	Correct palatal area of maxillary tray with modeling plastic; after modeling plastic chilled, trim to provide 5 to 7 mm of clearance for alginate.

REFERENCES

Boucher, C.O., editor: Swenson's complete dentures, ed. 6, St. Louis, 1970, The C.V. Mosby Co.

De Van, M.M.: The transition from natural to artificial teeth, J. Prosthet. Dent. **11**:677-688, 1961.

House, M.M.: Full denture technique, prepared from the notes of Study Club #1 by Conley, F.J., Dunn, A.L., Quesnall, A.J., and Rogers, R.M., Sept., 1950.

Sonis, S.T., Sonis, A.L., and Lieberman, A.: Oral complications in patients receiving treatment for malignancies other than of the head and neck. J. Am. Dent. Assoc. **97**:468-472, 1978.

BIBLIOGRAPHY

Anderson, J.N.: Flow and elasticity in alginates, Dent Prog **1**:63-70, 1970.

Ayers, H.D., Jr., and others: Detail duplication test used to evaluate elastic impression materials, J. Prosthet. Dent. **10**:374-380, 1960.

Beumer, J., III, and others: Radiation complications in edentulous patients, J. Prosthet. Dent. **36**:193-203, 1976.

Cottone, J.A., and Kafrawy, A.H.: Medication and health histories: A survey of 4,365 dental patients, J. Am. Dent. Assoc. **98**:713-718, 1979.

Craig, R.G., editor: Restorative dental materials, ed. 6, St. Louis, 1980, The C.V. Mosby Co.

Crawford, J.J.: New light on the transmissibility of viral hepatitis in dental practice and its control, J. Am. Dent. Assoc. **91**:829-834, 1975.

Deneen, L.J., and others: Effective interpersonal and management skills in dentistry, J. Am. Dent. Assoc. **87**:878-880, 1973.

Department of Prosthodontics Junior Complete Denture Clinical Manual, The University of Texas Health Science Center at San Antonio Dental School, 1980.

Glasser, S.P.: The problems of patients with cardiovascular disease undergoing dental treatment, J. Am. Dent. Assoc. **94**:1158-1162, 1977.

Harris, W.T., Jr.: Water temperature and accuracy of alginate impressions, J. Prosthet. Dent. **21**:613-617, 1969.

House, M.M.: Full denture technique, Notes of House Study Club No. 1, 1960.

House, M.M.: An outline for examination of mouth condition, Dominion Dent. J. **33**:97-100, 1921.

Kaiser, D.A., and Nicholls, J.I.: A study of distortion and surface hardness of improved artificial stone casts, J. Prosthet. Dent. **36**:373-381, 1976.

Katberg, J.W.: Cross-contamination via the prosthodontic laboratory, J. Prosthet. Dent. **32**:412-419, 1974.

Kerr, D.A., and others: Oral diagnosis, ed. 5, St. Louis, 1978, The C.V. Mosby Co.

Krol, A.J.: A new approach to the gagging problem, J. Prosthet. Dent. **13**:611-616, 1963.

Merchant, H.W., and Carr, A.A.: Blood pressure measurements; problems and solutions, J. Am. Dent. Assoc. **95**:98-102, 1977.

Morrow, R.M., and others: Compatibility of alginate impression materials and dental stones, J. Prosthet. Dent. **25**:556-566, 1971.

Nassif, J.: A self administered questionaire—an aid in managing complete denture patients, J. Prosthet. Dent. **40**:363-366, 1978.

Peyton, F.A.: Restorative dental materials, 4th ed., St. Louis, 1971, C.V. Mosby.

Phillips, R.W., and others: Detail duplication test used to evaluate elastic impression materials, J. Am. Dent. Assoc. **46**:393-403, 1953.

Phillips, R.W.: Elements of dental materials, ed. 3, 1977, W.B. Saunders Co.

Phillips, R.W.: Skinner's science of dental materials, ed. 7, 1973, W.B. Saunders.

Plainfield, S.: Communication distortion. The language of patients and practioners of dentistry, J. Prosthet. Dent. **22**:11-19, 1969.

Rahn, A.O.,, and others: Prosthetic evaluation of patients who have received irradiation to the head and neck regions, J. Prosthet. Dent. **19**:174-178, 1968.

Rudd, K.D., and others: Accurate alginate impressions, J. Prosthet. Dent. **22**:294-300, 1969.

Rudd, K.D., and others: Accurate casts, J. Prosthet. Dent. **21**:545-554, 1969.

Rudd, K.D., and others: Comparison of effects of tap water and slurry water on gypsum casts, J. Prosthet. Dent. **24**:563-570, 1970.

Rudd, K.D., and Morrow, R.M.: Premedication: an aid in obtaining accurate complete denture impressions, J. Prosthet. Dent. **18**:86-89, 1967.

Sauser, C.W.: Pretreatment evaluation of partially edentulous patients, J. Prosthet. Dent. **11**:886-893, 1961.

Tolentino, A.T.: Prosthetic management of patients with pemphigus vulgaris, J. Prosthet. Dent. **38**:254-260, 1977.

6 Examination and evaluation of diagnostic data

THE SECOND DIAGNOSTIC APPOINTMENT

The second diagnostic appointment is used to complete the gathering and the evaluation of the diagnostic data. The patient's occlusion is evaluated intraorally and by means of mounted diagnostic casts. The radiographs are evaluated and correlated with the definitive oral examination, which is completed at this appointment. Medical or dental consultations are requested if needed.

MOUNTED DIAGNOSTIC CASTS

Mounted diagnostic casts are fundamental diagnostic aids in dentistry (Fig. 6-1). They assume an extremely important role in the evaluation of the partially edentulous patient, and they should be used as carefully as are the roentgenographic survey and the visual and digital examination of the oral cavity. Their uses include the following:

1. They supplement the examination of the oral cavity. Extruded teeth, low-hanging tuberosities, lack of interarch space, malposed teeth, and defective restorations, are readily apparent if accurate casts are correctly mounted on a suitable articulator.
2. They provide for a detailed analysis of the patient's occlusion. Whereas the lips, cheeks, and skull block out good visual access to the patient's teeth and the relationships between the teeth in various occlusal positions, accurately mounted diagnostic casts provide good visual access from all directions. The information gained can be used in determining the design of the removable partial denture and in selecting appropriate treatment for the restoration of the mouth.
3. They are a tremendous aid in the education of the patient and in the presentation of the treatment plan.
4. They provide a permanent dental record of the patient's condition before treatment. This record can be of great value if a conflict should arise during the treatment phase or after the completion of treatment.

The objective of the diagnostic mounting is to position the casts of the dental arches on an articulator so that the casts have the same relationship as do the mandible and maxilla in the patient's skull. There are three distinct phases to the procedure:

1. Orientation of the maxillary cast to the condylar elements of the articulator by means of a face-bow transfer.
2. Orientation of the mandibular cast to the maxillary cast at the patient's centric jaw relation by means of an accurate centric jaw relation record.
3. Verification of these relationships by means of additional centric jaw relation records and comparison of occlusal contacts on the articulator with those in the mouth.

Face-bow transfer

The first step in the diagnostic mounting procedure is the mounting of the maxillary cast on a semiadjustable articulator. A fully adjustable articulator could be used but would involve a more complicated and time-consuming procedure. Relating the maxillary cast to the condylar elements of a suitable articulator at the same orientation that the maxillary teeth have to the mandibular condyles of the patient allows a more accurate and meaningful analysis of the occlusion. A face-bow transfer provides this orientation.

EQUIPMENT AND SUPPLIES

The following equipment and supplies are needed for the face-bow transfer:

1. Semiadjustable articulator
2. Conventional face-bow and bite fork compatible with the articulator to be used
3. Baseplate wax or red modeling compound
4. Millimeter ruler and marking pencil
5. Accurate maxillary cast
6. Bunsen burner
7. Dental stone, mixing bowl, and spatula
8. Stone-separating medium*
9. Petroleum jelly or Masque†

---

*Super Sep, Kerr Manufacturing Co., Romulus, Mich.
†Masque, The Harry J. Bosworth Co., Chicago, Ill.

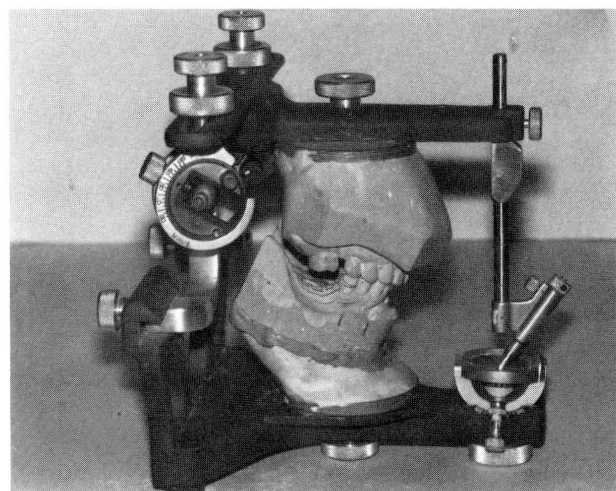

Fig. 6-1. Mounted diagnostic casts have an important role in the evaluation of a partially edentulous patient.

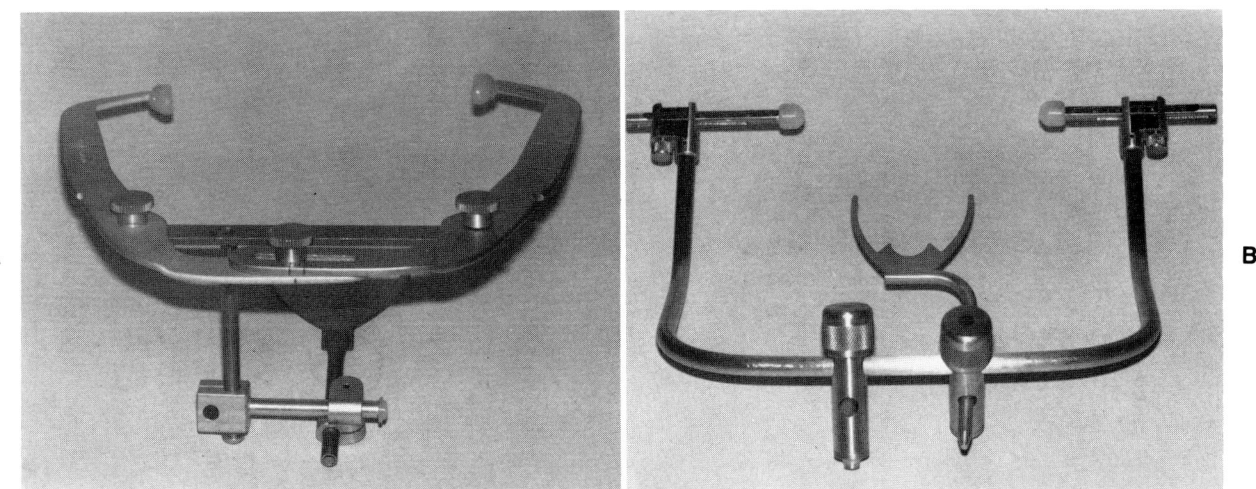

Fig. 6-2. A, Whipmix ear type face-bow. **B,** Hanau ear type face-bow.

Location of hinge axis

The most accurate method of making a face-bow transfer is to determine the patient's true hinge axis kinematically and to use the axis in positioning the face-bow. However, the determination of the actual hinge axis requires additional time-consuming procedures and is not necessary for most patients. Arbitrary hinge axis points will be within acceptable limits for more than 90% of patients. If the interocclusal records used for mounting the mandibular cast are made with minimal separation of the teeth, the errors in the occlusal contacts of the mounted casts because of the use of an arbitrary hinge axis will usually be negligible.

Arbitrary hinge axis. The selection of the arbitrary hinge axis points will depend on the type of face-bow and articulator being used. The styli of an "ear type" face-bow such as the Whip-Mix* are placed into each external auditory meatus (Fig. 6-2). Other face-bows such as the Hanau SM† require that the styli be placed on selected points that have been marked on the face (Fig. 6-3). Several arbitrary points have been described. A convenient point to use is Beyron's point, which is located 13 mm anterior to the posterior margin of the tragus of the ear on a line to the outer canthus of the eye (Fig. 6-4). The line running through the marks placed on both sides of the face is the arbitrary hinge axis.

*Whip-Mix, Whip-Mix Corp., Louisville, Ky.

†Hanau SM, Teledyne Dental Products Co., Hanau Division, Buffalo, N.Y.

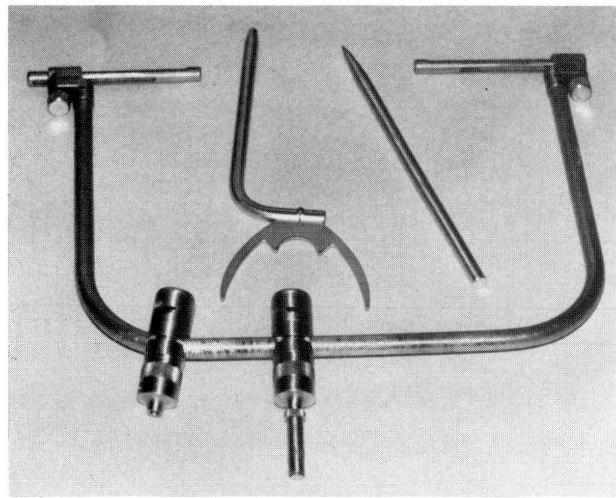

Fig. 6-3. Components of Hanau SM face-bow.

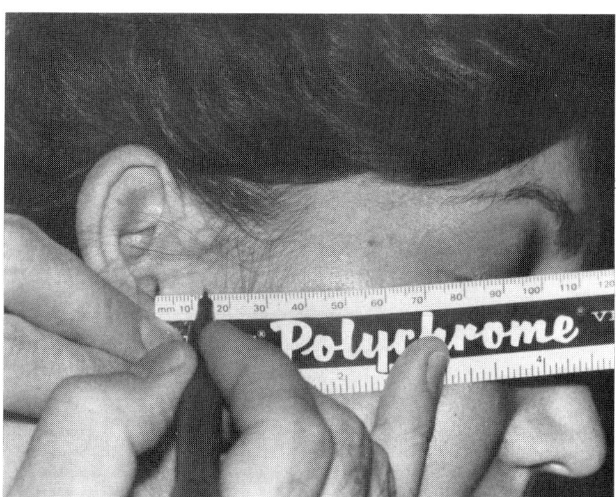

Fig. 6-4. Marking an arbitrary axis point.

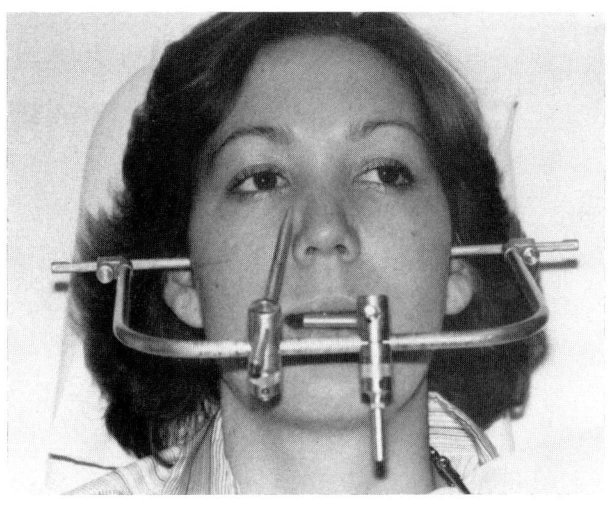

Fig. 6-5. Hanau SM face-bow assembly with third point of reference at level of infraorbital notch.

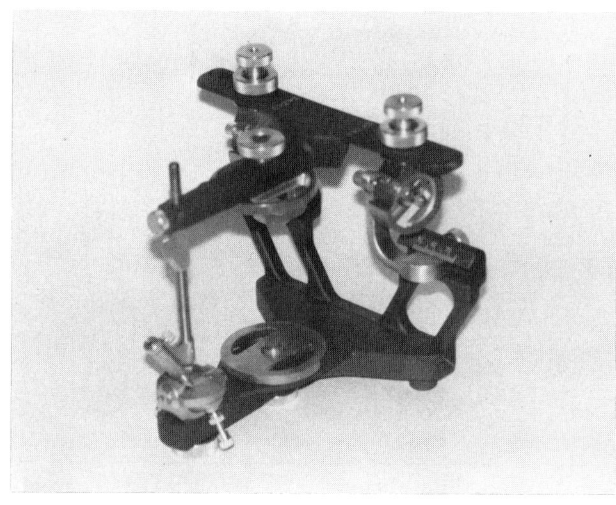

Fig. 6-6. Hanau 130-28 articulator.

Anterior point of reference

An anterior or third point of reference is also needed for positioning the face-bow on the patient's face. Different articulator and face-bow combinations require different anterior points of reference so it is important to use the point recommended in the descriptive literature provided by the manufacturer of the articulator being used. As an example, the infraorbital notch is selected when a Hanau SM face-bow is used with the Hanau 130-28 articulator (Fig. 6-5). The plane contacting the anterior reference point and the two arbitrary hinge axis points is parallel with the Frankfort horizontal plane in the head. This plane will properly orient the occlusal plane of the maxillary cast to the condylar elements of the articulator. Failure to use the anterior point of reference correctly may result in errors in the analysis of eccentric occlusal interferences.

Technique

The technical steps involved in making a face-bow transfer vary somewhat depending on the face-bow and articulator that are being used. However, the following basic steps apply for any of the combinations:

1. Selection of reference points
2. Preparation of bite fork
3. Orientation of face-bow to bite fork and reference points
4. Orientation of face-bow to articulator

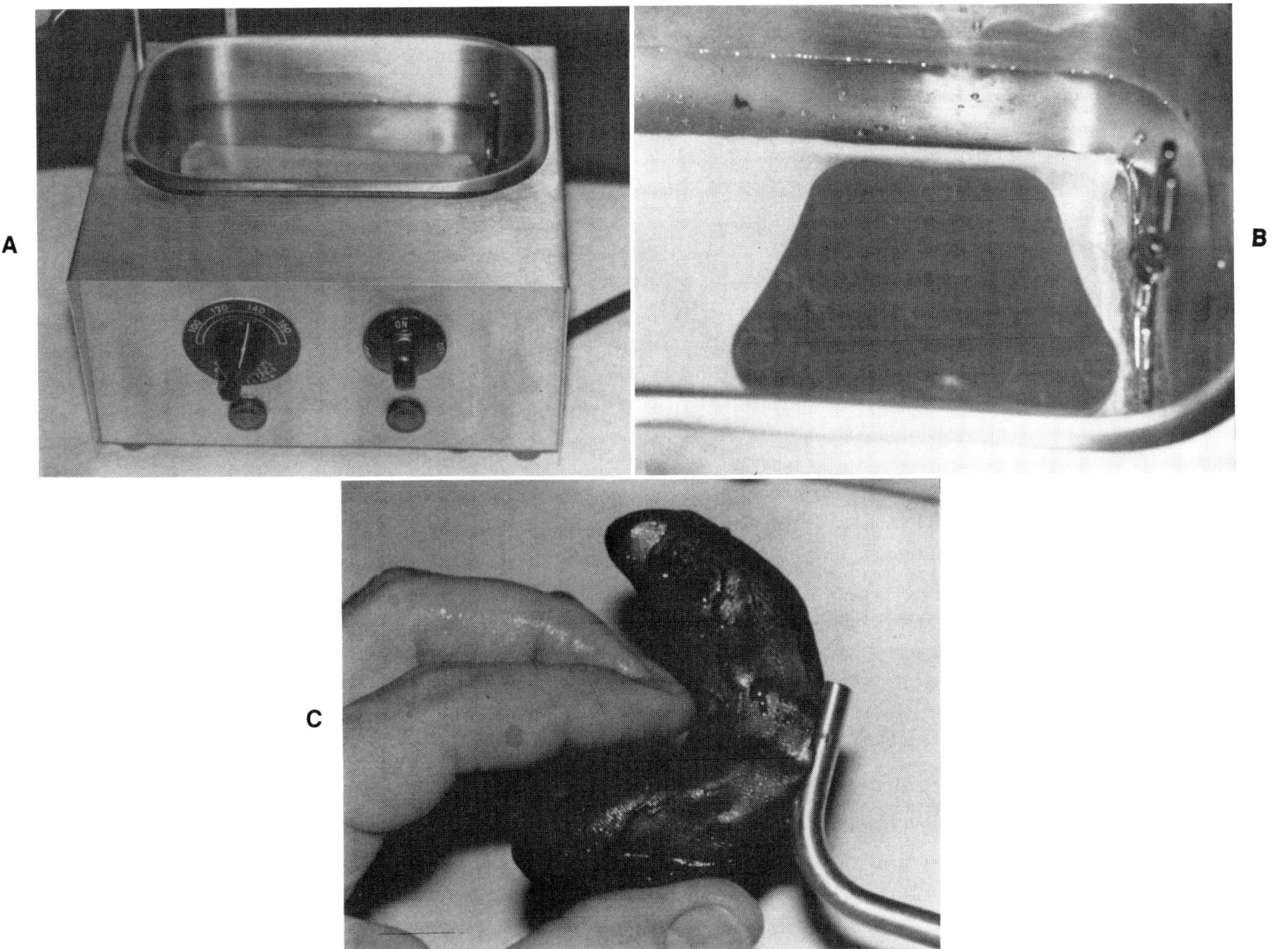

Fig. 6-7. A, Hanau water bath set at 60°C (140°F). **B,** Cake of red modeling plastic being softened in water bath. **C,** Softened modeling plastic adapted to bite fork.

5. Attachment of maxillary cast to articulator

The steps involved in making the face-bow transfer for the Hanau SM face-bow and Hanau 130-28 articulator (Fig. 6-6) are described. If another combination is to be used, appropriate departures from this description will be necessary.

Selection of reference points. With the use of a millimeter ruler, Beyron's point (13 mm anterior to the posterior margin of the center of the tragus of the ear on a line to the outer canthus of the eye) is marked on each side of the face. The third point of reference is palpated and marked below the right orbit at the level of the infraorbital notch.

Preparation of bite fork. One sheet of baseplate wax is thoroughly softened over the Bunsen burner, formed into a cylinder, and adapted around both sides of the bite fork. A cake of red modeling compound softened in a water bath is equally effective (Fig. 6-7). While the wax is still soft, the bite fork is positioned in the mouth with the projecting attachment arm to the left side of the patient, and the midline mark on the fork corresponding to the midline of the patient. Imprints of the maxillary teeth are accurately recorded (Fig. 6-8).

The mandibular teeth are allowed to close lightly into the soft wax to stabilize the face-bow. Occasionally the patient may not be able to stabilize the fork with the mandibular teeth. In this case the dentist must hold the bite fork with the wax record firmly in place with finger pressure. The wax is allowed to cool in the mouth, removed, and chilled with cold water. Then the face-bow record is trimmed so that only indentations of the maxillary cusp tips remain and all soft tissue contacts are removed (Fig. 6-9). There should be no metallic show-through of the bite fork.

If there are insufficient teeth in the maxillary arch to stabilize the bite fork (a widely separated tripod of support), a baseplate with a wax occlusion rim is used to provide the necessary occlusal contacts with the bite fork record (Fig. 6-10).

After the record has been trimmed, the maxillary cast

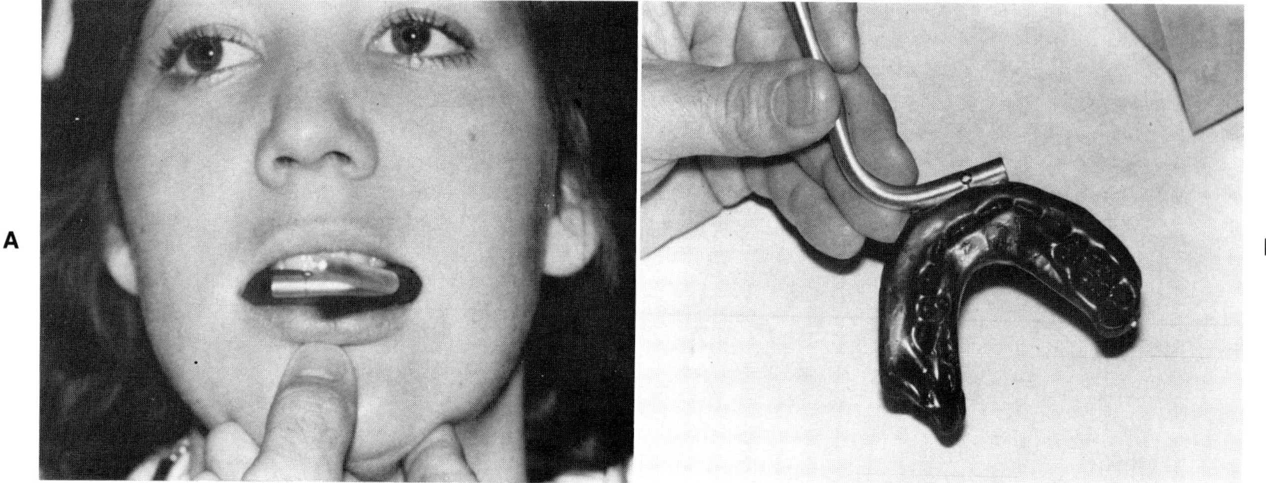

Fig. 6-8. A, Bite fork positioned with bite fork arm on patient's left side. **B,** Bite fork with imprint of maxillary teeth.

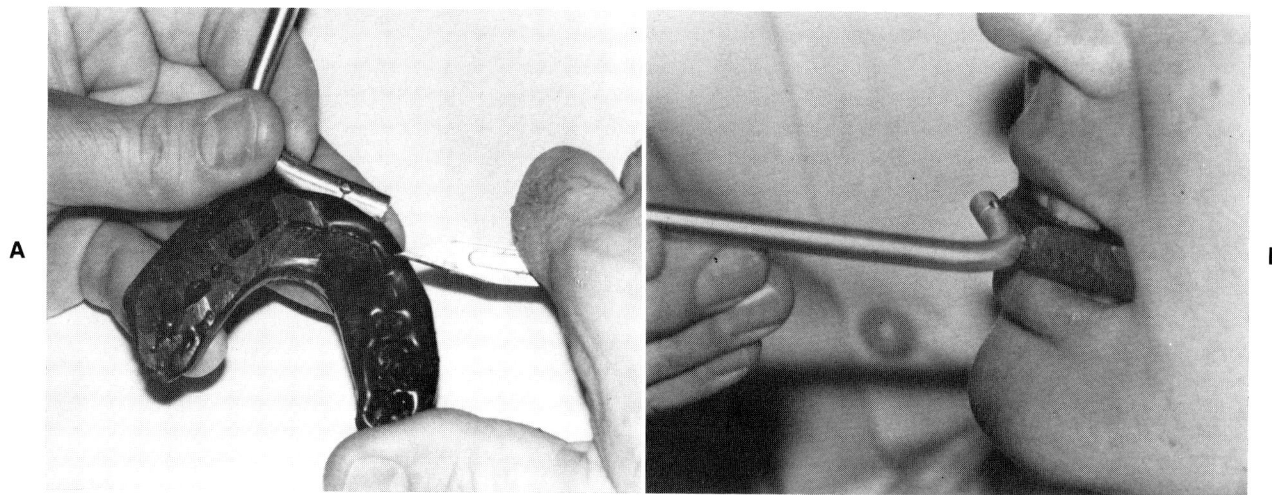

Fig. 6-9. A, Modeling plastic trimmed, leaving only indentations of cusp tips. **B,** Checking stability of bite fork in mouth.

should be seated in the record to verify fit and stability (Fig. 6-11). Before the cast is placed into the wax record, all nodules on the occlusal surfaces of the teeth on the cast that resulted from voids in the impression must be removed. If the accuracy of the record is doubtful (for example, if the cast is not completely seated or if it rocks), the cuspal imprints may be corrected by placing zinc oxide–eugenol impression paste into the cuspal imprints and reseating the record in the mouth. Another method is to place low-fusing Alu-wax* in the imprints, temper it in warm water, and reseat the bite fork record. Either technique will result in an accurate bite fork record. This procedure may also serve as a check on the accuracy of the cast. If the cast does not now seat firmly in the corrected cuspal imprints, there may be nodules on the occlusal surfaces of the teeth or the cast may be distorted. One should be certain the cast is accurate before proceeding.

Orientation of face-bow to bite fork and reference points. Before the transfer is made, the styli of the face-bow should be adjusted so that their readings are the same. This is best done by locking one stylus at 7.0 and placing the face-bow in position on the patient's face. With the fixed stylus centered over one arbitrary hinge

*Alu-wax, Aluwax Dental Products Co., Grand Rapids, Mich.

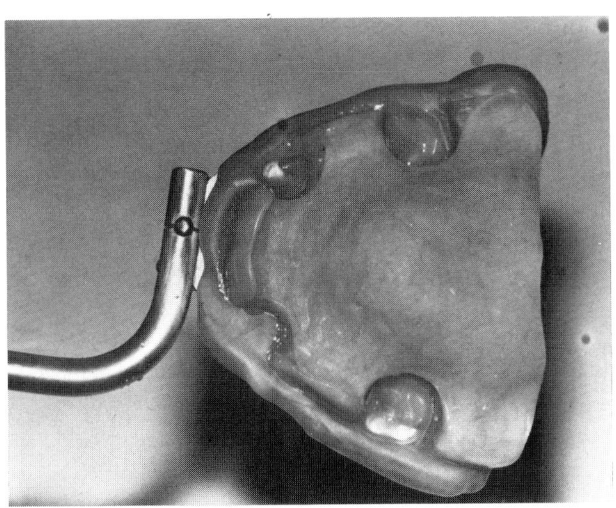

Fig. 6-10. Baseplate with wax occlusion rim provides stabilizing contacts when an insufficient number of teeth is present.

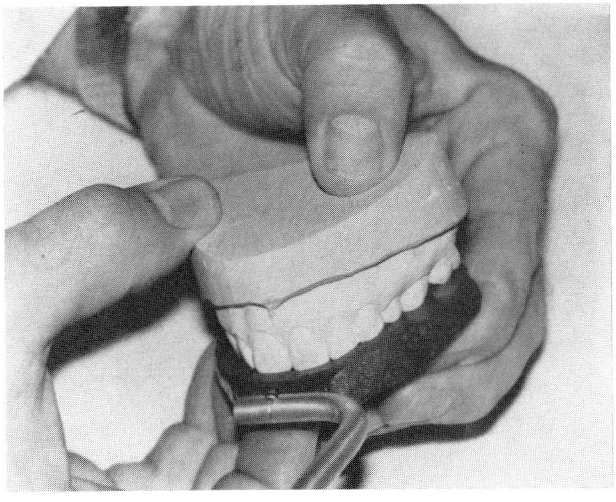

Fig. 6-11. Checking stability of bite-fork on cast.

axis mark, the other stylus is adjusted until it lightly contacts the hinge axis mark on the opposite side of the face. The reading on that stylus is averaged with the 7.0 reading on the fixed stylus, and the result is the setting at which both styli are now locked. For example, if the reading on the second stylus were 7.6, both styli would be adjusted to 7.3:

$$\begin{array}{r} 7.6 \\ \underline{7.0} \\ 2\overline{)14.6} \\ 7.3 \end{array} \text{ on each side}$$

This procedure equalizes the readings on the styli and simplifies the orientation of the face-bow to the articulator.

The bite fork with its record is positioned on the maxillary teeth and supported by the mandibular teeth. The face-bow is centered and loosely attached to the handle of the fork. The styli rods are adjusted so they lightly touch the skin over the arbitrary hinge axis points with the readings equal on both sides. The axis styli and screw clamps are secured (Fig. 6-12). The orbital pointer is attached as the final step. The pointer is carefully passed through its attachment, and its tip is placed in contact with the anterior reference mark at the infraorbital notch. The screw clamp is tightened (Fig. 6-13). The face-bow is checked to make certain that both condylar extensions and the orbital pointer are in contact with the three reference points. The face-bow is removed by grasping the end of the orbital pointer with one hand to prevent accidental injury to the eye and by grasping the face-bow itself with the other hand. The patient is instructed to open, and the face-bow is gently removed.

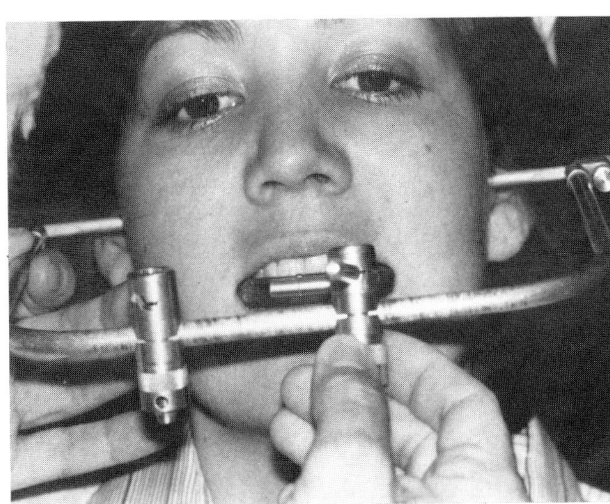

Fig. 6-12. Face-bow centered on patient's face and attached to bite-fork.

Orientation of face-bow to articulator. The Hanau 130-28 articulator has a variable intercondylar distance that can be set to simulate the patient's intercondylar distance. However, a semiadjustable articulator is adequate for the diagnostic procedure, and in this description the Hanau 130-28 will be used as though it were a fixed intercondylar distance instrument. This will simplify the technique. The technique would be similar for the Hanau H-2 series or the Dentatus* articulators.

The following steps are used for preparing the articulator and orienting the face-bow to the articulator.

---

*Dentatus ARH, Almore International Inc., Portland, Ore.

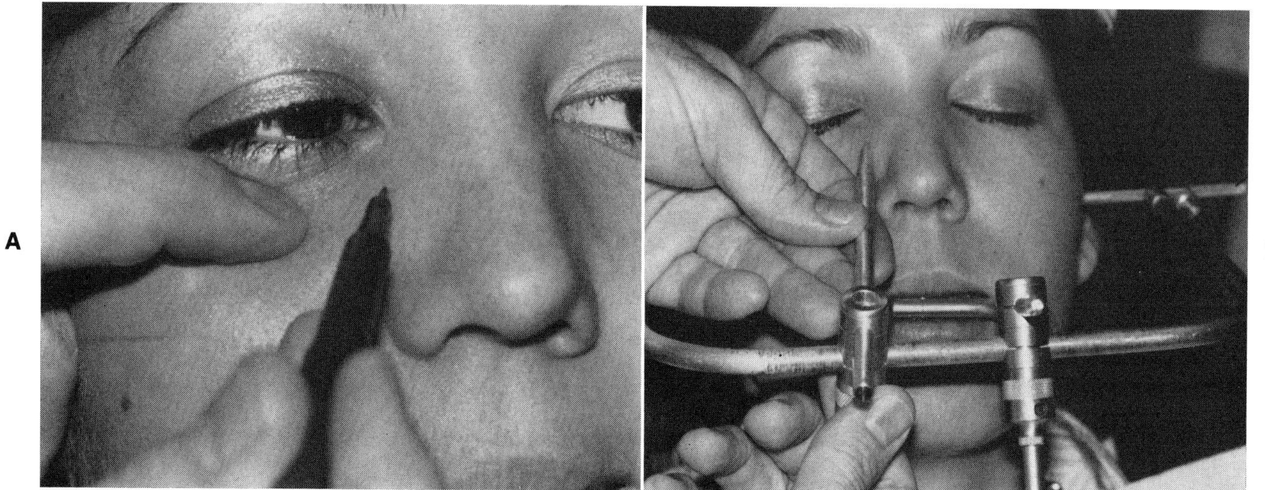

Fig. 6-13. A, Anterior reference point marked at level of infraorbital notch. **B,** Anterior reference pointer attached to face-bow.

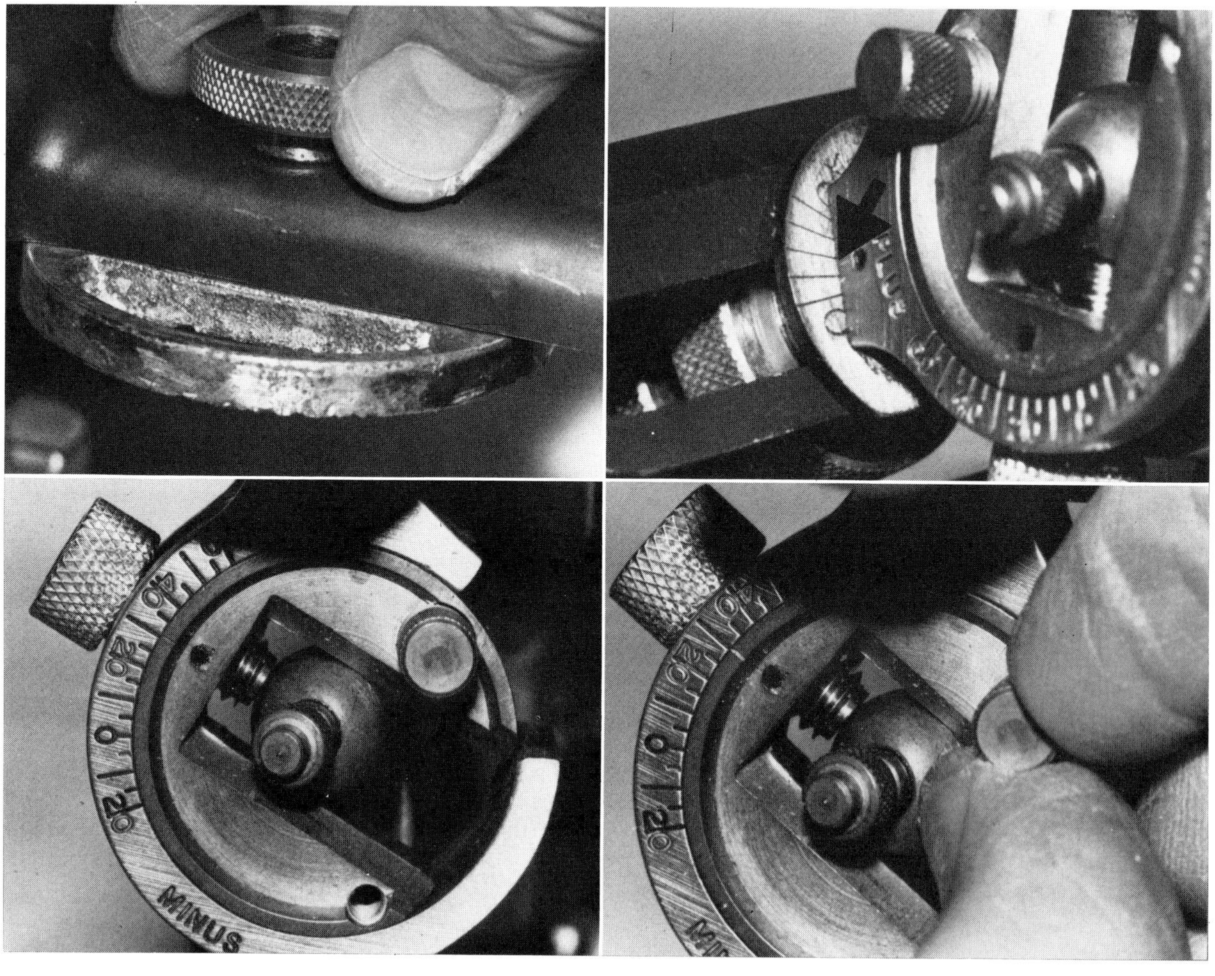

Fig. 6-14. A, Mounting ring attached to upper member. **B,** Lateral condylar inclination set at 15 degrees (arrow). **C,** Horizontal condylar guidance set at 30 degrees. **D,** Condylar elements locked.

1. The under surface of the upper member of the articulator that will be contacted by mounting stone is lubricated, and a mounting ring is attached to the upper member of the articulator (Fig. 6-14, *A*).
2. The cast support is attached to the lower member.
3. The adjustable incisal guide pin is replaced with the L-shaped mounting pin.
4. The orbital indicator is attached to the under surface of the upper member with the indicator on the patient's or articulator's right side.
5. The condylar shaft supports should be set at 55 mm on each side. (The articulator has an adjustable intercondylar distance. Frequently the face-bow will be positioned on the articulator with the face-bow styli rods locked at the intercondylar width taken from the patient, and the articulator intercondylar distance guides adjusted to contact the face-bow rods. However, in this mounting the articulator intercondylar distance will remain set at 55 on each side, and the face-bow styli rods will be adjusted so that the readings remain equal on both sides.) The lateral condylar inclination should be set at 15 degrees on each side, and the protrusive inclination of the condylar guide should be set at 30 degrees on each side (Fig. 6-14, *B* and *C*).
6. The condylar elements are locked in their most posterior position (Fig. 6-14, *D*).
7. The face-bow is attached to the articulator, and the styli are adjusted so that they contact the extension of the condyles firmly and so that the readings on the styli are equal (Fig. 6-15, *A*).
8. The incisal guide lock screw that is retaining the L-shaped pin is loosened, and the upper member

A

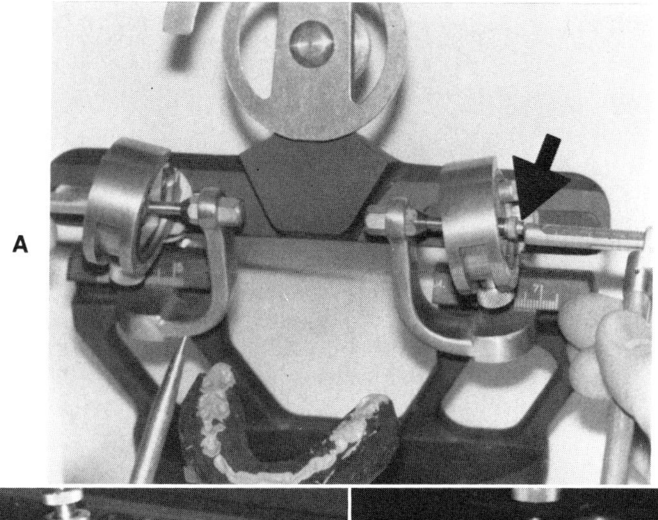

B

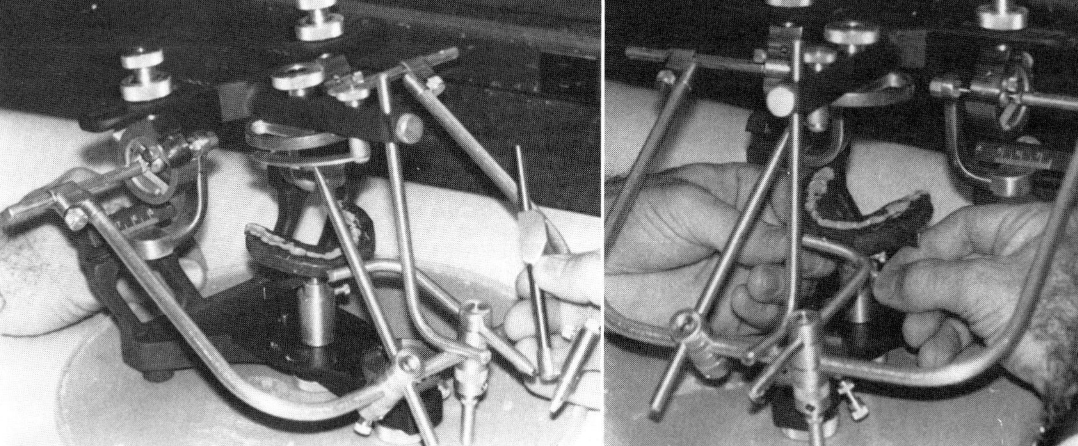

C

Fig. 6-15. A, Styli adjusted to contact condylar extensions (arrow) with equal readings on styli. **B,** L-shaped pin replaces incisal pin and contacts face-bow. Anterior reference pointer contacts under surface of infraorbital indicator, which is attached to upper member of articulator. **C,** Cast supports adjusted to contact undersurface of bite-fork record.

is raised or lowered so that the tip of the orbital pointer contacts the under surface of the orbital indicator. The L-shaped pin is positioned so that it rests on the stem of the bite fork, and the incisal guide lock screw is tightened. The L-shaped pin should maintain the position of the orbital pointer's contact with the under surface of the orbital indicator (Fig. 6-15, *B*).

9. The height of the cast support is adjusted to contact the under surface of the bite fork record (Fig. 6-15, *C*).
10. The face-bow assembly is now related to the upper member of the articulator in the correct position. When the maxillary cast is seated on the bite fork, it will be in the same relation to the condylar elements of the articulator as are the maxillary teeth to the condyles of the patient.

Attachment of maxillary cast to articulator

1. The base of the maxillary cast is indexed by cutting two intersecting V-shaped grooves approximately 2 to 3 mm deep across the base.
2. A dental stone–separating medium is placed in the grooves of the cast, after which the cast is soaked in clear slurry water for approximately 2 to 3 minutes.
3. The upper member of the articulator is raised, and the cast is placed on the bite fork record. The cast must be checked for stability on the record.
4. A mix of low-expansion dental stone and concentrated slurry water is placed on the base of the cast, and the upper member is closed to contact it. The dentist should make certain that the L-shaped pin returns to its position resting against the stem of the bite fork, that the orbital pointer touches the under surface of the orbital indicator, and that dental stone fills the retentive areas of the mounting ring. Only enough stone to attach the cast is used (Fig. 6-16). Additional stone can be added to the mounting to improve its appearance.

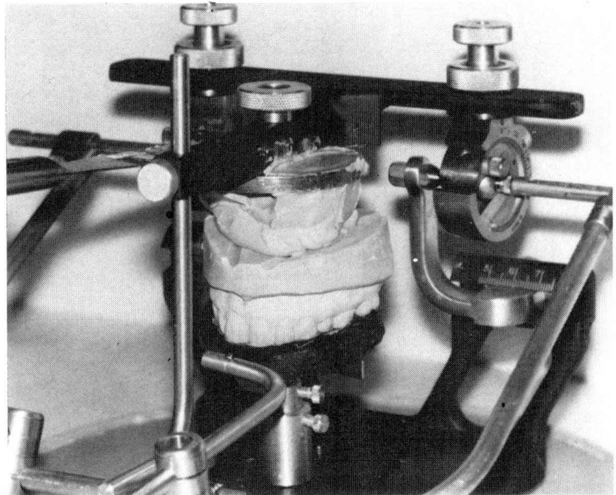

Fig. 6-16. Maxillary cast attached to mounting ring with mix of dental stone.

Centric jaw relation record

Centric jaw relation is the most posterior relation of the mandible to the maxilla at the established vertical relation. It is a bone-to-bone relation of the mandible to the maxilla in terminal hinge closure. This most retruded relation of the mandible to the maxilla is fundamental to any diagnostic evaluation of the patient's occlusion.

More than 90% of patients do not routinely close their jaws at this most retruded position. The point of closure is usually anterior or anterior and lateral to the retruded position at which the occlusal surfaces of the teeth make maximum contact. This position is called the centric occlusal position or centric occlusion.

In spite of this phenomenon, diagnostic casts are mounted at the patient's centric jaw relation for several reasons. Centric jaw relation is the only relationship of the jaws that can be recorded repeatedly and verified on an articulator. Wear facets that are invariably present between centric jaw relation and centric occlusion attest to the fact that all patients, at least part of the time, do close at centric relation. It is the best reference position for studying the other relationships of the jaws. The importance of centric jaw relation as a reference position is magnified by the fact that interferences between the patient's centric jaw relation and centric occlusion are the most common cause of bruxism and severe occlusal trauma. These interferences are present to a much greater degree in the partially edentulous patient because of the tipping, drifting, and extrusion of teeth that commonly occur when the continuity of the dental arch is lost.

The decision whether to construct the prosthesis at the patient's centric jaw relation or centric occlusion must be made on the basis of all the diagnostic data.

With the exception of the small percentage of patients whose centric jaw relation and centric occlusion coincide, the patient must be assisted or guided when the centric jaw relation is recorded. For this position to be recorded consistently, the muscles controlling the movements of the mandible must be relaxed. Because patients exhibit varying degrees of muscle relaxation, the difficulty encountered will vary considerably from patient to patient. The determination of centric jaw relation is difficult if there is splinting of the muscles associated with pain, hypertonicity of the muscles associated with occlusal interferences, or any degree of psychologic tension.

The accurate recording of centric jaw relation is impossible if the patient is suffering from acute temporomandibular joint or muscle disturbances. Usually the use of an occlusal splint is indicated to aid in the relief of the symptoms of these disturbances before an attempt is made to record centric jaw relation.

Ramfjord and Ash (1971) have stated that the following three factors must be controlled in order to succeed in determining centric jaw relation: psychologic or emotional stress; pain in the temporomandibular joints or the musculature concerned with mandibular movement; and "muscle memory," or the proprioceptive reflex resulting from occlusal interferences. Because patients will exhibit varying degrees of muscle and emotional relaxation, knowledge of more than one method of determining centric jaw relation is necessary.

Recommended method of determining centric jaw relation

This method should always be attempted initially because it is designed to control the three factors just described.

1. The patient is comfortably seated in the dental chair. The backrest or chair is tilted to about 60 or 70 degrees to provide patient comfort and better visibility for the dentist. The patient's head should be well supported so that there is no tension in the neck muscles (Fig. 6-17). The patient is asked to relax and to breathe through the nose. All distraction should be avoided, and the dentist's manner should be as relaxed as possible.
2. The patient is asked to open widely and to maintain that position for about a minute in an attempt to deprogram the "muscle memory." An alternative approach is to have the patient close lightly on large cotton rolls, one on each side of the dental arch, for 4 to 5 minutes.
3. If mandibular anterior teeth are present, the dentist's thumb is placed on the labial surface of these teeth with the index finger under the chin. The thumb must be placed high enough on the mandibular incisor teeth to prevent contact of the opposing teeth if the patient should attempt to close or swallow (Fig. 6-18). The thumb and the index or middle finger of the other hand are placed on each side of the maxillary arch opposite the premolars.
4. The dentist must speak to the patient and give all instructions in a soft monotone. The patient is told that the dentist will guide the movements of the jaw. The instructions to try to relax the entire body and to breathe through the nose should be repeated throughout the entire procedure. The dentist must do nothing to cause pain or create anxiety in the patient. The patient must not be criticized regardless of the difficulty encountered in this procedure.
5. Slight backward and downward pressure is applied as the patient's jaw is guided in opening and closing movements over a short arc. The teeth are not allowed to touch because their contact may activate proprioceptive receptors in the periodontal ligament and cause the mandible to deviate into learned patterns of closure.

   Success in achieving the desired retrusion of

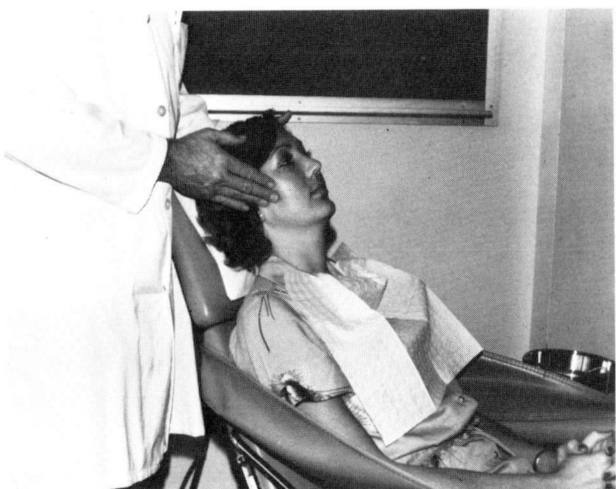

Fig. 6-17. Dental chair tilted at approximately 60 degrees and head well supported by headrest.

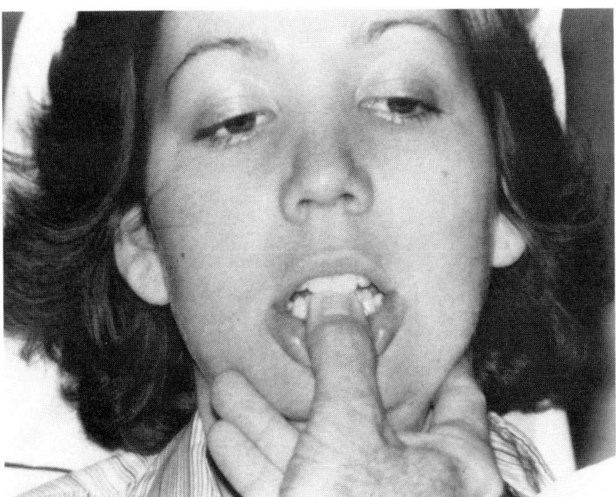

Fig. 6-18. Thumb placed to prevent contact of posterior teeth when guiding mandible.

the mandible is signified by a freely moving mandible and the feel of the mandible rotating in its most retruded position. Wide opening of the jaws should not be allowed once the mandible is in its most retruded position because it will cause translation of the condyles and meniscus.

6. The thumb should be gradually moved down on the mandibular incisors once the ability to guide the mandible in the retruded position is achieved. This is continued until the first occlusal contact occurs. Once this initial contact is established, subsequent guiding of the mandible is more easily achieved.
7. When the patient has been rehearsed sufficiently to cooperate and remain relaxed, the centric jaw relation record is made.

If a freely rotating mandible under control of the operator cannot be achieved, one of the alternative methods of retruding the mandible should be attempted.

Alternate method one: bilateral manipulation of the mandible

Some dentists prefer to use bilateral manipulation of the mandible for recording centric jaw relation. This method is said to place the condyles in their most superior rather than most retruded position. All four fingers of each hand are placed on the lower border of the mandible, and the thumbs are placed over the symphysis (Fig. 6-19). When the mandible is rotating freely, the dentist exerts firm pressure in an upward direction with the fingers and downward and backward pressure with the thumbs. Reproducible results can be attained, and it is an acceptable method of positioning the mandible.

Alternate method two: alternation of protrusion and retrusion

Frequently the lateral pterygoid muscle prevents relaxation and free rotation of the mandible. This method attempts to fatigue this muscle sufficiently so that it will reduce its contraction and allow retrusion of the mandible.

1. Using the same finger position as in the recommended method, the dentist instructs the patient (in understandable terminology) to protrude and retrude the mandible alternately. This procedure is repeated until the operator can feel that the mandible "falls back" into its most retruded position. At this point the mandible is assisted in a rotational closure.
2. This procedure is practiced until the patient can follow the instructions and the dentist can feel that complete retrusion has been achieved. At this time the centric jaw relation record is made.

Alternate method three: use of an occlusal splint

Patients with severe splinting or hypertonicity of the muscles or with acute symptoms of temporomandibular joint dysfunction will usually provide inconsistent and inaccurate results. The construction of an occlusal spint to be worn for a time in an attempt to relieve symptoms and to precondition the neuromuscular system is usually indicated for this type of patient (Fig. 6-20).

Media for recording centric jaw relation

A number of media can be used to record centric jaw relation, including wax, which is the most commonly used; impression and recording pastes such as zinc ox-

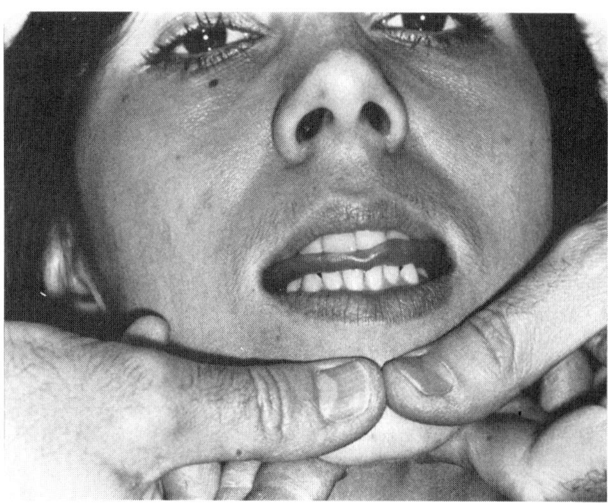

Fig. 6-19. Finger position for bilateral manipulation of mandible.

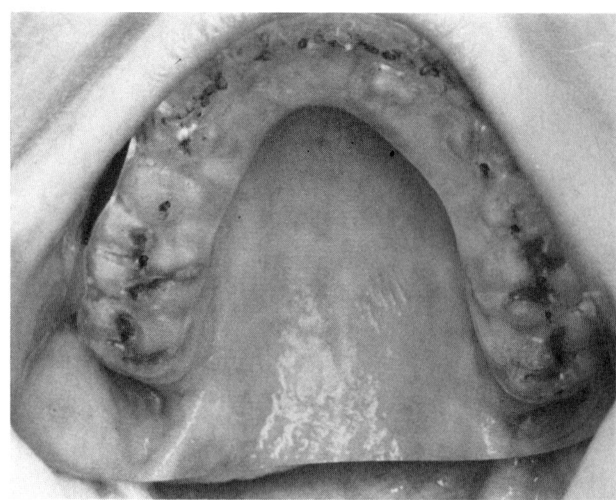

Fig. 6-20. Acrylic resin occlusal splint for patient with severe splinting or hypertonicity of musculature.

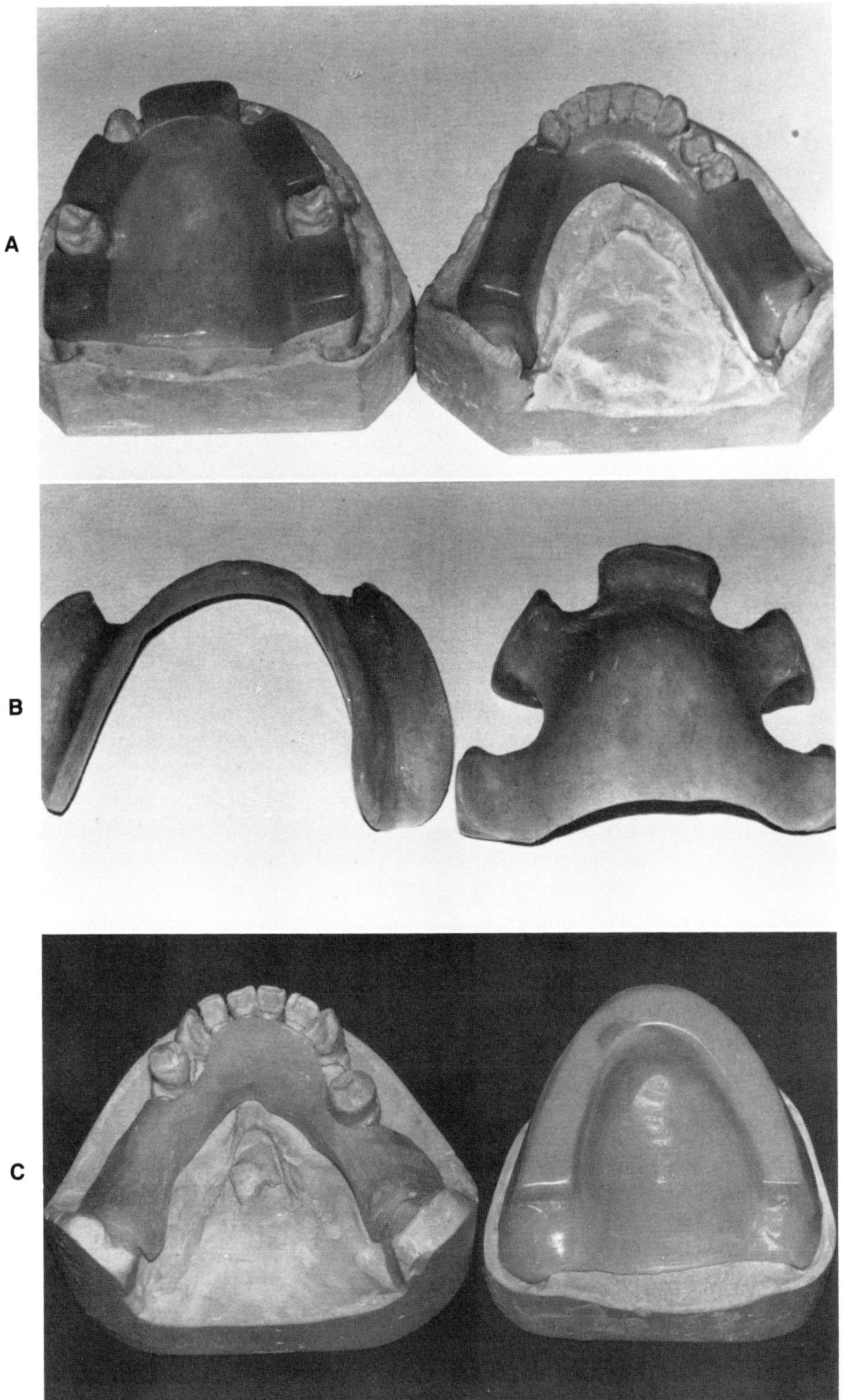

Fig. 6-21. A baseplate (record base, temporary base, or trial base), according to Boucher's *Current Clinical Dental Terminology,* is "a temporary form representing the base of a denture and used for making maxillomandibular (jaw) relation records, for arranging artificial teeth, or for trial placement in the mouth." **A,** Maxillary and mandibular baseplates with wax occlusion rims. **B,** Tissue surface of baseplates pictured in **A. C,** Baseplates for completely edentulous maxillary arch and partially edentulous mandibular arch.

ide–eugenol paste; plaster of paris; dental stone; acrylic resin; and modeling plastic.

The material selected for recording centric jaw relation in the diagnostic mounting depends on the number and location of the remaining teeth. If there are a sufficient number of widely spaced occlusal contacts (at least three widely separated areas of contact), baseplates are not needed and wax is indicated for making the interocclusal record. However, wax distorts easily with changes in temperature and careless handling, so the record should be stored in cool water until it is needed. If the edentulous areas are extensive or if one or both of the posterior segments are edentulous, a baseplate is needed for accurately relating the mandibular cast to the maxillary cast (Fig. 6-21). If baseplates are used, the selection of a suitable recording medium becomes critical because of the ease with which baseplates constructed for the partially edentulous arch can be displaced. A free-flowing medium such as accelerated dental stone or one of the impression or recording pastes is indicated to minimize the danger of displacing the baseplates.

Vertical dimension of occlusion

With the exception of the completely edentulous opposing arch, there is usually at least one tooth that will have occlusal contact with an antagonist at the patient's original vertical dimension of occlusion. However, there are exceptions, and it is necessary to use such guides as the physiologic rest position and phonetics to determine an appropriate vertical dimension of occlusion at which the centric jaw relation is to be made. A more in-depth discussion of vertical dimension is included in Chapter 14.

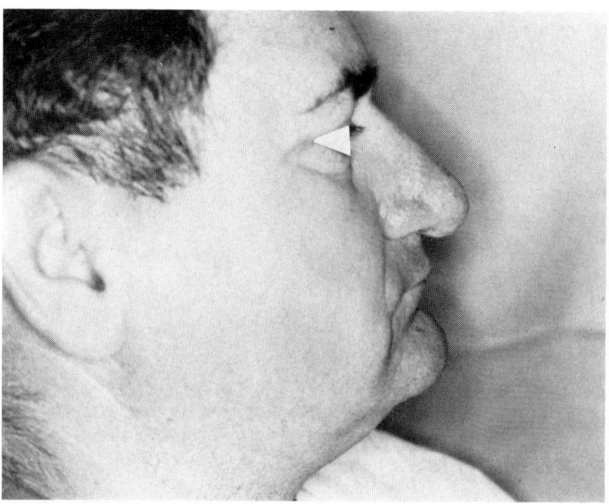

Fig. 6-22. Patient with apparent overclosure of vertical dimension of occlusion.

The mounted diagnostic casts are of critical importance even when there is no opposing occlusion. Casts mounted at a physiologically acceptable vertical dimension of occlusion will provide essential information such as the presence of interfering tuberosities, lack of interarch space, abnormal jaw relationships, or an unacceptable plane of occlusion. Baseplates are obviously needed in these situations.

Probably the most difficult diagnostic decisions relative to the vertical dimension of occlusion occur when there is occlusal contact but with an apparent overclosure caused by drifting or extreme occlusal wear of the remaining teeth (Fig. 6-22). The opening or restoring of the vertical dimension of occlusion by means of a removable prosthesis must be approached with extreme care. The diagnostic period is lengthy because the patient must learn to tolerate the wearing of a diagnostic removable splint at the new vertical dimension of occlusion. The splint should be worn for several months before definitive treatment is attempted. Procedures for this treatment are described in Chapter 18.

Procedure for making a centric jaw relation record using wax

Wax is used as the recording medium when there are sufficient teeth present to make the record and relate the casts without the use of a baseplate. Although wax is the most widely used recording medium, it is also the most unreliable and unpredictable; thus its use necessitates excellent technique and great care. Distortion can occur when the record is made, when the records are stored, and when the cast is mounted. The dentist must understand the problems involved and how to avoid them. Probably the greatest problem is the "memory" exhibited by most waxes. The warpage factor is the most difficult and most important factor that must be overcome. The method of heating the wax and the way the wax is handled after the recording are critical.

Two distinctly different types of waxes are used for interocclusal records. One type is a soft wax that has a metallic filler such as aluminum or bronze powder. An example is Alu-wax. The filler allows more rapid and uniform heating of the wax, provides for retention of heat for a longer working time, and contributes to uniform cooling of the wax. These properties decrease warpage of the record. A major disadvantage is that the wax is soft. Deeper penetration into the record can occur from force used in placing the record on the cast or from the weight of the mounting stone and the cast itself in the mounting procedure.

Hard baseplate wax has the advantage of being hard after the record is made. This property minimizes the error that occurs if the teeth of the cast penetrate deeper into the wax when the cast is placed into the record or when it is mounted. The major disadvantages are the difficulty in uniformly heating the wax to a "dead" condition and the comparatively greater degree of "memory" this wax exhibits.

Considerable care must be exercised when either wax is used. A method of using each type is described. Both methods attempt to minimize the effect of the potential problems inherent in the materials.

Use of metal-impregnated wax. The following equipment and supplies are needed to make the interocclusal record with metal-impregnated wax:

1. Water bath at 43° C (110° F)
2. Bowl of cool water
3. Alu-wax—2 sheets (or similar metal-impregnated wax)
4. Ash metal No. 7—2 pieces
5. Sticky wax
6. Bunsen burner
7. No. 7 wax spatula
8. Diagnostic casts
9. Semi-adjustable articulator
10. Rubber bowl and plaster spatula
11. Dental stone
12. Bard Parker knife

Two thicknesses of metal-impregnated wax are shaped to fit the arch form of the maxillary cast by passing the sheet of wax through the flame until it is slightly softened, folding it over on itself, and placing it over the occlusal surfaces of the maxillary cast. The wax is trimmed with a sharp Bard Parker knife so that the wax extends 2 to 3 mm buccal and labial to the teeth (Fig. 6-23). The wax should not extend distally beyond the remaining teeth.

The soft wax should be reinforced to help prevent warpage. A piece of Ash No. 7 soft metal is cut that is approximately 15 mm wide and 50 mm long. The metal is folded over the center of the posterior margin of the

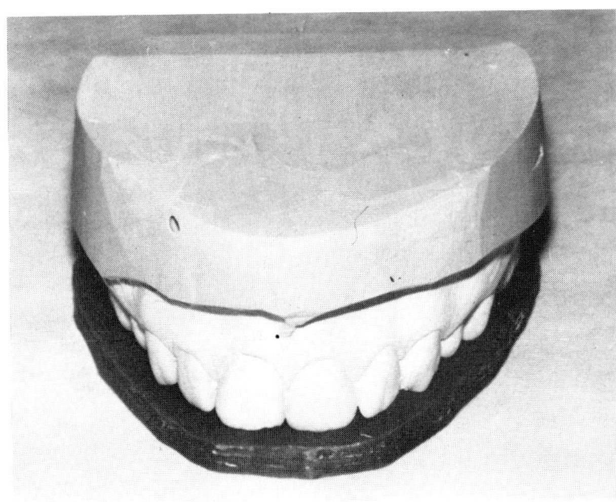

Fig. 6-23. Two thicknesses of Alu-wax trimmed 2 to 3 mm buccal and labial to maxillary teeth.

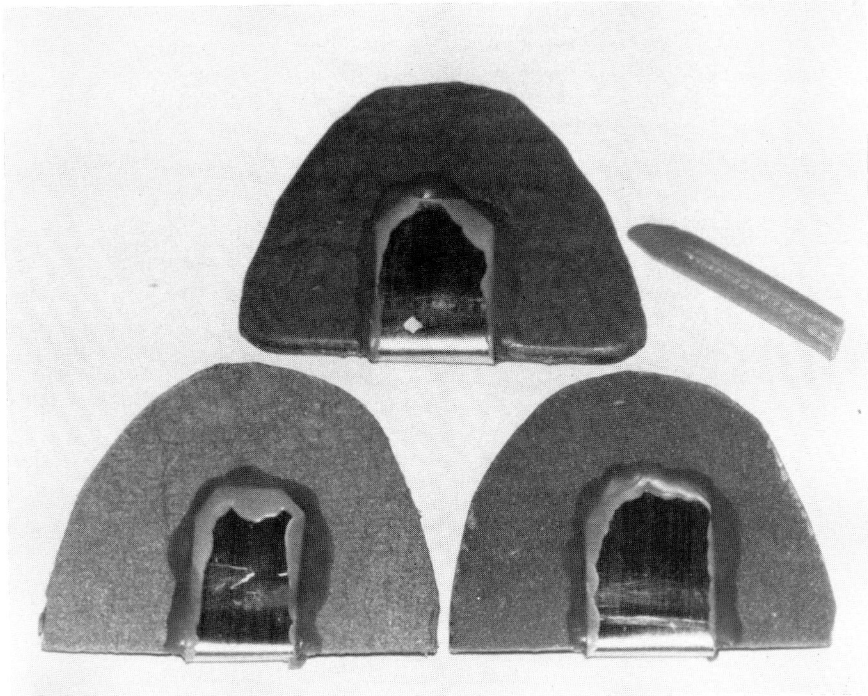

Fig. 6-24. Alu-wax records reinforced with No. 7 Ash metal and sticky wax.

wax so that it extends anteriorly an equal distance on both sides of the wax. There should be a minimum of 5 mm clearance between the edge of the metal and the teeth. The metal is secured to the wax by a small amount of sticky wax along the margins of the metal (Fig. 6-24).

The use of a rubber dam punch to punch several holes into the soft metal wax record also effectively secures the metal to the wax. A final check is made to ensure adequate clearance between the metal or sticky wax and the teeth.

The prepared wax jaw relation record of wax and Ash metal is softened uniformly in warm water (approximately 43° C, or 110° F) (Fig. 6-25).

The softened record is aligned over the maxillary teeth and adapted lightly (Fig. 6-26). The record is supported by the thumb and index finger of the left hand (for a right-handed operator) on each side of the arch at the premolar region. The right hand guides the mandible into terminal hinge closure (Fig. 6-27). Only light contact of the cusp tips with the softened wax is desired. The teeth must not penetrate the wax.

The record is carefully removed from the mouth to avoid distortion, after which it is chilled and examined (Fig. 6-28). Areas of soft tissue contact should be removed, and the record returned to the mouth, and the patient again helped to close in terminal hinge position. This second closure serves to correct any slight distortion that may have occurred and to check whether the patient is closing repeatedly into the same contacts. The patient is guided into several light contacts with the record. The interocclusal record should be checked for accuracy and stability on both the maxillary and mandibular casts (Fig. 6-29).

If any of the following errors are present, the centric jaw relation record must be corrected or reaccomplished:

1. Deep indentations of the mandibular teeth into the wax record.
2. Contact of the wax record with any area of the cast other than the cusp tips of the teeth.
3. Penetration of the cusp tips through the wax record.
4. Contact of the cusp tips with either the Ash metal or the sticky wax that reinforce the record.
5. Instability or rocking of either the maxillary or mandibular cast on the wax record. (The possibility also exists that the wax record is accurate and that nodules are present on the occlusal surfaces of the cast, or the cast itself is inaccurate, or both.)
6. Shadow or double image appearance, indicating that the patient does not close into the original indentations in the wax record.
7. Inability to orient the cast with the record.

An additional record should be made using the same technique and meeting the same criteria. This record will be used in verifying the accuracy of the mounting.

When the records have been completed, the mounting record is carefully seated on the mandibular cast. It must fit accurately with light pressure. With as much care as possible, the maxillary cast is lightly seated into the record. The two casts with the record interposed are luted together by wood or metal strips that extend to the bases of both casts. Sticky wax or modeling plastic is flowed on the ends of the strips to firmly attach the strips to the bases of the casts (Fig. 6-30). This procedure helps avoid distortion of the record during storage and the mounting procedure.

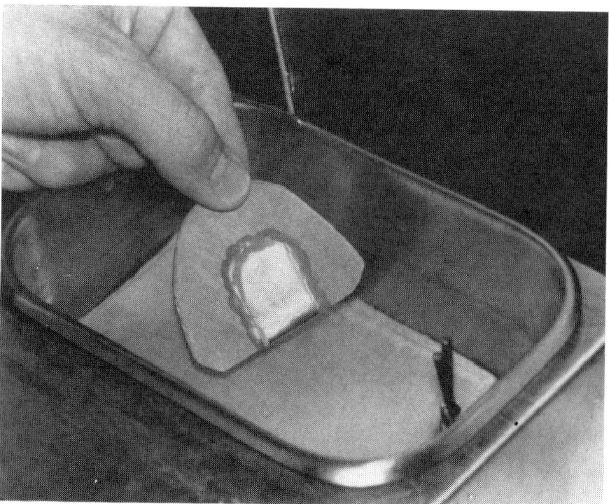

Fig. 6-25. Prepared record is softened in 43°C water bath.

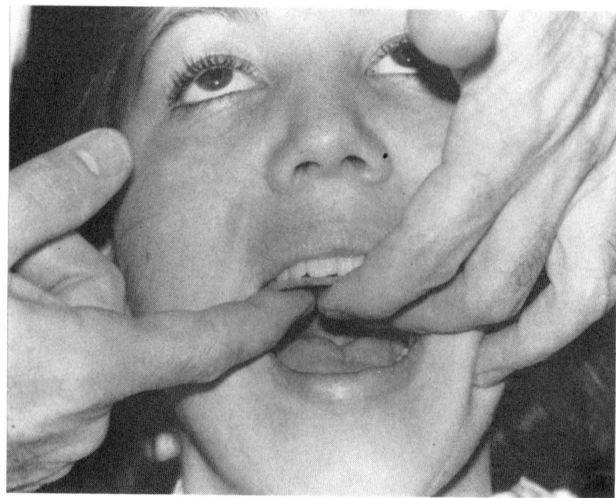

Fig. 6-26. Softened record positioned on maxillary teeth.

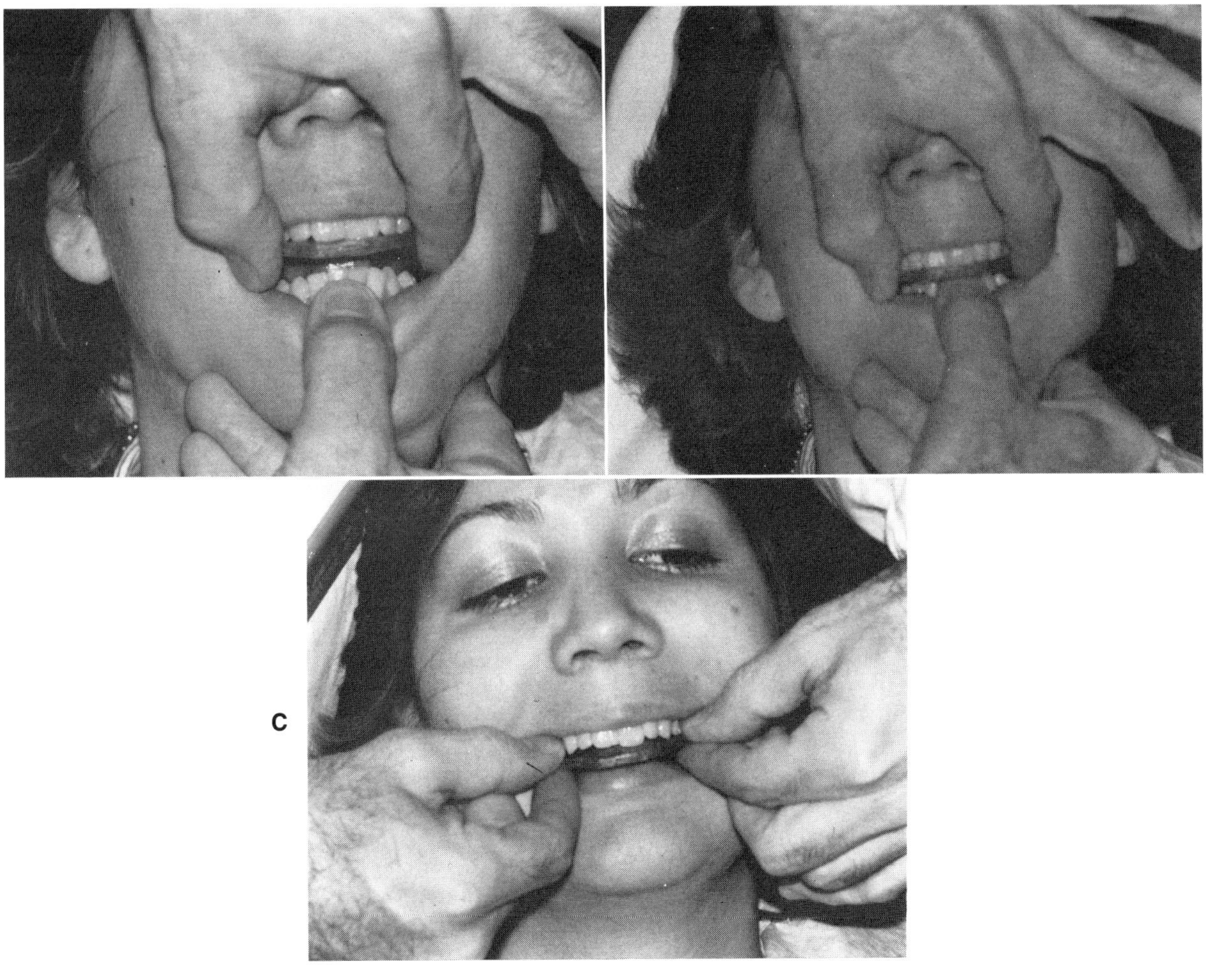

Fig. 6-27. A, Mandible guided into terminal hinge closure. **B,** Mandibular teeth closed into light contact to register indentations of cusp tips. **C,** Record held in contact with maxillary teeth while patient opens and then removed with a downward snap.

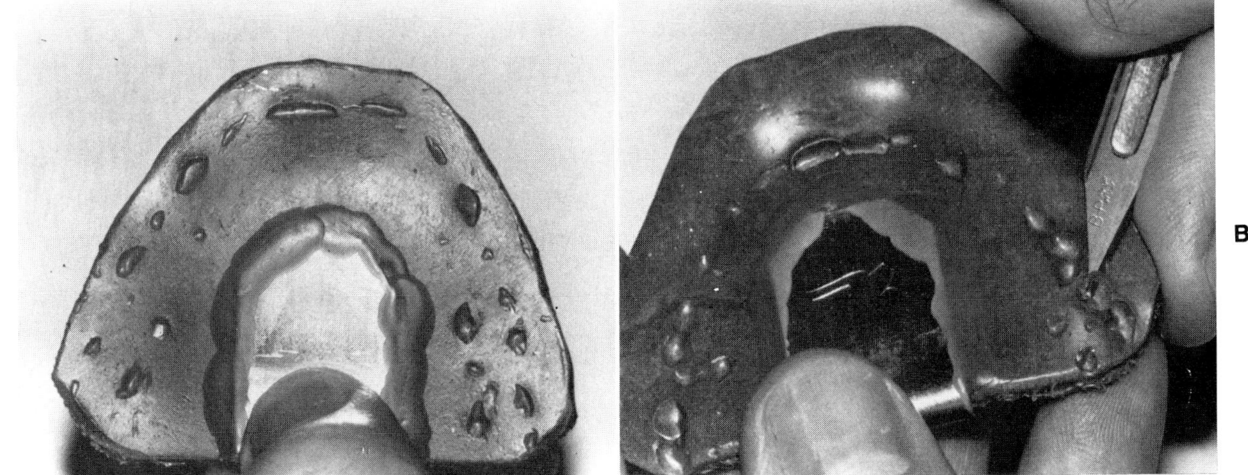

Fig. 6-28. A, Chilled record inspected for penetration through wax or contact with soft tissue. **B,** Wax trimmed in areas of deep cuspal penetration, and all soft tissue contacts removed.

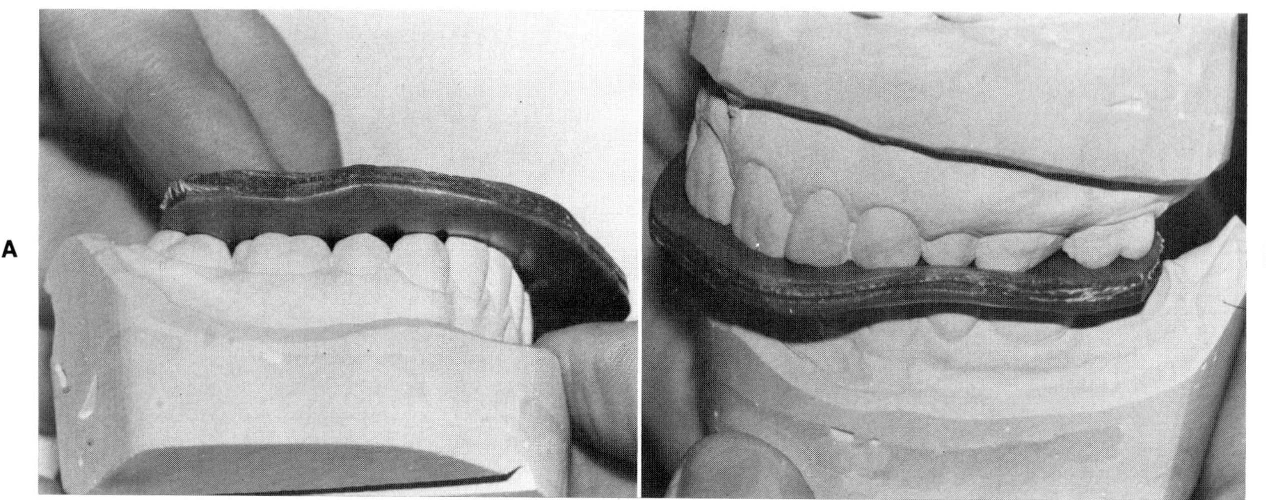

Fig. 6-29. Record placed on mandibular cast, **A,** and maxillary cast placed into record, **B,** to check accuracy of fit.

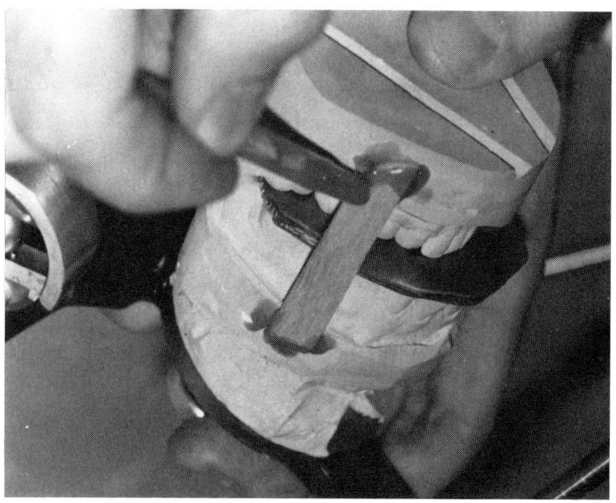

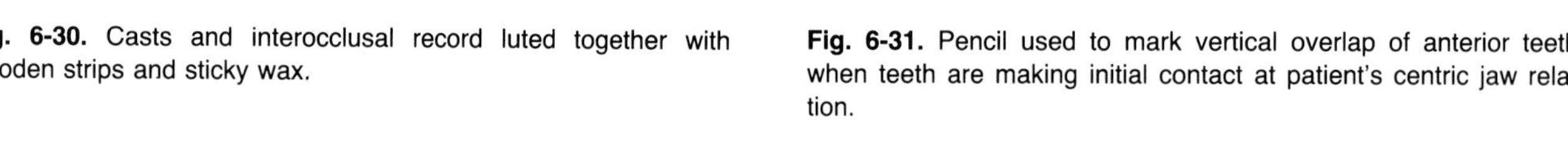

Fig. 6-30. Casts and interocclusal record luted together with wooden strips and sticky wax.

Fig. 6-31. Pencil used to mark vertical overlap of anterior teeth when teeth are making initial contact at patient's centric jaw relation.

Use of hard baseplate wax. The following equipment and supplies are needed to make the interocclusal record with hard baseplate wax:

1. Water bath at 60° C (140° F)
2. Bowl of cool water
3. Hard baseplate wax—2 sheets
4. Diagnostic casts
5. Articulator
6. Rubber bowl and plastic spatula
7. Dental stone
8. Bard Parker knife

The patient is seated comfortably. Centric jaw relation is located as described previously. With the jaws closed to the point of initial occlusal contact, an orientation mark is placed on one of the mandibular anterior teeth (Fig. 6-31). This mark indicates the vertical overlap of the anterior teeth at the initial contact; it will serve as a guide when the interocclusal record is made.

A 100 × 25 mm (4 × 1 inch) strip of wax is placed in a hot water bath at 60° C (140° F). When the wax is uniformly soft, it is folded lengthwise (Fig. 6-32). While the wax is still soft, it is adapted to the patient's maxillary teeth (Fig. 6-33). The mandible is guided into centric jaw relation and tapped into the soft wax (Fig. 6-34). The closure should result in a thickness of 1.0 mm of wax between the teeth that were involved in the ini-

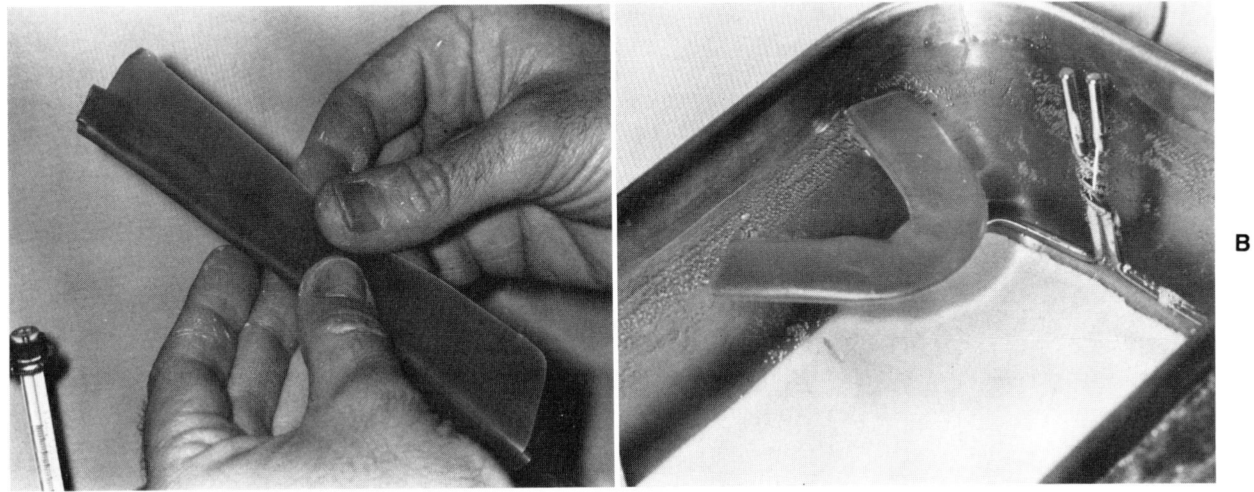

Fig. 6-32. A, A sheet of baseplate wax is softened in a water bath set at 60° C (140° F) and is folded to make a strip 100 mm (4 inches) long and 13 mm (½ inch) wide. **B,** Wax is shaped and trimmed to follow arch form of patient and is placed back in water bath to develop uniform softness.

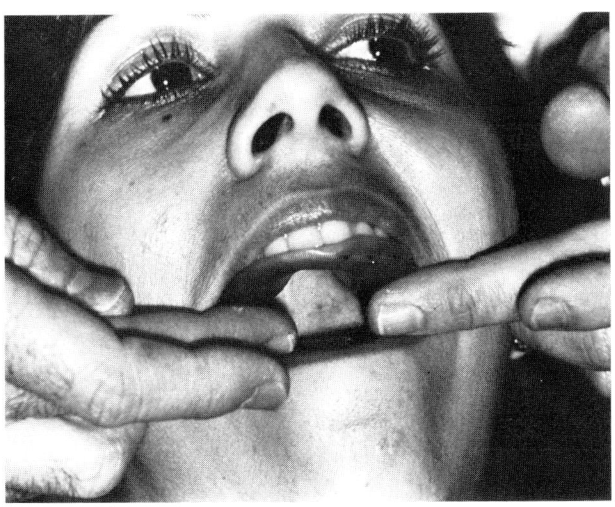

Fig. 6-33. Softened wax is adapted over maxillary teeth.

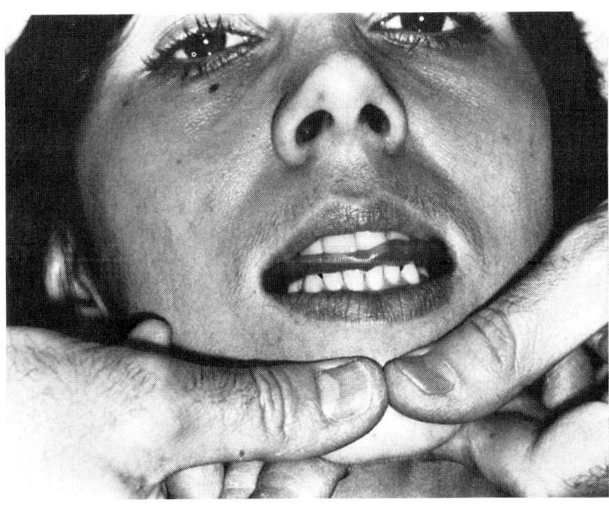

Fig. 6-34. Mandible is guided into centric jaw relation and is tapped into softened wax.

tial occlusal contact at centric jaw relation. The previously placed orientation mark serves as a guide; an opening of 1.0 mm at this mark will provide the appropriate clearance of the posterior teeth.

Excess wax is trimmed to expose the buccal cusp tips while maintaining the mandible in its retruded position with light pressure. While the mandible is held in the record, the patient is asked to open, and cold water or compressed air is used to cool the occlusal and lingual aspects of the record. Wax must be removed from areas where it has made contact with the soft tissue.

The record is removed from the mouth and inspected for thickness. Any penetration of the wax would indicate contact of opposing teeth. The thinnest areas of the record should not be appreciably thicker than 1.0 mm. The record should be repeated if either of these criteria is not satisfied.

The record is placed back on the patient's maxillary teeth, and the patient is guided into centric jaw relation (Fig. 6-35). The teeth are lightly tapped into the record to verify its accuracy.

The record is carefully removed from the mouth and placed on the maxillary cast (Fig. 6-36). The record must fit the cast accurately without the evidence of contact with soft tissue areas or rocking on the cast. The mandibular cast is carefully placed into the record.

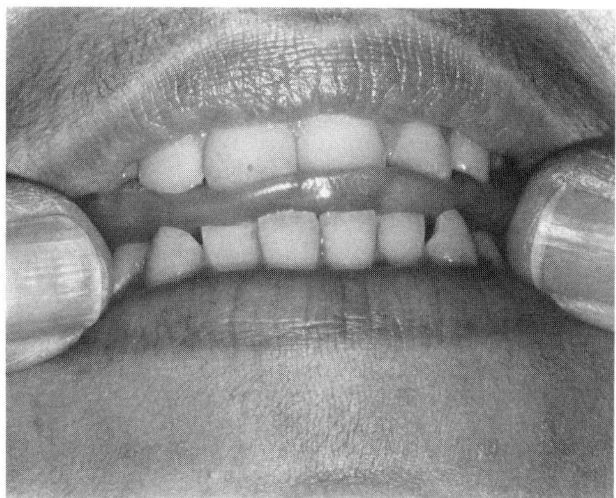

Fig. 6-35. Record is placed back into mouth to verify accuracy of record.

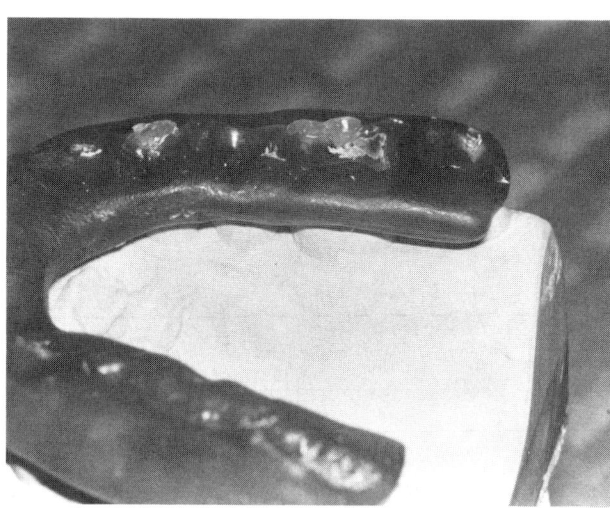

Fig. 6-36. Record is checked on maxillary cast for stability and accuracy of fit.

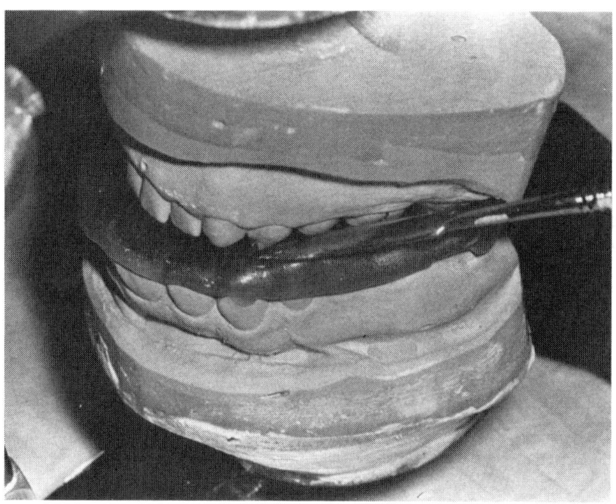

Fig. 6-37. Mandibular cast is placed in record to check for accuracy of fit.

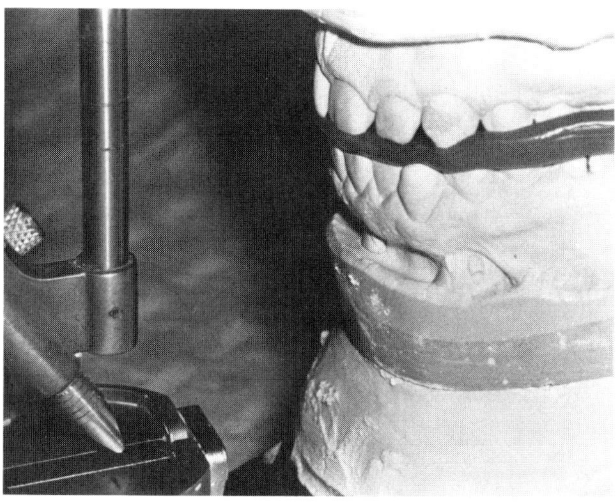

Fig. 6-38. Wax interocclusal record used for mounting mandibular cast.

Again the cusp tips must fit the indentations of the record perfectly (Fig. 6-37). If the record fails to fit either cast, the record may be distorted, or one or both casts may be inaccurate. In this situation the record is placed back in the mouth and its accuracy is again verified. If either cast is found to be inaccurate, a new impression is made and a new cast is poured.

When an acceptable record has been made, a second record is made following the same technique. The mounting record is placed on the casts, and the casts are luted together using wood or metal strips and sticky wax. The casts are then mounted on a semiadjustable articulator (Fig. 6-38).

Procedure for making a centric jaw relation record using baseplates with occlusion rims

This method is used when one or more distal extension areas are present, when a tooth-bounded edentulous space is large, or when opposing teeth do not meet.

A baseplate, or a record base, is a temporary form representing the base of a denture and used for making jaw relation records. It may be constructed of gutta-percha baseplate material or of autopolymerizing acrylic resin. (Refer to Chapter 9 for detail on construction of baseplates.)

The baseplates must fit well and be comfortable,

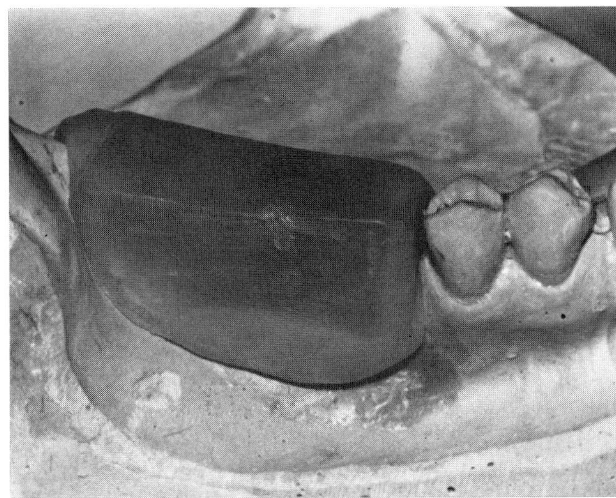

Fig. 6-39. Mandibular baseplate with wax occlusion rim. Borders are underextended to avoid interference with surrounding tissues.

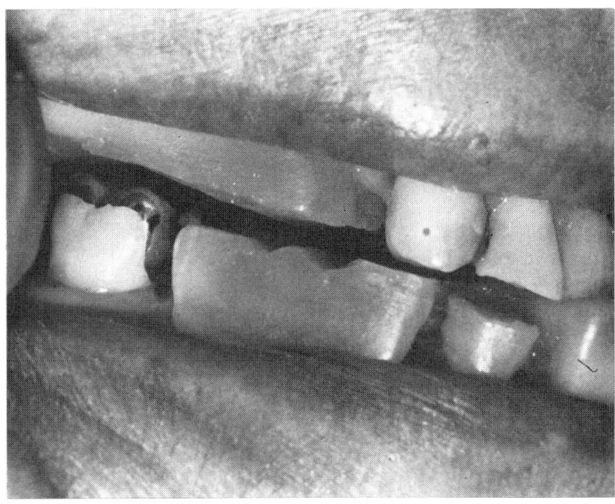

Fig. 6-40. Wax occlusion rim trimmed to avoid contact with opposing teeth.

rigid, and stable in the mouth. The accuracy of the jaw relation records is affected by the adaptation of the bases on the casts.

All surfaces that contact the lips, cheeks, and tongue should be smooth, rounded, and polished. The borders of the baseplates must not interfere with the functional activity of the surrounding tissues. For this reason the borders should always be underextended (Fig. 6-39).

The baseplate with the occlusion rim provides the necessary artificial occluding surfaces to record the position of the jaws in centric relation and a vehicle by which this relationship may be accurately transferred to the articulator. Without the use of an occlusion rim it would be impossible to position the casts on the articulator in the identical horizontal and vertical relationship found on the patient in centric relation.

When interocclusal records are obtained by means of baseplates with occlusion rims, it is important to avoid excessive pressure on the displaceable tissue of the denture-bearing area. If interocclusal records for a distal extension partial denture are recorded under pressure, the soft tissue will be compressed as the baseplate is forcibly depressed toward the tissue. When the pressure type of occlusal record is placed on the stone cast, the baseplate cannot depress the stone cast. This results in an inaccurate relationship of the two stone casts. This problem may be avoided by using a uniformly soft recording medium such as dental stone or zinc oxide–eugenol bite registration paste. The wax occlusion rim must not contact the opposing teeth.

Accurately fitting baseplates are essential to the success of this technique.

The baseplate is tried in the patient's mouth to verify that the patient is comfortable, the borders are not overextended, and the baseplate is stable. If a wax occlusion rim has been added, it should be trimmed to provide 1 to 2 mm clearance between the wax and the opposing teeth (Fig. 6-40).

A free-flowing recording medium such as zinc oxide–eugenol paste or accelerated dental stone is mixed and placed on the occlusion rim. (A complete discussion of recording media is included in Chapter 10.) The baseplate and recording medium are placed in the mouth. Frequently, dental adhesives are necessary to ensure stability and retention of the baseplate. The patient is guided into centric jaw relation until the first occlusal contact is reached. The patient is helped to maintain light contact at this position until the recording material has set. If the patient cannot maintain the position of initial contact at centric jaw relation, an anterior stop of acrylic resin or modeling plastic must be developed. The teeth should contact the stop when the jaw is retruded and the remaining teeth are barely separated.

The record is removed and is trimmed until only the imprints of the tips of the cusps remain. The wax occlusion rim must not show through the recording medium indentations because this would indicate contact of the wax with the opposing occlusion.

The record is placed back in the mouth, and the patient is again guided into the retruded position to verify that the patient is closing into the same position as when the record was made.

The baseplate is placed on the cast, and the opposing cast is placed into the record (Fig. 6-41). The opposing teeth should fit into the indentations, and the opposing teeth of the casts should contact the same as in the mouth.

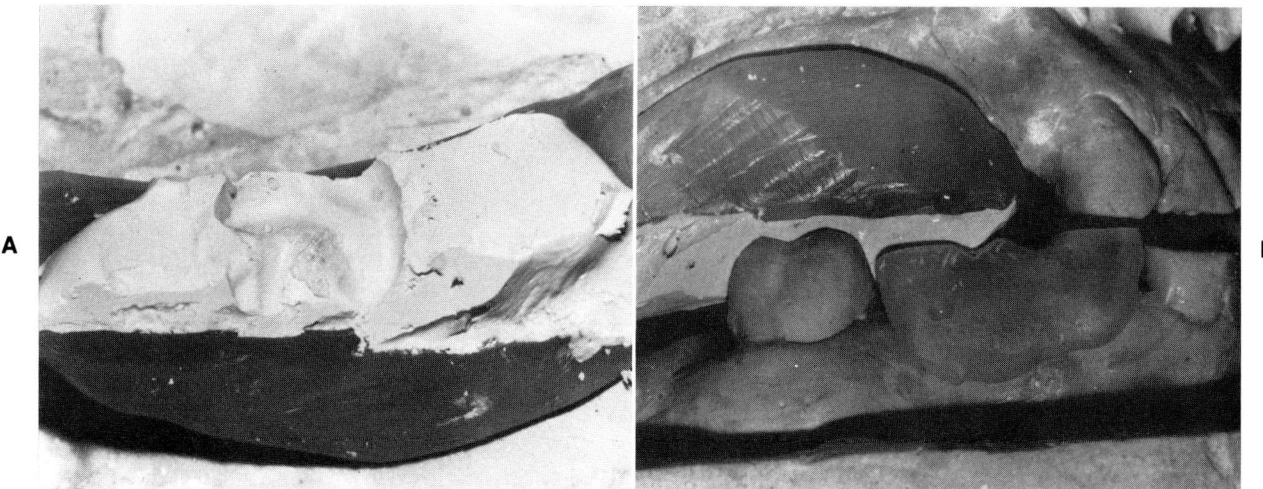

Fig. 6-41. A, Imprints of opposing tooth and wax occlusion rim in zinc oxide–eugenol paste registration. **B,** Cast and occlusion rim seated in record.

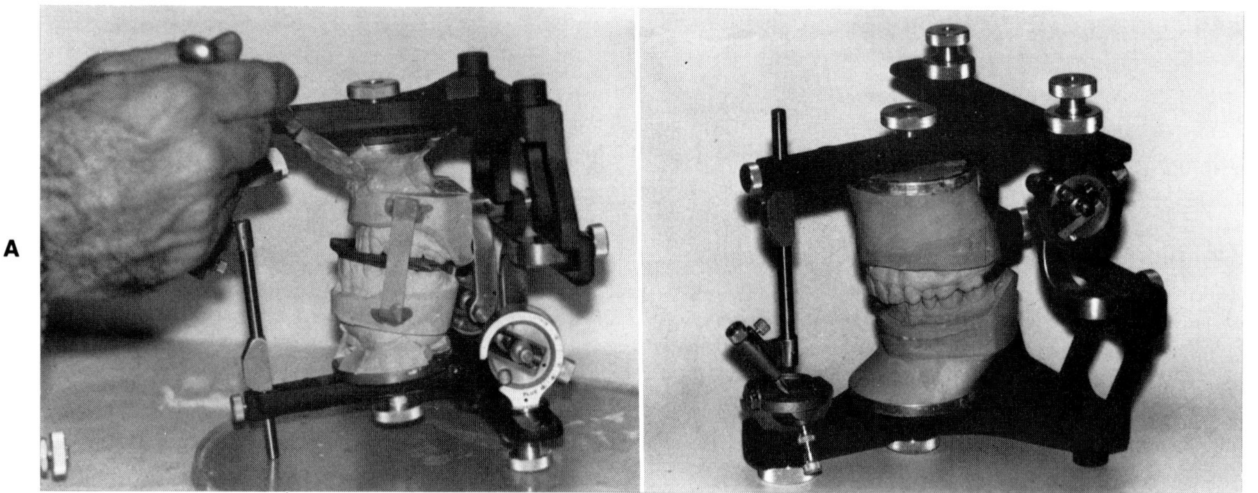

Fig. 6-42. A, Mandibular cast is attached to mounting ring with a mix of dental stone. **B,** Once accuracy of mounting has been verified, additional dental stone is used to smooth the mounting.

If any of the following errors are present, the centric jaw relation record should be reaccomplished:

1. Evidence of contact between the baseplate or occlusion rim with the opposing teeth.
2. Inability to verify fit of record in the mouth or on the cast.

Preparation of articulator and mounting of mandibular cast (maxillary cast has been mounted with face-bow transfer)

1. The face-bow assembly and cast support are removed from the articulator.
2. The L-shaped pin is replaced with the incisal pin. The thumbscrew of the incisal guide control is loosened, and the pin is opened 3 mm from the neutral, or 5, setting. This vertical pin opening will approximately compensate for the thickness of the wax interocclusal record. (The pin is not opened if baseplates were used and record was made at the initial occlusal contact.)
3. The surface of the lower member of the articulator that will be contacted by mounting stone is lubricated. A mounting ring is attached to the lower member of the articulator.
4. The articulator is inverted, and the mandibular cast with its record is placed on the mounted max-

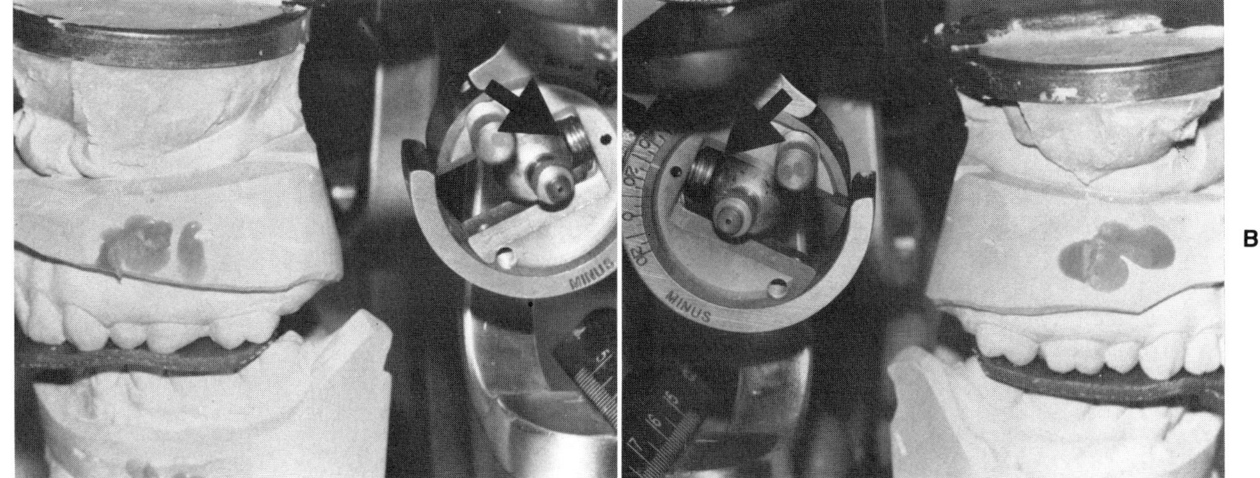

Fig. 6-43. A, Mounting considered correct if teeth of both casts fit indentations of interocclusal record and condylar balls on both sides remain in contact with posterior stops of condylar paths (arrow) when the second record is seated between the casts. **B,** Mounting appears in error because space is present between condylar ball and condylar stop (arrow).

illary cast. The cusp tips must be seated accurately in the record, and the mandibular cast should be completely stable. (If the cusp tips fit the wax record accurately but the mandibular cast is not stable, a tongue blade broken into pieces approximately 75 mm long and sticky wax can be used to lute the casts together. This procedure should be accomplished before the cast is soaked because sticky wax will not adhere to a wet cast.) If wax interocclusal records were used, the casts should have been luted together immediately after the records were completed.

5. The base of the mandibular cast is indexed, the grooves are painted with gypsum-separating medium, and the cast is soaked in clear slurry water for 2 to 3 minutes.
6. A light to medium mix of dental stone and concentrated slurry water is made. (If the mix is too thick, the record may be distorted or displaced when the articulator is closed.) A mound of the mix is placed on the base of the cast, and some is forced into the mounting ring openings. Only enough dental stone to attach the cast to the articulator should be used. After the accuracy of the mounting has been verified, additional stone can be used to fill in voids and to smooth the mounting (Fig. 6-42).

Verification of mounting

No diagnostic mounting is complete until the centric relation registration has been verified. Equilibration or analysis of occlusion should *never* be attempted on an articulator until the mounting has been proved correct.

The additional interocclusal record that was taken is used to verify the accuracy of the mounting. Before the second record is placed in the articulator, the incisal guide pin should be removed and the centric condylar locks released. The record is seated between the casts, and the position of the condyle ball in the condyle slot is observed.

The mounting can be considered correct if (1) the cusp tips of both casts fit the jaw relation record accurately and (2) the condylar ball remains in contact with the posterior stop of the condylar path on both sides.

If, however, the condylar ball moves forward when the record is tried, or if the cusp tips do not fit the record, then either the original mounting or the additional record is incorrect. Additional interocclusal records must be made. Frequently the mandibular cast must be removed and remounted with a new record. This procedure must be repeated until the articulator will accept at least one additional record with the condyle balls remaining in contact with the posterior walls of the condylar paths (Fig. 6-43).

Another method of verification is to compare the initial contact of the mounted casts with the patient's initial occlusal contact at centric jaw relation. They should be identical.

Improving appearance of mountings

If the mounting is shown to be correct in the verification procedure, both mountings should be removed from the articulator by loosening the thumbscrews that secure the mounting rings. The mountings should be soaked in clear slurry water for at least 5 minutes, after which a mix of dental stone and concentrated slurry water is used to fill in the voids and smooth the mounting in general. The mounting stone should not extend onto the lateral surfaces of the cast or onto the outer surface of the mounting rings. Stone must not be added to the surface of the mounting ring that contacts the articulator because this would prevent the mounting rings from going to place.

Setting condylar elements of articulator

Either a protusive record or wear facets on the teeth can be used as a guide for setting the condylar elements of the articulator. Both techniques are briefly described.

Use of protrusive wax record

After the patient has been taught to make a straight protrusive movement of 4 to 5 mm, a wax record of several thicknesses of baseplate wax is softened in a water bath and positioned over the maxillary teeth. The patient is instructed to make the straight protrusive movement. When the mandible has moved forward 4 to 5 mm, the patient is instructed to close into the wax (Fig. 6-44, *A* and *B*). The anterior teeth should be about 1 mm apart. When the wax is hardened, the record is removed and chilled. It is checked for stability in the mouth and on the cast. The record should be repeated if any of the following errors are present:

1. Patient's protrusion less than 3 mm. (This degree of movement is too small to accurately set the instrument.)
2. Patient's protrusion greater than 6 mm. (This degree of movement will carry the condyle too far down on the articular eminence.)
3. Lateral component in the protrusive movement.
4. Incisal contact of the anterior teeth.
5. Instability of record in the mouth or on the cast.

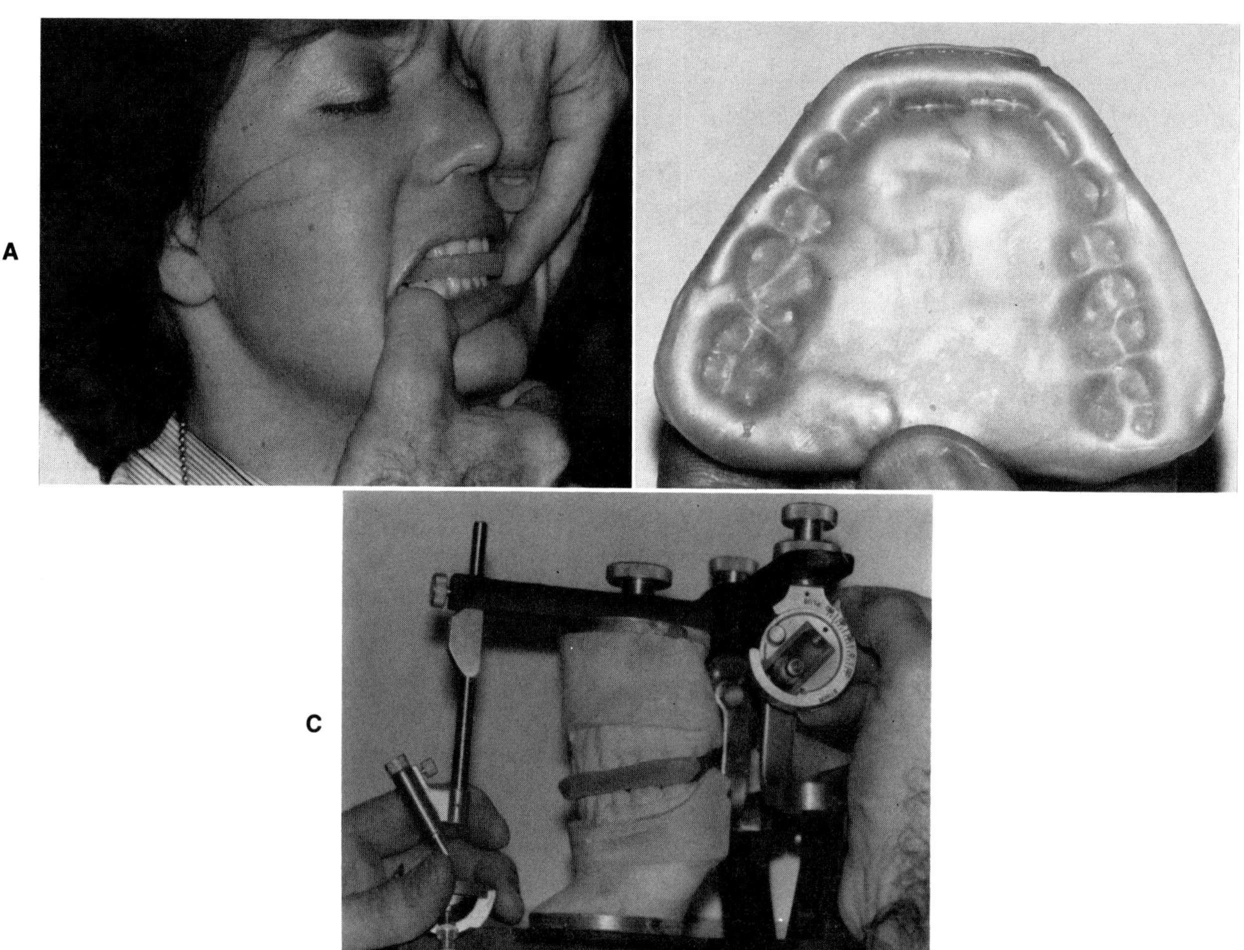

Fig. 6-44. A, Protrusive record made by patient closing into softened wax with the mandible protruded 4 to 5 mm. **B,** Protrusive wax record. **C,** Condylar mechanism rotated until teeth fit indentations of wax record.

6. Difference of more than 10 degrees when condylar elements are set.

When an accurate protrusive wax record has been made and verified, the condylar guidance is set by the following procedure.

The incisal pin is removed, and the centric locks and the condylar inclination locking mechanism are loosened.

The record is placed on the mandibular teeth, and an attempt is made to place the maxillary teeth into the indentations. The condylar inclination mechanism should be rotated until the maxillary teeth fit accurately into the indentations of the record (Fig. 6-44, C). The condylar inclination locking mechanism is then tightened.

This procedure is repeated, and the results of the two settings are compared. They should be within 2 to 3 degrees for each condyle. The condylar inclination reading on one side should be within 10 degrees of the opposite side. Usually the readings will be within 2 to 5 degrees on the opposite side.

Use of wear facets

The incisal pin is removed, and the centric lock and the condylar inclination locking mechanism are loosened.

The opposing teeth are lightly occluded in eccentric positions. The condylar inclinations are adjusted to allow the articulator to follow the wear patterns on the remaining natural teeth (Fig. 6-45).

The casts should now be correctly mounted on the articulator and ready for analysis of the patient's occlusion and other diagnostic procedures.

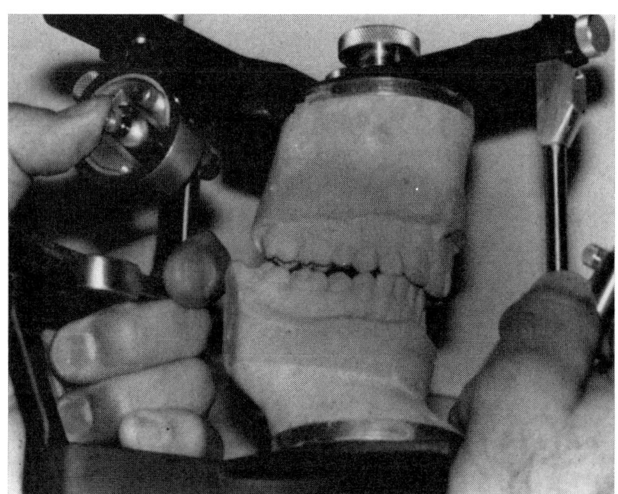

Fig. 6-45. Condylar mechanism adjusted to allow articulator to follow wear facets of remaining teeth.

DEFINITIVE ORAL EXAMINATION

The oral examination must be thorough. It should include the following:

1. A thorough explorer examination is made of a dry field in good light. Carious lesions and defective restorations are correlated with radiographic and other diagnostic findings.
2. All teeth that appear questionable clinically or radiographically are tested for pulp vitality. An electric pulp tester is used in conjunction with thermal tests.
3. The teeth are tested for sensitivity to percussion.
4. The teeth are tested for mobility.
5. A periodontal examination that includes determination of pocket depth, examination for evidence of infection or inflammation, and determination of the amount of attached gingiva of the prospective abutment teeth is made.
6. The oral mucosa is examined visually and with palpation for evidence of pathologic change.
7. The oral cavity is examined for the presence of tori, exostoses, sharp or prominent bony areas, soft or hard tissue undercuts, and enlarged tuberosities.

Other diagnostic steps that must be completed follow:

1. An examination is made of the radiographic survey with special attention focused on the abutment teeth and the residual ridge areas.
2. The mounted casts are examined for the presence of extruded teeth, malposed teeth, reduced interarch space, unfavorable occlusal plane, and any other potential problems.
3. The occlusion is examined and evaluated.
4. A suitable measuring device such as a periodontal probe is used to determine the distance from the active floor of the mouth to the gingival margins of the mandibular teeth.
5. The diagnostic casts are analyzed on a dental surveyor, and the design of the removable partial denture is drawn on the cast.

EVALUATION OF DIAGNOSTIC DATA

All the diagnostic data must be collected before an effective evaluation can be made. Frequently it is necessary to correlate the intraoral findings with those of the radiographic survey, the mounted casts, the survey and analysis of the diagnostic casts, and other phases of the diagnostic procedure. Collection of data is meaningless unless a thorough evaluation of the data is made and used in the development of the treatment plan.

Evaluation of caries and existing restorations

The selection of a suitable restoration for the partially edentulous patient encompasses more factors than the size of the carious lesion and the extent of a defective restoration. The relationship of the tooth to the occlusal plane and the overall contours of the tooth must also be considered. A simple two-surface intracoronal restoration may be adequate for restoring a carious tooth. However, if the tooth has extruded above the occlusal plane because of the lack of an antagonist, the choice may be an extracoronal restoration to improve the occlusal plane (Fig. 6-46). Or if a tooth that does not possess adequate contours for clasping is to serve as an abutment, a full coverage restoration may be necessary. Therefore it would be imprudent to initiate restorative treatment for the patient before the diagnostic mounting and the design of the diagnostic cast have been completed. Inadequate contours for clasping may dictate the placement of restorations on teeth that are noncarious or that have satisfactory restorations (Fig. 6-47). In addition, the selection of teeth to receive rest seats must be made before restorative procedures are begun. If the tooth requires a restoration because of caries or a defect in the existing restoration, the choice of restorative material is a metallic casting. Amalgam and tooth-colored restorative materials other than porcelain are more likely to fail under the forces of occlusion than is a cast metallic restoration. If an otherwise satisfactory amalgam restoration is present in the area of a tooth that is to receive the rest seat, it must be evaluated to determine whether it is strong enough to withstand the forces it will receive. The occlusion should be examined to help determine how deep the rest seat will have to be. The radiograph is examined to determine the thickness of the restoration in the area to be prepared. The outline of the restoration is examined to determine whether the entire rest seat will be in amalgam or whether part of the rest will contact soundly supported tooth structure. Another factor to be considered is whether the rest seat is on a tooth next to an edentulous space or whether the rest will serve as an indirect retainer, which would apply less force to the restoration. After all these factors have been considered, the most conservative decision may be to replace the amalgam with a metallic casting.

Satisfactory amalgam or tooth-colored restorations on the buccal or labial surfaces of prospective abutment teeth must be carefully evaluated. Excessive wear of the restoration may occur if the retentive area of the clasp arm will contact the restoration or cross its margin while moving in and out of the undercut. This wear can result in loss of retention of the prosthesis or failure of the restoration. Care must be taken in the placement of margins of cast metallic restorations as well. The frequent movement of the retentive area of a clasp arm across the margins of a restoration will contribute to early failure of the restoration.

Not every tooth that can be saved through restorative procedures should be retained. The more prudent treatment may be removal of the tooth (for example, if its retention would complicate the design of the prosthesis because of its position or if it would have limited value to the overall prognosis and greatly increase the cost for the patient). Preventive dentistry for the partially edentulous patient does not mean the retention of every retainable tooth.

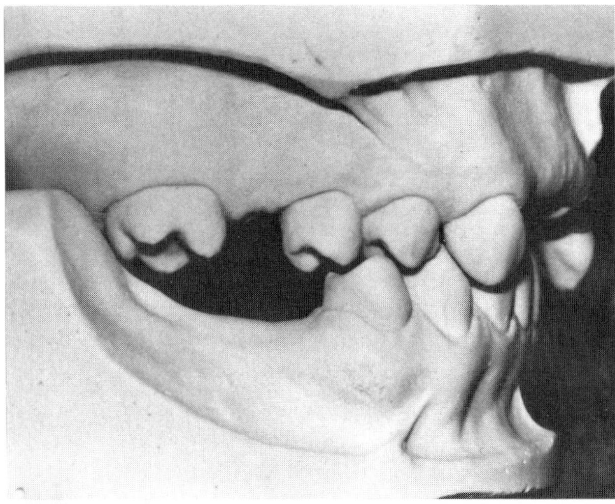

Fig. 6-46. Cast restoration necessary to improve occlusal plane and create interarch space.

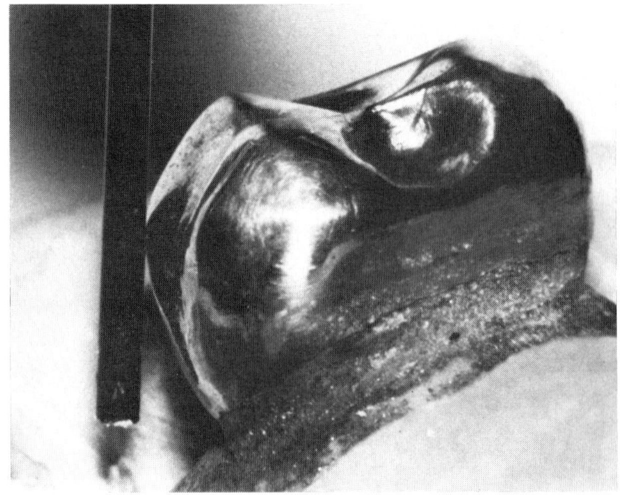

Fig. 6-47. Crown placed to create contours for clasping.

Evaluation of pulp

An electric pulp tester in conjunction with thermal tests, if needed, should be used to detect pulpal necrosis or pulpitis. The success of endodontic treatment must be assured before an affected tooth is selected as an abutment. It can be inconvenient and expensive for the patient as well as embarrassing for the dentist if a pulpal problem is overlooked and at a later date it is discovered that an abutment tooth has to be treated endodontically or removed.

Endodontically treated teeth tend to become more brittle with time; and an abutment tooth for a removable partial denture is subjected to considerable stress. However, the selection of an endodontically treated tooth as an abutment is not contraindicated. If the tooth has a relatively large access opening or an extensive intracoronal restoration, it is vulnerable to fracture and an onlay or full crown is indicated to protect the tooth. A prospective abutment tooth with a large intracoronal restoration or a large restoration at the cervical area of the tooth may require a post and core type restoration to ensure a successful prognosis.

Evaluation of sensitivity to percussion

All remaining teeth are tested for sensitivity to percussion. Special attention is focused on the prospective abutment teeth. The following conditions can contribute to the irritation of the periodontal ligament fibers, making the tooth sensitive to percussion testing:

1. Tooth movement caused by a prosthesis or the occlusion
2. A tooth or restoration in traumatic occlusion
3. Periapical or pulpal abscess
4. Acute pulpitis
5. Gingivitis or periodontitis
6. Cracked tooth syndrome

The exact cause must be determined through the evaluation of other diagnostic data. A removable partial denture should not be constructed until the cause is discovered and the sensitivity is eliminated. The use of a percussion-sensitive tooth as an abutment would result in early failure of the treatment.

Evaluation of mobile teeth

Teeth with detectable mobility are evaluated to determine the cause. A mobile tooth used as an abutment tooth will have a poor prognosis unless the cause of the mobility is eliminated and the mobility is markedly decreased. The cause of mobility may be one of the following:

1. Trauma from occlusion
2. Inflammatory changes in the periodontal ligament
3. Loss of alveolar bone support

Tooth mobility that is the result of traumatic occlusion is usually reversible provided the cause of the occlusal trauma is eliminated. The mounted diagnostic casts are evaluated to help determine the cause of trauma. A judgment should be made as to whether the occlusal discrepancy causing the trauma can be corrected by occlusal equilibration or whether a restoration will be necessary.

Tooth mobility caused by inflammatory changes in the periodontal ligament may be reversed if the inflammation is eliminated.

Tooth mobility caused by a loss of alveolar bone support is not reversible. A tooth with less than a 1:1 crown/root ratio is not suitable as an abutment tooth for a removable partial denture (Fig. 6-48). In this case the tooth adjacent to the mobile tooth should be evaluated as an abutment. The radiographic findings are correlated with the clinical findings. If the adjacent tooth is capable of serving as a strong abutment tooth, the best choice of treatment may be removal of the weak tooth. Splinting of a weak tooth to a strong tooth must be approached cautiously because such splinting frequently weakens the strong tooth rather than strengthening the weak one. Buccal or lingual forces applied to the weaker tooth by the prosthesis may cause rotational forces to be applied to the stronger tooth through the lever arm effect (Fig. 6-49).

An alternative to removal of the weak tooth is its use as an overdenture abutment. Overdenture abutments in the design of removable partial dentures can significantly help to support the vertical load applied to a prosthesis and contribute to the denture's stability. The tooth is treated endodontically, and the clinical crown

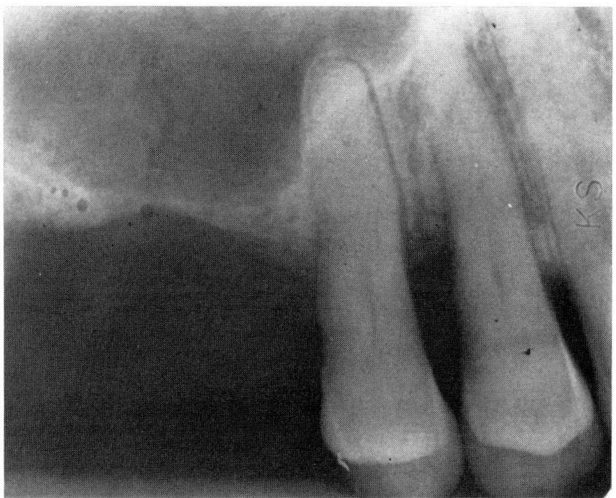

Fig. 6-48. Tooth adjacent to edentulous space has less than a 1:1 crown/root ration; it is unfavorable as an abutment tooth.

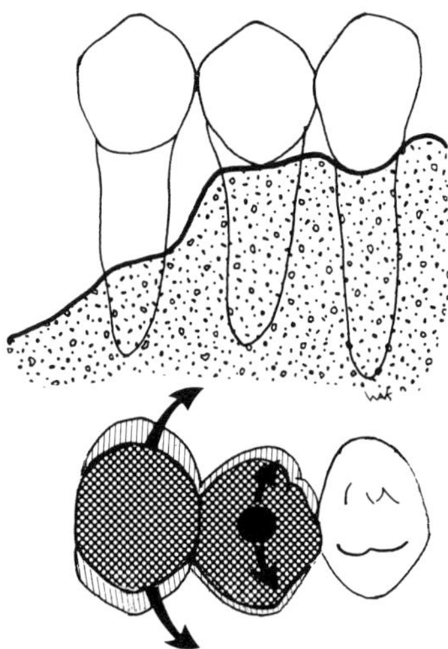

Fig. 6-49. Splinting of a weak to a strong tooth is likely to weaken the strong tooth rather than strengthen the weak tooth because of rotational movement allowed by weaker tooth.

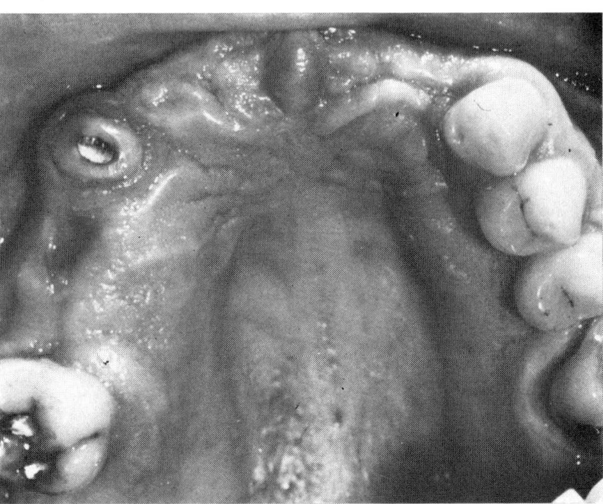

Fig. 6-50. Tooth with a poor crown/root ratio used as overdenture abutment to provide support for a removable partial denture.

reduced to approximately 2 to 3 mm above the gingival margin. This procedure greatly improves the crown/root ratio of a mobile tooth and usually eliminates the mobility (Fig. 6-50). This concept of treatment should always be considered when the removal of several teeth will result in a large edentulous area. A single overdenture abutment is extremely valuable in providing support, particularly in large anterior edentulous areas and distal extension situations.

Indications for splinting of abutment teeth

Splinting of two or more teeth is necessary when all the remaining teeth have reduced support. Teeth that have lost support through periodontal disease and teeth with short, tapered roots have a poor prognosis as abutment teeth. Splinting of two or more teeth with crowns will provide an abutment with greater total periodontal support than that provided by one of the teeth serving alone (Fig. 6-51). It is imperative that the crowns used to splint the teeth be constructed in harmony with the occlusion of the remaining teeth, the temporomandibular joint, and the musculature. The removable partial denture must be designed and constructed to place minimum stress on the splinted teeth.

Another indication for splinting is the presence of only two or three widely spaced retainable teeth. An example is the splinting of two strong mandibular canines pictured in Fig. 6-52.

Splinting with a fixed partial denture is indicated when the first premolar and the molars have been lost and the second premolar is to serve as the abutment tooth. The premolar standing alone is likely to succumb quickly to the forces applied by a distal extension removable partial denture. The placement of a fixed partial denture will restore the continuity of the arch and will create a more favorable prognosis for the abutment tooth and the removable prosthesis (Fig. 6-53).

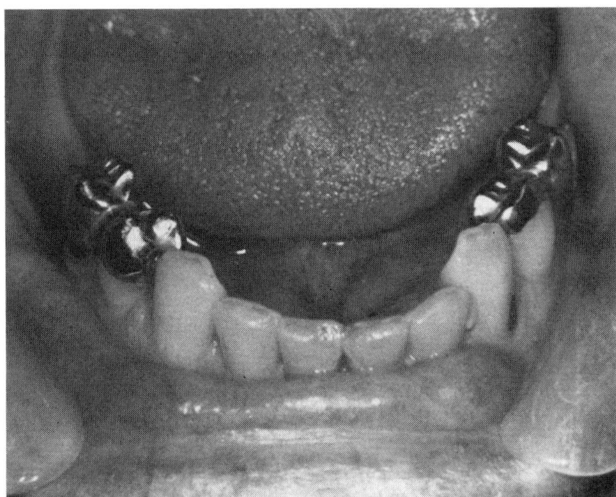

Fig. 6-51. Splinted premolars provide greater total periodontal support than would be supplied by a single abutment tooth.

Evaluation of periodontium

Periodontal disease is one of the main etiologic factors in the loss of teeth. It follows that a large percentage of partially edentulous patients seeking treatment will have evidence of gingivitis and periodontal disease. A removable partial denture placed in the presence of active periodontal disease will contribute significantly to the rapid progression of the disease and the loss of

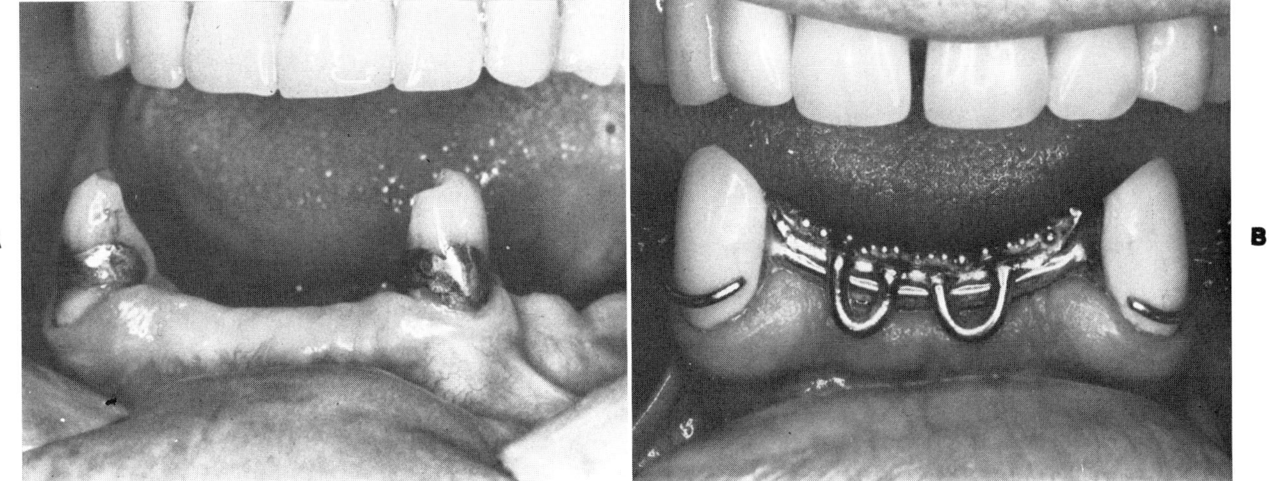

Fig. 6-52. A, Only canine teeth remain in mandibular arch. **B,** Rotational movements of prosthesis and subsequent stress on abutment teeth have been reduced by splinting the two teeth with a cast bar. Framework of prosthesis rests on bar, which prevents partial denture from moving toward tissue and distributes force applied to one abutment tooth between periodontal ligament support of both canines.

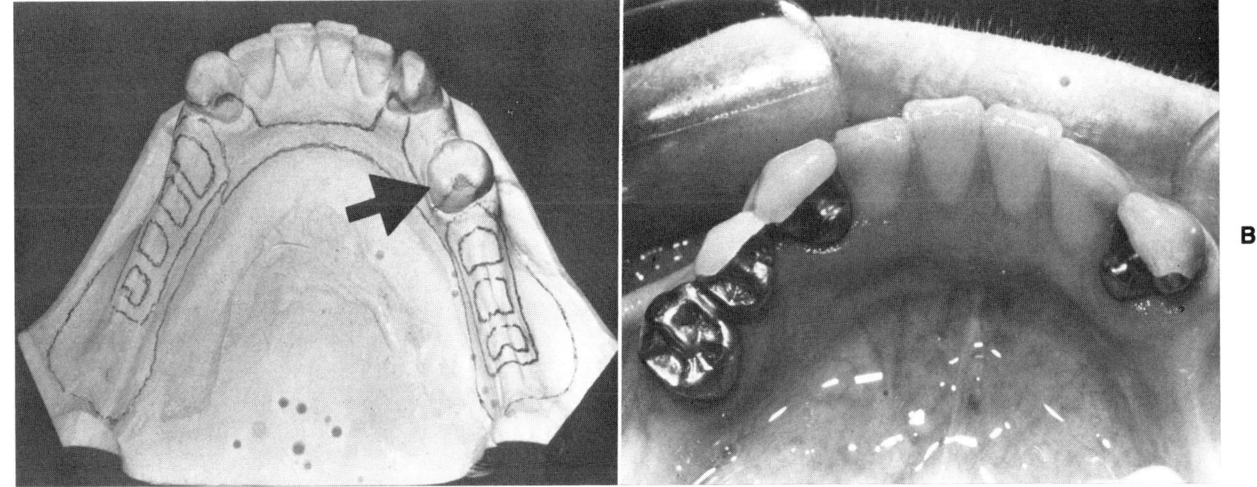

Fig. 6-53. A, Premolar standing alone (arrow) is vulnerable to stress created by a removable partial denture. **B,** Fixed partial denture splints second premolar to canine and restores continuity of arch. Lingual rest seats have been created on canine crowns.

the remaining teeth. The causative factors must be eliminated, the disease processes must be controlled or reversed, and the effects of the disease must be corrected if treatment with a removable partial denture is to achieve any success.

The periodontium of partially edentulous patients must be evaluated if any type of prosthodontic treatment is contemplated. The evaluation of the periodontium must be based on a systematic, thorough examination to disclose any significant pocket depth, infection, inflammation, furcation involvement, and absence of sufficient attached gingiva (Fig. 6-54).

The health of the periodontium is determined by careful, systematic probing with a calibrated periodontal probe; by observation of the color, texture, and architecture of the gingiva; by observation of any crevicular exudate revealed through digital pressure or probing; by determination of the width of the attached gingiva; and by observation of any tension placed on the attached gingiva by muscle or frena attachments.

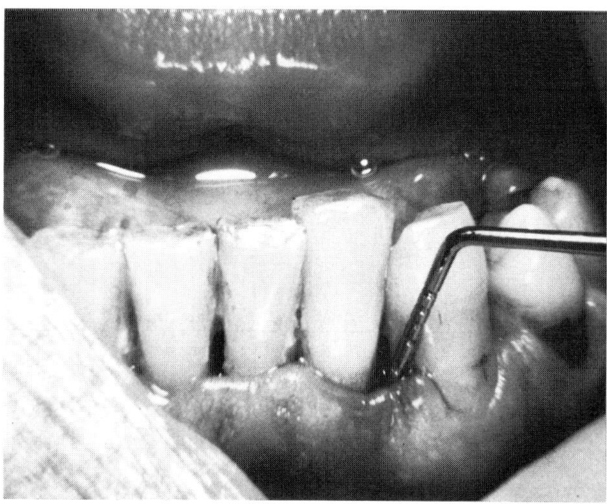

Fig. 6-54. Definitive examination must include periodontal probing of pocket depth.

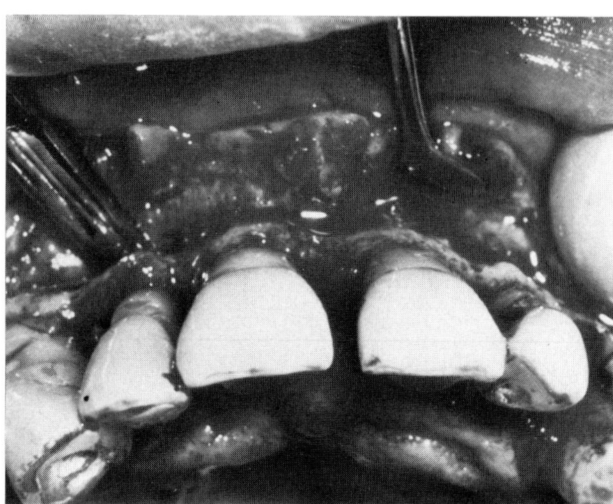

Fig. 6-55. Periodontal flap procedures have a wide range of indications.

The complete radiographic survey supplements the clinical findings but cannot be substituted for a thorough clinical evaluation.

Examination findings that indicate possible need for periodontal treatment include the following:

1. Pocket depth in excess of 3 mm
2. Furcation involvement
3. Deviations from normal color and contour in gingiva, indicating gingivitis
4. Marginal exudate
5. Potential abutment teeth with less than 2 mm of attached gingiva
6. Pulling of muscle or frena on attached gingiva

The selection of abutment teeth in the presence of periodontal disease can be a real diagnostic challenge. Many times clear-cut choices are not available. The decisions to be made in evaluating the periodontal condition go beyond simply determining whether the etiologic factors can be eliminated and the progression of the disease reversed. Pocket elimination and osseous recontouring will not make a tooth a good abutment if the tooth is left with an inadequate crown/root ratio. Root size, root form, the amount of root in alveolar bone, the number and distribution of remaining teeth, the patient's age, the type of opposing occlusion, the nature of the residual ridge, and the patient's interest and desire are as important as the pocket depth in the selection of a suitable abutment tooth. Frequently it is advantageous to sacrifice an involved tooth if the tooth adjacent to it would serve as a better abutment. A tooth with furcation involvement is not a good candidate for service as an abutment. A better prognosis may result from the use of one of the roots for vertical support through endodontic treatment, hemisection, and placement of a crown.

From the prosthodontic standpoint, the objective of periodontal treatment of abutment teeth is restoration of the periodontium to optimum health and creation of contours that will allow the patient through appropriate oral hygiene measures to preserve this state of health. Periodontal therapy that falls short of this objective will severely compromise the prognosis of overall treatment.

Several types of periodontal treatment are effective in restoring the abutment teeth, as well as the other remaining teeth, to optimum health.

Root scaling and planing in conjunction with good home oral hygiene procedures can dramatically improve the health of the periodontium.

Gingivectomy has limited use, although it can increase clinical crown length in selected situations. The treatment may allow the use of a tooth undercut that was hidden by the gingival tissue. It can also create a longer clinical crown when retention becomes a problem in crown preparation (a frequent problem with teeth that have extruded above the occlusal plane). Gingivectomy is ineffective treatment if the pocket extends to the mucogingival junction or if the osseous contours are unacceptable.

Periodontal flap procedures have the widest range of indications in the surgical treatment of periodontal disease (Fig. 6-55). By allowing access to the underlying osseous structures, these procedures provide good visibility of the defect and allow corrective osseous procedures to be accomplished. Flap procedures may also be used to correct pocket depth that extends to or beyond

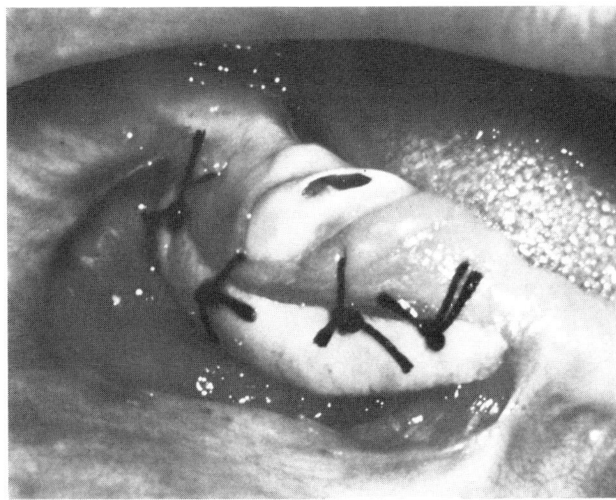

Fig. 6-56. Free gingival graft used to provide adequate zone of attached gingiva.

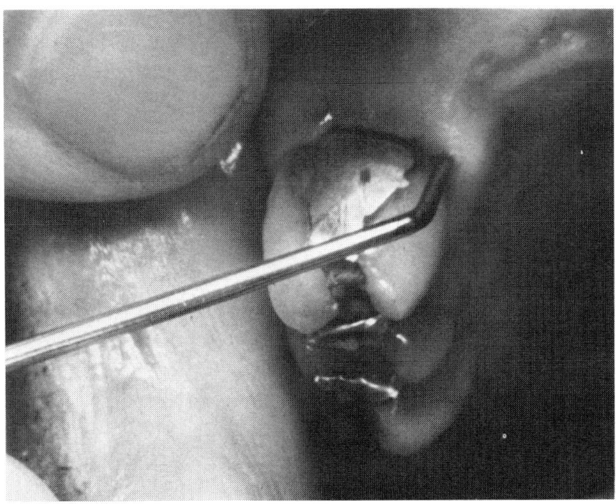

Fig. 6-57. Poorly fitting prosthesis and inadequate oral hygiene are likely cause of buildup of redundant tissue on proximal surface of abutment tooth.

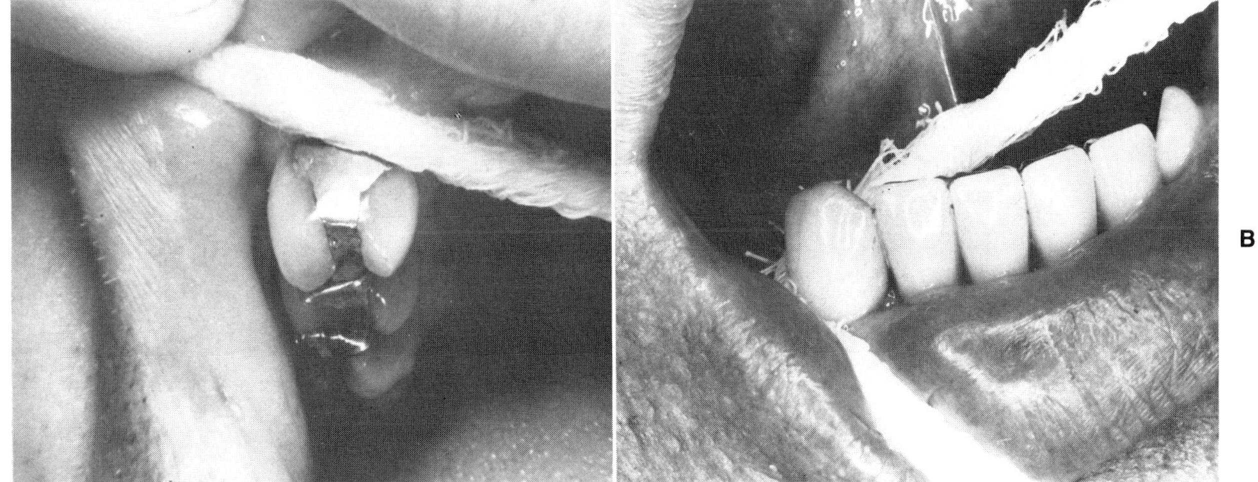

Fig. 6-58. A, Rolled and dampened 1-inch gauze used with a shoeshine motion will contribute toward resolution of redundant tissue. **B,** This gauze is an excellent adjunct to oral hygiene procedures for maintenance of abutment teeth supporting a removable prosthesis.

the mucogingival junction and to correct muscle or frena pull on the attached gingiva.

Free gingival grafts can provide adequate attached gingiva when an abutment tooth has an insufficient zone of gingival attachment (Fig. 6-56). The use of a graft extending beyond the involved tooth is effective for increasing the vestibular depth.

The wear of an ill-fitting prosthesis or continuous wear of a removable partial denture coupled with inadequate oral hygiene frequently contributes to accumulation of redundant tissue on the proximal surfaces of the abutment teeth (Fig. 6-57). The initiation of good oral hygiene measures and tissue rest 6 to 8 hours per day (preferably at night) will usually allow some resolution of the redundant tissue. Rolled and dampened 1-inch gauze used with a shoeshine motion against the proximal surfaces and gingival margin areas of the abutment teeth can be a good adjunct to other oral hygiene procedures (Fig. 6-58). If there is not sufficient resolution of the redundant tissue in 2 to 3 weeks, surgical intevention may be required.

Patients who have been the victims of the ravages of

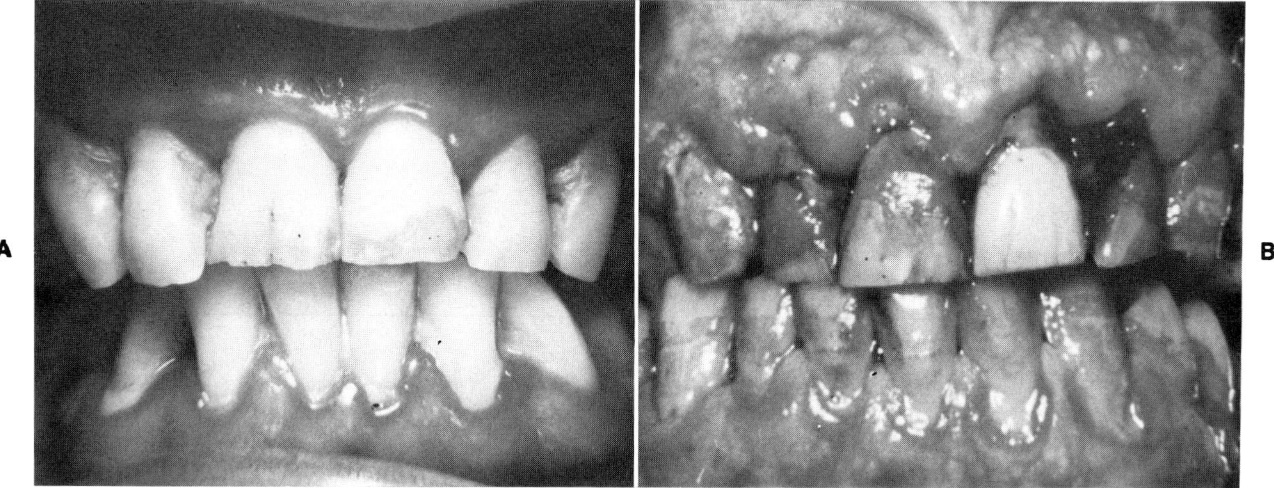

Fig. 6-59. Patients with long-standing periodontal disease, **A,** and neglect, **B,** present difficult diagnostic challenges.

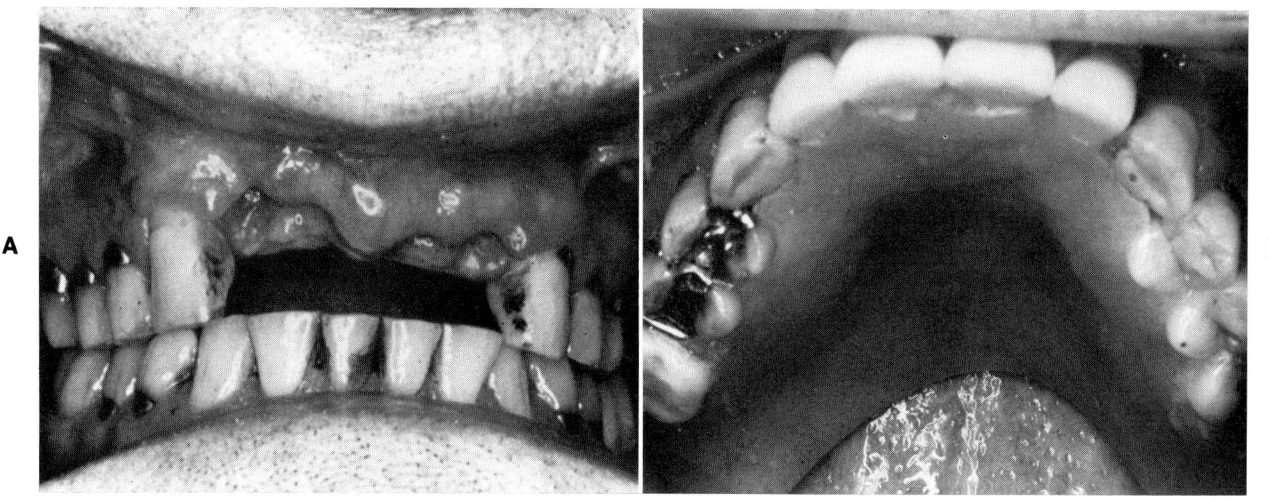

Fig. 6-60. A, Unsalvageable anterior teeth have been removed. **B,** Immediate interim prosthesis satisfies patient's esthetic requirements and serves as a diagnostic prosthesis.

long-term periodontal disease can present an extremely difficult diagnostic challenge (Fig. 6-59). Examination findings often include extremely long clinical crowns, root caries, complaints of pain, discomfort or an inability to chew, and inadequate oral hygiene. Most patients have given up trying to maintain a satisfactory level of oral hygiene and ask for complete dentures. The dentist must not be too hasty in consenting to the patient's request. The physiologic and psychologic trauma of becoming completely edentulous can be devastating to some patients. The dentist must evaluate all factors that contribute to the patient's ability to wear complete dentures successfully, including the patient's age, psychologic makeup, neuromuscular capability, the presence of a retracted tongue, the anticipated size of the residual ridge, and habits. The removal of the unsalvageable teeth and the construction of an interim or transitional removable partial denture can be a useful diagnostic tool (Fig. 6-60). Once their discomfort has been relieved, many patients change their attitude toward becoming completely edentulous and show a great improvement in their motivation and performance in oral hygiene. Frequently, sufficient teeth can be retained to support a conventional removable partial denture, or at least two or three suitable teeth can be selected to support an overdenture. Even when this is impossible, the patient usually benefits because the transitional period between the dentulous and the edentulous state usually enhances the patient's ability to adapt to complete dentures.

Evaluation of oral mucosa

Pathologic changes

Any ulceration, swelling, or color change that might indicate malignant or premalignant changes should be recognized and properly evaluated through biopsy or referral. In spite of the frequency with which the oral cavity is examined by dentists and physicians, 60% of intraoral carcinomas are well advanced at the time of discovery. The surgical morbidity of oral cancers is high, and the 5-year survival rate is low, only about 30%.

Erythematous (red) lesions seem to be much more indicative of oral cancer than white lesions, as was formerly believed. Any persistent (14 days or more) red velvety lesion of the floor of the mouth, ventrolateral tongue, and soft palate complex should be considered carcinoma in situ or invasive carcinoma unless these entities are ruled out by biopsy. Heavy smokers and drinkers (the oral cancer high-risk group) are particularly vulnerable to these tissue changes. Red lesions may be speckled with white or may be present in conjunction with white patches. If the reddened tissue is dried gently with gauze, it will often have a granular appearance.

Partially edentulous patients usually fall within the cancer-prone age group (40 to 60). Diligent examination and evaluation of the oral mucosa are absolute requirements in the diagnostic procedure for these patients.

Tissue reactions to the wearing of a prosthesis

Tissue reactions to the wearing of a prosthesis should be recognized, evaluated, and treated if necessary. Four types of tissue reaction are discussed.

Palatal papillary hyperplasia. Palatal papillary hyperplasia is a lesion of the mucosa that occurs most often on the hard palate but may extend onto the residual ridges. The lesion, which is caused by an inflammatory response in the submucosa, consists of numerous small wartlike or papillary growths (Fig. 6-61). Food debris, fungi, and bacteria collect in the crevices and may give rise to secondary infection.

The hyperplasia is associated most often with a poorly fitting prosthesis that has been worn for prolonged periods, generally 24 hours per day. Inadequate oral and prosthesis hygiene are likely contributors to this condition.

Although at one time the lesion was considered a possible premalignant state, recent studies have failed to find evidence of premalignancy. However, a premalignant or malignant lesion may occupy the same area of the palate.

Inflammatory papillary hyperplasia can occur under removable partial dentures as well as complete dentures. It is best visualized by directing a soft stream of air on the affected area to remove the saliva and separate the papillae (Fig. 6-62). Tissue conditioning and tissue rest may help resolve some of the edema and inflammation, but only surgical, abrasive, or cryogenic removal will eliminate the papillae. The hyperplasia must be evaluated to determine whether it presents an oral hygiene problem for the patient. If the patient will not be able to keep the papillary hyperplasia adequately clean, it should be removed.

Epulis fissuratum. Epulis fissuratum is a tumorlike hyperplastic growth caused by an ill-fitting or overextended border of a removable prosthesis. It may occur as a double fold of tissue with one fold on the tissue side and one fold on the polished side of the denture border (Fig. 6-63). The sulcus between the folds may

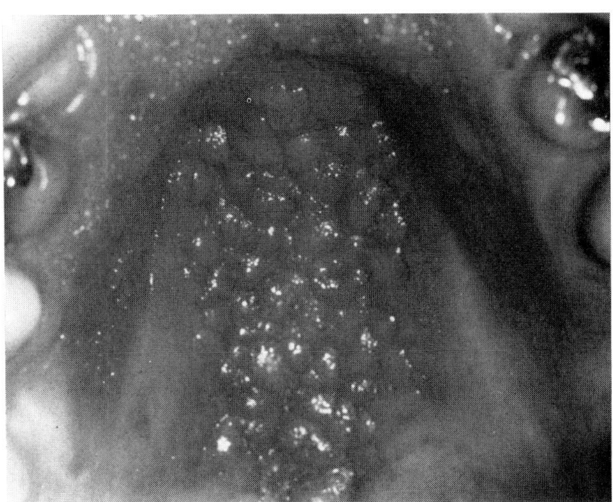

Fig. 6-61. Palatal papillary hyperplasia. Prosthesis worn for 24 hours per day with infrequent removal for cleaning.

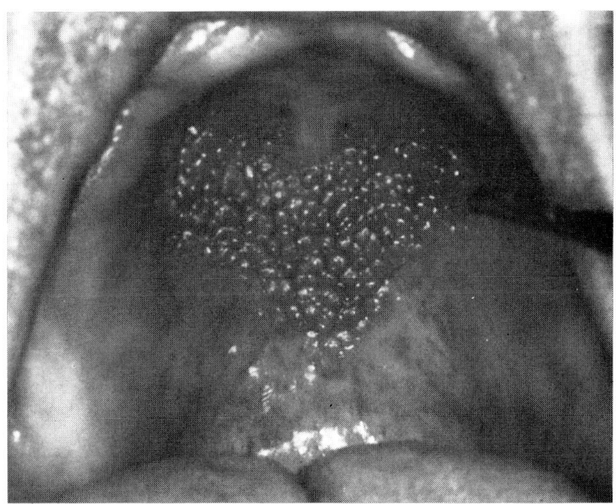

Fig. 6-62. Papillary hyperplasia is best examined by blowing soft stream of compressed air on lesion. Depth of crevices between papillae is easily visualized when saliva and debris are removed by the stream of air.

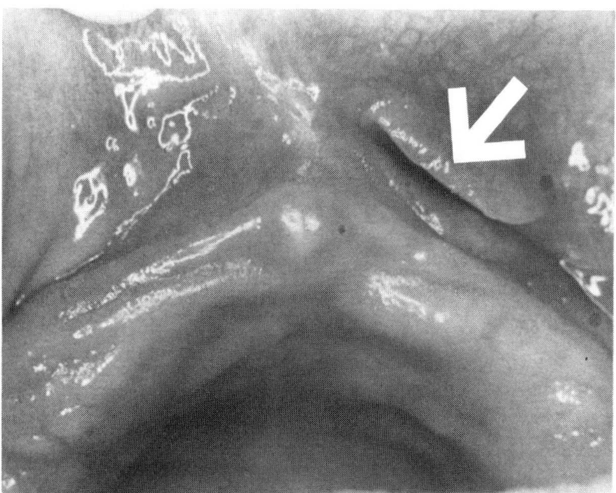

Fig. 6-63. Epulis fissuratum (arrow) caused by ill-fitting border of denture.

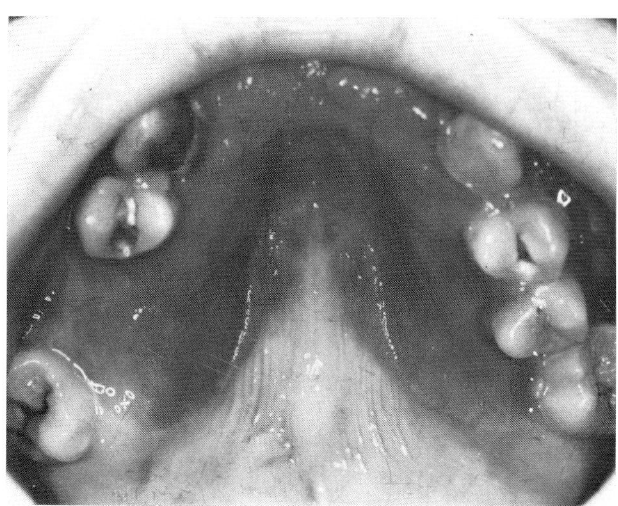

Fig. 6-64. Denture stomatitis under a maxillary removable partial denture.

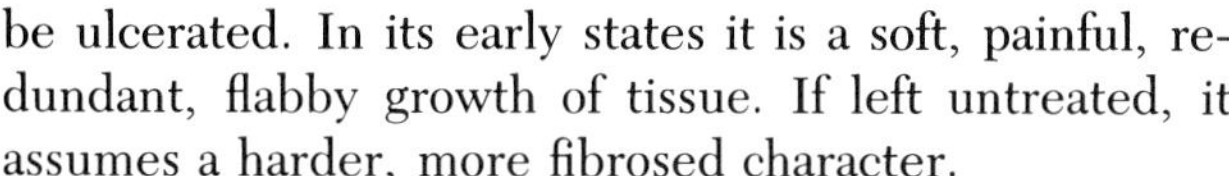

be ulcerated. In its early states it is a soft, painful, redundant, flabby growth of tissue. If left untreated, it assumes a harder, more fibrosed character.

In the past the lesion has generally been surgically excised. Surgical removal results in the formation of scar tissue in the depth of the vestibule, which is not conducive to the development of a good border seal. If the epulis is large, primary closure may decrease the depth of the vestibule.

If an epulis has developed at a denture border, its consistency should be evaluated. A relatively soft epulis may resolve if the irritation is removed. The offending border should be adjusted until it is completely out of contact with the lesion. The more fibrosed the epulis, the longer the resolving period. Even badly fibrosed epuli will decrease in size, thereby decreasing the size of the surgical area if excision becomes necessary.

Denture stomatitis. Denture stomatitis is characterized by generalized erythema, usually including all the tissues covered by the prosthesis (Fig. 6-64). It occurs under metal as well as acrylic resin denture bases, usually under maxillary prostheses. Frequently the oral mucosa is swollen and smooth. At times the patient complains of burning or itching. Although the tissues appear raw and inflamed, the patient rarely complains of pain.

Research indicates denture stomatitis to be an endogenous infectious disease that invades the tissues and causes the lesion. *Candida albicans* has been shown to be present in much higher percentages of denture stomatitis patients than normal patients. However, treatment with nystatin alone will not cause resolution of the stomatitis.

Trauma from occlusion, poor fit of the prosthesis, poor oral hygiene, and continuous wearing of the prosthesis have all been suggested as contributing to this condition.

Complete tissue rest and tissue conditioning procedures have been effective in treating denture stomatitis. A treatment prosthesis is usually necessary if tissue conditioning procedures are to be used. Generally the existing prosthesis will not allow adequate room for the tissue conditioning material. (Refer to Chapter 18 for discussion of treatment dentures and tissue-conditioning material.)

Soft tissue displacement. Displacement of the soft tissues underlying ill-fitting or poorly designed removable partial dentures occurs frequently. Some tissue displacement is usually present in the beaded areas of even a well-fitting prosthesis (Fig. 6-65). The soft tissues must be allowed to return to normal contours through tissue rest before impressions for master casts are made.

Evaluation of hard tissue abnormalities

The presence of a torus, exostosis, or bony undercut can severely compromise the prognosis of treatment of the partially edentulous patient. All areas to be covered by the prosthesis should be palpated to reveal sharp bony protuberances that could interfere with the placement and removal of the prosthesis as well as the comfort of the patient. The diagnostic cast should be examined at the selected path of insertion to reveal potential hard tissue problems.

Torus palatinus

Torus palatinus is a benign, slowly growing protuberance of the palatine processes of the maxilla (Fig. 6-66). It occasionally involves the horizontal plates of the palatine bones. Palatal tori occur twice as often in women

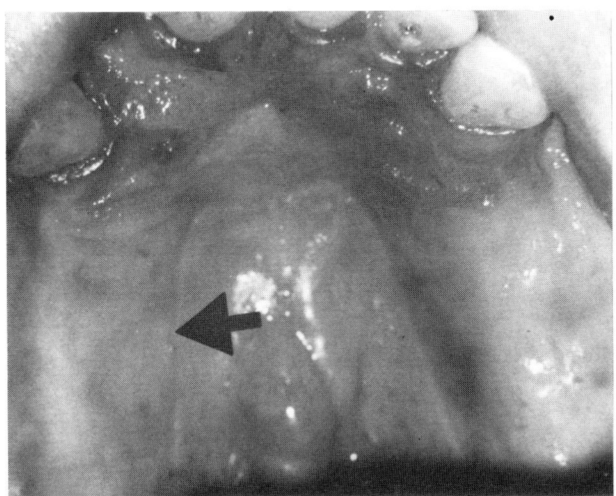

Fig. 6-65. Tissue displacement caused by bead on borders of framework (arrow). Severe gingival inflammation is also apparent.

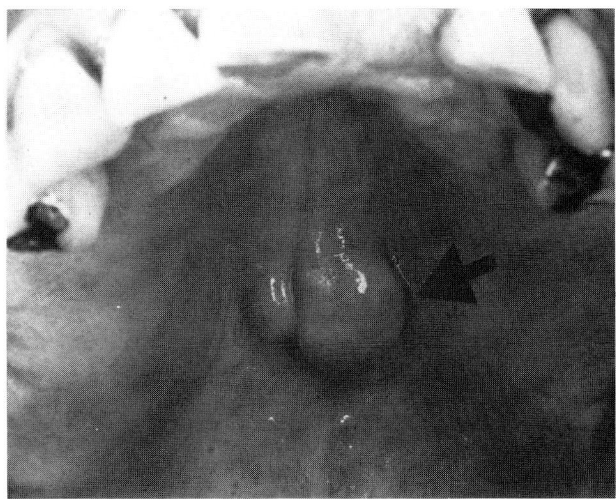

Fig. 6-66. Torus palatinus (arrow).

as in men and can be observed in approximately 20% to 25% of the adult population. They serve no useful purpose. Removal of a torus palatinus is not necessary unless it is so large that it interferes with the design and construction of the prosthesis. Usually a major connector can be selected and designed to circumvent the torus.

If removal of the torus is deemed necessary, an acrylic resin surgical splint should be constructed preoperatively (Fig. 6-67). The splint is used to adapt and support the mucosal flaps in contact with the bone. Hematoma and displacement of the flaps can occur if the flaps are not supported. (Construction of the surgical splint is discussed in Chapter 18.)

Torus mandibularis

The torus mandibularis is an exostosis, usually occuring bilaterally, on the lingual surface of the body of the mandible (Fig. 6-68). Mandibular tori occur in about 5% to 10% of the adult population and are equally distributed between the sexes. The mucoperiosteum covering the torus is very thin and easily traumatized.

Mandibular tori should be removed if the patient is to wear a removable partial denture with any degree of comfort. Severe compromises have to be made in the design, rigidity, and placement of the major connector if the tori are not removed. Patient satisfaction with a removable partial denture constructed in the presence of a mandibular torus is rare. Most patients discontinue wearing the prosthesis in a short time. Removal of mandibular tori is not difficut; and complications are rare if good technique and proper instrumentation are used. Tori can be removed with the patient under local anesthesia and in conjunction with teeth extractions or periodontal surgery.

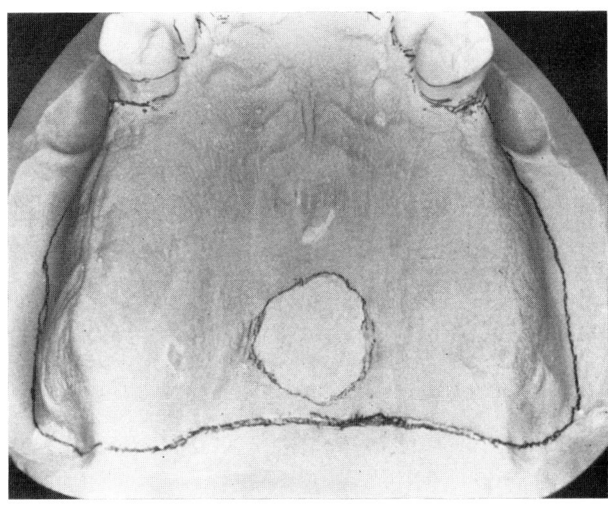

Fig. 6-67. Surgical splint outlined and torus trimmed from cast in preparation for construction of splint.

Exostoses and undercuts

Exostoses and undercuts in residual ridge areas that prevent the proper extension of the denture borders should be evaluated and, if necessary, surgically corrected (Fig. 6-69).

Exostoses of the buccal surface of the alveolar process are common in the maxilla. They occur less frequently in the mandible. The soft tissue covering the bony protuberance is usually thin. Pressure from the placement and wear of a removable partial denture can cause the patient a considerable amount of discomfort. Exostoses should be removed. The technique for removal is similar to that for a simple alveolectomy.

The maxillary tuberosities, the distolingual areas in

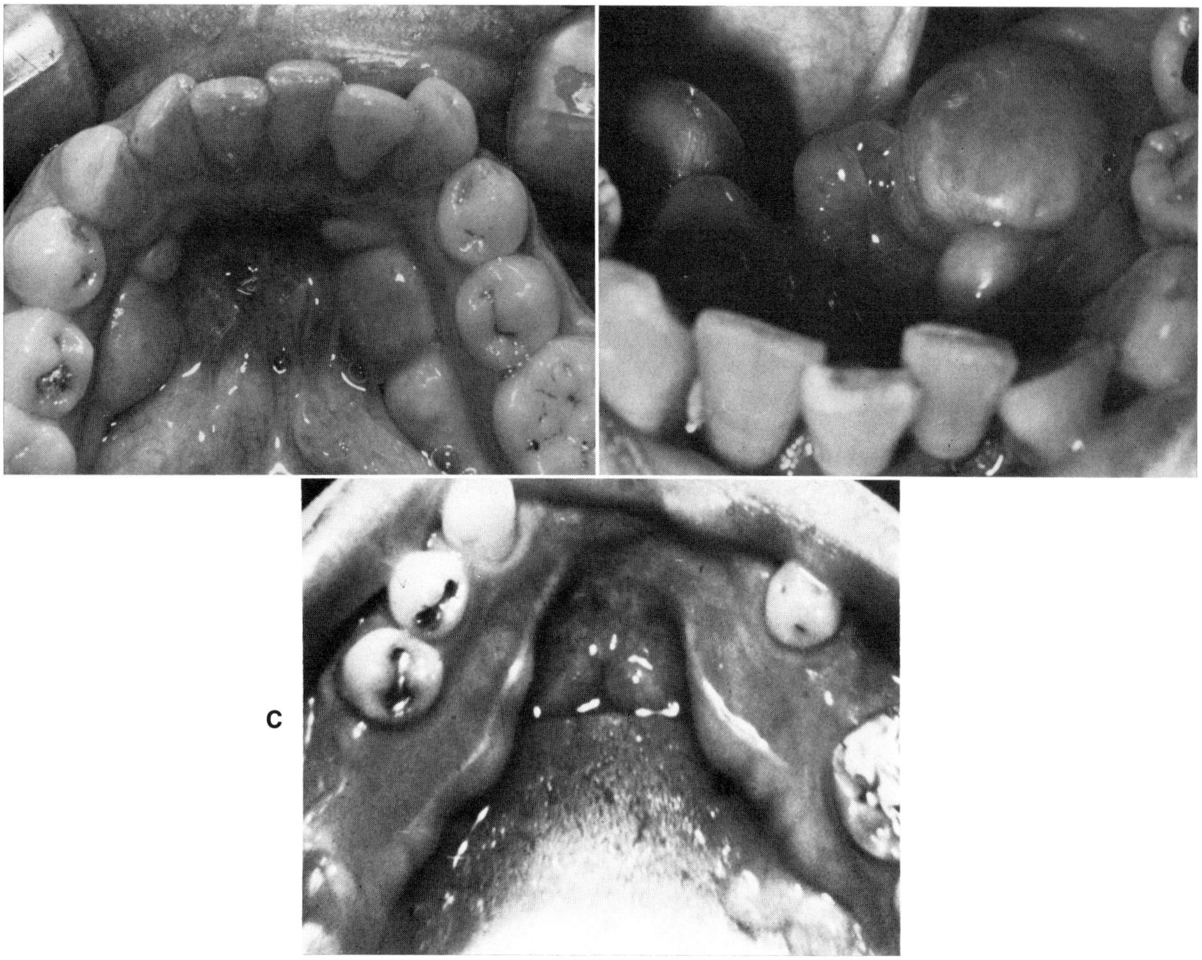

Fig. 6-68. A, Bilateral mandibular tori. **B,** Massive mandibular tori. **C,** Inflammation and tissue displacement over tori caused by mandibular prosthesis.

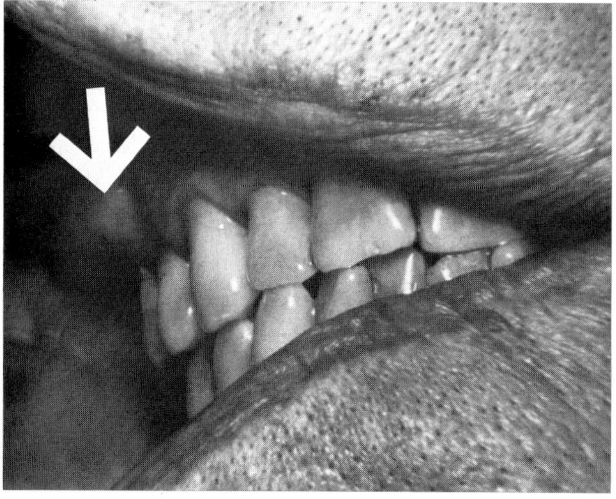

Fig. 6-69. Maxillary buccal exostosis (arrow).

the mandibular arch, and recent extraction sites are the most common undercut areas.

The effect of some, but not all, undercut areas may be minimized by a change in the path of insertion of a removable partial denture. Only those undercuts that would seriously compromise the prognosis should be surgically corrected. This decision should be based on whether the denture base can be effectively relieved to accommodate the undercut areas.

Surgical correction of undercuts should be accomplished if relieving the denture base or reducing the length of the denture border would (1) signigicantly reduce the support for and stability of the prosthesis, (2) create a bothersome food impaction area, or (3) cause a denture border to be so far away from the underlying tissue that it may affect function, compromise esthetics, or cause discomfort for the patient.

Mandibular tuberosity

The mandibular lingual shelf, or lingual tuberosity, is a bony protuberance at the distal end of the mylohyoid ridge in the third molar area (Fig. 6-70). The soft tissue covering is thin, and the area is easily traumatized by the insertion and removal of a removable partial denture. Many times the protuberance precludes the proper extension of the distal extension base of a removable partial denture.

A prominent lingual tuberosity can be easily recognized by palpation. Surgical reduction is indicated.

Evaluation of soft tissue abnormalities

Various soft tissue conditions can present problems in the design and construction of a removable partial denture. Labial and lingual frena as well as unsupported and hypermobile gingiva should be evaluated to determine whether surgical correction will improve the prognosis of treatment.

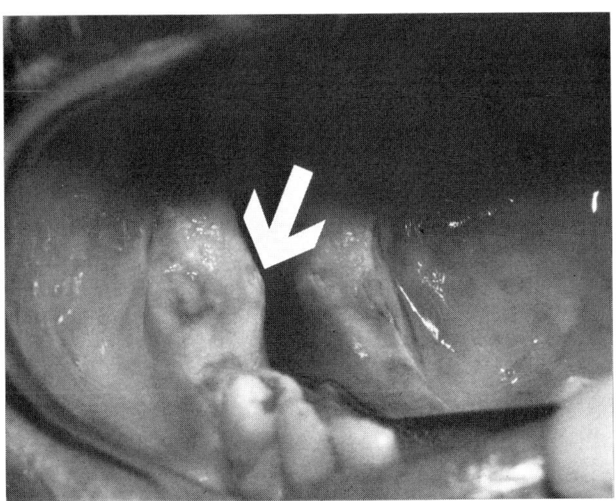

Fig. 6-70. Sharp and irritated mandibular lingual tuberosity (arrow).

Labial frenum

The maxillary labial frenum occasionally presents problems when anterior teeth are replaced with a removable partial denture (Fig. 6-71). If the frenum is attached near the crest of the ridge or if it is hypertrophic, the notch that must be placed in the denture base to accommodate the frenum may be unsightly. A patient with a short or a highly mobile upper lip is most likely to need a frenectomy to correct the condition. A better result is achieved if the patient wears a prosthesis, which serves as a surgical splint, during the healing process.

Hypertrophic lingual frenum

Only rarely is a hypertrophic lingual frenum observed in the adult patient. When it is present, it can greatly compromise the rigidity and the placement of the major connector (Fig. 6-72). A frenectomy should be accomplished. The procedure is more involved than for a labial frenectomy, and the postinsertion course is more difficult.

Unsupported and hypermobile gingiva

Unsupported and hypermobile gingiva occurs more frequently in the completely edentulous patient. However, severe atrophy of the residual ridge does occur occasionally in the edentulous areas of the partially edentulous patient. The gingiva loses its bony support

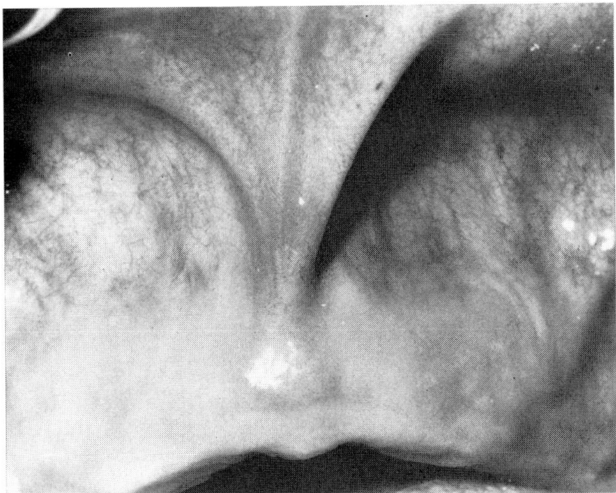

Fig. 6-71. Large maxillary labial frenum attached near crest of residual ridge.

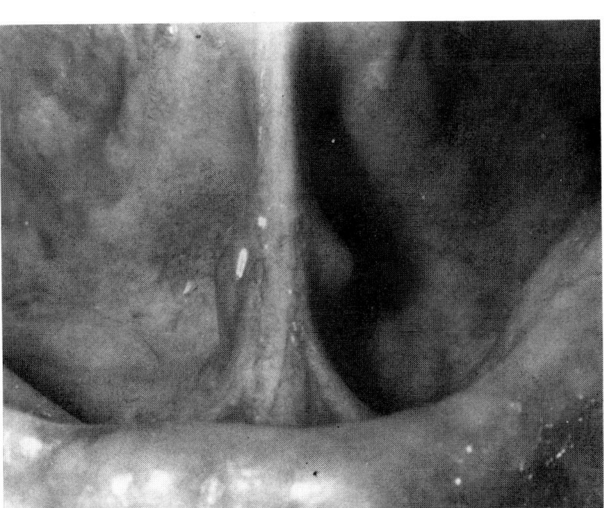

Fig. 6-72. Large mandibular lingual frenum.

and becomes freely mobile. Adequate support is not provided for the denture base. The area should be evaluated to determine whether removal of the soft tissue would result in an excessively short residual ridge. Vestibular extension or ridge augmentation procedures may be indicated.

Evaluation of quantity and quality of saliva

If the mouth is dry, the patient will probably be uncomfortable wearing a removable partial denture. The denture bases will drag across the tissues during placement and removal if the lubricating effect of the saliva is not present. Nervousness, age, drugs, systemic disturbances, and radiation can markedly reduce the salivary output. A lubricating saliva substitute* can help make the prosthesis more tolerable for the patient.

Thick and ropy saliva or copious amounts of serous saliva present problems in the impression procedure. These problems and their solution are discussed in Chapter 5.

Evaluation of space for mandibular major connector

A properly constructed lingual bar major connector is approximately 5 mm wide from its inferior to its superior border. The superior margin of the connector should be located 3 mm below the free gingival margins of the mandibular teeth to avoid damage to the gingival tissues. The inferior border of the connector should be positioned at or slightly above the position of the active floor of the mouth to prevent interference with the functional movements of the floor of the mouth and to help avoid the packing of food under the major connector. Therefore a minimum of 7 to 8 mm of space should be available if a lingual bar major connector is to be used. A lingual plate major connector should be used if less than 7 mm of space is available.

It is not possible to accurately "read" the position of the active floor of the mouth on a cast because most casts are overextended in this area. The selection of the major connector and the determination of the location of its inferior border can be accomplished most effectively when the distance from the free gingival margins to the active floor of the mouth is measured in the mouth.

Available space is measured with a suitable calibrated instrument (Fig. 6-73). A periodontal probe with millimeter markings works well. The patient is instructed to raise the tongue toward the palate. This raises the floor of the mouth to its highest level. The tip of the probe is placed to contact the floor of the mouth lightly. The millimeter depth is read at the point where the probe contacts the gingival margin. Readings are made and recorded at several positions. The probe is then used to transfer the measurements to the diagnostic cast (Fig. 6-74). The points are connected by drawing a line that will indicate the position of the active floor of the mouth.

*Xero-Lube, Scherer Laboratories, Inc., Dallas, Tex. 75234.

Evaluation of radiographic survey

An evaluation of the complete radiographic survey is made with special attention focused on the residual ridge areas and the prospective abutment teeth.

All radiolucent and radiopaque areas that vary from normal ranges should be evaluated to determine whether a pathologic condition is present.

The radiographic findings are correlated with the clinical examination to reveal the presence and extent of caries and the relation of the carious lesion to the dental pulp. Existing restorations are evaluated to determine the adequacy of proximal contours and the presence of overhanging or deficient margins and recurrent caries.

Root fragments and other foreign bodies are evaluated to determine whether their removal is indicated. Not all retained roots have to be removed. If the roots are deeply embedded without evidence of pathologic changes, it is frequently more advisable to keep them under observation than to remove them. Removing deeply embedded root tips may necessitate the removal of a large quantity of bone, resulting in a decrease in the size of the residual ridge. Root tips not completely enclosed in bone and any retained root or foreign body that shows radiographic evidence of pathologic changes should be removed.

Unerupted third molars are evaluated to determine whether they should be retained or removed (Fig. 6-75). Consideration should be given to retaining the third molar as a posterior abutment if its size, shape, and position appear favorable. The greater comfort and stability provided by a tooth-borne compared with a distal extension removable partial denture make the retention of a possible posterior abutment extremely important. Surgical uncovering of the clinical crown can hasten the eruption process. It can be hazardous to retain an unerupted third molar if it is to be covered by a prosthesis. Subsequent eruption of the tooth under the prosthesis can contribute to considerable occlusal and tissue trauma if the erupting tooth is ignored. If an unerupted third molar is retained under a prosthesis, the patient must understand the potential problems and must report the first signs or symptoms of eruption of the tooth. Frequent clinical and radiographic examination is also essential.

Root canal fillings are evaluated with special emphasis on those in prospective abutment teeth. Root canal

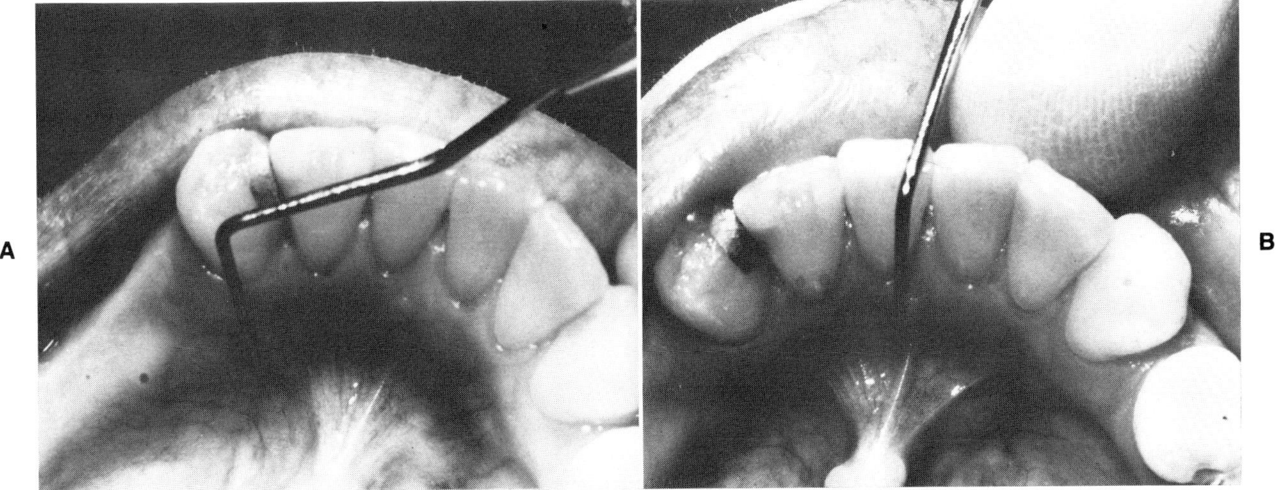

Fig. 6-73. A, Tip of calibrated periodontal probe contacting elevated floor of mouth. **B,** Measurement in midline.

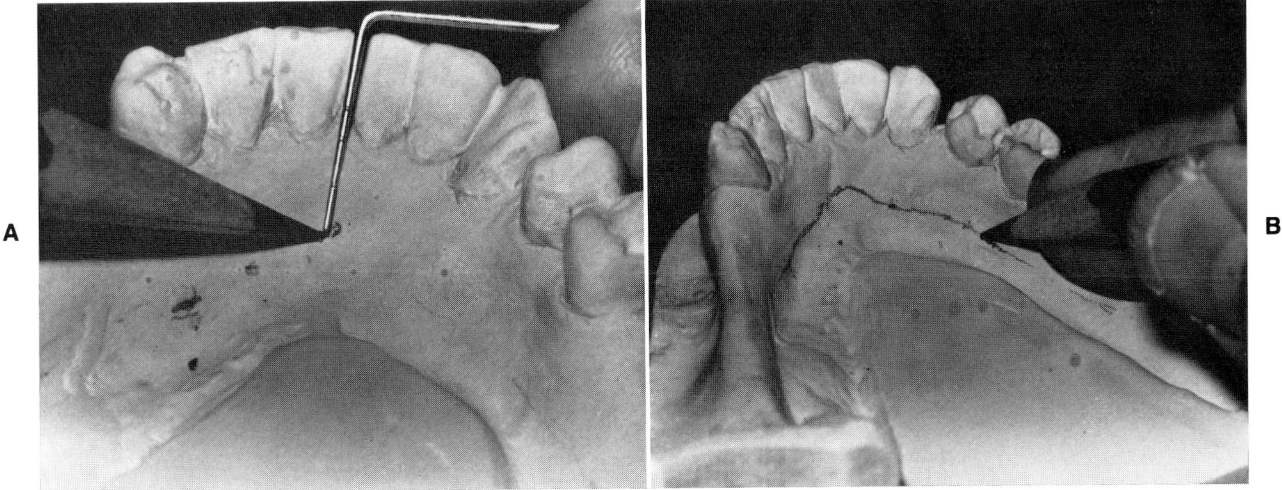

Fig. 6-74. A, Position of elevated floor of mouth is indicated on the cast. **B,** Marks are connected to indicate position of inferior border of major connector.

Fig. 6-75. Unerupted third molars should be evaluated for potential use as abutment teeth.

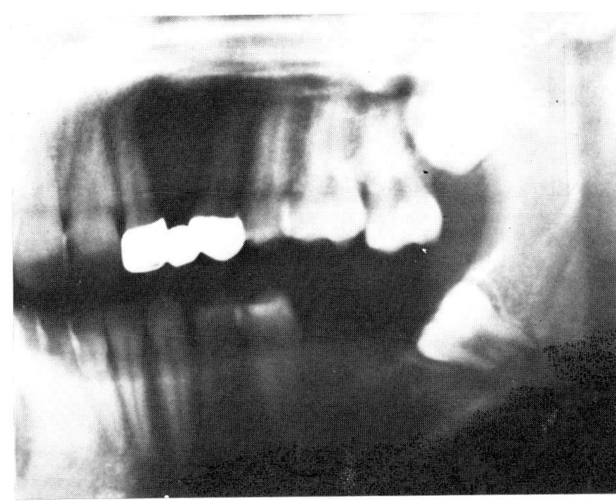

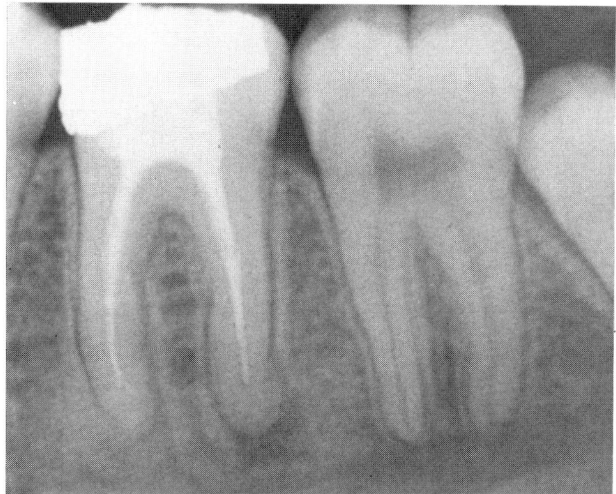

Fig. 6-76. Radiolucent area at apex of endodontically treated tooth.

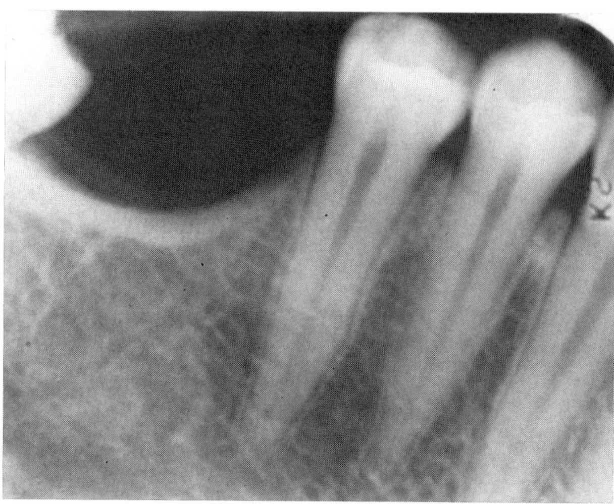

Fig. 6-77. Premolars with large, long roots and good crown/root ratio are good prospective abutment teeth.

fillings should be reaccomplished if the quality or completeness of the fill is questionable. Radiolucent areas on the lateral or apical aspects of the root require further evaluation (Fig. 6-76). Pretreatment radiographs should be consulted to determine whether the radiolucency indicates a new pathologic condition or fibrous healing. The placement of an extracoronal restoration is usually indicated on abutment teeth that have received endodontic treatment, particularly if a large access opening has been made or if the tooth has extensive intracoronal restorations.

Radiographic evaluation of prospective abutment teeth

All prospective abutment teeth must be critically evaluated as described in the following discussion.

Root length, size, and form. Teeth with large or long roots are more favorable abutment teeth because of the greater potential area for periodontal ligament support (Fig. 6-77). However, the relationship between the length of the clinical crown and the amount of root embedded in bone is the most critical factor.

The form of the root of a prospective abutment tooth has a significant influence on its possible effectiveness. Tapered or conical roots are unfavorable because even a small loss of bone height can greatly diminish the attachment area (Fig. 6-78). Multirooted teeth whose roots are divergent or curved are stronger abutment teeth than single-rooted teeth or multirooted teeth whose roots are fused.

The position of roots of adjacent teeth is also important. If the roots of the approximating teeth are close together with little interproximal bone separating them, even moderate irritation or force may be destructive.

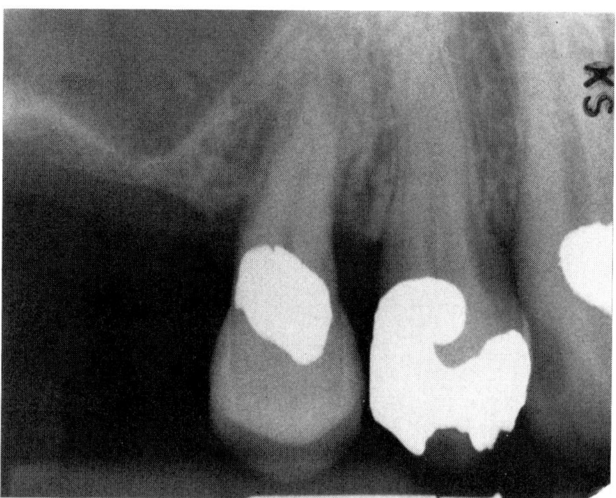

Fig. 6-78. Second premolar with tapered root and bone loss has poor prognosis as abutment tooth.

Crown/root ratio. The angulation factor of the radiographs can cause a considerable degree of interpretive error in estimating the bone height of prospective abutment teeth. This error can be greatly reduced by use of the long-cone paralleling technique in making the radiographs. The amount of tooth embedded in bone is related to the length of the tooth out of bone. If the crown/root ratio is greater than 1:1 or if furcation involvement of a multirooted tooth is present, the tooth has a poor prognosis as an abutment tooth. However, a tooth with a poor prognosis as an abutment can be used in other ways to provide support for the prosthesis: endodontic, periodontic, and restorative treatment can be used to retain one or two roots of a multirooted tooth by

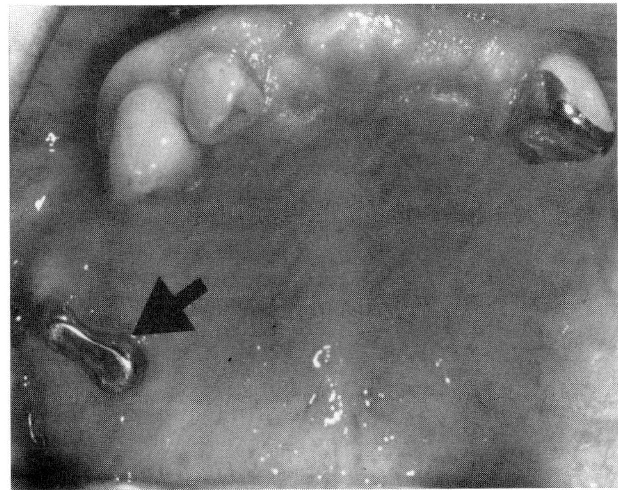

Fig. 6-79. Mesial and palatal root of maxillary molar used as overdenture abutment (arrow).

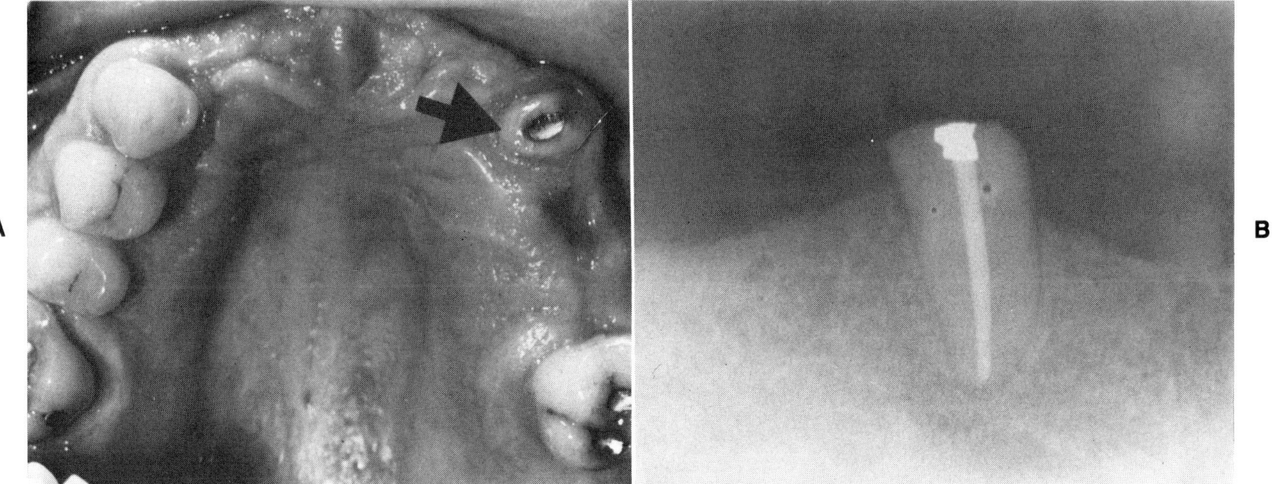

Fig. 6-80. A, Canine with poor crown/root ratio prepared as an overdenture abutment (arrow). **B,** Preparation of endodontically treated tooth as overdenture abutment creates a good crown/root ratio.

a hemisection procedure; or endodontic treatment can be used to prepare a tooth with a poor crown/root ratio as an overdenture abutment (Figs. 6-79 and 6-80).

Lamina dura. Partial or total absence of the lamina dura may be found in systemic disorders such as hyperparathyroidism and Paget's disease. Thus systemic disease must be considered whenever this condition is noted. Changes in the lamina dura are more frequently caused by function, however. Resorption or loss of lamina dura occurs where there is pressure, and apposition occurs where there is tension. A tooth that is in the process of tipping because of loss of an adjacent tooth will show evidence of both resorption and apposition. A thickening of the lamina dura may occur if the tooth is mobile, has occlusal trauma, or is under heavy function. Occlusal trauma can also cause partial or total loss of the lamina dura. Evidence of changes in the lamina dura should be correlated with findings of the clinical examination and evaluation of the occlusion. Destructive forces or disease processes causing changes in the lamina dura must be corrected or the abutment tooth will have a poor prognosis.

Periodontal ligament space. Changes in the width of the periodontal ligament space must be considered when prospective abutment teeth are evaluated. A widening of the periodontal ligament space with a thickening of the lamina dura indicates mobility, occlusal trauma, and heavy function (Fig. 6-81). To evaluate

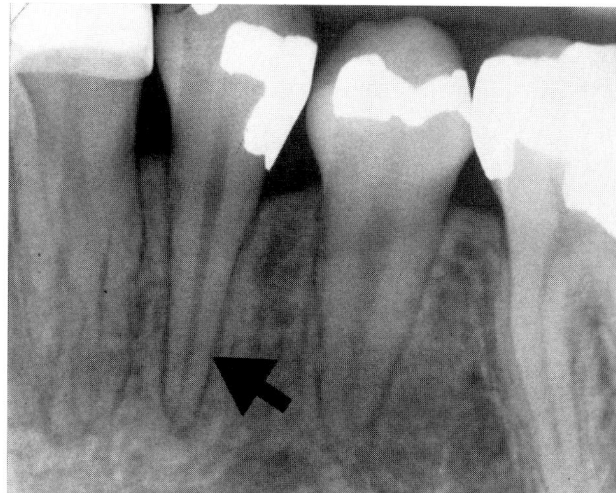

Fig. 6-81. Widening of periodontal ligament space of premolar (arrow) caused by occlusal trauma.

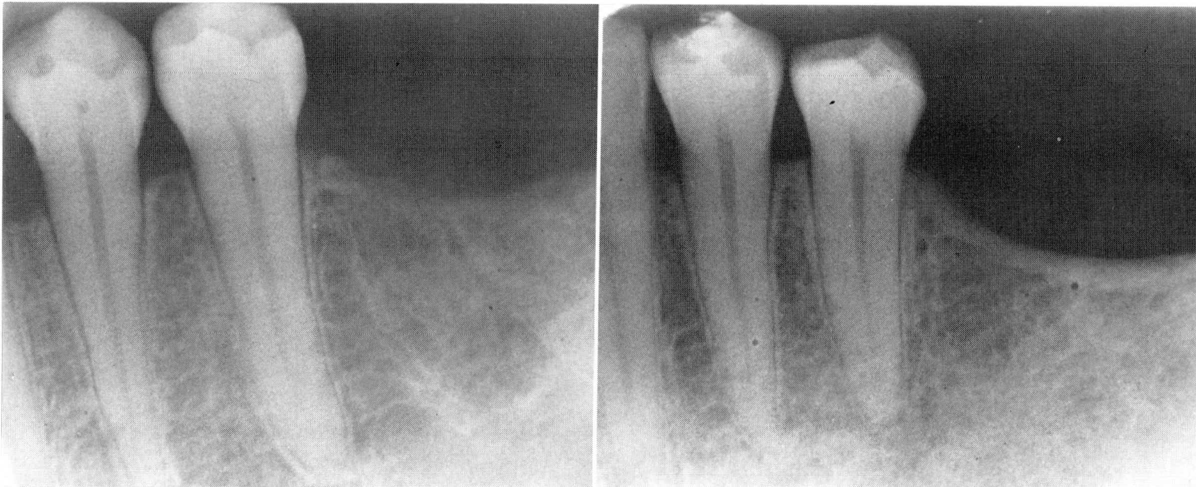

Fig. 6-82. Premolars with a positive bone factor such as these can serve as abutment teeth for a removable partial denture.

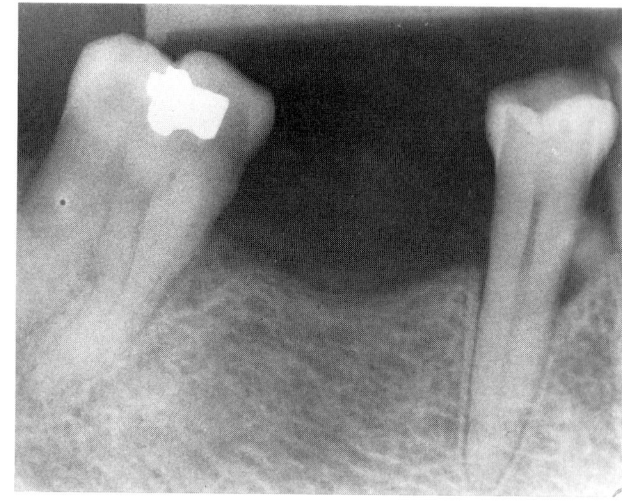

Fig. 6-83. Signs of retrograde changes indicate patient has a negative bone factor.

these radiographic findings, it is necessary to correlate them with the clinical mobility of the tooth. If the tooth is mobile, these radiographic signs indicate destructive changes. If the tooth is not mobile, these signs may indicate a favorable response to increased occlusal forces. However, the added stress of serving as an abutment tooth or a decreased resistive capacity of the bone in the future may result in failure of the abutment tooth. Therefore every effort should be made to eliminate the traumatic occlusal forces and to reduce the heavy functional forces on the prospective abutment tooth.

Occlusal trauma can also widen the periodontal ligament space with a partial or total loss of the lamina dura. These findings must be correlated with the evaluation of the occlusion. Retrograde changes and the potential for destructive changes must be ruled out before a tooth with thickened periodontal ligament space is accepted as an abutment.

Bone index areas. Bone index areas are areas of alveolar bone that support teeth known to have been subjected to a larger than normal workload. If there is a positive response of the alveolar bone and the periodontal ligament to the increased forces, the patient has a "positive bone factor" (Fig. 6-82). Other teeth in the dental arch can also be expected to react favorably to the additional stress. Signs of a positive response include a supportive trabecular pattern, a heavy cortical layer, dense lamina dura, normal bone height, and a normal periodontal ligament space.

If retrograde bone changes occur, the patient has a "negative bone factor" (Fig. 6-83). The prognosis is poor because the additional stresses created by a removable partial denture may hasten destructive processes and cause failure of the abutment teeth. Signs of retrograde changes include loss of lamina dura, loss of bone height, widening of the periodontal ligament space, and apical or furcation radiolucency.

Teeth that are subjected to greater than normal stress and provide good index information include the following:

1. Abutment teeth of a fixed or a removable partial denture
2. Teeth involved in occlusal interferences
3. Teeth receiving greater occlusal stress because of loss of adjacent teeth
4. Tipped teeth with occlusal contact

Evaluation of mounted diagnostic casts

The mounted diagnostic casts can provide important information that may be difficult to obtain by intraoral examination alone. Potential problems such as insufficient interarch distance, irregularity or malposition of the occlusal plane, extruded or malposed teeth, and unfavorable maxillomandibular relationships are more apparent in accurately mounted casts because the lips, cheeks, and skull block out good visual access to the teeth in the mouth. The mounted diagnostic casts provide visual access from all directions and enable the dentist to make a detailed analysis of the patient's occlusion.

Interarch distance

A fairly common finding is lack of sufficient interarch distance for the placement of artificial teeth. Frequently the problem is caused by a maxillary tuberosity that is too large in vertical height (Fig. 6-84). A segment of teeth that has been unopposed for a prolonged period will frequently overerupt, carrying the alveolar process with it. Subsequent removal of the teeth will produce a situation in which it is impossible to establish a functionally and esthetically acceptable plane of occlusion. The surgical reduction of the vertical height of the tuberosity and at times the adjacent residual ridge is necessary if satisfactory replacement of the missing teeth is to be accomplished. The area and amount of tissue that should be removed can be indicated on the diagnostic cast. This provides an excellent guide for the oral surgeon or dentist who performs the surgical correction. The radiographs are a valuable aid in planning the surgical procedure. The shadow on the radiographs that indicates the thickness of soft tissue overlying the tuberosity and residual ridge will help determine whether the procedure can be accomplished by soft tissue correction alone or whether removal of bone is also necessary (Fig. 6-85). By far the majority of tuberosity interferences can be corrected by removal of a wedge

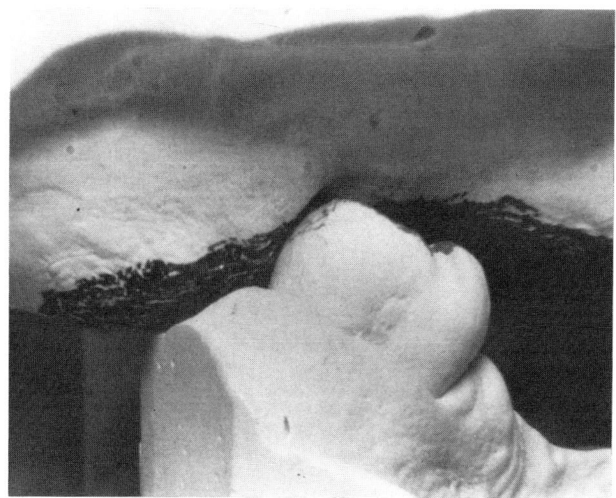

Fig. 6-84. Enlarged maxillary tuberosity precludes development of adequate occlusal plane.

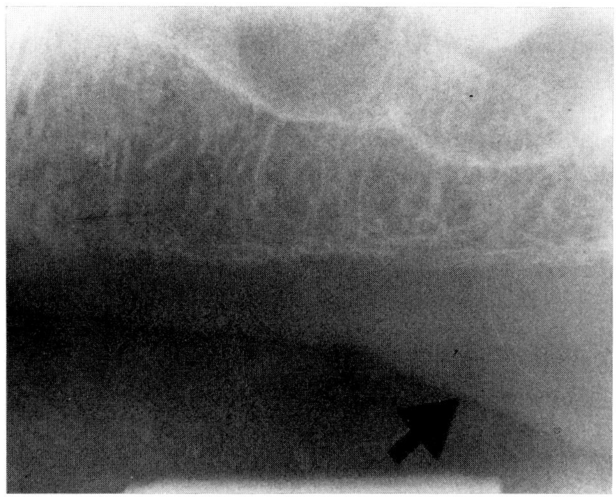

Fig. 6-85. Shadow on radiograph indicates thickness of soft tissue overlying bone (arrow).

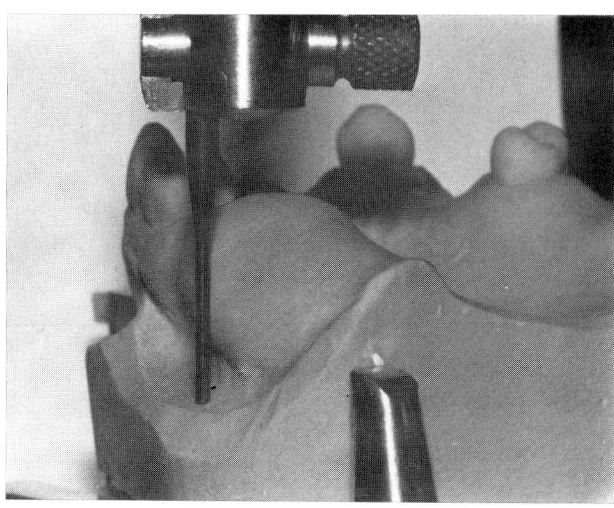

Fig. 6-86. Diagnostic cast on surveyor is used to analyze depth of tuberosity undercut.

of fibrous tissue. Healing is usually complete in 7 to 10 days. The healing period is extended to 2 to 3 weeks when bone removal is necessary.

The maxillary tuberosity area may be undercut on one or both sides. The path of insertion of a complete denture can usually be compatible with an unilateral tuberosity undercut, but a removable partial denture, with a more controlled path of insertion, presents greater problems. The undercut must be evaluated with the aid of the dental surveyor. With the cast on the surveying table at the predetermined path of insertion, a determination is made as to the amount of relief that will be required in the denture if the undercut is not reduced (Fig. 6-86). Moderate to severe tuberosity undercuts usually require surgical correction with bone removal.

Occasionally the tuberosities are so bulbous that there is no space for the denture base during mandibular movements. The coronoid process of the mandible may actually rub against the tuberosity during functional movements. Surgical reduction of such a tuberosity is necessary if the patient is to wear a removable partial denture.

Occlusal plane

The occlusal plane may be irregular (because of extrusion of one or more unopposed teeth) or malposed (because of extrusion of an entire segment of an arch with concomitant drop of the alveolar process). Both conditions require corrective procedures if an acceptable occlusion is to be developed.

Irregular occlusal plane. Several courses of treatment are available for correction of an extruded tooth. The treatment will vary depending on the degree of extrusion and the condition of the tooth.

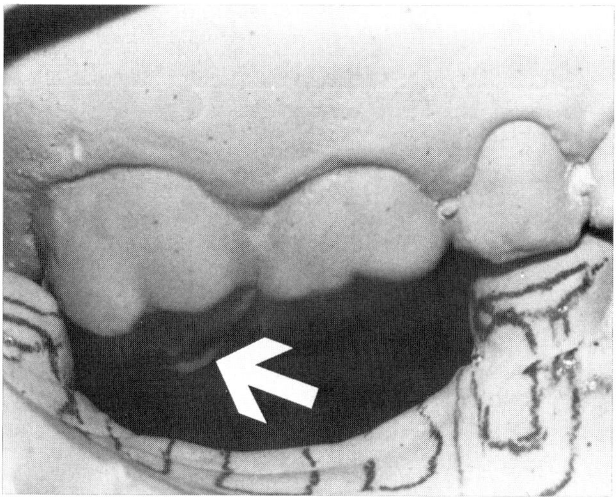

Fig. 6-87. Maxillary molar in buccoversion with lingual cusp below occlusal plane. Line drawn on cusp indicates area for correction by enameloplasty (arrow).

Enameloplasty can effectively reduce a moderately extruded tooth. Approximately 2 mm of enamel can be removed in many situations. At times the reduction of a single cusp improves the occlusal plane (Fig. 6-87).

If the extrusion is greater than 1 or 2 mm or if the tooth does not lend itself to enameloplasty, the placement of an extracoronal cast metallic restoration is indicated (Fig. 6-88). The degree of reduction is limited as much or more by the clinical crown length of the tooth as by the size of the dental pulp. The clinical

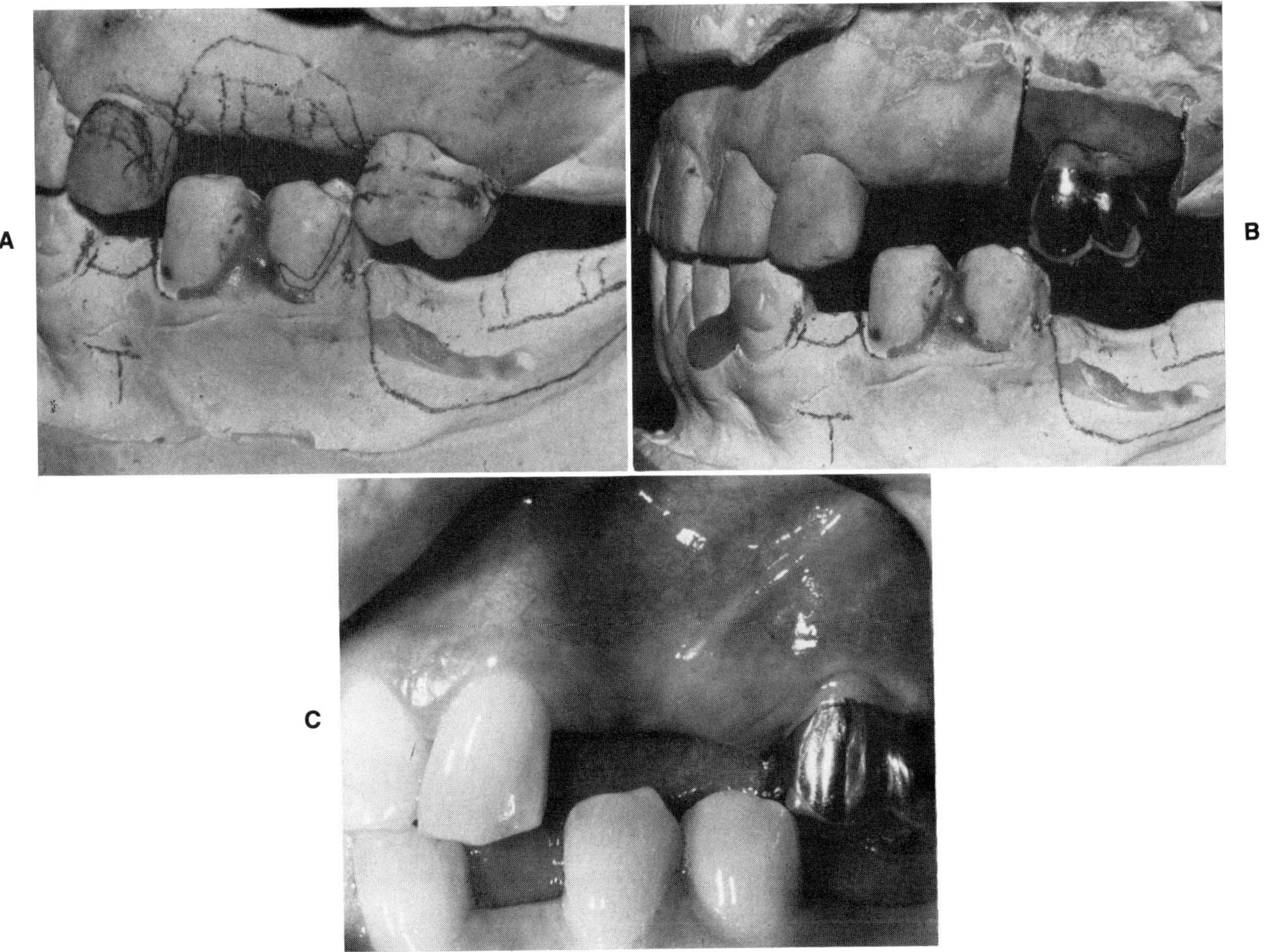

Fig. 6-88. A, Extruded maxillary molar. **B,** Cast crown constructed after gross reduction in clinical crown length. **C,** Improved occlusal plane.

crown length can often be increased by appropriate periodontal therapy if crown lengthening is needed to obtain adequate retention for the restoration. Useful crown lengthening procedures include tissue shrinkage, gingivectomy, apical positioning flaps, and osseous surgery. Extruded teeth can also be repositioned through minor tooth movement procedures (Fig. 6-89).

Severely extruded teeth such as those contacting the opposing ridge present greater problems. If the alveolar bone has followed the eruption of the offending tooth, it may be necessary to remove the tooth and the surrounding bone. At times endodontic treatment and drastic reduction of the tooth will enable it to be used as an overdenture abutment. This treatment can provide valuable support for a distal extension base. Extruded teeth must always be evaluated with the occlusal plane in mind. Retention of a tooth that will jeopardize the development of a functional and esthetic occlusal plane is rarely justified.

Malposed occlusal plane. A not uncommon finding is the extrusion of maxillary molars or premolars, or both, with a concomitant drop of the alveolar process when this segment of teeth is left unopposed (Fig. 6-90). The teeth may contact the opposing residual ridge, causing obvious space problems and malposition of the occlusal plane.

One approach to treatment is the removal of the extruded teeth in conjunction with an extensive alveolectomy. However, consideration should be given to the use of one of the newer orthognathic surgical procedures. A posterior segmental osteotomy can be effective in correcting the problem (Fig. 6-91). Close cooperation and communication between the prosthodontist or dentist and the oral surgeon are essential. Because the den-

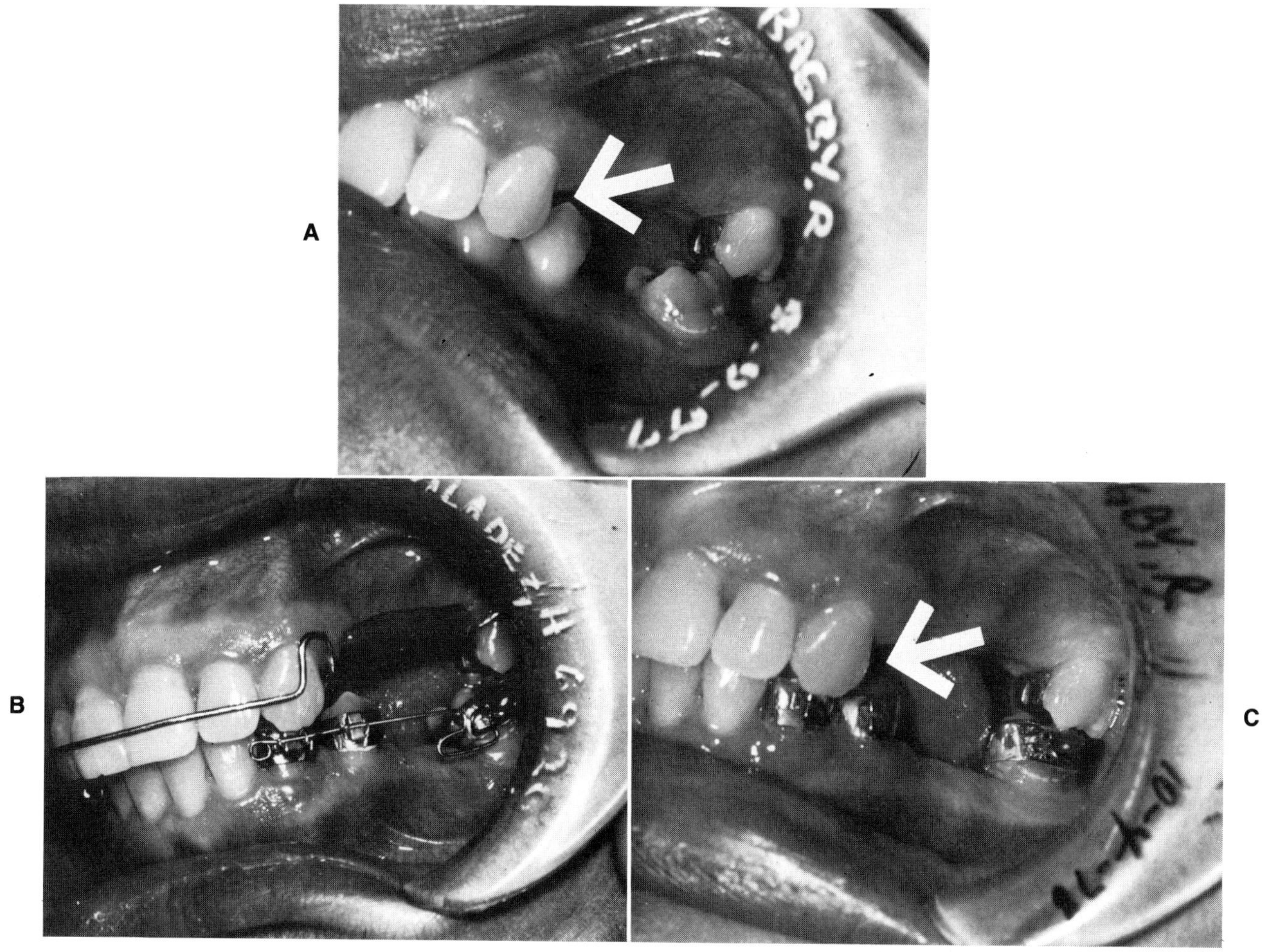

Fig. 6-89. **A,** Mandibular molar has tipped mesially, and extruded first premolar is in close proximity with maxillary ridge (arrow). **B,** Removable and fixed orthodontic appliances have been placed to correct position of both teeth. **C,** Uprighted molar is in good occlusion. Increased space is available between premolar and maxillary ridge (arrow). (Courtesy Undergraduate Orthodontics, University of Texas Health Science Center at San Antonio.)

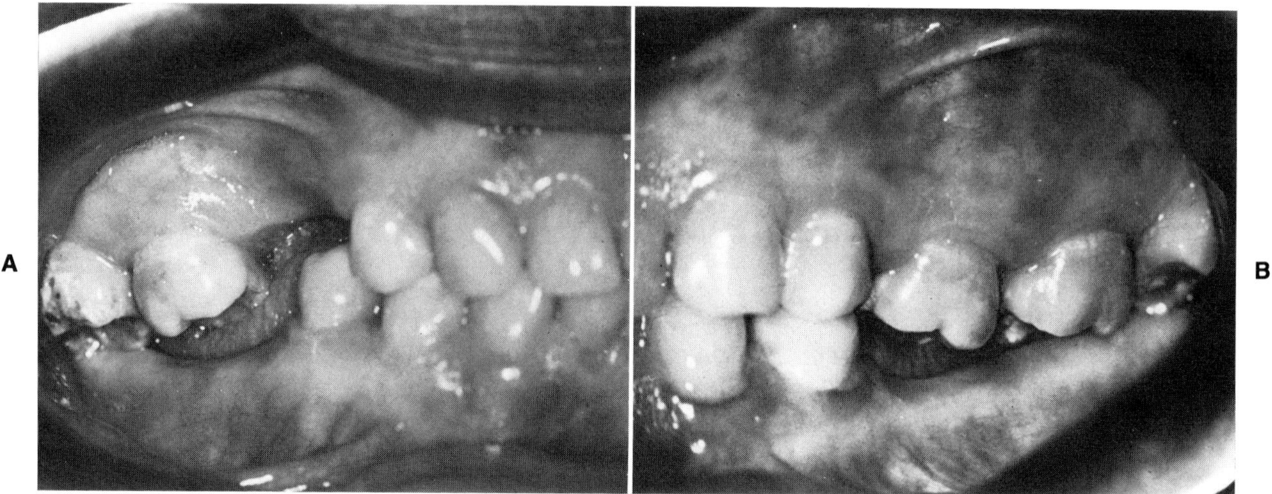

Fig. 6-90. Extrusion of maxillary molars and drop of alveolar processes on right side, **A,** and left side, **B.**

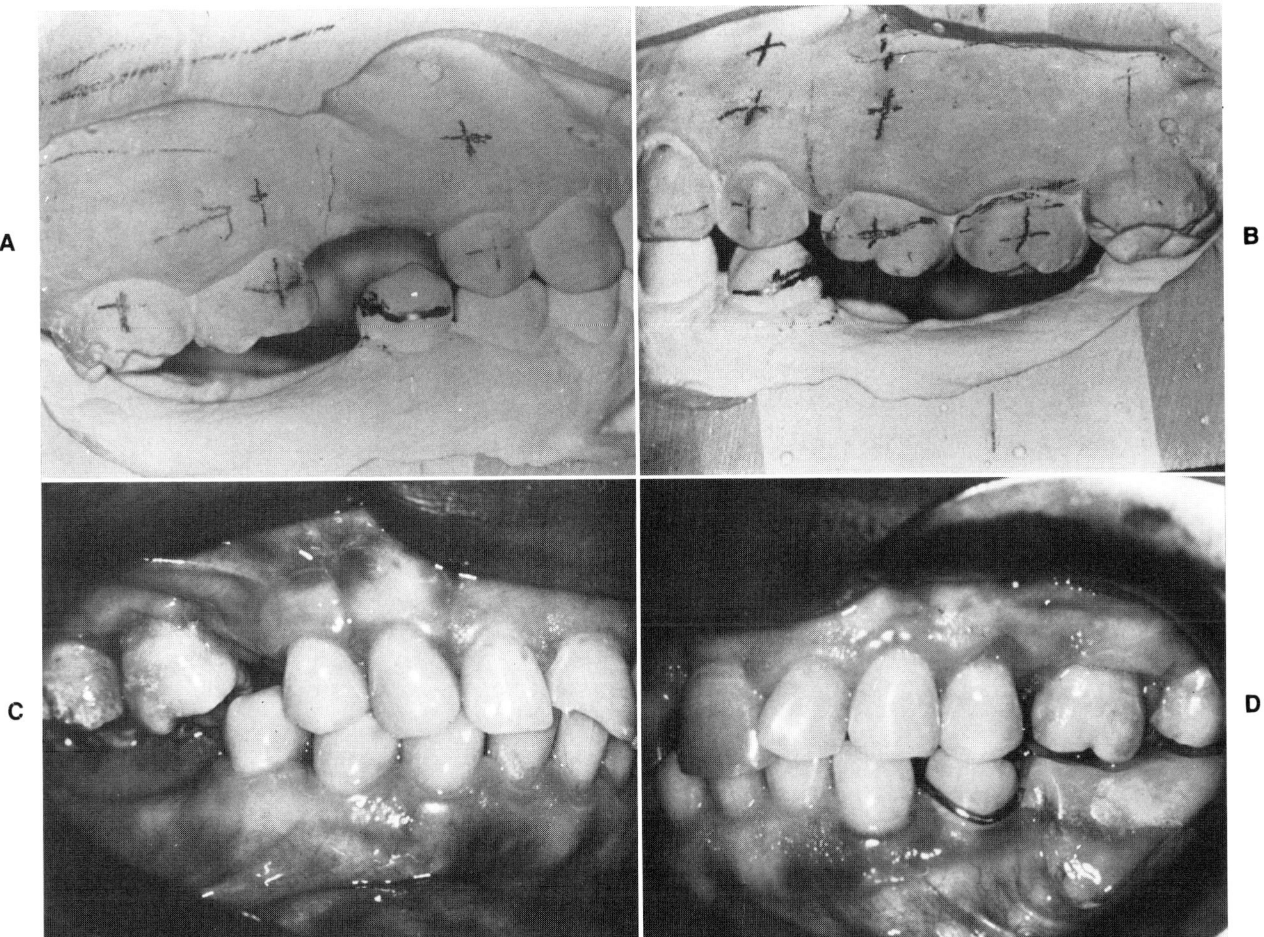

Fig. 6-91. This 36-year-old patient was treated by bilateral posterior segmental osteotomy. **A,** Diagnostic cast, right side, with plan to remove segment of bone and place posterior segment upward. **B,** Diagnostic cast, left side. **C,** Right side, 6 weeks after surgery. Surgical splints have been removed. **D,** Left side, 2 months after surgery, with splint in position to prevent extrusion of teeth. (Courtesy Dr. Frank Dolwick, University of Texas Health Science Center at San Antonio.)

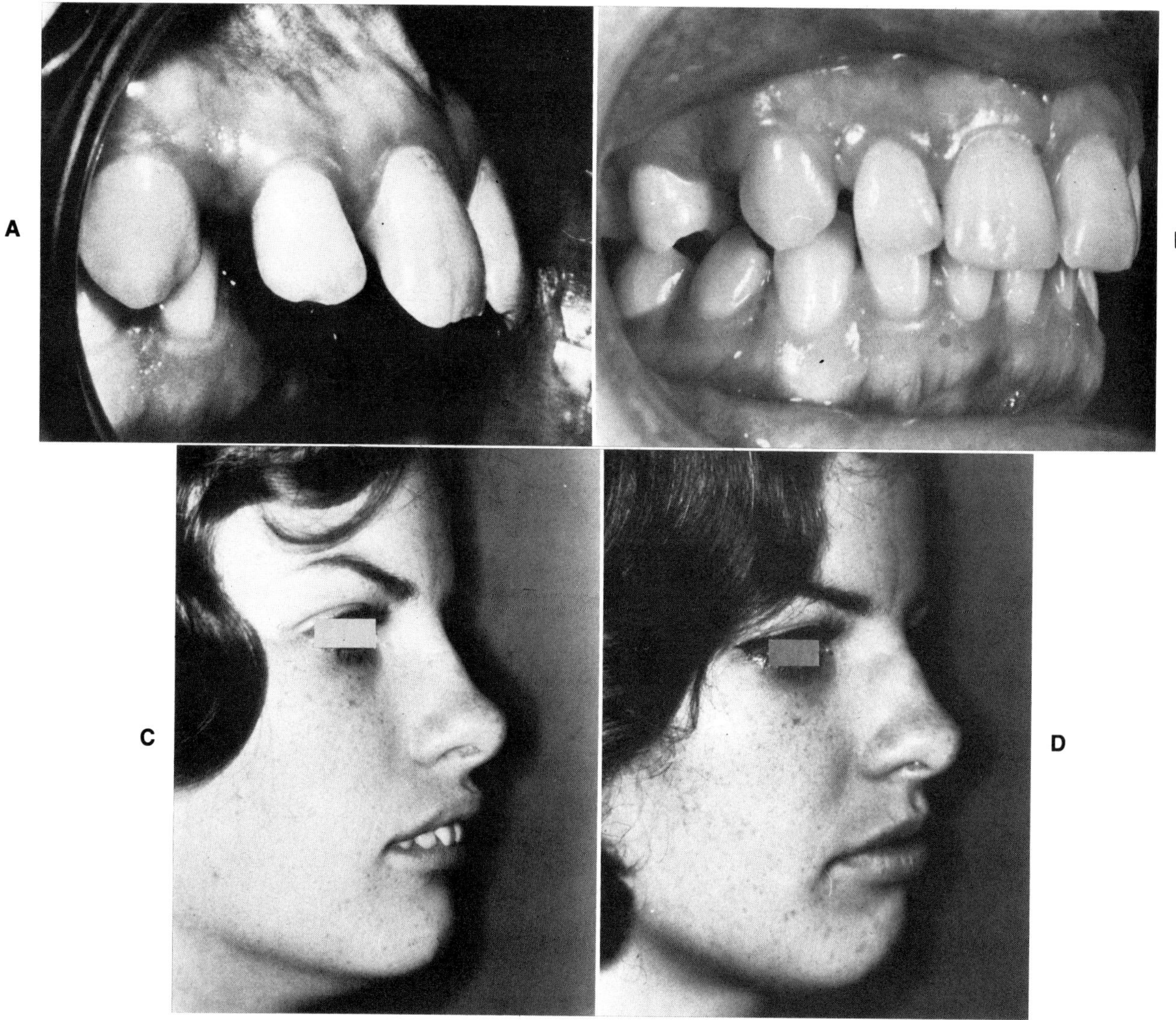

Fig. 6-92. This 23-year-old patient was treated by anterior maxillary osteotomy. **A,** Procumbunt maxillary incisors before treatment. **B,** Maxillary incisors after treatment. **C,** Patient's profile before, and after, **D,** surgical correction. (Courtesy Dr. Robert Johnson.)

tist must construct the prosthesis for the postsurgical tooth and ridge relations, he should determine the ideal position of the segment. The oral surgeon must determine the procedures and techniques to employ in making the correction.

Anterior maxillary osteotomy can also be effective in repositioning the anterior teeth and alveolar ridge for patients with severe protrusion of the anterior teeth or deep vertical overlap (Fig. 6-92). The psychologic as well as the functional and esthetic factors must be evaluated before this type of treatment is initiated. Close cooperation between the dentist and oral surgeon is essential.

Acute temporomandibular joint and associated neuromuscular problems must be resolved before the ideal position of the segments to be repositioned is determined. Elimination of the symptoms can greatly change the occlusal relationships of the remaining teeth.

Traumatic vertical overlap

Akerly (1977) has classified traumatic vertical overlap into the following four basic types (Fig. 6-93):

Type I—The mandibular incisors extrude and impinge into the palate.

Type II—The mandibular incisors impinge into the gingival sulci of the maxillary incisors.

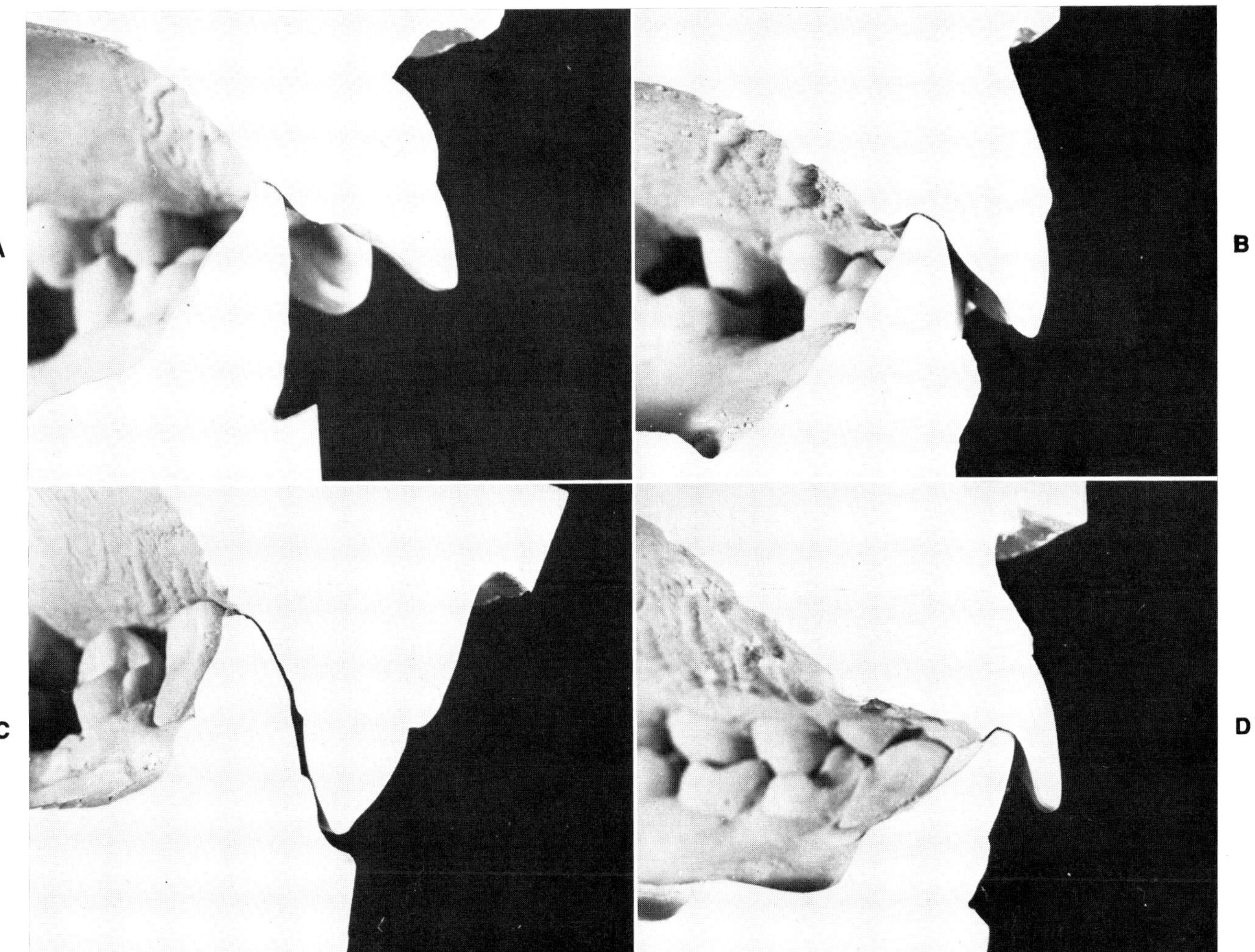

Fig. 6-93. Akerly's classification of traumatic vertical overlap. **A,** Type I: Mandibular incisors extrude impinging into palate. **B,** Type II: Mandibular incisors impinge into gingival sulci of maxillary incisors. **C,** Type III: Maxillary and mandibular incisors lingually inclined with impingement of gingival tissues of each arch. **D,** Type IV: Mandibular incisors move or extrude into abraded lingual surfaces of maxillary anterior teeth. (From Akerly; W.B.: J. Prosthet. Dent. **38:** 26-34, 1977.)

Type III—Both maxillary and mandibular incisors incline lingually with impingement of the gingival tissues of each arch.

Type IV—The mandibular incisors move or extrude into the abraded lingual surfaces of the maxillary anterior teeth.

Clinical symptoms of traumatic vertical overlap include abrasion, mobility, and migration of the teeth, as well as inflammation and ulceration of the gingiva and palatal mucosa.

Early recognition of the problems and treatment with orthodontic or combined orthodontic and orthognathic surgical procedures are the treatments of choice (Fig. 6-94). However, many patients have advanced clinical symptoms.

The removal of teeth is indicated if the periodontal disease and migration of the teeth have progressed to the hopeless state. The replacement teeth will have to be placed with a fairly deep vertical overlap because the skeletal problem will still be present. Alveolectomy at the time of removal of the teeth will help provide space for some improvement.

Other treatment options are available if the teeth are retainable. Reduction of the length of the mandibular anterior teeth that close into the palatal or gingival tissues will relieve symptoms. However, the effect will be

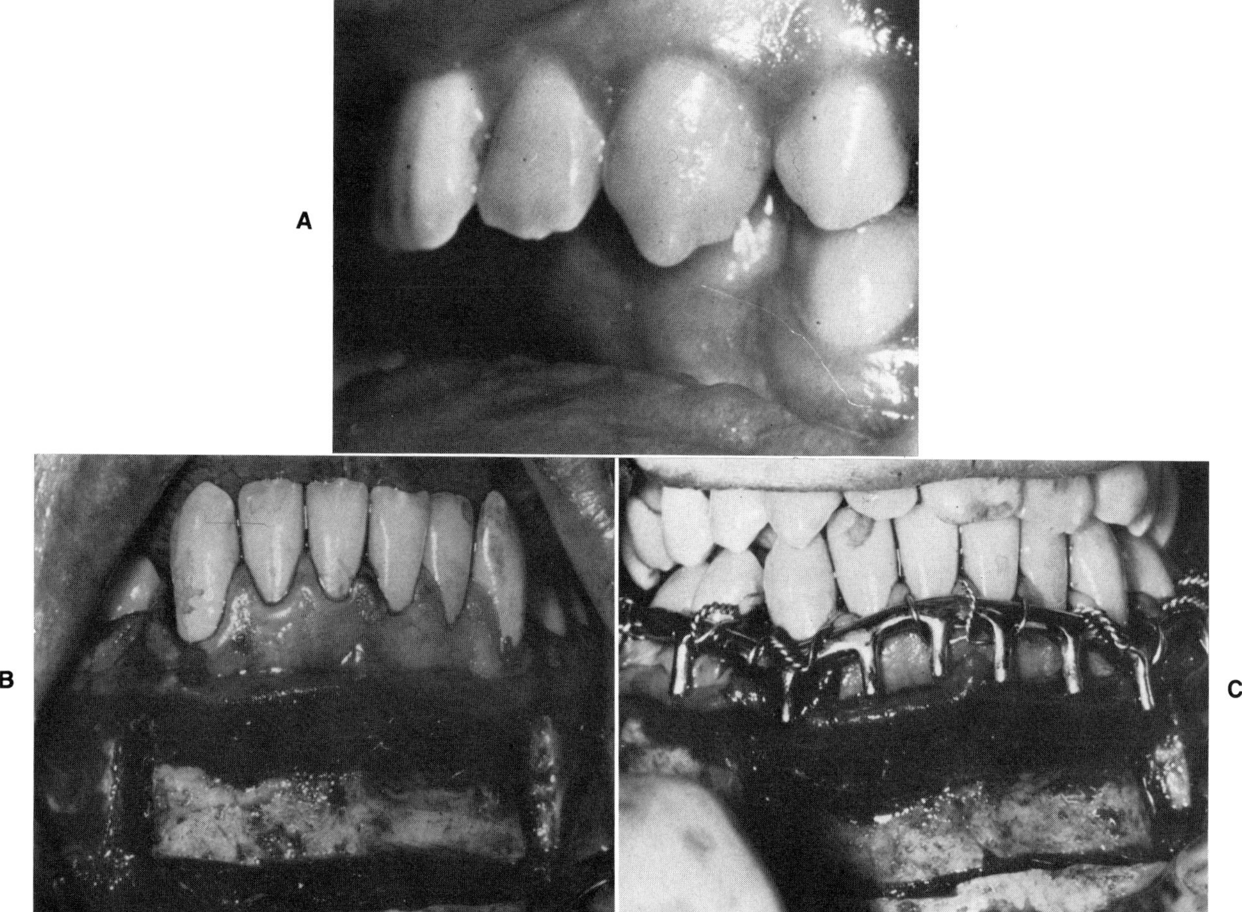

Fig. 6-94. A, Extruded mandibular anterior teeth impinge into gingiva of maxillary anterior teeth. **B,** Six anterior teeth to be lowered by mandibular subapical osteotomy with removal of 5-mm strip of bone below apices of teeth. **C,** Mandibular anterior teeth in new position and arch bar in place. (Courtesy Dr. Donald Steed, University of Texas Health Science Center at San Antonio.)

only temporary because the mandibular teeth will continue to erupt unless they are put into function. Unfortunately a common treatment history is that of reduction of the length of the teeth, leading to a vicious cycle of extrusion, grinding, and then further extrusion.

A treatment prosthesis that plates the lingual surfaces of the maxillary anterior teeth can be used to prevent further extrusion of the mandibular incisors until more definitive treatment can be accomplished. Using the prosthesis as a guide plane appliance will apparently cause intrusion of the mandibular incisors or allow some extrusion of the posterior teeth. In either case, space can frequently be created that will allow the construction of a definitive prosthesis to prevent extrusion of the mandibular anterior teeth and allow normal contact of the posterior teeth.

The type of definitive treatment must be based on the degree of horizontal overlap, the number and the occlusal relationships of the remaining teeth, and the health of the supporting structures. If all the maxillary teeth are present and have healthy support, it may be possible to build up the cingula of the anterior teeth with cast restorations (Fig. 6-95). This choice of treatment is not feasible if the horizontal overlap is too great.

If a maxillary removable partial denture is indicated, the major connector can be extended onto the lingual surfaces of the anterior teeth with a thin plate of metal. This will provide a vertical stop to prevent further eruption of the mandibular anterior teeth (Fig. 6-96).

If only a mandibular removable partial denture is required for replacement of teeth, a lingual plate major connector can be designed to prevent continued eruption of the anterior teeth. The plating should cover the

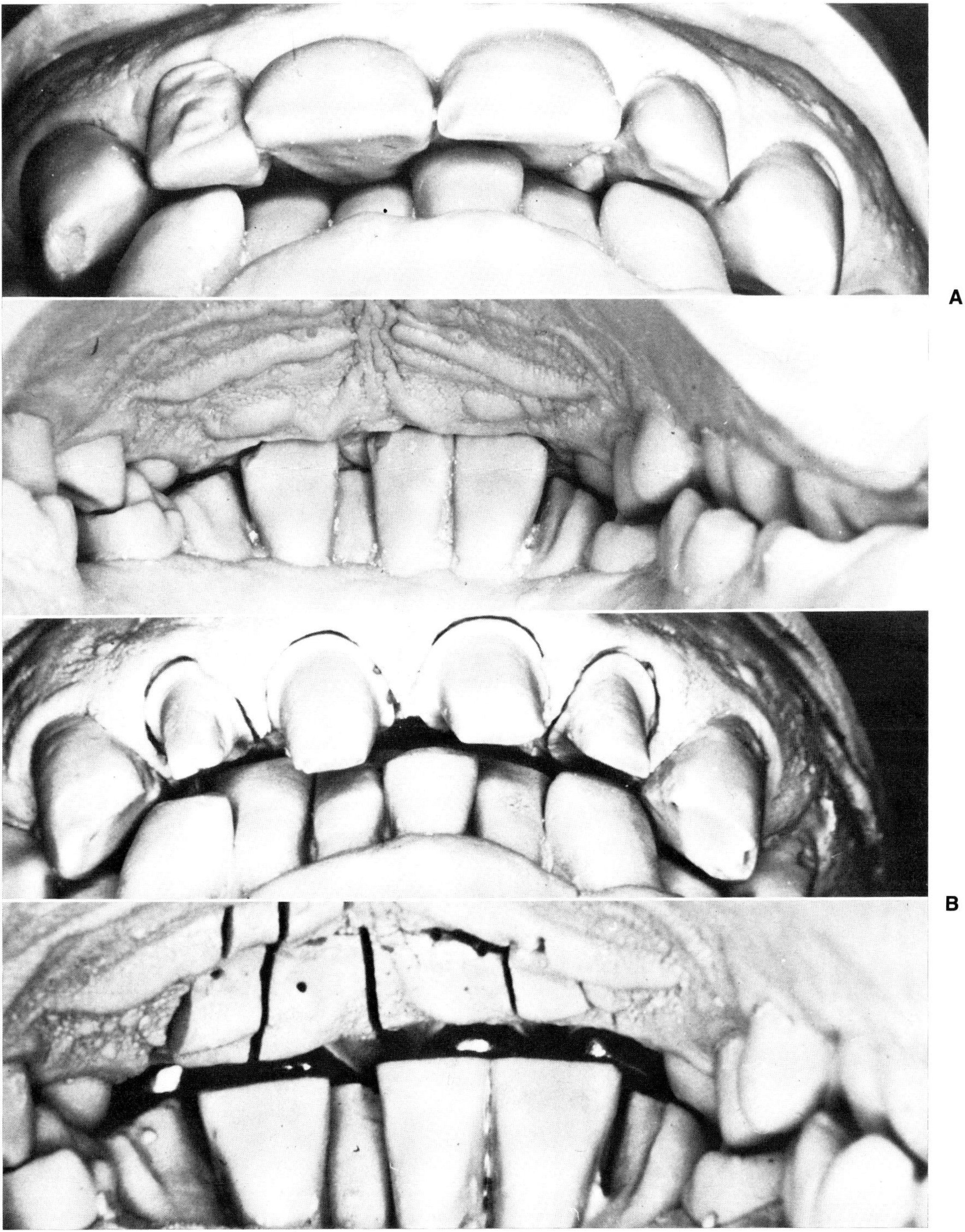

Fig. 6-95. A, Mandibular anterior teeth impinging into maxillary gingival tissues and palatal mucosa. Problem in **B** treated by building up cingula of maxillary crowns to contact and prevent extrusion of mandibular anterior teeth which have been shortened by grinding. (From Akerly, W.B.: J. Prosthet. Dent. **38:**26-34, 1977.)

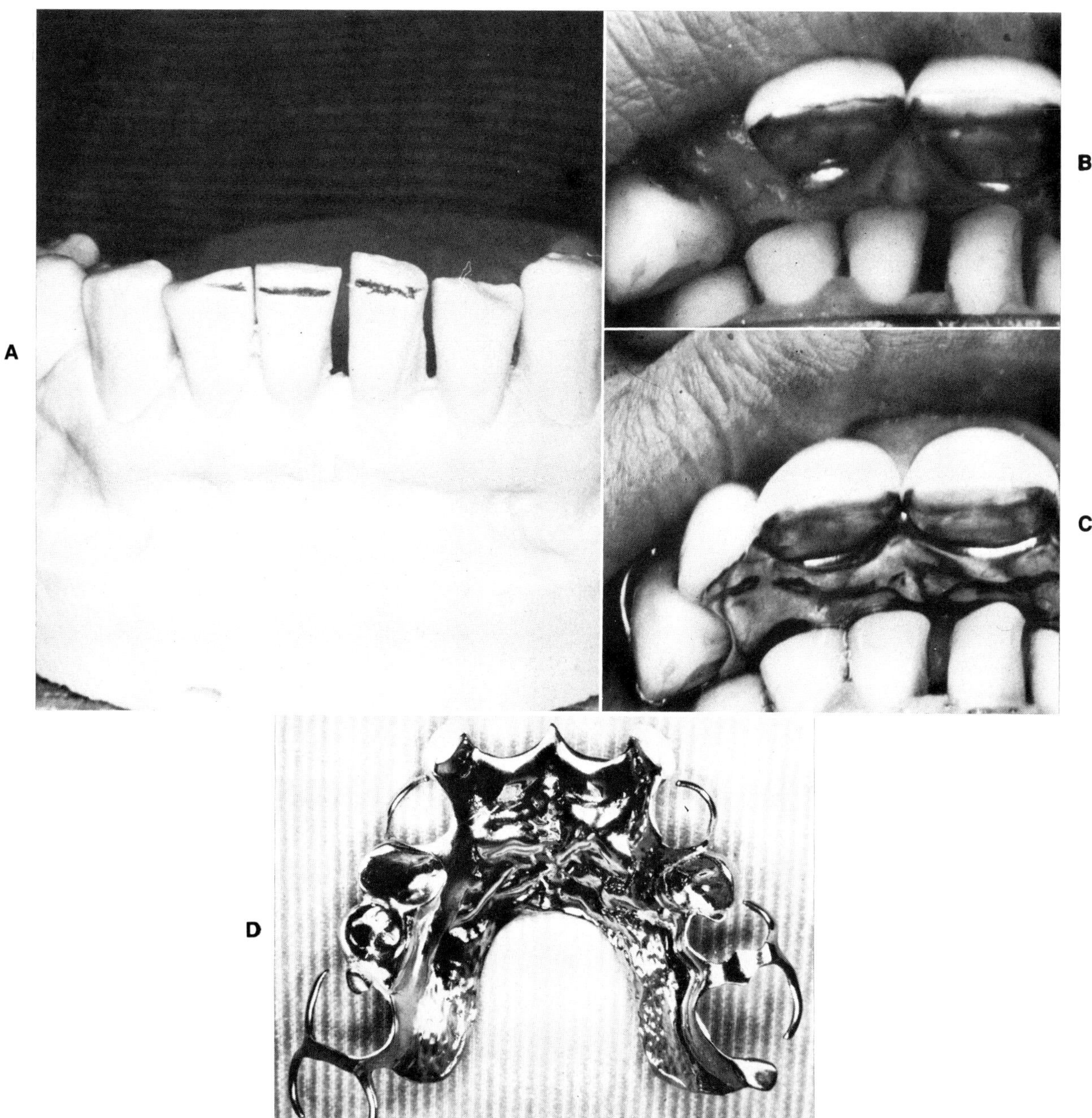

Fig. 6-96. A, Extruded mandibular teeth with line drawn to indicate area to be reduced by grinding. **B,** Note horizontal and vertical overlap. **C,** Maxillary anterior teeth plated on lingual surface with extension from major connector of removable partial denture. Mandibular anterior teeth have been shortened; they contact the metal of major connector to prevent extrusion. Lingual rests in crowns on central incisors provide vertical support and prevent potential anterior flaring of maxillary anterior teeth. **D,** Removable partial denture with area for contact of mandibular anterior teeth. (**A, B,** and **C** from Akerly, W.B.: J. Prosthet. Dent. **38:**26-34, 1977.)

cingula of the teeth with projections extending to the contact points. Rest seats should be placed on the canines or first premolars to prevent labially directed forces from being applied to the teeth.

The vertical dimension of occlusion may appear to be decreased because of the severe vertical overlap or the extensive abrasion of the anterior teeth. It may appear that the posterior teeth have migrated or that an insufficient number of teeth have been present to maintain the vertical dimension of occlusion. The opening or restoring of an apparent loss of vertical dimension of occlusion must be approached cautiously.

Deflective posterior occlusal contacts can cause or aggravate anterior traumatic occlusion. Removal of deflective contacts that cause a significant anterior slide is essential. Establishing stable occlusal contacts at centric jaw relation will often reduce or eliminate traumatic contacts between the anterior teeth.

Malrelation of jaws

Severe malrelation of the jaws can preclude the restoration of adequate function and esthetics. Several maxillary and mandibular osteotomy procedures are useful in correcting these problems (Figs. 6-97 to 6-99). Close cooperation, consultation, and communication between the prosthodontist or dentist and the oral sur-

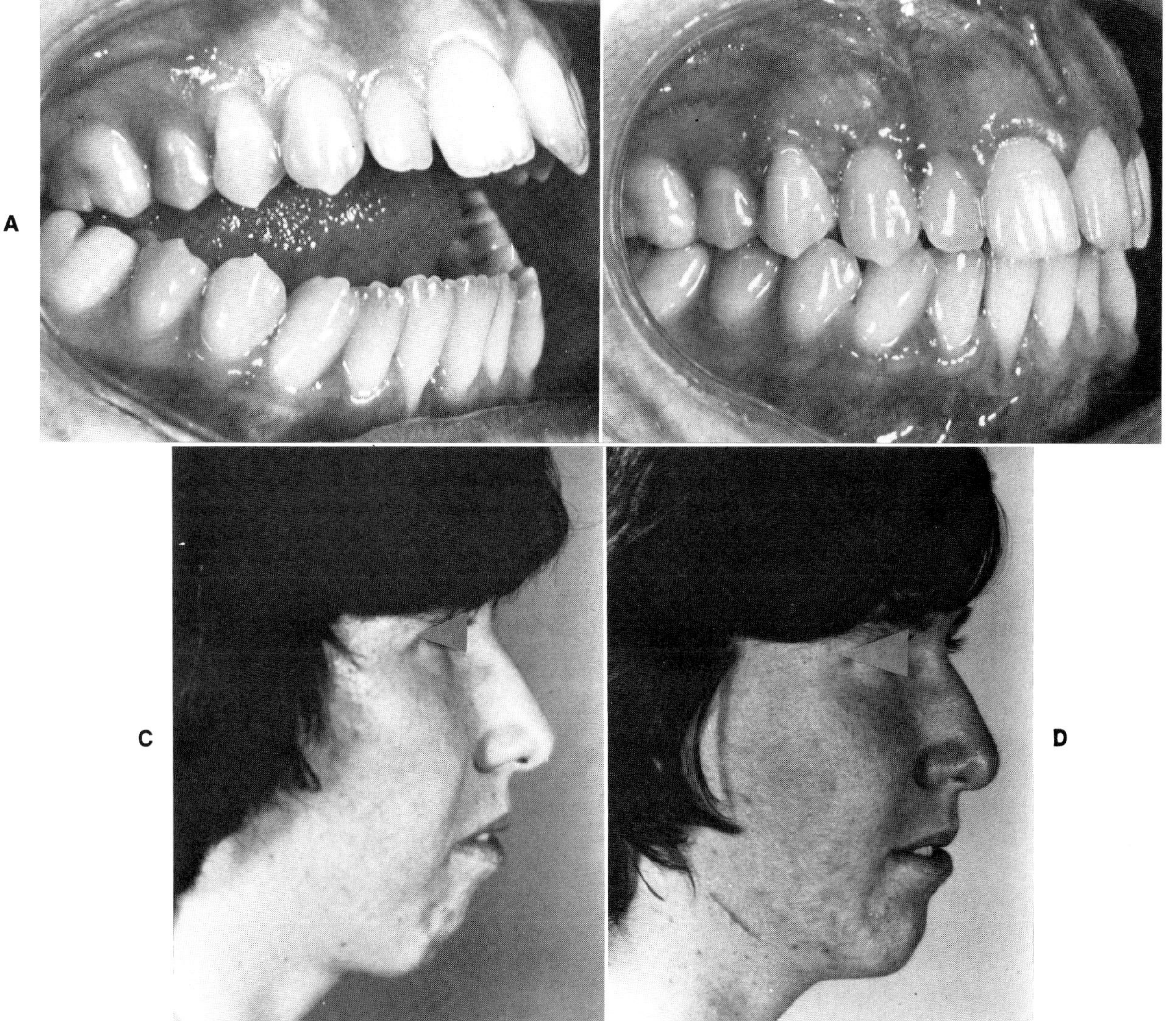

Fig. 6-97. A, Retrognathic mandible and severe apertognathia of 23-year-old patient. **B ,** Appearance 2 months after an intraoral sagittal split procedure to advance mandible and point chin up; and a bilateral posterior maxillary osteotomy with approximately 3 mm impaction of posterior segments from distal aspect of canines to include second molars. Patient's profile before, **C,** and after, **D,** surgery. (Courtesy Dr. Donald Steed.)

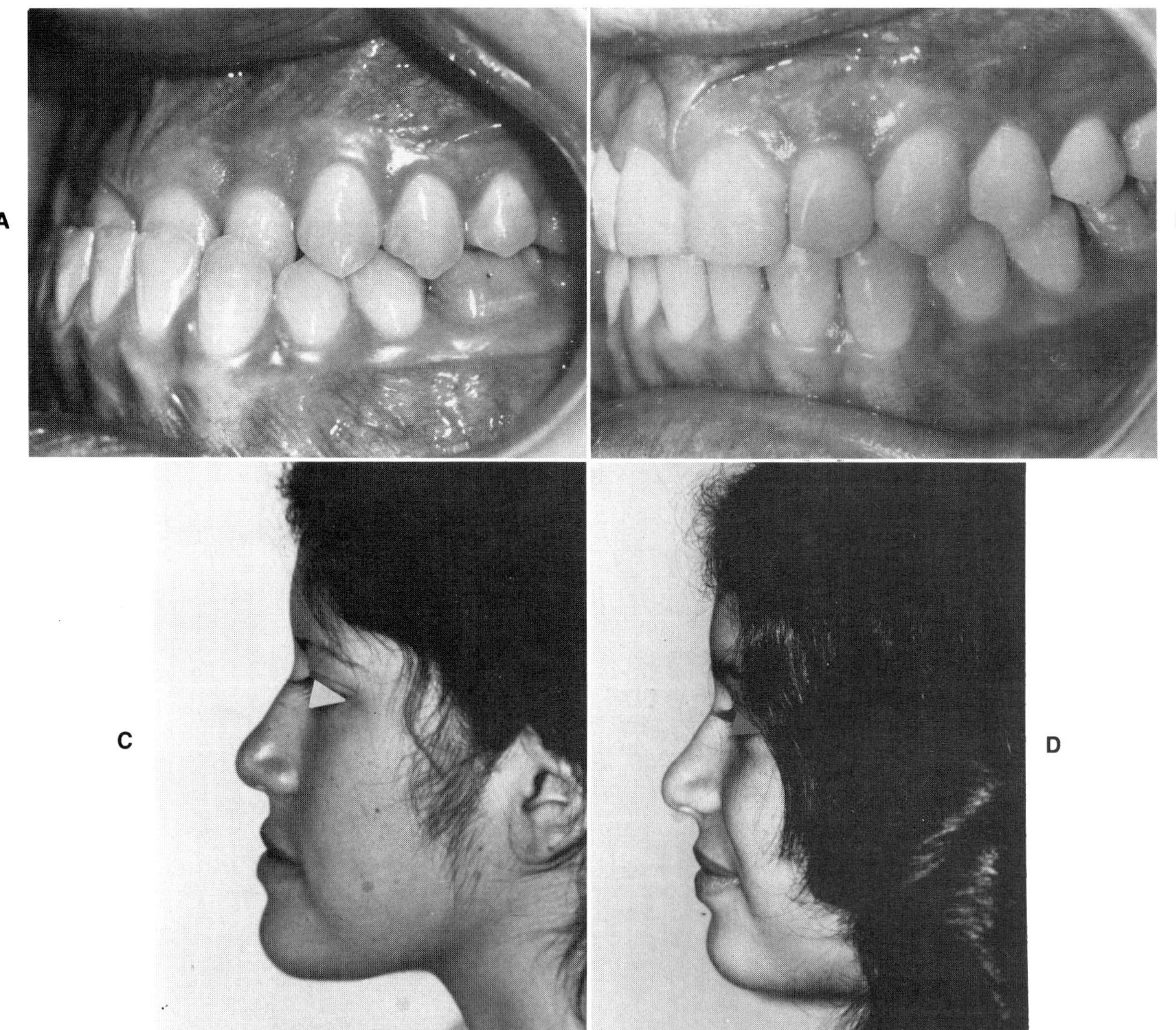

Fig. 6-98. A, Prognathic mandible and retrognathic or hypoplastic maxilla in 17-year-old patient. **B,** Occlusion 2 months after mandibular bilateral vertical subcondylar osteotomy and Le Fort I maxillary osteotomy. Profile before **C,** and after, **D,** surgery. (Courtesy Dr. Donald Steed.)

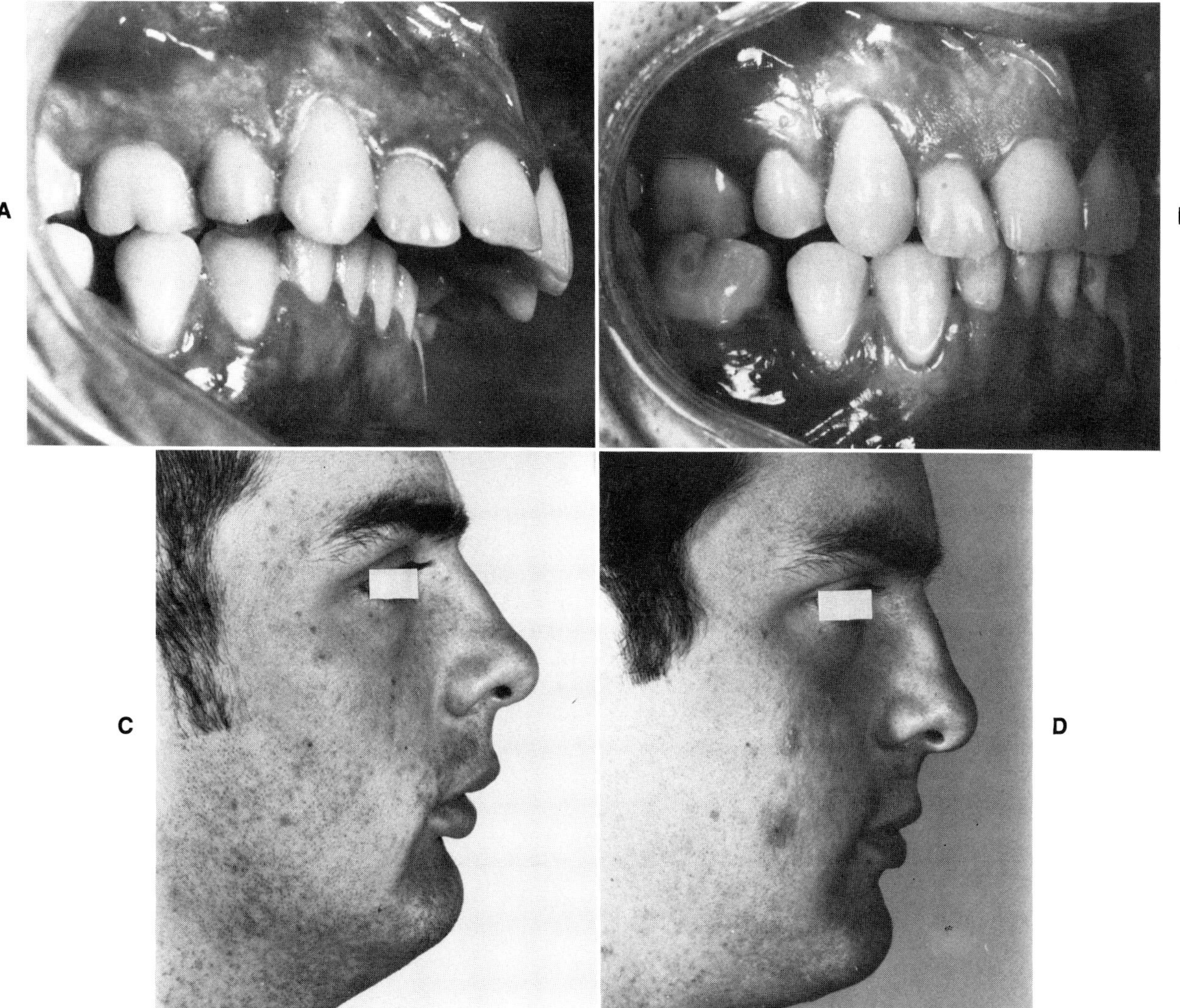

Fig. 6-99. A, Retrognathic mandible in 20-year-old patient. **B,** Occlusion 2 months after intraoral sagittal split of mandible with advancement of mandible. Profile before, **C,** and 2 months after, **D,** surgery. (Courtesy Dr. Donald Steed.)

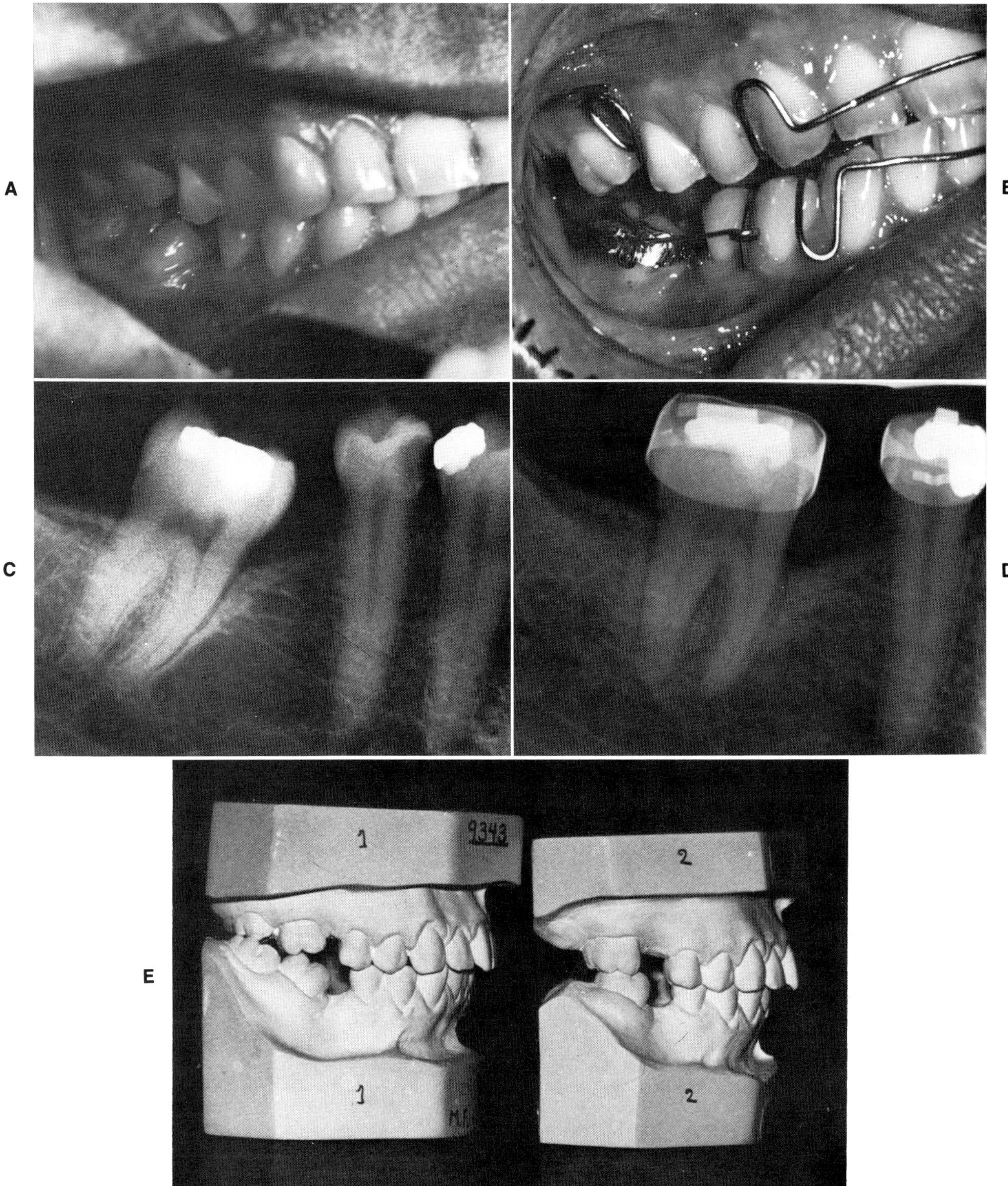

Fig. 6-100. A, Mandibular second molar tipped lingually and mesially into first molar space. Maxillary second molar tipped mesially. **B,** Maxillary and mandibular orthodontic appliances for uprighting teeth. Third molars have been removed. Mandibular molar before **C,** and after, **D,** treatment. **E,** Diagnostic casts before and after treatment. (Courtesy Undergraduate Orthodontics, University of Texas Health Science Center at San Antonio.)

geon are essential in treating patients with malrelation of the jaws.

Tipped or malposed teeth

A posterior tooth tends to drift forward into the space created by the removal of the tooth mesial to it. Limited orthodontic procedures for minor tooth movement can be used to upright the tipped tooth to allow the placement of an artificial tooth of more normal size (Fig. 6-100).

Teeth in severe buccoversion or linguoversion should be evaluated. At times the removal of the malposed tooth will simplify the design of the prosthesis. At other times the retention of the malposed tooth will significantly improve the prognosis of treatment. Limited orthodontics for minor tooth movement can be used to move the tooth to a more favorable position (Fig. 6-101).

Occlusion

The mounted diagnostic casts are also used for an evaluation of the patient's occlusion. The information obtained from the analysis of the occlusion should be correlated with other clinical findings.

A common finding is the presence of occlusal interferences (Fig. 6-102). Over 90% of the population has a discrepancy between centric jaw relation and maximum occlusal contact, or centric occlusion. Partially edentulous patients have an even greater probability of having premature occlusal contacts because of the drifting and migration of teeth that usually accompany the loss of continuity of the dental arch (Fig. 6-103). Most patients can adapt to imperfections in the occlusion so that the premature contacts do not become traumatic factors. However, there is a limit to physiologic adaptation to the imperfections or disharmony of occlusion. This limit may be surpassed if additional discrepancies

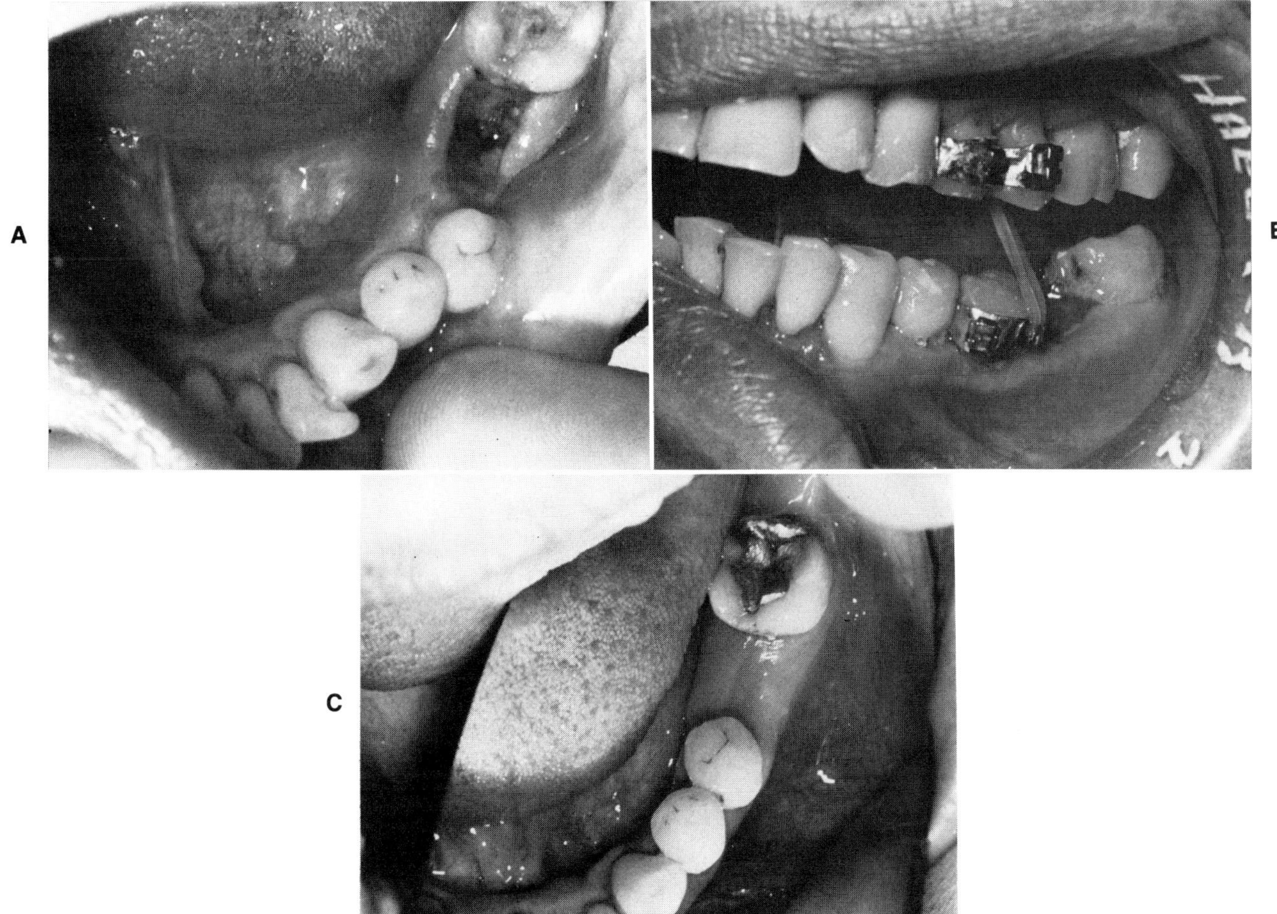

Fig. 6-101. A, Second premolar in buccoversion and rotated. **B,** Rubber ligature used to correct position. **C,** After treatment. (Courtesy Undergraduate Orthodontics, University of Texas Health Science Center at San Antonio.)

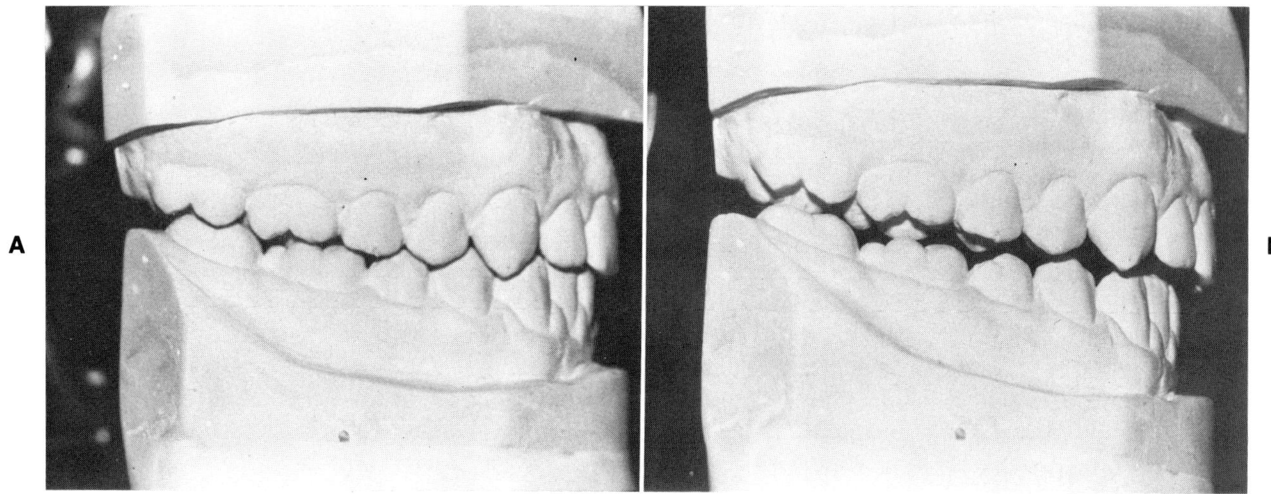

Fig. 6-102. A, Casts at maximum occlusal contact, or centric occlusion. **B,** Initial occlusal contact with casts related with mandible at most retruded position, or patient's centric jaw relation.

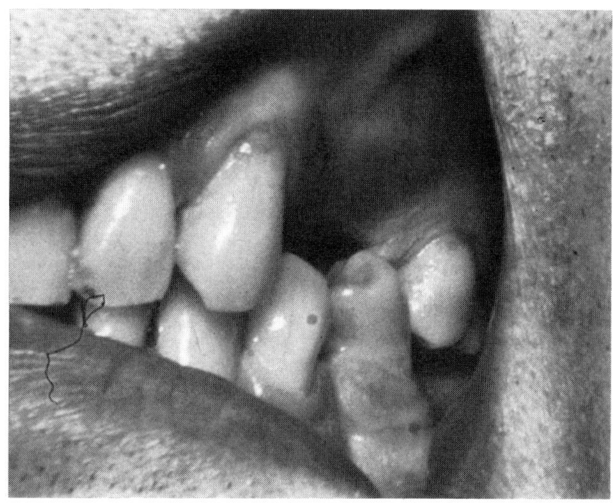

Fig. 6-103. Severe tipping, rotation, and overeruption of teeth into edentulous areas of opposing arches.

are added to the occlusion or if central nervous system tension increases. The result may be increased hypertonic muscular response leading to bruxism. Severe bruxism can injure the teeth, the periodontium, and the temporomandibular joint and may initiate muscle spasm, pain, or discomfort. The most common causes of bruxism are (1) occlusal interferences between centric jaw relation and centric occlusion and (2) balancing side contacts.

Efforts to overcome occlusal interferences may become traumatic and cause clinical symptoms and radiographic signs.

The clinical symptoms of traumatic occlusion follow:
1. Excessive wear of the teeth, which may include chipping or fracture of the teeth (Fig. 6-104).
2. A change in, or a loss of, the supporting structures, which may include increased mobility, tooth migration, and pain during and after occlusal contact.
3. Involvement of the neuromuscular mechanism of the temporomandibular joint, which may include muscle spasm, muscle pain, and joint symptoms.

The radiographic signs of traumatic occlusion follow:
1. Widening of the periodontal ligament space with either thickening or loss of lamina dura.
2. Periapical or furcation radiolucency.
3. Resorption of alveolar bone.
4. Root resorption.

Role of occlusal equilibration. Occlusal equilibration is the selective grinding or coronal reshaping of teeth with the intent of equalizing occlusal stress, producing simultaneous occlusal contacts, or harmonizing cuspal relations.

It would seem logical that the solution to the problem of occlusal interferences would be to equilibrate the teeth of every patient whose centric jaw relation and centric occlusion do not coincide. However, occlusal equilibration should not be accomplished for every patient with occlusal interferences. Many patients have a great enough resistive capacity that occlusal forces are not destructive regardless of the occlusal relationships of the teeth. If occlusal equilibration were accomplished on these individuals, an "occlusal sense" or continued "awareness of the occlusion" may be developed

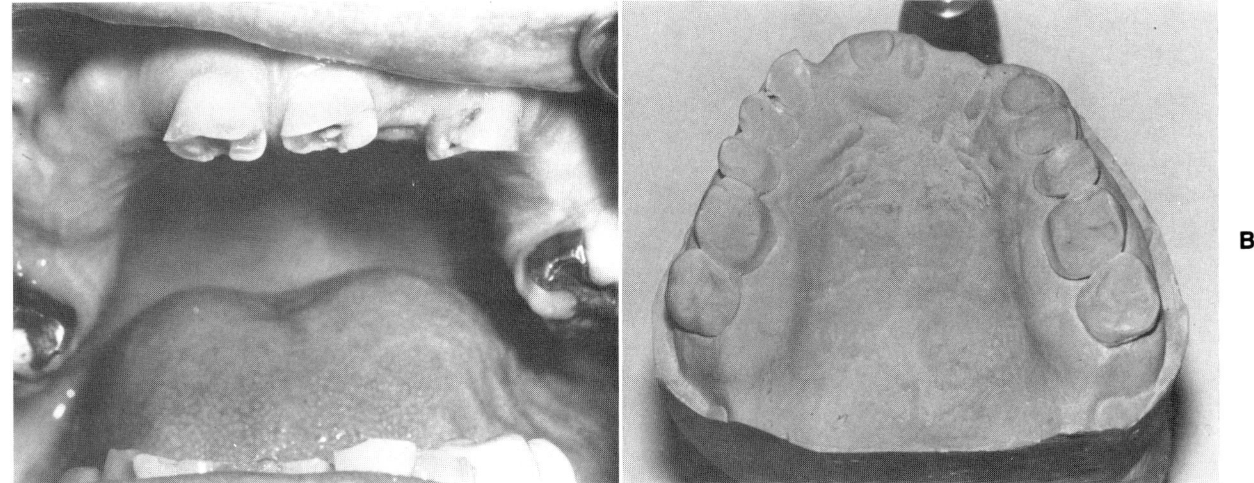

Fig. 6-104. A, Excessive occlusal abrasion of anterior teeth caused by severe bruxism. **B,** Extensive occlusal abrasion of all remaining teeth caused by bruxism.

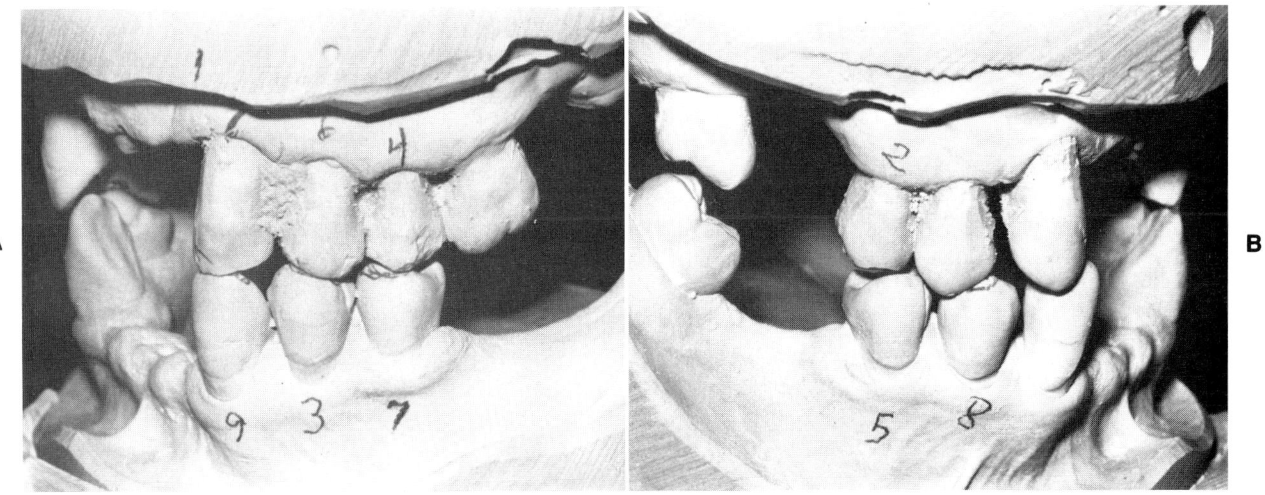

Fig. 6-105. Mounted duplicate casts equilibrated to determine whether equilibration of teeth is feasible and to serve as a blueprint for grinding in mouth. Numbers indicate sequence in which areas on teeth are ground. Ground areas are circled in red. **A,** Left side. **B,** Right side.

and could lead to destructive neuromuscular activity. Faulty occlusal equilibration may induce severe trauma from occlusion. In addition, extensive occlusal equilibration should never be initiated on a patient with acute temporomandibular joint dysfunction. The symptoms and muscle spasm should be eliminated through the use of an occlusal splint before occlusal adjustment is initiated.

Occlusal equilibration should be accomplished only for those individuals who have a definite need for this treatment, such as those with symptoms of traumatic occlusion. Balancing side or nonchewing side interferences, which are usually the most destructive eccentric interferences, should always be eliminated.

If the decision is made to equilibrate the occlusion, the equilibration should be accomplished before any definitive restorative procedures. Usually it is beneficial to perform the equilibration on a duplicate set of diagnostic casts to determine whether equilibration is feasible and what the final result may be. This trial equilibration can serve as a blueprint for the grinding in the mouth if the sequence of the grinding is recorded (Fig. 6-105). The diagnostic equilibration may indicate the need for the placement of cast restorations, repositioning of teeth, removal of teeth, or a combination of these procedures to achieve an acceptable result.

Treat at centric jaw relation or centric occlusion?

The decision whether to construct a prosthesis at centric jaw relation or centric occlusion must be made in the diagnostic phase of treatment. The following clinical situations indicate construction of the prosthesis at centric jaw relation:

1. Coincidence of centric jaw relation and centric occlusion.
2. Absence of posterior tooth contacts because the opposing arch is completely edentulous or because of the pattern of missing teeth.
3. Situation in which all posterior tooth contacts are to be restored with cast restorations.
4. Only a few remaining posterior contacts.
5. Minimum alveolar support for all the remaining teeth that can be made acceptable with minimum occlusal equilibration.
6. Anterior slide from centric jaw relation and symptoms of traumatic occlusion of the anterior teeth.
7. Clinical symptoms of occlusal trauma.

In the absence of these indications, the removable partial denture should be constructed at centric occlusion. Special care must be taken in the construction and fitting of the prosthesis to make certain that no new interferences are built into the occlusion at centric jaw relation or between centric jaw relation and centric occlusion.

Diagnostic wax-up

A diagnostic wax-up is a valuable diagnostic tool, especially if multiple crowns or fixed partial dentures need to be constructed in conjunction with a removable partial denture (Fig. 6-106). Problems involving the po-

A

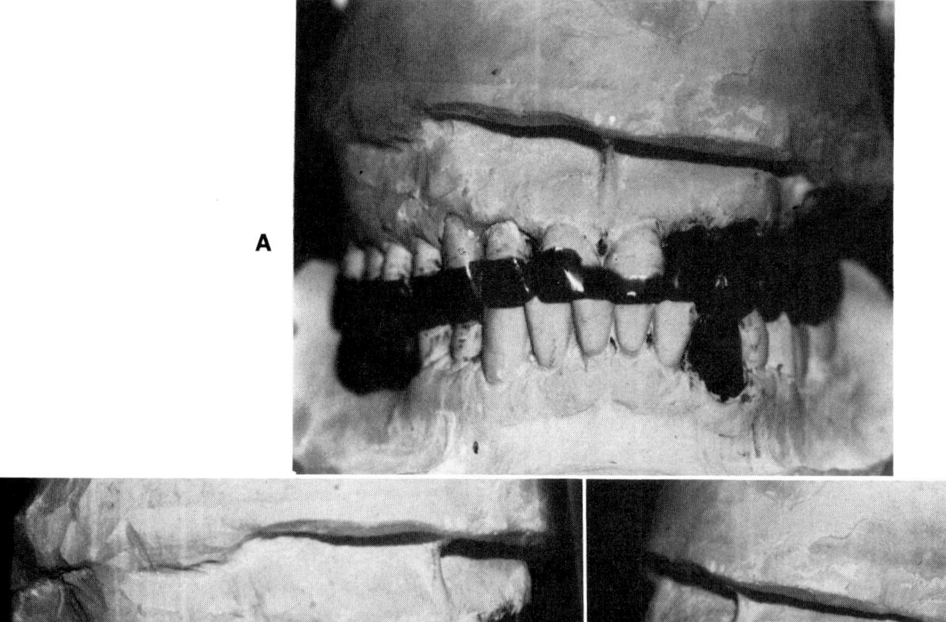

B

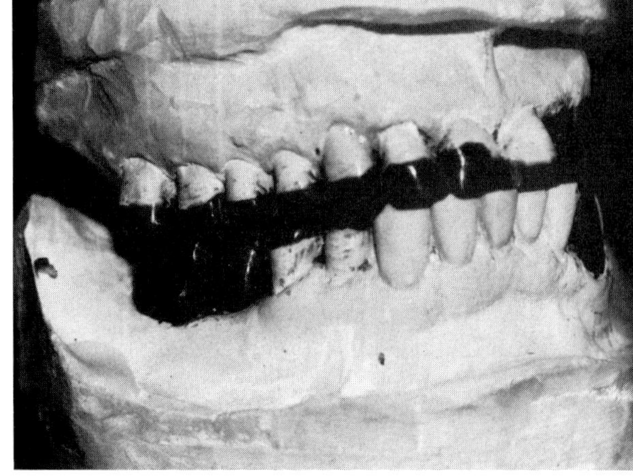

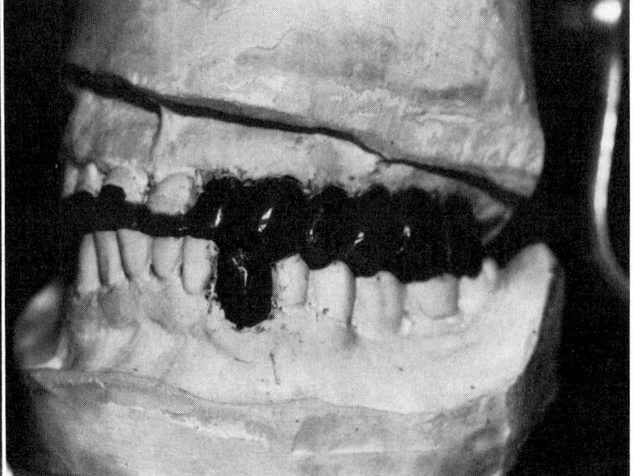

C

Fig. 6-106. Diagnostic wax up accomplished for patient whose treatment includes multiple crowns, fixed partial dentures, and a maxillary and mandibular removable partial denture. **A,** Anterior view. **B,** Right side. **C,** Left side.

sition and relationship of the remaining teeth become apparent. The diagnostic wax-up provides a guide for tooth preparation and helps indicate problems that may be encountered in positioning cusps and in establishing acceptable occlusal contacts.

CONSULTATION REQUESTS

Consultation with appropriate medical or dental specialists is often necessary to ensure the safety and efficiency of the patient's treatment. Consultation requests and reports should always be written to avoid errors or misunderstanding in communication. The written consultation becomes a permanent part of the patient's record and will be available for future reference if needed.

The request for medical consultation should include information about the patient's oral condition and should indicate the dental procedures to be used in treatment. Specific questions concerning the need for premedication or supportive medical care may be appropriate.

Consultation requests to dental specialists should indicate whether the patient is being referred for an opinion or for specific treatment. The dentist's evaluation of the present oral condition and the tentative sequence of treatment should also be included. Close communication and cooperation are essential whenever more than one dentist is responsible for the treatment of the patient.

DEVELOPMENT OF TREATMENT PLAN

The development of an appropriate treatment plan for a partially edentulous patient can be extremely difficult. A great number of factors influence the ultimate success of treatment. An adequate level of oral hygiene is one of the most important factors, and yet is one of the most elusive.

The patient with insufficient teeth for adequate function or esthetics and poor oral hygiene presents a dilemma for the dentist. Possible treatment plans range from not treating the patient to removing all the teeth and constructing complete dentures. The extremes of treatment, are not always appropriate, and some degree of compromise between the ideal and practical considerations becomes necessary. It is in these gray areas of decision making that the dentist's clinical judgment is put to its greatest test. It is essential that the judgments and decisions be based on complete evaluation of all appropriate diagnostic data. Diagnostic casts that have been mounted and designed are essential in the planning for treatment for the partially edentulous patient. The procedures required to treat the patient should then be placed into a logical treatment sequence.

The treatment of the partially edentulous patient can be divided into five phases. Two phases may overlap, but the overall treatment plan should reflect the sequence of these five phases of treatment. Procedures within each phase should be completed on a priority basis depending on the patient's needs.

Phase I

1. Collection and evaluation of the diagnostic data, including a diagnostic mounting and the analysis and design of diagnostic casts
2. Immediate treatment to control pain or infection
3. Biopsy or referral of patient
4. Development of a treatment plan
5. Initiation of education and motivation of patient

Phase II

1. Removal of deep caries and placement of temporary restorations
2. Extirpation of inflamed or necrotic pulp tissues
3. Removal of nonretainable teeth
4. Periodontal treatment
5. Construction of interim prosthesis for function or esthetics
6. Occlusal equilibration
7. Reinforcement of education and motivation of patient

Phase III

1. Preprosthetic surgical procedures
2. Definitive endodontic procedures
3. Definitive restoration of teeth, including placement of cast metallic restorations
4. Fixed partial denture construction
5. Reinforcement of education and motivation of patient

Phase IV

1. Construction of removable partial denture
2. Reinforcement of education and motivation of patient

Phase V

1. Postinsertion care
2. Periodic recall
3. Reinforcement of education and motivation of patient

LENGTH OF APPOINTMENT

The length of this appointment can vary greatly, depending on the complexity of the problems presented by the patient. A good estimate of the time requirement can be made at the first appointment. If consultations with medical or dental specialists are needed, it is obvious that not all the necessary diagnostic procedures can be accomplished at this appointment. Using shortcuts or omitting diagnostic procedures is based on false economy because failure of treatment may be the ultimate price.

The dental student should plan on using 3 or 4 hours to complete the procedures required for this appointment.

REFERENCES

Akerly, W.B.: Prosthodontic treatment of traumatic overlap of anterior teeth, J. Prosthet. Dent. **38**:26, 1977.

Ramfjord, S.P., and Ash, M.M., Jr.: Occlusion, ed. 2, Philadelphia, 1971, W.B. Saunders Co.

BIBLIOGRAPHY

Alexander, J.M., and Van Seckels, J.E.: Posterior maxillary osteotomies: an aid for a difficult prosthodontic problem, J. Prosthet. Dent. **41:** 614-617, 1979.

Applegate, O.C.: An evaluation of the support for the removable partial denture, J. Prosthet. Dent. **10**:112-123, 1960.

Bhaskar, S.N.: Synopsis of oral pathology, ed. 5, St. Louis, 1977, The C.V. Mosby Co.

Bollender, C.L., Swenson, R.D. and Yamane, G.: Evaluation of treatment of inflammatory papillary hyperplasia of the palate, J. Prosthet. Dent. **15**:1013-1022, 1965.

Brasher, W.J., and Rees, T.D.: The medical consultation: its role in dentistry, J. Am. Dent. Assoc. **95**:961-964, 1977.

Carranza, F.A., Jr.: Glickman's clinical periodontology, ed. 5, Philadelphia, 1979, W.B. Saunders Co.

Christiansen, R.L.: Rationale of the facebow in maxillary cast mounting, J. Prosthet. Dent. **9**:388-398, 1959.

Epker, B.N., and Bronson, J.: Surgical-prosthetic correction of dentofacial deformities, J. Am. Dent. Assoc. **97**:184-192, 1978.

Goldman, H.M., and Cohen, D.: Periodontal therapy, ed. 6, St. Louis, 1980, The C.V. Mosby Co.

Langland, O.E., and Sippy, F.H.: Textbook of dental radiography, Springfield, Ill., 1973, Charles C Thomas.

Mashberg, A.: Erythroplasia: The earliest sign of asymptomatic oral cancer, J. Am. Dent. Assoc. **96**:615-620, 1978.

McCarthy, P.L., and Shklar, G.: Diseases of the oral mucosa, ed. 2, Philadelphia, 1980, Lea and Febiger.

McNeill, C., and others: Craniomandibular (TMJ) disorders—the state of the art, J. Prosthet. Dent. **44**:434-437, 1980.

Miller, E.L.: Clinical management of denture induced inflammations, J. Prosthet. Dent. **38**:362-365, 1977.

Miller, E.L.: Sometimes overlooked, preprosthetic surgery, J. Prosthet. Dent.**36**:484-490, 1976.

Millstein, P.L., and others: Determination of the accuracy of wax interocclusal registrations, Part II, J. Prosthet. Dent. **29**:40-45, 1973.

Mopsik, E.R., and others: Surgical intervention to reestablish adequate intermaxillary space before fixed or removable prosthodontics, J. Am. Dent. Assoc. **95**:957-980, 1977.

Palomo, F., and Kopczyk, R.A.: Rationale and methods of crown lengthening, J. Am. Dent. Assoc. **96**:257-260, 1978.

Pruden, W.H. II: The role of study casts in diagnosis and treatment planning, J. Prosthet. Dent. **10**:707-710, 1960.

Reynolds, J.M.: Occlusal wear facets, J. Prosthet. Dent. **24**:367-372, 1970.

Scott, A.S., and Frew, A.L., Jr.: Orthognatic surgery: combined maxillary and mandibular osteotomies with variations of surgical modalities, J. Am. Dent. Assoc. **93**:98-104, 1976.

Sheppard, I.M., and Sheppard, S.M.: Characteristics of temporomandibular joint problems, J. Prosthet. Dent. **38**:180-191, 1977.

Stafne, E.C., and Gebilisco, J.A.: Oral roentgenographic diagnosis, Philadelphia, 1975, W.B. Saunders Co.

Starshak, T.J.: Preprosthetic oral surgery, St. Louis, 1971, The C.V. Mosby Co.

Turner, C., and Shaffer, F.W.: Planning the treatment of the complex prosthodontic case, J. Am. Dent. Assoc. **97**:992-993, 1978.

Weinberg, L.A.: An evaluation of basic articulators and their concepts, I and II. J. Prosthet. Dent. **13**:622-633, 1963.

Weinberg, L.A.: An evaluation of the face-bow mounting, J. Prosthet. Dent. **11**:32-42, 1961.

Wood, C., Jr., Harrison, B., Ackerson, D., and McCurdy, T.: Coordination of the goals of orthodontic, surgical, and prosthetic dentistry, anterior maxillary osteotomy, J. Am. Dent. Assoc. **97**:650-655, 1978.

Wood, N.K.: Treatment planning: a pragmatic approach, St. Louis, 1978, The C.V. Mosby Co.

Zarb, G.A., and others: Prosthodontic treatment for partially edentulous patients, St. Louis, 1978, The C.V. Mosby Co.

7 Survey and design

CAST SURVEYOR

The current clinical practice of removable partial prosthodontics is more accurate, physically less tiring, and certainly more enjoyable than when impressions were made in plaster of paris, sectioned to be removed from the mouth, and reassembled to produce a cast on which a removable partial denture was then constructed. Until the 1950s most removable partial dentures were designed and constructed by the time-honored method of "eyeballing." A prosthesis made on the basis of educated guesses as to the location of interferences and beneficial undercuts required many hours of additional work as the dentist tried to fit it to the remaining teeth. Offending parts of metal were cut away and pieces of the framework were cut and reassembled until finally the removable denture would, or would nearly, fit in the mouth. The forces such a prosthesis would exert on the remaining teeth and soft tissues are not difficult to imagine. During this period a removable partial denture was considered by many to be a stepping stone on the path to complete dentures, and unfortunately this was too often true.

The turning point in the change of partial denture construction from guesswork based on clinical experience to scientifically based procedure was the appearance of the dental surveyor in 1918. Many advances made in the field of removable partial dentures have made the practice more accurate, but the one piece of equipment without which the modern clinical practice of removable partial prosthodontics would not be possible is the surveyor.

The surveyor is essentially a parallelometer, an instrument used to determine the relative parallelism of surfaces of teeth or other areas on a cast of the jaws. The partially edentulous mouth consists of groups of natural teeth interspersed with spaces where the residual ridge may be complicated with bony exostoses or undercuts. In the planning of a removable partial denture, the shapes of teeth that will serve as abutment teeth must be analyzed and coordinated with the shapes of the other teeth that will play a part in supporting the partial denture. The contour of adjacent soft tissue and edentulous ridges that will be covered by, or help support, the prosthesis must also be considered in the planning process. The best and most accurate way this can be accomplished is through the use of the dental surveyor.

Dr. A.J. Fortunati is thought to be the first person to employ a mechanical device to determine the relative parallelism of tooth surfaces. At a clinic in Boston in 1918 he demonstrated a method for charting correct clasp placement by using a parallelometer. The first such device to be produced commercially, the Ney instrument, was made available in 1923; it remains the most widely used surveyor in the dental field (Fig. 7-1). There are other surveyors on the market today, many of them rather complicated machines, but in the long run they all accomplish the same purpose. The Wills surveyor by Jelenko is the second most widely used (Fig. 7-2).

Surveyors may vary somewhat as to construction, but most have the following parts:

1. A level platform that is parallel to the bench top and on which the cast holder is moved.
2. A vertical arm that supports the superstructure.
3. A horizontal arm that extends at a right angle from the vertical column from which extends the other part of the superstructure, the surveying tool. (In the Ney surveyor the horizontal arm is fixed, whereas in the Wills instrument it may revolve horizontally around the vertical column.)
4. A surveying tool that drops vertically from the horizontal arm. The surveying tool is capable of movement in a vertical direction. (In the Wills surveyor the surveying tool is spring loaded. When the tool is not in use, it is held at its most vertical position by spring tension. In the Ney instrument the tool is completely passive, dropping to its lowest position unless secured at another height by a locking device.) The lower end of the surveying tool contains a mandrel, in which the special tools used in the surveying procedure may be locked.
5. A cast holder, or surveying table, to which the cast to be studied is attached. The table, equipped with a clamp to lock the cast in place, is mounted on a ball-and-socket joint that permits the cast to be oriented in various horizontal planes so that

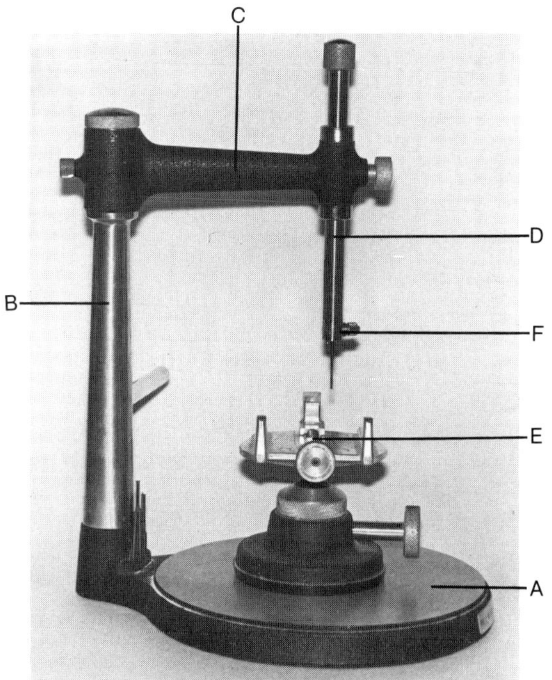

Fig. 7-1. Ney dental surveyor. **A,** Surveying platform. **B,** Vertical column. **C,** Horizontal arm. **D,** Surveying arm. **E,** Cast holder, or surveying table. **F,** Mandrel with attached analyzing rod.

the axial surfaces of the teeth as well as other areas of the cast can be analyzed in relation to the vertical plane (Fig. 7-3).

6. An analyzing rod, or paralleling tool. This tool contacts the convex surface of the object being studied in the same way a tangent contacts a curve. In this way the parallelism of one surface to another may be determined (Fig. 7-4). If a carbon rod or marker is substituted for the analyzing rod and the objects being studied are rotated in contact with the marker, as the horizontal plane of the cast is maintained by the cast holder, a survey line indicating *the height of contour* will be transferred to those surfaces (Fig. 7-5).
7. Additional tools that may be attached to the vertical surveying arm and used in conjuction with the surveyor.
   a. Undercut gauges. These gauges are used to identify the specific amount and location of desired retentive undercut on the surface of an abutment tooth (Fig. 7-6).
   b. Wax knife. This instrument is used in late stages of removable partial denture construction to eliminate or block out areas of undesirable undercuts with wax on the cast before the framework is made (Fig. 7-7).
   c. Carbon marker. The marker may be used to scribe the survey line and to delineate an undercut area of the soft tissue or ridge.

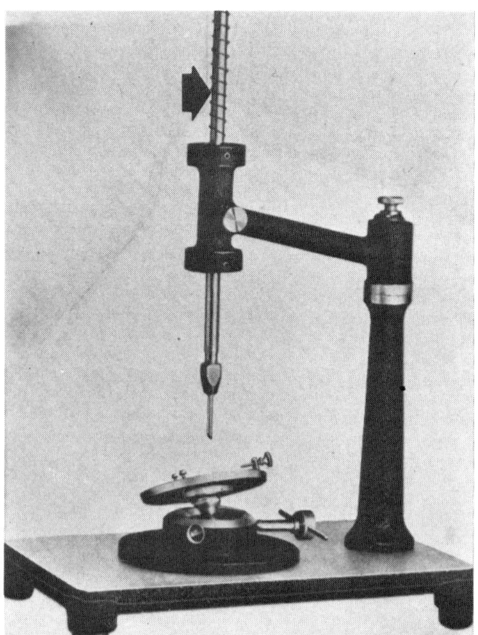

Fig. 7-2. Wills dental surveyor. It is basically the same as the Ney surveyor except that (1) the surveying arm remains in the up, or lifted, position by the action of a spring (arrow), and (2) the horizontal arm is capable of revolving horizontally around the vertical column.

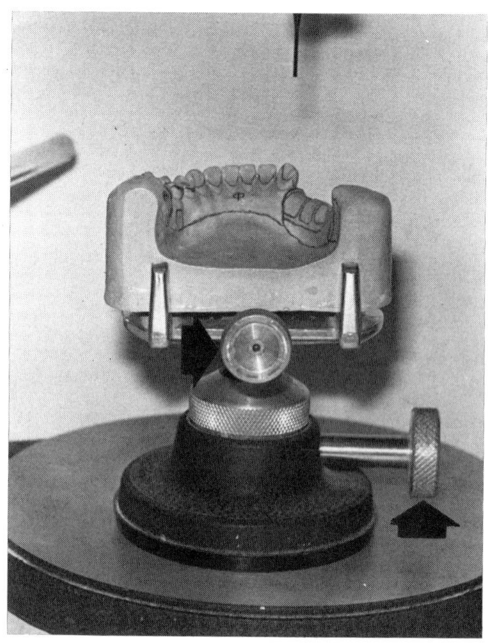

Fig. 7-3. The cast holder, or surveying table. The top locking device (horizontal arrow) locks the cast in place. The lower locking device (vertical arrow) controls the tilt or angle at which the cast is mounted.

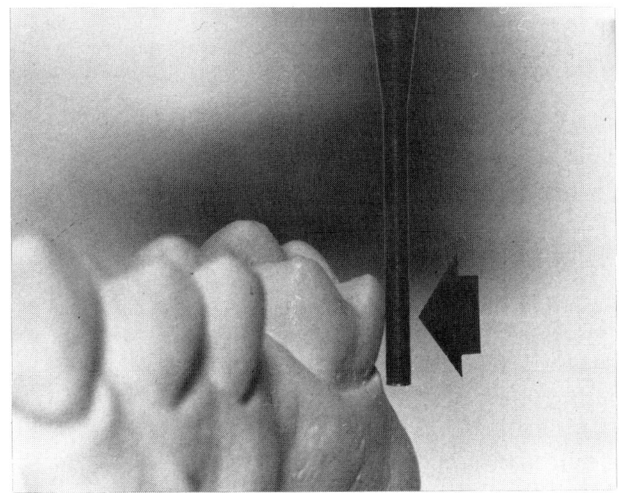

Fig. 7-4. The analyzing rod, or paralleling tool, is fixed in the mandrel of the surveying arm. By holding the analyzing rod against the teeth on a cast, the relative parallelism of the tooth surfaces can be evaluated.

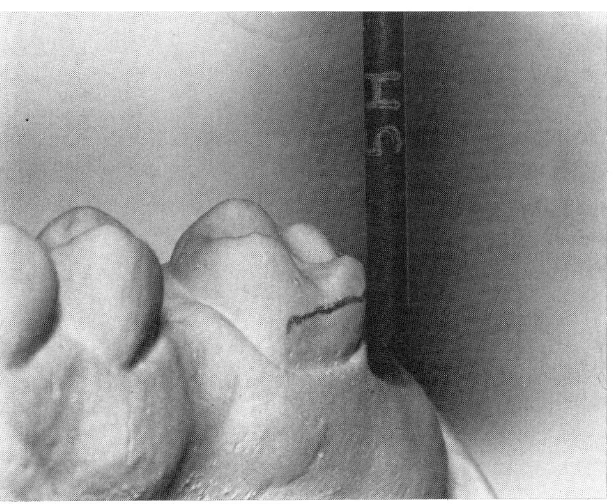

Fig. 7-5. By replacing the analyzing rod in the mandrel with a carbon rod or marker, a line indicating the greatest bulge of the teeth at that horizontal tilt of the cast may be transferred to the teeth of the cast. The line is referred to as the survey line.

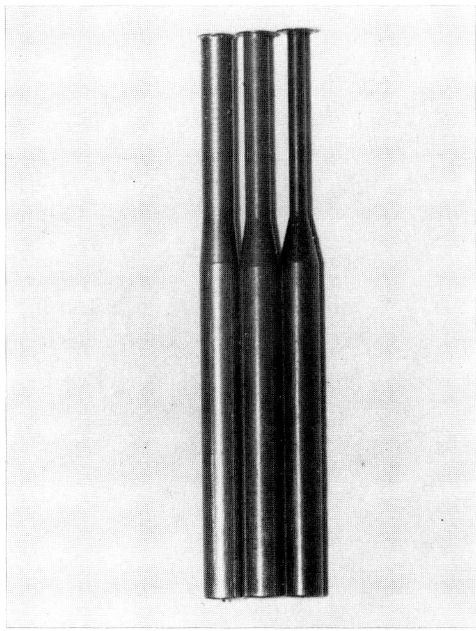

Fig. 7-6. Undercut gauges inserted in the mandrel of the surveying arm are used to locate and measure retentive undercuts on abutment teeth.

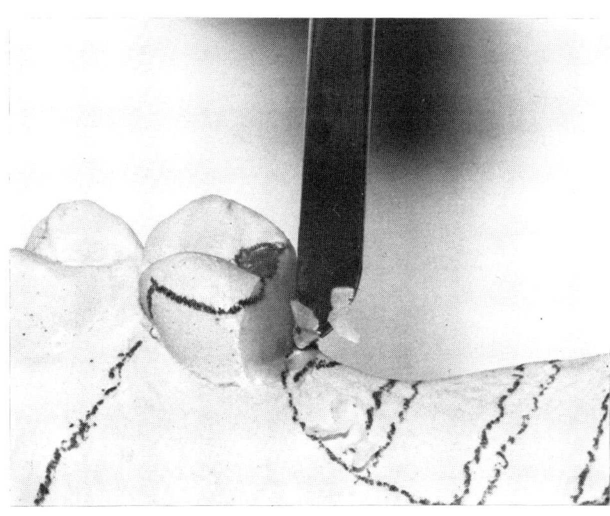

Fig. 7-7. With the wax knife held in the mandrel and the cast firmly secured on the cast holder, the cast may be rotated against the knife so that wax, previously placed in undercuts on the teeth or cast, can be shaved away to eliminate undesirable undercuts. This procedure must be accomplished in the late stages of partial denture construction.

Uses

Surveying diagnostic cast

The diagnostic cast must be surveyed before the treatment plan for the patient can be formulated. The physical characteristics of the mouth recognized through the use of the surveyor influence or dictate the design to be used. Some structures may need to be modified. For example, the relative parallelism of the abutment teeth must be analyzed to learn whether modification of the tooth surfaces by either contouring the enamel surfaces or by the placing of restorations is required. Soft tissue contours must also be studied to determine what effect they may have on the partial denture that is being planned. Undercuts in the soft tissue areas may require surgical removal before the prosthesis will go to place in the mouth.

The position of the cast being studied can be changed on the surveying table to allow the designer to analyze what effect this changing of the tilt will play on the relative parallelism of the structures. The tilt of the cast is spoken of from the viewpoint of a person looking at the cast holder from the rear. Thus if the anterior of the cast is lowered, the cast is said to have an anterior tilt; if the posterior is lowered, the cast has a posterior tilt; if the right side is lowered, as viewed from the rear, the cast has a right tilt; and if the left side is lowered, a left tilt (Fig. 7-8). Any combination of tilts may be used, but excessive tilts must be avoided.

The surveyor is also used to scribe the survey line on the teeth after the final tilt of the cast has been determined. The significance of the survey line is that all rigid components of the partial denture must be kept occlusal to it. Normally only the terminal third of the retentive clasp arm is placed gingival to the survey line. The survey line also helps locate areas of undesirable tooth undercuts that must be avoided or eliminated by contouring or placing restorations on the teeth.

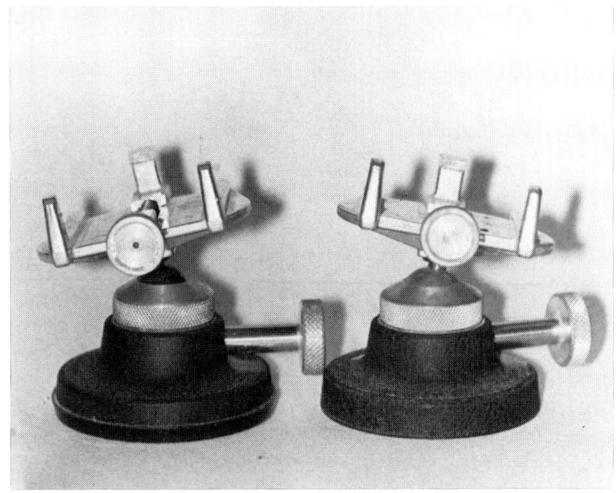

Fig. 7-8. In referring to the tilt of the cast on the cast holder, the designer views the cast from the rear. The cast holder on the left has a left tilt; the one on the right, a right tilt.

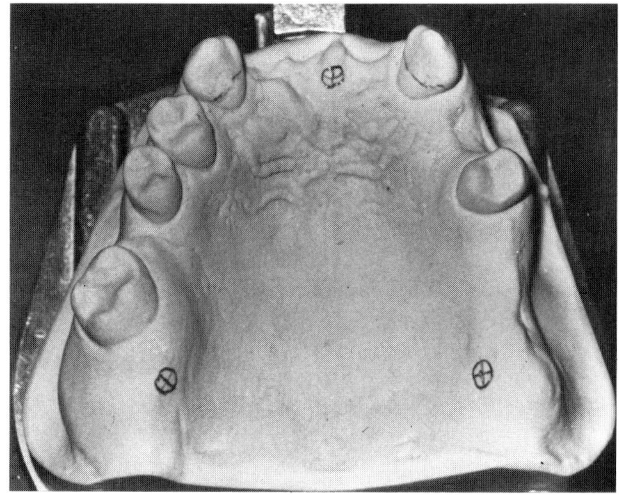

Fig. 7-9. Tripod marks, circled crosses on the cast surface, indicate three points located in the horizontal plane at the selected tilt for the cast. When these points are realigned in the horizontal plane, the cast is in the correct position.

Tripoding the cast

After the final tilt of the cast has been selected, it must be recorded so that the cast may later be repositioned precisely. This procedure is referred to as *tripoding*. The simplest method consists of placing three crossmarks on the tissue portion of the cast, lingual to the remaining teeth, at widely separated points while the cast and the vertical arm of the surveyor are held at fixed positions. This will establish three points on the same horizontal plane and permit the cast, through trial and error, to be repositioned precisely (Fig. 7-9). The tip of the carbon maker should be trimmed at an angle of 45 degrees. This angle prevents unnecessary duplicate marks by the tip of the marker. (Normally all marks or lines made by the carbon marker are made by the side of the marker and not by the tip).

Transferring tripod marks to another cast

It is often necessary to place a second cast of the same mouth on a surveyor at the same tilt the diagnostic cast had originally. This can most accurately be accomplished by using the analyzing rod to select three widely separated and easily identifiable points on the *teeth* of the diagnostic cast that are on the same horizontal plane, with the cast at the correct tilt as determined by use of the tripod marks. These points must not have been altered since the diagnostic cast was made. The second cast may now be placed on the surveying table. The three points selected from the diag-

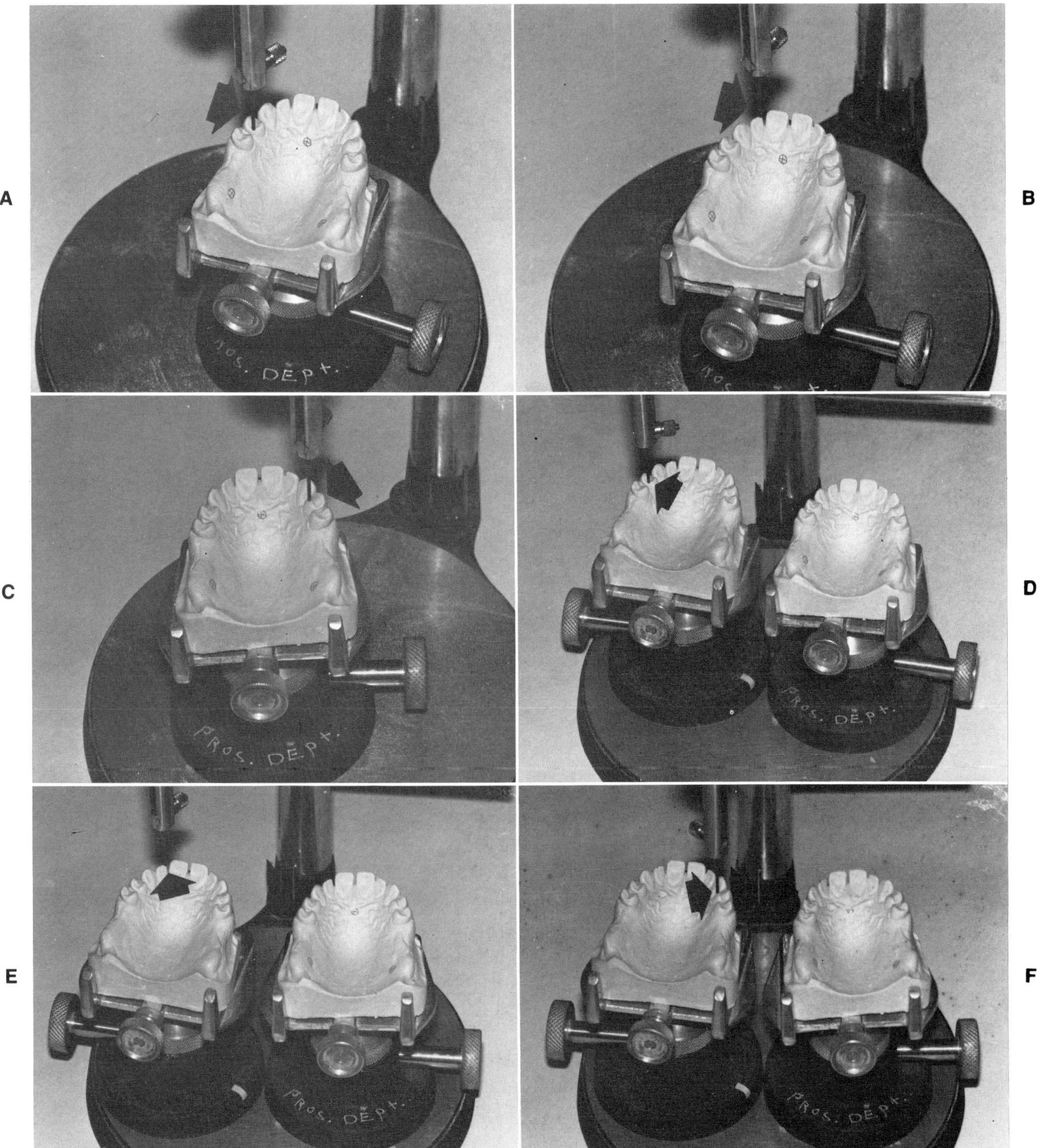

Fig. 7-10. With the original cast mounted on the cast holder at the correct tilt as determined by the tripod marks, three additional points on one horizontal plane must be selected on the surfaces of the teeth to make it possible to mount another cast of the same mouth on the cast holder at the identical tilt. **A,** The analyzing rod touches the distal marginal ridge of the first premolar of the original cast. With the vertical surveying arm remaining fixed, two other points on the same horizontal plane are identified: the incisal edge of the lateral incisor, **B,** and the lingual cusp tip of the left first premolar, **C. D, E,** and **F,** the original cast is at the right, mounted on the cast holder at the proper tilt as verified by the tripod marks. The second cast is shown at the left. The left cast is moved and the tilt of it adjusted until the analyzing rod contacts the three selected points on the same horizontal plane. Once this has been accomplished, the two casts are at the same tilt.

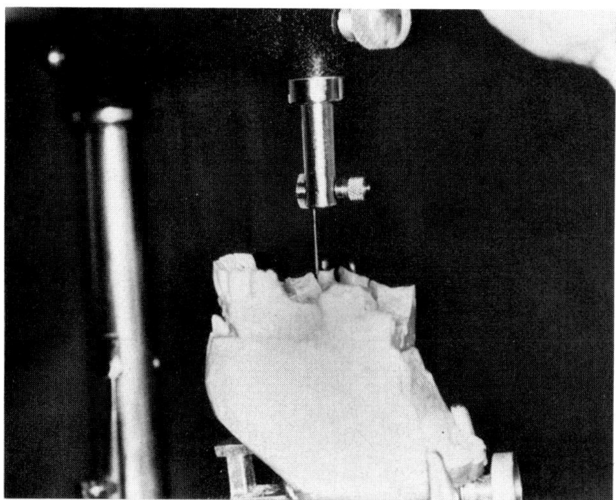

Fig. 7-11. Wax patterns for restorations on abutment teeth, such as crowns, inlays, and onlays, can be shaped to harmonize with the planned partial denture. The working cast with the dies can be positioned on the surveyor, and the wax pattern shaped to accommodate the prosthesis.

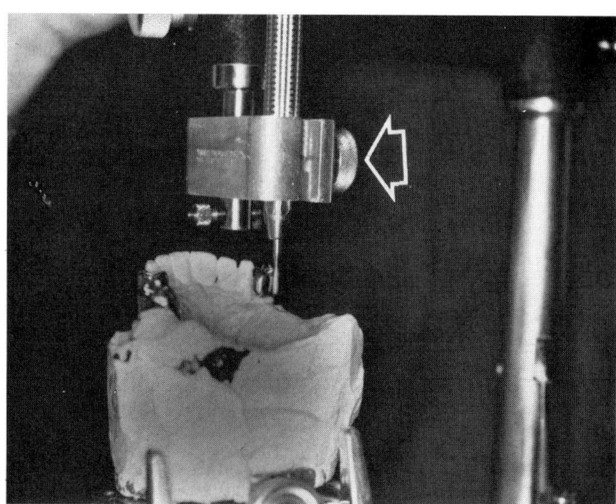

Fig. 7-12. A handpiece holder can be attached to the surveying arm, and a straight handpiece locked in the holder. The cylinder stone in the handpiece will be parallel to the selected path of insertion of the partial denture; it can be used to contour the guiding planes prepared in wax patterns or on cast restorations to be parallel to the path of insertion.

nostic cast must be identified, and, with the analyzing rod held at a fixed vertical position, the cast is tilted in various ways until the tip of the analyzing rod contacts the points on the same horizontal plane. The tilt of the two casts is now exactly the same (Fig. 7-10).

Contouring wax patterns

Cast restorations are frequently required on abutment teeth or other teeth that will be contacted by the partial denture to restore lost portions of the crown following the removal of dental caries or fracture of the tooth or simply to improve the contour of the crown for the placement of the prosthesis. As the restorations are being waxed, the working cast with the dies and wax pattern in position should be placed on the surveying table, and the tilt of the table adjusted to that used when the removable partial denture was designed. Then guiding planes parallel to the path of insertion of the prosthesis may be prepared in the wax patterns. The height of contour of the wax pattern may also be adjusted to the most desirable position for placement of retention and reciprocal clasp arms (Fig. 7-11).

Contouring crowns and cast restorations

The shape of a wax pattern for a cast restoration is usually altered to some degree during the casting and finishing procedures. It is essential that the contours planned in the wax pattern be returned to the completed crown or restoration. This should be accomplished before the final polishing.

The working cast with the restorations in place on the dies is placed on the surveying table at the same tilt as originally used. A handpiece holder is attached to the vertical arm of the surveyor, and a straight handpiece holding a true running mounted cylinder stone is attached to the holder. The handpiece will be parallel to the selected path of insertion, and the guiding planes can be refined by moving the surveying table so that the mounted stone contacts the guiding plane of the crown or restoration (Fig. 7-12). A final check may also be made with the analyzing rod to determine that the height of contour and retentive undercuts remain as planned.

Placing internal attachments and rests

The surveyor is used to position the intracoronal retainers, or internal attachments, in the wax crown pattern on abutment teeth as the patterns are being formed. Absolute parallelism among all the attachments is essential. (The indications and use of internal attachments are discussed in Chapter 22.)

Internal rests, exaggerated occlusal rests with vertical walls and flat floors, can be created by using the surveyor as a form of drill press. A handpiece is attached to the vertical arm of the surveyor by means of a handpiece holder. With appropriate burs in the handpiece, the internal rests can be machined in the wax patterns for crowns on the abutment teeth. After the crowns are cast, the same handpiece and burs are used to refine the rests in the gold castings (Fig. 7-13).

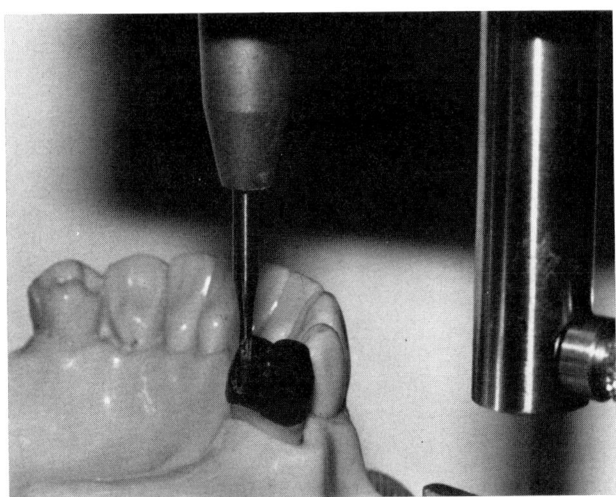

Fig. 7-13. Internal rests can be prepared in wax patterns of restorations by using a straight handpiece in the handpiece holder on a surveyor. The cast must be adjusted to the proper tilt for the path of insertion. A tapered fissure bur is used to cut the internal rest in harmony with the path of insertion.

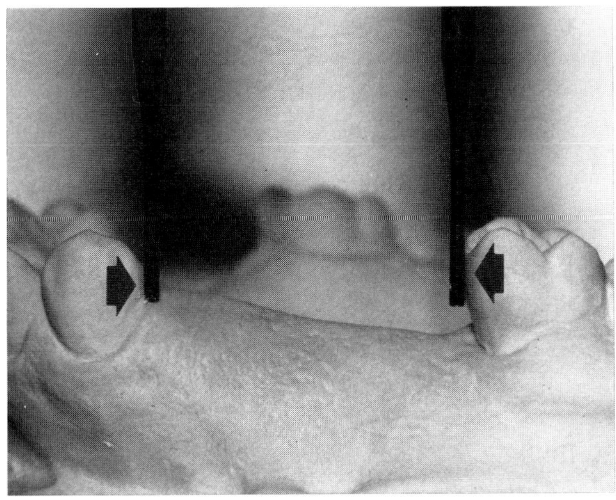

Fig. 7-14. After mouth preparation for the construction of the partial denture has been accomplished, the master cast should be examined on the dental surveyor to verify that the reshaping of the teeth has been done correctly. The master cast must be mounted on the surveying table at the same tilt at which the diagnostic cast was designed. The guiding planes shown here on the molar and premolar must be parallel to each other and to the path of insertion.

Surveying the master cast

The master cast for a removable partial denture is made following the completion of the mouth preparation that was indicated from the design drawn on the diagnostic cast. The mouth preparation may have included the placement of crowns or other restorations on abutment teeth, the development of guiding planes, the contouring of enamel surfaces, and the placement of rest seat preparations. Before the master cast is sent to the laboratory for construction of the removable partial denture framework, it must be surveyed to determine whether the mouth preparation accomplished all it was supposed to. With the master cast mounted on the surveying table at the same tilt at which the diagnostic cast was designed, the dentist checks the parallelism of the guiding planes, the height of contour, and the retentive undercuts (Fig. 7-14). In the event the mouth preparation did not produce the desired results, either the mouth preparation must be reaccomplished and new impressions made or a slight change in the tilt of the master cast may bring about an acceptable solution.

Important considerations in use of dental surveyor

The dental profession as a whole has been slow in accepting the routine practice of using the dental surveyor. Too often the profession has relegated the use of this diagnostic tool to the hands of the laboratory technician. It should be remembered that when a laboratory technician receives a cast from a dentist on which he is to construct a removable partial denture, there is nothing the technician can do but accept that cast as it is. He cannot alter the slope of the stone teeth to improve the position of the height of contour so that a retentive clasp may be located in the gingival third of the tooth for better esthetics and mechanical advantage. He cannot cut away a bony exostosis on the edentulous ridge to permit greater ridge coverage by the denture base. Thus it is essential that the dentist use the surveyor before planning the treatment for the patient.

All the many variables that occur on each diagnostic cast must be weighed before the design of the prosthesis is begun. The ultimate goal is a partial denture that will go to place smoothly over the teeth and soft tissue, will function as it was planned, and will remain in place by resisting dislodging forces. The problems faced in designing such a prosthesis are both biologic and mechanical.

The problems that a technician faces by not being able to alter the surfaces of a master cast are ones the dentist should not have to face if the planning process is carried out at the start of treatment. By altering the horizontal tilt of a cast on the surveying table, the technician may be able to eliminate or control some difficulties with undesirable undercuts, but the solution he arrives at is seldom the best possible plan of treatment or design. It must be considered a compromise and too often not one that enhances the health of the patient. The dentist, on the other hand, if he studies the diagnostic cast with the surveyor, can identify tooth con-

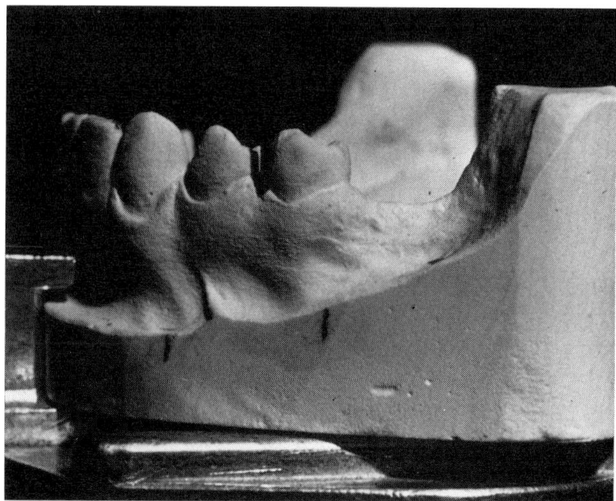

Fig. 7-15. Examination of a cast on the dental surveyor should always be started with the plane formed by the occlusal surfaces of the remaining teeth horizontal (parallel to the base of the surveyor).

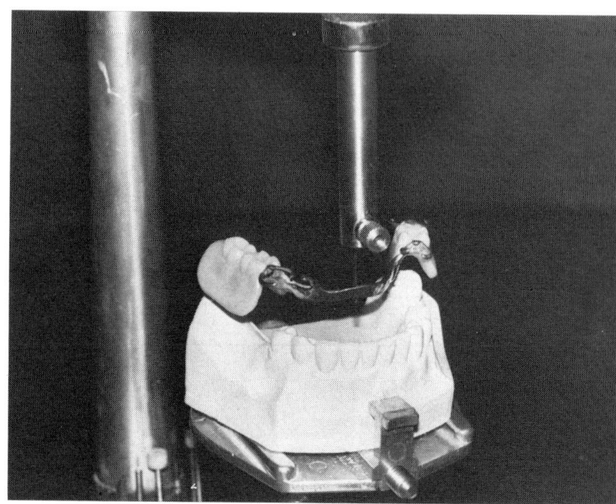

Fig. 7-16. The path of insertion is the direction in which the removable partial denture is placed on or withdrawn from the abutment teeth. It will always be parallel to the vertical arm of the surveyor.

tours or soft tissue irregularities that should be corrected (for example, by surgery, enameloplasty, or the placement of restorations) before the construction of the prosthesis is begun.

A surveyor, then, makes it possible to design a removable partial denture so that the resilient and nonresilient sections go to place in the mouth as a single unit, free from interferences from either tooth or soft tissue convexities, which, when in place in the mouth, will resist dislodging forces that would tend to unseat it.

To arrive at this ideal partial denture design, certain steps in the use of the surveyor must be followed. The cast to be studied is attached to the cast holder so that the occlusal surfaces of the remaining teeth are as nearly in a horizontal plane, or as parallel to the base of the surveyor, as possible. This horizontal position must always be used as a starting point (Fig. 7-15). The tilt may be changed to accomplish specific purposes, but exaggerated tilts (more than 30 degrees from the horizontal) must be avoided.

PATH OF INSERTION

The tilt of the cast on the surveyor is contemplated to determine at what angle the partial denture will seat over the remaining teeth and any other obstructions that may be present. This angle that the prosthesis takes as it goes to place is referred to as the *path of insertion*, or path of withdrawal, of the denture (Fig. 7-16). Any exaggerated tilt must be avoided because a patient would be unable to open the mouth sufficiently to accommodate a tilt that is too far from the horizontal.

As the numerous factors inhibiting or influencing the seating of the restoration are considered, the tilt of the cast on the cast holder is varied until the most usable compromise position—the one that least complicates the treatment plan—is determined. The simplest position should not be accepted unless all factors influencing the tilt are most nearly satisfied.

The path of insertion will always be parallel to the vertical arm of the surveyor and is determined by the tilt of the cast on the surveying table. The path of insertion is referred to most often as if it were a single entity. In actuality it is only when the denture has been constructed under rigid conditions that a denture will have only one path of insertion. Most dentures have two or more paths of insertion.

The most influential factor as to whether a partial denture will have one or more paths of insertion is whether the edentulous space or spaces are tooth bounded or are of the distal extension type (Figs. 7-17 to 7-19). If the edentulous space is tooth bounded and if guiding planes have been created on the proximal surfaces of all abutment teeth, the prosthesis will have a single path of insertion, because it can move in no other direction than along the created guiding planes.

If the prosthesis is of the single distal extension type with a tooth-bounded space on the opposite side of the arch, the path of insertion will be determined by the modification space. If guiding planes exist on the proximal surface of the abutment teeth on the tooth-bounded side, there will be a single path of insertion because the path of the distal extension side will be controlled by the rigid major connector and must follow the path of the tooth-bounded side.

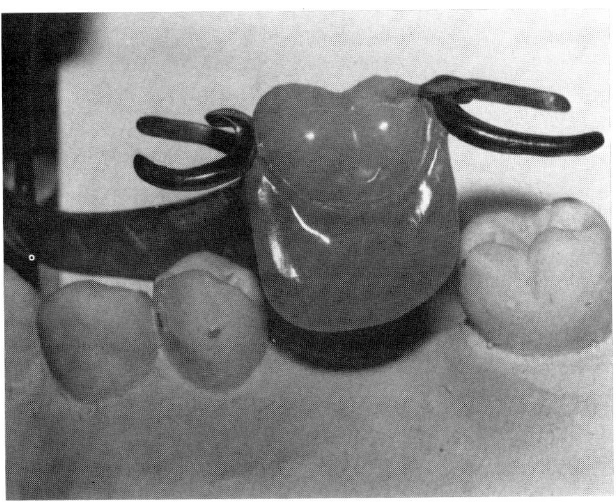

Fig. 7-17. A single path of insertion will exist for a removable prosthesis if the edentulous space is bounded by teeth at each end. The guiding planes on the proximal surfaces of the abutment teeth permit the denture to be inserted along a single path.

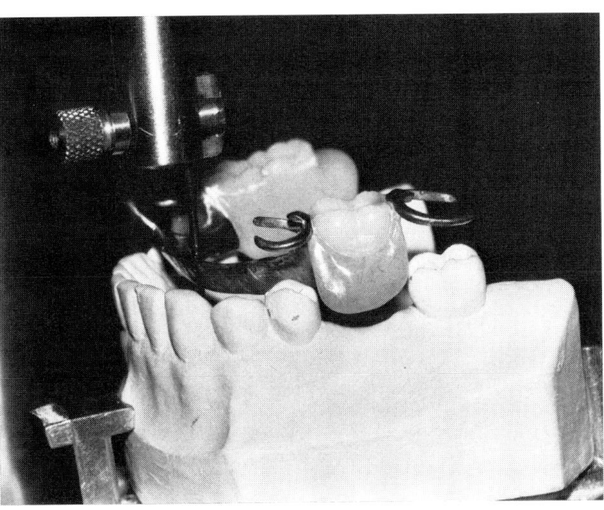

Fig. 7-18. The path of insertion for a Class II partial denture with a modification space is determined by the modification space. This will result in a single path of insertion.

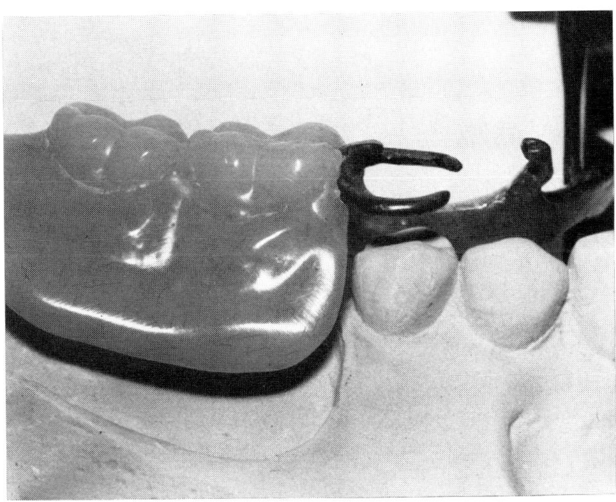

Fig. 7-19. For Class I partial dentures multiple paths of insertion may exist. The path is controlled only by the two terminal abutment teeth. Additional guiding planes may be developed on the lingual surfaces of other teeth to limit the number of paths of insertion.

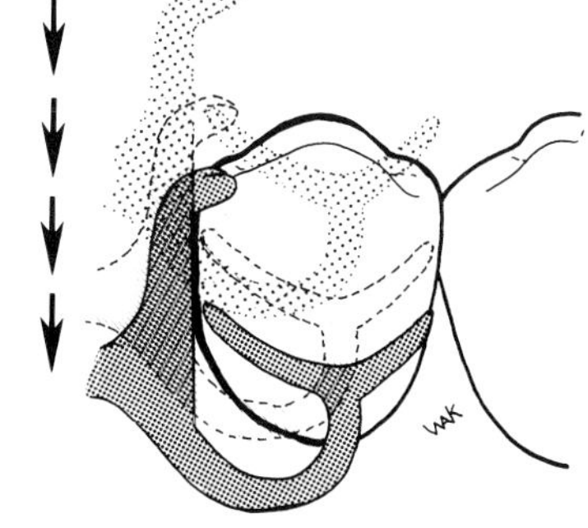

Fig. 7-20. The path of insertion is controlled by the minor connector that joins the clasp assembly to the major connector. The minor connector should contact the guiding planes on the abutment teeth during the entire process of insertion or withdrawl.

Multiple paths of insertion occur in Class I partial dentures in which the two distal extension bases are controlled only by the two terminal abutment teeth. A prosthesis of this type may enter or exit its position on the abutment teeth in a variety of angles. Additional guiding planes on the lingual surfaces of other teeth may be developed to control the number of paths of insertion.

If the partial denture has an anterior edentulous space, it will usually have a single path of insertion. The path will be parallel to the guiding planes on the proximal surfaces of the teeth on either side of the space.

The component of the denture that governs the path of insertion is the minor connector that joins the clasps to the major connector. The minor connector is normally the only portion of the prosthesis that contacts the guiding planes on the teeth; it should be in continual contact with the guiding planes throughout the processes of seating and removing the partial denture (Fig. 7-20).

The body and the shoulders of the clasps may exert

some influence on the path of insertion. However, the effect is limited because the clasps are usually positioned above the guiding planes and lie on sloping tooth surfaces.

In the event that guiding planes have been created on the lingual surfaces of the teeth, the reciprocal clasps, or lingual plate acting as reciprocal arms, can exert a definite influence on the path of insertion. The action of these components will be the same as that of the minor connector.

Factors influencing path of insertion

The following four factors must be considered before the path of insertion is selected; retentive undercuts, interferences, esthetics, and guiding planes. Rarely, if ever, will it be possible to achieve the optimum in all four factors; rather one factor is compromised against another. Clinical judgment, which time, dedication, and knowledge eventually produce, is extremely important in the decision as to which factor can best be compromised without sacrificing the quality of the service being rendered. In the preceding list and the following discussion these factors are given in order of their descending relative importance to help dentists with less clinical experience make correct decisions regarding compromise.

Retentive undercuts

The first, unchangeable rule to remember when surveying diagnostic casts for removable partial dentures is that retentive undercuts must be present on the abutment teeth at the horizontal tilt.

The surveying procedure is always started with the cast to be analyzed positioned in the cast holder so that the occlusal surfaces of the remaining teeth are parallel to the surveying table or base of the surveyor. This is an essential step. With the analyzing rod attached to the vertical arm, each abutment tooth is examined for the presence of retentive undercuts. The desired location of the undercut on the tooth will depend on the philosophy of design that the designer chooses to follow. This book will emphasize, but not be limited to, a concept referred to as *broad stress distribution,* in which a number of teeth are selected to bear the stress created by the partial denture in function (Fig. 7-21). It is from this philosophy that the discussion of locating and equalizing retentive undercuts will be broached. The technique of using the surveyor and the factors that must be satisfied remain the same for practically all other philosophies.

The occlusal surfaces of the teeth must be viewed first in the horizontal plane because dislodging forces applied to the partial denture (for example, the pull of sticky foods, the force of gravity on a maxillary denture) are always perpendicular to the occlusal plane. Resistance to this dislodging force must be present when the cast is at a horizontal position (see Fig. 3-5). Changing the tilt to produce undercuts is an illusion and one that is too often relied on (Fig. 7-22). Unfortunately in the harsh world of reality the illusion will vanish, and all that will be left is a nonretentive and nonusable prosthesis.

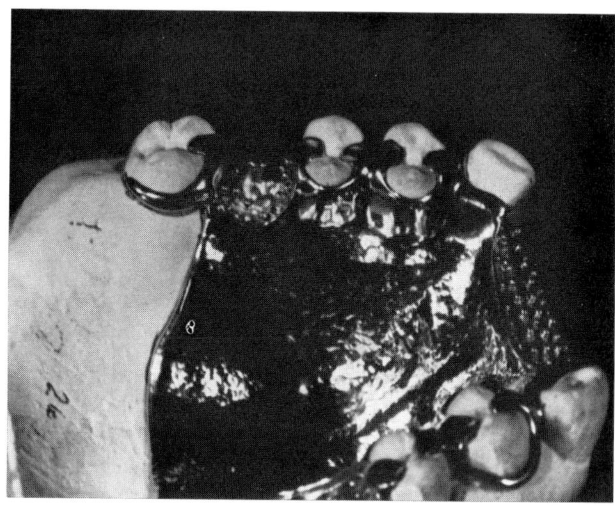

Fig. 7-21. In the broad stress distribution philosophy of design a number of teeth are selected as rest seat–bearing areas to distribute the forces acting on the prosthesis over as great an area as possible. Multiple rests and clasps are frequently included in this design concept.

If retentive undercuts are not present, they must be created. The most obvious method is by the use of a full crown, usually a full gold crown or a porcelain-bonded-to-metal full veneer crown. If either of these types of crowns is planned, it must be placed on the surveyor as it is being formed and contoured to satisfy the requirements of the partial denture. Other restorations such as Class V inlays or direct gold restorations may occasionally be used to create retentive undercuts, but they are not as common as full or partial crown restorations.

Enamel surfaces may be contoured in limited circumstances to produce or improve retentive undercuts, but this procedure should not be embraced in favor of other potentially less dangerous approaches. Careful analysis of the teeth on the diagnostic cast will usually reveal whether an undercut can be prepared without penetrating the enamel surface. Awareness of the oral hygiene status of the patient must also be weighed. This procedure of producing undercuts is discussed in detail in Chapter 9.

Ideally each of the proposed abutment teeth should have 0.010 inch of undercut at the most desired location, either the distobuccal or mesiobuccal line angle

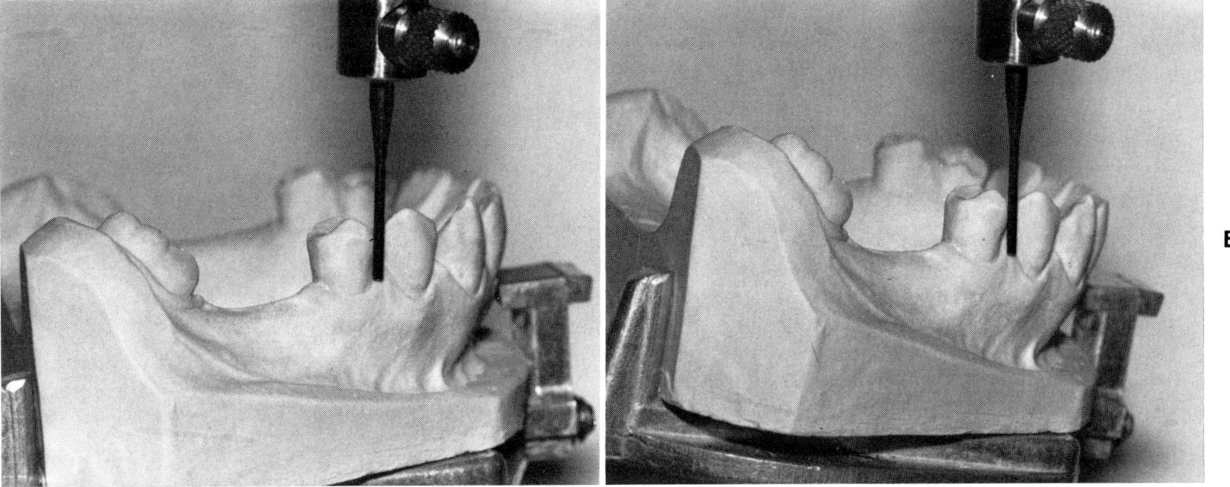

Fig. 7-22. A, The cast, mounted on the surveying table at a horizontal tilt, reveals no retentive undercut at the mesiobuccal line angle. **B,** Giving the cast an anterior tilt produces an apparent undercut at the mesiobuccal line angle of the premolar. It is not a functioning retentive undercut, because dislodging forces will occur on the prosthesis on a line perpendicular to the occlusal plane. A partial denture designed at this tilt would not be successful.

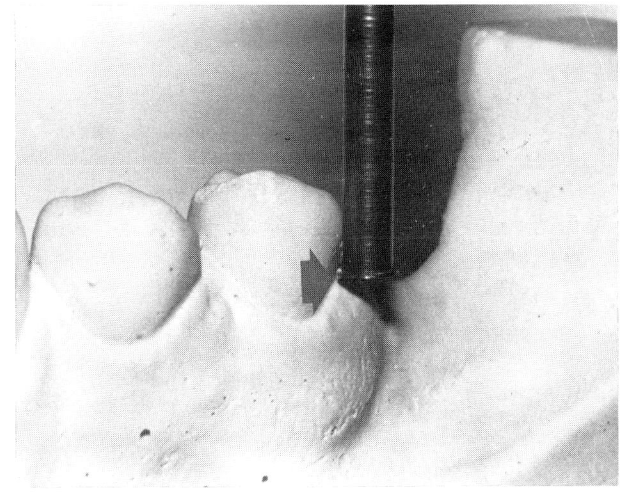

Fig. 7-23. To find a 0.010-inch undercut, the 0.010-inch undercut gauge is held perpendicular to the tooth (in this case at the distobuccal line angle of the terminal abutment tooth, the second premolar) with the shank contacting the tooth at the height of contour. The point on the tooth where the lid at the end of the shank contacts the tooth measures the exact amount of retentive undercut, in this case 0.010 inch.

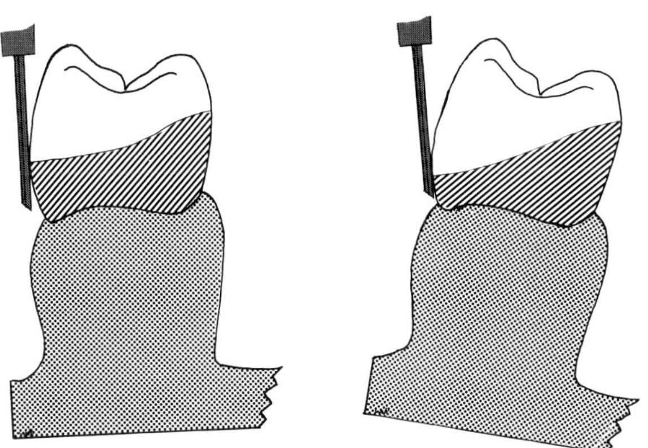

Fig. 7-24. The tilt of the cast may be altered to change the position of the survey line. This is most often done to position a clasp more favorably on an abutment tooth. *Changing the tilt to improve clasp placement does not alter the requirement that the retentive undercut must be present at the horizontal tilt of the cast.*

and in the gingival third of the clinical crown of the tooth (Fig. 7-23). (The RPI design concept, discussed in Chapter 8, prefers the retentive undercut to be more nearly in the center of the facial surface rather than on the line angle.)

The 0.010-inch undercut is desired when cast chrome alloy is used for the framework. Slightly more undercut may be needed if the abutment teeth are large molars or canines or if gold is to be used instead of chrome. If a wrought wire combination clasp (18 gauge) is planned, a retentive undercut of 0.020 inch is needed because of the greater flexibility of the wrought wire.

Once retentive undercuts have been found at the horizontal tilt, the tilt may be changed to alter the amount of undercut on any given tooth. It must be kept in mind that changing the tilt to alter the amount of undercut on one tooth will affect the undercuts on the remaining teeth. The tilt is normally changed to lower the height of contour on an abutment tooth so that a clasp, either retentive or reciprocal, can be positioned no more occlusal than the junction of the gingival and middle third of the tooth (Fig. 7-24). This position not only produces a more esthetic result, but also improves the mechanical advantage by lowering the torquing or rotational forces the clasp transmits to the tooth. The lowering of the clasp in effect shortens the length of the lever arm acting on the tooth, thus reducing instead of magnifying the applied force.

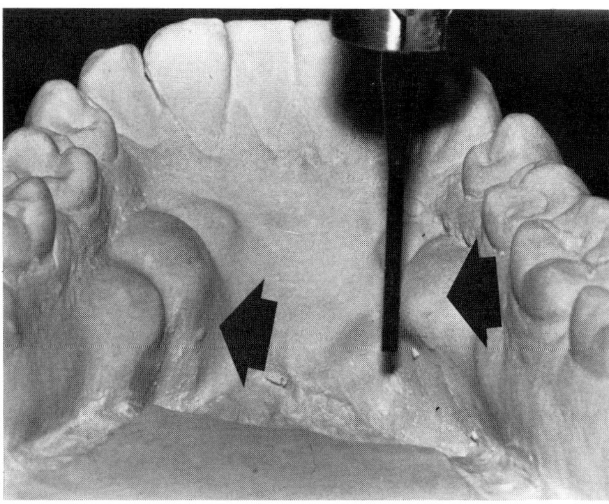

Fig. 7-25. Torus mandibularis may be so large as to contraindicate the construction of a mandibular removable partial denture until surgical removal has been accomplished. Rarely may the path of insertion be changed to avoid prominent tori. Surgery is generally indicated.

Interferences

Certain areas of the mouth—the teeth, soft tissue undercuts, and bony exostoses—frequently interfere with the insertion of the partial denture. These areas have to be eliminated either by altering the tilt of the cast on the surveying table or by surgery. It should be the goal of the designer to submit the patient to as little surgical intervention as possible, but never to compromise the success of a prosthesis because interferences that rendered the prognosis less than favorable were not recognized. Interferences in the mandible and maxilla are discussed separately.

Interferences in mandible. Tissues lingual to the remaining teeth that will be crossed by the major connector during insertion frequently cause problems. One of the greatest errors in treatment planning is attempting to position the major connector to avoid a lingual torus, especially if a lingual bar is planned as the major connector. If the torus is of any size, it is almost impossible to avoid it except by providing so much relief space between the bar and the bone that either the function of the tissues of the floor of the mouth or the activities of the tongue are interfered with. The thickness of the lingual bar may also be compromised, resulting in a nonrigid major connector that is damaging to the remaining teeth. Surgery must be seriously considered in cases of lingual tori. The general health of the patient

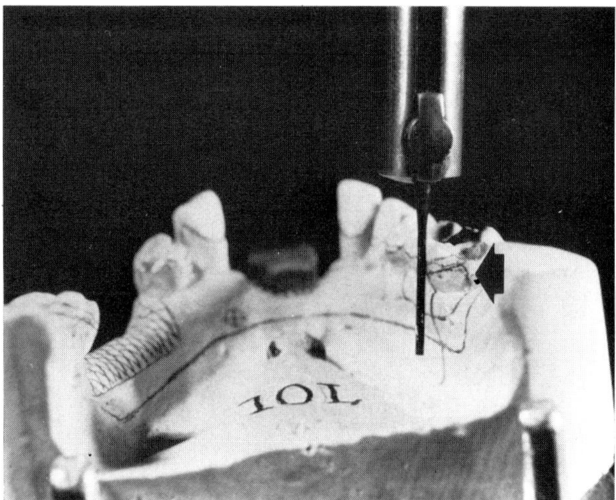

Fig. 7-26. Mandibular posterior teeth, if unsupported by adjacent teeth, tend to drift mesially and lingually. This lingual tipping (arrow) complicates the placement of reciprocal clasps, lingual plating, and the major connector.

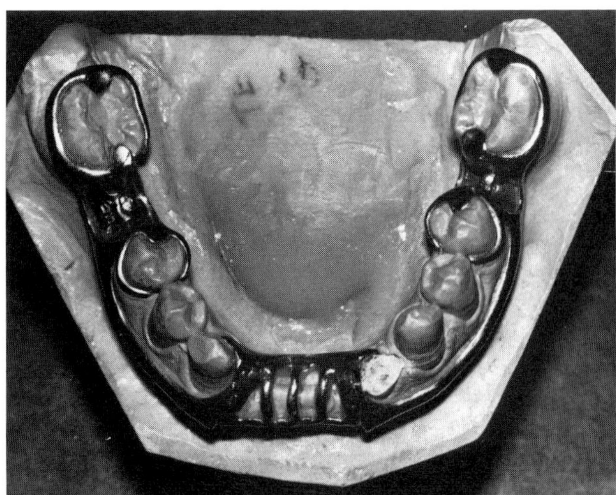

Fig. 7-27. It is difficult for a patient to accept a labial bar major connector. The metal bar placed labial to the anterior teeth frequently distorts the lip because the bulk is too great for the space available.

should be the governing factor in deciding whether to remove the tori. It is a certainty that not removing prominent tori will complicate patient treatment (Fig. 7-25).

The remaining teeth in the mandible are frequently lingually inclined. These unsupported or partially supported remaining premolar and molar teeth tend to drift in a mesiolingual direction (Fig. 7-26). Anterior teeth are not as often involved in this drifting movement. If the lingually inclined teeth are bilateral, the space available for a lingually positioned major connector will be greatly reduced. This could result in a major connector that would encroach on the tongue space. The major connector would have to be designed to stand well away from the lingual mucosa. This would result not only in tongue interference, but also in an undesirable space where food and other debris would tend to collect. It would overall be unacceptable for the patient.

One answer to this problem would be to plan a labial bar major connector in place of the lingual one. Experience has shown, however, that the labial bar has poor patient acceptance because of the bulk of metal necessary to maintain rigidity. The bulk causes an uncomfortable and unattractive plumping of the lower lip. Only on rare occasions should a labial bar be selected as the major connector (Fig. 7-27). The most acceptable answer to this problem is either contouring the enamel of the lingual surface or placing restorations on the teeth to eliminate the undercuts.

Another area of the mandible that frequently causes interference to the path of insertion is the area lingual to the pear-shaped pad. A lateral tilt of the cast on the surveying table may help to eliminate some, if not all, of a unilateral undercut in this area (Fig. 7-28). Fortunately the portion of the partial denture that will usually have to engage an undercut of this nature is the denture base. The acrylic resin can be relieved to avoid the interference much easier than can a metallic component. In relieving the denture base, some resistance to lateral movement of the prosthesis will be sacrificed, but this may still be the method of choice in avoiding the interference.

Bony exostoses or simple bony undercuts in the alveolar ridge of the mandible buccal to premolar and canine teeth are not unusual. These will interfere with the denture base if the teeth are missing, or can interfere with positioning of the approach arm of a vertical projection clasp (Fig. 7-29). If the teeth are missing and lateral tilting of the cast on the surveying table cannot produce a path of insertion that avoids these undercuts, surgical recontouring of the edentulous ridge should be considered. If the undercuts interfere with positioning an approach arm of a clasp, the use of that type clasp would be contraindicated. For example, the approach arm of a vertical projection clasp cannot cross a soft tissue undercut because it would produce a food trap that is unacceptable to most patients.

Interferences in maxilla. One of the major sources of interference in the maxilla is a torus palatinus. The torus interferes with the placement of the major connector. As a general rule, changing the tilt of the cast on

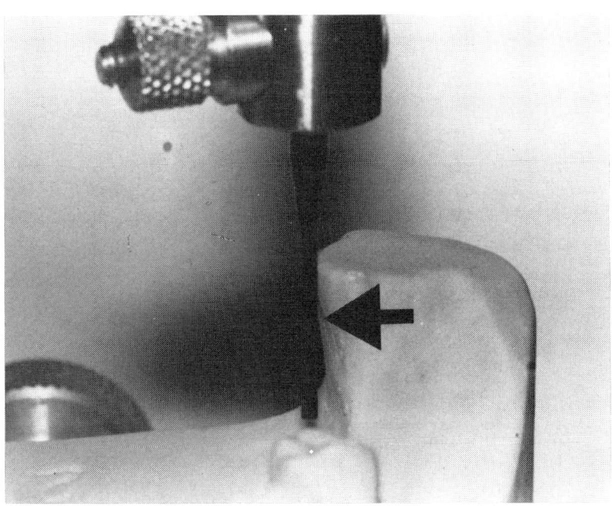

Fig. 7-28. A frequent area of interference to the path of insertion in the mandibular arch is the area lingual to the pear-shaped pad. If the condition is unilateral, a slight lateral tilt of the cast on the surveying table may eliminate the problem.

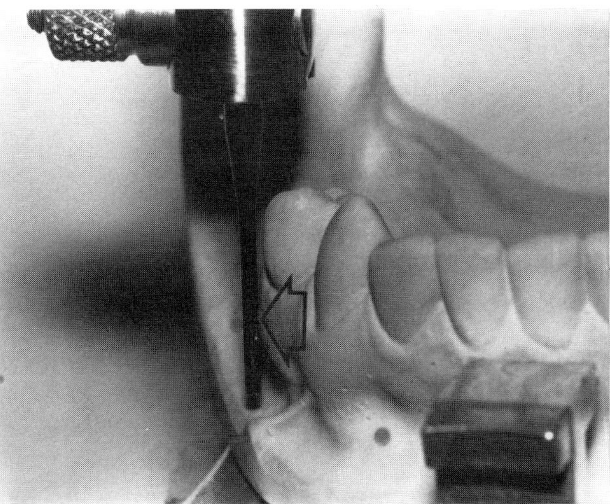

Fig. 7-29. Bony exostosis of the alveolar ridge buccal to the mandibular premolar teeth can interfere with the path of insertion of the denture base or the approach arm of vertical projection clasps. A change in the lateral tilt of the cast may avoid these interferences.

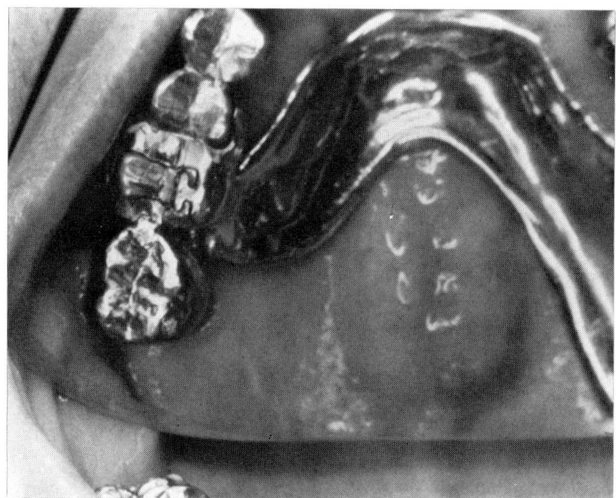

Fig. 7-30. A torus palatinus interferes with the placement of the maxillary major connector. An internal attachment removable partial denture with a horseshoe major connector was designed to avoid the broad torus. The horseshoe major connector would not be indicated for a Class I partially edentulous arch.

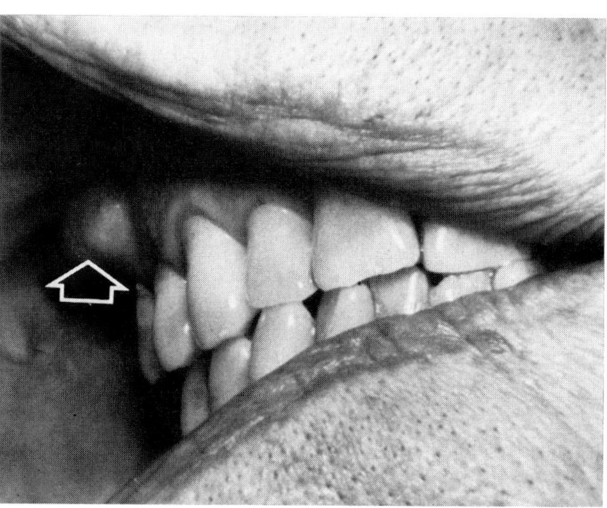

Fig. 7-31. Bony exostosis buccal to the posterior edentulous ridge complicates the placement of the maxillary partial denture. Surgical removal of these undercuts before construction of the prosthesis is usually indicated.

the surveying table will not give the needed relief. Usually the design of the major connector must be changed to avoid the torus; if this is not possible, surgical intervention must be accomplished (Fig. 7-30).

Bony exostoses or undercuts buccal to the posterior edentulous ridge are encountered frequently. Their surgical removal is not a complicated procedure and should be done to provide better support for the denture base (Fig. 7-31).

Just as lingually tipped teeth are a problem in the mandible, buccally, or facially, tipped teeth are a source of interference in the maxillary arch. As a result of the buccal tipping, the height of contour on the facial surface of these teeth will be very close to the occlusal surface (Fig. 7-32). This makes positioning of buccal clasp arms difficult for esthetic and mechanical reasons. Because of the high clasp position, undesirable tipping forces are created too near the occlusal surface of the tooth. These forces are much more damaging than would be those occurring nearer the center of the tooth.

The buccal tipping also may cause the entire area gingival to the tooth to be in an undercut when viewed from a vertical or occlusal direction. This situation would contraindicate the use of a vertical projection clasp because the approach arm for this clasp must contact the mucosa.

If these bucally inclined teeth are located on one side of the arch only, tilting the surveying table away from the teeth may lower the height of contour sufficiently to permit the clasps to be located in a nearly ideal position (Fig. 7-33). If these inclined teeth are located on both sides of the arch, changing the tilt of the cast will have no helpful effect. If the tipping is not too severe, contouring the enamel surfaces to lower the survey line may be attempted. Most often, however, full crown restorations will be required to produce a height of contour that will satisfy the requirement for clasp placement (Fig. 7-34).

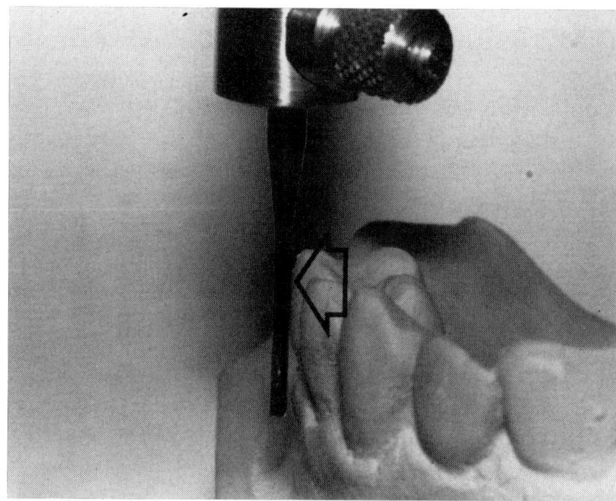

Fig. 7-32. Maxillary posterior teeth in the partially edentulous patient tend to tip buccally. As indicated by the analyzing rod, this tipping causes the height of contour to be close to the occlusal surface. This complicates the positioning of buccal clasp arms from both a mechanical and an esthetic standpoint.

An anterior edentulous ridge in the maxilla frequently presents an undercut situation, at times severe

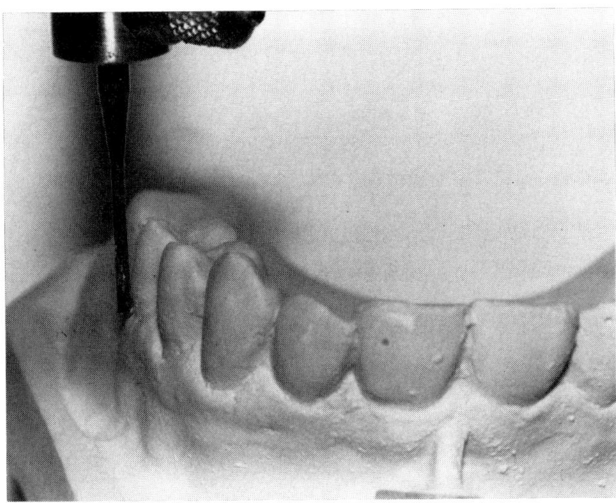

Fig. 7-33. If buccally inclined teeth are present on only one side of the arch, it may be possible to lower the height of contour to a more acceptable position by changing the cast on the surveying table to a slight lateral tilt. The effect of this change of tilt must be evaluated on other factors being considered.

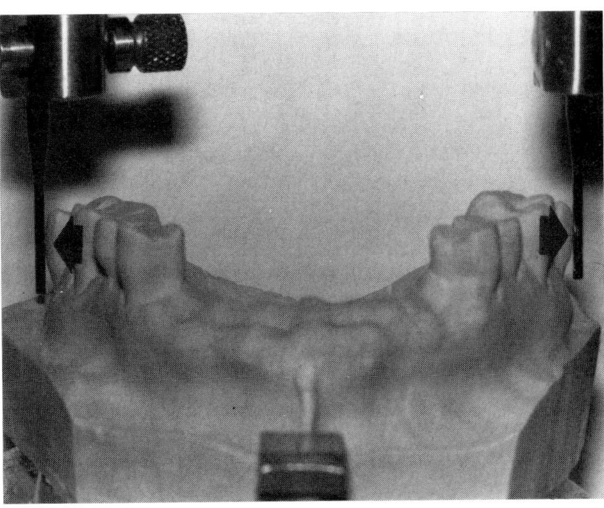

Fig. 7-34. If buccally inclined teeth are located on both sides of the arch, changing the tilt will not improve the problem. Either enamel surfaces must be recontoured or full crown restorations must be placed to lower the height of contour.

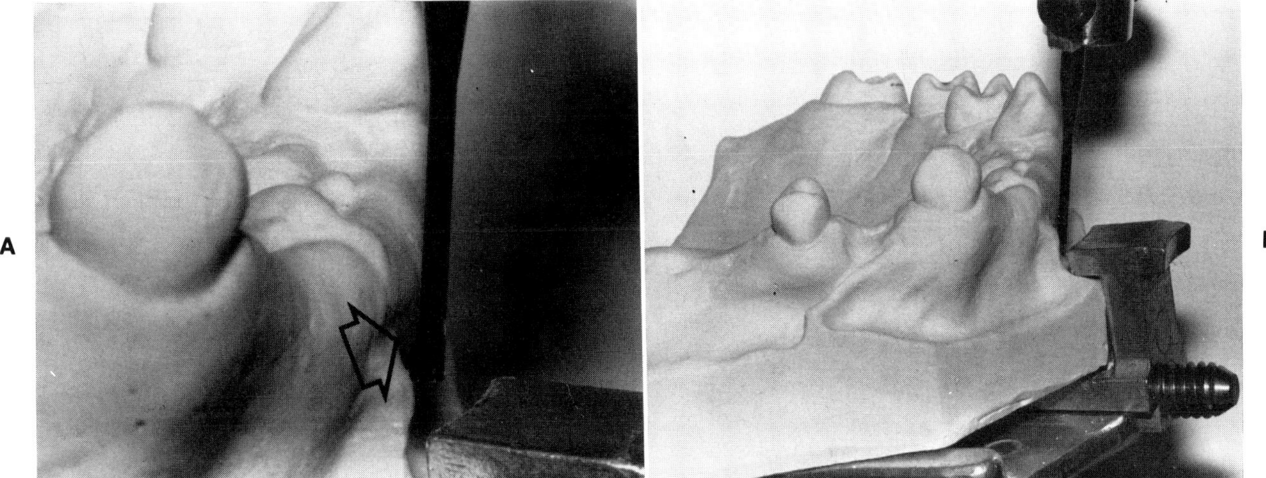

Fig. 7-35. A,The anterior edentulous ridge of the maxillary arch frequently presents an undercut situation unless considerable bone loss has occurred. It is rarely desirable to eliminate these anterior undercuts surgically. Maintenance of bone on the anterior ridge must be given high priority. B, Most undercuts of the maxillary anterior ridge can be controlled by giving the cast a slight posterior tilt.

(Fig. 7-35). Most of these undercuts can be controlled by giving the cast a slight posterior tilt. This posterior tilt not only helps reduce the undercut, but also may place the artificial anterior teeth in a more natural position. This anterior undercut may also be controlled at times by modifying or even eliminating the anterior flange of the denture base and butting the replacement teeth directly against the edentulous ridge. This can produce an excellent esthetic result.

Esthetics

To obtain optimum esthetics, (1) the metal, usually in the form of clasp arms, must be concealed as much as possible without compromising the necessary support and stability of the prosthesis and (2) the artificial anterior teeth must be placed in the most natural position possible. The desire to produce the ultimate in patient acceptance of the appearance of the partial denture must not be placed above the requirement that the

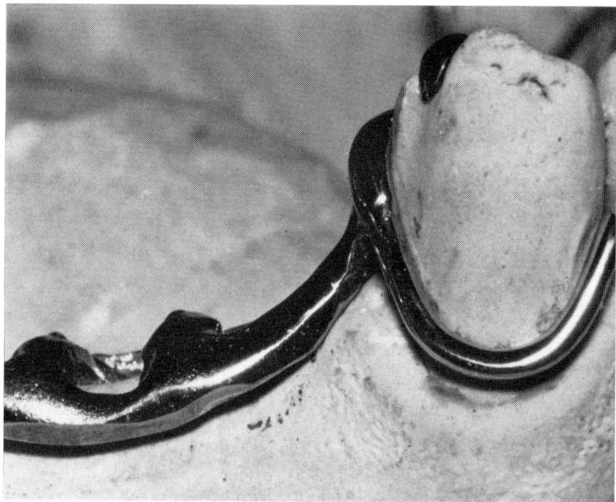

Fig. 7-36. The ideal position for a retentive clasp, the gingival third of the crown of the abutment tooth, is desirable from an esthetic view because the clasp is hidden as much as possible and from a mechanical view because the forces created by the flexing action of the clasp are located closer to the axis of rotation of the abutment tooth.

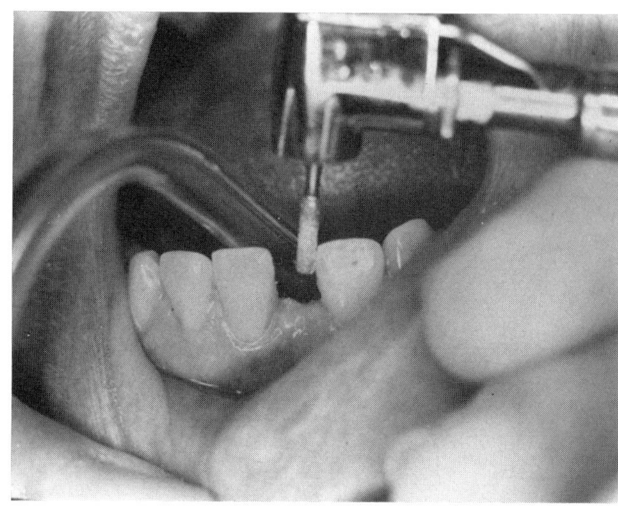

Fig. 7-37. In the event that a missing anterior tooth is to be replaced by a removable partial denture, the proximal surfaces of the teeth bordering the space should be contoured to restore the original mesiodistal dimension of the missing tooth and to produce guiding planes that will be compatible with the path of insertion.

prosthesis not damage the remaining oral tissues. If esthetics is the patient's primary concern, replacement of missing teeth by fixed partial dentures, internal attachment partial dentures, or overdentures must be given priority. These approaches should all be considered during the treatment planning process.

To satisfy the first requirement of avoiding unnecessary display of metal, the tilt of the survey table should be such that the survey lines on teeth that will be visible be as close to the gingival margin as is compatible with maintaining periodontal health. The ideal clasp position for retentive clasps is in the gingival third of the clinical crown (Fig. 7-36). Selection of types of clasps for purposes of concealment is discussed at greater length later in this chapter when design procedures are considered.

If the tilt of the cast is changed to satisfy this third of the four factors, the effect of this change on the other factors that have been previously satisfied must be determined. If changing the tilt has adversely affected the retentive undercuts, compromise between the two tilts must be arrived at. Compromise among the four factors is a constant problem in the surveying process.

The second requirement in obtaining optimum esthetics is placing the artificial anterior teeth in the most natural position.

When lost anterior teeth are not replaced immediately (which unfortunately is too often the case), the space remaining is frequently less than the space occupied by the missing teeth because of mesial drifting of the remaining teeth. It is axiomatic that teeth with spaces anterior to them will drift mesially, except mandibular premolars and canines, which will move distally if not supported adequately.

Unless something is done to correct this closing of anterior spaces, the tooth used as a replacement will be smaller in the mesiodistal dimension than the original tooth and than its counterpart on the opposite side of the arch. This result is not pleasing, even to the untrained eye.

To counter this esthetic shortcoming, the use of the surveyor is a necessity. In determining the final tilt of the cast, the space of missing anterior teeth must be given high priority. As mentioned previously, a missing anterior tooth or teeth almost always signals that the prosthesis will have a single path of insertion. This means that the surveyor must be used to determine whether contouring, or disking, the proximal surfaces of teeth bordering the space or spaces can be accomplished not only to restore the original mesiodistal dimension of the missing tooth, but also to produce an acceptable path of insertion (Fig. 7-37). If disking the proximal surfaces can accomplish the desired results, it is the procedure of choice. If contouring the enamel surfaces is not possible, crowns or other types of restorations must be planned.

Large undercuts may also be present next to the proximal surfaces of the teeth adjacent to the anterior edentulous space. These undercuts are caused by either the bell shape of the crown of the tooth or by tipping of the tooth toward the edentulous space. The spaces not only detract from the esthetic value of the restoration, but also tend to act as food traps that can be annoying to the patient. They should be eliminated or de-

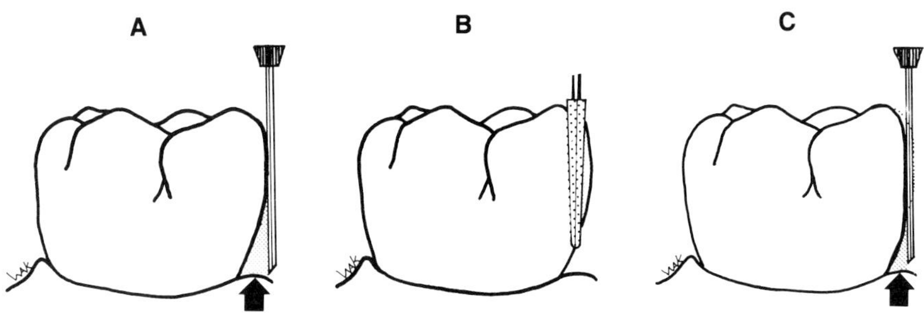

Fig. 7-38. Large undercuts adjacent to proximal surfaces of abutment teeth, **A,** should be reduced in size. The reduction can be accomplished by altering the tilt of the cast or by selective grinding of the enamel surface, **B.** The result of either technique is the reduction of the undesirable undercut, **C.** An extra advantage gained by selective grinding is that an additional guiding plane is produced.

creased in size by altering the tilt of the cast, usually giving it a slight posterior tilt. In addition, some disking of the proximal surfaces is usually beneficial in reducing the undercut and in producing guiding planes (Fig. 7-38). The surveyor is a necessity in determining the amount of recontouring that will be needed to reduce these undesirable undercuts and to reestablish the space required for optimum esthetics.

Guiding planes

Guiding planes are formed from the proximal or axial surfaces of the teeth and are contacted by the minor connectors or other rigid elements of the partial denture. These planes guide the prosthesis in and out of the mouth without causing undesirable forces against the teeth. When the denture is completely seated in the mouth, the guiding planes, in intimate contact with the minor connectors, help stabilize it against lateral forces. They also help protect weakened teeth from potentially destructive lateral forces. In most cases, except where some of the periodontal support of the teeth have been lost and the teeth must be supported rigidly, the guiding plane does not need to be more than 2 or 3 mm in occlusogingival height.

The surveyor is used to locate existing or potential surfaces of teeth that can be converted to guiding planes by selective grinding. These planes are always developed parallel to the path of insertion.

Of the four factors considered in determining the final tilt of the cast on the surveying table, or the path of insertion, the development of guiding planes is the one that can be most easily compromised. Guiding planes can usually be readily prepared in enamel surfaces. If teeth for which guiding planes are planned are to receive cast restorations, the wax patterns should be shaped by the surveyor with their surfaces parallel to the path of insertion.

PRINCIPLES OF DESIGN

Authorities in the field of removable partial denture design may differ on their approach in developing the design of each individual prosthesis. There is, however, complete agreement that the correct design incorporates proper use and application of mechanical and biologic principles. These principles enable the supporting teeth and the soft tissues to withstand the forces that will be created by the movement and stress placed on the prosthesis during function.

It would be gratifying to be able to say that partial denture design is based on the results of scientific achievement accomplished under rigid and repeatable conditions. Regretfully this is not so, although this is not to say that there are not now nor have there been in the past a number of research activities that have contributed greatly to the knowledge of partial denture design.

Removable partial denture design does not lend itself readily to scientific methods of study because the variables in the partially edentulous mouth are so many, and the time before true clinical research yields results that can be interpreted as reliable or meaningful is so great.

Much laboratory research has been and is being done that helps expand our knowledge. However, the results yielded from a laboratory bench must be evaluated and assessed carefully before they are applied to a similar clinical condition. The biologic response may not follow totally the inanimate response of the laboratory. An observer has remarked, after assessing the results of an abutment tooth mobility test on teeth mounted in a Thiokol rubber socket, that until Thiokolclasts and Thiokolblasts are developed, such results may be looked upon as a mechanical answer to a test situation and not as a biologic response.

In considering the design, the dentist should bear in

mind the following basic principles of removable partial denture construction. If these principles are acknowledged and adhered to, the many complexities that appear to be present in the field of dentistry will be reduced. The principles were first expounded by A.H. Schmidt in 1956. Chances are they were not totally original with him, but he did stress them strongly in his teaching. The principles remain as true and unassailable today as the day they were proposed.

1. *The dentist must have a thorough knowledge of both the mechanical and biologic factors involved in removable partial denture design.* The dentist must have a background in the basic and applied sciences, and a working knowledge of the laws of physics and engineering, particularly as they relate to levers.
2. *The treatment plan must be based on a complete examination and diagnosis of the individual patient.*
3. *The dentist must correlate the pertinent factors and determine a proper plan of treatment.* This is an area in which the profession has functioned poorly in the past. The tendency, all too often, has been to submit casts to a laboratory and allow the technician to produce a removable partial denture. The dentist alone can modify the conditions in the mouth to enhance the success of the treatment.
4. *A removable partial denture should restore form and function without injury to the remaining oral structure.* In restoring occlusion, the prosthesis should also restore a normal or desirable facial contour and not impede the normal movement of the tongue and other tissues. The prosthesis must be so planned that the remaining oral structures are not stressed beyond their physiologic capability.
5. *A removable partial denture is a form of treatment and not a cure.* The responsibility of the dentist to the patient does not end with the final placement of the prosthesis in the patient's mouth. Oral tissues never remain static, but are constantly undergoing change reflecting the general health and age of the patient. The patient should be recalled periodically to prevent any deleterious change from taking place. The denture should be planned with the knowledge that future corrections may be required. The design should be such that modifications may be made to compensate for changes that can be expected in oral tissues.

These principles are indeed basic, but if they are referred to as problems arise during the design and planning procedure, the chances of successful treatment will be greatly increased.

PHILOSOPHY OF DESIGN

Of the various philosophies, or schools of thought, relating to removable partial denture design, none is backed by scientific research or statistics. They are rather the ideas of dentists who, by means of extensive clinical experience, have formulated rules by which they produce a design for a removable partial denture. Little or no evidence is available that any of the philosophies has a real advantage over another except in the mind of the follower. This is not to say that none of the various methods of design has proved to be clinically acceptable. On the contrary, all have produced excellent clinical results if attention to detail has been observed. It is not so much the theoretical side of partial denture design that is critical, but rather the carrying out of that design with competent clinical and laboratory procedures. Nearly any removable partial denture design can be made to work successfully if respect for the physiologic limits of the supporting structures is observed.

In partial denture design, the main concern is for the part tooth-borne and part soft-tissue–borne prosthesis. For the Class III arch the design is generally straightforward. Because the denture will be all tooth supported, a single impression may be used to record the teeth and soft tissue. The edentulous ridge does not offer support, so it may be recorded in its anatomic form. Because rotational forces do not occur, indirect retention or flexible direct retention is not required. Retentive clasping is done for convenience, that is, the simplest clasp possible is used for undercuts on the abutment teeth. It is generally not necessary to restore the abutment teeth with crowns or other restorations to improve the tooth contour. The challenge in design, then, lies primarily in Classes I and II arches and to some extent in the Class IV arch.

Great controversy continues to exist as to what constitutes correct design and adequate support for the free end, or distal extension, removable partial denture. The method of using and equalizing support from the edentulous ridge and the remaining teeth is the main issue. The different methods used have given rise to the various design philosophies.

The variations in the concept of design are multitudinous. However, there are three basic, underlying approaches to distributing the forces acting on a partial denture between the soft tissue and the teeth:

1. Stress equalization
2. Physiologic basing
3. Broad stress distribution

There are obviously some design concepts that may attempt to take advantage of more than one of these basic goals, but nearly all can be grouped into one of the three. Internal attachment removable partial dentures are considered to be in a separate category; they are discussed in Chapter 22.

The three basic design philosophies will now be discussed. The reader should note that the advantages presented for the different concepts are those *cited by the advocates of that particular school of thought.*

Stress equalization

The advocates of the stress-equalizing, or stress-directing, approach to partial denture design emphasize that the resiliency of the tooth secured by the periodontal ligament in an apical direction is not comparable to the greater resiliency and displaceability of the mucosa covering the edentulous ridge. Because of this great disparity, forces are transmitted to the abutment teeth as the denture bases are displaced in function.

It is the belief of this school of thought that the rigid connection between the denture bases and the direct retainer on the abutment teeth is damaging and that some type of stress director or stress equalizer is essential to protect the vulnerable abutment teeth (Fig. 7-39).

The stress director may take several forms. The most commonly used ones are composed of a hinge device interposed between the minor connector of the abutment tooth and the denture base. The hinge is designed to permit vertical movement of the denture base as occlusal forces are applied to the artificial teeth. Most can be adjusted to control the amount of vertical movement that is permitted—usually the estimated thickness of the mucosa covering the ridge.

Advantages

The stress director design usually calls for minimal direct retention, because the denture base operates more independently than in a conventional denture.

Internal attachments for retention of the stress-broken prosthesis are widely used. Advocates of this theory find that the stress director is mandatory on Class I and II partial dentures because of the positive lock on the abutment tooth created by the internal attachment. Forces against the abutment tooth are magnified greatly because of the internal attachment. Theoretically, at least, the stress director eliminates the tipping strain on the tooth, thus preventing bone resorption about the tooth (Fig. 7-40).

It is proposed that the stress equalizer is successful because the sum of its resiliency and that of the periodontal ligament is equal to the resiliency of the mucosa. Thus forces are distributed equally between the teeth and the soft tissue.

Intermittent pressure against the mucosa caused by the movement of the bases has a massaging or stimulating effect on the underlying bone and soft tissue. This stimulation, it is claimed, minimizes tissue change and reduces the necessity of relining or rebasing the denture to compensate for tissue change as is required for most distal extension partial dentures.

Disadvantages

The stress director is comparatively fragile, and its construction is complex and costly. It requires constant maintenance and may be difficult or impossible to repair.

Although attempts are usually made to strengthen the hinge to prevent lateral movement of the denture base, its lack of ability to prevent damaging lateral stresses from occurring on the edentulous ridge can re-

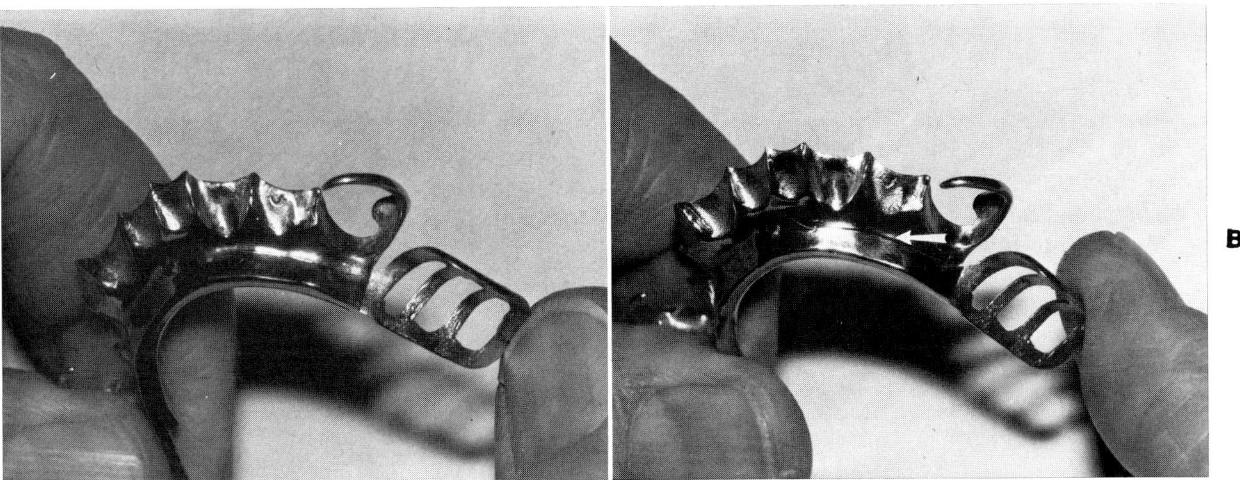

Fig. 7-39. A, The purpose of the stress director is to equalize forces transmitted by the partial denture. The split lingual bar shown is in the relaxed state, and the split is not evident. **B,** Downward force on the acrylic resin retention activates the split lingual bar (arrow). The bar separates, thus dissipating forces that would otherwise be transmitted to the abutment tooth.

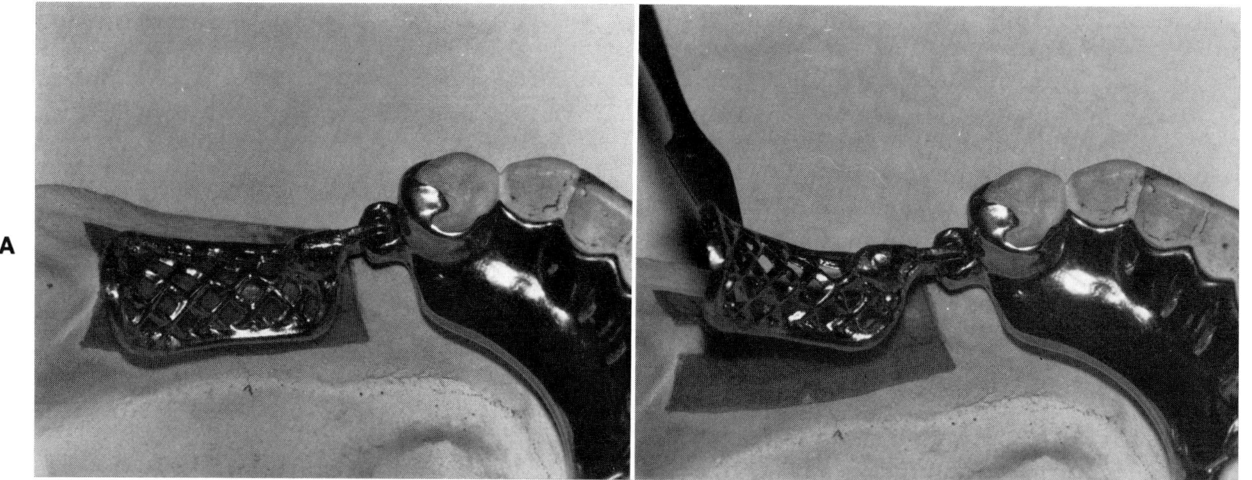

Fig. 7-40. A, Stress directors are indicated in the Class I and II arches. Shown is a hinge device that permits vertical movement of the acrylic resin retention areas. The hinge is in the normal, or down, position. **B,** The hinge is activated by a lifting force and is raised upward away from the ridge. This lifting action removes torquing force from the abutment tooth.

sult in rapid resorption of bone and settling of the denture. If sufficient thickness of metal in the hinge is used to prevent lateral movement, the prosthesis becomes heavy, bulky, and annoying to the patient.

Of the three schools of thought of partial denture design, the stress-equalizing school has the fewest advocates. It may appeal to the more experienced or sophisticated practitioner. Details on the use and construction of the stress director are presented in Chapter 22.

Physiologic basing

This philosophy of design agrees in part with the first school about the relative lack of movement of the abutment teeth in an apical direction but denies the necessity of using stress directors to equalize the disparity of vertical movement between the tooth and mucosa. The belief is that the equalization can best and most simply be accomplished by some form of physiologic basing, or lining, of the denture base. The physiologic basing is produced either by displacing or depressing the ridge mucosa during the impression-making procedure or by relining the denture base after it has been constructed.

The reason for displacing the mucosa during the impression procedure is to record the soft tissue in its functioning, not anatomic, form (Fig. 7-41). The feeling of this group is that if the tissue is recorded in its functioning form when occlusal forces take place on the denture, the denture base, formed over displaced tissue, will adapt more readily to the depressed tissue and will be better able to withstand the force that is generated. The technique for making this impression is covered in detail in Chapter 13.

It seems obvious that the artificial teeth of a removable partial denture constructed from a tissue-displacing impression will be positioned above the plane of occlusion when the denture is in the mouth and not in function (Fig. 7-42). To permit vertical movement of the partial denture from the rest position to the functioning position, the direct retainers or retentive clasps must be designed with minimal retention and the number of direct retainers must be limited. The occlusal rests and direct retainers will also be slightly unseated at rest; they will be completely seated only when the mucosa beneath the denture base is displaced to its functional form.

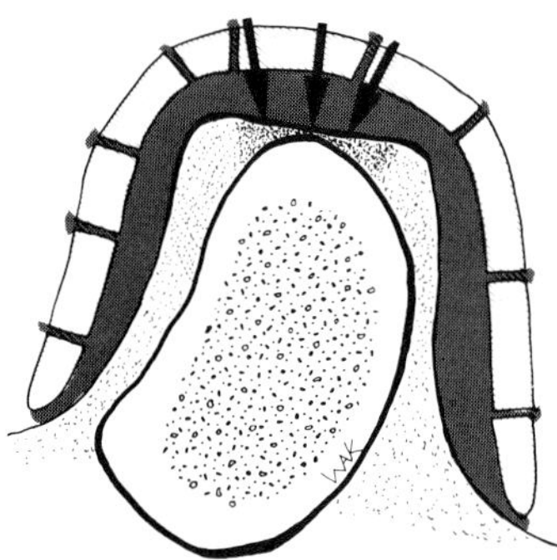

Fig. 7-41. During the impression procedure for the physiologic-basing philosophy of partial denture design, the mucosa covering the edentulous ridge is displaced to its functioning form.

Advantages

The intermittent base movement that occurs as occlusal loads are applied and removed has a physiologically stimulating effect on the underlying bone and soft

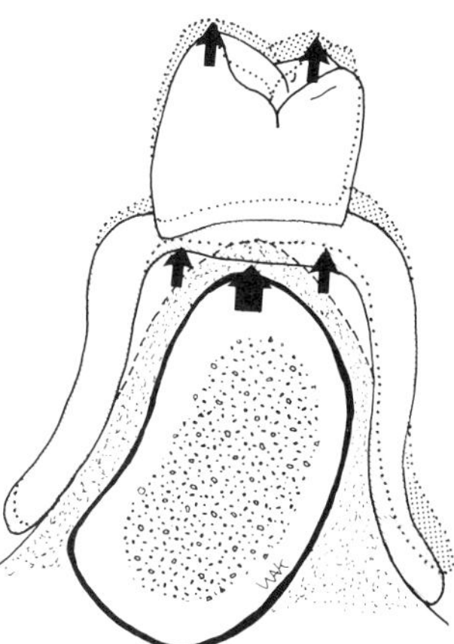

Fig. 7-42. When the partial denture is at rest in the mouth, the artificial teeth will be positioned slightly above the plane of occlusion of the remaining natural teeth because of the rebound of the compressed mucosa to its normal architecture.

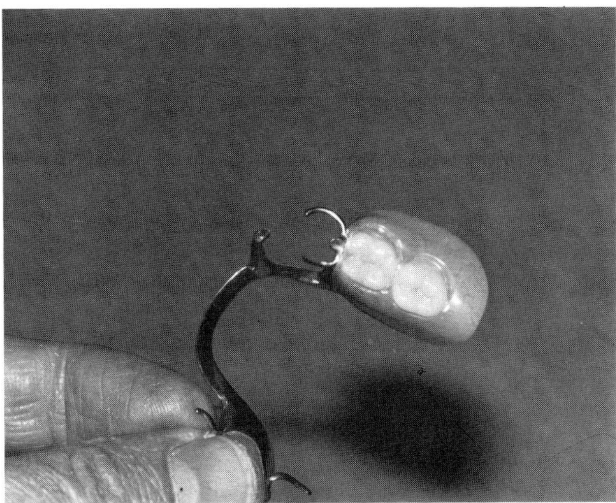

Fig. 7-43. The simplicity of design and construction of the physiologically based removable partial denture makes it a light weight prosthesis.

tissue, which is said to reduce the frequency of the need to reline or rebase the prosthesis to correct for tissue change caused by resorption.

The simplicity of design and construction because of the minimal retention requirements results in a lightweight prosthesis needing minimal maintenance and repair (Fig. 7-43).

An additional advantage is gained by the minimal direct retention used. The looseness of the clasp (combination clasp with wrought wire retentive arms) on the abutment tooth reduces the functional forces transmitted to the tooth. The proponents of this theory claim that abutment teeth are preserved because of this.

Disadvantages

The denture is not well stabilized against lateral forces because of the minimum number and flexibility of the direct retainers. The residual ridge receives a greater proportional amount of the forces that are transmitted by the denture. Many critics of the physiologic-basing philosophy believe that the tooth, in its periodontal ligament, is better able to withstand lateral forces than is the residual ridge. The load of stabilizing and supporting the denture is limited to a few teeth instead of being shared by a number of remaining teeth as in other design philosophies.

Because the artificial teeth are always slightly above the occlusal plane when the denture is not in function, there will always be slightly premature contacts between the opposing teeth and the denture teeth when the mouth is closed. This is an uncomfortable sensation for many patients and may result in a sense of insecurity.

It is difficult to produce effective indirect retention because of the vertical movement of the denture and the minimal retention of the direct retainer. By the time the indirect retainer engages a rest seat to prevent the denture base from being dislodged, the direct retainer will have lost contact with the abutment tooth.

Broad stress distribution

Advocates of this school of partial denture design believe that excessive trauma to the remaining teeth and residual ridge can be prevented by distributing the forces of occlusion over as many teeth and as much of the available soft tissue area as possible. This is accomplished by the use of additional rests, indirect retainers, clasps, and broad coverage denture bases (Fig. 7-44).

Advantages

Following this philosophy, the forces of occlusion are reduced on any one tooth or area of the ridge because all the teeth and the entire available ridge collectively bear the load. For example, occlusal forces distributed among five or six teeth may physiologically stimulate them to a state of health, whereas the same load applied to two teeth may exceed the physiologic limit of these teeth, with resulting resorption of alveolar bone.

It is also recommended that multiple tooth contacts by direct retainers, additional rests, and minor connectors be planned so that lateral forces may be distributed over as many teeth as possible.

The occasional use of multiple clasps in this design concept does not cause overretention. Clasps may be used on some teeth not for retention but to aid in lateral stability—not only for the prosthesis, but also for

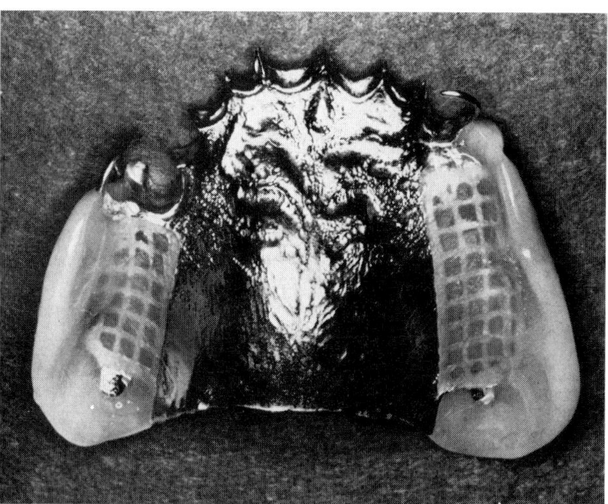

Fig. 7-44. The typical broad stress distribution partial denture features maximum coverage of teeth and soft tissue. This prosthesis shows full palate coverage by the major connector and lingual plating of the remaining teeth. The main purpose is to distribute forces generated by the partial denture over as wide an area as possible.

teeth that may have lost some periodontal support. This approach constitutes a form of removable splinting and can be very helpful in instances where fixed splinting is not indicated because of a guarded prognosis or for economic reasons.

In addition to the advantages already listed, proponents of this philosophy believe that the prostheses are easier and less expensive to construct. There are no flexible or moving parts, so there is less danger of distorting the denture. It is also less subject to breakage. The indirect retainers and other rigid components prevent rotational movements of the denture and provide excellent horizontal stabilization. Because of this increased stability and decreased movement, the broad stress distribution partial denture does not require relining as frequently as the other types because the residual ridge does not bear as much of the occlusal load.

Disadvantages

The greater amount of tooth and soft tissue coverage and the increased bulk, in some cases, may cause the prosthesis to be less comfortable and less well accepted by the patient than some simpler designs.

An increased amount of tooth surface coverage is associated with this design philosophy. Preventive dental programs to monitor caries must be instituted and carefully followed for each patient. The mouth must be kept meticulously clean. With today's increased dental awareness and the currently available aids such as fluoride rinses, this factor may not be as critical as it might once have been.

Summary

It must be remembered that any of these philosophies can be successful if applied to the correct partially edentulous situation and that all will fail if used under the incorrect circumstances. The specific indications for the use of each are subjects for additional research.

Practitioners and technicians presently have outstanding materials and techniques with which to fabricate removable partial dentures. There are also numerous designs than can be used for any given partially edentulous arch. To achieve success, nothing can replace good judgement coupled with the knowledge of basic fundamental principles of partial denture design.

Essential considerations to partial denture design are summarized here to help the student remember what components must be used as each class of partially edentulous arch is being prepared for treatment. The outline most closely follows the broad stress distribution philosophy, but it is also valid for the other concepts.

Essentials of design

A. Classes I and II
  1. Direct retention
    a. Retention should *not* be considered the prime objective of design.
      (1) The main objectives should be the restoration of function and appearance and the maintenance of comfort, with great emphasis on preservation of the health and integrity of all the oral structures that remain.
    b. Close adaptation and proper contour of an adequately extended denture base and accurate fit of the framework against multiple, properly prepared guide planes should be used to help the retentive clasp arms retain the prosthesis.
  2. Clasps
    a. The simplest type of clasp that will accomplish the design objectives should be employed.
    b. The clasp should have good stabilizing qualities, remain passive until activated by functional stress, and accommodate a minor amount of movement of the base without transmitting a torque to the abutment tooth.
    c. Clasps should be strategically positioned in the arch to achieve the greatest possible control of stress.
      (1) A Class I prosthesis usually requires only two retentive clasp arms: one on each terminal tooth.
        (a) If a distobuccal undercut is present,

the vertical projection retentive clasp is preferred. A reverse circumferential clasp would be the next best selection.

(b) If a mesiobuccal undercut is present, a wrought wire clasp is indicated. A cast circumferential type clasp *should not* be used.

(c) The reciprocal or bracing arm must be rigid. This component of the clasp system can be replaced by lingual plating.

(2) A Class II prosthesis should usually have three retentive clasp arms.

(a) The distal extension side should be designed with the same considerations as for a Class I prosthesis.

(b) The tooth-supported, or modification, side should usually have two retentive clasp arms: one as far posterior and one as far anterior as tooth contours and esthetics permit. If a modification space is present, it is usually most convenient to clasp a tooth anterior and a tooth posterior to the edentulous space.

(1) The type of clasp and position of the retentive undercut can be selected for convenience.

(2) Rigidity is required for all bracing arms. Lingual plating may be substituted.

3. Rests

a. Teeth should be selected for rest preparation to provide maximum possible support for the prosthesis.

b. Rest seats should be prepared so that stress will be directed along the long axis of the teeth.

c. Rests should be placed *next to the edentulous space* with few exceptions.

4. Indirect Retention

a. Indirect retention should be employed to neutralize unseating forces.

(1) The indirect retainer should be located as far anterior to the fulcrum line as possible.

(2) Two indirect retainers should generally be used in a Class I design, whereas one placed on the side opposite the distal extension base may be adequate in a Class II design.

(3) The indirect retainers should be positioned in teeth prepared with positive rest seats that will direct forces along the long axis of the tooth.

b. Lingual plating can be used to extend the effectiveness of indirect retention to several teeth. It must always be supported by positive rest seats.

5. Major Connector

a. The simplest connector that will accomplish the objectives should be selected.

(1) The major connector must be *rigid*.

(2) It must not impinge on gingival tissue.

b. Support from the hard palate should be used in the design of the maxillary major connector when it would be beneficial.

c. Extension of the major connector onto the lingual surfaces of the teeth may be employed to increase rigidity, distribute lateral stresses, improve indirect retention, or eliminate potential food impaction areas. Lingual plating should always be supported by adequate rest seats.

6. Minor Connectors

a. Minor connectors must be rigid.

b. Minor connectors should be positioned to enhance comfort, cleanliness, and the placement of artificial teeth.

7. Occlusion

a. Centric occlusion and centric relation should coincide.

b. A harmonious occlusion should be established with no interceptive contacts and with all eccentric movements dictated by, or in harmony with, the remaining natural teeth.

c. Artificial teeth should be selected and positioned to minimize stresses produced by the prosthesis.

(1) Smaller and/or fewer teeth, and teeth that are narrower buccolingually may be selected.

(2) For mechanical advantage teeth should be positioned over the crest of the mandibular ridge when possible.

(3) Teeth should be modified if necessary to produce sharp cutting edges and ample escape-ways.

8. Denture base

a. The base should be designed with broad coverage so that the occlusal stresses can be distributed over as wide an area of support as possible.

(1) The extension of the borders must *not interfere* with functional movements of the surrounding tissues.

b. A *selective* pressure impression should record the residual ridge in a functional form.

c. The polished surfaces should be contoured to enable the patient to exercise maximum neuromuscular control.

B. Class III
  1. Direct retention
    a. Retention can be achieved with much less potential harmful effect on the abutment teeth than with the Class I or II arch.
    b. The position of the retentive undercut on abutment teeth is not critical.
  2. Clasps
    a. The quadrilateral positioning of direct retainers is ideal.
    b. The type of clasp selected is not critical.
      (1) Tooth and tissue contours and esthetics should be considered, and the simplest clasp possible selected.
      (2) If restorations are required to correct tooth contours, the wax patterns must be shaped with the surveyor.
    c. Bracing arms must be rigid.
  3. Rests
    a. Rest seats should be prepared next to the edentulous space when possible.
    b. Rests should be used to support the major connector and lingual plating.
  4. Indirect retention
    a. Indirect retention is usually not required.
    b. If one or both of the terminal abutment teeth are used for vertical support alone without retentive clasp arms, the entire design must follow the requirements of a Class I or II design.
  5. Major and minor connectors
    a. They must be rigid and meet the same requirements as for a Class I or II design.
  6. Occlusion
    a. The requirements for occlusion are the same as for a Class I or II design.
  7. Denture base
    a. A functional type impression is not required.
    b. The extent of coverage of the residual ridge areas should be determined by appearance, comfort, and the avoidance of food impaction areas.

C. Class IV
  1. The movements of this type of removable partial denture and the resulting stresses transmitted to the abutment teeth are unlike the pattern seen in any other type of prosthesis.
  2. The esthetic arrangement of the anterior replacement teeth may necessitate their placement anterior to the crest of the residual ridge, resulting in potential tilting leverage. Every effort should be made to minimize these stresses. Some possibilities follow:
    a. As much of the labial alveolar process should be preserved as possible.
    b. A central incisor or other tooth should be retained to serve as an intermediate abutment or as an overdenture abutment.
    c. A critical evaluation of each remaining tooth in the arch should be made with the intent of retaining as many teeth as possible.
      (1) The shorter the edentulous area, the less will be the harmful tilting leverage.
  3. Strategic clasp position should be used. The quadrilateral configuration, with the anterior clasps placed as far anterior and the posterior clasps placed as far posterior as possible, would be the ideal.
  4. The major connector should be rigid, and broad palatal coverage should be used in the maxillary arch.
  5. Indirect retention should be used as far posterior to the fulcrum line as possible.
    a. An ideal quadrilateral configuration of clasping may preclude the need for an additional indirect retainer.
  6. A functional type of impression may be indicated if the edentulous area is extensive.

DESIGN PROCEDURE

The past reluctance on the part of the dentist to survey and design removable partial dentures has been caused in part by lack of knowledge of the step-by-step sequence involved. A great deal of mystery and, at times, controversy has surrounded the act of designing. It is the goal of this text to present the rudiments of producing a *usable* design. Simplicity is of prime concern in the following discussion, but it will never be the goal at the expense of mechanical and biological standards that are necessary for maintenance of the patient's health.

Criticism may come from proponents of other design philosophies. Criticism is to be expected, and it is welcome if alternate methods of design are proposed and defended. Criticism for the sake of controversy, however, is perhaps the main reason that dentists have avoided the practice of designing removable partial dentures. It does not require an astute student to prove that a removable partial denture can do nothing but destroy the remaining oral structures. In the same way students of aeronautical engineering can prove absolutely that the bumblebee cannot fly, and the bee flies.

For these reasons it is up to the designer to know about components of the partial denture, to understand the functions of the parts, and to select the ones that will counter the forces generated around fulcrum lines by levers or by inclined planes.

There are only a few absolute taboos when it comes to designing removable partial dentures. Seldom, if ever, is there a single best way to design any one partial denture. More often than not several completely acceptable designs may be used for a given partially edentulous arch with the same prognosis.

It must be stressed once again that knowledge of the components of the partial denture is essential before meaningful decisions can be made as to what component to select for a given situation. For example, each major connector has definite indications and contraindications, and each retentive clasp or clasp assembly is capable of performing certain functions well and others not so completely. These must be known, or the design process will be more of a guessing game than a scientific process.

This is a good time to make a plea for the dental laboratories. Before casts, either diagnostic or master, are forwarded to a laboratory, they should be checked carefully for accuracy and neatness. The casts should be thin enough that they can be handled easily but not so fragile as to be subject to breakage. (The requirements for accurate casts are covered in Chapter 5.) The more presentable the work submitted to the laboratory, the better are the chances for quality work being returned.

Armamentarium

The armamentarium needed to accomplish the survey and design procedure is shown in Fig. 7-45. The equipment required should be available to prevent unnecessary waste of time and effort.

The surveyor, in this case a Ney surveyor, should be maintained in a usable condition. The surface of the platform tends to oxidize over time. This oxidation prevents the surveying table from sliding smoothly over its surface and makes the surveying process unnecessarily difficult. This can be corrected by wiping the surface with a gauze pad wet with a cleansing agent such as acetone. To ease the movement of the cast holder, a small amount of fine acrylic resin polymer may then be spread on the surface of the platform (Fig. 7-46). The base of the cast holder should also be cleaned with the acetone sponge.

The vertical arm of the surveyor tends to collect debris over time and become difficult to move. It may be cleaned with acetone to improve its action. Lubricants such as oil or grease should not be used because the sleeve within which the vertical arm rides will collect the oil, and the problem of sticking will be aggravated.

Other essential items in the armamentarium are the cast holder, analyzing rod, carbon marker (5-H), and undercut gauges (0.010, 0.020, and 0.030 inch). The 0.010-inch gauge is used to position most retentive cast chrome alloy clasps. The 0.020-inch gauge may be used to locate the position of the retentive clasp tip for a combination or wrought wire clasp. The 0.030-inch undercut gauge is used mainly to locate retentive undercuts for a temporary removable partial denture with very lightweight wrought wire clasps.

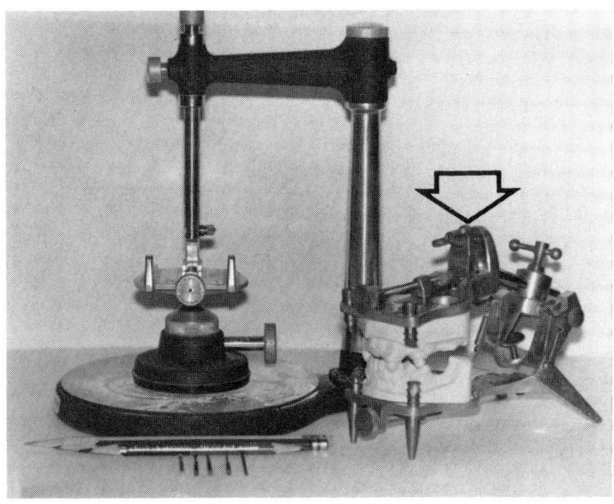

Fig. 7-45. The armamentarium needed to accomplish the survey and design procedure. The surveyor and cast holder are shown. In front of the surveyor are the colored pencils and the surveying tools. At the right is the plasterless Galetti-Luongo articulator.

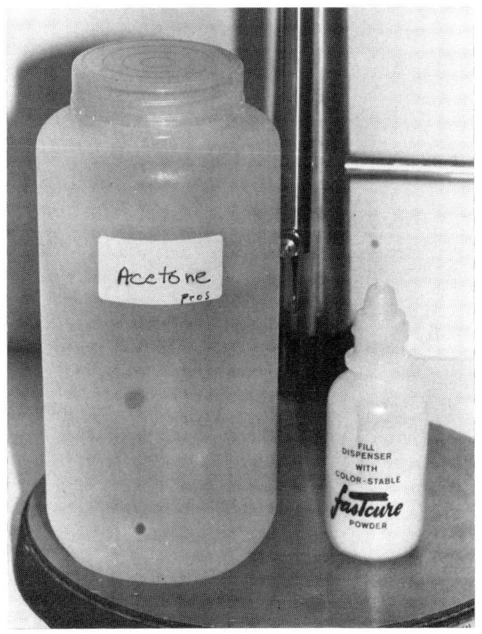

Fig. 7-46. To keep the surveyor in its most usable condition, the platform surface must be cleaned of rust. This is best done by wiping the platform occasionally with gauze pads soaked in acetone. Sprinkling the platform, after it has been cleaned, with acrylic resin polymer will provide a surface over which the surveying table will slide freely.

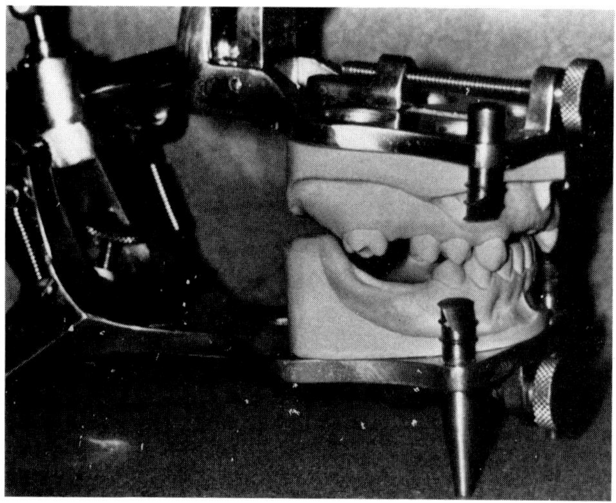

Fig. 7-47. The Galetti-Luongo articulator locks the casts firmly in place without the use of plaster of paris or dental stone. This articulator is an excellent diagnostic tool, but should not be used for patient treatment.

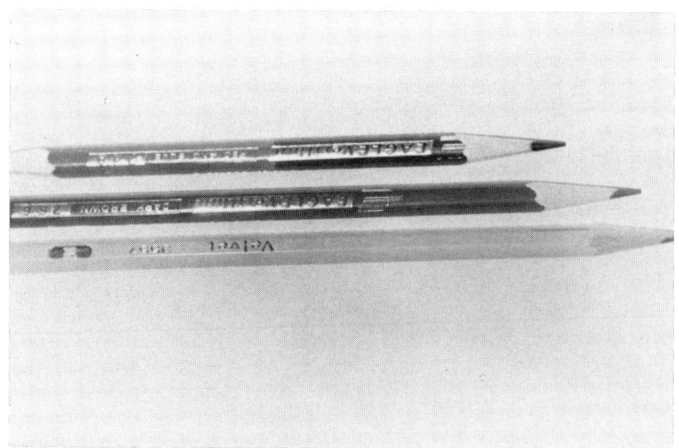

Fig. 7-48. The use of red, blue, brown, and black pencils in the design process helps differentiate the various components of the partial denture.

The articulator included in the armamentarium is a plasterless type, the Galetti-Luongo (Fig. 7-47). It is an excellent diagnostic tool, and its use should be limited to that purpose. The casts are held in place by adjustable clamps. The casts are occluded by means of a jaw relation record. When the controls of the articulator are released, the casts move independently in three dimensions. Once the casts are properly aligned, the controls are locked. the occlusion may be studied in either centric occlusion or centric relation, whichever was decided during the diagnostic phase of treatment.

It is essential that the occlusion of the patient be known and possible problems be observed before and during the design procedure. The amount of space between opposing teeth will influence and may at times even dictate the positioning of various components, particularly occlusal rests and lingual plating. Failure to be aware of occlusal interferences most often results in problems becoming magnified as treatment progresses. Occlusal rests or lingual plating positioned so that occlusal interferences between the metal and opposing teeth cannot be corrected without mutilating either the metal or the teeth can necessitate construction of a new framework. A few minutes spent in the planning phase of treatment can save many hours of frustrating attempts to correct errors that should not have been made.

Color coding

A color coding system for the various parts of the removable partial denture as well as for other items of information that should be included on the diagnostic casts helps prevent confusion on the part of a dental laboratory technician or anyone trying to understand the design being proposed. The need for color coding becomes obvious when it is realized that many large commercial dental laboratories process as many as a hundred partial dentures in a single day. Well-designed diagnostic casts are not only the clearest way of illustrating to the technician what is desired, but also serve as blueprints for the dentist during the mouth preparation appointment.

There is not at present a universally accepted color coding system* As a result, any system agreed to and understood by a dental laboratory and a submitting dentist is considered acceptable.

We have long used the system that will be presented in this chapter. Red, blue, and brown crayon pencils and a black lead pencil, two H or three H hardness, are used (Fig. 7-48). The accompanying photographs are not in color, but the difference in brightness is distinguishable.

The brown crayon pencil is used to outline the metallic portion of the partial denture; the blue crayon pencil, to outline the acrylic resin portion of the prosthesis; and the red crayon pencil, to indicate areas on the teeth that will be prepared, relieved, or contoured. Rest seats are drawn in solid red, whereas tooth surfaces that are to be recontoured are outlined in red. The black pencil and the carbon marker in the surveyor are used to denote survey lines, tripod marks, soft tissue undercuts, and other information that must be included, such as the type of tooth replacement or the use of wrought wire for retentive clasps.

*A color coding system is currently being standardized by the Army, Navy, and Air Force Dental Corps. They are using the system presented here with the exception that green is used in place of brown for the outline of the metal portion to avoid possible confusion between brown and black. This change has merit and certainly can be incorporated in any system.

Step-by-step procedure

The following list presents a step-by-step technique for designing a removable partial denture.* The accompanying photographs, Fig. 7-49 to 7-103, illustrate the design process for one pair of casts.

Too often the mechanical aspects of dentistry have been belittled as being subprofessional. Nothing could be further from the truth. The biologic aspects of dentistry are all greatly influenced by the mechanical phases. It is essential that a wedding of the two occur in order to produce the quality of care the patient deserves.

1. Examine the occluded diagnostic casts (Fig. 7-50 to 7-52).
   a. Indicate the proposed rest areas by a short vertical line on the cast below the tooth with the black pencil (Fig. 7-53 to 7-57). (The reason for indicating the location on the base of the cast at this time is that, in the event a change in rest seat location is indicated, corrections will not have to be made on the teeth. Incorrect lines placed on the cast may be removed by lightly scraping the cast surface with an excavator, but an excessive amount of erasing will change the appearance of the cast.)
   b. Indicate by *outlining* in red any cuspal relief that will be needed to provide adequate occlusal clearance for rest spaces (Fig. 7-58 to 7-60).
   c. Examine the lingual aspect of the occluded casts for adequate space for cingulum rests, indirect retainers, and so on. Using the black pencil from the rear of the casts, draw a line on the lingual surfaces of the maxillary anterior teeth using the incisal edges of the mandibular teeth as a guide. This line shows the incisal limit of proposed metal extensions (rests or lingual plating) onto those teeth (Fig. 7-61).
2. Indicate with a pencil, using the following symbols, the type of tooth replacement desired (Fig. 7-62 and 7-63).
   Denture teeth on a denture base—no symbol
   Tube tooth—T
   Facing—F
   Metal pontic—M
   Reinforced acrylic pontic—RAP
   Place these symbols on the soft tissue portion of the cast, adjacent to the edentulous area. One symbol should be used for each tooth replacement.
3. Place the cast on the cast holder at a horizontal tilt. Examine the teeth to be clasped for favorable retentive undercuts. Examine anterior edentulous areas for esthetic considerations. Examine proximal and lingual tooth surfaces for guiding planes. Be aware of soft tissue undercuts that may interfere with the placement of the partial denture. After considering these factors, select the best tilt, or path of insertion. Outline in red pencil those surfaces that will require recontouring or reshaping to produce the desired result (Fig. 7-64 to 7-81).
4. Tripod the cast (Fig. 7-82).
5. Place a carbon marker in the vertical arm of the surveyor and scribe the survey line on the teeth that will be contacted by the partial denture (Fig. 7-83 and 7-84).
6. With a red pencil draw in the extent of rest areas to be prepared in the mouth (Fig. 7-85).
7. Outline the exact position and extent of the denture base area (Figs. 7-86 and 7-87). Blue pencil indicates acrylic resin denture base; brown indicates a metal denture base.
8. With a brown pencil outline the framework design to harmonize and join the major connectors, rest areas, indirect retainers, minor connectors, denture bases, and replacement teeth. Use the carbon marker to outline soft tissue undercuts that will influence the design (Figs. 7-88 to 7-93).
9. Replace the carbon marker with the appropriate undercut gauge. (For most clasps of chrome cobalt alloy a 0.010-inch undercut is adequate. In unusual cases, large molars or long canines, 0.015 inch may be used. For wrought wire retentive clasps 0.020 inch is usually indicated. If gold is used, the amount of undercut should be increased slightly.) Place the gauge on the desired retentive undercut area so that the head and shank of the gauge touch the tooth simultaneously. With the red pencil mark the spot that the head touches the tooth. This mark represents the gingival edge of the clasp tip in the desired retentive undercut (Fig. 7-94).
10. With the brown pencil draw the clasp arms to the actual shape, size, and location desired. If wrought wire clasps are to be used, place the symbol *WW* on the soft tissue below the tooth (Fig. 7-95 to 7-102).
11. The design should now be complete (Fig. 7-103). Reexamine for accuracy and clarity.
12. Most state dental laws require that a written Work Authorization Order accompany all work submitted to a laboratory.

*This procedure was originally proposed by Dr. Benjamin W. Dunn in Treatment planning for removable partial dentures, J. Prosthet. Dent. **11**:247-255, 1961.

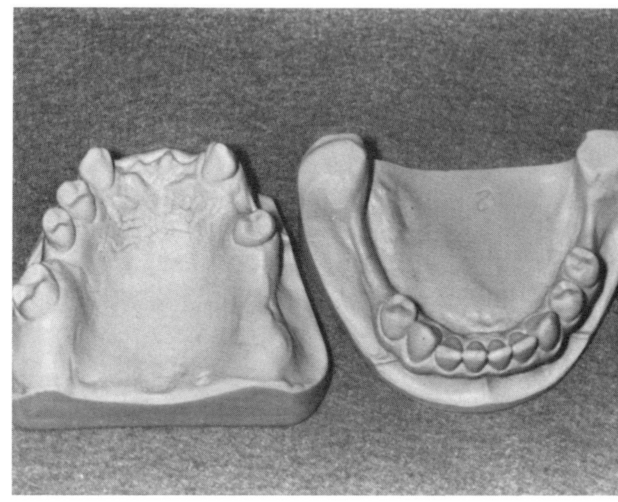

Fig. 7-49. The diagnostic casts that are to be designed are shown. The maxillary cast is a Class II, Modification 3. The mandibular cast is a Class I. These casts were selected not because they are typical but because a variety of conditions that may be encountered are included. It can be defended that a combination of fixed and removable partial dentures would be the treatment of choice for this patient. (Unless otherwise stated the oral and general health conditions, including periodontal support and bone height, are to be considered satisfactory.) However, removable partial dentures have been planned for this patient.

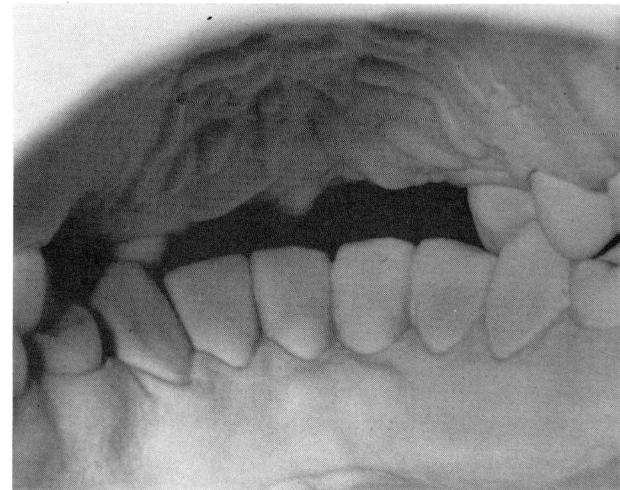

Fig. 7-50. A lingual view of the occluded casts indicates the amount of vertical and horizontal overlap of the anterior teeth. This will be an important consideration when the position of the lingual plating of the maxillary teeth is considered. The only way this can accurately be determined is by the use of mounted diagnostic casts.

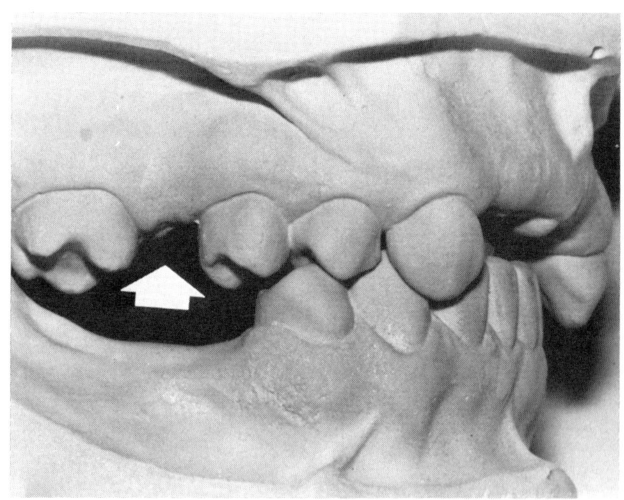

Fig. 7-51. The right lateral view of the occluded casts reveals that the edentulous space of the maxillary first molar is restricted because of drifting of the teeth. This may require special planning as the type of tooth replacement is selected.

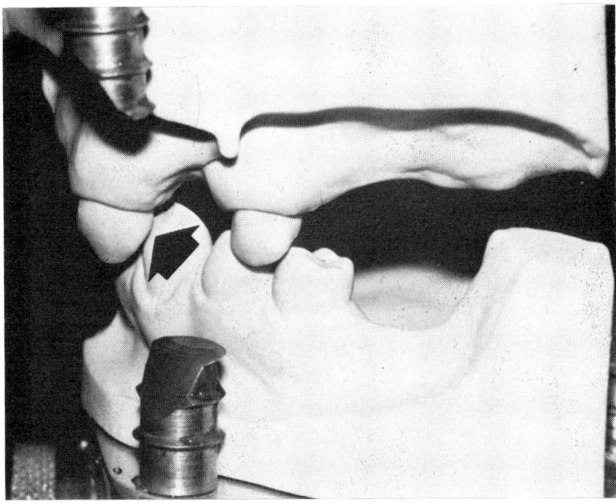

Fig. 7-52. The left lateral view shows a deep vertical overlap of the canine teeth. This will play a role in later considerations. A decrease in interarch space is always a problem in design procedures.

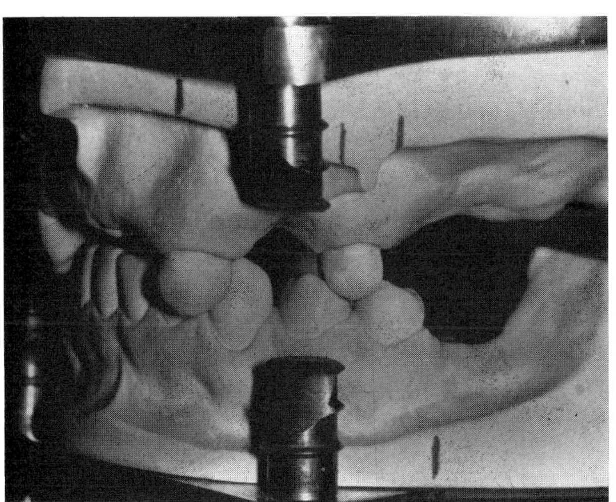

Fig. 7-53. A vertical mark is placed on the base of the cast directly below the area of the tooth on which a rest seat will be prepared. The philosophy described here will place a rest seat adjacent to all edentulous spaces. In this case, rest seats will be placed on both the mesial occlusal and distal occlusal surfaces of the maxillary left second premolar, on the lingual surface of the maxillary left canine, and on the distal occlusal surface of the mandibular left second premolar.

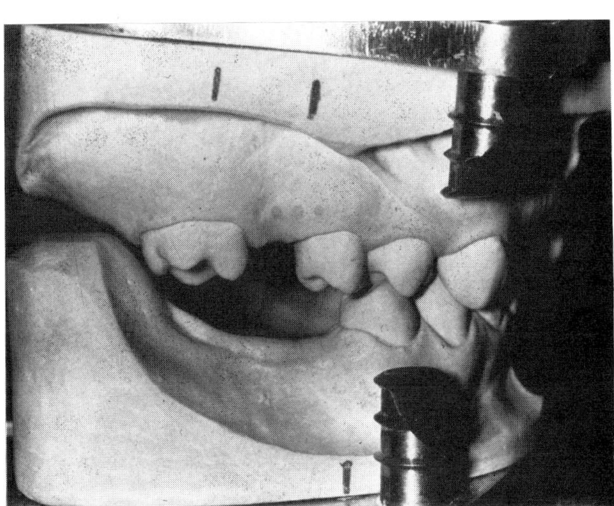

Fig. 7-54. On the right side of the maxillary cast rest seat preparations are indicated for the mesial occlusal surface of the second molar and the distal occlusal surface of the second premolar. On the right side of the mandibular cast a rest seat is indicated for the distal occlusal surface of the second premolar.

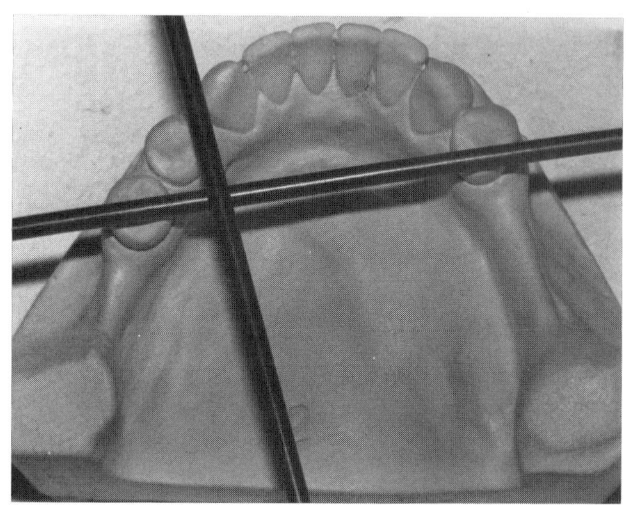

Fig. 7-55. Indirect retention is required for all Class I and II partial denture designs. The fulcrum line is depicted as a rod running from the distal occlusal rest of one premolar to the distal occlusal rest of the premolar on the opposite side of the arch. A line perpendicular to the fulcrum line, bisecting its center, and extended anteriorly should locate the most mechanically sound position for an indirect retainer (in this case a rest seat to act as the indirect retainer). In this instance the line falls on the left lateral incisor, a tooth that cannot tolerate additional stress, so a compromise in the position of the rest seat must be made. It would be logical to accept the canine as the tooth to support the indirect retainer. Normally it has a large root surface and can tolerate additional stress. However, to prepare an adequate rest seat in a mandibular canine, an incisal rest must usually be used. The shape of the lingual surface of most mandibular canines is such that by the time sufficient tooth structure is removed to establish a preparation that would support a cingulum rest, the enamel will have been penetrated. An incisal rest as an indirect retainer concentrates the forces created against the canine, resisting the lifting tendency of the denture base caused by the action of sticky foods or rebound of the mucosa, at the tip of the canine. This greatly magnifies the force that the tooth is called on to resist. To avoid this undesirable result, a second compromise in the position of the indirect retainer is necessary. The mesial fossa of the left first premolar is the next logical position to be considered. In most mouths the mesial fossae of lower first premolars are nonfunctioning, that is, an upper cusp does not occlude into them. The root of the first premolar is large enough to accept additional stress. The rest preparation of the mesial fossa, being spoon-shaped, allows the forces to be directed down the long axis of the tooth. Therefore, after several compromises, the indirect retainer is placed in the mesial fossa of the first premolar.

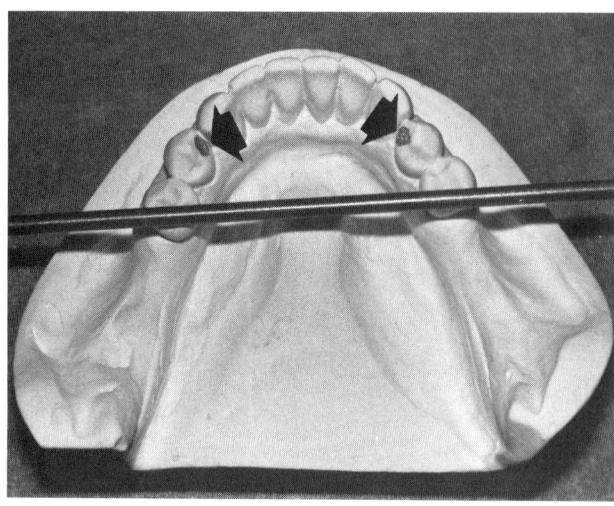

Fig. 7-56. Class I partially edentulous arches should normally have two symmetric indirect retainers, one on each side of the arch as far anterior from the fulcrum line as can practically be positioned. The locations are indicated at the mesial fossae of the two first premolars. This is an ideal solution. In the practical case being designed here a compromise has been reached using a single indirect retainer. This is an exception, not the rule.

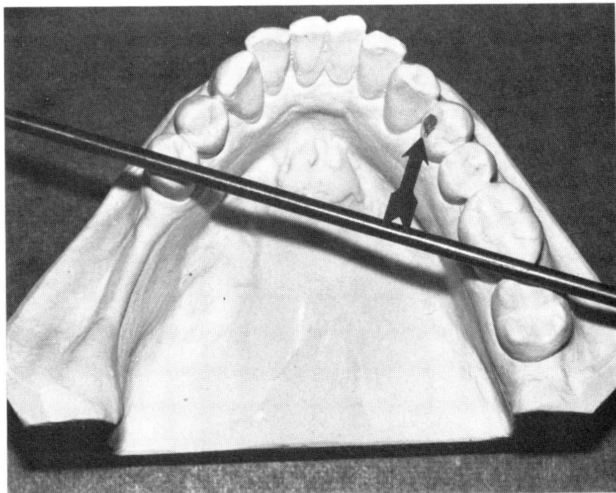

Fig. 7-57. The Class II arch normally requires one indirect retainer. The fulcrum line, as shown by the rod, runs between the most posterior rest seats on each side of the arch. A perpendicular to this rotation line falls, as the most usable location, in the mesial fossa of the first premolar on the side of the arch opposite the distal extension edentulous area.

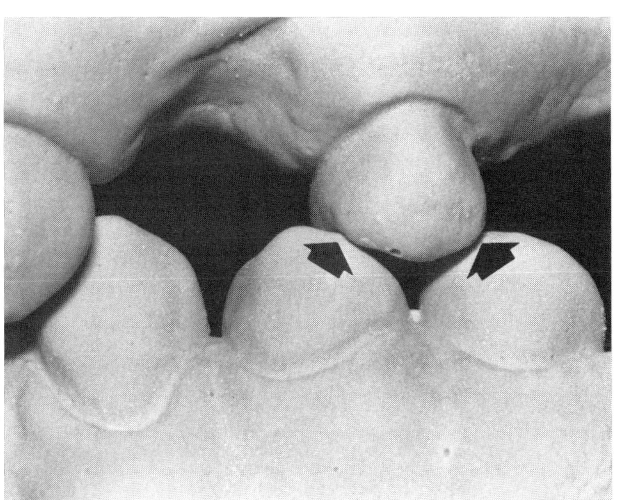

Fig. 7-58. Examination of the occlusal contacts of the premolar teeth on the left side of the arch reveals that both marginal ridges of the maxillary premolar are in intimate contact with the distal incline of the buccal cusp of the lower first premolar and the mesial incline of the buccal cusp of the second premolar. Interocclusal space in addition to that provided by rest seat preparations may be needed to provide adequate thickness of metal without overcutting the enamel surface over the marginal ridge of the maxillary premolar.

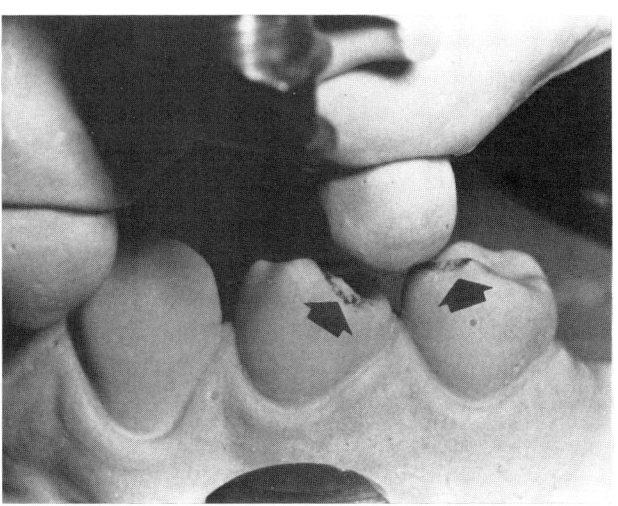

Fig. 7-59. The buccal cuspal inclines of the mandibular first and second premolars are circled in red to remind the dentist that during mouth preparation these enamel surfaces will be slightly reduced to provide space for adequate thickness of metal for the rest seat. (A reminder that should be made at this time that under most circumstances a lone standing second premolar, either mandibular or maxillary, makes a poor terminal abutment for a distal extension removable partial denture. It is being used in this exercise only to demonstrate problems that may be encountered in this or other similar design situations. Do not consider that this configuration of abutment tooth selection, particularly in the maxillary arch, is one that should be used for most patients.)

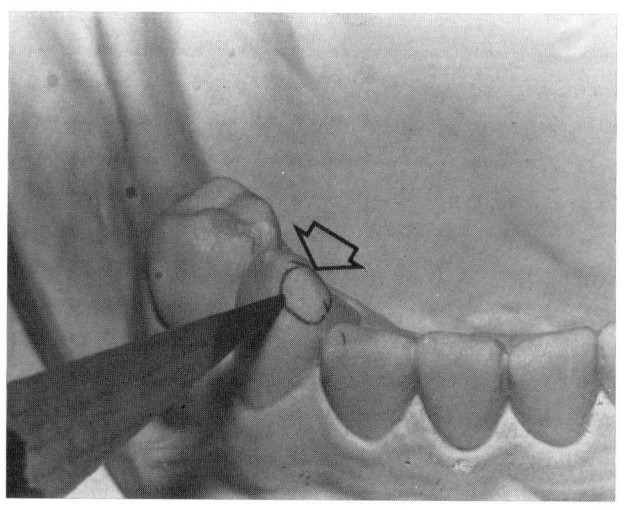

Fig. 7-60. The mesial incline of the mandibular right canine contacts the lingual surface of the maxillary canine. To gain space for the metal of the cingulum rest on the upper canine, a slight reduction of the enamel surface is indicated. The incline has been circled in red.

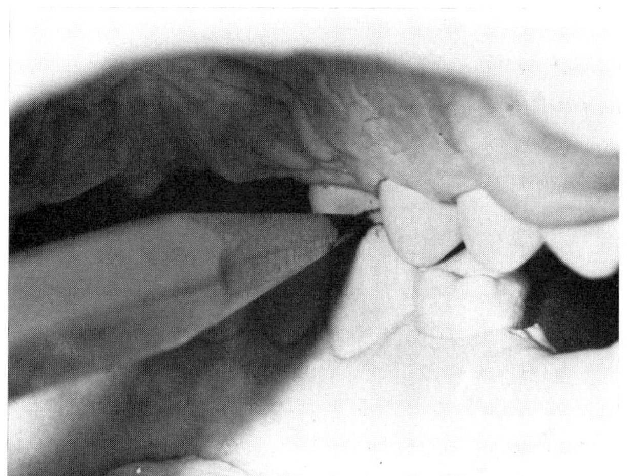

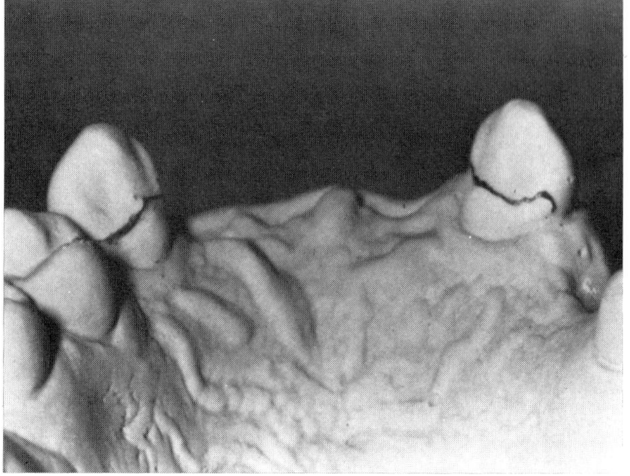

Fig. 7-61. A, With the diagnostic casts occluded, the black pencil is used from the posterior aspect of the casts to scribe a line on the lingual aspect of the maxillary anterior teeth. The position of the line is dictated by the incisal edges of the mandibular anterior teeth. **B,** The line is shown as scribed on the lingual surfaces of the maxillary canines. No metal component of the partial denture can extend incisal to the line without producing occlusal interference with the mandibular anterior teeth. The relief to be provided on the mandibular right canine will allow a slight extension of the metal without ill effect.

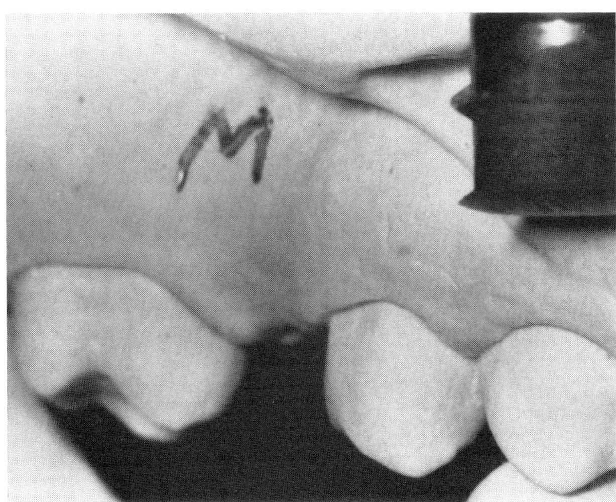

Fig. 7-62. The replacement for the missing first molar is considered first. Because the space is restricted, strength of the replacement tooth is important. If a porcelain or acrylic resin tooth were shaped to conform to the size of the space, it would be too weak to function. For this reason and also because the replacement will be opposed by artificial teeth, a metal pontic has been selected.

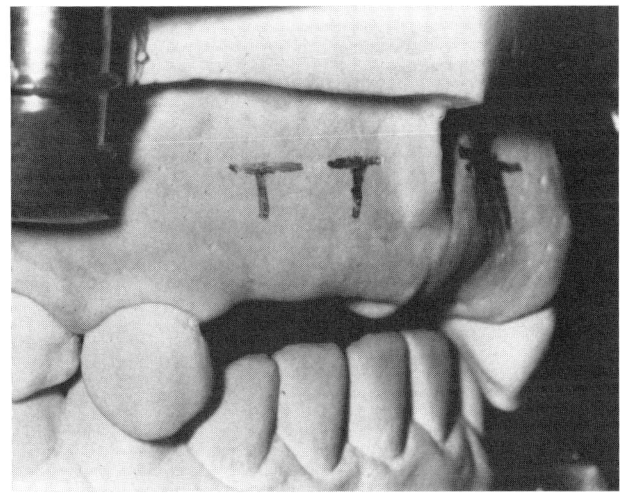

Fig. 7-63. The maxillary anterior replacement teeth are the next consideration. The possible options are facings, tube teeth, reinforced acrylic pontics (RAP), and denture teeth on a denture base. As was noted in Chapter 3, the single greatest indication for facings is where strength is an overwhelming requirement. In this case special strength is not needed and the limited esthetic quality of facings makes them a poor choice. The maxillary anterior ridge appears to be well healed with little resorption—an excellent indication for either tube teeth or the RAP. There is little to choose between these two replacements. The RAP may be slightly the stronger of the two. The last possible anterior selection would be denture teeth, normally acrylic resin teeth, on a denture base. This choice is seldom incorrect, but in this patient, where little bone resorption has occurred, a better result can be obtained by using tube teeth butted against the broad edentulous ridge. A decision has been made to replace the missing maxillary anterior teeth with tube teeth. This is indicated on the cast by placing the symbol T for each tooth to be replaced.

The other missing teeth will be replaced as follows (not shown): the maxillary left first premolar will be replaced with a tube tooth; the missing maxillary left molars and the missing mandibular teeth will be replaced by acrylic resin denture teeth on a denture base. When the latter replacement is selected, no symbol need be used. The acrylic resin retention minor connector and the denture base will be drawn in the design.

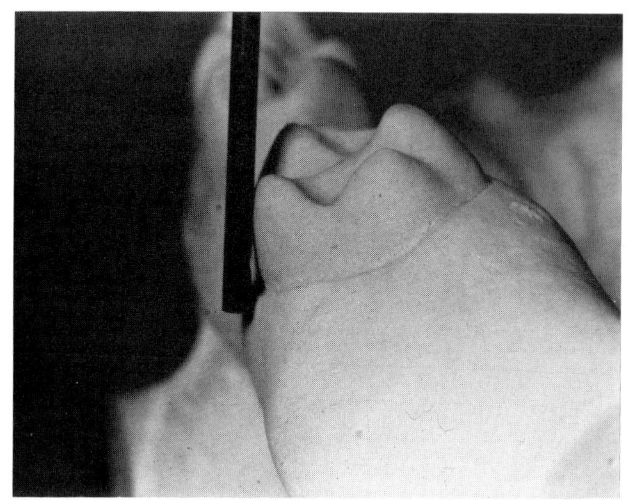

Fig. 7-64. In the maxillary arch retentive clasps should be placed on the right second molar and second premolar on each side of the edentulous space and on the left canine and second premolar. These positions provide for as widely spaced clasping as possible. In this illustration the presence of a distobuccal undercut on the facial surface of the second molar is verified by the analyzing rod. An ideal retentive clasp for this tooth would be a simple circlet clasp originating from the mesial occlusal rest and running across the facial surface into an undercut on the distobuccal line angle of the tooth. This is the simplest clasp as far as construction and maintenance are concerned; and since this side of the partial denture is tooth supported, the position of the retentive clasp tip is not significant. The point is once again emphasized that retentive undercuts must be present at this horizontal tilt or the partial denture will not be retentive.

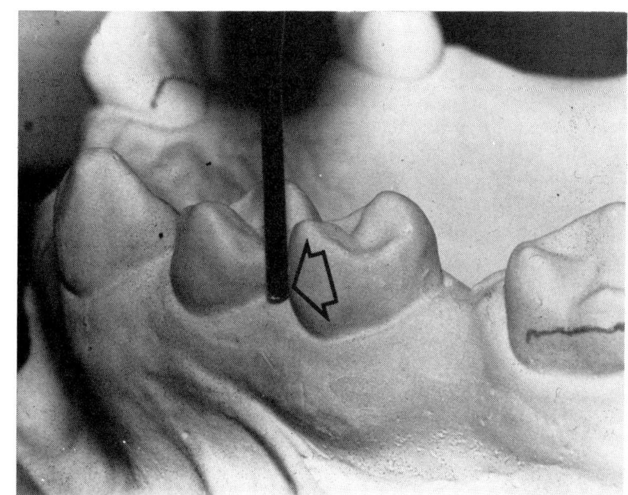

Fig. 7-65. The right second premolar is analyzed next. The clasping of choice here would be a simple circlet clasp running from the distal occlusal rest across the facial surface and engaging in mesiobuccal undercut. The analyzing rod reveals, however, that no undercut is present.

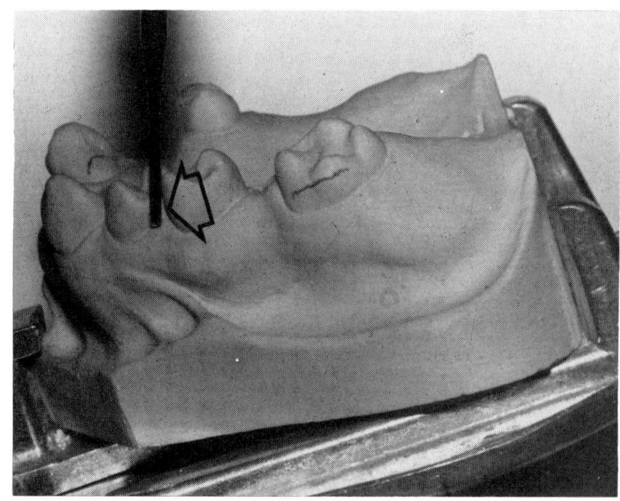

Fig. 7-66. The cast is moved to an anterior tilt. There now appears to be an undercut at the mesiobuccal line angle. This is a false retentive undercut; it is present only at this exaggerated tilt.

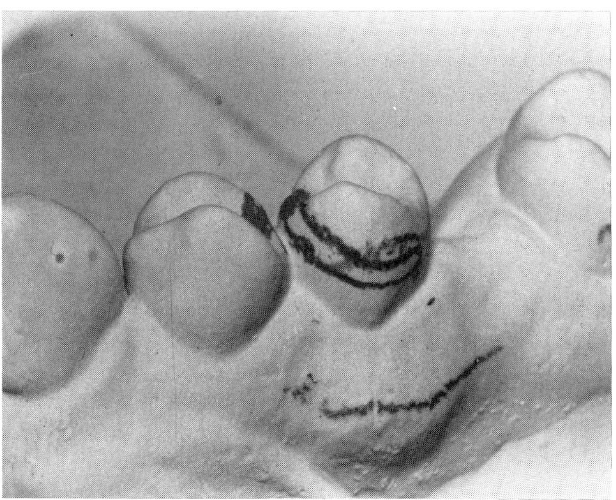

Fig. 7-67. The remainder of the facial surface of the premolar is examined and an undercut is found to be present at the distobuccal line angle. The reverse circlet clasp is a possible consideration, but there are several disadvantages to its use. A large amount of tooth structure must be removed to provide occlusal space for its use, and it is an unesthetic clasp on premolars.

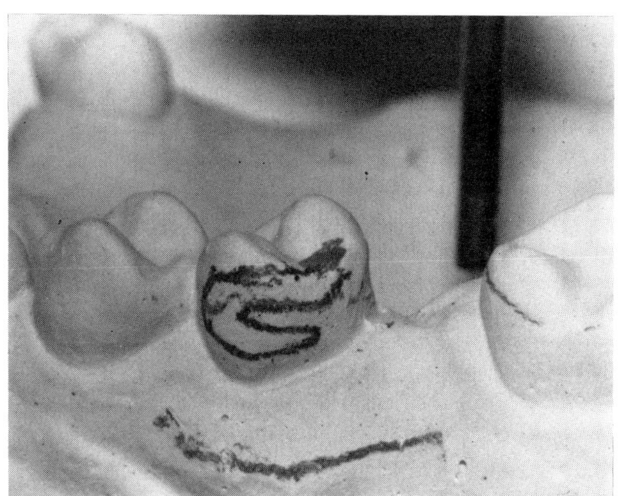

Fig. 7-68. A circumferential C, or fishhook, clasp may be considered for the second premolar. The retentive undercut, the distofacial surface, is adjacent to the edentulous space, one indication for the C clasp. The clasp has several disadvantages. It covers a large amount of tooth structure and tends to be unesthetic.

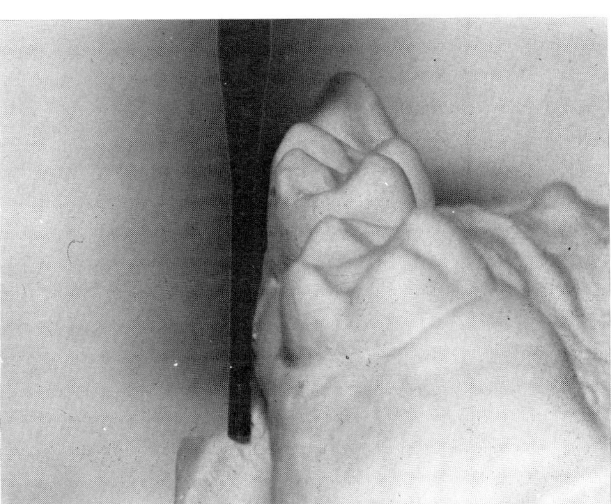

Fig. 7-69. Perhaps the best method of engaging a distobuccal retentive undercut when a distal occlusal rest is planned is by a vertical projection T clasp. If this clasp is to be planned, the soft tissue below the abutment tooth must not be undercut in relation to the path of insertion. The analyzing rod reveals that the soft tissue gingival to the abutment tooth is not in an undercut area relative to the path of insertion. Thus the approach arm of a vertical projection clasp could be inserted and remain in contact with the mucosa.

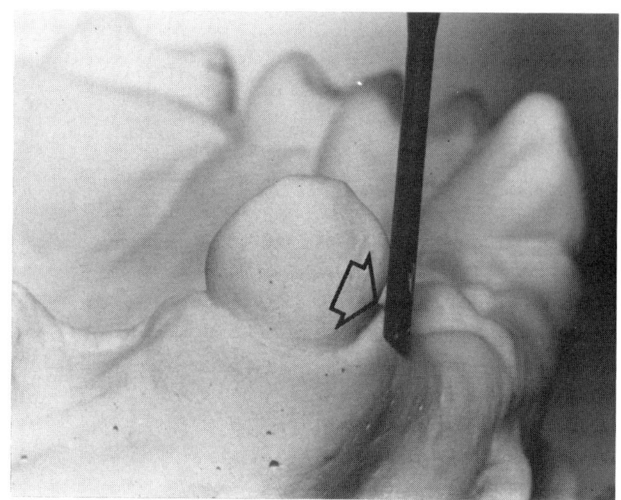

Fig. 7-70. The third retentive abutment tooth to be considered is the maxillary left canine. Several special considerations must be faced when the decision on the type and position of the retentive clasp is made. Esthetics and the release of stresses that will occur on this tooth because of its position in the arch are of concern. It is the anterior abutment tooth on the distal extension side, and stresses that are deliberately released from the posterior abutment tooth on that side will tend to be magnified on it. The analyzing rod reveals that a mesiolabial undercut is located in the gingival third of the crown of the canine (arrow). This position is ideal from an esthetic point of view because the clasp will be as unobtrusive as possible. Because forces resulting from the downward movement of the denture base during function will tend to pull the canine posteriorly, a wrought wire retentive clasp arm is indicated. The greater flexibility of the wrought wire clasp produces a stress-equalizing action that will dissipate some of these undesirable forces.

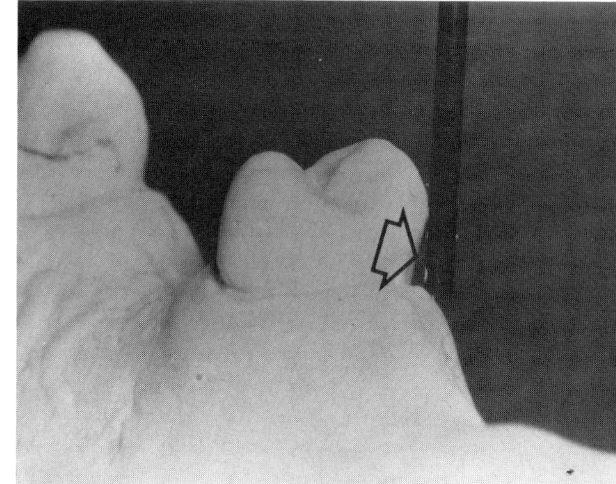

Fig. 7-71. The fourth and final abutment tooth in the maxillary arch, the left second premolar, actually is the abutment tooth of principal concern, because it will bear most of the forces generated during function. The type of clasp and position of the retentive clasp tip cannot be varied to the extent that those on abutment teeth on tooth-supported segments can. The ideal location for a retentive clasp tip on a terminal abutment tooth on the distal extension edentulous ridge is at the distobuccal line angle. Analysis of the buccal surface of the premolar shows that a distobuccal retentive undercut is present at this horizontal tilt (arrow). The clasp of choice in this situation is the T clasp. If only a mesiobuccal undercut were present, a combination clasp with wrought wire retentive arm would be planned.

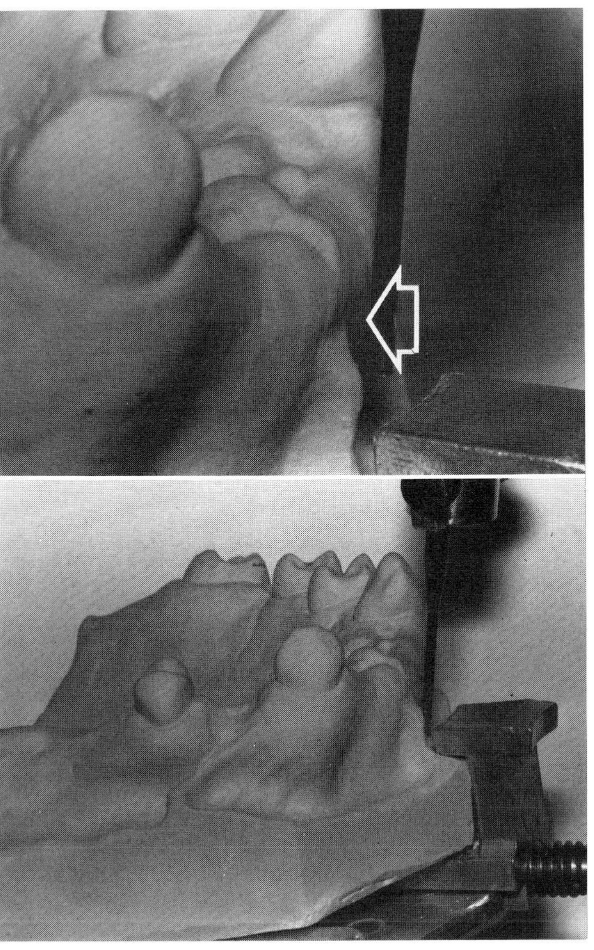

Fig. 7-72. A, The anterior ridge is examined with the analyzing rod. The undercut (arrow) could interfere with the placement of the artificial anterior teeth. **B,** A slight posterior tilt of the cast eliminates the anterior undercut. The analyzing rod shows that the retentive undercuts are still present and usable, so the tilt change did not interfere with the retention.

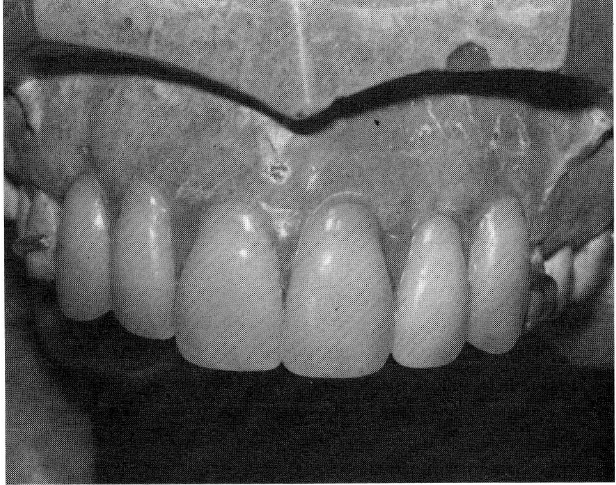

Fig. 7-73. The change to a slight posterior tilt permits the necks of the artificial teeth to be butted closely against the edentulous ridge. This results in a natural appearance of the replacement teeth.

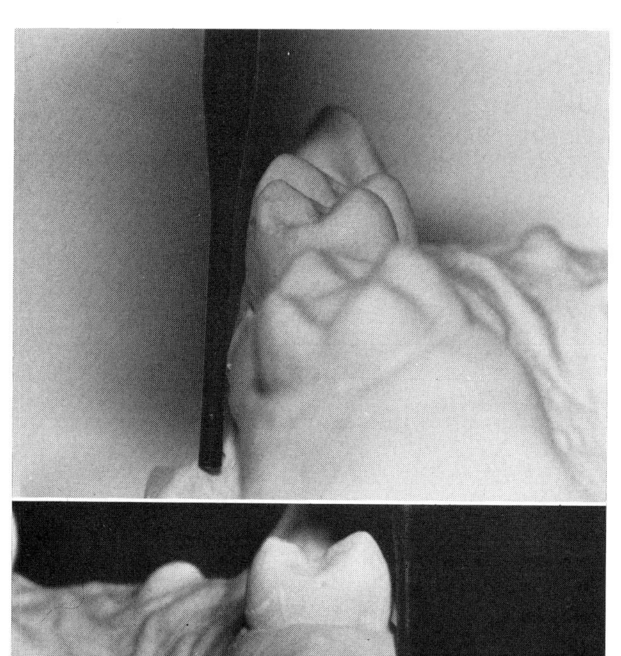

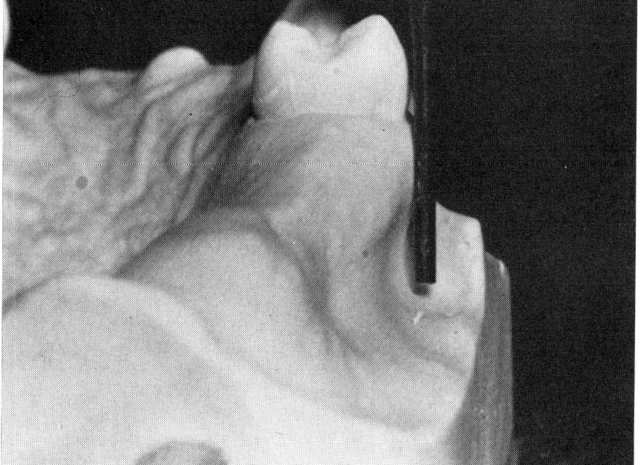

Fig. 7-74. The second consideration for possible interference is the soft tissue buccal to the second premolars. **A,** The analyzing rod shows that no interference to the path of insertion is present facial to the right second premolar. **B,** There is no soft tissue interference facial to the left second premolar. Thus the vertical projection clasp can be positioned properly.

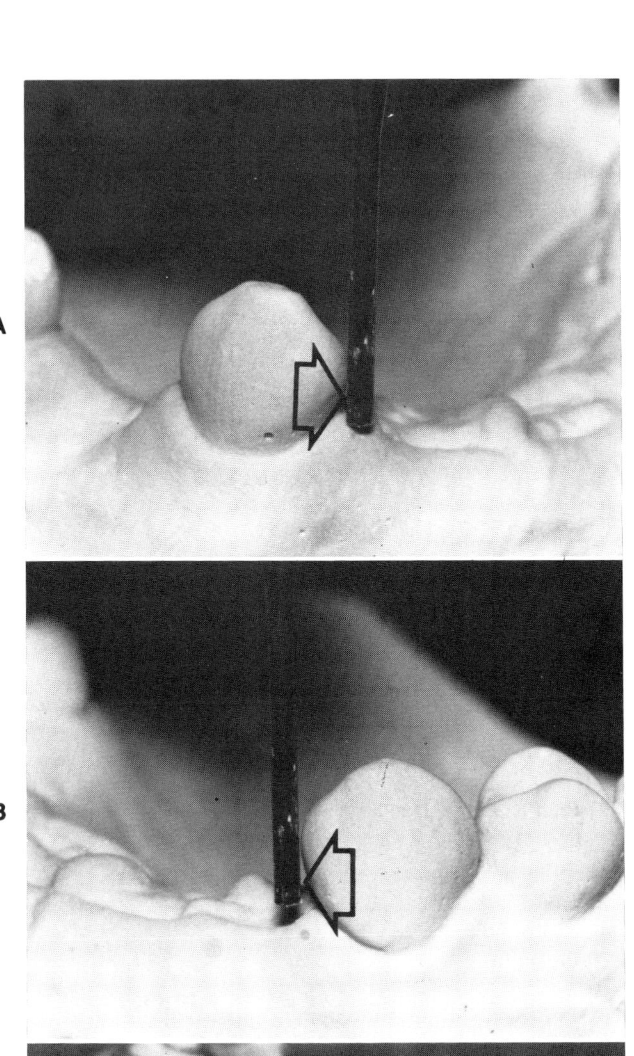

Fig. 7-75. A remaining consideration is the size of the interdental space that will exist adjacent to the mesial surfaces of the right and left canines when the artificial teeth are in position. **A,** The analyzing rod, resting against the mesial proximal surface of the left canine, shows that only a small interproximal space will exist between the canine and the artificial lateral incisor. **B,** Examination of the right canine shows that at this tilt a comparatively large interproximal space exists between the mesial surface and the analyzing rod. This would produce an unsightly and unhygienic result. **C,** To solve this problem, the tilt of the cast may be changed slightly to alter the path of insertion. However a change in tilt at this point could modify the previously determined undercuts and esthetic considerations. To avoid this possibility, a simpler solution is to recontour the mesial surface of the right canine and eliminate most of the undesirable undercut. This is indicated on the cast by circling the area in red crayon pencil.

Fig. 7-76. The proximal surfaces of the maxillary abutment teeth must be examined as potential guiding planes. It is desired that the surfaces be parallel or nearly parallel to the path of insertion, represented by the analyzing rod. The proximal surface of the second molar, **A,** the distal proximal surface of the second premolar, **B,** the distal surface of the left canine, **C,** and the mesial surface of the left second premolar, **D,** have acceptable guiding planes. If any of these surfaces is not parallel to the path of insertion, the surface should be circled with red to indicate that it must be made parallel by recontouring the enamel surface during the mouth preparation appointment. Indicating the need to prepare the guiding planes satisfies the last of the four factors needed to establish the path of insertion. The present tilt of the cast is the one at which the maxillary design will be drawn. The cast holder should be locked tightly at this position.

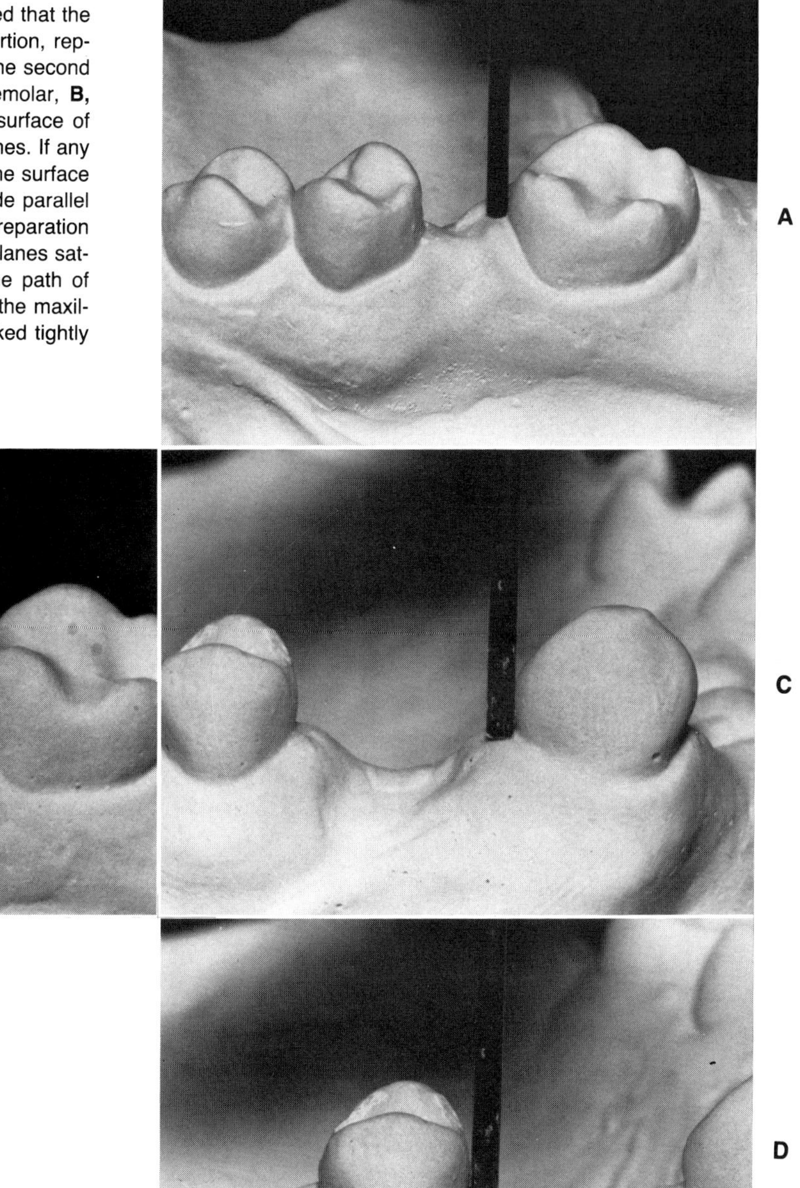

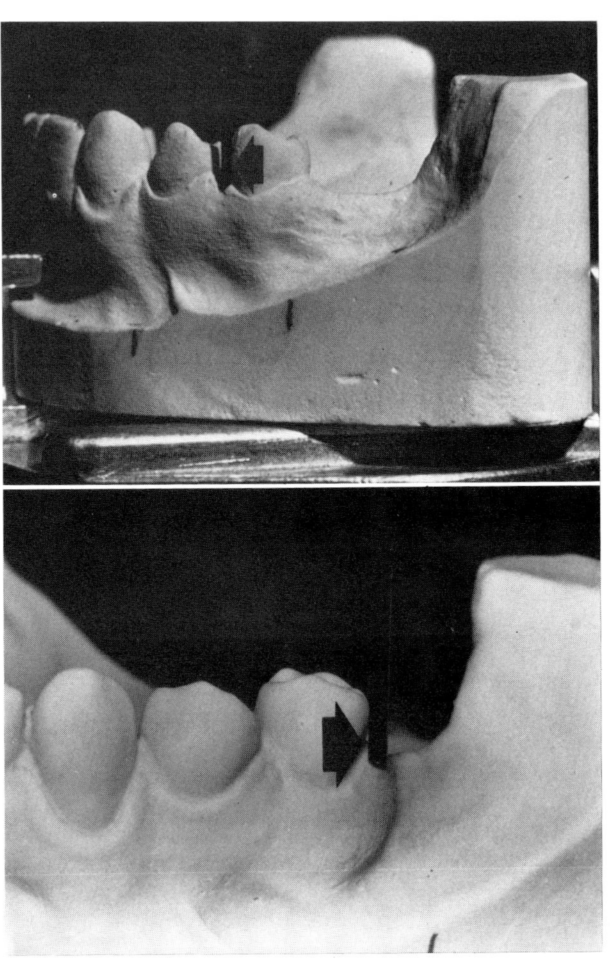

Fig. 7-77. The mandibular abutment teeth are examined for retentive undercuts. **A,** The left second premolar shows no undercut on the mesiobuccal line angle as demonstrated by the analyzing rod. **B,** The cast is moved on the surveying table to bring the distobuccal surface of the abutment tooth in contact with the analyzing rod. An acceptable retentive undercut can be visualized below the contact of the rod with the tooth. This is the most desirable location of retentive undercut for this Class I partial denture. If no contraindications are encountered, this retentive undercut and the one on the facial surface of the right first premolar (not shown) will be used with vertical projection T clasps.

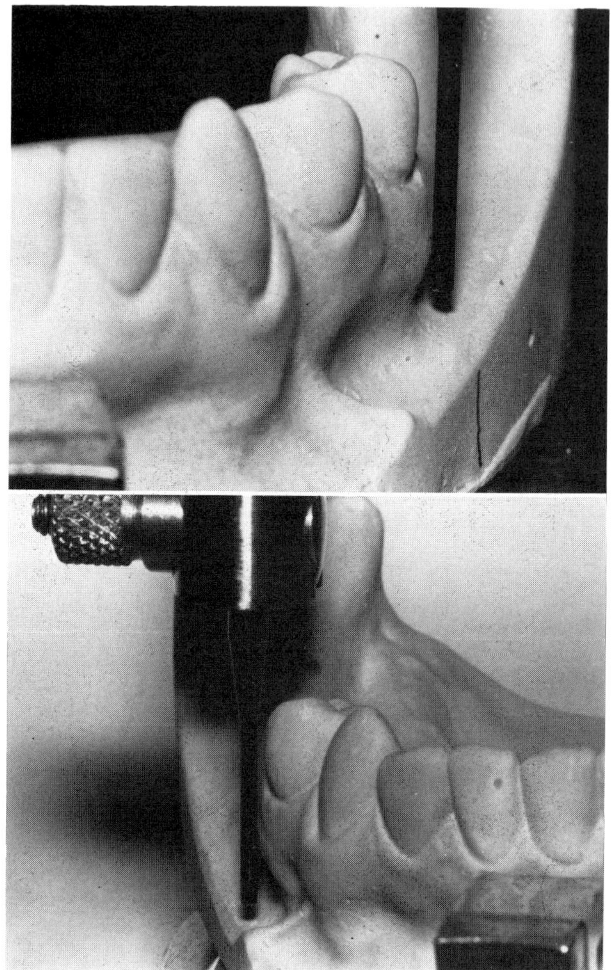

Fig. 7-78. Potential areas of interference for this mandibular partial denture are the soft tissue areas facial to the two abutment teeth, the right and left premolars. **A,** Analysis of the left premolar shows that the soft tissue area is not in an undercut. This will permit the use of a vertical projection T clasp. **B,** The same situation holds true for the right abutment tooth.

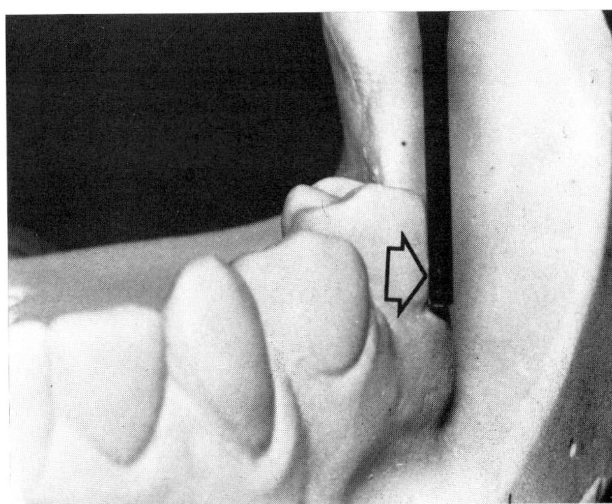

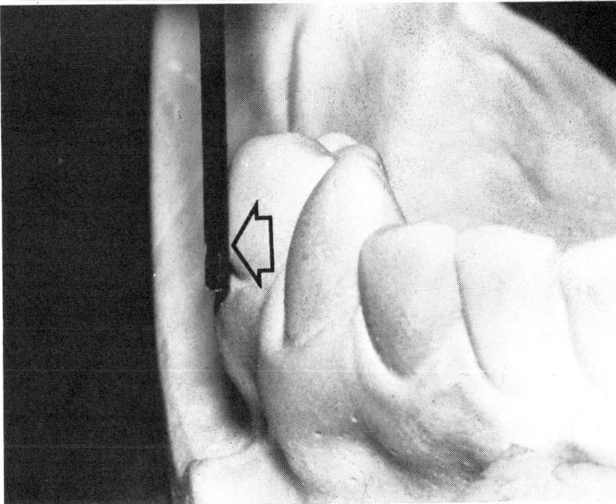

Fig. 7-79. To obtain optimum esthetics, the retentive clasp should be kept as low on the abutment teeth as possible to avoid unnecessary display of metal. The analyzing rod, held against the facial surfaces of the two abutment teeth, indicates that the height of contour will fall between the gingival and middle third of the facial surface. This is an ideal position; not only is the metal concealed as much as possible, but the mechanical advantage of the clasp is improved.

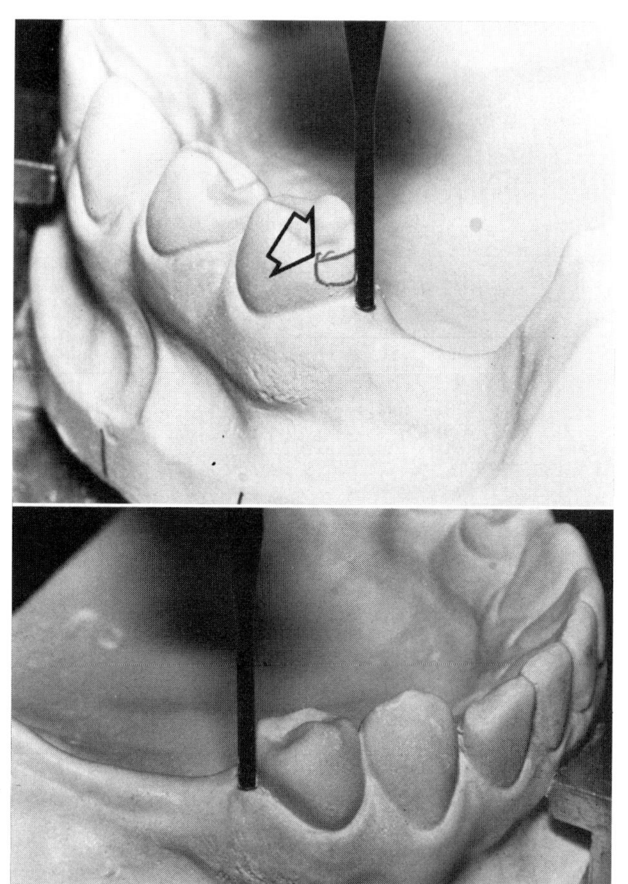

Fig. 7-80. The proximal surfaces of the two abutment teeth, adjacent to the edentulous spaces, are examined for use as guiding planes. **A,** The left second premolar has a bell-shaped surface. It is circled in red to indicate that a guiding plane must be created in this enamel surface. **B,** The right first premolar displays a surface that is parallel to the path of insertion. It can be accepted as is.

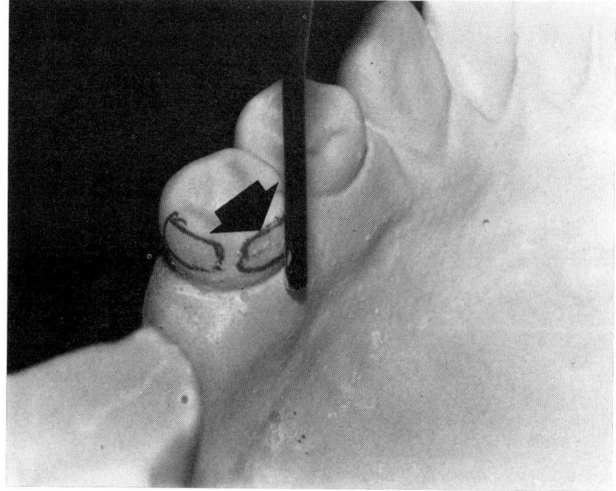

Fig. 7-81. The lingual surfaces of the premolar must be analyzed. The height of contour of the left premolar lies close to the occlusal surface, which is undesirable because the reciprocating clasp should be no higher than the middle third of the crown of the tooth. To lower the height of contour, the surface should be recontoured. This is indicated by circling the lingual surface in red. The four factors influencing the tilt of the mandibular diagnostic cast have now been satisfied. The cast should now be locked securely in the cast holder and the next step in the design sequence accomplished.

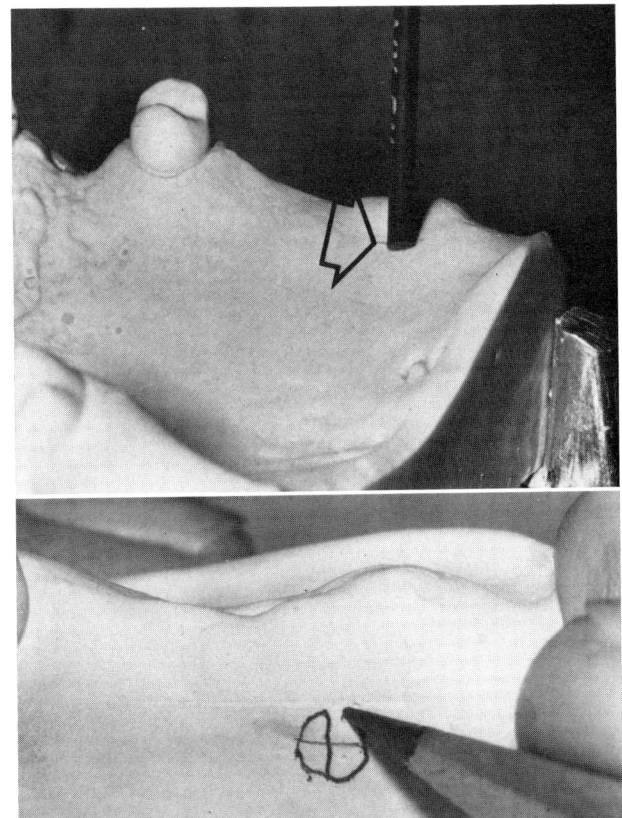

Fig. 7-82. A, To tripod the cast, the tip of the carbon marker must contact the cast at three widely separated points while the cast remains at a fixed tilt and the marker remains at a constant height. The carbon marker scribes a 4- to 5-mm horizontal line at the three selected points. **B,** The line made by the carbon marker is crossed and circled. This makes the three tripod marks easy to identify. The cast can be repositioned to the original tilt by referring to these tripod marks.

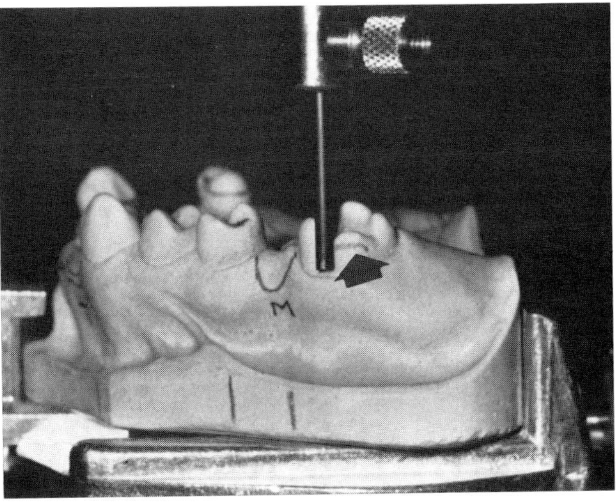

Fig. 7-83. Survey lines may be transferred to the teeth or other structures on the cast by releasing the vertical arm of the surveyor and rotating the cast while the side of the carbon marker remains in contact with the tooth. The survey line, being transferred to the second molar here, represents the height of contour of the tooth. Everything gingival to the survey line will be undercut to the path of insertion.

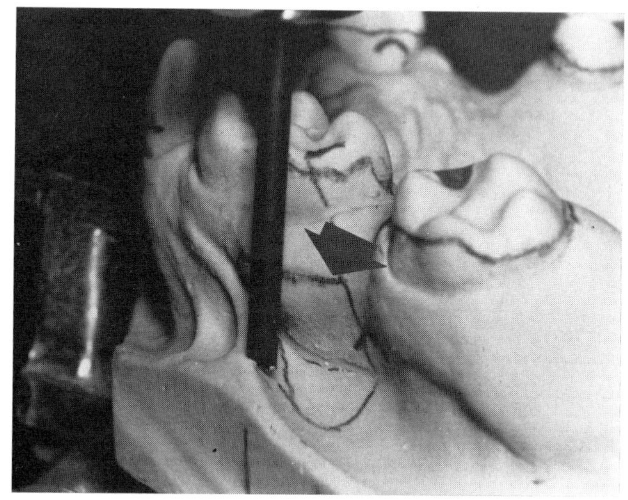

Fig. 7-84. The survey line is also transferred to soft tissue areas that will be contacted by the partial denture (arrow). The most common of these areas are soft tissue contours buccal or labial to teeth that are to be clasped with bar clasps, and also tissue lingual to the mandibular teeth. No rigid component of the prosthesis can lie below the survey line. In this case, the approach arm of the vertical projection clasp being planned for the second premolar cannot be positioned below the survey line being transferred to the soft tissue area.

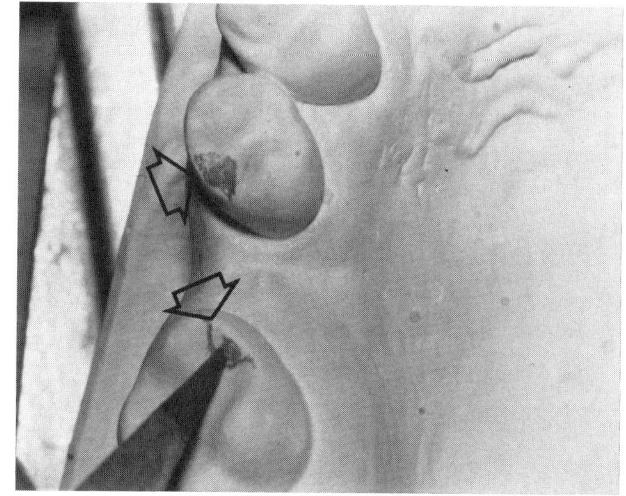

Fig. 7-85. The location of the rest seat preparations has been determined and indicated by a short vertical mark on the base of the cast adjacent to the tooth surface to be prepared. The full extent of the rest seat should now be colored solid red. It is important that the rest seats be drawn to actual size so that the effect of the rest seat on surrounding and opposing structures can be accurately forecast. Interferences between the rest and other structures should be known at this time so plans to correct or prevent them may be made.

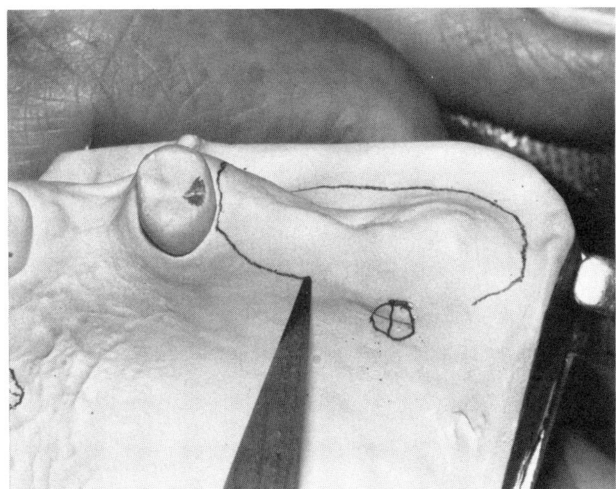

Fig. 7-86. The maxillary denture base is next outlined with the blue pencil. The palatal extensions of this denture base should be positioned 2 mm. lingual to what will eventually be the lingual surfaces of the artificial teeth. This will become the external finish line, or the juncture between the major connector and the acrylic resin denture base. The buccal extent should be to the soft tissue reflection. The posterior extension on the distal extension side should always be to the hamular notch. The maxillary tuberosity on a distal extention partial denture must *always* be *completely covered.* If interferences prevent this complete coverage, they must be surgically removed or a special thin metal casting must be designed to provide the coverage required.

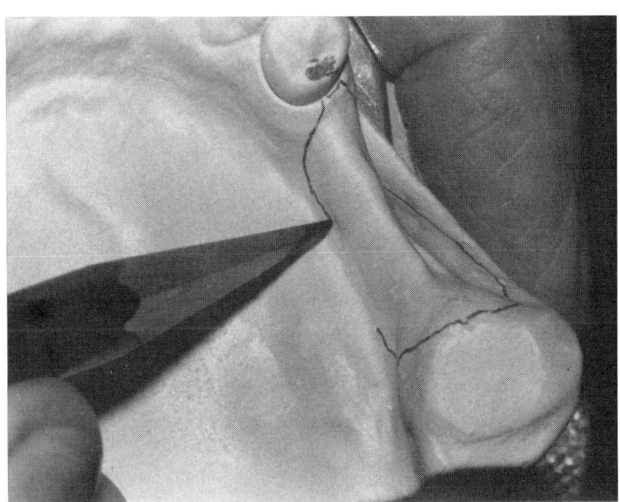

Fig. 7-87. The denture bases for both sides of the mandibular arch are indicated in blue. The denture base begins at the distal lingual line angle of the posterior abutment tooth and extends downward and slightly posteriorly on the lingual surface of the edentulous ridge to the reflection of the tissues of the floor of the mouth. This line establishes the external finish line on each side of the arch. The lingual extension of the denture base should be short of the floor of the mouth. Posteriorly the denture base must cover two thirds of the pear-shaped pad. Buccally the extension is to the soft tissue reflection. These components must be drawn to actual size and position because other components are influenced by them.

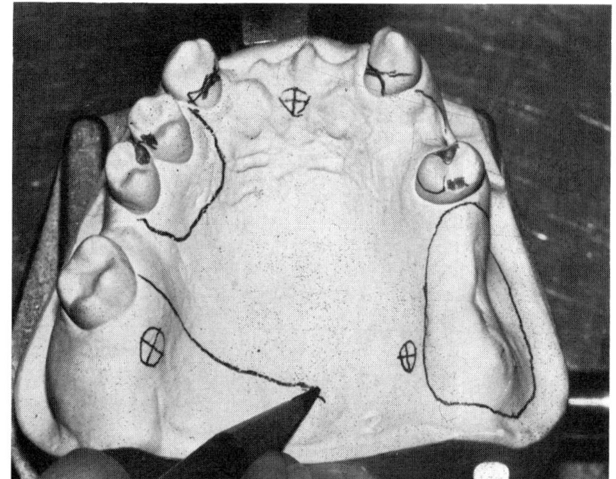

A

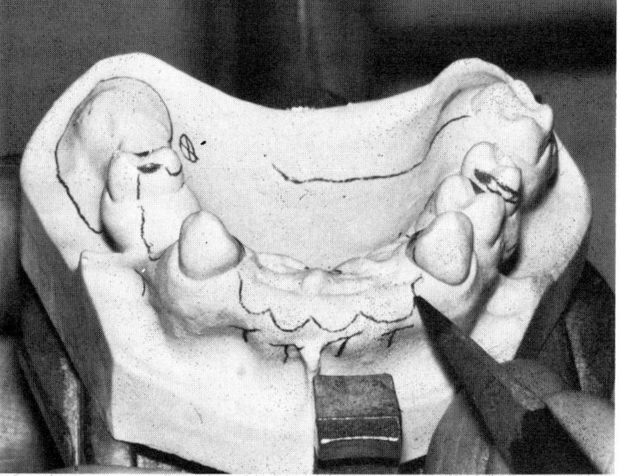

B

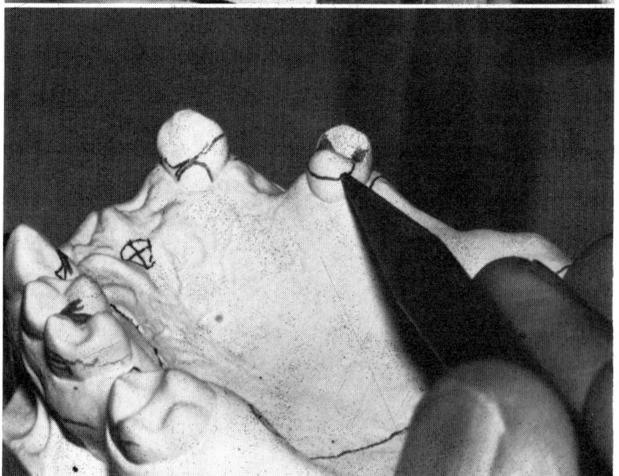

C

Fig. 7-88. For the patient for whom the design is being accomplished, maximum support from the hard palate should be the goal. For this reason a modified complete palate is selected. **A,** The posterior extent of the major connector is drawn from the mesiolingual line angle of the right second molar directly across the palate to the hamular notch. The outline is continued anteriorly on the right side to include the metal tooth replacement of the first molar. The lingual surfaces of the two premolars are avoided. This is an optional choice in design. These teeth could receive a lingual plate, or the major connector can step back from them. Factors such as oral hygiene and the need for additional stabilization should be considered when deciding whether to use lingual plating or to avoid contact with the teeth. The main point to remember is that if a maxillary major connector is not going to contact the lingual surfaces of the teeth, it must stay a minimum of 6 mm from the gingival crevice. **B,** The anterior extent of the major connector is scalloped to simulate the necks of the tube teeth. **C,** The left premolar receives a lingual plate. This will provide the tooth with additional horizontal stabilization.

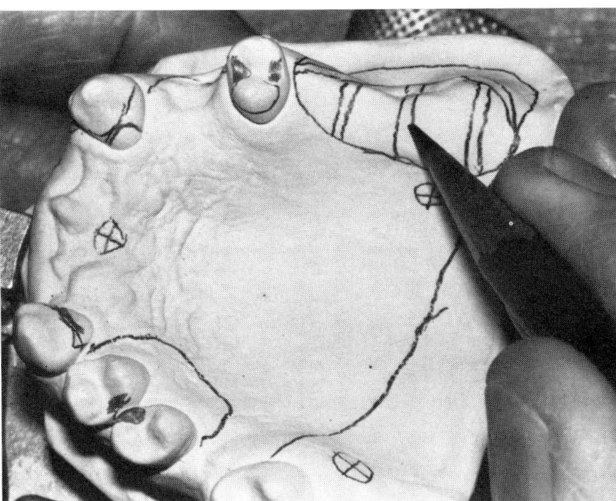

Fig. 7-89. The acrylic resin retention minor connector is added to the maxillary design. In this instance open latticework is selected for the obvious reason that relining of the denture base must be considered inevitable because of the normal resorption process of the distal extension ridge. The horizontal straps extend outward from the major connector. The longitudinal strap lies buccal to the crest of the ridge. The retention minor connector must cover the tuberosity.

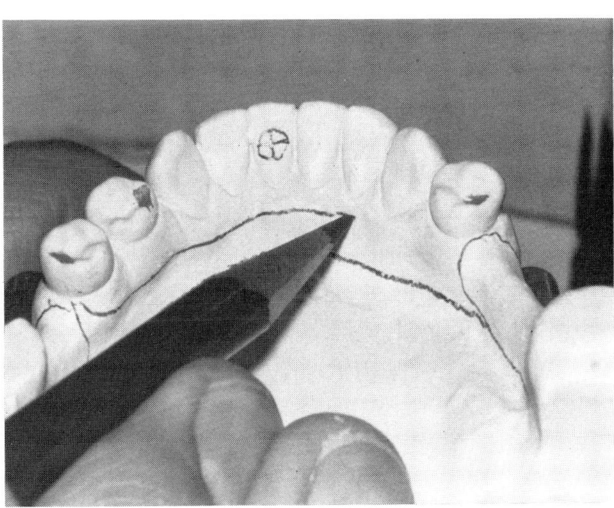

Fig. 7-90. The lingual bar has been selected as the a mandibular major connector. The superior margin of the bar must not be closer than 3 mm to the gingival margin of the teeth (see Fig. 7-91).

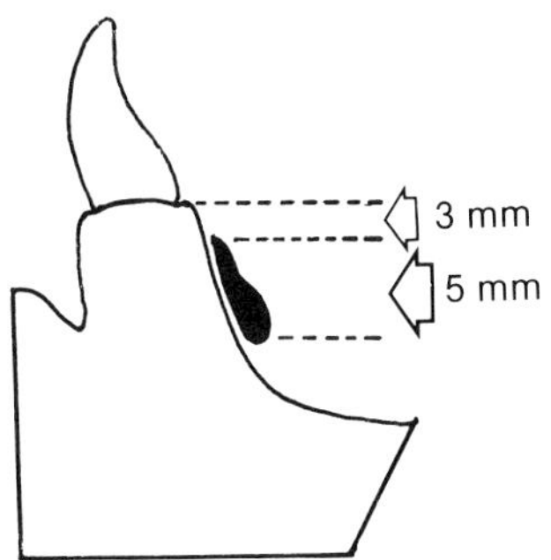

Fig. 7-91. To ensure rigidity a lingual bar must be a minimum of 5 mm in occlusogingival height. With the 3 mm of space required between the bar and the gingival crevices of the teeth, a minimum height of 8 mm must be available between the teeth and the floor of the mouth.

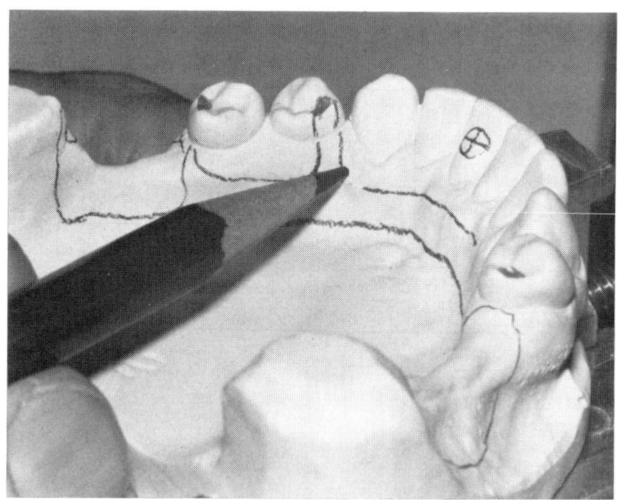

Fig. 7-92. The minor connector for the indirect retainer is added. It should project from the major connector at a 90-degree angle, and its junction with the major connector should be smooth and rounded.

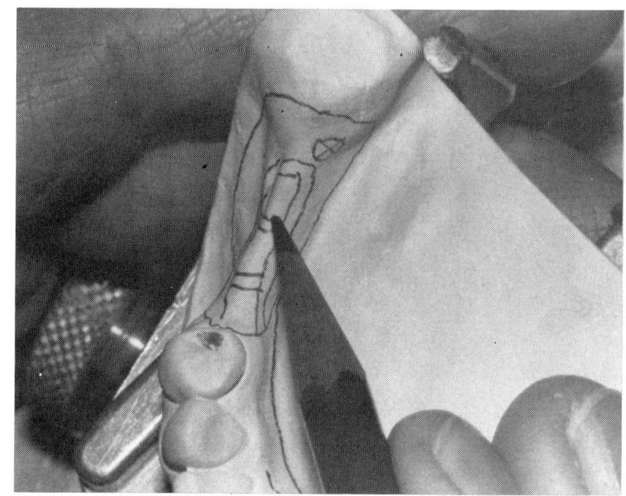

Fig. 7-93. The acrylic resin retention minor connector is added to both sides of the mandibular design. Open latticework is planned because relining of the bilateral distal extension ridge will be inevitable. Note that the horizontal lingual strut originates from the major connector several millimeters above the inferior border of the lingual bar. The buccal strut is positioned facial to the crest of the ridge. Posteriorly the acrylic resin retention extends only two-thirds the length of the edentulous ridge. With the exception of the clasps, the outline of the metallic portion of the partial denture is now complete.

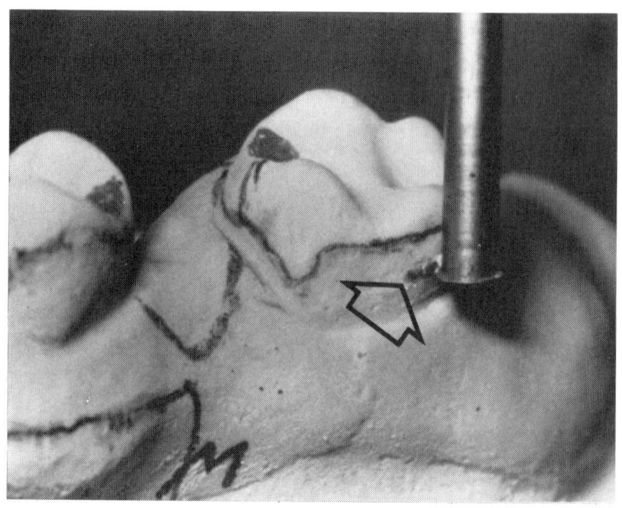

Fig. 7-94. The 0.010-inch undercut gauge is used to position the lower border of the tip of the retentive clasp. The shank contacts the molar at the survey line as the lid of the gauge contacts the tooth. This point should be marked with the red pencil. The undercut mark should be at the *line angle* of the tooth (for example, mesiobuccal, distolingual)—not in the center of the facial or lingual surface.

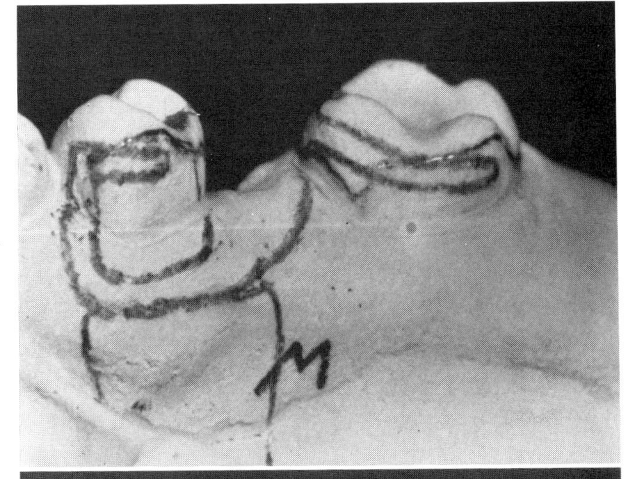

A

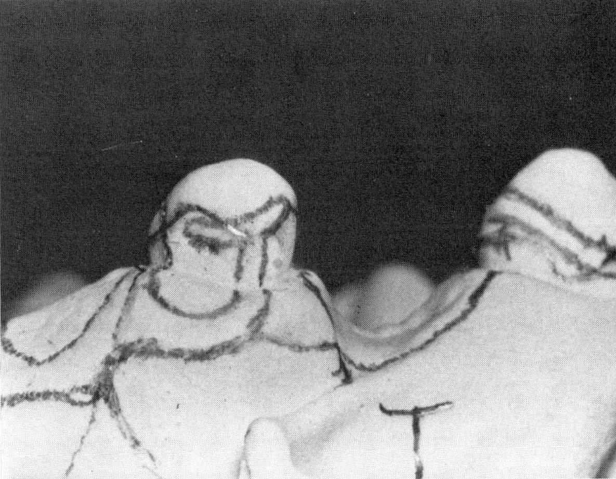

B

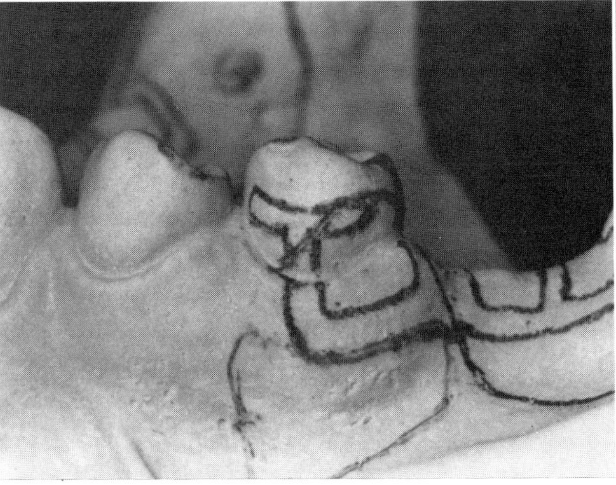

C

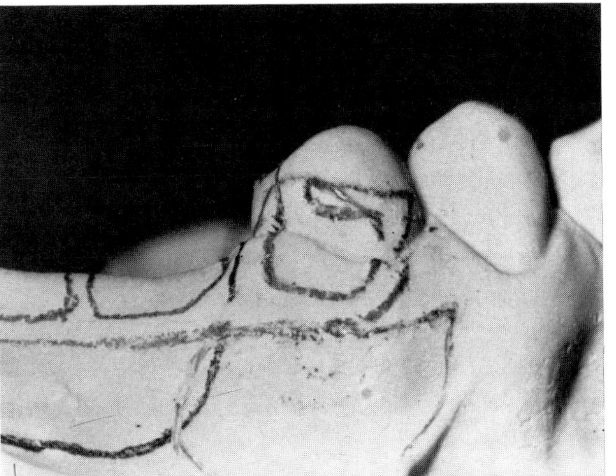

D

Fig. 7-95. The retentive clasps selected earlier are now added. The size, position, and contour of the clasps should be drawn accurately so that possible interferences with the opposing occlusion can be detected. The designer must always bear in mind that the clasps and other components of the partial denture are actually three dimensional. **A,** The circumferential clasp on the molar is positioned so that only the terminal third of the clasp arm is below the survey line. The approach arm of the modified T clasp is positioned superior to the soft tissue undercut. Only the distal terminal finger of the clasp enters the undercut. **B,** On the left side of the maxillary arch the T clasp on the premolar avoids the soft tissue undercut. The body and mesial terminal of the clasp are above the survey line. The circumferential clasp on the canine is positioned as low on the tooth as the survey line permits. Only the terminal tip enters the undercut. **C,** The T clasp on the mandibular left premolar avoids the soft tissue undercut. The approach arm is smoothly tapered from the origin to the body of the clasp. **D,** A modified T clasp is designed for the mandibular right premolar. The position of the survey line dictates the type of clasp in this case. Because the survey line is low on the mesial half of the tooth, the clasp must be positioned as low on the tooth as possible.

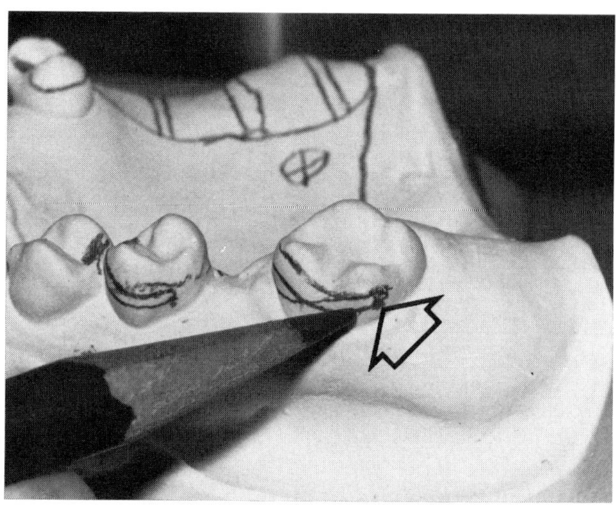

Fig. 7-96. The inferior border of the tip of the retentive clasp should rest on the red mark that indicates the measured depth of retentive undercuts.

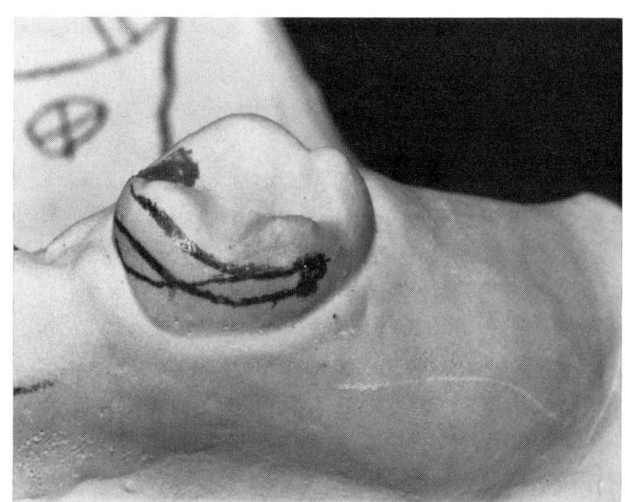

Fig. 7-97. The retentive clasp should be smoothly tapered and should be curved as it crosses the tooth surface. The clasp should never run straight across the tooth.

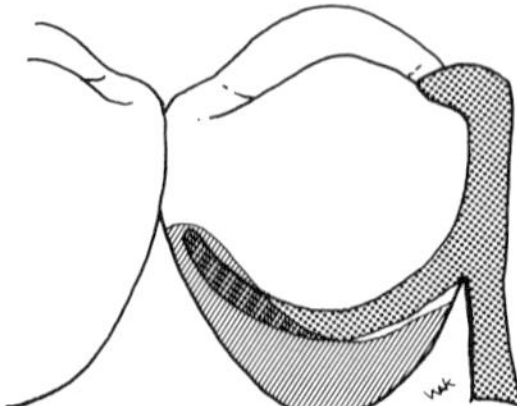

Fig. 7-98. Retentive clasps should be kept as low on the crown of a tooth as the survey line permits, preferably in the gingival third.

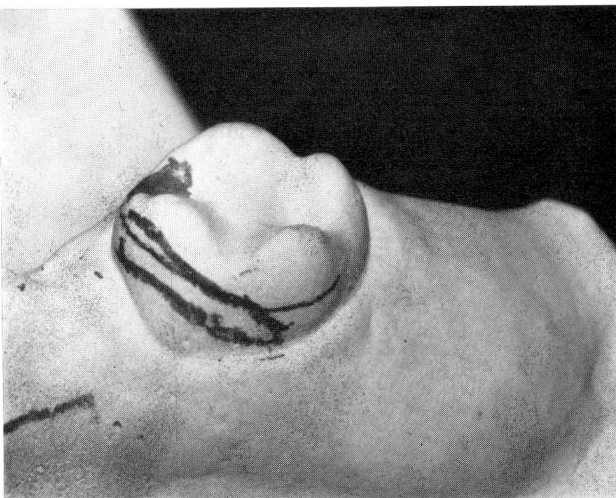

Fig. 7-99. The tip of the retentive clasp arm should terminate pointing occlusally, *not* gingivally as shown here.

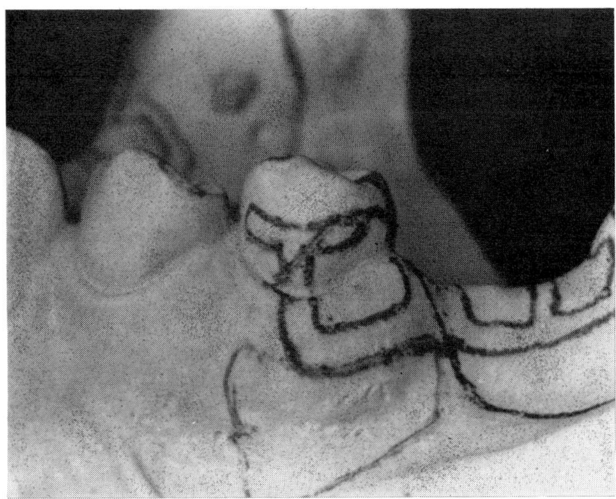

Fig. 7-100. The approach arm of the bar clasp should be tapered, should not cross soft tissue undercuts, and should cross the gingival margin at right angles, generally in the middle of the facial surface.

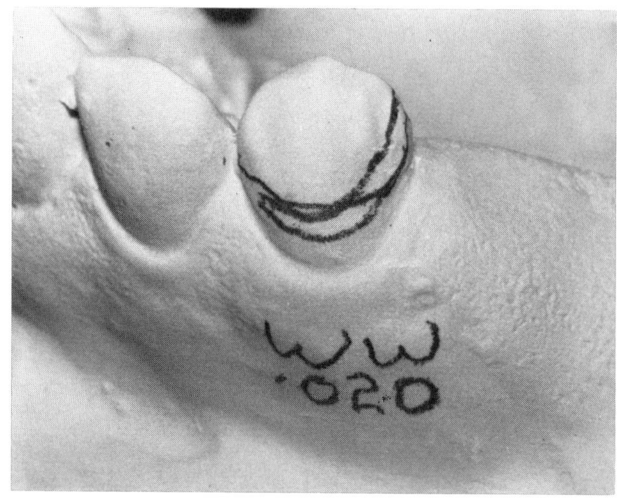

Fig. 7-101. If a wrought wire clasp is being included in the design, the symbol WW must be placed on the soft tissue portion of the cast below the abutment tooth. The measured amount of undercut should also be indicated.

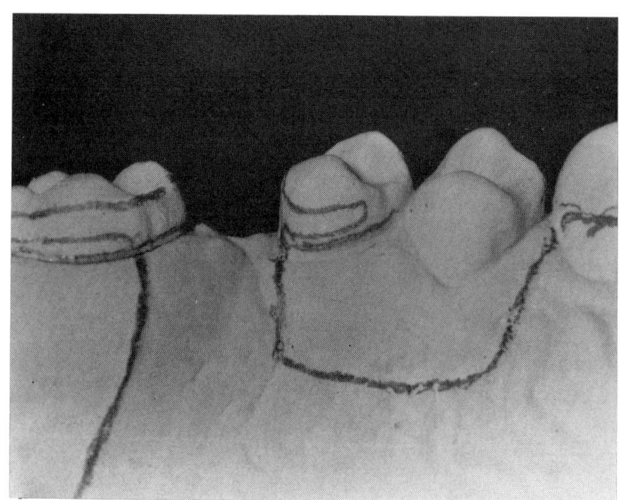

Fig. 7-102. The final components to be added to the design are the reciprocal clasp arms, the components most often inadvertently omitted. The arms should not be tapered because flexibility must be avoided. Reciprocal clasp arms must always be positioned above the survey line, at the junction of the gingival and middle thirds of the crown. If the survey line is too high to permit this, the enamel surface must be recontoured to lower the survey line.

Fig. 7-103. A, Right lateral view of the completed design. Each component can be visualized accurately by the dentist or the laboratory technician. **B,** Left lateral view of the final design. **C,** Occlusal view of the removable partial denture design.

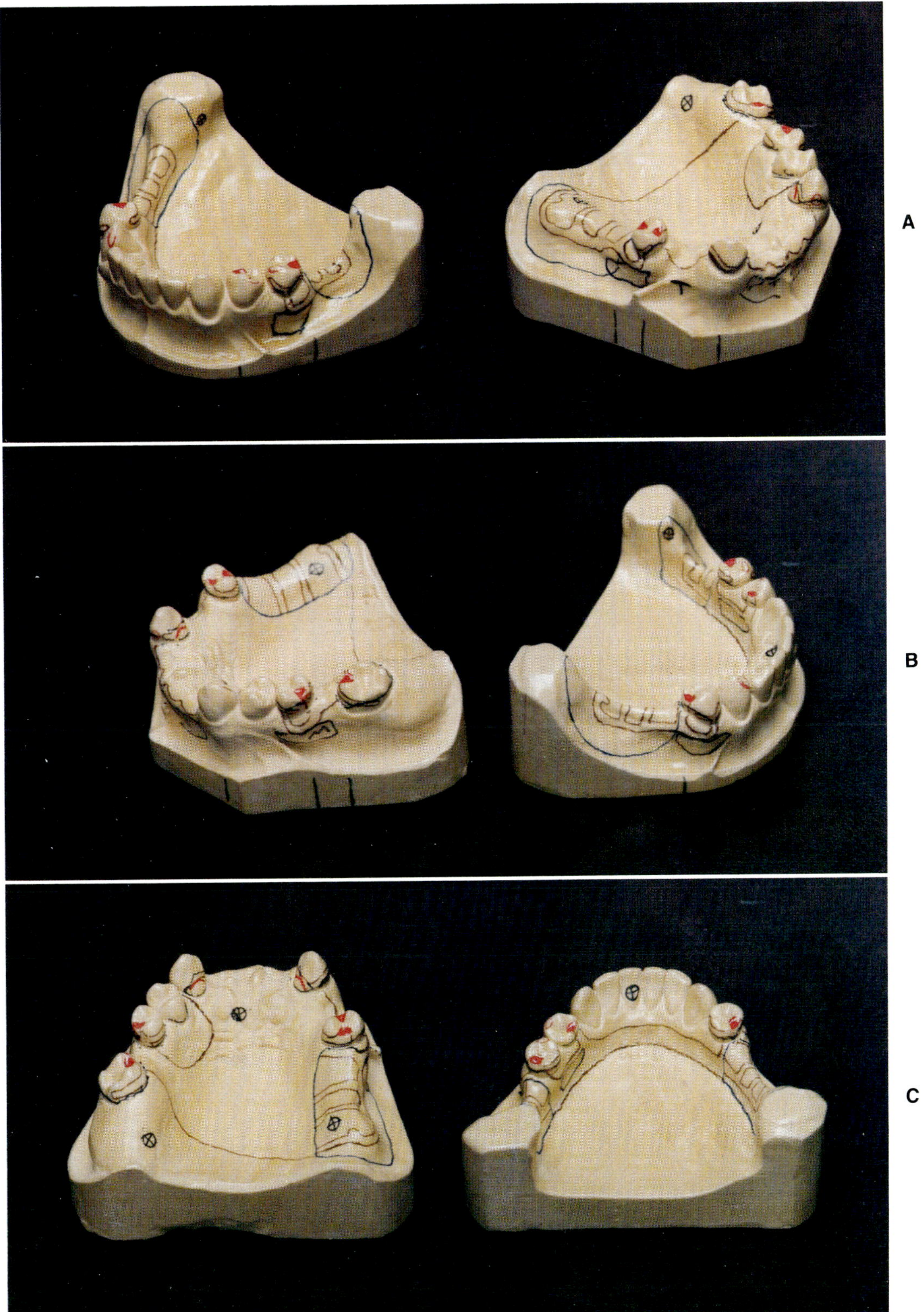

BIBLIOGRAPHY

Applegate, O.C.: Use of paralleling surveyor in modern partial denture construction, J. Am. Dent. Assoc. **27**:1317-1407, 1940.

Atkinson, H.F.: Partial denture problems: surveyors and surveying, Aust. J. Dent. **59**:28-31, 1955.

Atkinson, H.F.: Partial denture problems: designing about a path of withdrawal, Aust. J. Dent. **37**:187-190, 1953.

Atkinson, R.A., and Elliot, R.W.: Removable partial denture designed for laboratory fabrication by recent dental school graduates, J. Prosthet. Dent. **22**:528-543, 1969.

Black, G.V.: A work on operative dentistry, ed. 4, Chicago, 1920, Medico-Dental Publ. Co.

Blatterfein, L: A new approach to partial denture design for unilaterally remaining lower teeth, J. Prosthet. Dent. **28**:145-163, 1972.

Boero, E., and Forbes, W.G.: Considerations in design of removable prosthetic abutments, J. Prosthet. Dent. **28**:253-263, 1972.

Boitel, R.H.: The parallelometer, a precision instrument for the prosthetic laboratory, J. Prosthet. Dent. **12**:732-736, 1962.

Bolouve, A.: Removable partial denture design for a few remaining natural teeth, J. Prosthet. Dent. **39**:346-348, 1978.

Chistner, S.B.: A methodical approach to the analysis of study casts, J. Prosthet. Dent. **4**:622-624, 1954.

Christidon, T., and others: The effects of partial denture design on the mobility of abutment teeth, Br. Dent. J. **135**:9, 1973.

Coy, R.E., and Arnold P.D.: Survey and design of diagnostic casts for removable partial dentures, J. Prosthet. Dent. **32**:103-106, 1974.

Craddock F.W.: Clasp surveying and mysticism, Aust. J. Dent. **59**:205-208, 1955.

Dental Laboratory Technician's Manual, Department of the Air Force, Washington, D.C., 1959, U.S. Government Printing Office.

Dunn, B.W.: Treatment planning for removable partial dentures, J. Prosthet. Dent. **11**:247-255, 1961.

Elliot, F.C.: A method that simplified the design of partial dentures, J. Am. Dent. Assoc. **27**:1263-1268, 1940.

Fish, E.W.: A new principle in partial denture design, Br. Dent. J. **92**:135/144, 1952.

Frantz, W.R.: Variations in a removable maxillary partial denture design by dentists, J. Prosthet. Dent. **34**:625-633, 1975.

Frechette, A.R.: The influence of partial denture design on distribution of force to abutment teeth, J. Prosthet. Dent. **6**:195-212, 1956.

Giradot, R.I.: History and development of partial denture design, J. Am. Dent. Assoc. **28**:1399-1408, 1941.

Goodkind, R.J.: The effects of removable partial dentures on abutment tooth mobility: a clinical study, J. Prosthet. Dent. **30**:139-145, 1973.

Hanson, J.G.: Surveying, J. Am. Dent. Assoc. **91**:826-828, 1975.

Hardy, I.: Partial lower denture design, Dent. Digest. **44**:57-71, 1938.

Jordan, L.G.: Designing removable partial dentures with external attachments, J. Prosthet. Dent. **2**:716-722, 1952.

Kaires, A.K.: A study of partial denture design and masticatory pressure in a mandibular distal extension case, J. Prosthet. Dent. **17**:472-478, 1967.

Katulski, E.M., and Appleyard, W.N.: Biological concepts of the use of the mechanical cast surveyor, J. Prosthet. Dent. **9**:629-634, 1959.

Kelley, E.K.: The physiologic approach to partial denture design, J. Prosthet. Dent. **3**:699-710, 1953.

Kratochvil, F.J.: Influence of occlusal rest position and clasp design on movement of abutment teeth, J. Prosthet. Dent. **13**:114-124, 1963.

LaVere, A.M.: A simplified procedure for survey and design of diagnostic casts, J. Prosthet. Dent. **37**:680-683, 1977.

Lazarus, A.H.: Partial denture design, J. Prosthet. Dent. **1**:438-442, 1951.

McCracken, W.L.: Contemporary partial denture designs, J. Prosthet. Dent. **8**:71-84, 1958.

McCracken, W.L.: Survey of partial denture designs by commercial dental laboratories, J. Prosthet. Dent. **12**:1089-1110, 1962.

Maxfield, J.B., and others: The measurement of forces transmitted to abutment teeth of removable partial dentures, J. Prosthet. Dent. **41**:134-142, 1979.

Moore, D.S.: Some fundamentals of partial denture design to conserve the supporting structures, J. Ont. Dent. Assoc. **32**:238-240, 1955.

Neurohr, F.G.: Health conservation of the periodontal tissues by a method of functional partial denture design, J. Am. Dent. Assoc. **31**:58-70, 1974.

Osborne, J., and Lammie, G.A.: The bilateral free-end saddle lower denture, J. Prosthet. Dent. **4**:640-653, 1954.

Perry, C.: A philosophy of partial denture design, J. Prosthet. Dent. **6**:775-784, 1956.

Potter, R.B., and others: Removable partial denture designs: a review and a challenge, J. Prosthet. Dent. **17**:63-68, 1967.

Rudd, K.D., and Dunn, B.W.: Accurate removable partial dentures, J. Prosthet. Dent. **18**:559-570, 1967.

Ryan, J.: Technique of design in partial denture construction, J. Dent. Assoc. S. Africa **9**:123-133, 1954.

Ryback, S.A., Jr.: Simplicity in a distal extension partial denture, J. Prosthet. Dent. **3**:783-806, 1953.

Schmidt, A.H.: Planning and designing removable partial dentures, J. Prosthet. Dent. **3**:783-806, 1953.

Scott, D.D.: Suggested designs for metal partial dentures, Dent. Tech. **2**:21, 1954.

Sollé, W.: An improved dental surveyor, J. Am. Dent. Assoc. **60**:727-731, 1960.

Steffel, V.L.: Fundamental principles involved in partial denture design, J. Am. Dent. Assoc. **42**:534, 1951.

Steffel, V.L.: Current concepts in removable partial denture service, J. Prosthet. Dent. **20**:387-395, 1968.

Sykora, O., and Caliklsocaogln, S.: Maxillary removable partial denture designs by commercial dental laboratories, J. Prosthet. Dent. **23**:633-640, 1970.

Tench, R.W.: Fundamentals of partial denture design, J. Am. Dent. Assoc. **23**:1087-1092, 1936.

Thompson, W.D., and others: Evaluation of photoelastic stress patterns produced by various designs of bilateral distal extension removable partial dentures, J. Prosthet. Dent. **38**:261-273, 1977.

Trainor, J.E., and others: Removable partial dentures designed before and after graduate level instruction, J. Prosthet. Dent. **27**:509-514, 1972.

Trapozzano, V.R., and Winter, G.R.: Periodontal aspects of partial denture design, J. Prosthet. Dent. **2**:101-107, 1952.

Wagner, A.G., and Forgue, E.G.: A study of four methods of recording the path of insertion of removable partial dentures, J. Prosthet. Dent. **35**:267-272, 1976.

Wills, N.G.: Practical engineering applied to removable partial denture designing, Prosthet. Dent. Centenary pp. 319-331, 1940.

Yilmaz, G.: Optical surveying of casts for removable partial dentures, J. Prosthet. Dent. **34**:292-296, 1975.

8 I-bar removable partial dentures

Madeline Kurrasch

The I-bar removable partial denture, a subject of discussion since Kratochvil introduced the design in 1963, has achieved considerable status as a treatment modality in recent years. The logical mechanical approach that Kratochvil used in introducing and evaluating this design concept has encouraged others to apply sound engineering principles in challenging the design. As a result the design has been subjected to thorough evaluation and, in the process, has gained many followers and a few detractors.

The initial difficulty that was noted when the I-bar design was used resulted from the commercialization of the retentive element of the design and a disregard for other, equally important, components of the system.

Although the system can be applied easily to tooth-borne partial dentures, discussion here is limited primarily to the distal extension situation in order to demonstrate basic principles of design.

Distal extension partial denture components have the difficult assignment of making a transition from nonresiliant (tooth) to resiliant (mucosa) supporting structures without compromising either type of support. The clasp must provide vertical support, horizontal bracing, retention, and reciprocation and concurrently control movement of the abutment teeth. In this capacity the clasp determines the distribution of occlusal force between the two types of support, tooth and mucosa.

MESIAL REST, I-BAR, AND GUIDE PLANE

Kratochvil addressed his attention to the tooth-mucosa junction and developed a system that includes a mesial rest, I-bar retainer, and long guide planes that extend onto the tooth-tissue junction. The I-bar retainer is one element in the design equation and, as such, has been overemphasized (Fig. 8-1).

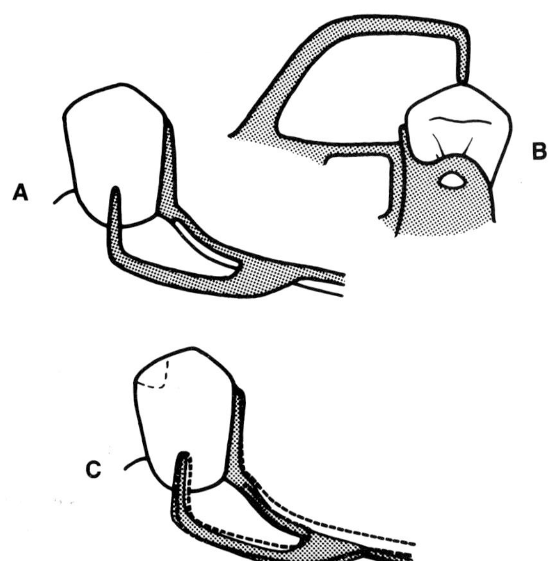

Fig. 8-1. I-bar clasp system. **A,** Mesial rest, I-bar retainer, and long guide plane. **B,** Occlusal view of system on maxillary canine. Note I-bar placement on mesiodistal height of contour and cingulum rest, which is advocated for anterior teeth. **C,** Occlusal force on distal extension base will cause rotation about the mesial rest; this disengages retentive tip into mesial undercut and eliminates abutment torquing that occurs with other distal extension clasp systems.

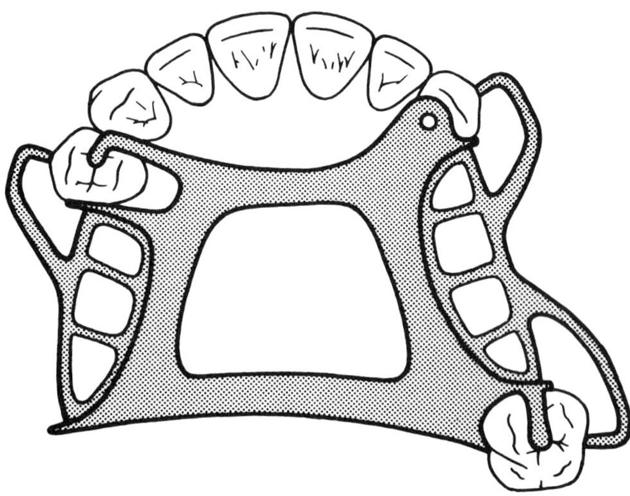

Fig. 8-2. Treatment planning phase includes a tentative ideal design with mesial rests on abutments adjacent to the extension base and rests on either side of tooth-borne segments. I-bar retention is reciprocated by long guide planes and minor connectors or a lingual plate as shown on molar.

DESIGN CONCEPTS

Successful partial denture treatment requires careful evaluation of the patient and an organized design sequence. Examination and diagnosis have been discussed in previous chapters, and the principles involved apply to I-bar designs. Essential information includes radiographs, a record of the periodontal status of all teeth, and diagnostic casts mounted on an articulator in centric relation.

In the treatment planning phase the ideal partial denture is designed and the casts are surveyed to determine whether this tentative design can be used without modification. Any tooth preparation necessary to implement the design is determined (Figs. 8-2 and 8-3).

Partial denture components are discussed in the order of the design sequence that is advocated: rests, proximal plates, major connectors, minor connectors, denture base connectors, and retainers (Kratochvil and Vig, 1979).

Rests

The function of rests is to provide vertical support against occlusal forces and control the relationship of the prosthesis to supporting structures. In order to perform this function, rests must be positive and of sufficient bulk to withstand direct occlusal force and also the indirect force that they are subjected to as fulcrum points for distal extension movement.

Anterior rests must meet the basic requirements of strength and positiveness. In addition, they are subjected to esthetic considerations. The ideal anterior rest is the crescent-shaped cingulum rest, which places vertical force low on the tooth and provides maximum stabilization (Berg and Caputo, 1978) (Fig. 8-4). The cingulum rest can be prepared directly in enamel on bulky canines and maxillary central incisors or can be implemented with a cast restoration (Fig. 8-5). The incisal rest is used on mandibular anterior teeth when esthetics allows (Fig. 8-6).

A 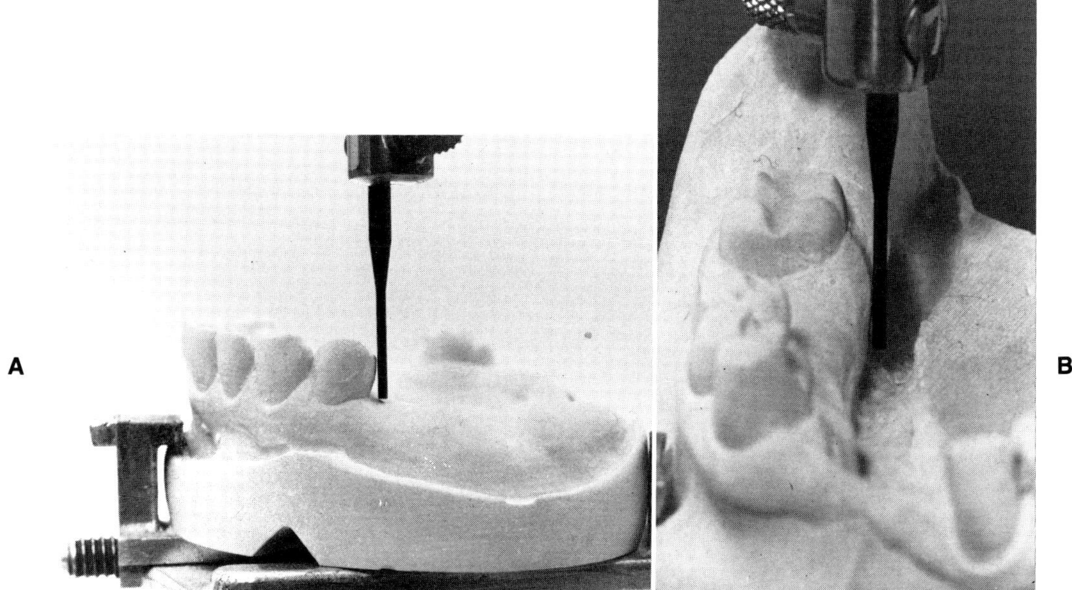 B

Fig. 8-3. A, Diagnostic casts are surveyed to determine amount of tooth modification necessary to provide retention and long guide planes. **B,** Excessive tipping of abutment teeth or soft tissue undercuts that interfere with ideal placement of retentive elements will dictate modification of "ideal" design.

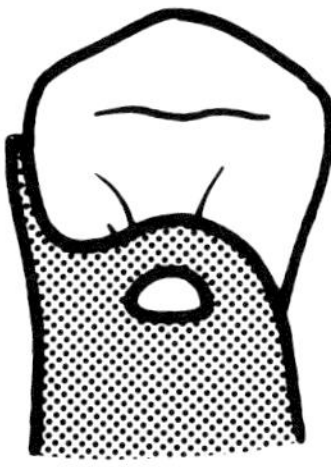

Fig. 8-4. Cingulum rest is advocated for both maxillary and mandibular anterior teeth. Framework is open to allow visualization of tip of rest to ensure seating and adaptation of framework in area.

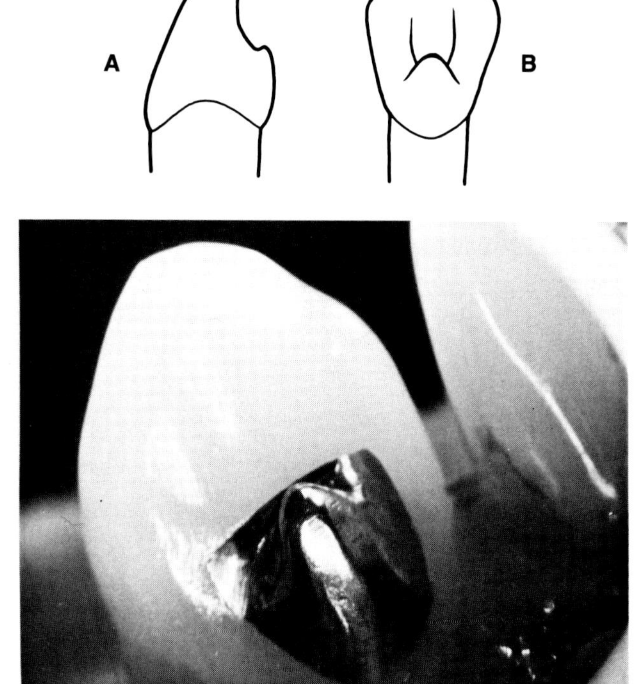

Fig. 8-5. Cingulum rest can be prepared in enamel if abutment is large enough to provide a rest with sufficient bulk to resist vertical forces of occlusion. The rest must be positive, **A**, and rounded, **B**, to allow rotation of framework if it is to be used as a distal extension rest. **C**, Cast pin inlay with ideal cingulum rest contour.

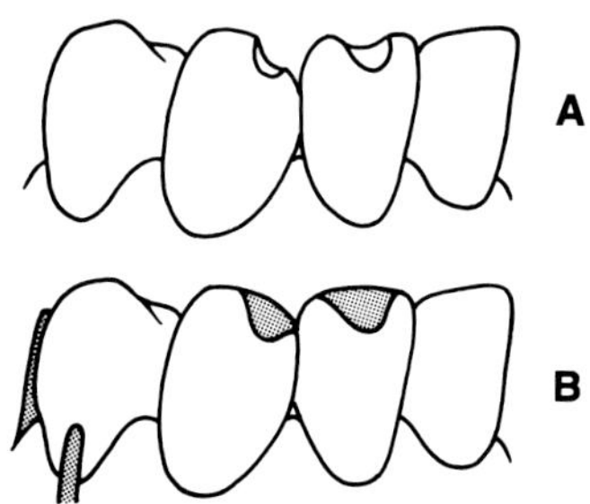

Fig. 8-6. Incisal rests can be used on mandibular anterior teeth when esthetics allows; they can also be used for splinting mobile, periodontally involved teeth. **A**, Tooth preparation is adequate (1.5 mm) to provide a sufficient bulk of metal for strength and to prevent overcontouring of incisal edges when prosthesis is in place, **B**. Preparation includes a short facial bevel to ensure tooth control.

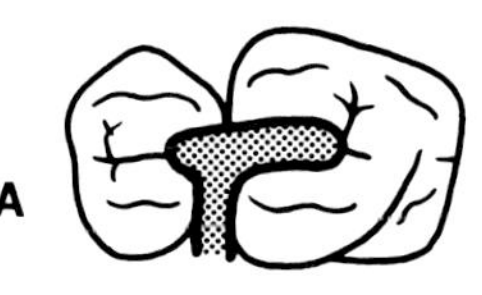

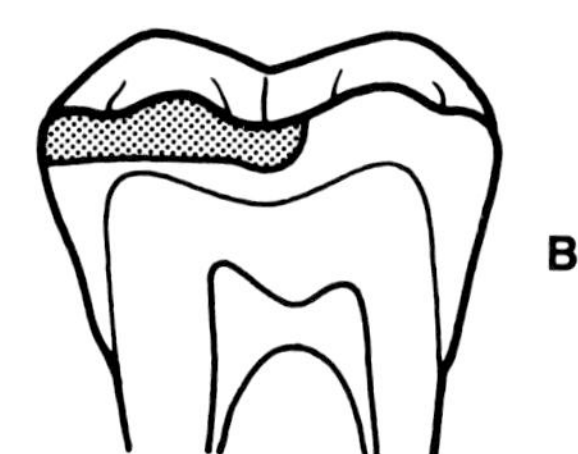

Fig. 8-7. Posterior rests are positive and direct vertical forces along the long axis of tooth. **A**, Thoughtless overpreparation of rests can weaken abutments and subject them to fracture. Ideally, rests should not cross triangular or oblique ridges. **B**, Preparation should be adequate (1.5 mm) to provide adequate strength of metal without causing interference with opposing occlusion.

Posterior rests are likewise designed to direct vertical forces along the long axis of the tooth; premolar rests are prepared in marginal and triangular ridges, and molar rests extend into the central fossa. The rests have a ball-shaped terminus that allows ball-and-socket movement around the axis of rotation (Fig. 8-7).

In distal extension cases the most distal rests are placed on the mesial aspect of the abutment teeth for the following two reasons (Kratochvil, 1963) (see Fig. 8-1):

1. Anterior placement of the rest (fulcrum) helps verticalize the forces of occlusion on bearing mucosa under the the denture base extension.
2. The mesial rest directs tipping forces on the abutment mesially and tends to move the abutment tooth into firm contact with the support of the anterior teeth.

Proximal plates

The retentive element has been overemphasized in the execution of Kratochvil's design, and the guide plane and proximal plate have been underemphasized. Parallel guide planes are prepared on all proximal tooth surfaces adjacent to edentulous spaces. The proximal plate covers the guide plane from marginal ridge to the tooth-tissue junction and extends onto the attached gingiva for 2 mm. This configuration serves many functions (see Fig. 8-1):

1. Provides horizontal stability.
2. Reunites and stabilizes the arch.
3. Increases retention because of parallelism and because dislodgement is limited to the path of insertion.
4. Protects the tooth-tissue junction by preventing food impaction and because of metal coverage in this area.
5. Provides reciprocation.
6. Distributes occlusal force throughout the arch (Berg, 1979; Berg and Caputo, 1978; Kratochvil, 1963; Kratochvil and Caputo, 1974).

In spite of the advantages offered by the long guide plane there is resistance to the amount of tooth preparation that is sometimes required (Krol, 1973). It is important to note that an underprepared guide plane compromises the stability of the I-bar partial denture and is an incorrect application of the design.

The path of insertion is chosen in deference to smaller anterior teeth that might otherwise require

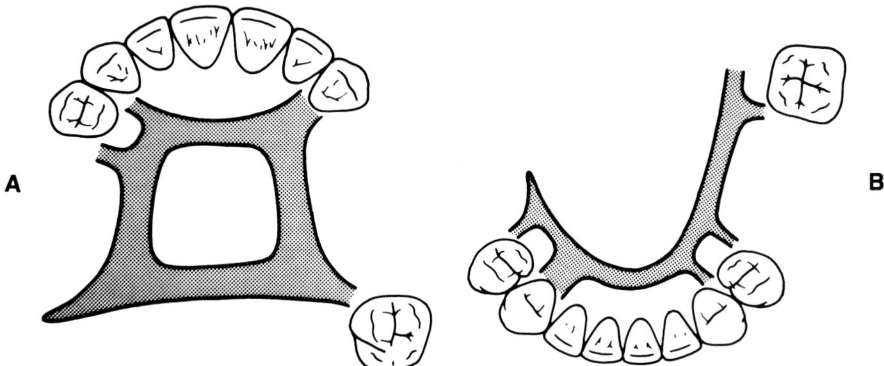

Fig. 8-8. Major connector. **A,** Anteroposterior strap is advocated for maxillary partial dentures. Connectors are placed 5 to 6 mm from tooth-tissue junctions to allow adequate stimulation of gingiva and to prevent gingival hypertrophy. **B,** Lingual bar is placed at least 4 mm from tooth-tissue junction for the same reason. If lingual tori are present or if lingual vestibule is too shallow to allow adequate space between bar and tooth-tissue junction, a lingual plate is provided.

unesthetic overreduction, and cast restorations are placed on teeth that require severe axial reduction because of buccolingual or mesiodistal tipping.

Major connectors

Major connectors are designed for maximum rigidity and gingival health. The combination anteroposterior strap is preferred for maxillary partial dentures, and a lingual bar is preferred for mandibular partial dentures (Fig. 8-8). Maxillary major connectors are placed 5 to 6 mm away from tooth-tissue junctions, and mandibular major connectors are placed on unattached mucosa or at least 4 mm away from the gingival crest. Modifications are made for anatomic variations such as a shallow anterior lingual sulcus with inadequate room for both a rigid lingual bar and 4 mm of space for gingival health. The lingual plate is advocated when space is inadequate for a lingual bar or when tooth or soft tissue contours promote food impaction. Major connectors are not relieved because close tissue adaptation is also important to prevent mucosal hypertrophy and food impaction. Tissue impingement by the major connector is avoided by providing adequate vertical support for long anterior connector segments. The mesial fossa of mandibular first premolars is a convenient place for anterior rests because of tooth form and because it is usually out of occlusion.

Minor connectors

Minor connectors connect rests, proximal plates, and retainers to the major connector. They also help provide horizontal stability. Because minor connectors are usually located in buccal or lingual embrasures, they have considerable potential for disrupting the food-deflecting morphology of the normal dentition. With this in mind, the connectors are designed to cross tooth-tissue junctions at right angles to minimize or eliminate food impaction. Embrasures that will be crossed by connectors are surveyed, and tooth contours are altered, if necessary, to eliminate gross undercuts and to allow an adequate bulk of metal for strength (Fig. 8-9).

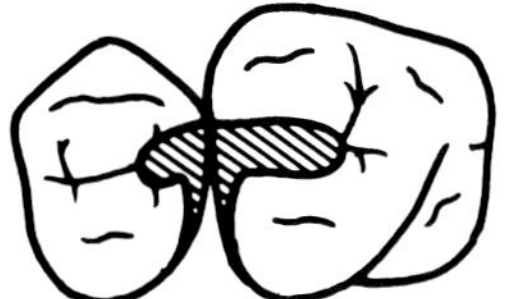
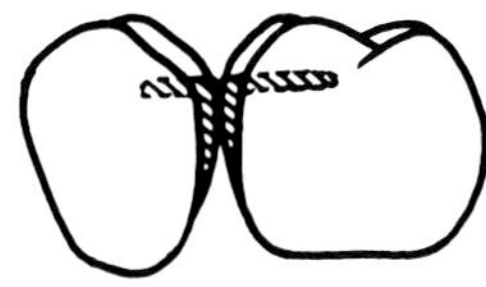

Fig. 8-9. Interproximal undercuts may necessitate enameloplasty to allow placement of minor connectors without creation of debris traps.

Denture base connectors

Denture base connectors are designed for strength and to adequately retain acrylic bases, yet not interfere with placement of denture teeth. One millimeter relief is provided for retention, and the retentive meshwork is placed on the lingual aspect of the ridge and extends only to the crest of the ridge to avoid interference with tooth placement on the facial side of the ridge (Fig. 8-2).

Acrylic resin is subject to deterioration under stress at the tooth-tissue junction, so this area is covered with metal, and the acrylic resin then forms a butt joint with metal 2 mm from abutment teeth (Kratochvil, 1963, 1979).

Altered cast impressions are made for all extension bases. The relationship of impression material to the metal that covers the tooth-tissue junction is an accurate indicator for proper framework orientation during the altered cast impression procedure.

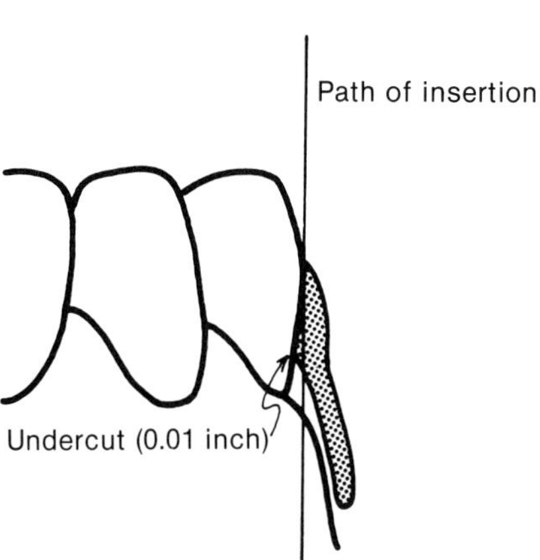

Fig. 8-10. The I-bar, which is long enough to allow flexure, engages a 0.01-inch undercut and terminates at or slightly above the height of contour to prevent it from snapping into undercut and abrading abutment during removal.

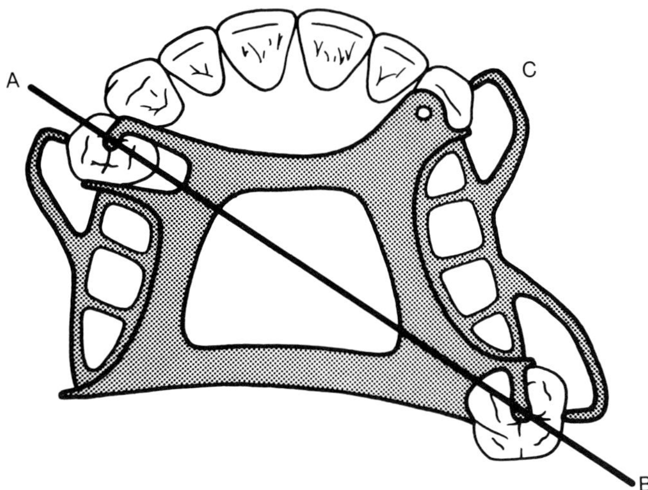

Fig. 8-11. Retentive I-bars, *A* and *B*, are placed at or mesial to mesiodistal height of contour. I-bars that are distant to axis of rotation, *C*, are not placed in retentive undercuts and are used for frictional retention and horizontal stabilization of prosthesis.

Direct retention

Retention in most partial denture clasps is achieved with a retentive arm that engages an undercut on an abutment tooth. In the conventional sense the I-bar provides retention against vertical displacement, but this retention is augmented considerably by the parallelism of guide planes that, in most situations, limit displacement to the path of insertion.

The I-bar is an infrabulge retainer with a configuration designed to minimize the deleterious effect that overcontoured retainers have on the health of both tooth and gingiva. The arm is long and tapering with a half-round cross section. The tip, which flexes, engages an undercut at the height of mesiodistal contour or mesial to it (Fig. 8-10). The position of the I-bar in relation to the height of contour is essential to this design because proper positioning allows the tip to move passively into the mesial embrasure space when the extension base receives occlusal loading. The retainer engages the undercut area and resists vertical displacement.

The following important advantages are gained with the I-bar configuration:

1. Because tooth contour is not altered, food accumulation against the tooth surface is minimized.
2. The I-bar is passive in its relationship to the abutment tooth except against vertical displacing forces.

The disadvantages of the I-bar are of consequence only if the design concept is not fully deployed:

1. Less horizontal stability than other retentive elements
2. Less retention

When used in the tooth-borne situation, the I-bar retainers can be placed for convenience relative to retentive undercuts and esthetics. In extension situations the retentive I-bars are placed with respect to the axis of rotation (Fig. 8-11).

Indirect retention

Indirect retention is provided by rests placed on secondary abutments as far from the axis of rotation and the edentulous area as possible to stabilize the major connector. Although recent studies have cast doubt on the effectiveness of indirect retention against displacing force (Frank and Nicholls, 1977), the indirect retainer has been shown to be effective in redistributing occlusal force more evenly throughout the entire dentoalveolar structure (McDowell, 1978).

PHYSIOLOGIC ADJUSTMENT OF EXTENSION BASE PARTIAL DENTURES

To allow movement of the partial denture around the axis of rotation, it is necessary to adjust the framework to reduce binding on guide planes and minor connectors.

Adjustment is a chairside procedure. A disclosing medium such as chloroform and rouge is placed on all parts of the framework that touch tooth surfaces (Fig. 8-12). The framework is placed in the mouth, and occlusal force is simulated by placing finger pressure on the extension base retention meshwork. Areas of binding, which are usually small, are relieved until the framework can move freely when the extension base is depressed. Initially, either the framework will have so much frictional retention from the guide planes and

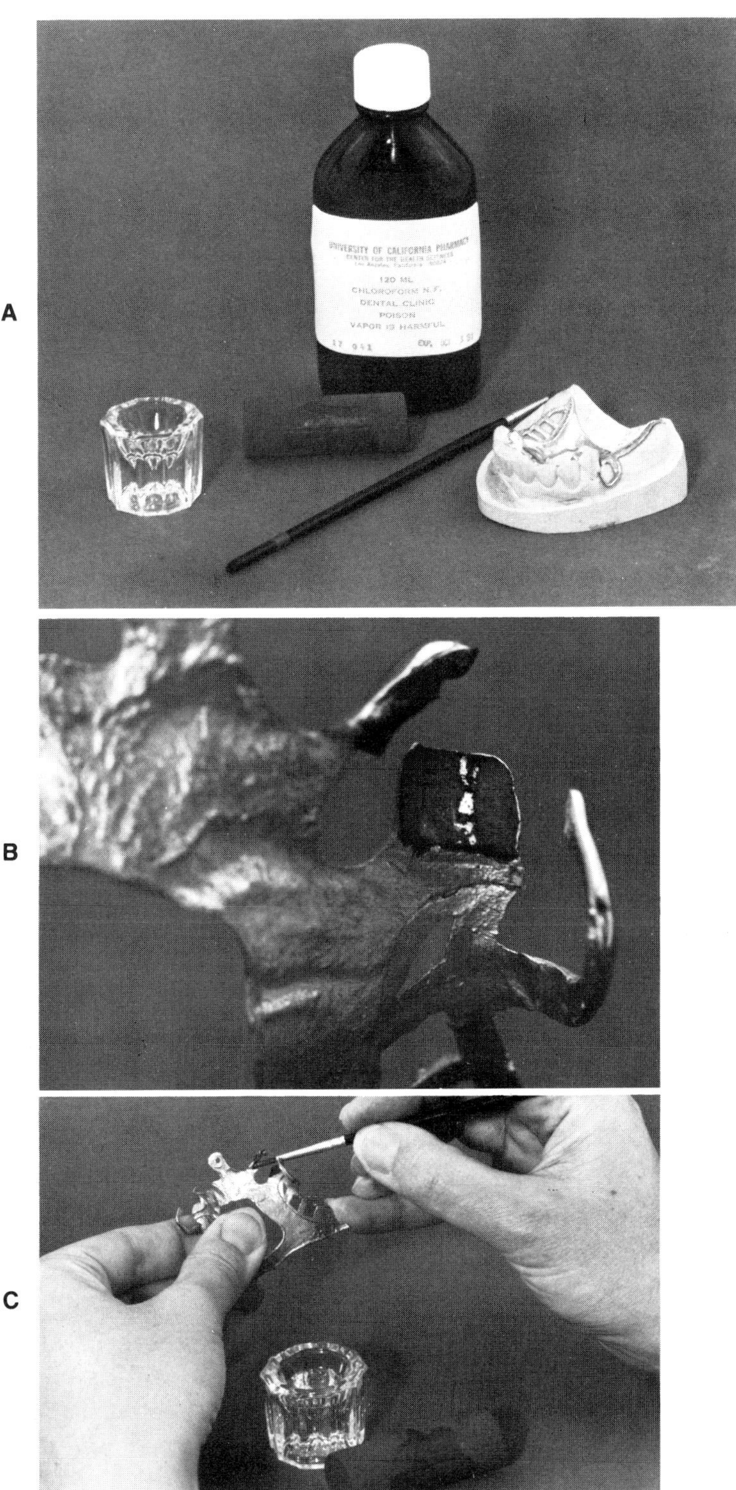

Fig. 8-12. A, Physiologic adjustment of framework allows free rotation about the axis of rotation, determined by most distal rests on distal extension partial dentures. Chloroform and rouge is used as a disclosing medium, **A, B.** Occlusal force is simulated by finger pressure on extension base, and framework is adjusted until movement occurs about axis of rotation, **C.**

minor connectors that rotational movement will not be possible, or the framework will bind or fulcrum on a portion of the framework that is not on the axis of rotation. Both situations subject primary and secondary abutments to destructive wrenching forces. The framework is adjusted until the rests that determine the axis of rotation become the actual fulcrum points for rotation. When the framework is properly adjusted, the extension can be depressed and the axis of rotation rests will rotate in their respective rest preparations without lifting away from them.

Altered cast impressions are made of all extension areas to provide maximum support from the edentulous ridge (Holmes, 1965; Leupold, 1966). In the passive state the rests make full contact with the rest preparations, and the distal extension base is adapted to the ridge. In function when the extension base receives occlusal loading, movement is limited to the resiliency of the supporting ridge tissues. Lack of tissue adaptation or support in the passive state indicates the need for a reline procedure.

DESIGN VARIATIONS

Physical considerations and alternate components

In spite of the versatility of the I-bar system, situations exist that defy successful application of the basic design. If the requirements for a clasp system are kept in mind, modification can be made that circumvents problems without compromising the treatment modality (Berg, 1979). Most problems in design application are related to tipped abutment teeth, soft tissue contours, or frenum attachments.

Tipping of abutment teeth affects retention in several ways. Buccolingual tipping frequently eliminates the necessary retention undercut or creates an excessive undercut that necessitates placing the retentive tip high on the tooth to obtain the desired 0.01-inch retention. The path of insertion in the case of buccal tipping of an abutment dictates that the retention arm be relieved excessively, creating a food trap and causing soft tissue irritation (Fig. 8-13). When tilting creates an excessive undercut, the solutions include enameloplasty to reduce the undercut or a cast restoration to provide ideal contours. When lack of retention exists, the solutions are preparation of an undercut or the use of a lingual undercut for retention. In tooth-borne partial dentures alternative treatment includes buccal or lingual rest extensions to provide retention, reciprocation, or both. The extension must be at least 3 mm long occlusogingivally to provide adequate frictional retention. Mesiodistal tipping affects the frictional retention provided by parallel-opposed guide planes and the indirect retention provided by the distal guide planes of distal extension partial dentures (Frank and Nicholls, 1977).

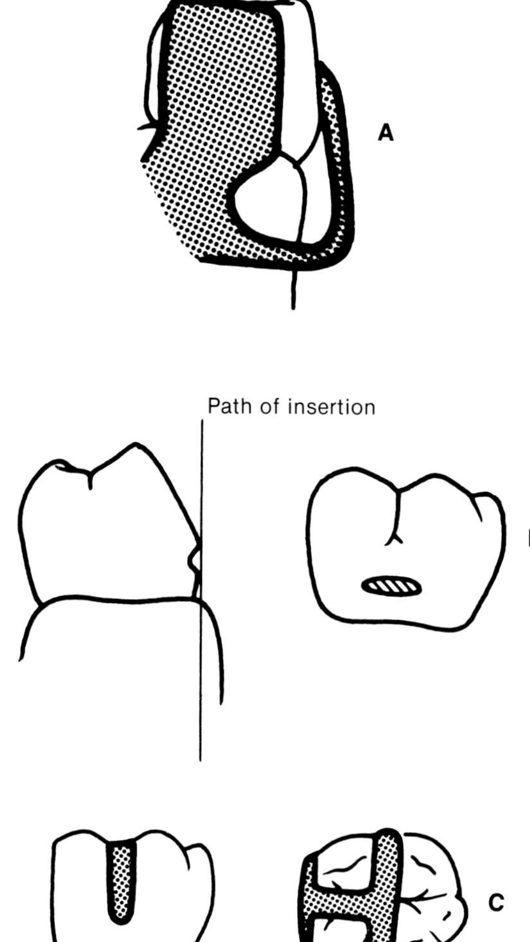

Fig. 8-13. Buccolingual tipping may dictate modification of basic clasp design. **A,** Excessive buccal tipping forces I-bar to stand out away from tooth and soft tissues. **B,** Lingual tipping eliminates retentive undercuts. **C,** If conservative enameloplasty cannot remedy these situations, buccal and lingual rest extensions can be used to provide frictional retention.

Severe tipping is most effectively controlled with a cast restoration. If adequate preparation of the guide plane risks pulpal exposure, one might be forced to consider the contribution of a single tooth to the overall retention of the framework. If adequate retention can be obtained from the other retentive elements in a design, one might consider sacrificing a guide plane on a tipped abutment. When this alternative is chosen, the framework should be kept well away from the tooth-tissue junction to prevent food impaction (Fig. 8-14). If retention is lacking because of the limited number of guide planes or because the guide planes are short, the tipped abutment can make a significant contribution to retention. Endodontic therapy and a cast restoration are then necessary for successful treatment.

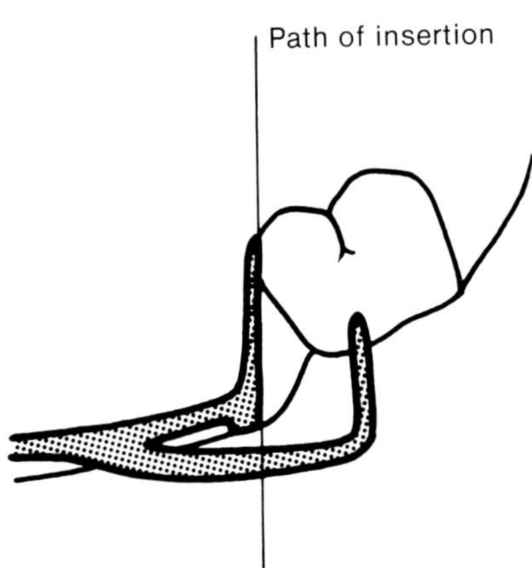

Fig. 8-14. Severely tipped molars occasionally require root canal therapy and cast restoration to provide ideal guide plane length. If restoration is not possible, guide plane should be short and proximal plate kept well away from the interproximal embrasure to prevent food impaction.

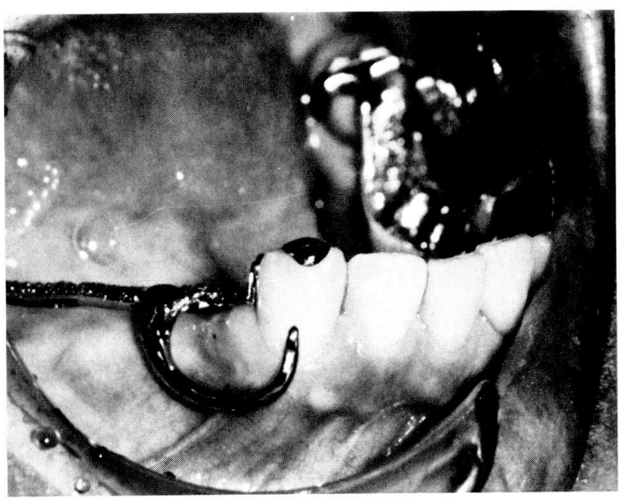

Fig. 8-15. Frenula attachments do not preclude the use of infrabulge retainers if the tissue is loose enough to allow vertical portion of the I-bar to be 5 mm long for flexure.

Frenula, high muscle attachments, lack of attached gingiva, and tissue undercuts all interfere with placement of infrabulge retentive elements. Frenula do not categorically preclude the placement of an I-bar. If the attachment is loose enough to allow the vertical portion of the I-bar to be at least 5 mm long for flexure and hygiene, I-bar placement is possible (Fig. 8-15). In many instances the frenulum can be avoided by using an alternative approach. When a frenulum attachment is also contributing to gingival recession, the patient's interests are best served with a frenectomy or graft procedure (Berg, 1979).

The attachment of the buccinator muscle adjacent to mandibular molars will occasionally obliterate the vestibule in this area. Lack of attached gingiva further aggravates the problem of I-bar placement. An alternative to placement of an I-bar in an inadequate vestibule is, again, the use of a lingual I-bar for retention and a buccal rest extension for reciprocation. In tooth-borne partial dentures an acceptable clasp alternative on molar abutments is the use of buccal and lingual rest extensions that are prepared parallel to the path of insertion and to each other (Fig. 8-13, *C*). The preparations are deep enough to avoid disrupting normal tooth contour with metal and long enough to provide frictional retention.

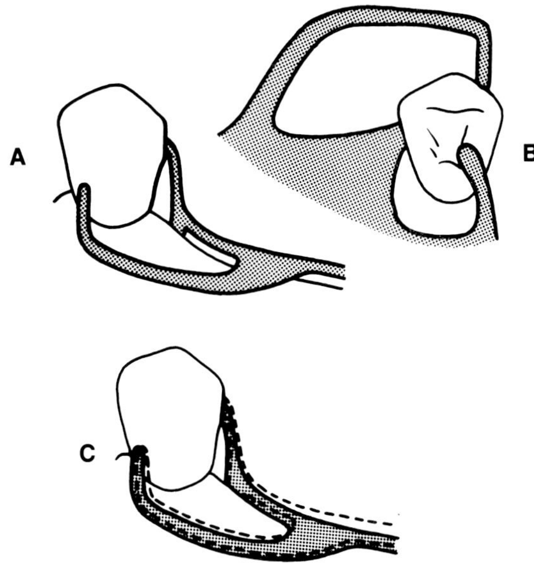

Fig. 8-16. The RPI system includes basic I-bar elements with modifications of each component. **A,** Rest is placed on mesial aspect of distal extension abutments, but is a circular concavity. **B,** Proximal plate is diminished in all directions, and I-bar retentive tips are placed mesial to the mesiodistal height of contour. **C,** Occlusal force on extension base disengages proximal plate into gingival concavity, and I-bar disengages into interproxial embrasure.

RPI (rest, proximal plate, and I-bar)

In agreement with Kratochvil's basic design, but unable philosophically to accept the amount of tooth preparation that is sometimes necessary to execute it, Krol developed a modification that studiously avoids tooth preparation. The stated emphasis in Krol's system is stress control with minimal tooth coverage and minimal gingival coverage (Krol, 1973).

The clasp system includes the three elements of Kratochvil's system: mesial rest, proximal plate, and I-bar (Fig. 8-16). Each element, however, has undergone significant change to meet Krol's criteria. Rest preparations are less extensive in the RPI system. The mesial rest extends only into the triangular fossa, even in molar preparations, and canine rests are often circular concave depressions prepared in the mesial marginal ridge.

The proximal plate makes the greatest departure from Kratochvil's design. The prepared guide plane is 2 to 3 mm high occlusogingivally, and the proximal plate contacts only 1 mm of the gingival portion of the guide plane. Relief is provided at the tooth-tissue junction to allow the proximal plate to disengage into the proximal undercut under occlusal loading.

Modifications in I-bar configuration and placement are needed to compensate for the loss of tooth contact on the proximal plate. The I-bar terminus is pod-shaped to allow more tooth contact, and placement tends toward the mesial embrasure space to achieve more efficient reciprocation from the diminutive proximal plate. Occlusal force on the extension base disengages the retentive tip into the mesial embrasure.

The stated purpose of reducing the proximal plate is to improve gingival health by opening up embrasure spaces as much as possible. A problem that might be anticipated is impaction of food into the space above the proximal plate (Berg, 1979), but Dr. Krol has not experienced problems related to food impaction interproximally, and the evolutionary tendency of the RPI system is toward an increasingly smaller proximal plate (Krol, 1980).

Tipped abutments and tissue impingement are treated with a further modification, the RPA clasp (rest, proximal plate, and Akers clasp). When the Akers clasp arm is used, careful attention is paid to relieving all undercuts except at the retentive tip (Krol, 1976).

CONCLUSION

The requirements of a partial denture clasp system (vertical support, horizontal stabilization, retention, reciprocation, and passivity) are all met by the I-bar system. Successful use of the system requires careful analysis of each component for the function that it provides and thoughtful execution of the system in abutment preparation. Nothing condemns a treatment modality as predictably as lack of commitment or lack of understanding on the part of the provider.

ACKNOWLEDGMENTS

Sincere thanks are extended to the UCLA School of Dentistry Art Department, Word Processing Center, and Media Center for their efforts in preparing the final manuscript.

REFERENCES

Berg, T.: I-bar: myth and countermyth, Dent. Clin. North Am. **23**:65-75, 1979.

Berg, T., and Caputo, A.A.: Anterior rests for maxillary partial dentures, J. Prosthet. Dent. **39**:139-146, 1978.

Frank, R.P., and Nicholls, J.I.: An investigation of the effectiveness of indirect retainers. J. Prosthet. Dent. **38**:494-506, 1977.

Holmes, J.B.: Influence of impression procedures and occlusal loading on partial denture movement, J. Prosthet. Dent. **15**:474-481, 1965.

Kratochvil, F.J.: Influence of occlusal rest position and clasp design on movement of abutment teeth, J. Prosthet. Dent. **13**:114-124, 1963.

Kratochvil, F.J., and Caputo, A.A.: Photoelastic analysis of pressure on teeth and bone supporting removable partial dentures, J. Prosthet. Dent. **32**:52-62, 1974.

Kratochvil, F.J., and Vig, R.G.: Principles of removable partial dentures, Los Angeles, 1979, UCLA School of Dentistry.

Krol, A.J.: Clasp design for extension-base removable partial dentures, J. Prosthet. Dent **29**:408-415, 1973.

Krol, A.J.: RPI (rest, proximal plate, I-bar) clasp retainer and its modification, Dent. Clin. North Am. 17(4):631-649, 1973.

Krol, A.J.: Removable partial denture design: an outline syllabus, ed. 2, San Francisco, 1976, Universtiy of the Pacific.

Krol, A.J.: Personal communication, 1980.

Leupold, R.J.: A comparative study of impression procedures for distal extension removable partial dentures, J. Prosthet. Dent. **16**:708-720, 1966.

McDowell, G.C.: Force transmission by indirect retainers during unilateral loading, J. Prosthet. Dent. **39**:616-621, 1978.

Potter, R.B., Appleby, R.C. and Adams, C.D.: Removable partial denture design: A review and a challenge, JPD**17**:63-68, 1967.

Thompson, W.D. and Kratochvil, F.J.: Evaluation of photoelastic stress patterns produced by various designs of bilateral distal-extension partial dentures, JPD 38:261-273, 1977.

BIBLIOGRAPHY

Benson, D., and Spolsky, V.W.: A clinical evaluation of removable partial dentures with I-bar retainers, Part I, J. Prosthet. Dent. **41**:246-254, 1979.

Potter, R.B., and others: Removable partial denture design: a review and a challenge, J. Prosthet. Dent. **17**:63-68, 1967.

Thompson, W.D., and Kratochvil, F.J.: Evaluation of photoelastic stress patterns produced by various designs of bilateral distal extension partial dentures, J. Prosthet. Dent. **38**:261-273, 1977.

9 Mouth preparation and master cast

The treatment plan for the patient who is to receive a removable partial denture can be finalized only after diagnostic casts have been mounted on an articulator and surveyed and the proposed partial denture has been designed. The design procedure will have disclosed procedures that are necessary to prepare the mouth to receive a removable partial denture (reshaping of enamel to produce more favorable contours).

After the examination, diagnosis, and treatment planning phase, the sequence of mouth preparation appointments must be planned with the goal of conserving as much time as possible. The following discussion is arranged in the order that the mouth preparation procedures are normally performed.

If extensive oral or periodontal surgery will be accomplished, interim partial dentures to maintain the position of the remaining teeth may be required. The indications for and the technique of constructing temporary partial dentures are discussed in Chapter 18.

RELIEF OF PAIN AND INFECTION

As early in the treatment process as possible all teeth that are causing pain or discomfort because of caries or defective restorations should be treated to eliminate the possibility of an acute episode of pain occurring during the treatment procedure. Asymptomatic teeth with advanced carious lesions should be treated in the same way and restored with an intermediate restorative material until definitive treatment is accomplished. Perhaps nothing is more discouraging to a patient under the active care of a dentist than to be suddenly subjected to a severe toothache. Such occurrences can change a patient's attitude toward the total treatment concept drastically.

The gingival tissues should also be treated early in the treatment sequence to eliminate the possibility of exacerbation of periodontal abscesses and other inflammatory responses. Definitive periodontal therapy need not be performed until the complete treatment plan is accomplished, but calculus accumulations should be debrided, plaque should be controlled, and a preventive dental hygiene program should be started and vigorously monitored.

Recent studies on the oral health care of partially edentulous patients reflect that the response to change in habits to maintain improved oral hygiene is not statistically significant. Habits learned over a lifetime are difficult to change. This fact does not relieve the dentist of the responsibility of attempting to alter the patterns of behavior, but it should alert the practitioner to be on guard and keep these patients on a frequent recall schedule.

Once the potential emergency-causing conditions have been controlled, the definitive treatment plan will be formulated.

ORAL SURGICAL PROCEDURES

As a general rule conditions requiring oral surgical intervention are treated first. Such conditions include teeth that have been ruled nonrestorable or nonusable because of position, impacted or unerupted teeth, and interferences such as palatal or mandibular tori or bony exostoses that would complicate partial denture construction. Preprosthetic surgical procedures such as ridge augmentation or vestibular extensions for which the healing time may be lengthy, must also be performed at the beginning so that the results of the surgical procedures may be observed before final treatment is begun to determine whether the intent of the surgery was achieved. The clinical procedures for this portion of the mouth preparation are described in many excellent textbooks on oral surgical procedures and on preprosthetic surgery.

PERIODONTAL THERAPY

The periodontal procedures necessary to restore the mouth to the state of health required for the definitive treatment also must be carried out early in the clinical sequence.

Periodontal surgical intervention may reveal that teeth originally expected to share the stress of the removable partial denture will be unable to support the increased load. Situations such as this could cause a reevaluation of the total treatment plan. For this reason the periodontal health must be ascertained before the patient is committed to other steps in the treatment plan.

The periodontal conditions that influence the removable partial denture design are covered in Chapters 5 and 6. Excellent texts on periodontal therapy are available and should be used as references. The general practitioner responsible for the total treatment of the patient must decide whether to carry out the treatment in these specialized areas or to refer the patient to a specialist.

CORRECTION OF THE OCCLUSAL PLANE

The occlusal plane in most partially edentulous mouths will be uneven. The severity of this irregularity will determine the extent of the treatment necessary to correct the condition. Teeth that have been unopposed for a time will tend to overerupt. Maxillary molars, if not opposed, tend to migrate downward, carrying the bony tuberosity along (Fig. 9-1). This makes the problem of reestablishing a usable occlusal plane more difficult because surgery to reduce the height of bone is indicated but the position of the maxillary sinus may not allow surgery to be performed. Problems such as this should have been recognized following the diagnostic mounting procedure, and the partial denture should have been designed to circumvent the problem if surgical correction is impossible. If space is extremely limited between the overerupted teeth and the opposing ridge, a thin metal casting may be designed to cover the ridge in place of an acrylic resin denture base (Fig. 9-2). Occasionally overeruption has occurred to the extent that extraction of the teeth will be the only possible solution (Fig. 9-3).

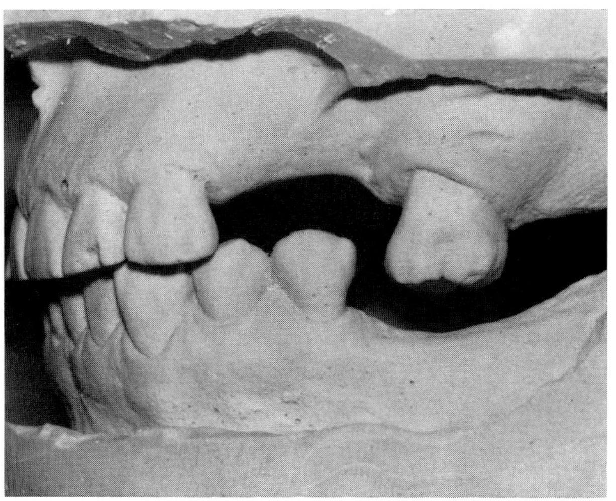

Fig. 9-1. Unopposed molar teeth will erupt beyond the ideal occlusal plane.

Normally the occlusal plane is corrected by reducing the height of overerupted teeth. There are times, however, when the clinical crown requires lengthening to restore the correct occlusal plane, such as when teeth fail to erupt fully because of interferences from other teeth or lack of stimulation. This condition is most often corrected by orthodontic treatment or the placement of cast onlays or crowns.

Tipped molars also present problems in establishing a harmonious occlusal plane. Loss of teeth anterior to the molars causes the molars to drift mesially and in doing so to tip. The ideal solution is to upright the teeth orthodontically. If orthodontic treatment is not possible, the occlusal plane may be reestablished by using crowns, onlays, or the removable partial denture itself in the form of onlay occlusal rests.

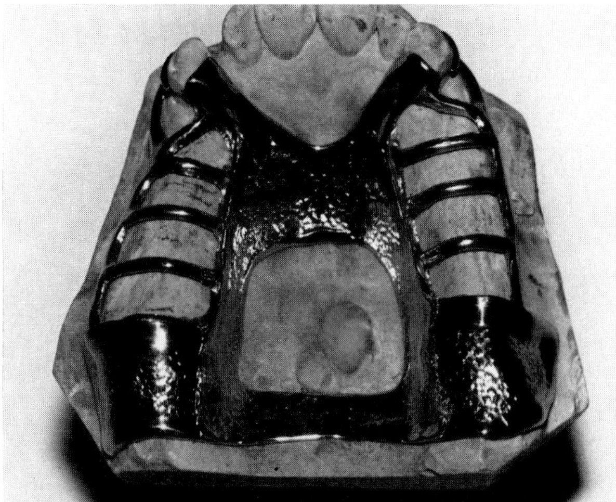

Fig. 9-2. Maxillary tuberosity must be completely covered by denture base. If interocclusal space is limited, a thin metal casting may be used.

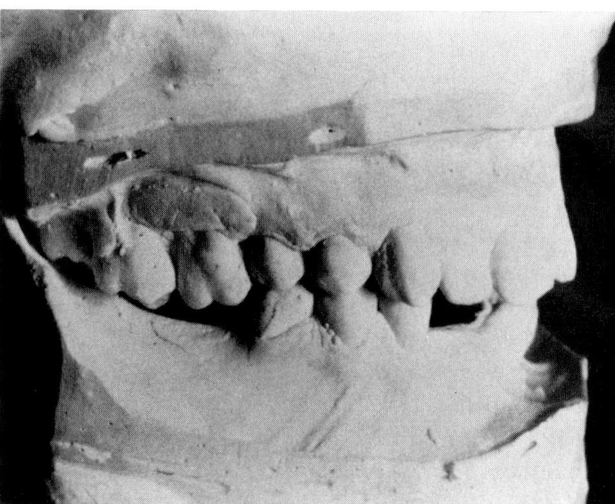

Fig. 9-3. Occlusal plane must be reestablished before partial denture construction can be undertaken. Extraction of teeth is at times indicated.

The methods of correcting an undesirable plane of occlusion are discussed from the simplest to the more complex.

Enameloplasty

Enameloplasty is a coined word used to describe the removal of a portion of the enamel surface of a tooth to accomplish specific purposes. For the correction of the occlusal plane, the enameloplasty consists of reducing cusp height in order to level or harmonize the curve of the occlusal plane.

It should be obvious that the amount of correction that can be accomplished by this technique is limited (Fig. 9-4). For most patients penetration through the enamel layer must be avoided. In older patients where considerable wear of the occlusal surfaces has taken place with resultant deposition of secondary dentin, slightly more tooth structure may be removed without endangering the tooth or producing sensitivity.

When cusp height is reduced, the anatomy of the occlusal surface should not be mutilated. Functional cusps with accessory grooves and sluiceways must be restored to the teeth once the necessary reduction has been made.

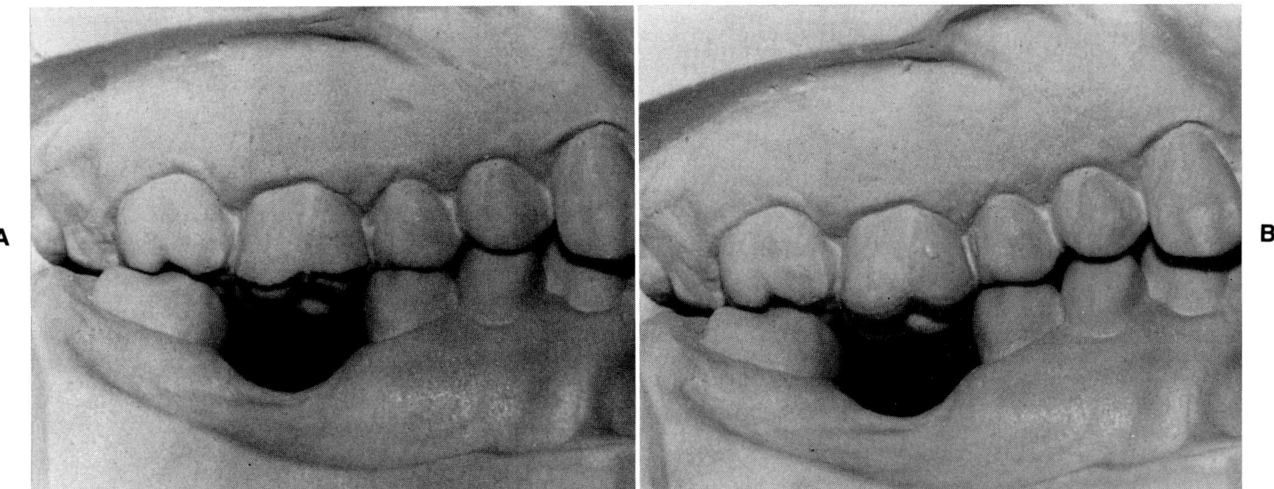

Fig. 9-4. A, Correction of occlusal plane by enameloplasty is limited by thickness of enamel layer. Cutting beyond level indicated may expose dentin. **B,** Proper anatomy should be restored to tooth after enameloplasty.

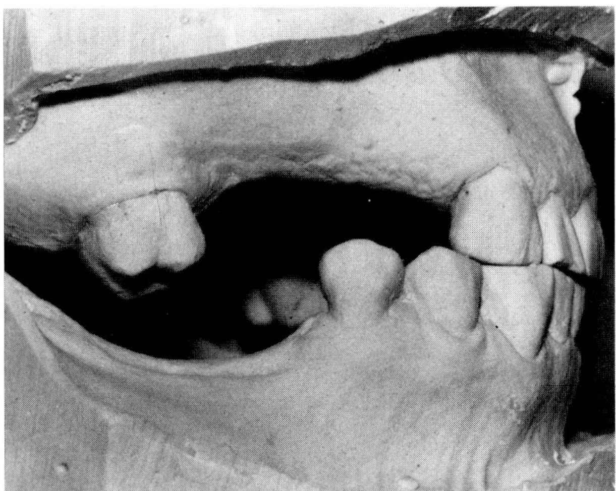

Fig. 9-5. Reduction of lingual cusp height on unopposed maxillary molars is often indicated.

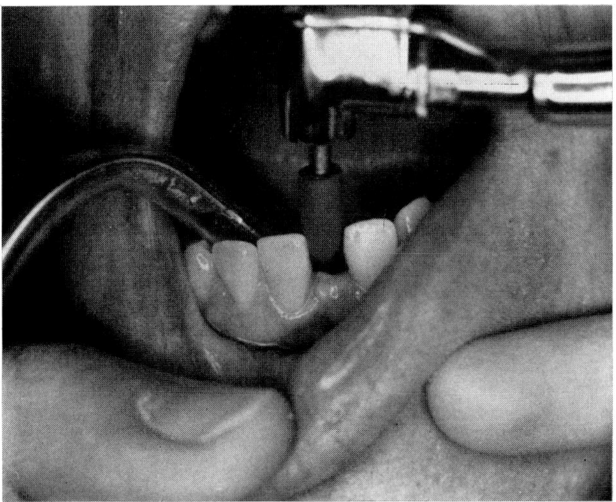

Fig. 9-6. Ground enamel surfaces must be restored to a smooth, polished state with Carborundum-containing rubber points or wheels.

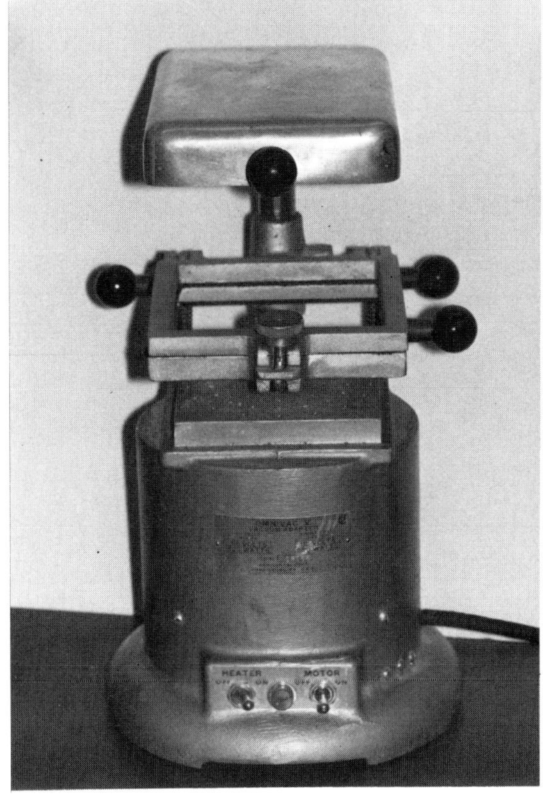

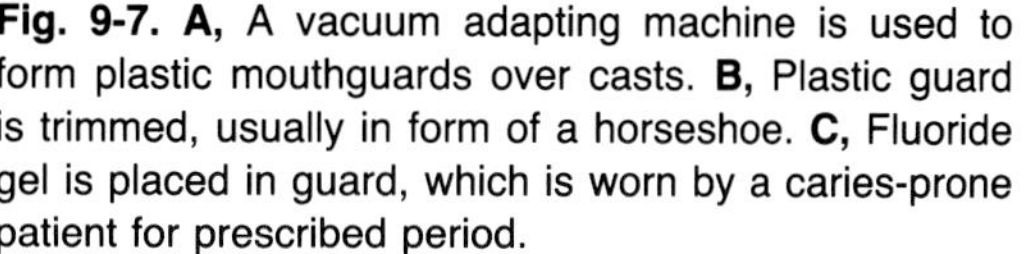

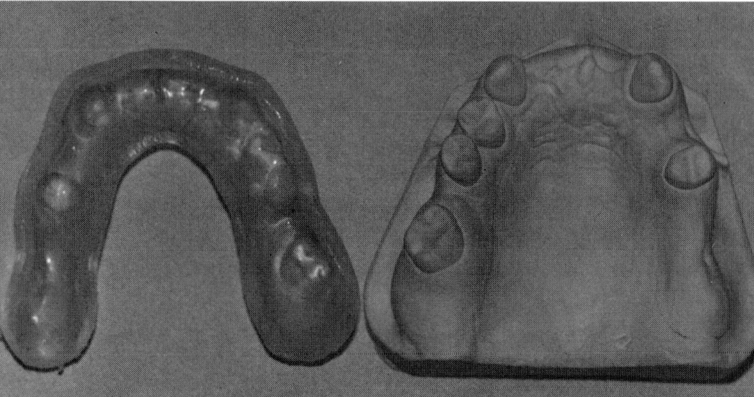

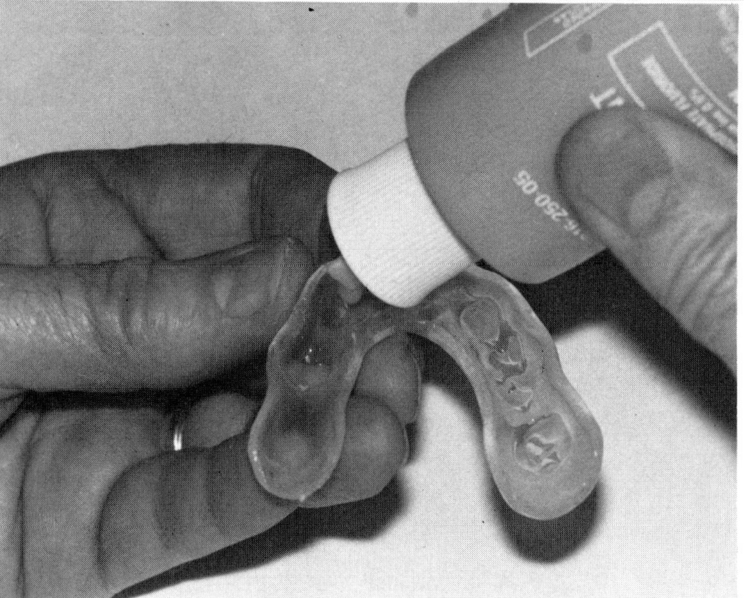

Fig. 9-7. A, A vacuum adapting machine is used to form plastic mouthguards over casts. **B,** Plastic guard is trimmed, usually in form of a horseshoe. **C,** Fluoride gel is placed in guard, which is worn by a caries-prone patient for prescribed period.

Unopposed maxillary molars tend to roll toward the facial surface as extrusion takes place. This rotation causes the lingual cusp in particular to drop below the occlusal plane. Reduction in height of these cusps often eliminates potential occlusal interferences (Fig. 9-5).

The actual reduction of the enamel surface is best accomplished by using tapered diamond cylinder stones in the high-speed handpiece. Air-water spray should always be used to prevent creating excess heat during the procedure.

Polishing the cut enamel surface is imperative. To remove the scratches in the enamel, Carborundum-containing rubber wheels or points must be used (Fig. 9-6).

Treatment of the tooth surfaces with a fluoride gel effectively raises the fluoride content of the enamel and increases the surface resistance to dental caries. One of the simplest and most effective techniques of applying the fluoride to the teeth makes use of a soft plastic mouthguard, as shown in Fig. 9-7.

Onlay

The use of onlay occlusal rests was rather common a number of years ago, before the advent of high-speed dental equipment, as a conservative method of correcting the plan of occlusion.

The occlusal surface of a tooth to be covered by an onlay rest should be free of pits and fissures or should be made so by eliminating the defects with small burs or stones. The smooth occlusal surface helps prevent caries caused by dental plaque and other debris being trapped and held against vulnerable tooth surfaces. Use of this rest in mouths with poor oral hygiene can lead to destruction of teeth.

The use of an onlay rest on a tooth that has been restored with a cast onlay or crown is redundant because the restoration itself should be used to restore the occlusal plane; the onlay rest would be superfluous.

If the onlay rest is to be constructed of chrome alloy, any opposing natural teeth should not occlude directly

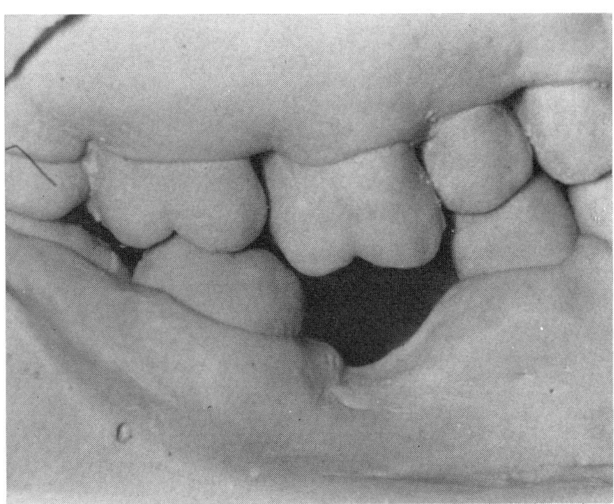

Fig. 9-8. Cast onlay is indicated for tooth that is above or below plane of occlusion to reestablish proper plane. (Courtesy Dr. Edmund Cavazos, Jr., University of Texas Health Science Center at San Antonio.)

against the rest. Chrome alloy, being extremely hard, will cause rapid wear of the opposing enamel surfaces. If the onlay rest must be used under these circumstances, the chrome metal should be constructed short of occlusal contact and the surface of the metal covered with projections of metal beads. Tooth-colored acrylic resin may be processed on the surface of the onlay rest with the beads used to retain the resin. Opposing natural teeth may then occlude against this resin without the danger of wearing the tooth surfaces. However, the acrylic resin will wear fairly rapidly and will require replacement more frequently than an acrylic resin denture tooth. The replacement can be accomplished as a chairside procedure with the patient developing the occlusal pattern by closing into the resin while it is still soft. After processing is complete, the resin surface can be shaped and finished with stones and polishing compounds.

One of the simplest methods of reestablishing the plane of occlusion is by the use of cast gold onlays, which can either lengthen or shorten the crown height of a tooth (Fig. 9-8).

One of the main advantages of the onlay is that the natural contours of the facial and lingual enamel surfaces can be maintained. This is normally an objective if the periodontal health of the tooth is optimal under the existing conditions. It is regrettable that there has been a tendency toward full crown restoration in preference to partial crown or onlay restorations in recent years, possibly because patient insistence on esthetics has become the primary consideration during the treatment planning phase. It should be remembered that conservative tooth preparation can help disguise unnecessary display of metal and that education in the realm of preventive dental treatment may convince the patient of the advantage of less than total crown coverage.

The cast onlay does present a problem of securing an adequate retention form for the restoration. Excellent books are available that describe techniques of securing additional retention through the use of pins, ledges, and other methods.

If the tooth bearing the onlay is also to be a primary abutment for the removable partial denture (that is, is to have a retentive extracoronal clasp), the retentive clasp tip should not engage an undercut in the onlay; it must be on the enamel surface. If this is not possible, the onlay is not indicated and a full crown should be planned for that tooth.

Crowns

When the crown height of the tooth must be changed to harmonize the occlusal plane, and the facial, lingual, or proximal surfaces must be altered to produce a more desirable height of contour, a guiding plane, or a retentive undercut, a full crown is normally the restoration of choice.

Before the tooth is prepared to receive the crown, mounted diagnostic casts should be measured to ascertain how much crown reduction is necessary to correct the occlusal plane. If the reduction of tooth structure will be so great as to endanger the dental pulp, a decision must be made as to whether endodontic treatment is indicated or whether this extent of treatment is not warranted and extraction would be the treatment of choice.

Endodontics with crown or coping

If strategically positioned teeth in the dental arch are retained, the prognosis of the partial denture is improved markedly. These teeth include mandibular second or third molars that may be used to serve as posterior abutment teeth so that the prosthesis may be all tooth supported. This greatly improves patient acceptance of the denture. Other vitally important teeth are those in the center of a long anterior edentulous span, either mandibular or maxillary. The presence of a usable abutment tooth in that location offers a great advantage in controlling vertical movement of the denture.

These important teeth are often overerupted and have lost some of the periodontal support needed to serve as an abutment. If this is the case, endodontic therapy and, if inter-occlusal space is available, construction of a crown will allow the teeth to serve as normal abutments.

If overeruption has been so gross as to nearly obliterate the remaining interarch space, the crown of the tooth can be removed at the gingival crest and a coping

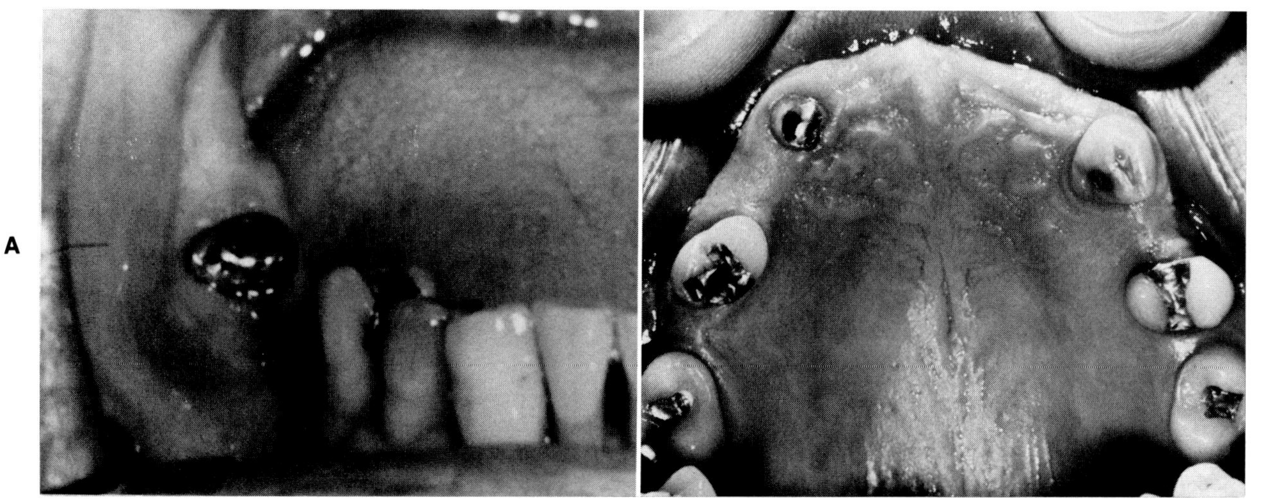

Fig. 9-9. A, Endodontically treated posterior teeth may be retained as a stop against vertical movement of a partial denture. B, An endodontically treated anterior tooth is beneficial in supporting a long-span denture base.

constructed. The tooth will serve as a vertical stop, preventing excessive vertical or horizontal movement of the prosthesis (Fig. 9-9).

The technique for preparing the abutment tooth to serve as an overdenture abutment is covered in detail in Chapter 20.

Extraction

It should be the goal of a designer of removable partial dentures to retain as many of the remaining teeth as possible. However, at times retaining certain teeth can greatly complicate or even compromise the success of the treatment.

For example, if orthodontic treatment cannot be accomplished to realign severely malposed molars or premolars, extraction must be considered. When the teeth interfere with the placement of the major connector and no other solution (such as crowning the tooth) is feasible, extraction must be planned (Fig. 9-10).

Leaving a lateral incisor as an anterior terminal abutment tooth when the central incisors and the opposite lateral incisor are missing frequently compromises not only the mechanical stability of the denture, but also the esthetic acceptance. This is not to condemn all lateral incisor teeth, but the benefit of the tooth to the finished denture must be carefully evaluated (Fig. 9-11).

Surgery

Surgical repositioning of one or both jaws or of segments of one or both jaws to correct malrelationship of teeth is not a new procedure.

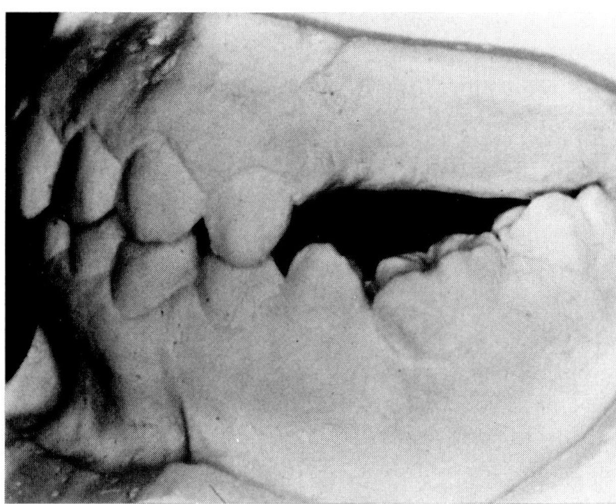

Fig. 9-10. Severely overerupted molars that interfere with placement of acrylic resin retention minor connector and artificial teeth must be considered for extraction.

Various forms of mandbuilectomies, usually to correct gross prognathic jaw relationships, have been performed with great success for a number of years.

Repositioning of the entire maxilla or segments of the bones has enjoyed increased success in recent years. The surgery is somewhat more complicated than repositioning of the mandible. This undoubtedly is the reason for the slower development of the techniques required for success.

Of particular interest in the area of reestablishing harmony of the occlusal plane is the procedure of

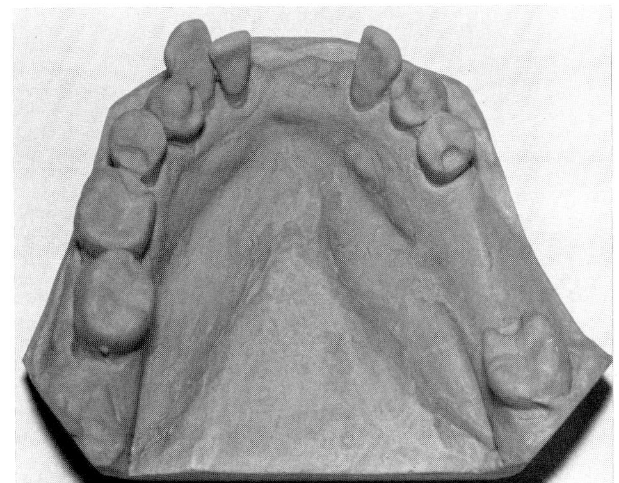

Fig. 9-11. Malposed lateral incisors frequently complicate design of prosthesis. Extraction of these teeth may be the treatment of choice.

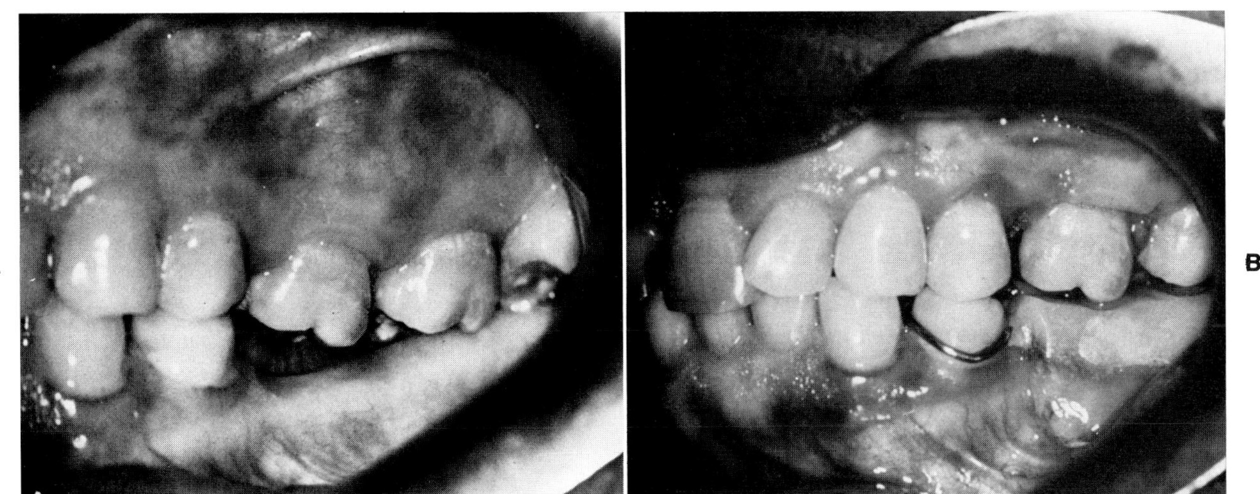

Fig. 9-12. A, Preoperative view of maxillary posterior teeth that have extruded to contact the mandibular edentulous ridge. **B,** View of the same mouth after a maxillary segmental osteotomy. The elevated segment of the maxilla is supported by a mandibular occlusion rim during the healing phase. (Courtesy Dr. Frank Dolwick, University of Texas Health Science Center at San Antonio.)

superiorly repositioning posterior segments of the maxillae containing the posterior teeth, a maxillary segmental osteotomy (Fig. 9-12). The segment (including the alveolar ridge, tuberosity, and teeth) is elevated into the maxillary sinus. This is one of the most effective methods of regaining interarch space lost because of downward migration of the teeth and tuberosity.

This type of surgical correction should be performed by a specialist, but the prosthodontist should be aware of what can be accomplished for the patient.

CORRECTION OF MALALIGNMENT

Teeth that are malposed facially or lingually are frequently more difficult to correct than overerupted or submerged teeth. There are definite limitations to the repositioning of these malposed teeth. Often it is the design of the removable partial denture that must be altered rather than the tooth position.

Orthodontic realignment

The technique of orthodontically moving the malpositioned tooth should be considered first (Fig. 9-13). Whenever it is possible, it is the treatment of choice.

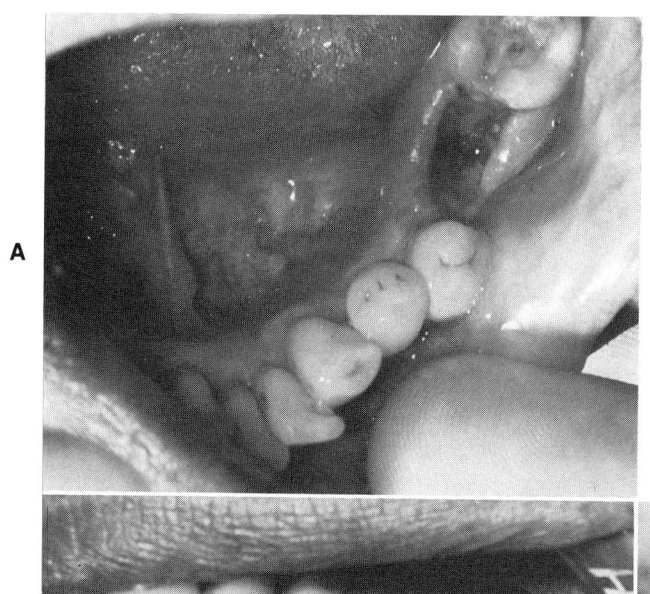

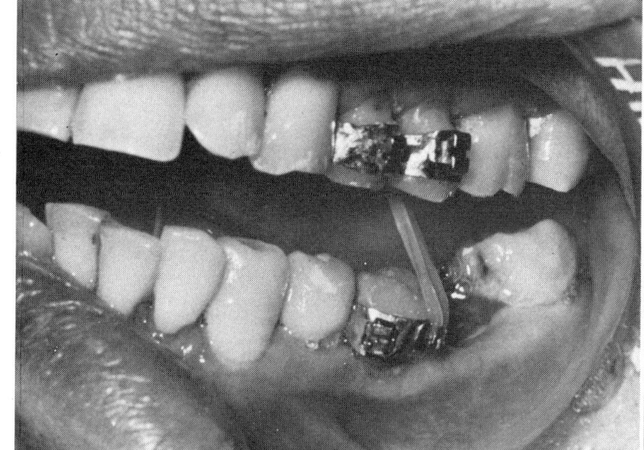

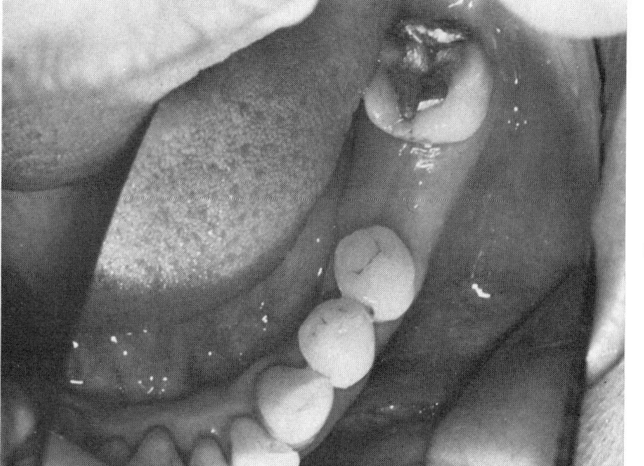

Fig. 9-13. A, A severely facially malposed second premolar. Orthodontic repositioning should be considered. The first molar has recently been extracted, so space for the tooth to be moved is present. **B,** Orthodontic bands with elastic in place. **C,** Second premolar in proper alignment. First molar may now be replaced. (Courtesy Department of Orthodontics, University of Texas Health Science Center at San Antonio.)

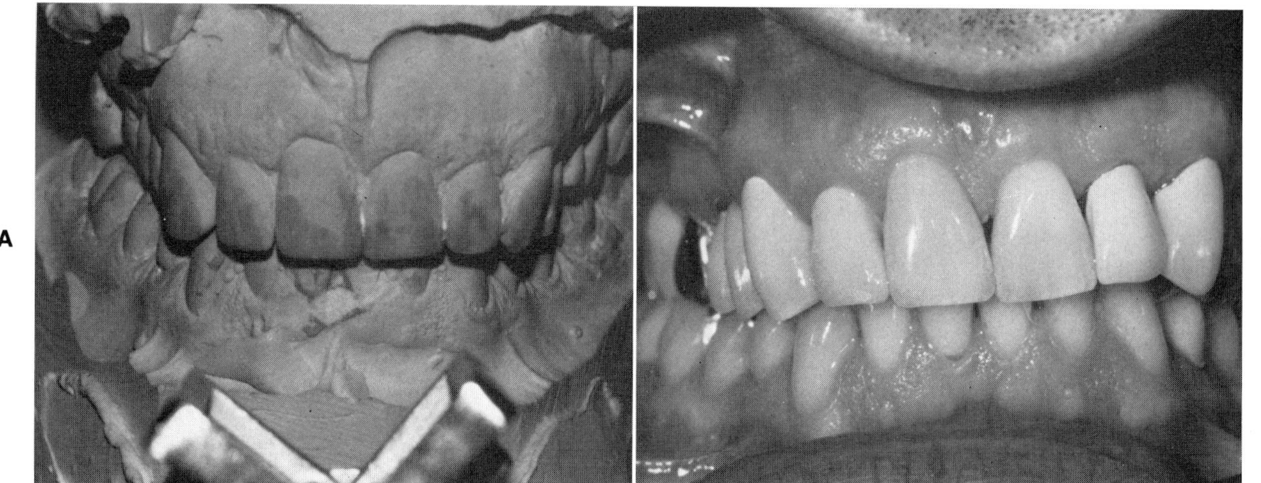

Fig. 9-14. A, Maxillary right premolars and first molar alignment is lingual to correct position. **B,** Placement of full crown restorations on these teeth reestablishes correct buccal position. (Courtesy Dr. D. Kaiser, University of Texas Health Science Center at San Antonio.)

Unfortunately it is often not possible to use this method. In many mouths where a large number of teeth are missing there may not be enough remaining teeth to serve as an anchor from where the moving force can be applied. There must be some means of applying force and resisting the equal and opposite counterforce that will be generated.

Crowns

Teeth that are not grossly out of position facially or lingually can occasionally be improved by a partial or full crown restoration (Fig. 9-14). The teeth to be considered for this form of correction are those that are tipped either buccally or lingually.

Normally it is the desire not to encroach on the dental pulp when preparing the tooth to receive a crown, so the amount of tooth structure that can be removed is minimal.

It is possible to treat the tooth endodontically and use a post and core to restore the crown in a nearly normal position. It must be remembered, however, that the long axis of the remaining root and the crown must not be too dissimilar or undesirable forces will take place on the structure supporting the root. Thus crown restorations may be used, but they will not cure severe malalignment.

Enameloplasty

The concept of reshaping or reducing enamel surfaces or cusps of teeth to correct the occlusal plane can be used to a lesser degree to correct malaligned teeth. It is possible to recontour buccal or lingual surfaces to eliminate interferences to the path of placement of a major connector. It is possible in certain instances to reshape the facial or lingual surfaces of tipped or malposed teeth to allow better placement of clasps or lingual plating (Fig. 9-15).

This approach to the correction of malaligned teeth should always be given first consideration when mouth preparation is planned, but it should be recognized that the amount of correction that can be achieved is limited.

The contoured enamel surfaces must be restored to a polished condition, as when enameloplasty is used to correct the occlusal plane.

PROVISION OF SUPPORT FOR WEAKENED TEETH

In many partially edentulous mouths some or all the remaining teeth have lost varying amounts of the supporting periodontal ligament and alveolar bone. To use these teeth to help support and stabilize a removable partial denture, it will be necessary to provide additional support for these teeth by splinting the teeth together or by using overdenture abutments.

Removable splinting

The premise behind splinting teeth with removable restorations is that the mobility will either decrease or remain the same. The tendency for tooth mobility to increase until the inevitable loss of the tooth will have been altered. The theory and technique of splinting weakened teeth by a removable prosthesis is covered in depth in Chapter 20.

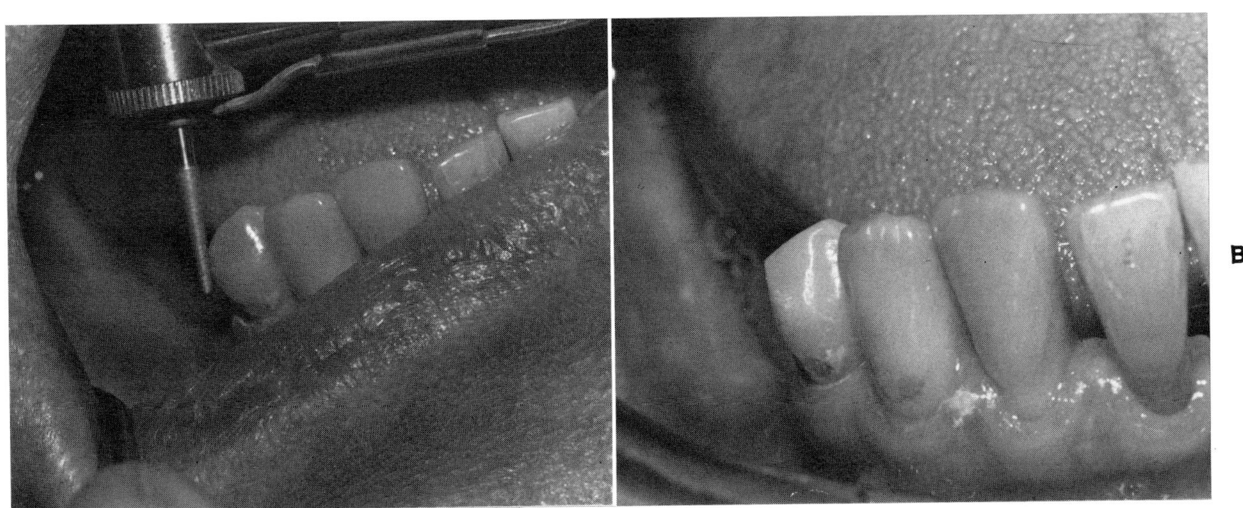

Fig. 9-15. A, Enamel surface of a facially tipped first premolar is recontoured to lower height of contour to a more favorable position. **B,** After enameloplasty, height of contour is now in an acceptable position.

Fixed splinting

There are times that an individual tooth or two adjoining teeth may have lost some periodontal support as a result of local conditions. The decision must be made as to the value of retaining such teeth as opposed to the extraction of the teeth and the inclusion of the teeth in the removable partial denture.

A tooth that has lost over 50% of its bony support (that is, has a crown/root ratio of less than 1:1) and is being considered as a terminal abutment tooth for a Class I or II partial denture would be a poor candidate for splinting to the adjacent tooth. In a situation such as this the usual result is that the stronger of the teeth is weakened by the splinting procedure rather than the weaker tooth being strengthened (see Fig. 6-49). If the difference in periodontal support of the teeth in question is great and the majority of the support and retention of the prosthesis is to be placed on the weaker of the two, the prognosis is poorer than if the teeth's support is similar or if the greater amount of work is borne by the stronger tooth.

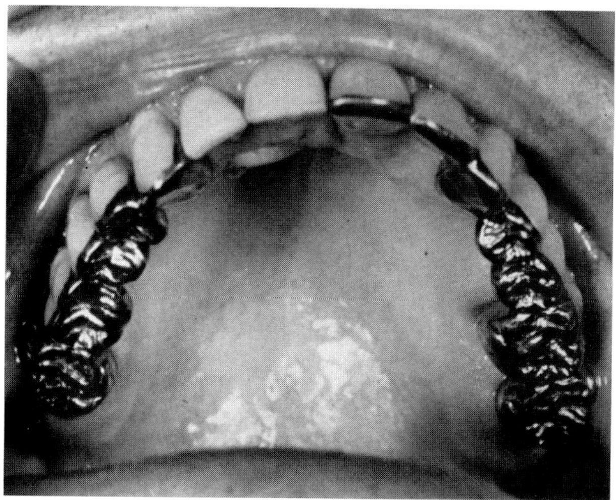

Fig. 9-16. Fixed splint on patient's right side offers little resistance to lateral forces because splint terminates at canine. On the left side the splint includes lateral and central incisor and will resist lateral forces to a greater degree. (Courtesy Dr. Fred Shaw, University of Tennessee Dental School.)

Splinting of weakened teeth in the partially edentulous arch located in a position where the partial denture will not require an unusual amount of support is highly desirable. It maintains the continuity of the arch and avoids additional modification spaces, thus simplifying the construction and fitting of the partial denture and improving the prognosis.

To be considered a permanent form of treatment, fixed splinting must be accomplished with full or partial coverage crowns soldered together or pin-ledge restorations that provide additional retention for the splint. Teeth that require splinting usually exhibit mobility. This mobility, if not completely controlled, may over time cause a break in the cementing medium with ultimate adverse effects on the tooth and surrounding tissues. To attempt to control mobility with inlay restorations is ill advised. If the teeth cannot be held totally immobile, splinting should not be attempted.

One of the most important points to consider when fixed splinting is contemplated is that joining adjacent teeth by means of crowns soldered together will pro-

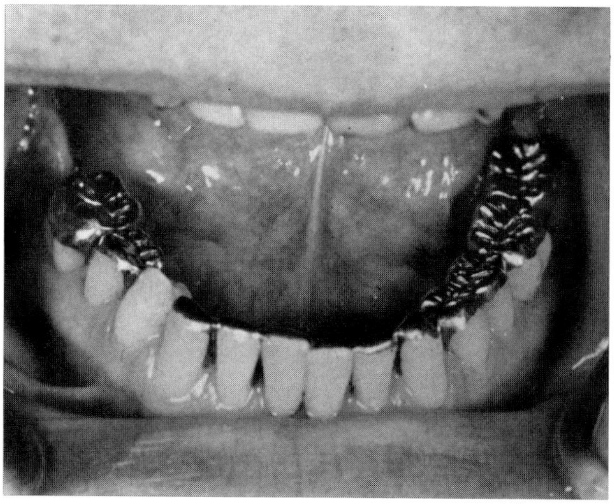

Fig. 9-17. Fixed splint shown extends from right canine to left second molar. This provides good cross-arch stabilization. (Courtesy Dr. Fred Shaw, University of Tennessee Dental School.)

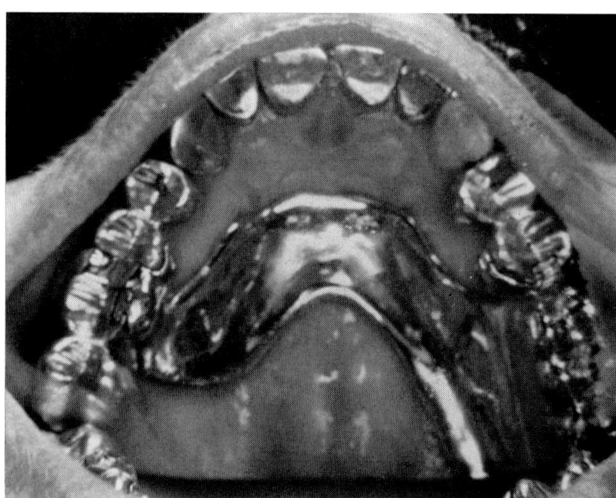

Fig. 9-18. This maxillary major connector retained by intracoronal attachments provides cross-arch stabilization for teeth that have lost some periodontal support.

vide additional resistance to anteroposterior stresses but offers little increased resistance to lateral forces.

To obtain resistance to lateral forces by fixed splinting, the splint must be extended anteriorly to include the canine teeth and beyond and must include not only the anteroposterior plane of the posterior teeth but also the turn of the arch, or the lateral plane (Figs. 9-16 and 9-17). This turn of the arch will incorporate the resistance to lateral forces as well as resistance to anteroposterior forces. One of the better methods of obtaining resistance to lateral forces when splinting periodontally weakened teeth is to be attempted is to obtain cross-arch stabilization by means of a removable prosthesis. This can be in the form of a wide palatal strap in the maxillary arch or a lingual bar or lingual plate in the mandibular arch. Fixed splinting on each side of the arch provides anteroposterior stability, and the removable major connector provides the cross-arch stabilization that is needed to resist lateral forces. The major connector may be retained with extracoronal attachments (clasps) or, as is commonly done, with intracoronal (internal) attachments (Fig. 9-18). Missing teeth may or may not be replaced with this cross-arch stabilizer.

Overdenture abutments

Certain teeth that have lost at least 50% of the supporting bone but are strategically positioned in the arch should be retained to provide support for a removable prosthesis (Fig. 9-19). The support provided will consist principally of resisting tissueward forces. If such teeth at the posterior end of an edentulous space are retained and used as vertical stops for the denture base, the prosthesis will be converted from a Class I or II partial denture to a functioning Class III prosthesis. This change improves the function of the denture, and the patient acceptance is consistently excellent.

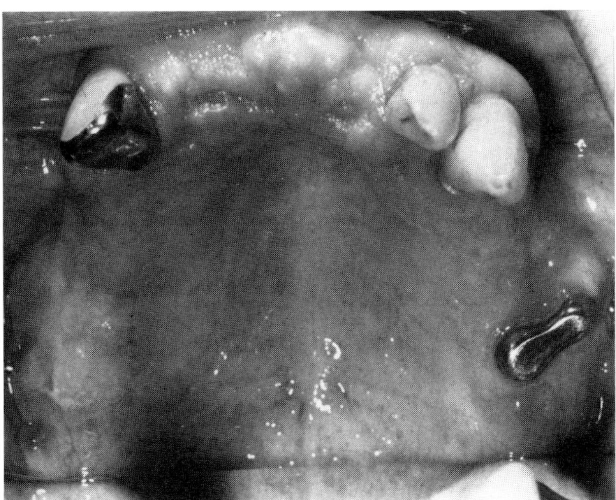

Fig. 9-19. A gold coping over endodontically treated roots provides vertical support and stabilization for a removable prosthesis.

RESHAPING TEETH

Tooth surfaces often need to be reshaped to accomplish specific purposes. This changing of tooth contour may be accomplished in the enamel, on the surface of an existing restoration, or by placing a new restoration.

Enameloplasty

Conservatism must be the rule when mouth preparation is to be accomplished on enamel surfaces for a removable partial denture. Sufficient tooth reduction must be accomplished to ensure adequate space or proper contour, but never at the expense of overcutting the tooth.

If the danger of overcutting is present, the preparations should first be accomplished on a diagnostic cast. This procedure will usually reveal whether restoration of the teeth by crowns or inlays is preferable to reshaping of enamel surfaces.

After tooth surfaces have been reshaped, the enamel must be highly polished. In the polishing procedure light intermittent pressure and moderate speed of the Carborundum-impregnated rubber wheel or point must be used. Dangerously high heat can be generated if care is not exercised.

The application of a fluoride gel to the reshaped surfaces may be beneficial. Oral hygiene techniques must be stressed and demonstrated to these patients.

Enameloplasty to develop guiding planes

Guiding planes are surfaces on proximal or lingual surfaces of teeth that are parallel to each other and, more important, to the selected path of insertion of the removable partial denture. The discussion of guiding planes in Chapter 4 should be reviewed to relate the requirements for guiding planes to the actual tooth reduction.

Guiding planes on abutment teeth adjacent to tooth-supported segments. The diagnostic cast, mounted on the surveying table at the tilt at which the design of the removable partial denture was drawn, should be available at the mouth preparation appointment. It should be placed on the bracket table in front of the patient, and the handpiece, with the appropriate diamond instrument in place, positioned over the cast so that the relationship of the handpiece and diamond stone to the teeth can be visualized. This same relationship can then be duplicated in the patient's mouth (Fig. 9-20). This procedure ensures that the guiding plane will be parallel to the planned path of insertion.

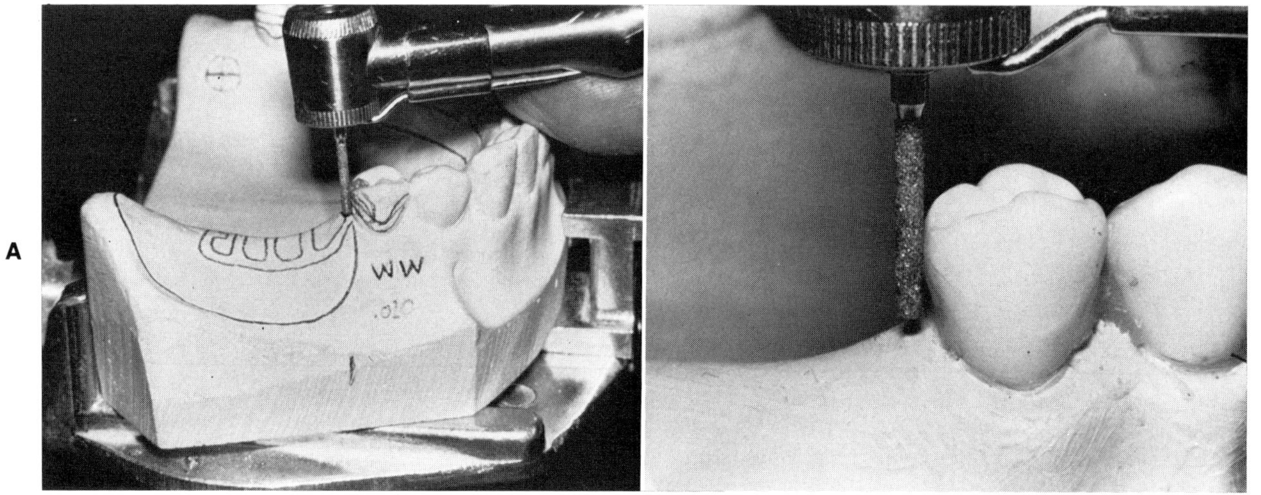

Fig. 9-20. A, The design cast, mounted on survey table at proper tilt, helps align handpiece at correct angle to develop a guiding plane. **B,** Handpiece is moved to mouth at same angle and guiding plane produced.

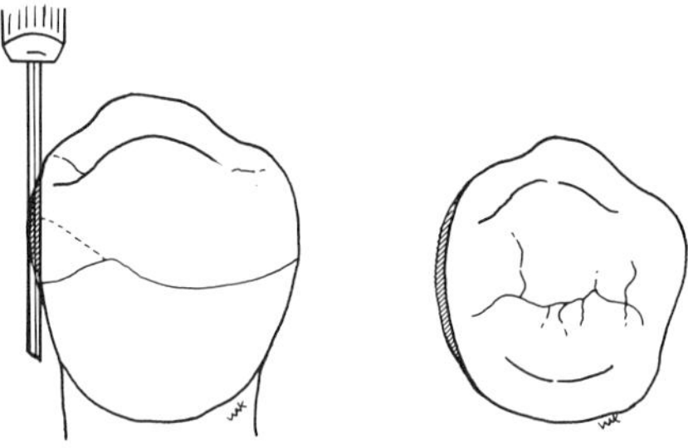

Fig. 9-21. The ideal guiding plane is 2 to 4 mm. in occlusogingival height. Normal contour of tooth surface is maintained.

A cylindric diamond point is generally the instrument used to make the preparation. A gentle, light, sweeping stroke from the buccal line angle to the lingual line angle should be used.

The flat surface created should ideally be 2 to 4 mm in occlusogingival height (Fig. 9-21). *Caution:* As a general rule five or six light strokes of the diamond stone are sufficient to produce the desired tooth reduction. More strokes usually will remove excessive tooth structure.

The reduction must not be a straight slice across the tooth surface; rather it should follow the curvature of the surface so that nearly uniform amounts of enamel are removed from throughout the buccolingual width of the preparation.

All prepared tooth surfaces must be polished with a Carborundum-impregnated rubber wheel or point when the contouring is complete.

Guiding planes on abutment teeth adjacent to distal extension edentulous spaces. The tooth preparation on the proximal surface of abutment teeth adjacent to distal extension edentulous spaces is accomplished in the same manner with a cylindric diamond stone held parallel to the path of insertion. The importance of maintaining parallelism in this instance is critical.

The principal difference between this guiding plane and the planes on teeth bordering a tooth-supported segment is that the occlusogingival height of the plane is reduced to 1.5 to 2 mm to permit the partial denture to rotate slightly around the distal occlusal rest as downward force occurs on the artificial teeth. This slight movement allows the release of the denture from the guiding plane, thereby avoiding the creation of torquing or twisting forces on the abutment tooth.

Guiding planes on lingual surfaces of abutment teeth. The purpose of guiding planes on lingual surfaces of teeth is to provide maximum resistance to lateral stresses. The more teeth involved in guiding plane preparation, the less will be the stress transmitted to each individual tooth.

Tooth preparation is accomplished in the same way as for the proximal surfaces of the tooth-supported and the distal extension abutment tooth. The cylindric diamond stone is used for this purpose (Fig. 9-22).

The occlusogingival height of the preparation is 2 to 4 mm. The plane ideally should be located in the middle third of the clinical crown of the tooth.

Special care must be shown to avoid changing the contour of the gingival third of the tooth because damage to the marginal gingiva through the improper

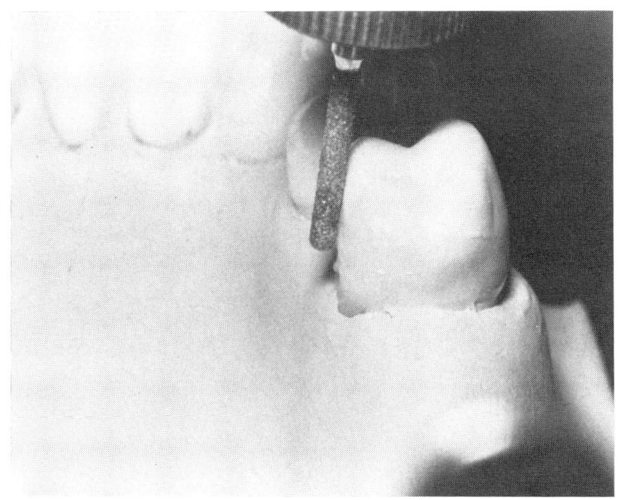

Fig. 9-22. Guiding planes are developed on lingual surfaces of teeth for additional stabilization.

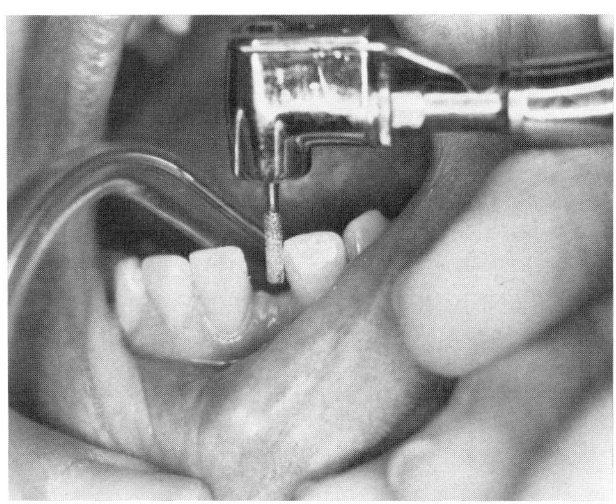

Fig. 9-23. Teeth adjacent to an edentulous space normally tip toward that space. This creates large interproximal undercuts that are reduced by enameloplasty.

shunting of food may occur if the normal morphology of the gingival third of the crown is lost.

Guiding planes on anterior abutment teeth. Guiding planes on anterior teeth adjacent to edentulous spaces provide the parallelism needed to ensure stabilization, minimize wedging action between the teeth, decrease undesirable space between the denture and the abutment tooth, and increase retention through frictional resistance.

Another special purpose of such guiding planes is to increase or restore the normal width of the edentulous space. As anterior teeth are lost and replacement teeth not provided immediately, teeth adjacent to the space will drift and tip into the space. Both actions reduce the size of the space and make the esthetic replacement of the missing teeth difficult. In addition, teeth that have tipped toward an edentulous space will exhibit a large undercut area below the height of contour on the proximal surface (Fig. 9-23). If the height of contour is not reduced as the guiding planes are established, the undercut will appear as a large, unsightly space between the artifical tooth and the restored tooth. The space not only detracts from the esthetic value of the denture, but also traps food.

A cylindric diamond stone is used to reduce the proximal surfaces of the adjacent teeth. If sufficient tooth structure cannot be removed to restore the space and to reduce the undercut without penetrating the enamel layer, a restoration must be planned.

The reduction of these proximal surfaces must be done with the path of insertion that has been planned for the prosthesis in mind. The reduction must be parallel to this path of insertion because the reduced proximal surface will act as a guiding plane. The denture in this case will have a single path of insertion.

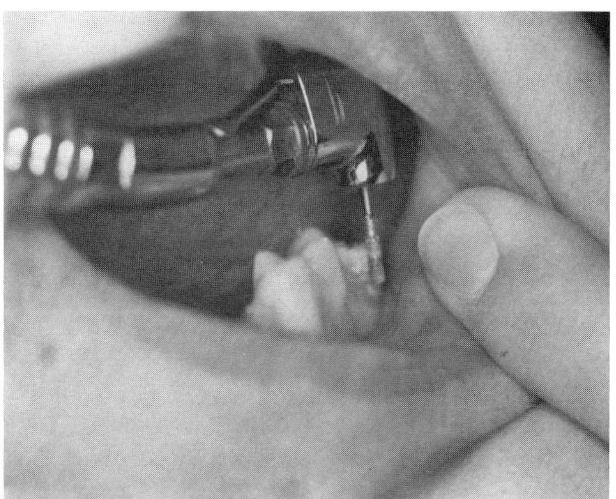

Fig. 9-24. Enamel surfaces of abutment teeth are reshaped to lower height of contour and provide a more ideal clasp position.

After reduction of the proximal surfaces, the original anatomy of these surfaces should be restored. As this is done, the parallel guiding planes must be maintained.

Enameloplasty to change height of contour

The height of contour is changed most frequently to provide better positions for clasp arms or for lingual plating (Fig. 9-24).

Ideally the retentive clasp arm should be located no higher on the crown of the abutment tooth than the juncture of the gingival and middle thirds. This position not only enhances the esthetic quality of the clasp, but also provides a definite mechanical advantage.

Maxillary molars and premolars, if unsupported in an arch that lacks continuity, tend to tip in a buccal direction. This causes the height of contour to be near the occlusal surface on the facial side of the abutment tooth. A clasp in this position on the maxillary molars or premolars is esthetically unacceptable (Fig. 9-25).

The reverse condition exists in the mandibular arch (Fig. 9-26). Premolar and molar teeth in this arch, if not supported, will tip lingually. This usually causes problems with positioning reciprocal clasps and lingual plating and, if the tipping is severe, with the placement of the lingual bar major connector.

The amount of correction that can be accomplished by recontouring the enamel surface is limited by the thickness of the enamel. Care has to be taken not to penetrate the enamel and expose dentin. In the event dentin is exposed, a restoration must be placed to protect the tooth.

The height of contour is best lowered by using tapered diamond stones. Minor reshaping of buccal and lingual surfaces can greatly improve mechanical and esthetic properties.

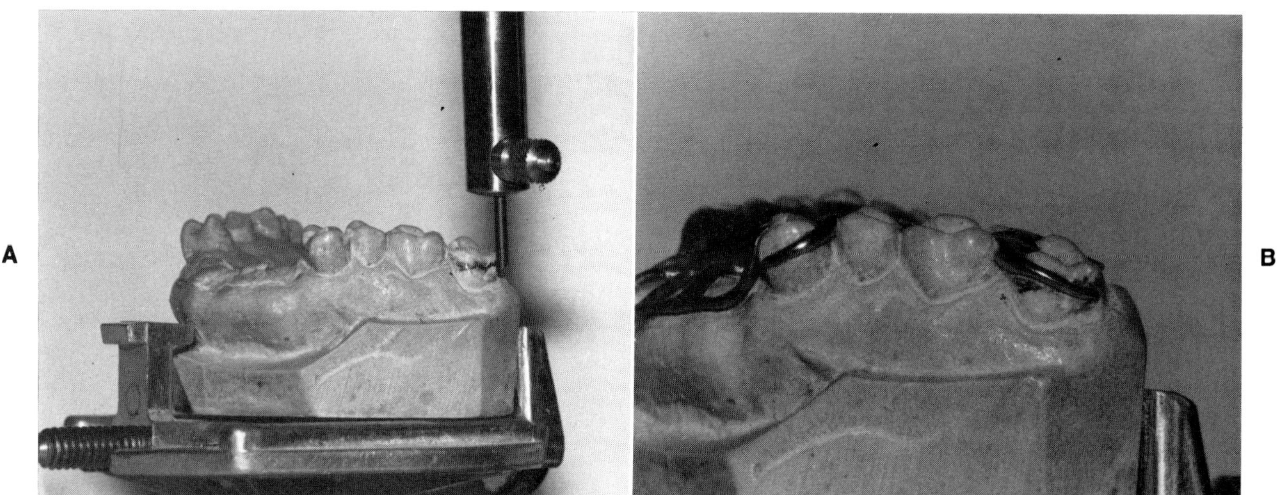

Fig. 9-25. A, Unopposed maxillary molars tip facially. This results in a high survey line and poor clasp position, **B.**

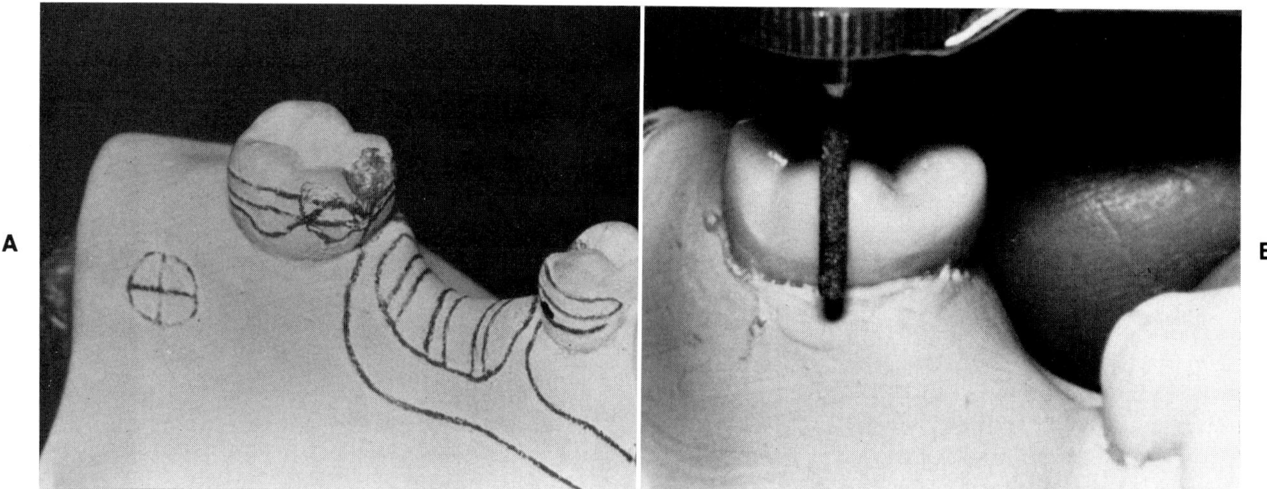

Fig. 9-26. A, Unopposed mandibular molars tend to drift mesiolingually. This causes survey line to be high on mesiolingual line angle. Area has been outlined in red to denote that it requires recontouring. **B,** With diamond stone held parallel to path of insertion, height of contour is reduced.

Enameloplasty to modify retentive undercuts

Occasionally a proposed abutment tooth has less than a sufficient retentive undercut. If the oral hygiene of the patient is adequate and if the caries index is low, some of these teeth may be treated to increase the amount of retentive undercut by contouring the enamel surface. This technique does not have universal application, but in a few instances it may be beneficial. This method of developing retentive undercuts should not be substituted for adequate design procedures. Retentive undercuts may exist on other surfaces that could be utilized by other forms of clasps. Relying on creating undercuts in enamel surfaces can lead to potentially damaging consequences for the patient.

In order for the technique of contouring the enamel surface to produce a retentive undercut to be successful, the buccal and lingual surfaces of the tooth must be nearly vertical. If either or both surfaces have a pronounced slope, the procedure is contraindicated. If the surface to receive the undercut is sloped, the indentation would have to be excessively deep to be effective. If the opposing surface is sloped, the reciprocal clasp arm could not brace the tooth sufficiently to prevent the retentive clasp tip from being dislodged from the undercut. (Fig. 9-27).

The retentive undercut must be created in the form of a gentle depression, not a pit or hole. The term *dimpling* has been applied to this technique, but the name appears to be misleading, implying a definite pit rather than a gentle depression.

The depression or undercut is prepared by using a small, round-ended, tapered diamond stone (Fig. 9-28). The end of the stone is moved in an anteroposterior direction near the line angle of the tooth. The preparation is made parallel to and as close as possible to the gingival margin without actually encroaching on the gingival crevice. The purpose is to create a slight concavity approximately 0.010 inch deep measured from a vertical line paralleling the path of insertion.

The depression should be approximately 4 mm in mesiodistal length and 2mm in occlusogingival height. Care must be taken not to develop a ledge or shoulder in the enamel (Fig. 9-29).

The preparation must be highly polished with a Carborundum-impregnated rubber wheel and point. Poor polishing technique may obliterate the depression.

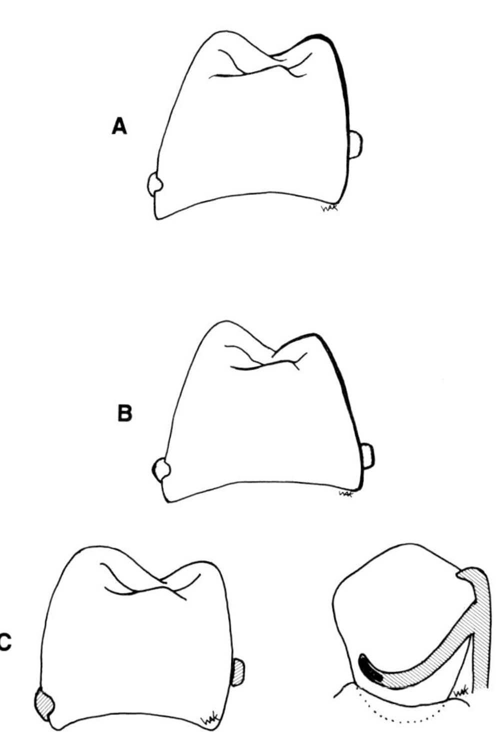

Fig. 9-27. A, If buccal or lingual surfaces of an abutment tooth are sloping, dimpling for a retentive undercut cannot be effective. **B,** If both opposing surfaces are sloping, dimpling will not be effective. **C,** Both opposing surfaces must be relatively vertical to create a retentive undercut by dimpling.

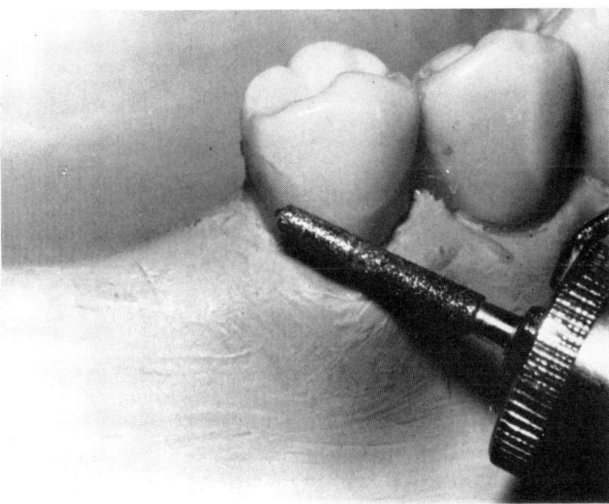

Fig. 9-28. A round-ended tapered diamond held parallel to gingival margin cuts a slight depression to produce a retentive undercut.

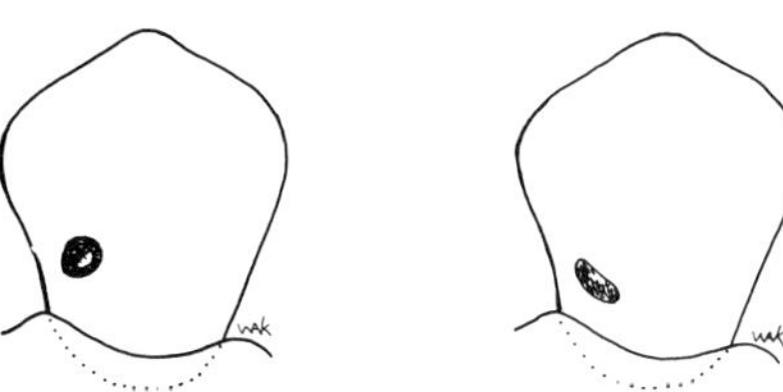

Fig. 9-29. Retentive undercut that is created is in form of depression, right, rather than dimple, as shown on left.

Inlays, onlays, and crowns

If the remaining teeth do not possess usable natural contours and the enamel surfaces cannot be corrected to produce these contours, cast restorations must be planned. The guiding planes, height of contour, and retentive undercuts can be placed in these restorations as the wax patterns are being developed. In addition, many teeth that are to serve as abutments for removable partial dentures will require restorations for more routine reasons such as the presence of caries or defective restorations, tooth fracture, or endodontic therapy. These restorations also must be planned to satisfy the requirements of the partial denture.

Before the teeth are prepared to receive the crown or other cast restorations, the articulated and designed diagnostic casts must be analyzed carefully. Lingually tipped teeth that are to be restored with crowns must be prepared so that a greater amount of tooth reduction takes place on the lingual surface and less on the buccal surface. This will allow the wax pattern to be developed so that the lingual surface is restored to a more ideal position (Fig. 9-30).

The same precaution must be taken for teeth tipped mesially or buccally. The ultimate aim in preparing and restoring malposed teeth with cast restorations is to produce a crown with the best possible alignment.

Tooth preparation on extruded teeth must reduce the crown height sufficiently so that the restoration will be on the correct occlusal plane. The actual amount of crown height reduction necessary to produce the ideal result should be measured on the diagnostic cast. Controlled tooth reduction can thus be accomplished by using diamond stones of known diameter. A series of cuts to the measured depth are made and then joined together to obtain the needed reduction (Fig. 9-31).

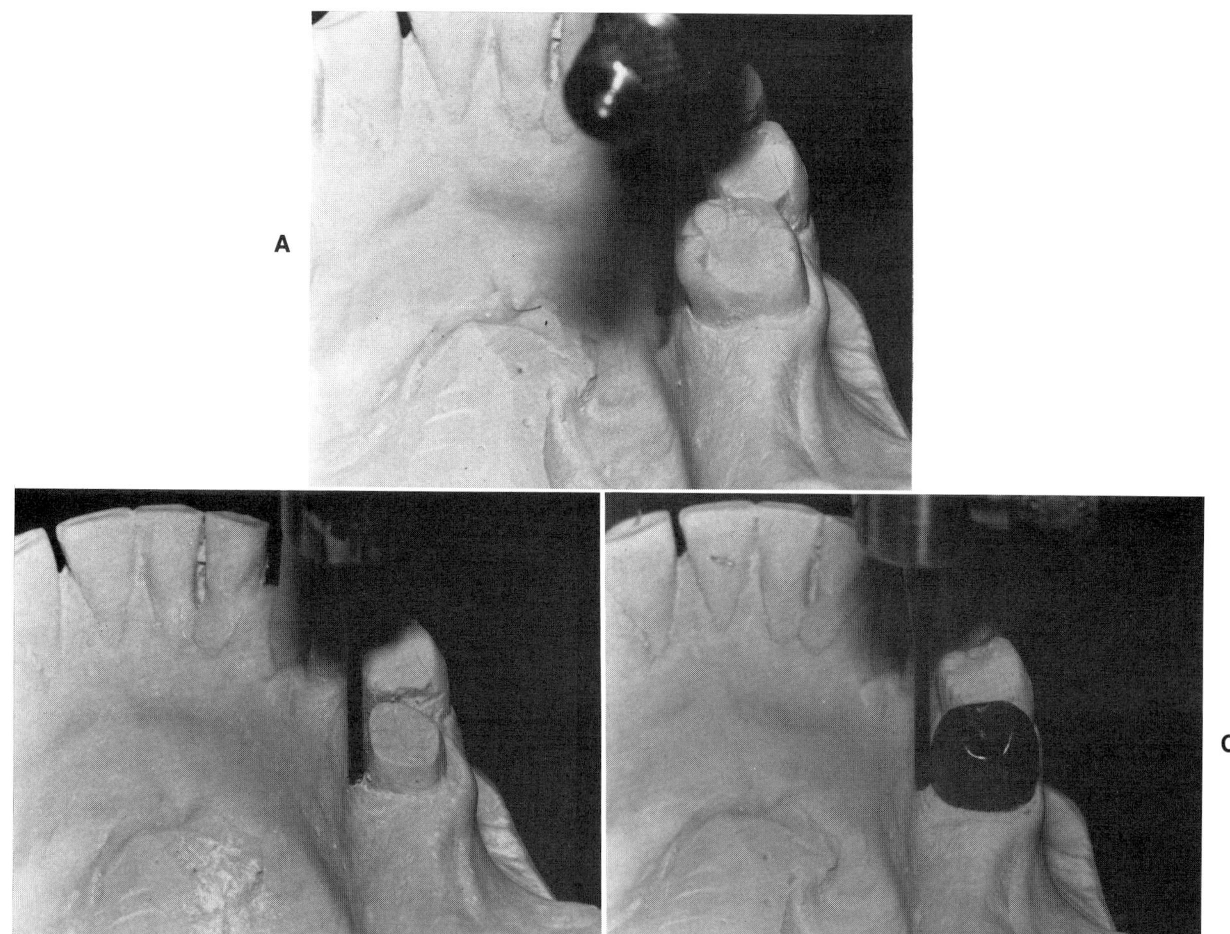

Fig. 9-30. A, Lingually tipped second premolar has a soft tissue undercut that would interfere with placement of major connector. **B,** Tooth prepared for a full crown. Lingual surface has been reduced more than normal. **C,** Wax crown has eliminated soft tissue undercut.

Shaping the wax pattern

To shape the wax pattern to the desired configuration, the die of the tooth preparation in a cast of the remainder of the arch must be analyzed on the surveyor.

The technique for mounting the working cast (the cast containing the die and wax pattern) on the surveyor at the same tilt that the diagnostic cast was mounted when the design for the removable partial denture was drawn is covered in detail in Chapter 7. Once the correct tilt has been established, the wax knife is substituted for the analyzing rod and the guiding plane is carved in the pattern by shaving the wax.

The height of contour of the crown can also be determined by use of the analyzing rod (Fig. 9-32). The pattern must be hand carved to place the height of contour in the middle third of the lingual surface of the abutment tooth if the tooth is to receive a reciprocal clasp and at the junction of the gingival and middle third if a retentive clasp has been planned.

The position and depth of the retentive undercut can be verified by use of an undercut gauge. The 0.010-inch gauge will be used for most cast chrome clasps. The measured undercut should fall at the distal or mesial line angle of the tooth, depending on the type of clasp that has been designed.

When cast restorations are planned for abutment teeth, all reshaping of natural teeth that will contribute to the support of the partial denture but will not receive cast restorations should be completed *before* the abutments are prepared for crowns, inlays, or onlays. This allows the guiding planes and contours of the wax patterns to be shaped to conform to the previously prepared enamel surfaces instead of the other way around. Better control of the completed mouth preparation can be maintained if this sequence is followed.

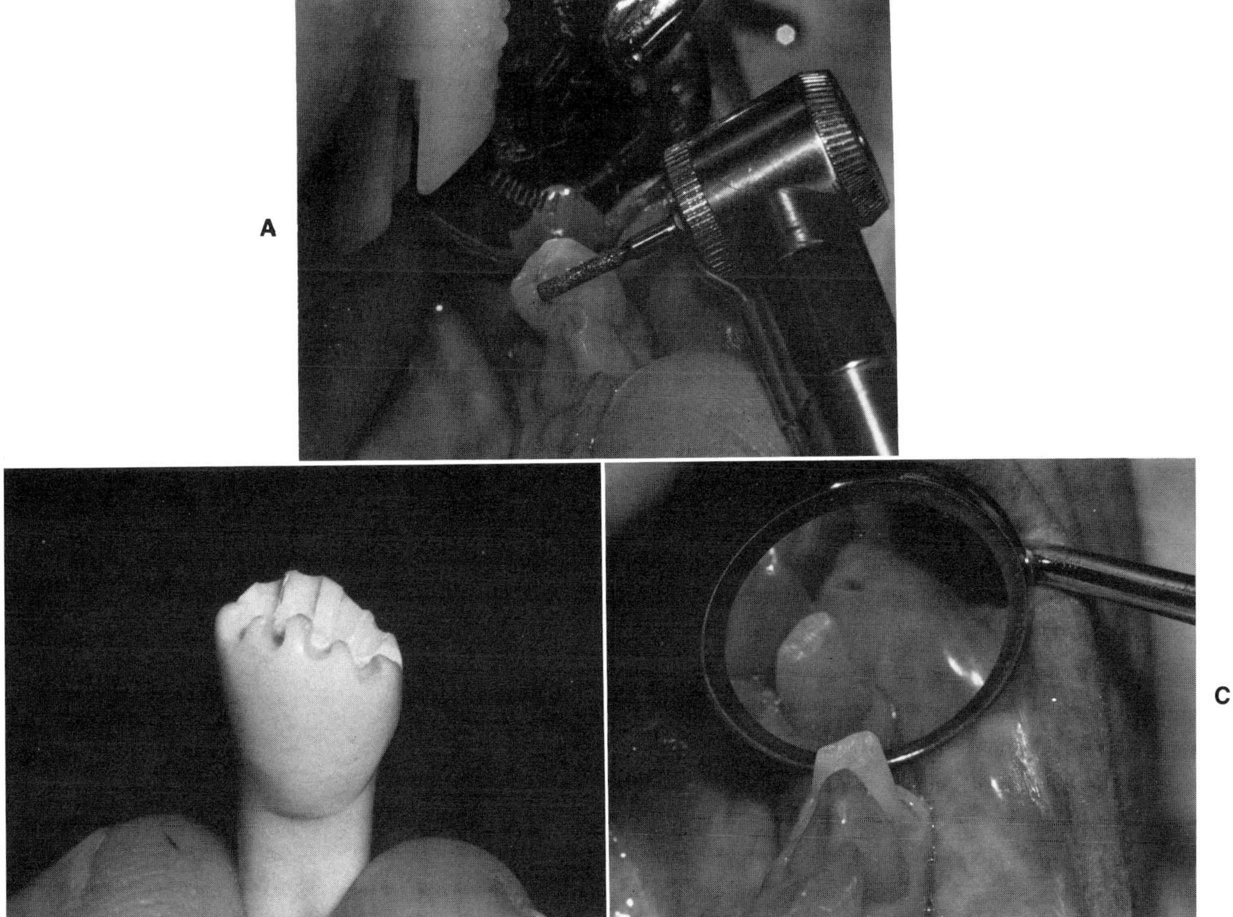

Fig. 9-31. A, A diamond cylinder stone of known diameter (1.5 mm.) is used to make a series of cuts on occlusal surface. **B,** Cuts are made to depth of diameter of stone. **C,** Cuts are connected, resulting in an occlusal reduction of 1.5 mm.

A B

C

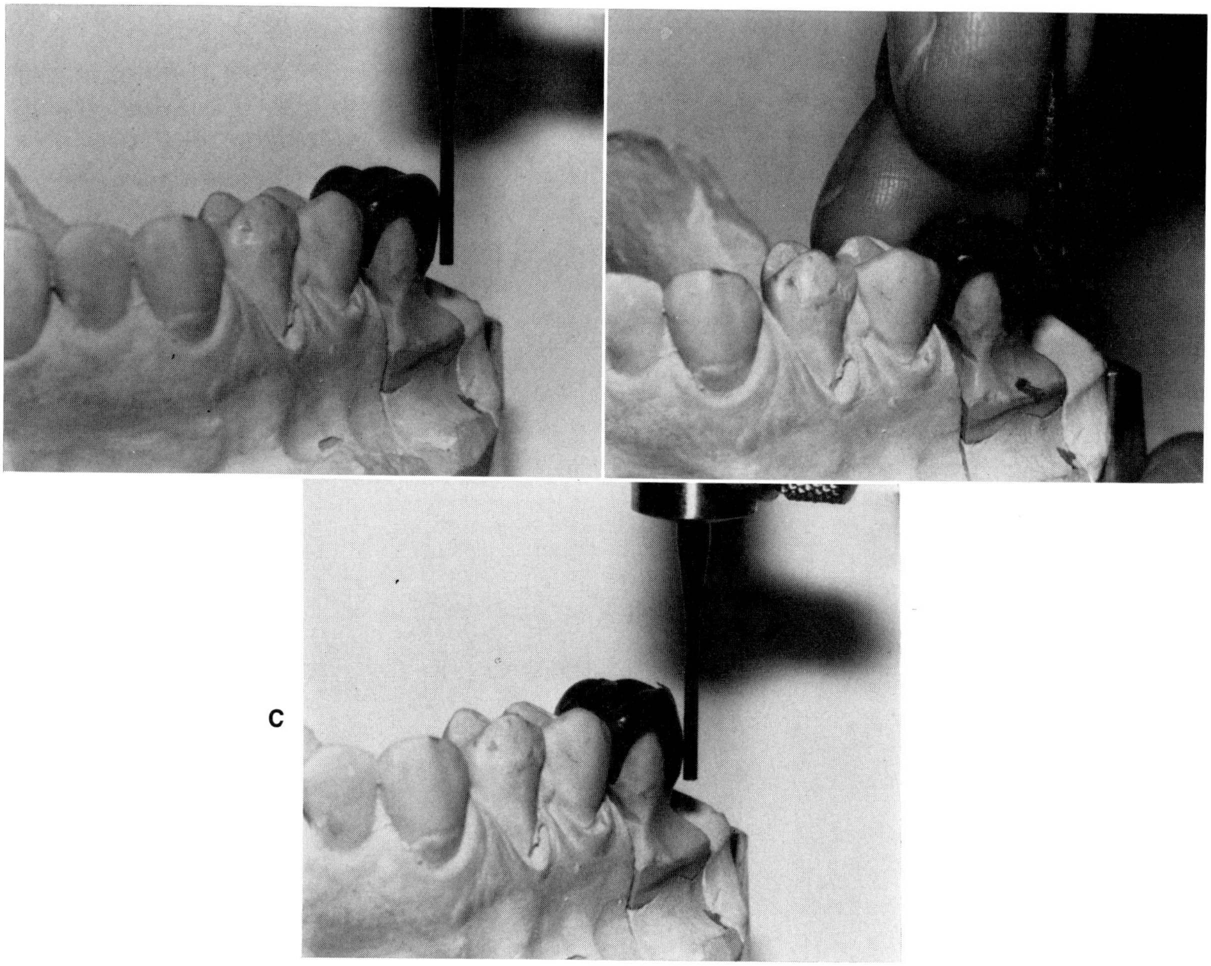

Fig. 9-32. Wax patterns for crowns of abutment teeth that will receive clasps must be properly contoured. A, Height of contour of this crown is too occlusal. B, Wax pattern is carved to lower survey line. C, An acceptable contour has been achieved.

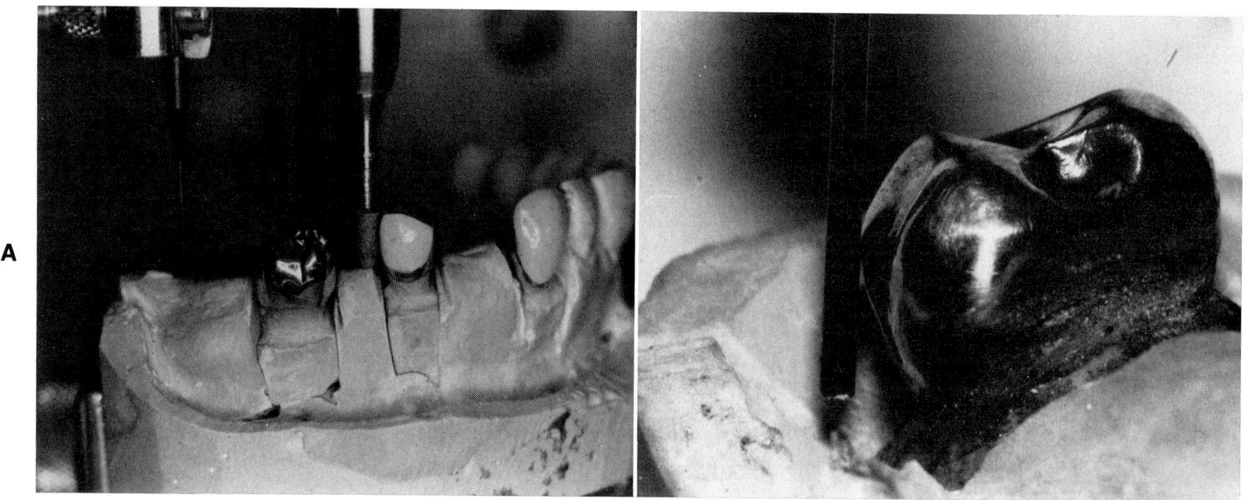

Fig. 9-33. A, Crowns on working cast are returned to surveying table at proper tilt. Surveyor, with handpiece holder attached, is used to machine the guide planes precisely. B, Analyzing rod is used to check that height of contour has not been changed.

Refining the cast restoration

Restorations are cast following techniques available in standard texts. After the casting has been made, it should be carefully finished. The contour that was carved in the wax pattern must be maintained. To be certain that the proper anatomy has not been lost in the finishing process, the working cast with the die and casting in position should be returned to the surveying table and surveyor before the final polish of the restoration is complete. The cast must be related in the same tilt at which the wax pattern was carved (Fig. 9-33). The position of the height of contour and the location and depth of the retentive undercut must be verified by using the analyzing rod. If either of these features has been lost, the casting will have to be recontoured. If the change has been so great that the casting cannot be ground to reestablish the correct contour, the wax pattern will have to be reaccomplished.

The guiding planes on the casting should also be refined before the final polish. This is done by using the surveyor as a machining device. A handpiece holder is attached to the vertical arm of the surveyor and a straight handpiece is attached to the handpiece holder. The handpiece holder aligns the handpiece parallel with the vertical arm of the surveyor. A straight cylinder mounted stone is used in the handpiece to accomplish the machining procedure. With the working cast mounted on the surveying table at the correct tilt, the table can be moved to bring the guiding plane of the cast restoration in contact with the mounted stone in the handpiece. This refining of the guiding plane is done exactly parallel to the path of insertion.

Shaping veneer crowns

The increase in the use of veneer, or porcelain-bonded-to-metal, restorations makes it essential that at-

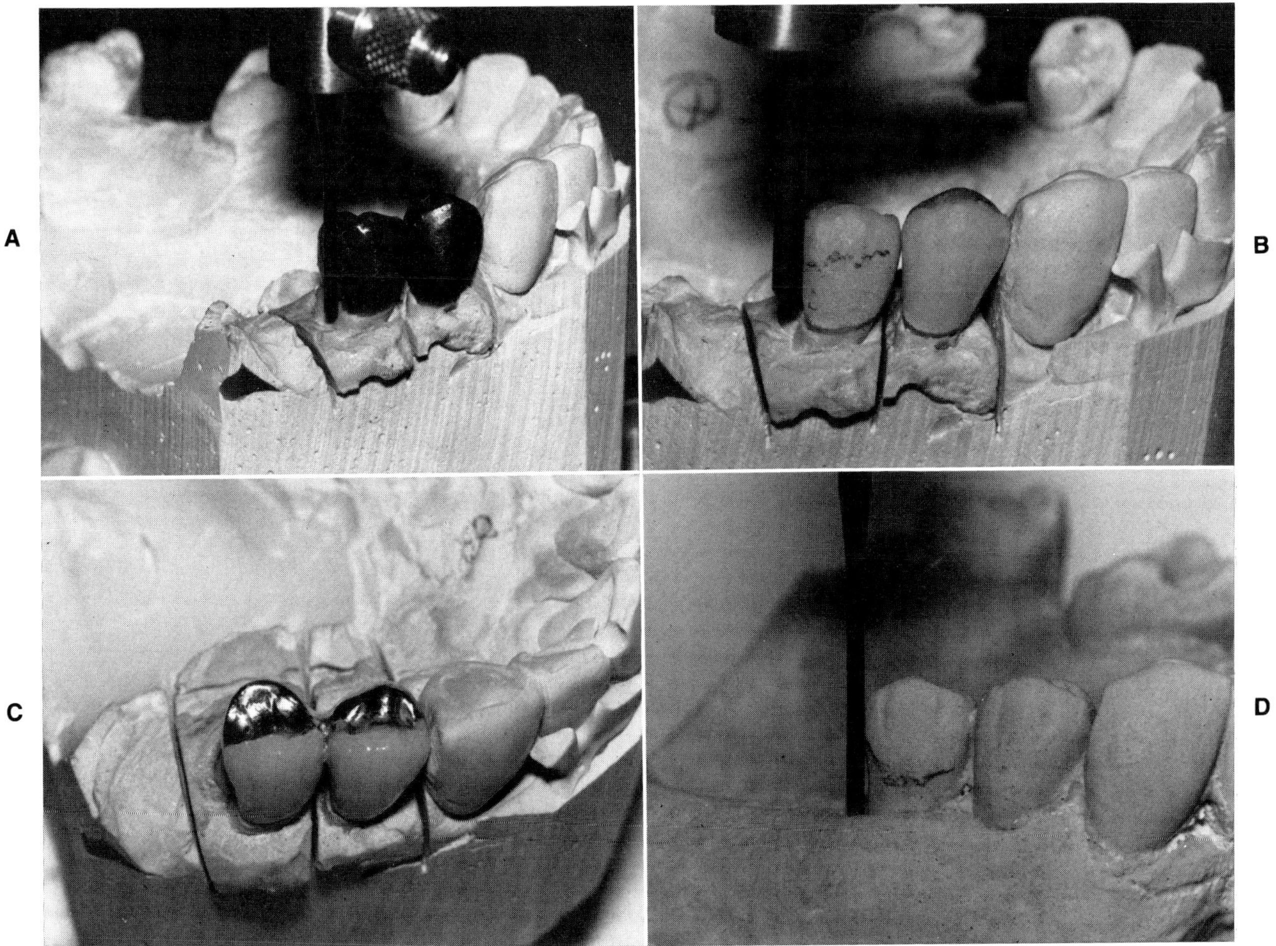

Fig. 9-34. A, Guiding planes in metallic portion of porcelain-fused-to-metal restorations must be developed in wax patterns. **B,** After porcelain is baked but before final glaze, height of contour must be developed in its correct position. **C,** Final glaze is added to porcelain. **D,** Master cast shows maintenance of survey line.

tention be devoted to providing the proper contour to these crowns if they are to be used in conjunction with a removable partial denture.

The wax pattern for the crown should be handled in the same way as previously described for any portion of the pattern that will eventually be contacted by the metal of the framework of the partial denture. If a guiding plane is to be designed for a part of the crown that will be in metal, it must be established in the wax pattern. If reciprocal clasps or lingual plating is to contact the lingual surface of the crown, the proper height of contour must be created in the wax pattern (Fig. 9-34).

After the casting is completed, the same verifying and refining procedures performed for any cast crown must be followed before the final polish and application of the porcelain.

Once the metal framework of the crown is verified as being complete, the porcelain can be added. The designed diagnostic cast should be available so that the ceramist may build the porcelain to the desired contour.

After the porcelain has been fired but before the final glaze is added, the crown on the working cast should be analyzed on the surveyor. With fine mounted stones in the handpiece, the porcelain can be adjusted to the proper height of contour and to the correct depth and location of retentive undercut if one is needed. When the final contour is complete, the final glaze can be added. A retentive clasp tip can function indefinitely against a glazed porcelain surface. Against an unglazed surface an excessive amount of friction may be created, making it difficult for the clasp to function properly.

The use of acrylic resin as a veneering material for crowns in general and for crowns used as partial denture abutments in particular should be discouraged. At best the life of the resin veneer is limited, and no clasp should be allowed to rest on the veneered surface (Fig. 9-35).

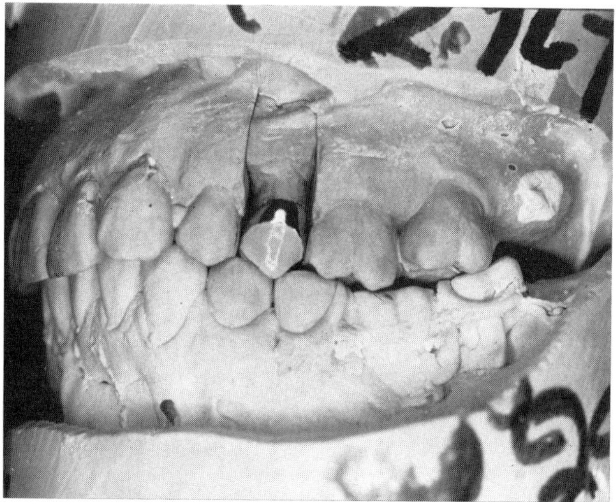

Fig. 9-35. If acrylic resin is used to veneer an abutment tooth crown, a collar of metal must be retained to support retentive clasp arm.

The main indications for the acrylic resin veneer crown are (1) economic purposes and (2) unavailability of equipment to fire porcelain. The first reason is difficult to justify, because the veneer will require replacing as wear takes place. The latter reason is becoming more uncommon.

OCCLUSAL REST SEAT PREPARATION

The purposes and functions of rests are detailed in Chapter 3. Basically, the function of a rest is to direct the forces of mastication parallel to the long axis of the abutment tooth. The form of the rest seat preparation helps carry out this function. The rest also acts as a stop against gingival displacement of the denture, maintains the clasp in its properly surveyed position, and will function as an indirect retainer in a distal extension partial denture. It may be used to close a small space between teeth, thus restoring the continuity of the arch and preventing food impaction between the minor connector and the proximal surface of an abutment tooth. A rest may also be used to onlay an abutment tooth to establish a more acceptable occlusal plane and to help prevent extrusion of teeth.

It is essential that a rest seat preparation be made for each rest before final impressions for master casts are made. If this is not done, the forces transmitted from the prosthesis to the abutment teeth will occur against inclined planes, resulting in a pushing action against the teeth and a sliding effect on the prosthesis. This represents an undesirable and damaging situation (see Fig. 2-78).

The rest seat must always be prepared *after* guiding planes have been established on abutment teeth.

Occlusal rest seat preparation in enamel

The outline form of an occlusal rest seat is basically triangular, with the base of the triangle at the marginal ridge and the apex pointing toward the center of the tooth. The apex of the triangle should be rounded as should all external margins of the preparation. The outline form of the occlusal rest essentially follows the shape of the mesial or distal fossa of the surface of the tooth in which the rest is prepared (see Fig. 2-74).

The tendency in preparing the teeth is to fail to extend the outline of the rest seat sufficiently and not obtain enough depth. An occlusal rest must be at least 1 mm thick at its thinnest point if chrome alloy is used for the framework, 1.5 mm if gold is to be used. The extension of the rest seat preparation should vary from one-third to one-half the mesiodistal diameter of the tooth, seldom less than 3 mm. The buccolingual extent should be half the distance between the buccal and lingual cusp tips.

The floor of the occlusal rest seat must be inclined toward the center of the tooth and must be spoon shaped. The enclosed angle formed by the inclination of the floor of the rest and the vertical projection of the proximal surface of the tooth must be less than 90 degrees. It is only by honoring this principle that occlusal forces can be directed along the vertical axis of the abutment tooth. If this concept is followed, the deepest part of the occlusal rest preparation will be approximately in the center of the preparation.

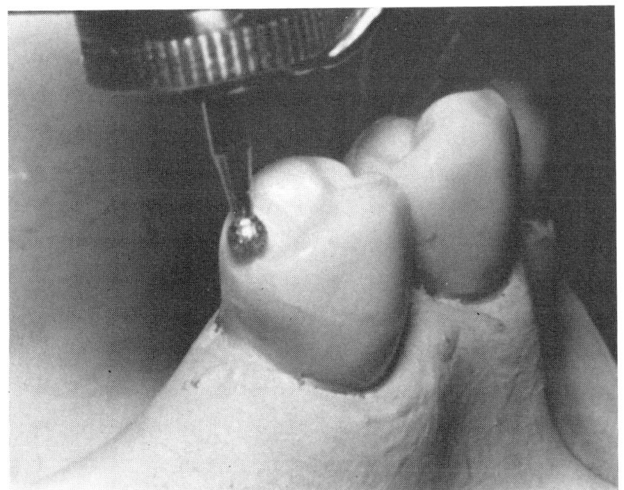

Fig. 9-36. A small round diamond stone is used to develop triangular outline form of occlusal rest.

Occlusal rest seats in enamel should be prepared with a round diamond stone approximating the size of a no. 4 round carbide bur. The entire preparation can normally be accomplished with this instrument. It is unfortunate that a larger round diamond stone is used on occasion to make a depression on the occlusal surface to act as a rest seat. This preparation may suffice, but it does not produce the outline form or the depth required at the critical points necessary for the success of an occlusal rest.

First a channel of the correct depth and at the desired outline of the preparation is created by using the small round diamond stone to lower the marginal ridge at either the buccal or lingual extent of the rest seat, to continue inward toward the center of the tooth, and to return to the marginal ridge (Fig. 9-36). With the same diamond stone the island of enamel that remains within the outline form can be removed and shaped so that sufficient tooth structure is removed to provide the thickness of metal required for strength of the rest. One must be careful not to carve an undercut to the path of insertion.

It is necessary to verify that the deepest portion of the rest seat is toward the center of the tooth, that the preparation rises gradually toward the marginal ridge, and that the preparation has adequate depth. The most accurate method of verifying the accuracy of the preparation is through the use of utility or red beading wax (Fig. 9-37 to 9-39).

The rest preparation must be highly polished. An excellent way to ensure that unsupported enamel rods

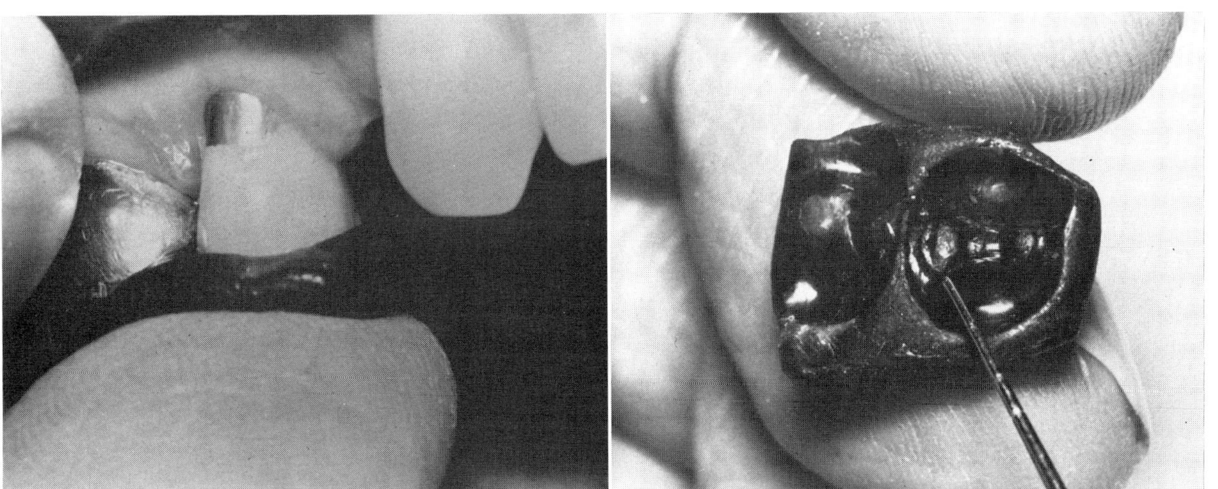

Fig. 9-37. A, Beading wax is pressed into rest seat preparation. **B,** Outline form of rest seat is read in wax impression. Properly prepared rest seat is round and smooth so rest in its rest seat can act as a ball-and-socket joint, as shown in Fig. 9-38.

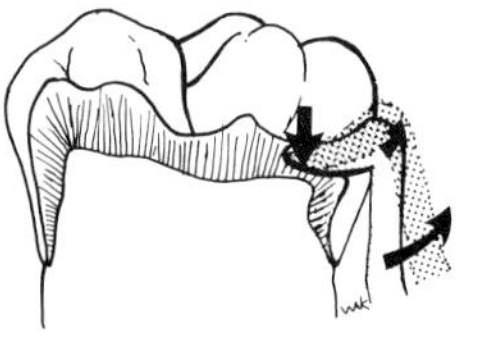

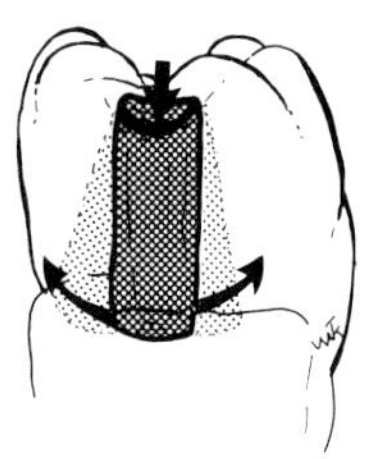

Fig. 9-38. Occlusal rest must be free to move in its rest seat to dissipate lateral forces transferred to abutment tooth. If there are vertical walls or angles to rest seat, torquing and twisting forces are transmitted to abutment tooth. This must never occur in a distal extension (Class I or II) prosthesis. If prosthesis is all tooth supported (Class III), form of occlusal rest is not as critical because torquing forces will not occur.

A

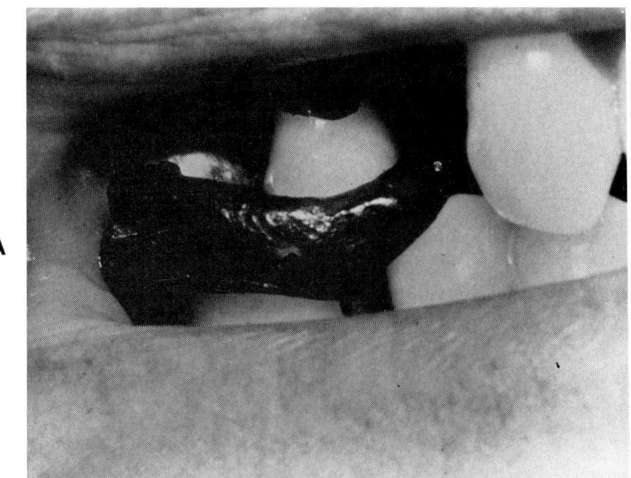

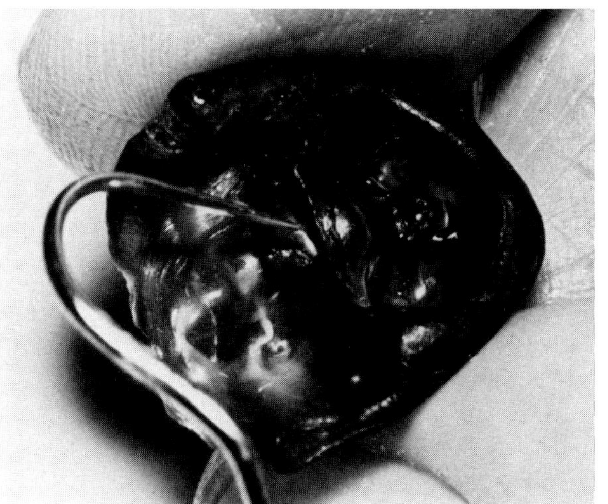

B

Fig. 9-39. A, Space available for occlusal rest can be measured by having patient close firmly in centric occlusion on a piece of beading wax. **B,** Thickness of wax remaining between opposing occlusion and rest seat (directly over marginal ridge) is measured with a Boley gauge. It must not be less than 1.0 mm. It should be remembered that it is good practice to remove a small amount of tooth structure from an opposing cusp or cuspal incline to obtain this space rather than overcutting surface of abutment tooth.

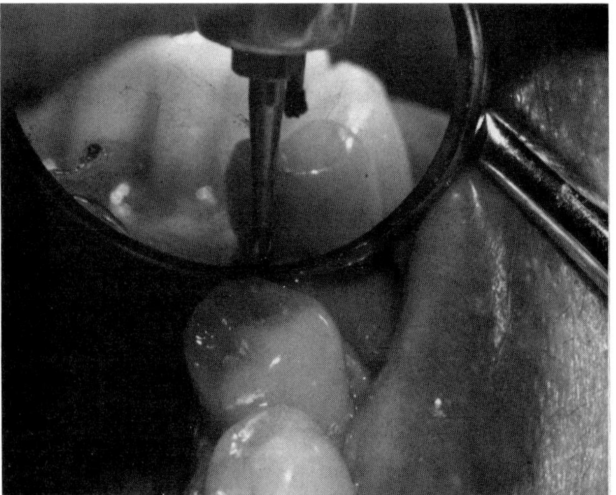

Fig. 9-40. A No. 4 steel bur rotating in reverse is used to remove unsupported enamel rods from rest seat preparation.

and any sharp angles are smoothed is through the use of a no. 4 round steel bur revolving in reverse at moderate speed. This will plane the surface of the preparation and produce a slightly beveled margin to the rest seat (Fig. 9-40).

Occlusal rest seat preparations in new gold restorations

Occlusal rest seats in cast gold restorations should always be placed in the wax patterns. The preparation for the rest seat must be carved in the wax after the establishment of guiding planes if guiding planes have been planned for the abutment tooth (Fig. 9-41).

It is essential that sufficient occlusal clearance be provided to permit proper dimensions of the rest seat. After the preparation for the restoration is complete, it is helpful to add a depression to the preparation to accommodate the depth of the occlusal rest (Fig. 9-42).

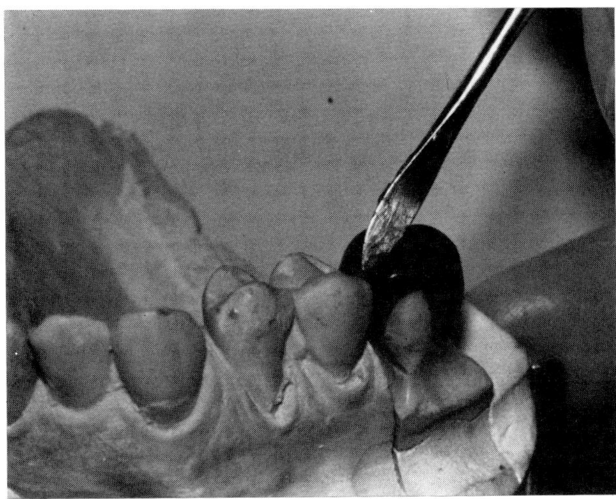

Fig. 9-41. Rest seats for cast gold restorations are carved in wax patterns.

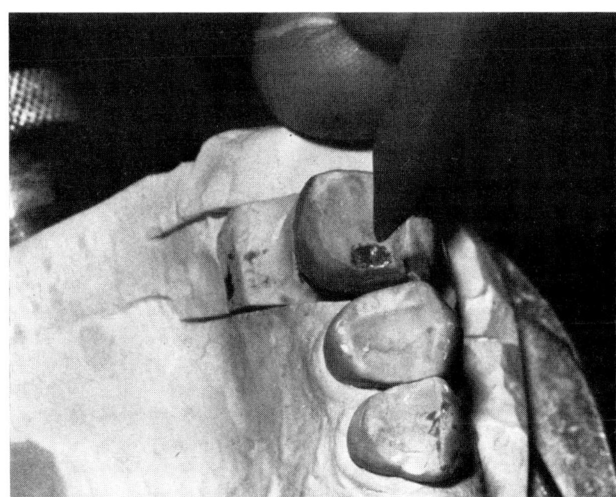

Fig. 9-42. To ensure that enough interocclusal space will be present to accommodate thickness of crown casting plus thickness of rest, a depression should be made in crown preparation.

To prepare the rest seat in the wax pattern, a no. 4 round steel bur can be used. The sequence is the same as that used to prepare the rest seat in enamel. Slow engine speed and light pressure must be used. The rest seat can also be carved with suitable wax instruments (small excavators or the cleoid and discoid). The path of insertion planned for the removable partial denture must be visualized as the preparation is being carved. If an unusual tilt, particularly a lateral tilt of the diagnostic cast, was selected, it is possible to carve an undercut to the path of insertion. This must be avoided.

After the restoration has been cast, the rest preparation must be polished. This may best be done with a small round finishing bur. The anatomy of the rest seat must not be destroyed during the polishing procedure.

Occlusal rest seat preparation in existing gold restorations

There will be times when a removable partial denture is indicated for a patient who has cast restorations on teeth that must serve as abutments for the prosthesis. Although it would be easier and more accurate to replace these restorations with ones specifically designed and prepared for the new prothesis, economically it would not be in the patient's best interest. If the existing restorations display marginal integrity and occlusal harmony, an attempt should be made to contour them to satisfy the requirements of the proposed prosthesis. It is usually not too difficult to prepare acceptable guiding planes in existing restorations. The necessary thickness of gold is normally present.

The greatest problem arises in developing adequate rest seats. If the concept that necessary space must be created *at all costs* is placed first on the priority list, the problems are greatly diminished.

Patients must always be thoroughly warned of the possibility of needing to replace existing restorations before mouth preparation. If an existing crown, onlay, or inlay is penetrated during the rest seat preparation, the restoration must be replaced.

If minimal penetration through a full crown occurs and all other aspects of the crown are acceptable, it is permissible to prepare the area of penetration to receive a direct gold restoration. This procedure will protect the tooth structure and will provide adequate support for the partial denture.

Occlusal rest seat preparation in amalgam restorations

An occlusal rest preparation in a multisurface amalgam restoration is less desirable than that in either sound enamel or a gold restoration (Fig. 9-43). Amalgam alloy tends to flow when placed under constant pressure. Care must be taken not to weaken the proximal portion of the amalgam restoration at the isthmus during the preparation. This may result in fracture during function.

Rest seats are prepared in the amalgam restoration the same as in enamel except that a no. 4 round bur is used instead of the diamond stone. The preparation is polished by reversing the revolutions of the no. 4 round bur. A final polish is obtained by polishing the amalgam as any other amalgam restoration.

Rest seat preparation for embrasure clasp

This preparation extends over the occlusal embrasure of two approximating posterior teeth, from the mesial fossa of one tooth to the distal fossa of the other tooth. There is probably more difficulty encountered in making this preparation correctly than with any of the others. The main problem is failure to remove sufficient tooth structure over the buccal slopes of the preparation. Insufficient tooth removal will generally lead to occlusal interferences between the metal of the clasp and the opposing cusps. Relieving the metal to gain occlusal freedom ultimately leads to breakage of the clasp during function. Repair of the embrasure clasp is usually difficult.

A small round diamond stone is used to establish the outline form for a normal occlusal rest in each of the approximating fossae (Fig. 9-44). Each marginal ridge should be reduced the same amount. If the marginal ridges are uneven because one tooth is extruded, the ridges should remain uneven after the preparation. No attempt should be made to even the ridges by overcutting one. The contact point between the teeth should not be broken because a wedging action and food impaction between the teeth may take place if the contact is lost.

The same round diamond stone is used to carry the buccal and lingual extensions of the occlusal rests over

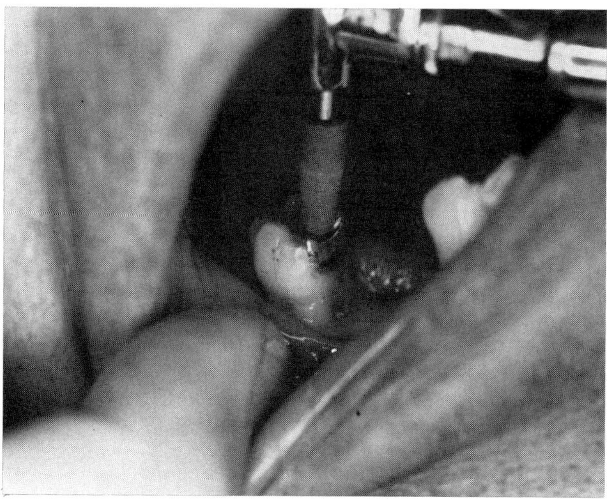

Fig. 9-43. Rests are not routinely placed in amalgam alloy restorations. When prognosis of a tooth is questionable, this may be done.

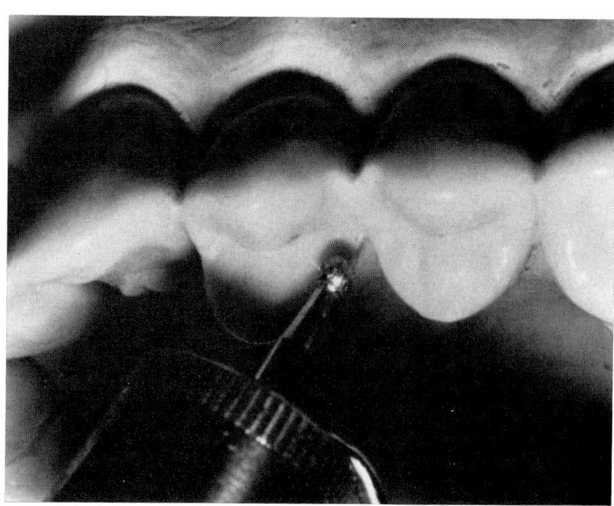

Fig. 9-44. A small round diamond stone is used to establish outline forms of two adjacent rests making up embrasure rest. Preparation must be carried over buccal and lingual surfaces.

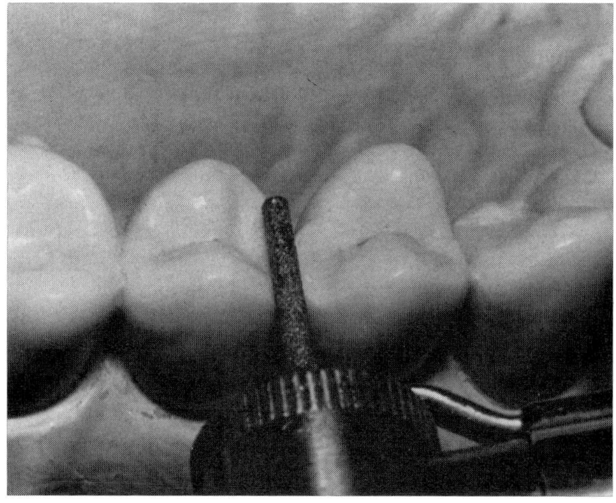

Fig. 9-45. A cylindric diamond stone held horizontally against distal and mesial inclines of buccal cusps may be used to obtain sufficient interocclusal space.

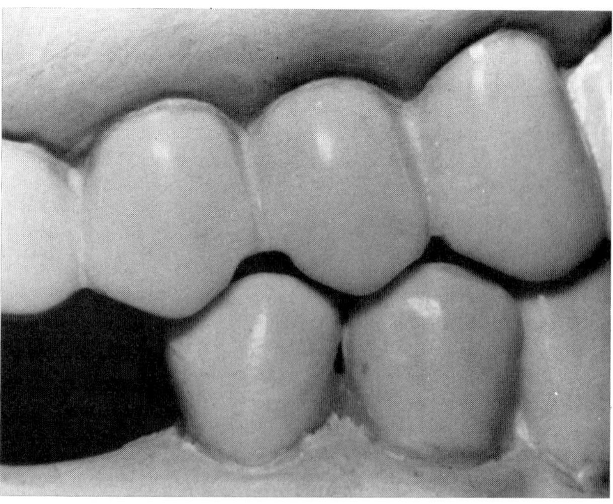

Fig. 9-46. Preparation for embrasure clasp must be 1.5 to 2 mm wide and 1 to 1.5 mm deep.

the buccal and lingual embrasures. As a general rule, obtaining sufficient occlusal clearance over the lingual embrasure is not as great a problem as it is over the buccal embrasure. An alternate method for obtaining clearance is by the use of a cylindric diamond stone held horizontally from the buccal surfaces of the teeth pointing toward the lingual surface (Fig. 9-45). The stone is held against the distal incline of the buccal cusp of one tooth and the mesial incline of the buccal cusp of the other tooth. The occlusal clearance may be checked by laying two pieces of 18-gauge wire side by side across the preparation. The patient should be able to close without contacting the metal. A normal verification of space available should be made by making an impression with red utility wax and measuring the thickness of the wax with a Boley gauge. As the preparation passes over the buccal and lingual embrasures, it should be approximately 1.5 to 2 mm wide and 1 to 1.5 mm deep (Fig. 9-46). The buccal inclines of the preparation must be rounded after the preparation is complete. There is a definite danger in producing undercut areas in the buccal inclines. The procedures used to finish and polish the preparation are the same as those used to polish the usual occlusal rests.

REST SEAT PREPARATION ON ANTERIOR TEETH

Lingual, or cingulum, rests on canine and incisor teeth

An occlusal rest on a molar or a premolar is preferred over a lingual or an incisal rest on anterior teeth to provide support for a partial denture. Forces are better directed down the long axis of the abutment tooth by an occlusal rest than by a lingual or incisal rest.

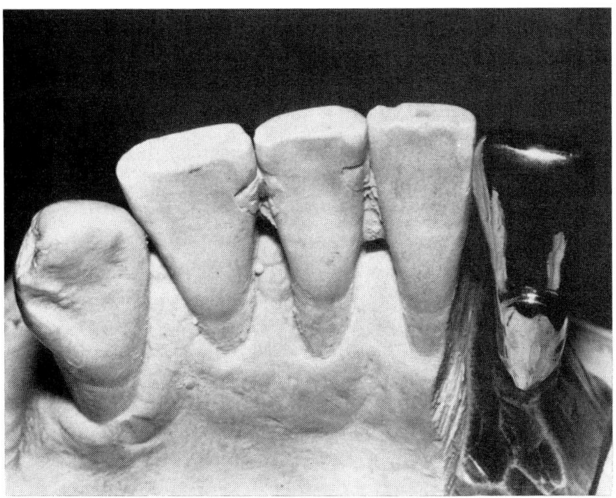

Fig. 9-47. A lingual rest on an incisor usually must be placed in a cast restoration.

A canine is preferred over an incisor for support of a denture. When a canine is not present, multiple rests on incisor teeth are needed in place of a single rest on a single incisor tooth.

A lingual rest is preferred to an incisal rest. The lingual rest can be prepared nearer the center of the tooth, preventing the tipping action that an incisal rest may produce. Lingual rests are also more acceptable esthetically and less subject to breakage and distortion (see Fig. 2-83).

The most satisfactory lingual rest from the standpoint of support is one that is placed on a prepared rest seat in a cast restoration. This should be used wherever possible. A lingual rest on a cast restoration may be used on any anterior tooth, either maxillary or mandibular. A lingual rest prepared in an enamel surface should be used primarily on maxillary canines and on a limited number of maxillary incisor teeth (Fig. 9-47).

The outline form of the lingual rest seat is half-moon shaped. It should form a smooth curve from one marginal ridge to the other, crossing the center of the tooth incisally to the cingulum. The deepest point of the rest seat will be over the cingulum. The rest seat itself is V shaped. The labial incline of the lingual surface of the tooth makes up one wall, and the other wall of the V-shaped notch starts at the top of the cingulum and inclines linguogingivally toward the center of the tooth to meet the other wall of the preparation. Sharp lines and angles must be avoided because they will interfere with the fit of the framework of the partial denture.

Lingual rest seat preparation in cast restorations

If a cast restoration is to be placed on the abutment tooth, the rest seat should be carved in the wax pattern and not cut in the cast restoration. The lingual form of the tooth should be restored with the cast framework of the denture. When the rest seat in the wax pattern is carved, a definite rest preparation can be developed that will direct the forces of occlusion through the long axis of the abutment tooth. Sharp angles or walls should still be avoided in the wax pattern (Fig. 9-48).

Lingual rest seat preparation in enamel

A lingual rest seat may be prepared in the enamel surface of an anterior tooth if the tooth is sound, the patient practices good oral hygiene, and the caries index is low. The cingulum should also be prominent to present a gradual slope to the lingual surface rather than a steep vertical slope. This is the principal reason why mandibular canines are poor candidates for a lingual rest. The lingual surface of the tooth normally has too great a vertical slope to permit the rest seat to be prepared without penetrating into dentin. In some instances a lingual rest can be placed on maxillary central

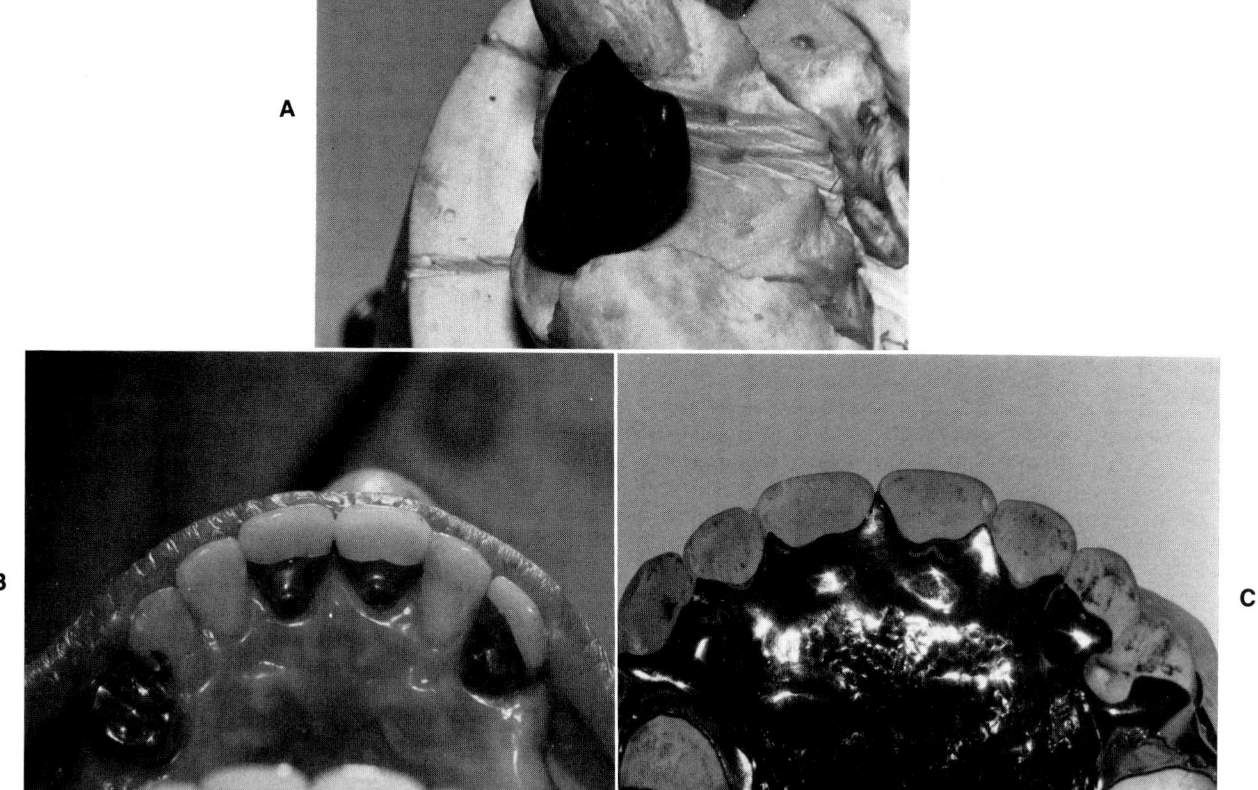

Fig. 9-48. A, Lingual rest preparations in wax patterns are rounded; angles and ledges are avoided. **B,** Roundness is preserved in completed crown. **C,** Framework restores lingual form to tooth.

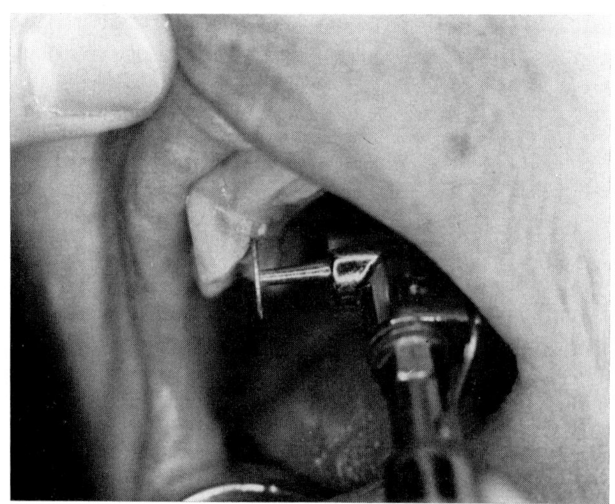

Fig. 9-49. Lingual rest is prepared in enamel with a safe-side diamond disk if space is available to accommodate disk. Angle at which disk is held is critical.

incisors that have prominent cingula, but most often this is a compromise effort unless it is placed in a cast restoration.

To prepare the lingual rest in enamel where space is available to properly manipulate the instrument, a safe-side $^1/_4$-inch diamond disk should be used (Fig. 9-49). The disk must be held so that it parallels or is inclined slightly labial to the path of insertion. An improperly held disk or other diamond instrument can produce undercuts in the preparation. The cut with the disk should start low on one marginal ridge, pass over the cingulum, and then pass gingivally to contact the opposite marginal ridge. This will produce the desirable half-moon shape.

Often the presence of the lateral incisor or the first premolar will preclude the use of the safe-side disc. When space is not available to permit the use of the instrument, a flat-end large diamond cylinder is the next best choice (Fig. 9-50). It must be held at the

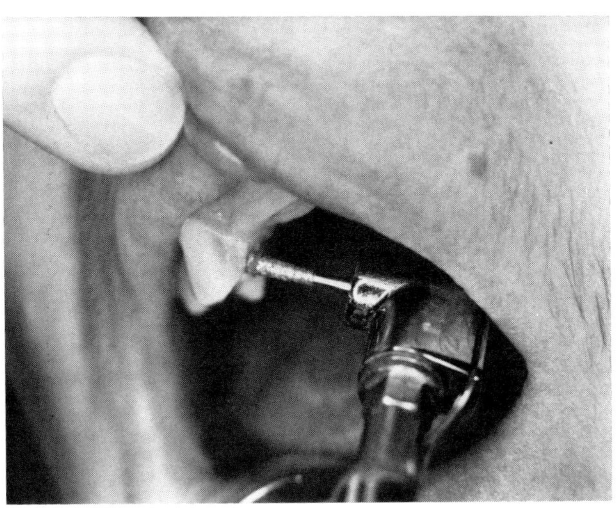

Fig. 9-50. If enough mesiodistal space is not present to use disk, a flat-end diamond cylinder stone may be used. This is more difficult to use than disk.

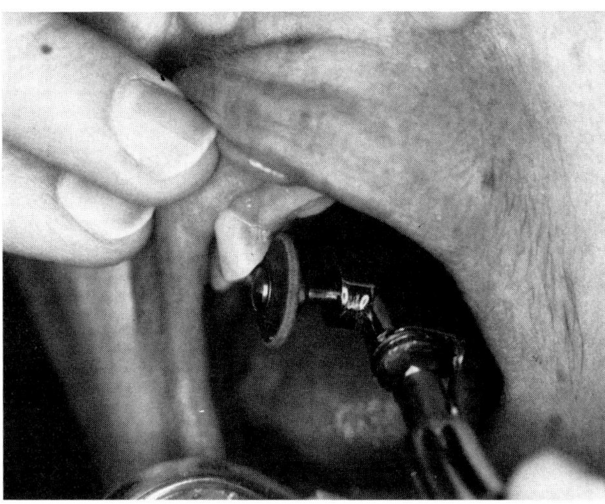

Fig. 9-51. A rubber wheel containing Carborundum is used to polish enamel surfaces and to round angles and corners.

proper angle, inclined slightly gingivally from the horizontal, so that the cutting is done by the flat end and side of the cylinder. An inverted cone diamond stone may be used, but it is more difficult to control and will tend to produce undercuts in the enamel surface.

It is extremely important that the occlusion be checked before the preparation is started to make certain that there will be adequate occlusal clearance. (This should be one of the first steps in the design sequence.) The rest seat must always be gingival to the contact level of the opposing tooth.

The preparation must be polished with the Carborundum-impregnated rubber wheels and points (Fig. 9-51). The rubber wheel can be used to round any sharp angles or corners on the preparation, but caution must be exercised not to remove the gingival incline of the lingual wall of the preparation, which is needed to direct the forces down the long axis of the tooth.

Incisal rest seat preparation

Incisal rest seats should be used only on enamel surfaces. If a cast restoration is planned for the abutment tooth, a lingual rest seat should be included in the restoration. Although incisal rests are the least desirable rests for anterior teeth, they may be used successfully on select patients if the abutment tooth is sound.

The incisal rest seat is usually placed near one of the incisal angles of canines. If the incisal rest is used in conjunction with a circumferential clasp, the rest should be placed at the distal incisal angle. If the rest is used in conjunction with a vertical projection or bar clasp that uses a distal buccal undercut for retention, the preparation should be made at the mesial incisal angle. In this position the mesial incisal rest will reciprocate the action of the bar clasp more effectively than if it were positioned at the distal incisal angle.

Although the incisal rest may be used on maxillary canines, it is not the rest of choice for that tooth because too much must be sacrificed in esthetics and in mechanical advantage.

On incisor teeth an incisal rest is usually used as a last resort to stabilize the removable prosthesis. The prognosis for these teeth is usually poor. If the denture is designed properly, artificial teeth may be added to the partial denture as the natural teeth are lost.

The incisal rest seat preparation is begun with a small safe-side diamond disk or a knife edge stone held parallel to the path of insertion (Fig. 9-52, *A*). The first cut is made vertically 1.5 to 2 mm deep in the form of a slice or notch and approximately 2 to 3 mm inside the proximal angle of the tooth.

A small flame-shaped diamond point is used to complete the preparation (Fig. 9-52, *B*). The notch created by the disk must be rounded. The enamel proximal to the notch should be reduced slightly but not to the level of the base of the notch. The enamel wall created by the disk toward the center of the tooth must be rounded with the flame-shaped diamond point. The base of the notch is also rounded with the tip of the flame-shaped diamond stone. The groove that results after the notch has been completely rounded must be carried slightly over onto the labial surface. This projection onto the facial surface provides a locking device to prevent the tooth from being tipped or moved facially. The groove should be continued partway down the lingual surface as an indentation. This indentation will

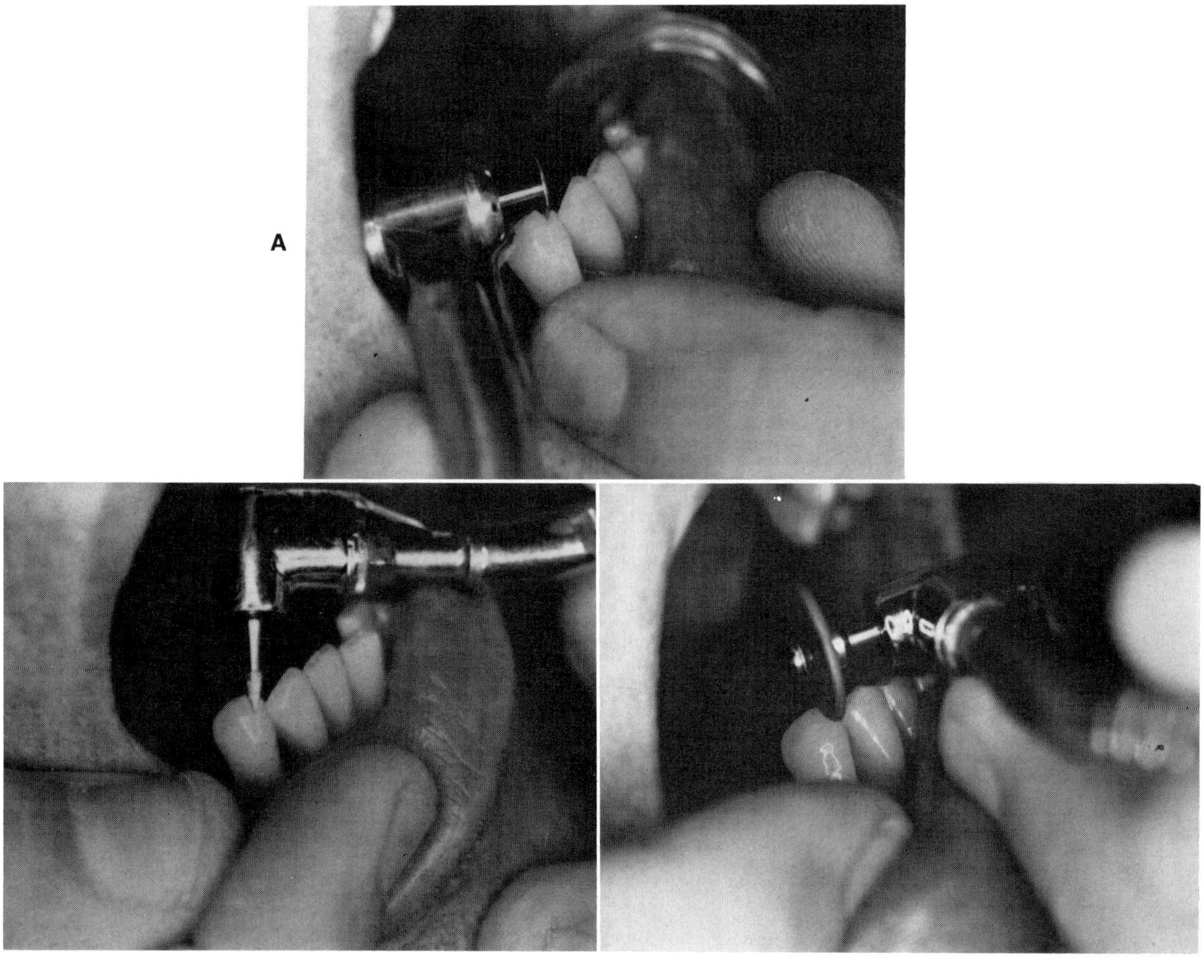

Fig. 9-52. Safe-side disk, A, and a pointed diamond stone, B, are used to create outline form of incisal rest preparation. C, Angles of rest seat are rounded with rubber wheel.

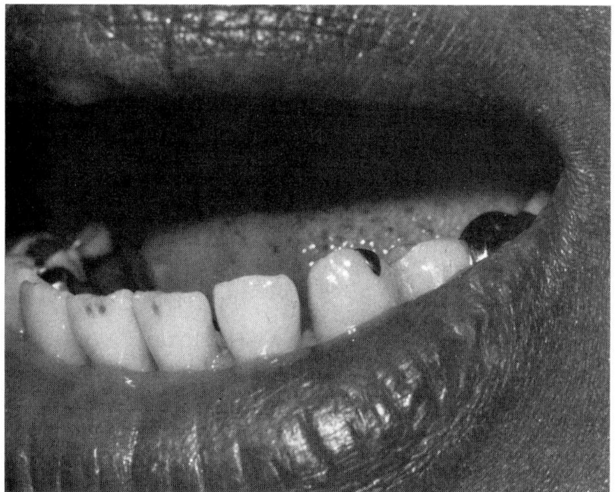

Fig. 9-53. Incisal rest will blend into normal anatomy of abutment tooth.

help accommodate the minor connector. The minor connector will not be as annoying to the tongue if it is partially concealed in this manner.

After all sharp angles and points have been reduced by the flame-shaped diamond point, the preparation is polished with Carborundum-containing wheels, which will provide the final rounding of any sharp angles (Fig. 9-52, *C*).

The incisal rest will restore the lost contour of the incisal edge. Although some metal will show, the display can be kept to a minimum without jeopardizing the effectiveness of the rest (Fig. 9-53).

MAKING THE FINAL IMPRESSION FOR THE MASTER CAST

For the production of an accurate master cast the impression technique far outweighs the selection of the impression material. Too often the practitioner is more concerned with what material to use rather than with how or where it should be used. No available impression material will produce results greater than the skill and knowledge of the person making the impression. *Good technique pays off* is not merely a motto to hang on a wall in the laboratory but words of wisdom; good technique will indeed result in better treatment and improved patient care.

Research has shown that all major classes of impression materials—irreversible hydrocolloid, reversible hydrocolloid, polysulfide rubber, and silicone rubber—are capable of producing accurate results if respect is shown for the properties of the particular material. However, no single impression material can be used for all impressions. For example, selection of polysulfide rubber to make an impression of an arch in which the remaining teeth have long clinical crowns and weakened periodontal support would be poor clinical judgment because the impression material would lock around the long clinical crown, making it difficult to remove the impression and tray from the mouth without endangering the remaining teeth. The same situation could be encountered if polysulfide rubber were used for an impression of a partially edentulous arch with splinted teeth or a fixed partial denture, in which case the impression would lock under the solder joint of the splinted crowns or under the pontic of the fixed partial denture. It is often necessary to section the tray to remove the impression. The impression, of course, is destroyed. It is possible to "block out" or obliterate, these undercuts in the mouth by pressing soft utility wax under the solder joint or under the pontic to prevent the impression material from becoming locked around these surfaces, but critical areas of tooth or soft tissue surfaces may be lost. In the circumstances just described, an impression material such as irreversible or reversible hydrocolloid, which is as accurate as polysulfide rubber but fragile, allowing the material to release from undercuts, is indicated.

The expression *making the impression* rather than *taking the impression* is used to refer to the impression phase of partial denture construction to indicate that this procedure is not a passive activity in which the impression material accomplishes the task and the operator is merely an observer. The operator must be in complete control of all aspects of the impression procedure: the position and intraoral condition of the patient, the size and position of the tray, and the selection of material and technique.

Impression materials

Irreversible hydrocolloid (alginate)

The properties and handling characteristics of alginate are covered in depth in Chapter 5. A few important points are repeated. Alginate impression material is the most widely used and possibly the most versatile of the impression materials available in the practice of removable partial prosthodontics. The ease of handling, the relative inexpense, the dimensional accuracy, the lack of need of additional items of equipment, and the cleanliness of the material contribute to its popularity.

The inability to store the impression safely is a true limiting factor in the use of alginate impression material. Although manufacturers and an occasional investigator may advocate storing the completed impression in a humid environment, alginate impressions *must* be poured no less than 12 minutes after being removed from the mouth. The impression should not be stored in anything during the 12-minute period.

Another advantage of irreversible hydrocolloid is that a custom-made tray is not required in making most impressions. The only time a custom-made tray is normally used is when the size of the arch will not accommodate a standard tray. This may be because the arch is too large or too small, or tooth alignment is such to preclude the use of a standard tray. The presence of tori or exostoses may occasionally interfere with the seating of a standard tray and will require the construction of a custom-made tray.

When a standard rim-lock or metal perforated tray is used for a final impression for a removable partial denture, the tray must be modified to reduce the bulk of alginate. If the impression material is not supported adequately it will tend to slump during the gelation process. This slumping may be severe enough, particularly in the palatal region of the maxillary arch, to produce an inaccurate impression. The simplest and most accurate method of modifying the tray is by the use of modeling plastic or cake compound (Figs. 9-54 to 9-56). The modeling plastic is softened in a water bath at 57° C (135° F), and molded over the area of the tray that requires modification, usually the palate and distal extension ridge in the maxilla or the distal extension edentulous ridge in the mandibular arch. The length of either tray may be modified by attaching the softened plastic to the rim lock or perforations at the end of the tray. While the plastic is still soft, the surface should be flamed briefly with an alcohol torch, tempered quickly in the warm water bath, and seated in the mouth. An accurate impression of the palate and/or the edentulous ridge will result. In the mandibular arch the reason for the modification is usually to displace the tissues of the floor of the mouth so an extension of the lingual slope of the edentulous ridge can be obtained. Normally a second final impression of the distal extension edentulous ridge in the mandibular arch will be made after the cast framework has been constructed and fitted to the mouth, but for the final impression to make the

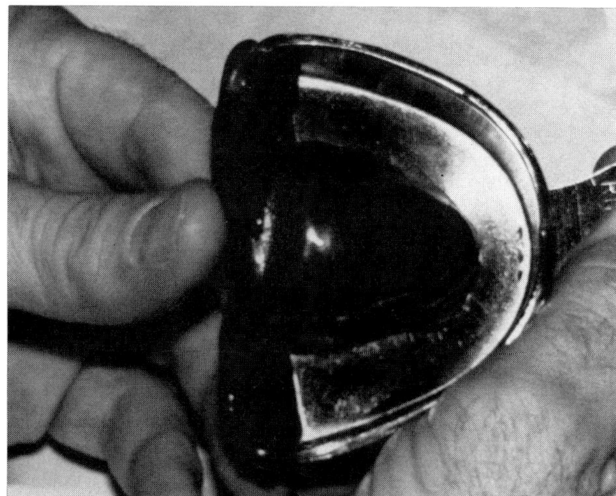

Fig. 9-54. Stock rim-lock impression tray modified with modeling plastic.

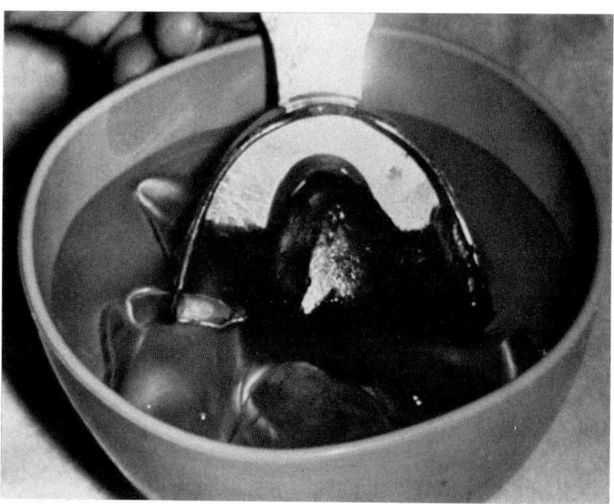

Fig. 9-55. Modeling plastic must be chilled in ice water before it is relieved.

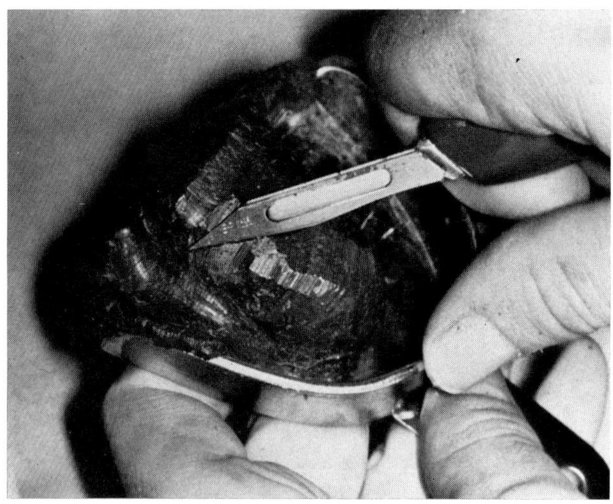

Fig. 9-56. Approximately 5 mm of relief is provided on surface of modeling plastic.

framework the lingual extent of the ridge must be visualized.

Wax is occasionally used to modify an impression tray. This is a hazardous method because if the wax is compressed during the impression procedure, it will rebound once the pressure is removed. This can cause an inaccurate impression. Therefore the use of beading or utility wax to gain peripheral extension of the impression is not good procedure for removable partial dentures, where dimensional accuracy is critical. Correct peripheral extension can be obtained by good impression technique.

Clinical use. The impression technique for a final impression for a removable partial denture is the same as for primary impressions, with the exception that special care must be shown in recording the rest seat preparations that have been made in the abutment teeth (Fig. 9-57).

Reversible hydrocolloid (agar-agar)

Agar hydrocolloid was the first successful elastic impression material to be used in dentistry. To this day it remains one of the most accurate and cleanest elastic materials. Its popularity among general practitioners has declined primarily because of the additional equipment required for its clinical application. Because of this additional equipment, the cost per impression is significantly higher than that of alginate.

The basic tray material is supplied as a gel in a collapsible tube. The lighter injectable material is supplied either in a small collapsible tube for injection into a disposable syringe for use or as a number of cylinders in a glass jar that are placed in a permanent syringe for use.

The tray material gel is composed of approximately 15% agar, 0.2% borax for strength, 0.1% benzoates as a preservative, and 1% to 2% potassium sulfate to obtain proper surface hardness of the master cast, which will be poured into the impression. Other additives control the flow of the material and modify the flavor. The water content is between 80% and 85%. The syringe materials have the same components but slightly lower agar content, 6% to 8%.

Agar gel is composed of a matrix of agar molecules that contain water in the intervening capillary spaces. This network of agar molecules is broken up following the application of heat, and the agar molecules become dispersed in the water, forming a sol. This conversion

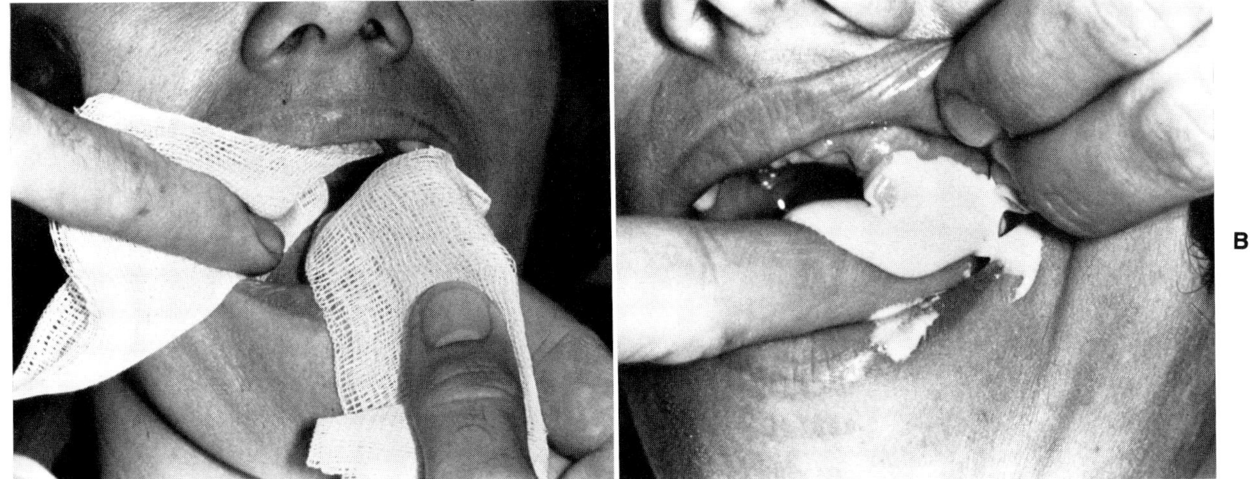

Fig. 9-57. After mouth is partially dried with gauze pads, **A,** and impression material is painted in vestibules, more is forcibly placed in rest seat preparations, **B,** to avoid air entrapment.

of the agar gel to a sol takes place by heating the collapsible tubes in a water bath at 100° C (212° F). The process may be reversed, as the name of the impression material implies, by cooling the sol below 43° C (110° F) to reform the agar. Sol may be stored in the fluid condition in a 65° C (150° F) water bath.

Like alginate impressions, agar hydrocolloid impressions must be poured immediately. If storing is necessary, it must be done in 100% humidity. This does not prevent dimensional change, only reduces it slightly. The storage should not be more than 10 minutes.

Another, more insidious weakness, is that reversible hydrocolloid, like irreversible hydrocolloid, tends to sag as the gel state is approached. The sagging is generally not significant except for impressions of the maxillary arch, particularly for removable partial dentures with a palatal major connector. Sagging of the impressions of the palate will produce a cast that is inaccurate, and the major connector will not be adapted to the palate even though other components of the denture may be acceptable. It is possible to modify the impression tray for an alginate impression to compensate for this sagging, but not for an agar hydrocolloid impression.

Clinical use. Hydrocolloid conditioning units are a must if the material is to be used as a primary impression material in a practice (Fig. 9-58). Most units consist of three controlled temperature water baths. One of the baths is used to liquefy the gel. It must be capable of reaching and sustaining a temperature of 100°C (212°F). Fifteen minutes' boiling time is usually adequate to liquify several tubes of the tray material. The second water bath is used to store the agar hydrocolloid at a temperature sufficient to maintain the liquid phase but nearer a clinically usable temperature. This bath should be maintained between 60° and 65° C, (140° and 150° F). The third bath is a tempering bath used to reduce the heat in a bulk of agar hydrocolloid to a temperature that can be tolerated by the oral tissues. An impression tray is normally filled with the agar hydrocolloid from the storing bath and transferred to the tempering bath (Fig. 9-59). The filled tray is left in the tempering bath long enough to lower the temperature to an acceptable degree but not so long as to cause sol-to-gel transformation, normally 5 minutes.

The injectable hydrocolloid is handled in similar fashion, except that the tempering bath is not used. When the injection material is needed, it is taken from the storage bath and used immediately. The passage of the hydrocolloid through the narrow orifice of the syringe is sufficient to reduce the temperature to an acceptable degree (Fig. 9-60).

In order not to burn the hard or soft tissues, the heat of the agar hydrocolloid must be dissipated rapidly. This is done by using a special water-cooled impression tray (Fig. 9-61). The tray has two tubes incorporated within the metal that transport the cooling medium. Hoses must be connected to the entering and exit tubes. Room-temperature water 21° to 22° C (70° to 72° F), is preferred to ice water because the latter can set up strains in the material that may be released when the hydrocolloid returns to room temperature. The selection of the size of impression tray for an agar hydrocolloid impression is the same as for an alginate impression except the tray cannot be modified safely. Any modification material will also serve as an insulator and interfere with the formation of the gel, influencing the accuracy of the impression.

The chairside impression technique remains the

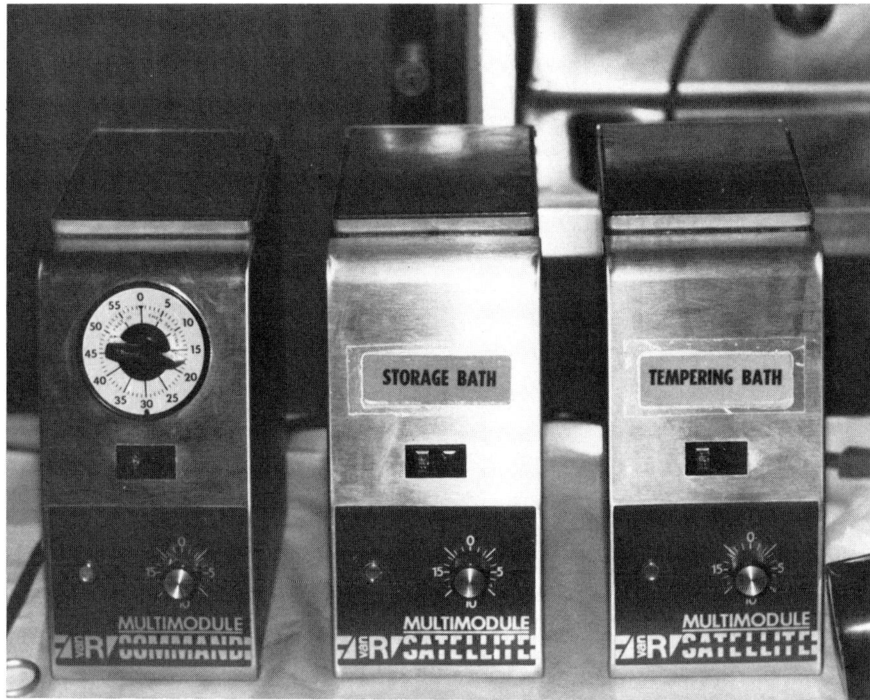

Fig. 9-58. Reversible hydrocolloid unit consists of three controlled-temperature water baths.

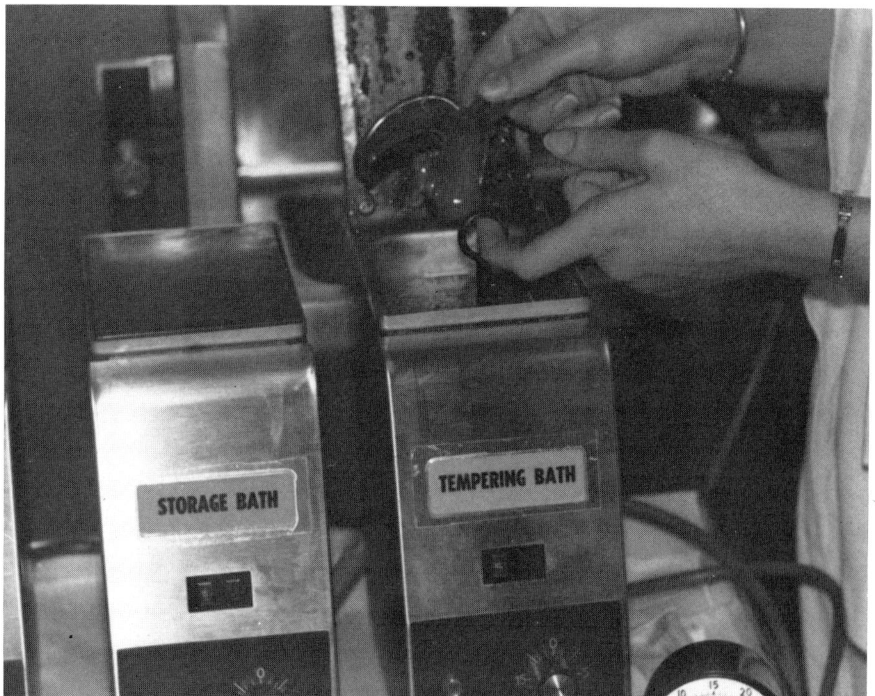

Fig. 9-59. Temperature of agar hydrocolloid is reduced to an acceptable mouth temperature (40° to 43° C, or 105° to 110° F) in a tempering bath.

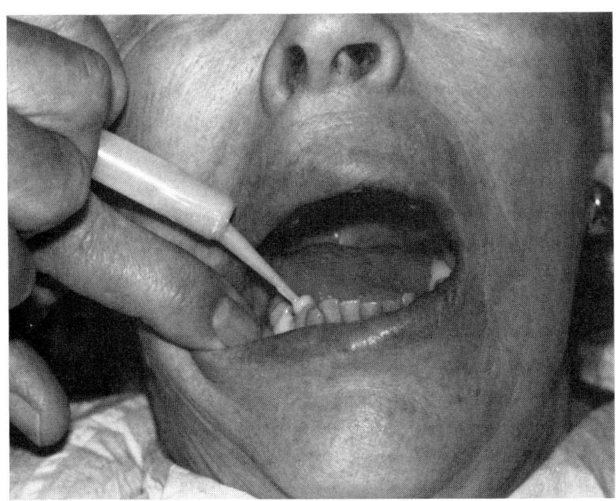

Fig. 9-60. Injection material is used without tempering. The entire preparation must be covered with hydrocolloid.

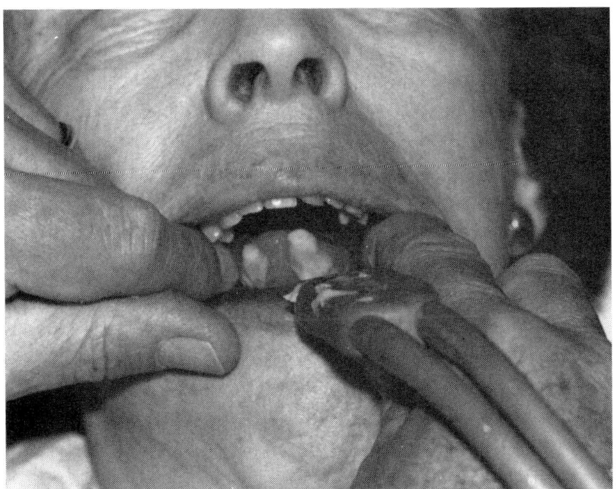

Fig. 9-61. Heated hydrocolloid is changed from sol to gel state by cool water passing through impression tray.

same except the mucosa does not need to be dried; however, pools of saliva should be removed or controlled. Also, instead of painting the impression into critical areas, rest seats, and vestibules, the syringe with the injectable material is used to deposit the lighter agar into these areas. The impression tray must be seated quickly after the injectable material is deposited to prevent this lighter agar from starting to gel before it combines with or is displaced by the heavier tray material.

Once the tray is seated, a pause of 30 seconds should be allowed before the cooling water starts to flow to cool the hydrocolloid. This pause permits the material to flow before gelation is begun. With 21° C (70° F) water flowing rapidly, a total of 3 minutes should be allowed to thoroughly cool and gel the tray material. The water is stopped, and the tray held steadily for an additional 30 seconds. This time allows the surface of the impression to return to body temperature and prevents the release of stress that may be built in the material as a result of the cooling.

The impression should be removed from the mouth with a single, quick, definite movement to prevent tearing or distorting the material.

After the impression has been poured with a minimal expansion dental stone, the cast should be separated within 45 to 60 minutes after the initial set of the stone. The impression material dehydrates, becomes stiff, and can damage the surface of the cast if not removed in that period of time.

Polysulfide rubber

The first rubber impression material introduced to dentistry was known as Thiokol, after the commercial manufacturer that produced it. Later the material became known as mercaptan rubber, because the unreacted base contained the —SH, or mercaptan, group. The group reacts during the setting process to form a rubber containing polysulfide group. For this reason the rubber material in general is referred to as polysulfide rubber impression material.

The impression material is supplied as two tubes of paste (Fig. 9-62). One tube contains the catalyst, or accelerator, and the other the base. The material is produced in several types and varies as to the viscosity and flow characteristics. The types are classified as being light, regular, or heavy bodied. The light-bodied is normally used in a syringe for injection purposes or for impressions for complete dentures where little tissue displacement is desired. The heavy-bodied is used in combination with the light-bodied injection material to capture the surface details essential for fixed prosthodontics or restorative dentistry. For removable partial prosthodontics the regular-bodied or a mix of regular with light-bodied is used for the impression.

The base material consists of 80% low-molecular-weight organic polymer containing the reactive mercaptan groups and 20% reinforcing agents. The catalyst tube contains the agent that activates the mercaptan groups to react and form the polysulfide rubber. The original and most common catalyst used, lead dioxide, results in the mixed paste being dark brown. Other catalysts have been developed, such as tert-butyl-hydroperoxide that produces a blue-green mix. Manufacturers now supply polysulfide in a variety of colors by adding dyes to the catalyst.

Clinical use. Equal lengths of the base and catalyst are extruded on a paper mixing pad. The two lengths

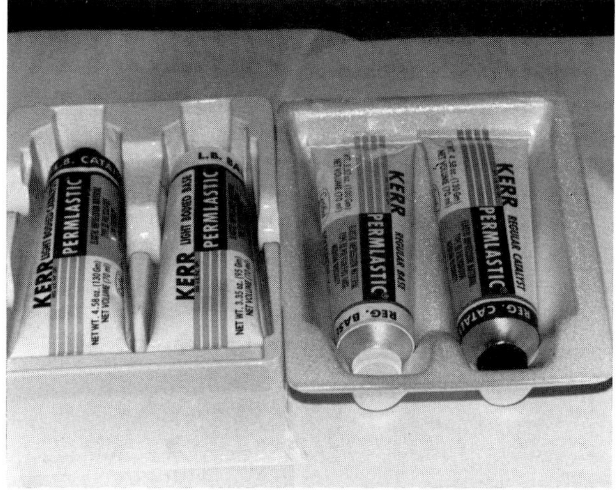

Fig. 9-62. Polysulfide rubber is supplied as two tubes of paste, catalyst and base.

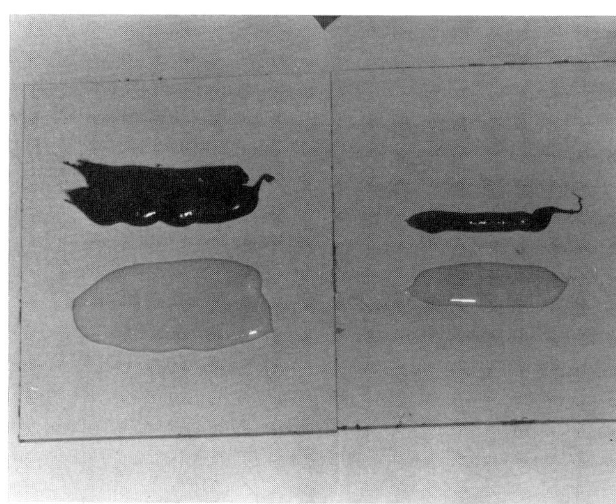

Fig. 9-63. Material is measured on mixing pad for tray (left) and injection (right).

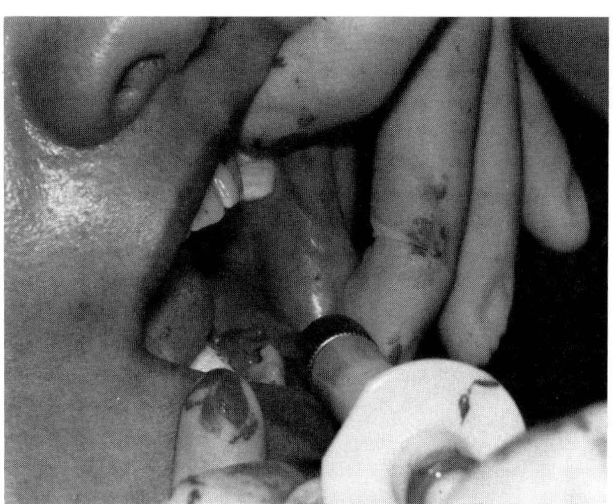

Fig. 9-64. Polysulfide rubber must be injected so that material precedes nozzle. This prevents air from being trapped in preparation.

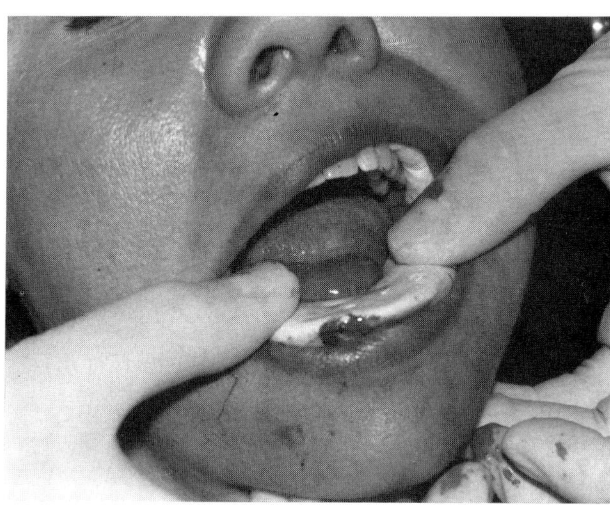

Fig. 9-65. Impression tray must be held firmly in place until material sets, 8 minutes.

should not be in contact because this could start the reaction before the mix is made. A stiff spatula is needed to make the mix (Fig. 9-63). If an injection with light-bodied material is to be made, the two mixes should be started simultaneously, so at least one assistant is needed. The mixing is accomplished with a circular sweeping motion. Because the base material is white and the catalyst colored, mix completion is evidenced by the absence of streaks and the uniformity of the color. This should take about 45 seconds. The injection material is loaded into the syringe and the tray material into the custom tray immediately. The injection material is deposited into rest seat preparations and other critical areas carefully with the syringe to avoid trapping air (Fig. 9-64). The loaded tray is seated by using the same technique as for any other impression. The tray must be held steady until the final set of the material has taken place, usually about 8 minutes (Fig. 9-65).

After removal from the mouth the impression is inspected for completeness and accuracy and cleansed by rinsing with cool tap water. The moisture should be removed by shaking the impression or by a gentle blast of air. Although reports are numerous that the pouring of the cast can be delayed, it is still a safe procedure to pour as soon as possible, because polymerization continues for a time and may cause dimensional change.

The pouring technique is the same as for alginate impression. Recovery of the cast from the impression should be delayed longer than when one of the hydrocolloids is used. Rubber will not damage the cast surface, and allowing extra time before recovering the cast will produce a harder cast. This will help prevent fracturing the stone teeth, particularly if there are isolated teeth in the arch. Polysulfide rubber is not as elastic as alginate or agar, and tooth breakage is not uncommon.

Silicone rubber

Some of the problems associated with the original polysulfide rubber material, such as the offensive odor and color, the staining of clothing caused by lead dioxide, and the effort required to mix the material, encouraged investigators to turn to silicone rubber for an alternate elastic impression material.

The first silicone rubber material had several major problems: short and unpredictable shelf life, short setting time, excessive dimensional change on setting, and a rough cast surface as a result of gas liberated by the silicone rubber after the cast was poured. These problems have been overcome for the most part, and silicone rubber is now an acceptable impression material.

The material is supplied as a base and a catalyst, or accelerator. The base paste contains a low-molecular-weight silicone liquid, dimethylsiloxane, which has the reactive —OH groups (Fig. 9-66). Silica or other agents are added to give the paste the proper consistency and provide stiffness to the set rubber. The catalyst, a tin octoate suspension and an alkyl silicate, is supplied as a liquid usually, but may be provided as a paste by the addition of thickening agents.

The silicone pastes are supplied in the same consistency as the polysulfide rubber—light-, regular-, and heavy-bodied—with the new addition of a very heavy bodied paste called a putty. The molecular weight of the dimethylsiloxane and concentration of silica determine the consistency of the paste. The higher the molecular weight, the heavier the paste. The concentration of silica or other reinforcing agents rises from 35% to 40% as the paste increases in consistency from light to heavy body. The concentration in the putty is 75%.

Silicone rubber impression materials usually are supplied as a white base material in a tube or occasionally in a jar. The catalyst normally comes as a liquid in a small bottle with a dropper. Less frequently the catalyst is provided as a paste in a collapsible tube. Caution is suggested in handling the catalyst because allergic reactions have been noted following direct contact with the skin. The color of the mixed silicone is controlled by dyes added to the colorless catalyst. Normally the various consistencies have different colors so they can be easily distinguished. This may be an important consideration when injectable material is used followed by a tray material.

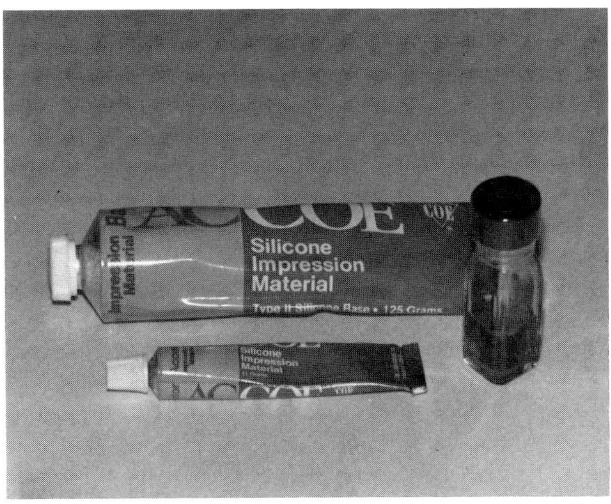

Fig. 9-66. Silicone impression material is supplied as a base and a catalyst.

The mixing technique is the same as that for polysulfide rubber. The mixing is continued until the material is free of streaks, normally 45 seconds. As a final step the mix should be spread in a thin layer to eliminate any trapped air bubbles. The syringe or tray is loaded, and the impression procedure followed as described for the polysulfide rubber material.

The use of the putty is seldom if ever indicated for an impression for a removable partial denture. The putty is used to make a loose fitting impression tray generally of a segment of an arch. The light-bodied, or injection, material is then used as a wash within the putty to refine the impression, usually of a crown or fixed partial denture.

The pouring of the impression should not be delayed. The material is compatible with improved stone. The tear strength for silicone rubber is less than that of the polysulfides, but care must be taken in recovering the cast to prevent breaking the teeth.

Custom impression tray

Highly filled powder-liquid self-polymerizing acrylic resins are used to construct custom impression trays when needed for a removable partial denture impression. Perhaps the most important requirement for a custom tray is that it be rigid. A flexible tray used to support an elástic impression material will inevitably lead to a distorted impression. Many disposable trays on the market suffer this lack of rigidity.

The custom tray is normally constructed on the diagnostic cast on which the design has been drawn (Fig. 9-67). Relief is required between the teeth and the tray to provide adequate thickness of impression material. For polysulfide or silicone rubber impressions a space of 2 mm is needed. For an alginate impression 5 mm is

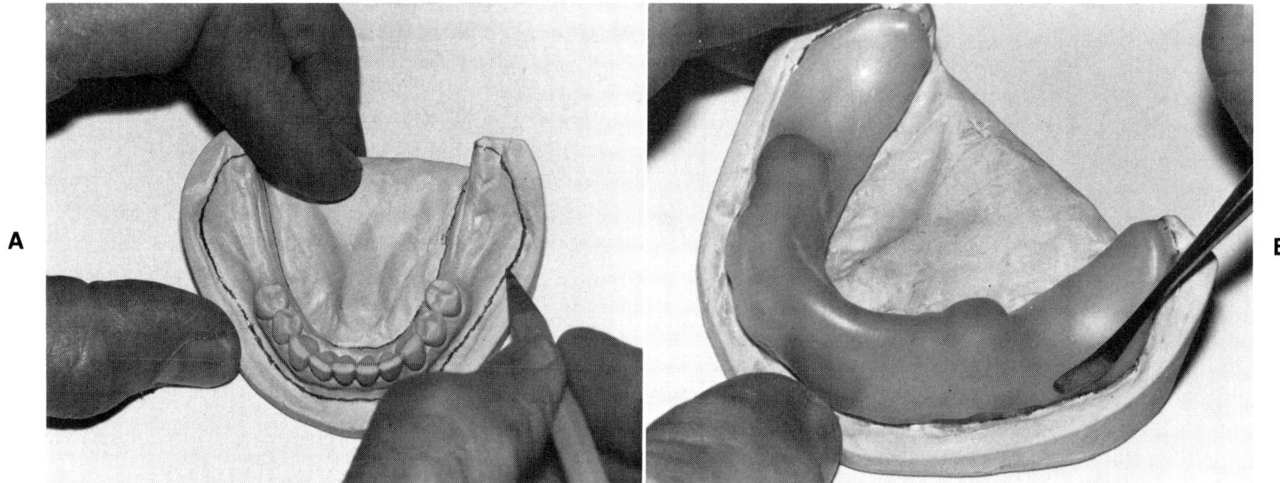

Fig. 9-67. A, Custom impression trays for polysulfide rubber or silicone impression material should cover only teeth and attached soft tissue. Outline should avoid muscle attachments, frena, and movable tissue. **B,** Two thicknesses of baseplate wax are adapted over outline form to provide 2 mm relief space in tray for polysulfide rubber or silicone impressions.

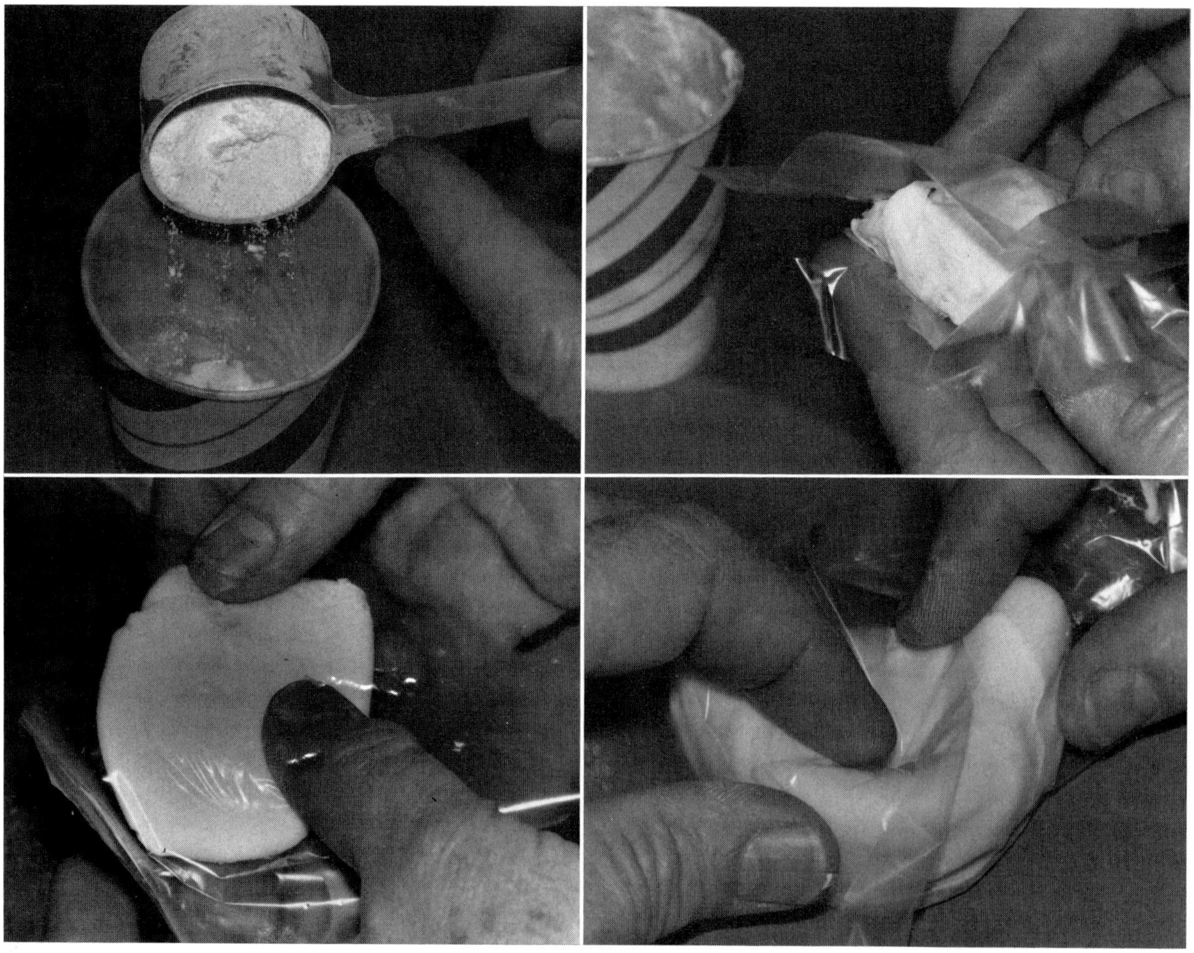

Fig. 9-68. A, Measured amount of powder (polymer) is added to liquid (monomer) in a disposable cup and mixed for about 1 minute, or until surface glaze disappears and mix becomes firm. **B,** Mix should be handled between sheets of plastic or cellophane. Mix is formed into a patty, **C,** and formed by light finger pressure over cast, **D.** Care must be taken not to thin the tray excessively during adapting process.

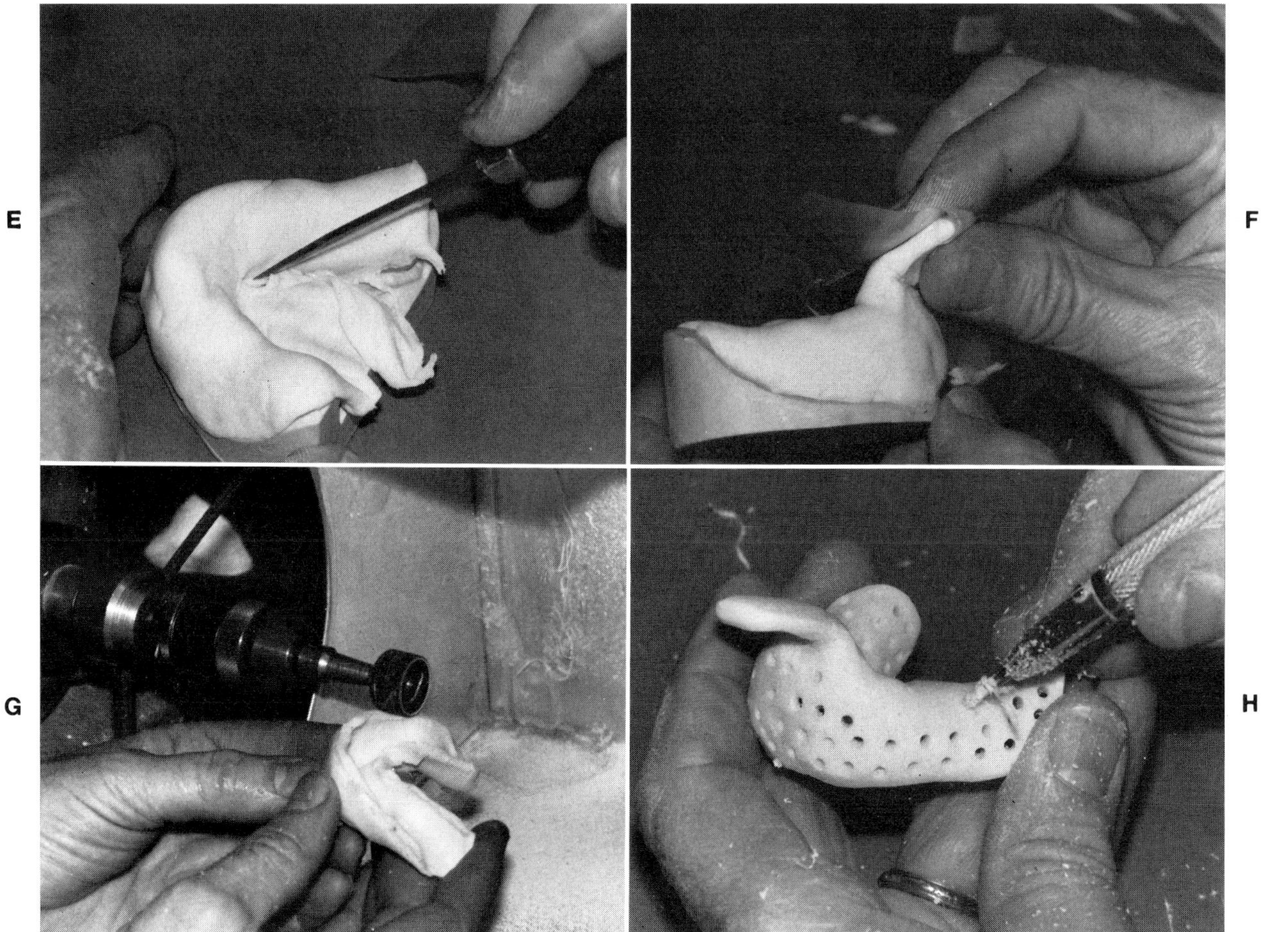

Fig. 9-68, cont'd. E, While material is still soft and workable, it is trimmed to outline form. **F,** A small piece of trimmed material is formed to make tray handle. Wetting end of handle in monomer will provide better attachment to tray. Tray should be undisturbed until polymerization has taken place. **G,** Tray is trimmed to desired outline with arbor bands. Sharp edges are rounded. **H,** If alginate is to be impression material, perforations are made in tray with a No. 8 round bur to ensure retention of impression material. In addition, an alginate adhesive should be painted on tray before impression is made. For silicone or polysulfide rubber impressions, perforations may be made if desired, but a rubber adhesive should be used routinely.

required to provide the necessary elasticity and strength of material.

The relief can be in the form of softened baseplate wax adapted evenly over the teeth and edentulous ridge. Although wet asbestos strips were frequently used in the past, their use has declined since the possible carcinogenic effect of asbestos has become known. In addition, the thickness of relief is more readily controlled with baseplate wax, because each strip is approximately 1 mm thick.

The tray acrylic resin is supplied as a liquid (monomer) and powder (polymer). Most manufacturers supply scoops and vials that will measure sufficient material to form one custom tray. The procedure is illustrated in Fig. 9-68.

Impression procedure

The impression procedure is the same as for the initial impression with the exception that the requirements of an acceptable impression are more demanding. Review Chapter 5 for the step-by-step procedure. The following are brief reminders of important points to observe:

1. Position the patient in the chair properly for the impression to be made.
2. After the tray has been modified, rehearse the operator position and the tray placement several times so that the patient will be aware of his responsibilities.
3. Prepare the mouth by having the patient rinse, and then pack with gauze pads.
4. Measure and mix the impression material according to directions, and load the tray in small increments to avoid trapping air.
5. Remove the packing and paint or inject impression material in critical areas: rest preparations, hard palate, and peripheral extensions.
6. Seat the tray as rehearsed, being careful not to overseat. Clear the lips and cheeks. For the mandibular impression be sure that the patient's tongue is raised and protruded gently.
7. Hold the tray steady until the material has set. *Never leave a patient unattended with an impression in the mouth.* Remove the tray with a sudden movement in a direction as near as possible to the long axis of the teeth.
8. Wash or clean saliva from the impression.
9. Examine the impression *critically* to determine whether all details are recorded accurately. If there is any doubt, reject the impression.

Reasons for rejecting impression

The following are specific reasons for rejecting and repeating an impression:

1. Bubbles or voids in and around rest preparations
2. Contact of cusps with the tray, especially when the teeth are involved in the framework design
3. Showthrough between teeth and modeling plastic or modeling plastic and hard palate if the tray has been modified for an alginate impression
4. Voids or bubbles in palatal vault when palatal major connectors are to be constructed
5. Peripheral underextension when a denture base has been designed and a corrected cast impression is not planned
6. Interproximal tearing of the impression material when coverage of those teeth has been designed
7. Lack of detail on the impression surface
8. *Any doubt* as to the accuracy of the impression

POURING THE MASTER CAST

The technique for pouring the master cast is the same as that for the diagnostic cast (described in Chapter 6) except that a minimal expansion improved artificial stone should be used.

1. After the impression has been cleaned of saliva and examined for defects, pour the cast immediately. Under no circumstances should a final alginate impression go unpoured for more than 12 minutes.
2. Never allow the impression to rest on a bench top or in a rubber bowl; suspend it by the tray handle.
3. Do not make the second, or opposing, impression before pouring the first.
4. Have preweighed stone available before the start of the appointment.
5. Make the stone mix, preferably under vacuum, according to directions and make the first pour.
6. Be certain all peripheries are covered by at least 6 mm ($^1/_4$ inch) of stone. Leave the stone surface rough.
7. After the initial set, 10 to 12 minutes, wet the base of the first pour with *slurry water* and add the second pour. Invert the impression with the first pour on a pad of stone and shape the base.
8. Between 45 and 60 minutes after the first pour separate the impression from the cast if either hydrocolloid material has been used.
9. Wet the cast thoroughly in slurry water by partially submerging it. Do not completely immerse the cast because this would prevent air from escaping from the stone and the cast will never be thoroughly wet.
10. Trim the cast (Fig. 9-69). The base of the cast should be trimmed so that the occlusal surfaces of the teeth will be as parallel to the base as possible. The thickness of the cast should be determined at this time also. The cast should be 10

mm thick at its thinnest point, usually the center of the hard palate for the maxillary cast and the depth of the lingual sulcus for the mandibular cast.

The posterior border of the cast is trimmed next. It must form an angle of 90 degrees with the base and should be perpendicular to a line passing between the central incisors.

The sides of the cast are trimmed so that they are parallel to the buccal surfaces of the posterior teeth or to the crest of the edentulous ridge. Do not trim so close as to obliterate the vestibule or the buccal shelf. A land area or periphery at least 3 mm wide should be maintained around the entire cast.

The sides and the posterior borders are joined by trimming just posterior to the hamular notch or retromolar pad. Be careful not to overtrim and thereby remove the hamular notch or the retromolar pad. These are essential landmarks and must be preserved.

The anterior borders of the maxillary cast are formed by trimming from the canine area on each side to a point anterior to the interproximal area of the central incisors, being careful again to maintain the vestibule and the land area.

The anterior border of the mandibular cast is formed by creating a curving wall from the canine on one side to the canine on the other. The curve should be kept constant, or harmonious.

The tongue space of the mandibular cast must be trimmed flat, but the integrity of the lingual frenum, sublingual fold space, and the lingual sulcus must be maintained.

11. Identify the casts with the patient's name. Do not put any foreign material on the master cast.
12. Casts must not be subjected to running water, brushing, or soaking in other than clear slurry water. If they are allowed to dry, they must be resoaked in clear slurry water before being shaped on the model trimmer.

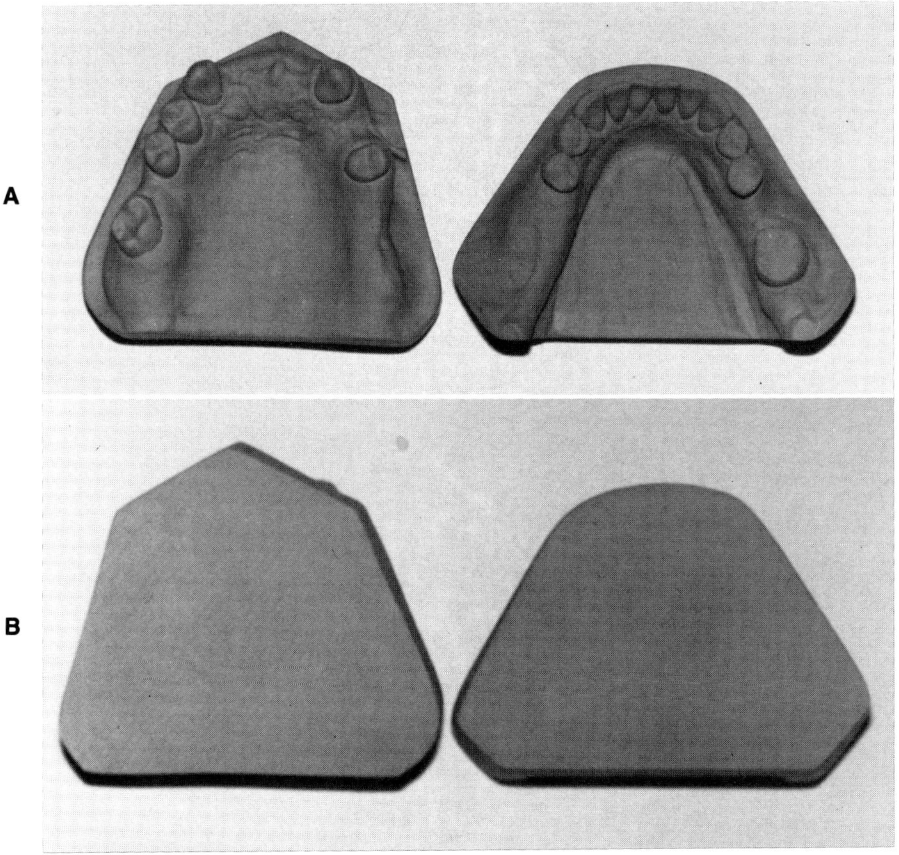

Fig. 9-69. Master casts should be trimmed to sharp clear outlines that can easily be handled by technician. **A,** Tissue surface. **B,** Base.

BIBLIOGRAPHY

Atwood, D.A.: Reduction of residual ridges in the partially edentulous patient, Dent. Clin. North Am. **17:** 747-754, 1973.

Axinn, S.: Preparation of retentive areas for clasps in enamel, J. Prosthet. Dent. **34:** 405-407, 1975.

Bailey, L.R.: Rubber base impression techniques, Dent. Clin. North Am. 1:156-166, March 1957.

Berg, T., Jr., and Caputo, A.A.: Anterior rests for maxillary removable partial dentures, J. Prosthet. Dent. **39:** 139-146, 1978.

Borkin, D.W.: Impression technique for patients that gag, J. Prosthet. Dent. **9:** 386-387, 1959.

Chase, W.W.: Adaptation of rubber-base impression materials to removable partial denture prostheses, J. Prosthet. Dent. **10:** 1043-1050, 1960.

Civjan, S., and others: Surface characteristics of alginate impressions, J. Prosthet. Dent. **28:** 373-378, 1972.

Craig, R.G., editor: Dental materials: a problem-oriented approach, St. Louis, 1978, The C.V. Mosby Co.

Fusayama, T., and Nakazoto, M.: The designs of stock trays and the retention of irreversible hydrocolloid impressions, J. Prosthet. Dent. **21:** 136-142, 1969.

Gaston, G.W.: Rest area preparations for removable partial dentures, J. Prosthet. Dent. **10:** 124-134, 1960.

Gilmore, W.H., and others: Factors influencing the accuracy of silicone impression materials, J. Prosthet. Dent. 9:304-314, 1959.

Glann, G.W., and Appleby, R.C.: Mouth preparations for removable partial dentures, J. Prosthet. Dent. **10:**689-706, 1960.

Hardy, I.: Partial dentures that function—partial dentures that fail, J. Am. Dent. Assoc. **25:**562-566, 1938.

Harris, L.W.: Boxing and cast pouring, J. Prosthet. Dent. **10:**390, 1960.

Holmes, J.B.: Preparation of abutment teeth for removable partial dentures, J. Prosthet. Dent. **20:**396-406, 1968.

Jochen, D.G.: Achieving planned parallel guiding planes for removable partial dentures, J. Prosthet. Dent. **27:**654-661, 1972.

Johnstone, J.F.: Preparation of mouths for fixed and removable partial dentures, J. Prosthet. Dent. **11:**456-462, 1961.

Kahn, A.E.: Partial versus full coverage, J. Prosthet. Dent. **10:**167-178, 1960.

Krokos, A.A.: Artificial undercuts for teeth which have unfavorable shapes for clasping, J. Prosthet. Dent. **22:**301-306, 1969.

Leupold, R.J.: A comparative study of impression procedures for distal extension removable partial dentures, J. Prosthet. Dent. **16:**708-720, 1966.

Mann, A.W.: A critical apprasial of the hydrocolloid technique: its advantages and disadvantages, J. Prosthet. Dent. **1:**733-749, 1951.

McCracken, W.L.: Mouth preparations for partial dentures, J. Prosthet. Dent. **6:**39-52, 1956.

Mills, M.: Mourth preparation for removable partial dentures, J. Am. Dent. Assoc. **60:**154-159, 1960.

Mitchell, J.V., and Dameles, J.J.: Influence of tray design upon elastic impression materials, J. Prosthet. Dent. **23:**51-57, 1970.

Paffenbarger, G.C.: Hydrocolloid impression materials: physical properties and a specification, J. Am. Dent. Assoc. **27:**373-388, 1940.

Perry, C.F., and Applegate, S.G.: Occlusal rest: an important part of a partial denture, J. Mich. Dent. Soc, **29:**24-25, 1947.

Craig, R.G., editor: Restorative dental materials, ed. 6, St. Louis, 1980, The C.V. Mosby Co.

Philips, R.W.: Factors affecting the surface of stone dies poured in hydrocolloid impressions, J. Prosthet. Dent. **2:**390-400, 1952.

Schorr, L., and Clayton, L.H.: Reshaping abutment teeth for reception of partial denture clasps, J. Prosthet. Dent. **4:**625-633, 1954.

Seiden, A.: Occlusal rests and rest seats, J. Prosthet. Dent. **8:**431-440, 1958.

Skinner, E.W., and Hoblit, N.E.: A study of the accuracy of hydrocolloid impressions, J. Prosthet. Dent. **6:**80-86, 1956.

Skinner, E.W., and Philips, R.W.: The science of dental materials, ed. 6, Philadelphia, 1967, W.B. Saunders Co.

Sollé, W.: The Parallelo-facere: a parallel drilling machine for use in the oral cavity, J. Am. Dent. Assoc. **63:**344-352, 1961.

Stern, W.J.: Guiding planes in clasp reciprocation and retention, J. Prosthet. Dent. **34:**408-414, 1975.

10 Preliminary jaw relation and esthetic try-in for some anterior replacement teeth

Before the master casts are sent to the laboratory for framework construction, they must be mounted on an articulator and studied from all angles to verify completeness of mouth preparation and sufficient space between the arches to accommodate the metal thickness of the framework. This procedure permits detection and correction of any possible occlusal interferences between natural teeth and the framework *before* the framework has been constructed, which can save considerable time and prevent frustration for the patient.

Also needed at this time is an esthetic try-in for any facings, tube teeth, or RAPs planned to replace anterior teeth or maxillary first premolars.

The casts must be mounted at either centric relation or centric occlusion, whichever position was selected for construction of the prosthesis. If the removable partial denture will be constructed in centric occlusion and the remaining teeth are so located that the casts can be accurately hand articulated, a jaw relation record is not required (Fig. 10-1). The casts should, however, be mounted on an articulator to be sent to the laboratory. Otherwise, if the denture is to be constructed in centric relation or if the denture is to be constructed in centric occlusion but the casts cannot be articulated by hand, a jaw relation record is needed to mount the casts accurately on the articulator.

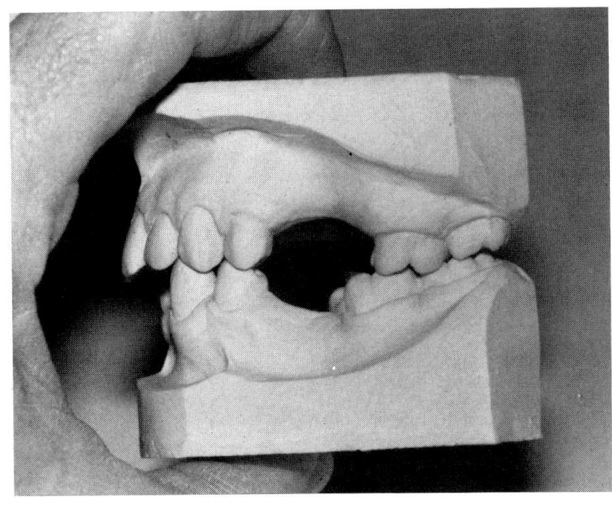

Fig. 10-1. If sufficient teeth remain, casts may be accurately hand articulated in centric occlusion.

Construction of baseplates

Baseplates used to record the jaw relation for partially edentulous patients may be made of gutta-percha or autopolymerizing acrylic resin. Either material can produce accurate results if proper technique is followed to construct the baseplate and record the jaw relation.

It must be remembered that a baseplate for a partial denture rests almost entirely on the soft tissue portion of the cast. Since the soft tissue areas of the mouth are constantly undergoing minor changes in position, shape, and size in response to physiologic stimulation, the baseplate must be constructed on the *master cast* and the master cast must be prepared and handled carefully before and during baseplate construction. If reinforcing wire is to be used to strengthen the baseplate, usually gutta-percha, the wire may be adjusted or formed on the diagnostic cast but must be incorporated into the baseplate on the master cast.

Gutta-percha baseplates

Gutta-percha is extracted from trees of the same family that are sources of the rubber hydrocarbon. Commercially available gutta-percha for dental use has compounding ingredients such as zinc oxide, chalk, carbon, or magnesium oxide added to improve the handling characteristics. The material is supplied in sheet form or in the shape of the maxillary or mandibular arch (Fig. 10-2). At room temperature it is comparatively hard, but when heated by open flame it softens to a plastic state and can be molded on a cast of the dental arch to the desired shape, which it will maintain on hardening as the material cools.

Among the advantages of the use of gutta-percha to form baseplates are that it is quicker and easier to use than autopolymerizing acrylic resin and offers less danger of damaging the cast on which it is molded. However, it is brittle and subject to breakage, is apt to distort if not used shortly after being constructed, and is not as accurate as the acrylic resin except perhaps in the hands of an experienced clinician.

The technique for constructing a gutta-percha baseplate is illustrated in Fig. 10-3.

Autopolymerizing acrylic resin baseplates

Autopolymerizing acrylic resin, often referred to as self-cure or cold-cure resin is supplied as a powder (polymer) and a liquid (monomer). Mixing of the two results in the formation of a hard resin. Whereas in heat-cured acrylic resin the stimulus that starts and

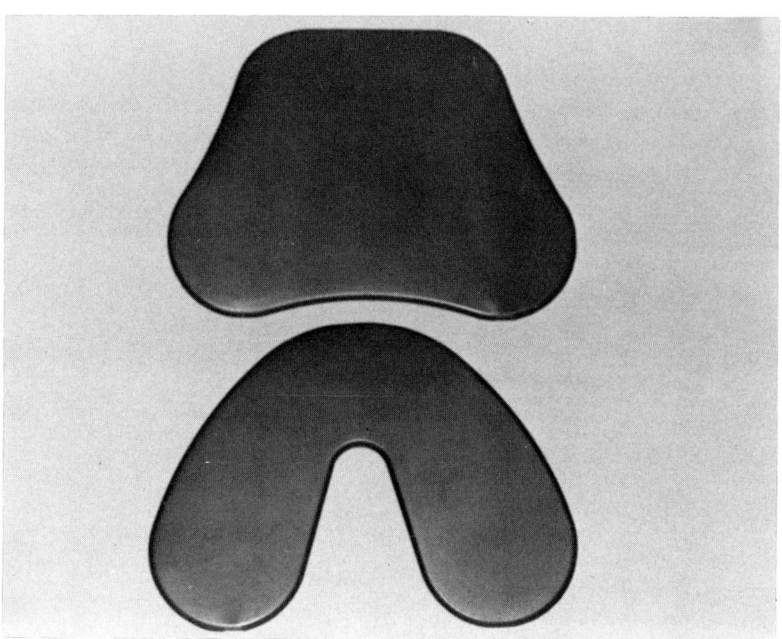

Fig. 10-2. Maxillary (top) and mandibular (bottom) gutta-percha baseplates.

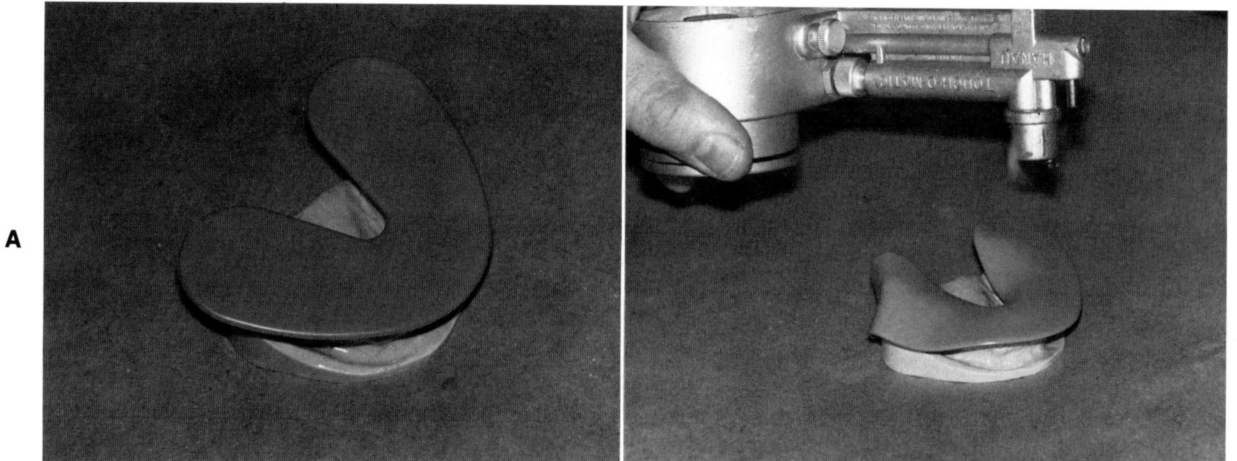

Fig. 10-3. Laboratory procedures to form a gutta-percha baseplate. **A,** Gutta-percha form is positioned to contact occlusal surfaces of remaining teeth on cast as it sits on bench. **B,** Flame from a Bunsen burner is passed over surface of gutta-percha until material starts to slump. Flame should be moved constantly to avoid burning or boiling the material.

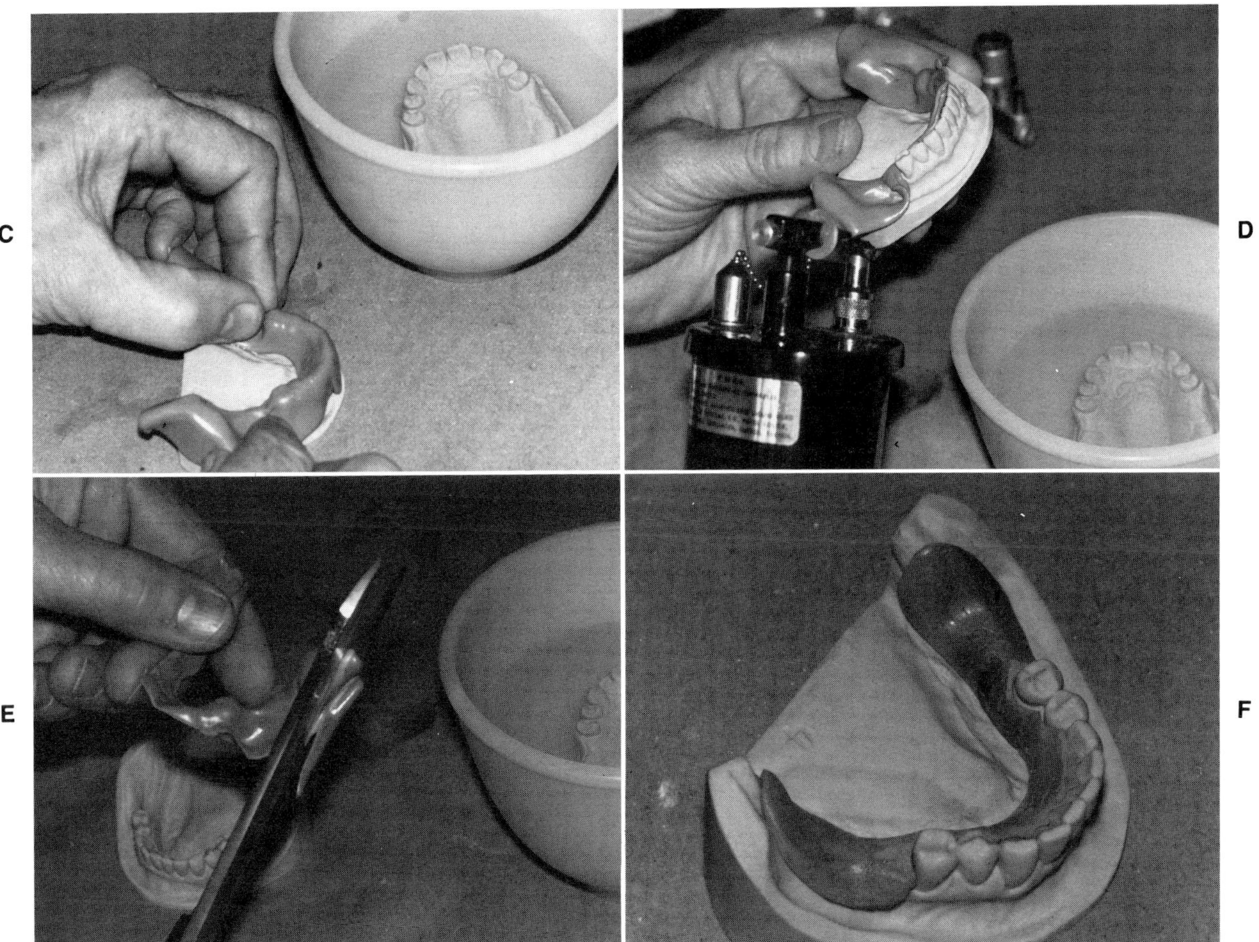

Fig. 10-3, cont'd. C, When gutta-percha begins to slump, finger adaptation should be started. To prevent heat injury, fingers should be dipped into room-temperature water before molding hot gutta-percha. Finger molding should cease before the material cools enough to become rigid. The baseplate must be removed from cast before it becomes so hard that its removal may damage cast. Overextended areas are heated with an alcohol torch, **D,** and cut away with scissors while soft, **E.** Process of heating baseplate and readapting it to desired outline on cast is repeated until baseplate conforms to necessary extensions, **F.**

Continued.

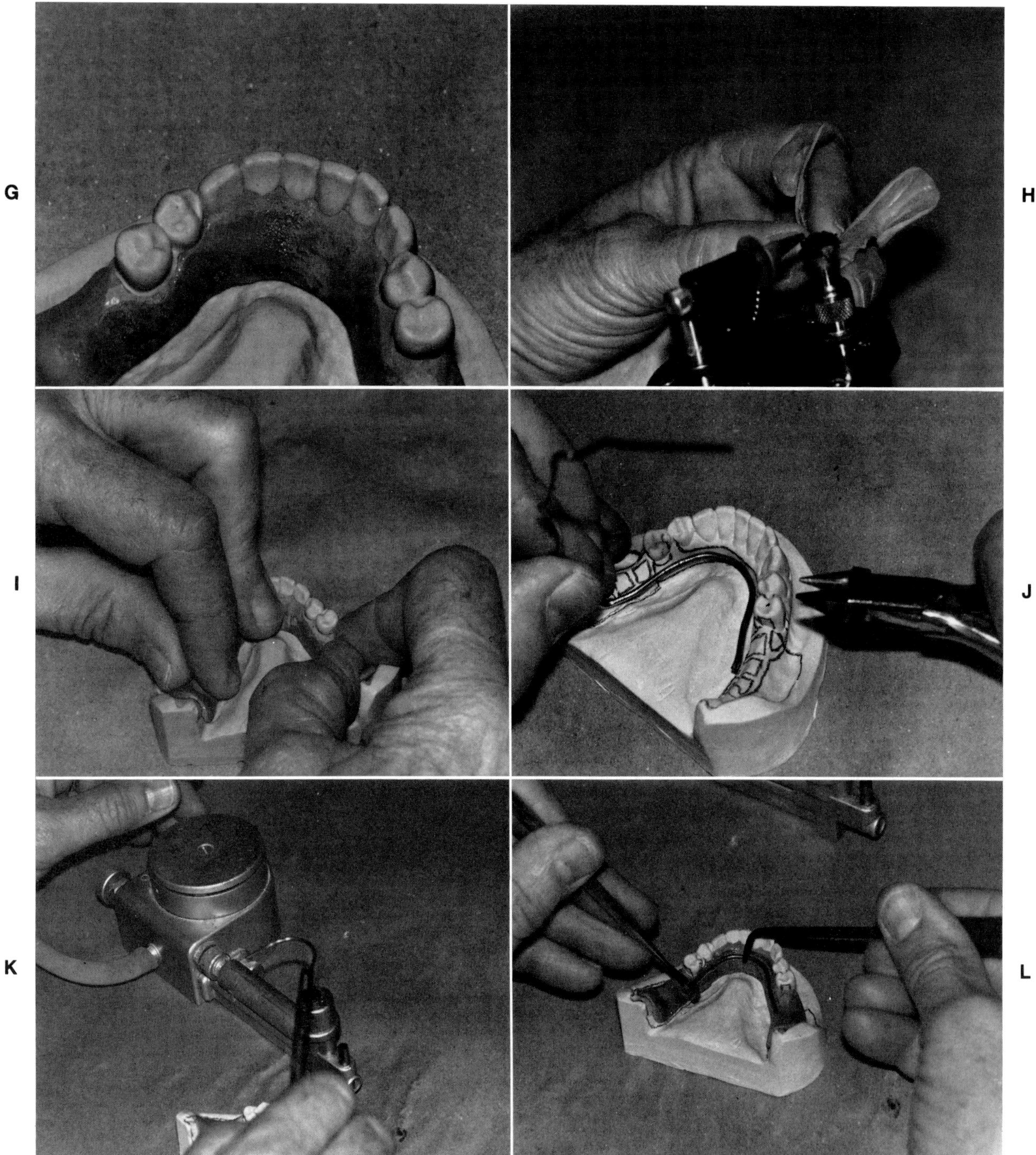

Fig. 10-3, cont'd. **G,** The baseplate should contact several anterior teeth so it can be replaced on cast and in mouth in same position. After correct borders are established, intimate contact with soft tissue areas must be developed. This is best accomplished by flaming tissue side of baseplate to soften gutta-percha, **H,** reseating it, and pressing it firmly against cast, **I. J,** Baseplate should then be reinforced with a piece of heavy-duty paper clip wire. For a mandibular baseplate, wire should be bent to conform to lingual slope of ridge from approximately second premolar to second premolar. (In maxillary arch, wire should be shaped to cross posterior extent of hard palate. All maxillary baseplates used to record jaw relations should be of complete palate type.) **K** and **L,** Once wire is shaped, gutta-percha is repositioned on cast. Wire, held with pliers and heated over a flame, is pressed into baseplate.

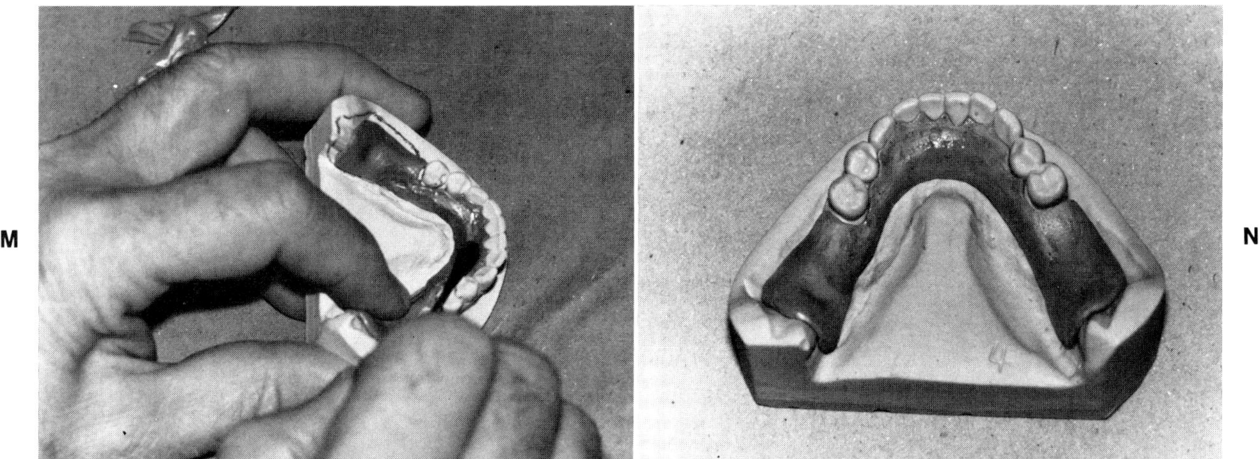

Fig. 10-3, cont'd. M, Wire should be completely covered with either softened gutta-percha or baseplate wax to prevent irritation to tongue. **N,** Completed baseplate should be totally passive in mouth.

continues the polymerization is external heat, in autopolymerizing resin a chemical stimulus starts the reaction. The monomer contains a small amount of tertiary amine such as dimethyl-p-toluidine. When this chemical promoter contacts the benzoyl peroxide in the polymer, a chain of events is started similar to that which occurs when heat is applied to heat-cured resin (free radicals liberated from benzoyl peroxide activate monomer molecules to form chains).

As much as 5% of a self-cure material may remain as monomer after polymerization (as compared with 0.2% to 0.5% for heat-cure resin). The remaining monomer is released slowly from the resin over a long period, causing a soft tissue inflammatory reaction in some patients wearing a prosthesis constructed from self-cure resin.

An acrylic resin baseplate or denture base constructed from self-cure resin will be dimensionally more accurate than one cured by heat. The heat-cured resin may shrink 3% to 7%, whereas the shrinkage of self-cure resin can be held to as low as 0.2%. The shrinkage of the self-cure resin will increase as the bulk of material increases.

Autopolymerizing acrylic resin can be applied to a cast to form a baseplate in one of two ways. The so-called patty technique in which the material is mixed and formed into a patty in a custom tray and adapted to the cast produces a baseplate that is reasonably accurate but not as well adapted as one formed by the "sprinkle-on" technique, illustrated in Fig. 10-4.

The cast may sit on the bench top while polymerization takes place. This method of curing the baseplate will produce a slightly porous baseplate surface because of evaporation of the monomer into the atmosphere. A second method of curing is to cover the cast with an inverted rubber bowl immediately after the sprinkling is complete. As initial evaporation of the monomer occurs, the evaporate is trapped and the atmosphere within the bowl becomes saturated with monomer. This prevents excessive loss of monomer and produces a denser baseplate surface. The densest, least porous, and most accurate baseplate is produced by placing the cast in a pressure pot under 20 pounds pressure for about 20 minutes (Fig. 10-4), *G*).

After polymerization is complete, the baseplate is finished. It should be teased or pried gently from the cast without marring the surface of the cast. Acrylic resin finishing instruments, arbor bands, acrylic stones, or vulcanite burs are used to establish the correct baseplate form. The edges of the baseplate should be rounded to prevent irritation of the surrounding tissues. The thickness of the baseplate is refined at the same time. Over the edentulous ridges the baseplate should be reduced to approximately 1 mm to allow space for the jaw relation record; elsewhere the baseplate should be 2 mm thick to ensure adequate strength. A slightly rough surface should be maintained on the external surface of the baseplate over the ridge so that the jaw relation record will adhere properly to the surface. The remainder of the external surface that will contact the surrounding tissues may be smoothed with flour of pumice and a wet rag wheel. Care should be taken to prevent even moderate heat from being generated during the finishing process because distortion of the acrylic resin may take place.

If the baseplate must be stored until the appointment for the jaw relation record, it is not necessary to store the baseplate in water.

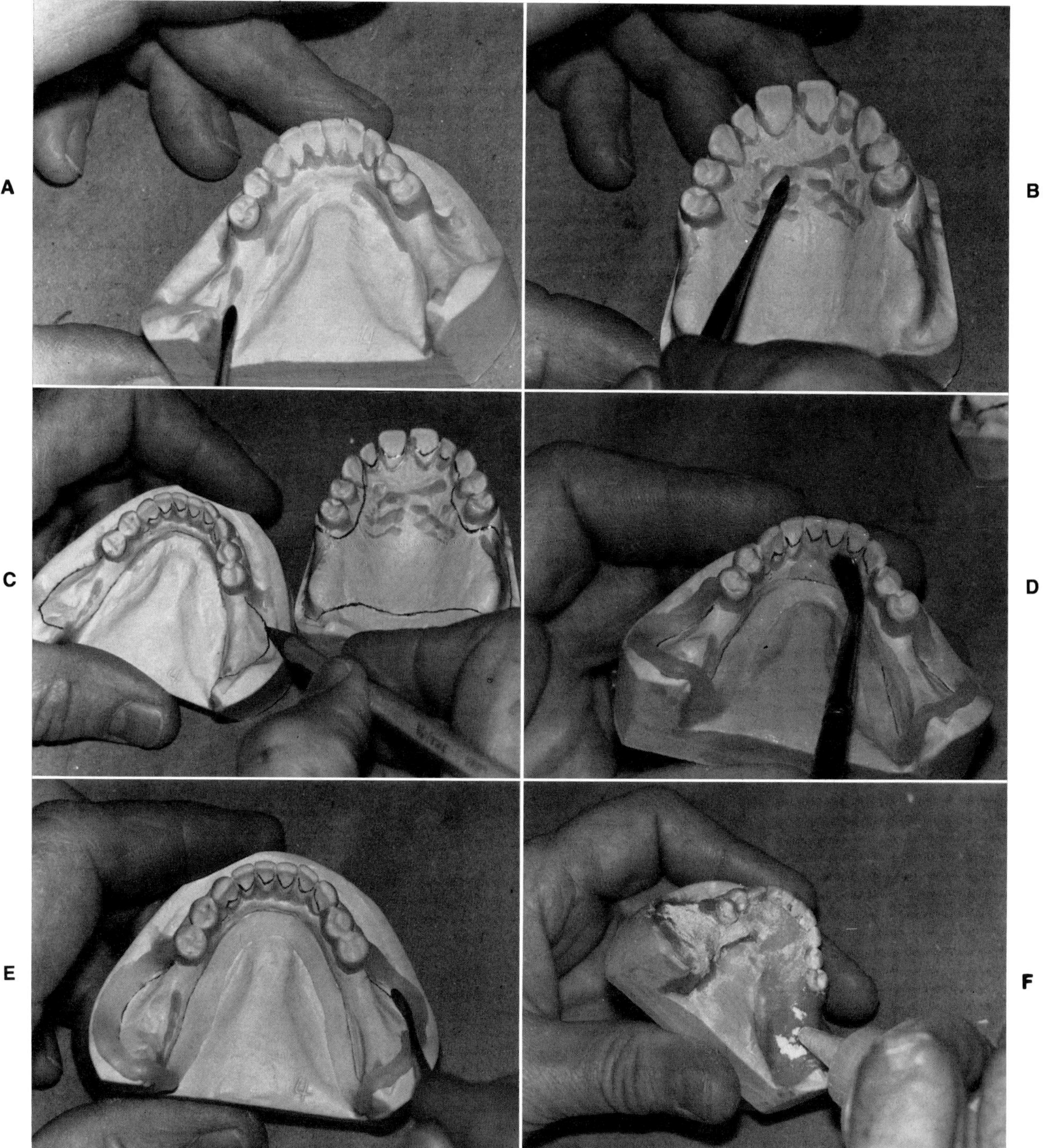

Fig. 10-4. Laboratory procedures to form an autopolymerizing acrylic resin baseplate by sprinkle-on method. **A,** Baseplate wax is flowed into all undercuts on cast, particularly areas between and around teeth. Excess wax should be avoided because it will compromise fit of baseplate. **B,** A thin film of wax is flowed over rugal area in palate. **C,** Desired limits of baseplate should be lightly drawn with a wax pencil on casts. Contact with posterior teeth should be avoided. Several anterior teeth are contacted to aid in repositioning. Peripheral borders should be slightly underextended, to ensure passivity of completed baseplate. **D,** Two coats of alginate separating medium are applied to cast. One coat should dry before second is added. **E,** A reservoir is formed around outline of baseplate with beading or utility wax. **F,** A small amount of dry polymer is sprinkled from a paper cup or a plastic container with a small orifice onto surface of cast, then wet with monomer, usually from an eyedropper. The polymer is added in small increments until entire outline of baseplate is covered with 2 to 3 mm of wet mix. Each addition of powder must be thoroughly wet with monomer, but an excessive amount of monomer should be avoided because it is difficult to control position of resin if it becomes too runny.

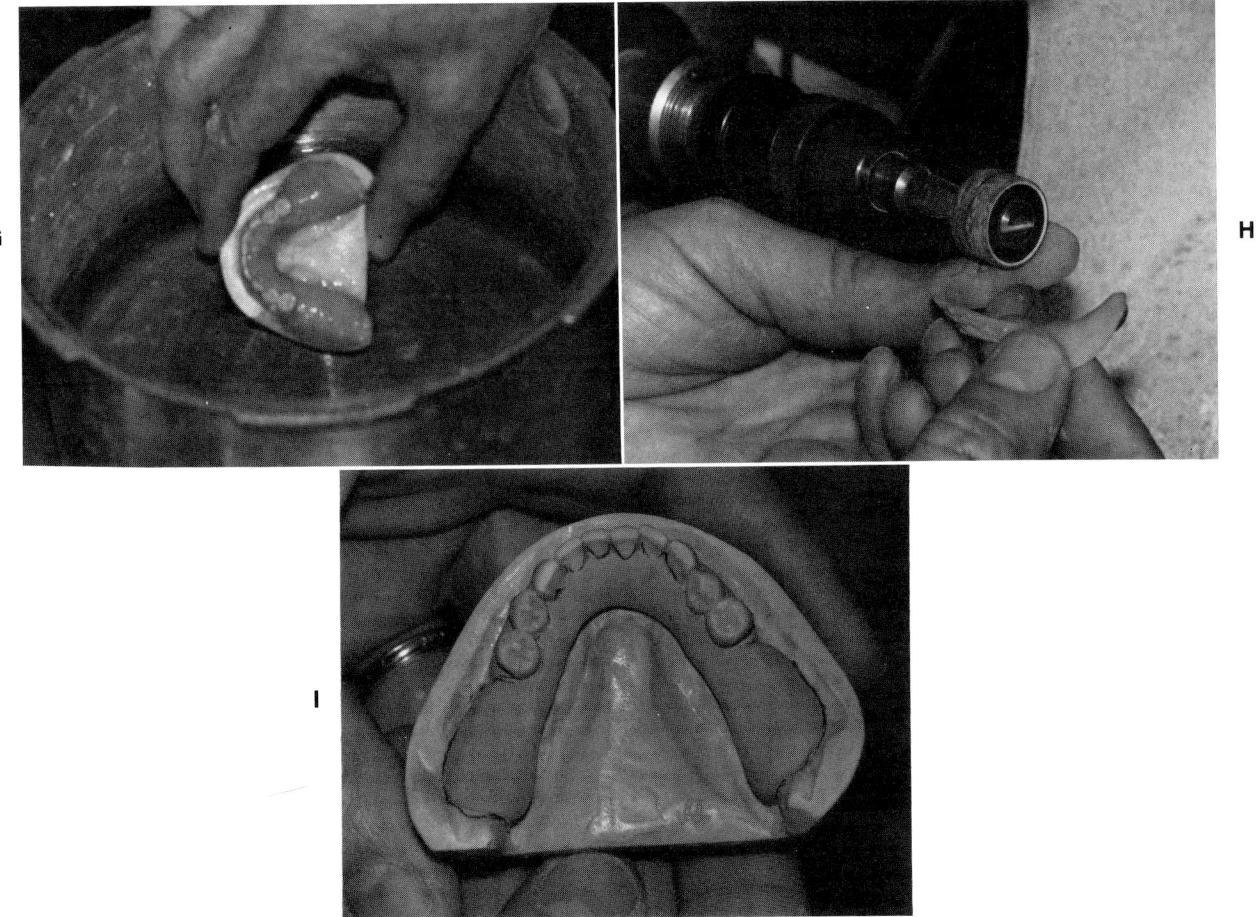

Fig. 10-4, cont'd. G, Densest baseplate is produced by allowing polymerization to occur under 20 pounds pressure for 20 minutes in a pressure pot. **H,** Baseplate is trimmed on a lathe with arbor bands. Edges are rounded, and thickness over edentulous ridge reduced to 1 mm; elsewhere 2-mm thickness is maintained. **I,** trimmed baseplate on cast.

Recording the jaw relation

As stated earlier, if casts can be unmistakeably hand articulated, there is no need to have a jaw relation appointment. The casts should be mounted on an articulator and forwarded to a commercial dental laboratory along with a work authorization order and the diagnostic casts. There will also be times when maxillary and mandibular partial dentures are being constructed for the patient so that baseplates for both arches will not be required. If when a single baseplate can be made for either arch and the opposing remaining teeth will contact either the recording media on the baseplate and/or other natural teeth in at least three widely separated points, that is usually sufficient to stabilize the casts as they are mounted on the articulator.

The most important point to observe when recording the jaw relation is that the recording must be accomplished completely free of pressure. The baseplate is supported only by the soft tissue covering the ridge. Even the slightest occlusal pressure will cause compression of the soft tissue with accompanying displacement of the baseplate. When the baseplate is returned to the noncompressible stone cast, an error will be present, sometimes of large magnitude.

Recording media that may be used to record other types of jaw relations, such as baseplate wax, softened modeling plastic, or even softer waxes, should not be used to record this type of jaw relation because some vertical force is required to produce indentations on the surface of all these media.

The recording material of choice is generally zinc oxide–eugenol paste or accelerated dental stone. Other pressure-free materials are available, but these two are simple to use, extremely accurate, and available in most dental offices.

The accuracy of the fit of the baseplate should be ver-

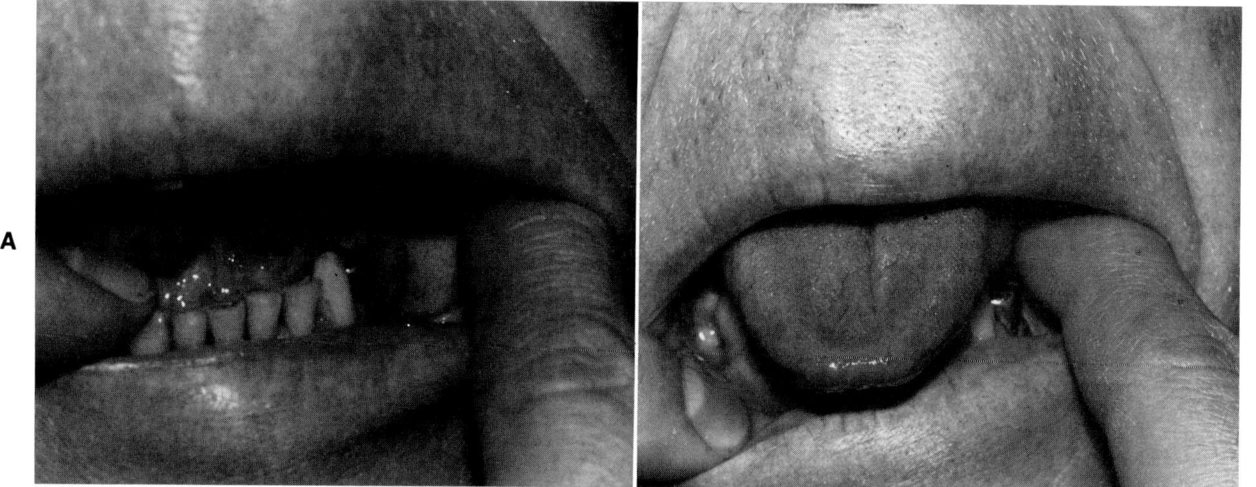

Fig. 10-5. A, Buccal peripheral extensions should be checked visually to be certain they are short of movable tissue. B, Lingual extension is checked by instructing patient to protrude tongue. Tissues of floor of mouth should not move baseplate.

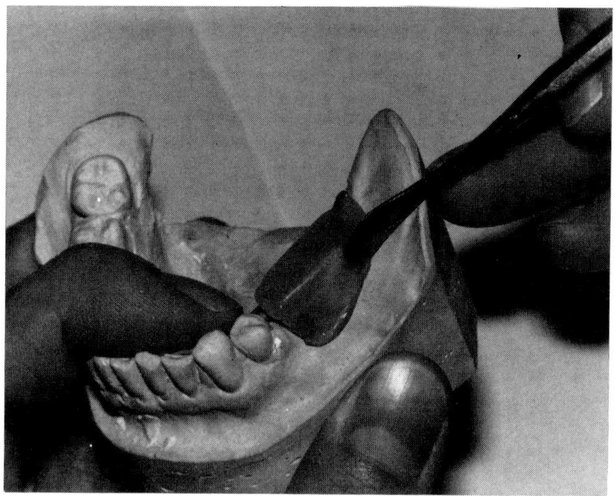

Fig. 10-6. A baseplate wax occlusion rim is added to edentulous ridge area of baseplate. It should be 7 mm wide and should not contact opposing teeth.

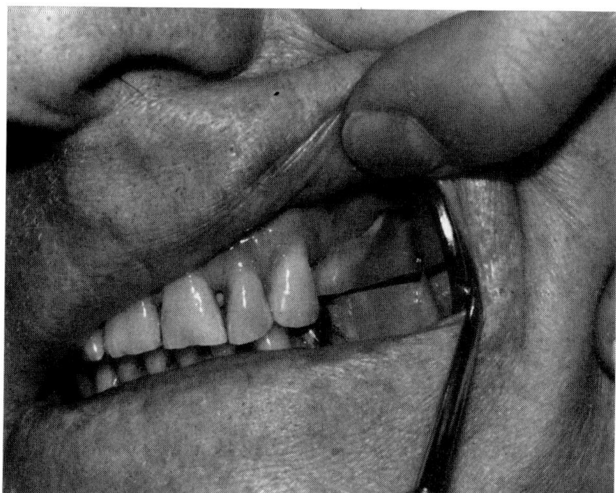

Fig. 10-7. A space of 1 to 2 mm between opposing occlusion rims or between opposing teeth and occlusion rim is desired.

ified at the start of the appointment. The baseplate should be tried on the cast to be certain that rocking does not take place, and it should be tried in the mouth to determine that the peripheral extensions of the base are short of movable tissues (Fig. 10-5). A well-constructed, accurately adapted base should not require denture adhesive for retention. The baseplate should remain passively in place when the patient is relaxed. The lingual surface of several anterior teeth should be contacted by the baseplate so that it may be repositioned accurately in the mouth.

It is necessary to provide some form of support for the recording medium. The support can best be provided by an occlusion rim constructed of baseplate wax. A sheet of wax is softened over a flame, adapted over the edentulous ridge portion of the baseplate, and sealed firmly to the base. The rim should be approximately 7 mm wide buccolingually, and its height should be adjusted so that it is just shy of contact with the opposing teeth, or with the opposing rim if two baseplates are being used (Figs. 10-6 and 10-7). *Any contact against the wax occlusion rim will result in an inaccurate jaw relation record.*

With the baseplate in the mouth the patient should

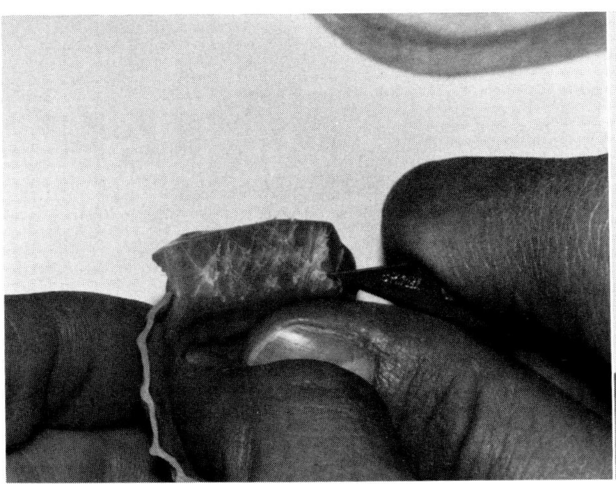

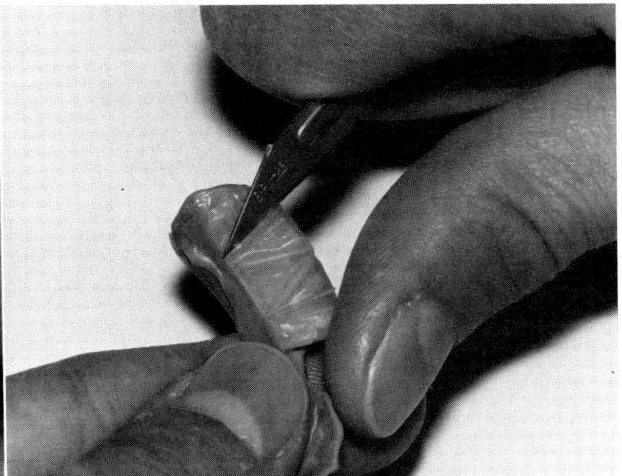

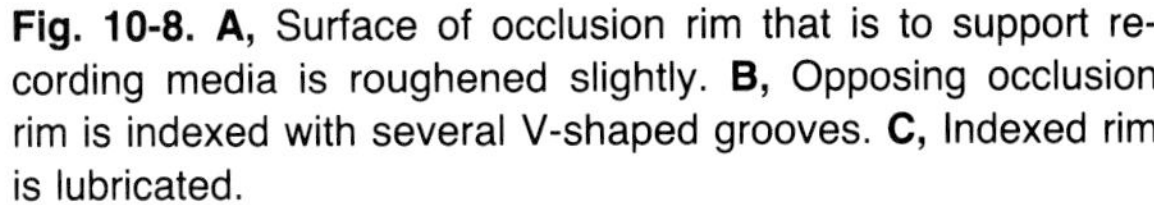

Fig. 10-8. A, Surface of occlusion rim that is to support recording media is roughened slightly. **B,** Opposing occlusion rim is indexed with several V-shaped grooves. **C,** Indexed rim is lubricated.

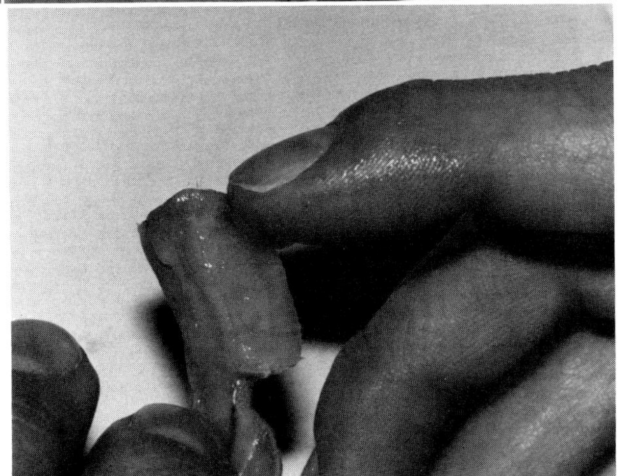

be rehearsed in closing to the proper position. It is helpful if the patient's lips are gently retracted so that visual verification of proper tooth contact can be made. The operator should maintain a slight backward and downward force on the patient's chin with either the thumb or forefinger. This force activates the elevator muscles of the mandible and maintains the head of the condyle in proper position in the glenoid fossa. If this pressure is not used and the condyle drops into a relaxed or rest position, the record will be incorrect.

The surface of the occlusion rim should be roughened slightly by either a series of scratches or several indentations so the recording medium will attach to it firmly. If occlusion rims are opposing each other, one, preferably the maxillary, rim should be indexed in the form of several V-shaped grooves cut approximately 2 mm wide and 2 mm deep to provide a definite seat for the record. The surface of the indexed rim should be lubricated with petrolatum or similar material to act as a separating medium (Fig. 10-8).

If zinc oxide–eugenol paste is the recording medium, it is mixed according to manufacturer's directions. If accelerated dental stone—made by mixing Hydrocal with concentrated slurry solution* (Fig. 10-9)—is the recording medium, it is mixed to a consistency of heavy cream. It must be thick enough not to run freely, but not so thick as to offer resistance to closure. Once mixed, the medium is placed on the rough surface of the occlusion rim. Sufficient material should be used to ensure contact with the opposing teeth or rim.

*Concentrated slurry solution is a supersaturated solution of calcium sulfate. It is made by collecting the liquid run-off from a model trimmer as a block of Hydrocal is being trimmed. The liquid containing the particles of Hydrocal is collected in a container and allowed to set for several hours. The stone particles will settle to the bottom of the container, leaving the supernatant liquid on top. The supernatant liquid should be poured off except for an amount equal to the layer of stone particles. Before this concentrated slurry solution is used, the container must be shaken to disperse the particles. This solution greatly decreases the setting time of dental stone, making it a feasible intraoral recording medium for the jaw relation. It also is a time-saver in mounting casts on an articulator. The resulting stone mixed with slurry solution is dimensionally as accurate but softer than normal dental stone. It should not be used in pouring casts because it does not produce surface detail as accurately as regular Hydrocal.

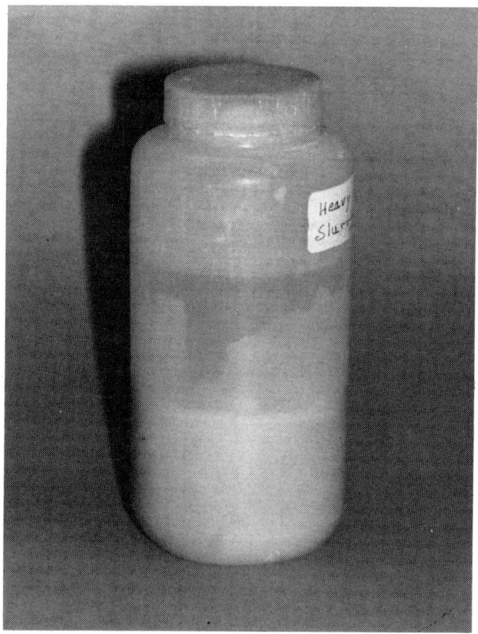

Fig. 10-9. Concentrated slurry solution should be composed of equal parts of supernatant liquid and settled particles.

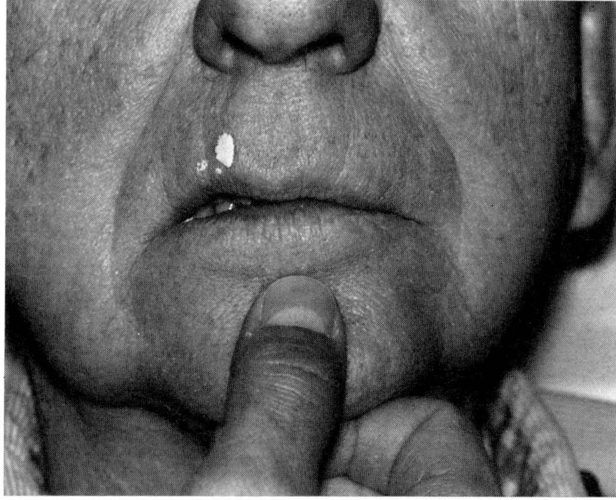

Fig. 10-10. Light thumb pressure should be maintained on chin until recording medium has set.

The baseplate is then positioned in the patient's mouth in contact with the lingual surfaces of the anterior teeth as it was designed. This ensures that the position can be duplicated on the cast. The patient is guided to the maximum intercuspal closed position with light pressure against the chin. The position must be maintained until the medium is completely set (Fig. 10-10).

Before the baseplate is returned to the cast, (1) the record should be trimmed with a sharp knife so that only the cusp tips or the surface of the indexed opposing rim is present on the record, (2) the record should be returned to the patient's mouth to verify accuracy, and (3) the record should be examined for signs of showthrough (Fig. 10-11).

If the record is acceptable, it should be placed on the cast and the opposing cast positioned on the record. Close examination of the occlusal surfaces of the teeth on the opposing cast should be made for bubbles or other defects that could prevent the accurate seating of the cast into the record. With the casts held together, the patient's occlusion and the occlusion of the teeth on the casts can be compared (Fig. 10-12). If any discrepancy can be found between the tooth contacts, the jaw relation record should be repeated.

Mounting the casts on the articulator

The question as to whether a fully adjustable, semiadjustable, or hinge articulator should be used to forward the mounted casts to the laboratory often arises. At this stage of partial denture construction, when the framework only is to be made, occlusal contacts in eccentric positions are not a major concern. A hinge articulator that maintains a solid centric occlusal position and has a vertical stop to protect the stone teeth from fracture is sufficient at this time (Fig. 10-13). A face-bow transfer will not be required if the casts are mounted on a hinge articulator. Later, when a jaw relation record is made to arrange the artificial teeth and complete the denture, a more adjustable instrument may be indicated and a face-bow transfer may be required.

Technique

Because the laboratory technician must remove the casts from the articulator for the framework construction, the bases of both casts should be indexed so that they can later be returned to the articulator in exactly the same relationship for correction of occlusal interferences. The index is in the form of bisecting V-shaped grooves at least 3 mm wide and 2 mm deep. A gypsum separating medium is then painted on the bases of the casts.

With the baseplates and jaw relation record in place on the cast or casts, the casts are hand articulated so that they are in the relationship desired, either centric occlusion or centric relation. In this position the casts must be stable; no rocking or tipping should be evident. The casts are luted together solidly and accurately with three pieces of tongue blade, two to the sides and one to the anterior edges, and sticky wax (Fig. 10-14).

The vertical stop of the articulator should be adjusted so that when the luted casts are set on the lower mem-

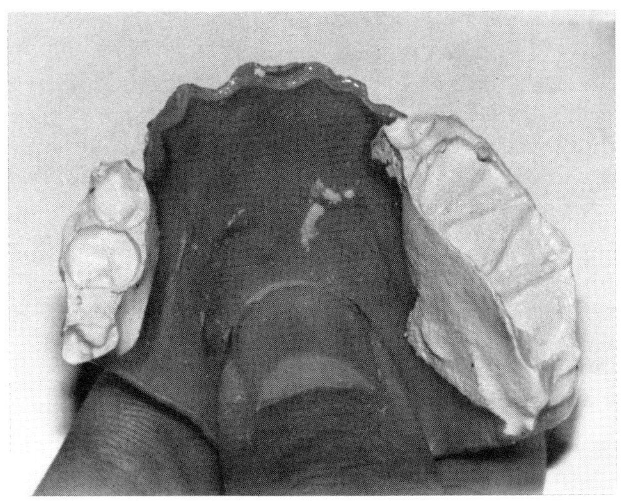

Fig. 10-11. Completed record is examined for evidence of contact between opposing occlusion rims or between opposing teeth and occlusion rim. If any showthrough is present, record is taken again.

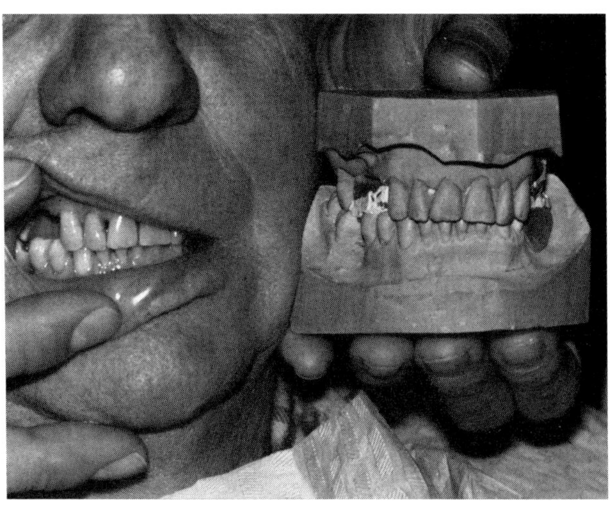

Fig. 10-12. Teeth on occluded casts must be exactly the same as patient's teeth in contact.

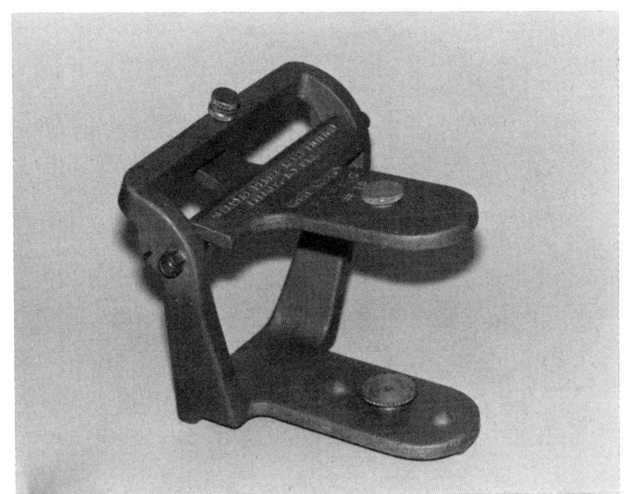

Fig. 10-13. A hinge articulator such as this Hanau LTD may be used to send mounted casts to laboratory for construction of framework.

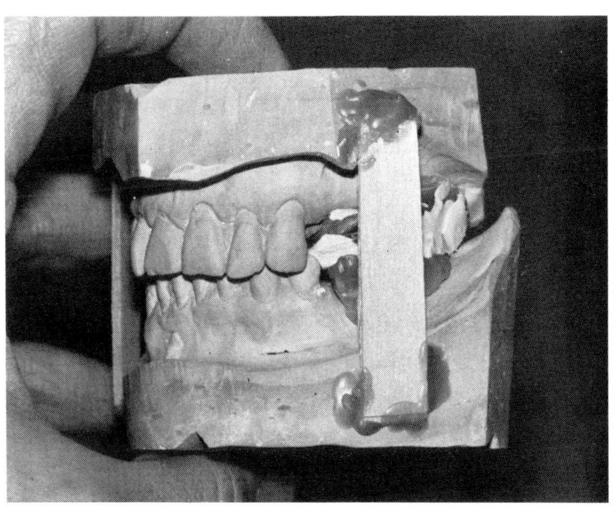

Fig. 10-14. Master casts, with jaw relation records in place, are luted together with tongue blades and sticky wax.

ber of the articulator there will be $^1/_2$ inch between the surface of the maxillary cast and the upper member (Fig. 10-15).

A mix of accelerated stone (Hydrocal and concentrated slurry solution) is made, and a mound is placed on the mounting device of the lower member. The base of the mandibular cast is centered on this mound with the occlusal plane parallel to the bench top and the midline of the casts centered in the articulator. Another mound of the mix is placed on the base of the maxillary cast, and the upper member of the articulator is closed to contact the stone. The vertical stop of the articulator should also be in contact at this time.

After the stone has set, the mountings are trimmed neatly and the mounted casts are examined carefully for accuracy (Fig. 10-16).

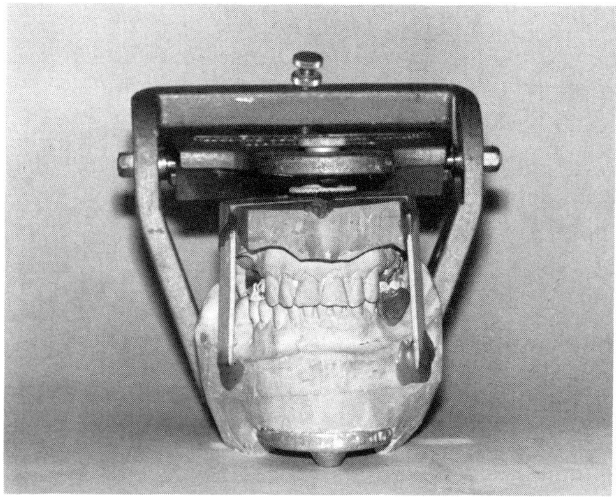

Fig. 10-15. Vertical stop of articulator is set so that 1/2 inch is present between surface of maxillary cast and upper member.

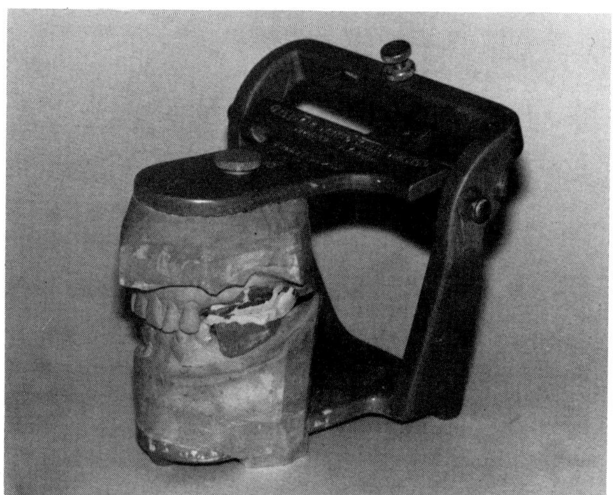

Fig. 10-16. Casts may be mounted on articulator with a single mix of stone, or two mixes may be used as shown here. Mounting stone is smoothed before casts are sent to laboratory.

ESTHETIC TRY-IN FOR ANTERIOR REPLACEMENT TEETH

If anterior teeth are to be replaced with facings, tube teeth, or RAPs, an esthetic try-in is needed at this time, because the support for the replacement tooth is waxed and cast as an integral part of the framework. Once the casting has been made, the replacement tooth cannot be altered without considerable trouble. A tube tooth to replace a maxillary first premolar should also have an esthetic try-in because the maxillary first premolar occupies a prominent esthetic position for most patients. (See Chapter 3 for a detailed discussion of the various types of artificial anterior teeth and the indications and limitations of each type.)

A single missing incisor tooth or even two missing incisors on the same side of the midline do not pose a major problem to most laboratory technicians as far as determining the size, shape, and position of the missing tooth or teeth. The remaining teeth on the opposing side of the arch can be matched to produce a natural appearance. However, the technician cannot match the shade. This the dentist must do and even with the wide variation of shade guides available, the shade cannot be confirmed until the artificial tooth or facing that will be used is actually tried in the mouth.

Clinical procedure for esthetic try-in

The master cast is used for the try-in appointment and must be handled carefully to prevent scratching or marring the surface.

A baseplate is needed to hold the artificial tooth or teeth in position during the try-in. A gutta-percha baseplate can be formed for this purpose; however, a single thickness of hard baseplate wax is usually sufficient. The baseplate wax is adapted to the hard palate of the master cast but extended only to the crest of the edentulous ridge (Fig. 10-17). It must be remembered that one of the requirements for, and one of the limiting factors governing the use of these replacement teeth is that the ridge be broad and nonresorbed because the necks of these replacement teeth must be butted against the ridge.

The teeth are contoured against the cast until the desired result is achieved and then attached to the baseplate for trial in the mouth (Figs. 10-18 and 10-19). If the baseplate is handled carefully and if the patient is cautioned against exerting force on the artificial tooth, the try-in can be successfully accomplished. Final shaping and positioning is done in the mouth.

When the patient is satisfied with the appearance of the teeth, a labial core of accelerated stone is made in the mouth (Fig. 10-20). A small mix of stone is made. The consistency of the mix should be such that it can be handled and molded with the fingers and yet not be so resistant as to displace the teeth being held by the baseplate wax. The stone is molded over the labial surfaces of the artificial teeth and the facial surfaces of at least two natural teeth on both sides of the space, so that the core can be repositioned accurately on the master cast (Fig. 10-21). The laboratory technician will use the core to hold the teeth as the framework is being waxed around them. When the wax-up is complete, the teeth will be removed and the framework cast. After the casting is complete and the framework finished and polished, the teeth can be cemented or attached to the partial denture.

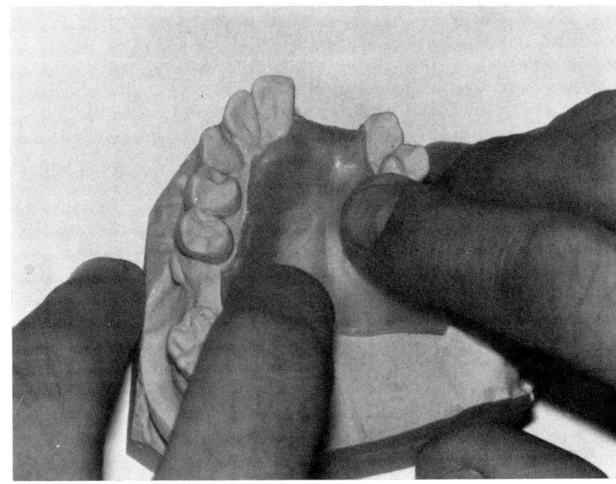

Fig. 10-17. A single layer of baseplate wax is adapted to palate.

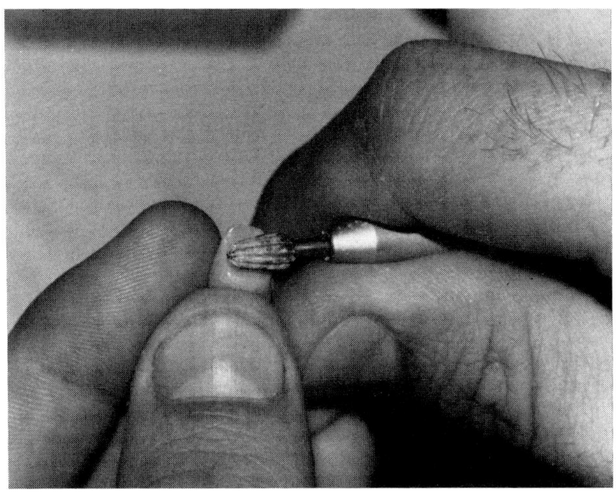

Fig. 10-18. Ridgelap of denture tooth is contoured to cast.

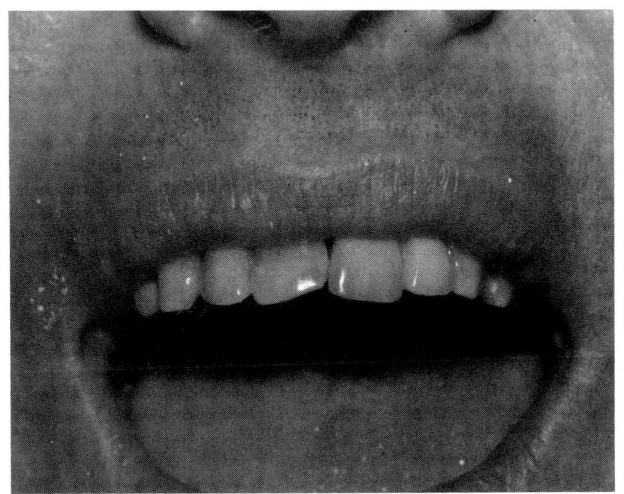

Fig. 10-19. Denture tooth is attached to baseplate wax and tried in mouth.

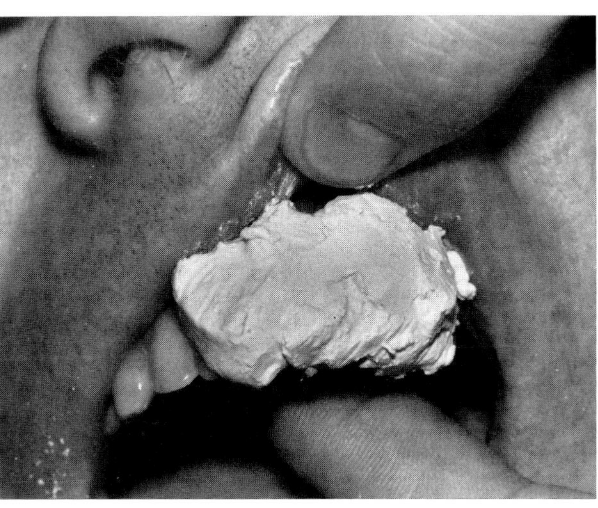

Fig. 10-20. After patient acceptance of esthetic quality of replacement, a labial matrix is made in quick-setting stone.

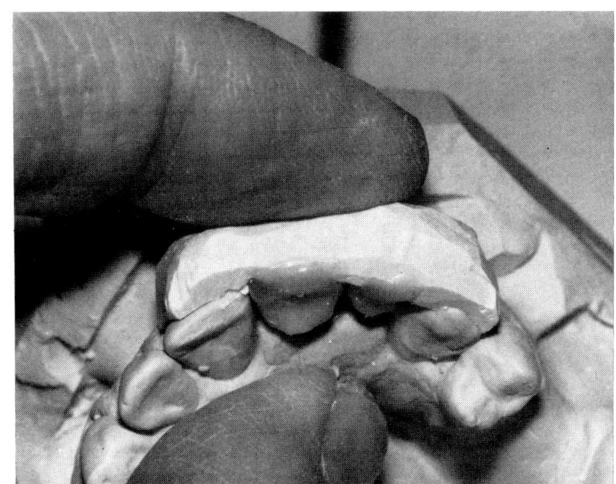

Fig. 10-21. Stone core is used to position artificial teeth on cast as framework is waxed.

FORWARDING CASTS TO LABORATORY

The mounted master casts, diagnostic casts, and work authorization order are submitted to the laboratory. The core and teeth or facings are also sent if anterior teeth will be replaced with tube teeth, facings, or RAPs.

BIBLIOGRAPHY

Askinas, S.W.: Facings in removable partial dentures, J. Prosthet. Dent. **33:** 633-636, 1975.

Beckett, L.S.: Accurate occlusal relations in partial denture construction, J. Prosthet. Dent. **4:** 487-495, 1954.

Coleman, A.J.: Occlusal requirements for removable partial dentures, J. Prosthet. Dent. **17:** 155-162, 1967.

Culpepper, W.D.: A comparative study of shade matching procedures, J. Prosthet. Dent. **24:** 166-173, 1971.

Heinlein, W.D.: Anterior teeth: esthetics and function, J. Prosthet. Dent. **44:** 389-393, 1980.

Hughes, G.A., and Regli, C.P.: What is centric relation? J. Prosthet. Dent. **11:** 16-22, 1961.

Jeffreys, F.E., and Platner, R.L.: Occlusion in removable partial dentures, J. Prosthet. Dent. **10:** 912-920, 1960.

Lytle, R.B.: Vertical relation of occlusion by the patients neuromuscular perception, J. Prosthet. Dent. **14:** 12-21, 1964.

McCracken, W.L.: Functional occlusion in removable partial denture construction, J. Prosthet. Dent. **8:** 955-963, 1958.

McCracken, W.L.: Occlusal relationships for removable partial dentures, J. Prosthet. Dent. **12:** 311-313, 1962.

Mehta, J.D., and Joglekar, A.P.: Vertical jaw relations as a factor in partial dentures, J. Prosthet. Dent. **21:** 618-625, 1969.

Reitz, P.V.: Technique for mounting removable partial dentures on an articulator, J. Prosthet. Dent. **22:** 490-499, 1969.

Robinson, S.C.: Equilibrated functional occlusions, J. Prosthet. Dent. **2:** 462-476, 1952.

Roraff, A.R., and Stansbery, B.E.: Errors caused by dimensional change in mounting material, J. Prosthet. Dent. **28:** 247-251, 1972.

Schuyler, C.H.: The function and importance of incisal guidance in oral rehabilitation, J. Prosthet. Dent. **13:** 1011, 1963.

Shanahan, T.E., and Leff, A.: Interocclusal records, J. Prosthet. Dent. **10:** 842-848, 1960.

Tench, R.W.: Dangers in dental reconstruction involving increase of the dimension of the lower third of the face, J. Am. Dent. Assoc. **25:** 566-670, 1938.

Thompson, J.R., and Brodie, A.G.: Factors in the position of the mandible, J. Am. Dent. Assoc. **29:** 925-941, 1942.

Waugh, D.B.: Arrangement of teeth in the natural and artificial dentures, Dent. Cosmos **78:** 1135, 1936.

11 Laboratory procedures for framework construction

James S. Brudvik

RESPONSIBILITY OF THE PROFESSION

The commercial dental laboratory is a business venture in the truest meaning of the word. Following instructions from a dentist, the laboratory produces a product for that dentist, never for a patient. For that product the laboratory owner is entitled to receive a fee. The amount of the fee is usually based on the quality of materials used, the degree of skill of the technician involved, and the time required to construct that product.

The relationship of the dentist and the laboratory should be one of mutual respect based on the knowledge and skill each displays in the performance of individual duties. The relationship begins to disintegrate when one or the other fails to carry out the assigned responsibility.

It is not only unfair for the dentist to expect the technician to perform tasks that are clinically oriented, it is also illegal. To ask a technician to design a partial denture on a cast is bordering on malpractice. Even if the technician is informed of the condition of the remaining teeth and soft tissue, he lacks the biologic background to recognize those areas of the mouth that can tolerate stress and those areas that must be protected. A dentist who accepts this help from a technician has abandoned the professional level of practice and has become merely a middleman in the selling of a product. This type of conduct has been tolerated for too long by the dental profession. It is difficult to fathom why a dentist could imagine that a technician is better qualified to design a partial denture than the dentist. The dentist has spent 4 years of intensive training studying the physiology of the oral cavity and the biomechanics of dental materials. This background provides the foundation required to make decisions that a technician simply is not capable of doing adequately. The technician, looking at a cast, cannot correctly select components of a partial denture to perform specific functions for definite purposes. The technician will logically use the same design for all similar partial dentures, which means the partial denture will be inadequate in a large percentage of cases.

The dentist must provide the clinical and professional aspect of patient treatment and let the technician perform those technical duties for which he has been trained.

Training of technicians

Dental laboratory technology education on a formal basis has increased rapidly during the past several decades. The great demand for dental care that resulted from the buildup of the military services during the 1940s and 1950s provided the impetus for an expanded dental laboratory need. The military services provided training for laboratory technicians, the first time this had been done on a large scale. Traditionally the technician learned the trade by on-the-job training, often beginning as the lowly plaster boy. The road to becoming an accomplished technician was long and often discouraging.

The advent of advanced technology, such as ceramics, porcelain bonded to metal, and internal attachments, required a different approach to training technicians, so formal education in the field resulted.

At present 55 *accredited* institutions offer formal dental laboratory training for 1600 students each year in the United States. Following training and a prescribed amount of experience, a technician may voluntarily be examined in one or more of five areas of expertise in the laboratory field—complete dentures, removable partial dentures, fixed partial dentures, ceramics, and orthodontics—to obtain certification. Certification is not required by any state; it serves primarily as a method whereby a technician can formally show that he or she has attained a level of proficiency greater than the average. It also may play a part in the job market, where a certified technician might be able to demand a higher salary than one who is not certified.

Registration of laboratories

Attempts have been made from time to time to certify dental laboratories. The purpose of the certification would be to control the quality of technicians and work that the laboratory performs. These attempts have never been successful, and the need for such control has never been demonstrated.

The dental laboratory business is self-policing. By self-policing it is meant that through competition laboratories are forced to maintain certain standards and to produce work of an acceptable quality. Where quality of work is inadequate, the laboratory suffers the same consequences as any business that cannot offer competition: ultimate failure.

Most states, however, do require that all laboratories that do business with a dentist licensed in that state be registered in that state. Technicians employed in the registered laboratories must also be individually registered.

Registration of technicians and laboratories is thought to be one method of combating the illegal practice of dentistry (denturism). Denturism is defined by the 1973 House of Delegates of the American Dental Association as the illegal fitting and dispensing of dentures to the public. Unfortunately, denturism is expanding primarily because of the political power of some uninformed but well-financed individuals and organizations who, behind the vote-getting battle cry of delivering economical denture care to the poor and needy, are in truth attempting to reap profits from the unsuspecting public.

Wherever the need for the denturist has been looked at in legal and legislative terms for the protection of the health and well-being of the public, the effort of permitting the nonprofessional to serve the public directly has failed. It is only after long and costly campaigns have been waged to appeal to the wallet of the uninformed voter that success has been achieved.

Campaigns to win voters to back the denturist movement by appealing to the financial aspect of denture care alone is akin to flooding the voter with misinformation and scare tactics in defeating referendums to establish fluoridation of public water supplies, a long-known and medically proven safe and effective means of controlling dental caries.

Work authorization order

All states now require that all work submitted to a dental laboratory by a dentist be accompanied by written instructions (Fig. 11-1). Few states have yet established a standard form that must be used, but most have listed in the state dental practice act the information that must be included on each work authorization order. The minimum information required by most states includes (1) the signature and license number of the dentist, (2) the date the authorization was signed, (3) the name and address of the patient (because of privacy laws, some states require only a patient identification number), and (4) a description of the kind and type of act or service or material ordered.

If the work authorization is used correctly, it represents an excellent line of communication between the dentist and the laboratory. The dentist should supply the laboratory with as much information, clearly phrased, as the technician will need to produce the requested prosthesis. The laboratory should never hesitate to contact the submitting dentist if the instructions are open to question or if further information is needed. Once this two-way avenue of communication is established, the quality of the work, both that submitted by the dentist and that returned by the laboratory, can be significantly improved.

In addition to providing instruction to the laboratory, the work authorization order also serves as a form of legal protection for both the dentist and dental laboratory technician if a lawsuit arises involving either party. For this reason most states require that both the dentist and the laboratory maintain a copy of each work authorization order on the premises for 2 years.

The work authorization order also serves to prove that the work was submitted to and accomplished by a legitimate and legal laboratory, another method of protecting the public from the illegal practice of dentistry. It also establishes clearly the separate responsibility of the dentist and the laboratory technician.

Design of work authorization order

Each teaching institution, each of the uniformed services, each large commercial dental laboratory, and each practicing dentist has designed and uses a form that suits the local requirement. Most forms are designed so that a carbon copy is made as the form is completed, one for the laboratory and one for the dentist.

The form should be designed so that it is easily read and so that a minimum of handwriting is required. An entry that cannot be deciphered or interpreted is worse than no entry at all. A series of boxes to indicate the desired components or the desired material that can be simply checked will save time and be completely understandable to the technician.

The form must be legible, concise, and clearly understood. Information that might be of interest to the dentist but carries little meaning to the technician should be avoided. However, the usual problem with work authorization orders is not extraneous information but lack of information. Too often such statements as "Make partial denture, keep it light" or "Don't use too many clasps" are the total instruction. Many dentists presume that the duties of the technician are more encompassing than they actually are. It is unfair to technicians to assume they will do things that are not part of their fair responsibility.

It is doubtful that a single form can be efficiently de-

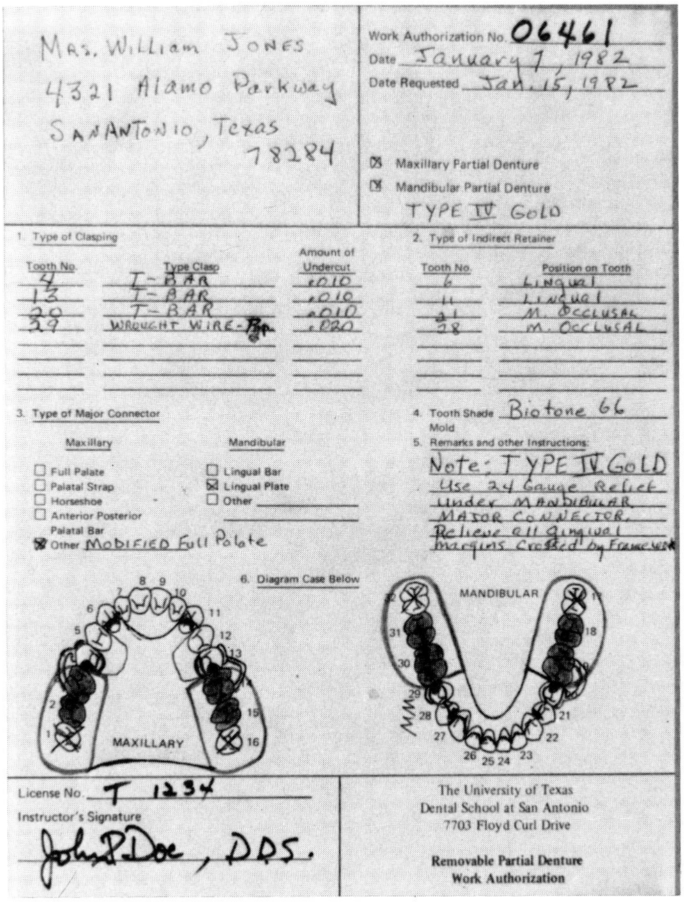

Mrs. William Jones
4321 Alamo Parkway
San Antonio, Texas
78284

Work Authorization No. 06461
Date January 1, 1982
Date Requested Jan. 15, 1982

☒ Maxillary Partial Denture
☒ Mandibular Partial Denture
TYPE IV GOLD

1. Type of Clasping

Tooth No.	Type Clasp	Amount of Undercut
4	T-BAR	.010
13	T-BAR	.010
20	T-BAR	.010
29	WROUGHT WIRE-[illegible]	.020

2. Type of Indirect Retainer

Tooth No.	Position on Tooth
6	Lingual
11	Lingual
21	M. Occlusal
28	M. Occlusal

3. Type of Major Connector

Maxillary
☐ Full Palate
☐ Palatal Strap
☐ Horseshoe
☐ Anterior Posterior Palatal Bar
☒ Other Modified Full Palate

Mandibular
☐ Lingual Bar
☒ Lingual Plate
☐ Other

4. Tooth Shade Biotone 66
Mold

5. Remarks and other Instructions:
Note: TYPE IV GOLD
Use 24 Gauge Relief under MANDIBULAR MAJOR CONNECTOR.
Relieve all gingival margins crossed by Framework

6. Diagram Case Below

MAXILLARY
MANDIBULAR

License No. T 1234
Instructor's Signature
John P. Doe, DDS.

The University of Texas
Dental School at San Antonio
7703 Floyd Curl Drive

Removable Partial Denture Work Authorization

Fig. 11-1. Work authorization order.

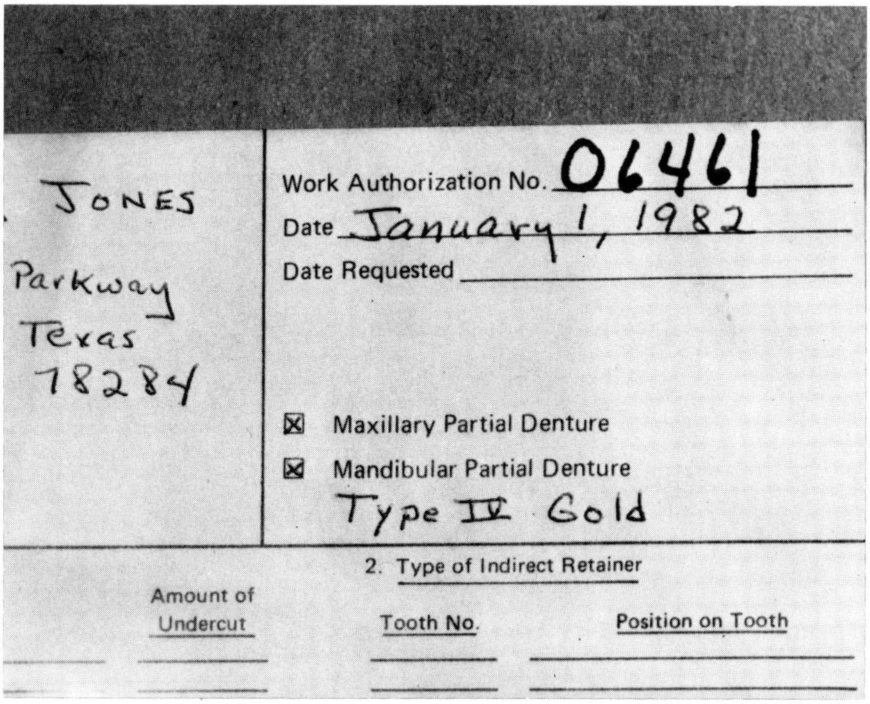

JONES
Parkway
Texas
78284

Work Authorization No. 06461
Date January 1, 1982
Date Requested

☒ Maxillary Partial Denture
☒ Mandibular Partial Denture
Type IV Gold

2. Type of Indirect Retainer

Amount of Undercut	Tooth No.	Position on Tooth

Fig. 11-2. Work authorization order number, the date, and the type of prosthesis requested must be included on order in most states.

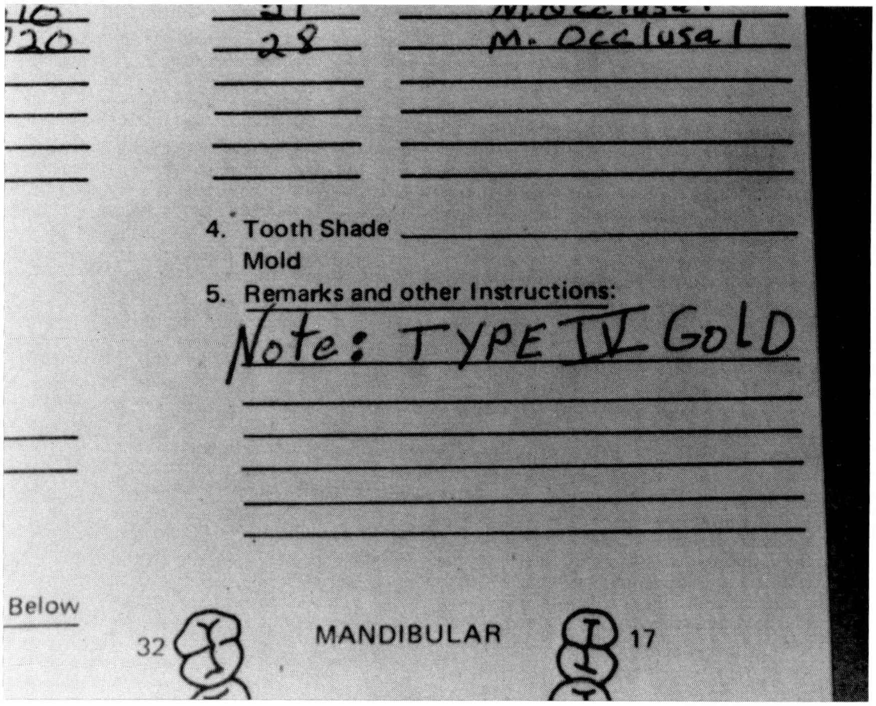

28 M. Occlusal

4. Tooth Shade
Mold
5. Remarks and other Instructions:
Note: TYPE IV GOLD

Below
32 MANDIBULAR 17

Fig. 11-3. Type of metal to be used in framework is included in Remarks section.

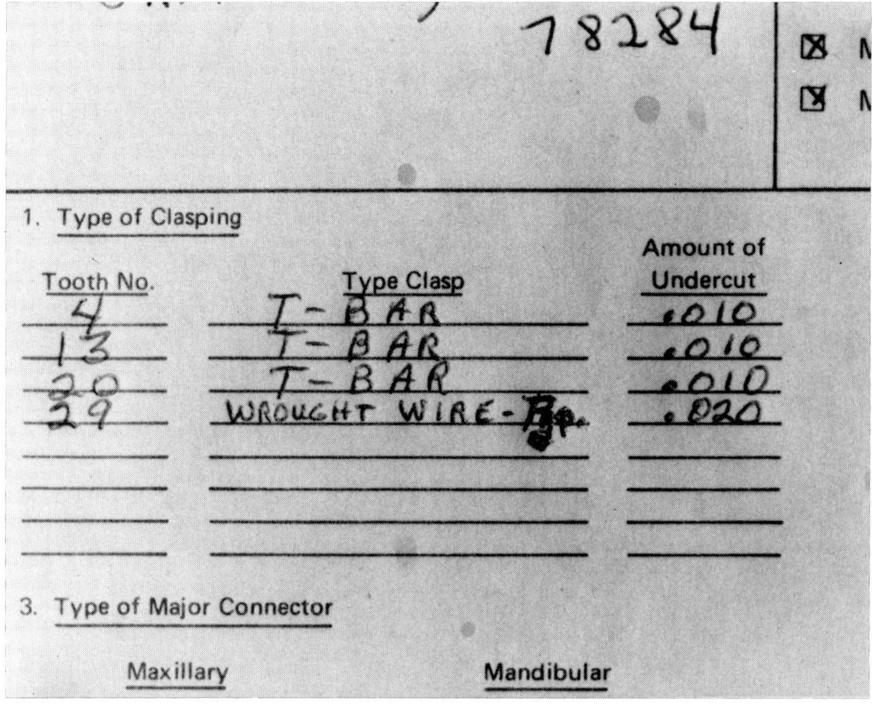

78284

1. Type of Clasping

Tooth No.	Type Clasp	Amount of Undercut
4	T-BAR	.010
13	T-BAR	.010
20	T-BAR	.010
29	WROUGHT WIRE-[illegible]	.020

3. Type of Major Connector

Maxillary Mandibular

Fig. 11-4. Types of retentive clasps are indicated clearly and briefly.

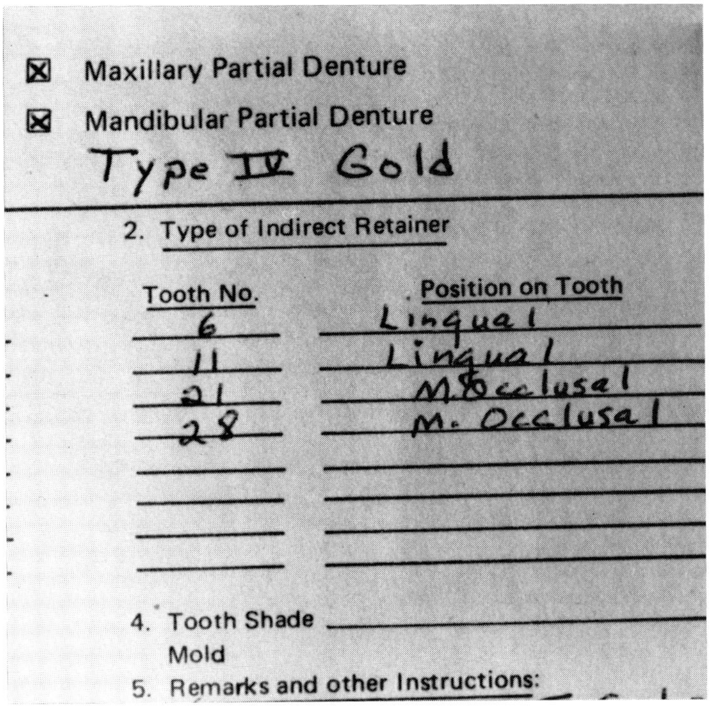

☒ Maxillary Partial Denture

☒ Mandibular Partial Denture

Type IV Gold

2. Type of Indirect Retainer

Tooth No.	Position on Tooth
6	Lingual
11	Lingual
21	M. Occlusal
28	M. Occlusal

4. Tooth Shade

Mold

5. Remarks and other Instructions:

Fig. 11-5. Indirect retainers are listed separately.

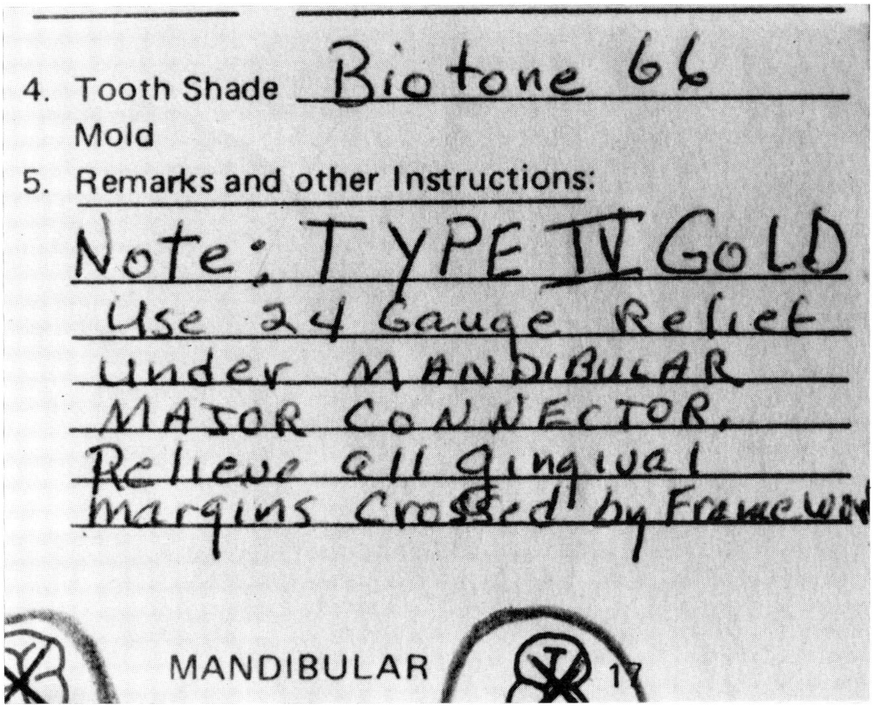

4. Tooth Shade Biotone 66

Mold

5. Remarks and other Instructions:

Note: TYPE IV GOLD
Use 24 Gauge Relief
under MANDIBULAR
MAJOR CONNECTOR.
Relieve all gingival
margins Crossed by Framew...

MANDIBULAR 17

Fig. 11-6. Remarks section is used for special instructions to laboratory technician.

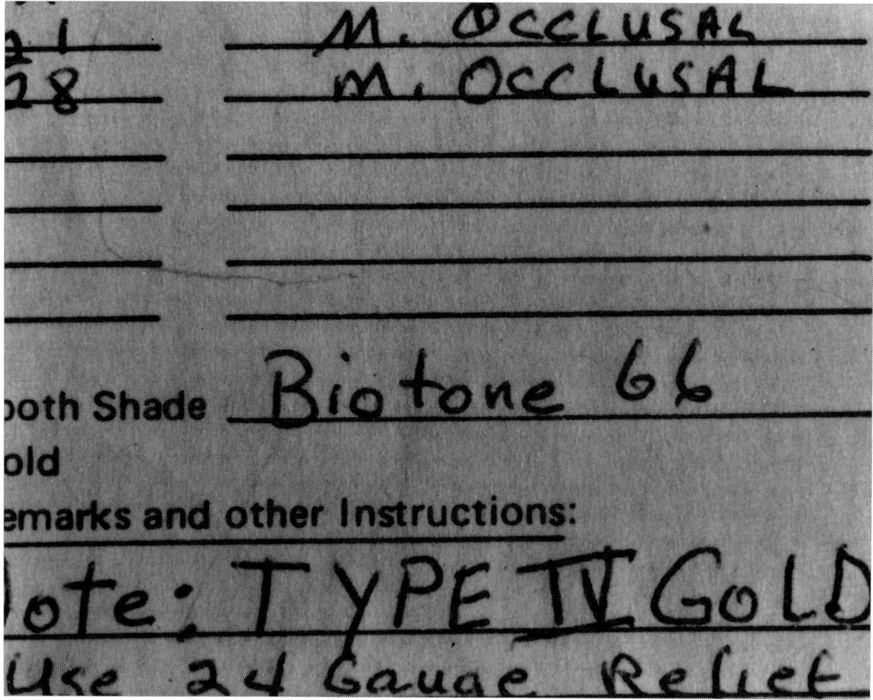

1 M. OCCLUSAL
28 M. OCCLUSAL

ooth Shade Biotone 66
old
emarks and other Instructions:
ote: TYPE IV GOLD
Use 24 Gauge Relief

Fig. 11-7. Type of shade guide used is included in instructions.

signed for instructions in all laboratory phases connected with the construction of removable partial dentures, complete dentures, crowns, fixed partial dentures, ceramics, and orthodontic laboratory procedures. Confusion would be apt to result if this were attempted. The safe approach is to develop an individual form for each phase of laboratory work.

During the course of patient treatment it is often necessary to submit to the laboratory the same prosthesis more than once. Casts for removable partial dentures may be submitted for framework construction, resubmitted for tooth set-up for try-in, and finally resubmitted for processing and finishing the denture bases. Attempting to use the same work authorization form for each of the steps is foolhardy because the technician will have difficulty relating the instructions to the correct phase. It is wiser to use a new work authorization order for each submission.

To help the laboratory identify the case as it passes through the laboratory, the form should have the doctor's and patient's names prominently displayed. The work authorization number assigned by the laboratory and the type of partial denture—maxillary or mandibular—should also be plainly indicated (Fig. 11-2).

Indication of the kind of metal desired for use in the framework construction is perhaps not as critical as it once was. The number of gold frameworks requested is going to be limited and for the few desired it might be better to add this in the Special Remarks section (Fig. 11-3). (Type IV gold is the type used in the construction of partial denture frameworks.) Most commercial dental laboratories that offer removable partial denture service are franchised to one of the major manufacturers of chrome-cobalt alloy and have the laboratory equipment needed to process that particular alloy. The casting of chrome alloy frameworks in the private dental laboratory is no longer feasible because of the special equipment and materials required.

It is good practice to list the teeth that are to be clasped along with the type of clasp (simple circlet, reverse circlet, T-bar) and also the amount of retention desired (Fig. 11-4). There will be times when it will be necessary to change the amount of retention, expressed in thousandths of an inch, from that which is normally used. This must be explained to the laboratory clearly and succinctly. There will also be times when bracing or stabilizing clasps only are wanted and no retention is desired. This is one area that is often misinterpreted by a technician.

The position of the critical components such as indirect retainers should be listed separately and distinctly (Fig. 11-5).

Perhaps the most important portion of the work authorization order is the Remarks and Special Instruc-

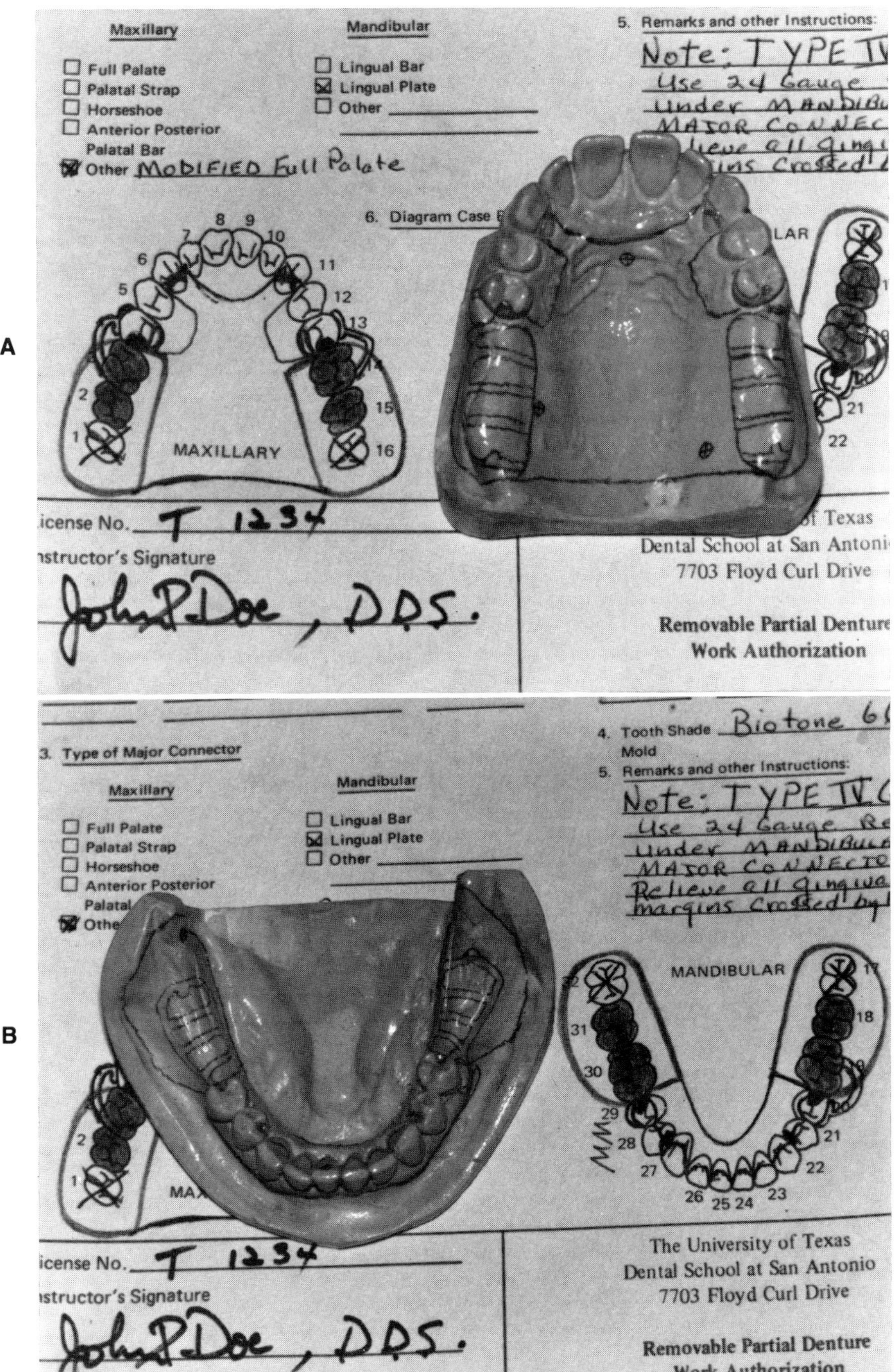

Fig. 11-8. A, The properly completed diagram of prosthesis helps laboratory identify case. **B,** Components of partial denture are drawn as to size and location.

tions section (Fig. 11-6). It is in this section that instructions that separate the removable partial denture designed to serve the special biologic conditions of each patient from the more routine partial denture must be included. Any portion of the design that deviates from the norm should be listed in this section.

The tooth selection portion of the form must be handled carefully. It is up to the dentist to determine the size and number of artificial teeth to be used as replacements. The type of artificial tooth and the material from which it is made, porcelain or plastic, must be indicated. Not only should the shade of tooth desired be listed, but also the shade guide that was used (Fig. 11-7). Shades from one guide to another can differ drastically.

In years past it was considered essential to inform the laboratory as to the thickness or width of major components of the partial denture. With the advent of the chrome-cobalt alloy systems this is not as critical as it once was. Manufacturers of each chrome-cobalt alloy system now supply to the laboratories plastic forms for major connectors, clasps, and lesser components of the correct thickness or bulk to ensure the proper degree of flexibility or total rigidity, whichever may be required. However, when special requirements exist for individual partial dentures, instructions should be added in the Remarks section. For example, if there is an extremely long lingual bar that might prove to be nonrigid, the instruction could be given to add a strip of 30-gauge wax to the plastic lingual bar form to increase rigidity.

The final section of the work authorization order to be completed is the diagram of the case submitted (Fig. 11-8). This should be done with care but should not be substituted for the completely designed diagnostic casts, which should always accompany the master casts to the laboratory. The design should include an indication of the missing teeth. The missing teeth that are to be replaced by the partial denture should be completely blacked out. Teeth that are missing but are not to be replaced (for example, the third molars) are indicated by an X through the teeth. The major connector, particularly the maxillary major connector, should be drawn to the extent desired. The configuration of the clasps should also be included.

One of the purposes of the diagrammed design, other than to remind the technician of the dentist's desire, is to serve as a verification that the proper casts are in the correct laboratory case pan in the event the casts and case pan become separated during the laboratory procedures.

The use of the work authorization order is essential for good dentist-laboratory communication and is required by the dental practice acts of most states. It should not be interpreted, however, as the absolute best in instruction in removable partial denture construction. It serves as a valuable adjunct to the completely designed diagnostic casts, which should always accompany the work authorization form. To the technician who transfers the design of the removable partial denture from the diagnostic cast to the master cast, the combination of the design on the diagnostic cast and the design and other information contained on the work authorization form should prove the ultimate in accurate instructions.

After all is said and done, whether the dentist assumes the proper degree of responsibility in designing and supervising the laboratory phases of partial denture construction or not, the legal weight of the consequences of patient treatment rests totally on the dentist, never on the technician.

In order for dentistry to maintain its status in the learned professions, it must cease delegating any of its professional activities to allied associates who are less qualified. The dentist is always responsible for all professional services.

LABORATORY PROCEDURES

There is no area of dentistry other than framework construction where a major part of patient treatment is delegated outside the dental office. The removable partial denture framework constructed in this manner requires a high level of communication between clinician and technician if a quality denture is to be achieved.

Knowledge of the laboratory phase of partial denture construction is essential for the clinician, who must assume total responsibility for the design and the quality control of all aspects of this construction. For the laboratory construction of the removable partial denture (1) a properly prepared and articulated master cast, (2) a diagnostic cast with a neat and specific design carefully drawn on it, and (3) a work authorization order covering all aspects of the desired denture are required. Anything less will compromise quality.

Design transfer

Before actual construction can begin, the design must be placed on the master cast. Since each laboratory employs its own system of design drawing, the best results can be expected when the laboratory technician transfers the design from the diagnostic cast.

A common color code in the dental lab industry has brown representing metal contours, blue for resin outline, red for areas requiring relief, and black to mark the height of contour on hard and soft tissue. These colors contrast sufficiently to eliminate confusion in design transfer.

Retripoding the master cast

When the clinician has determined a specific path of insertion and removal for the denture and has prepared both hard and soft tissues in harmony with this path, it is critical that this exact relation be maintained.

Three widely separated marks placed on the master cast with the dental surveyor vertical rod in a fixed position will allow rapid repositioning of the cast in the laboratory (Fig. 11-9). These marks must be placed in areas that are not involved with design outlines. To simplify this repositioning for the technician, the marks are placed on the lingual surfaces of the cast such that all three can be seen from the same view (Fig. 11-10). Should the technician *not* be able to view all three marks at once, the time required to regain the desired cast position is increased and may lead to frustration and indifference to the clinician's wishes. When the three marks are in the same horizontal plane, the table is securely locked.

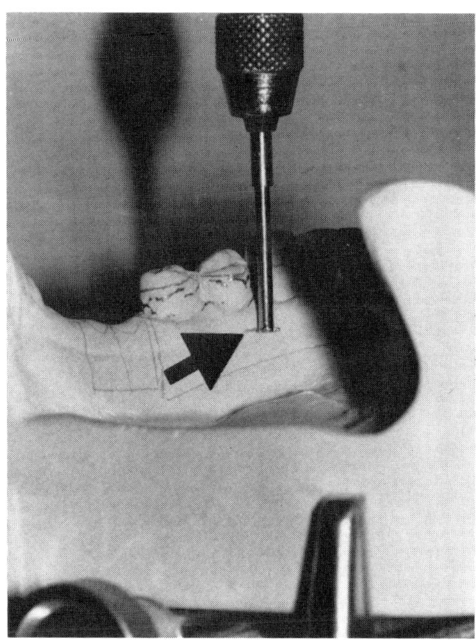

Fig. 11-9. Vertical rod in surveyor used to place reference mark on cast (arrow).

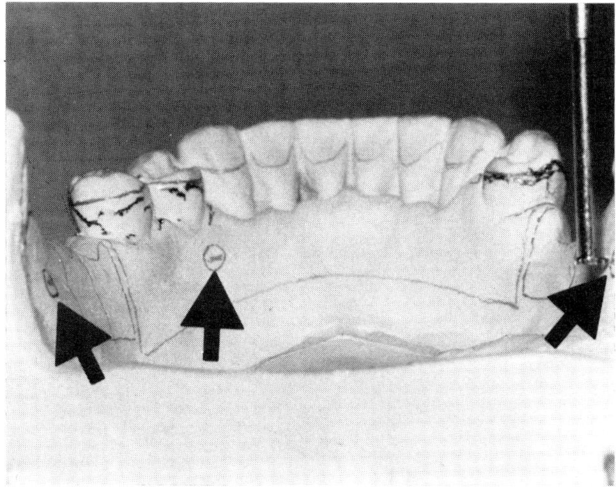

Fig. 11-10. Reference marks (arrows) placed so that all three are seen in same view.

Height of contour

With the master cast positioned on the survey table by the three tripod marks, the technician will substitute a pencil lead for the analyzing rod in the surveyor arm and place the height of contour line on involved teeth and soft tissue areas (Fig. 11-11). The survey table is moved smoothly along the surveyor base to contact the lead. Since the locked survey table maintains the predetermined special position of the cast, the vertical spindle of the surveyor can be released and the contour line scribed on the cast. Special care should be taken in the area of the retentive clasp tip. The lead must be replaced as soon as it begins to show wear so that the line it traces will always be sharp and clear.

Metal transfer

Without removing the master cast from the survey table or changing the tilt, the technician transfers the

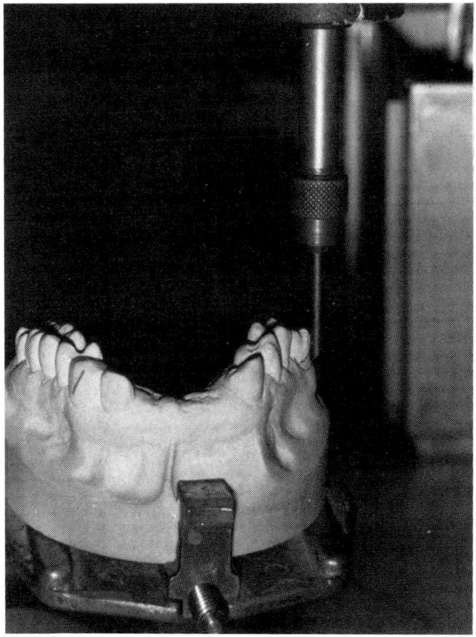

Fig. 11-11. Height of contour line is placed on cast with marking lead in surveyor.

design from the diagnostic cast (Fig. 11-12). Each laboratory has its own special schematics to identify finishing lines, resin retention, clasp position, and so on. Areas of special consideration (for example, undercut depths for retentive clasp arms, gauge of wrought wire clasps, cast clasp pattern size) and other critical items should be written in the work authorization order as well as drawn on the diagnostic cast. A dense cast of improved dental stone is unlikely to be damaged by the design transfer drawing. In those situations where the master cast is weak with a chalky surface, care must be taken to not abrade the cast surface with the pencil lead.

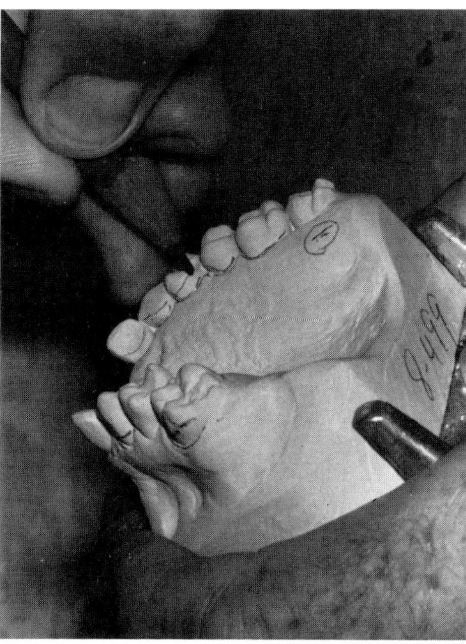

Fig. 11-12. Design of framework is transferred from diagnostic cast to master cast.

Blockout and relief

The elimination of undesirable undercuts on the master cast with wax is commonly referred to as *blocking out*. Both hard and soft tissue areas will require blockout so that the completed casting will go completely to place along the desired path of insertion. Should the metal engage some of these undercut areas, complete seating will not be possible without adjustment.

Cast preparation

Before the addition of the blockout wax, maxillary casts will be beaded (Fig. 11-13); that is, the outline of the major connector will be scraped into the master cast to half the diameter of a No. 2 round bur. This will result in a bead line on the finished maxillary casting that will ensure positive contact against the palatal tissues and greatly reduce the packing of food beneath the major connector. The bead line does not run all the way to the gingival margin but stops 3 to 4 mm from it. Beading is *not* done on the mandibular major connector, because it lies almost entirely on thin, unattached gingiva that cannot tolerate the positive contact.

The master cast must also be treated with a sealer (model spray). The model spray, an aerosol plastic, deposits a film on the cast that seals it and protects the design throughout the blockout and duplication process. The spraying must be done *after* the design is transferred because the pencil lines will not remain on

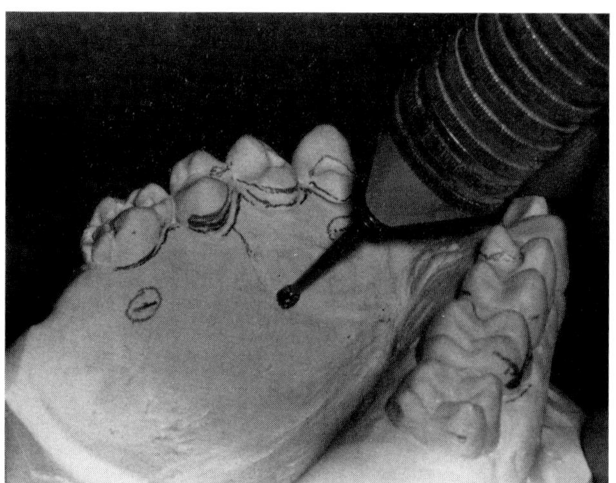

Fig. 11-13. No. 2 round bur is used to place bead on soft tissue area of cast to indicate outline of maxillary major connector.

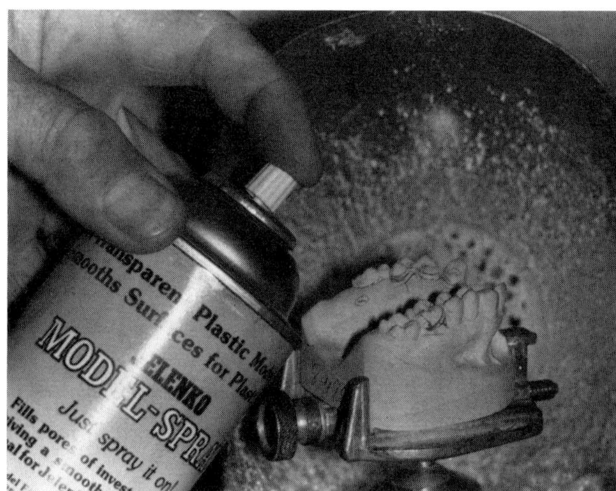

Fig. 11-14. Cast is sprayed with model spray in front of a suction vent to prevent inhalation of potentially harmful aerosol plastic.

a sprayed cast. The application of the model spray should be done in front of a suction vent because inhaling the aerosal is potentially dangerous (Fig. 11-14). The technician should wear a face (surgical) mask while spraying. It is not advisable to place any more spray on the master cast than is necessary to wet the surface. A buildup of spray will create a false contour, which will be carried into the refractory cast and result in an inaccurate casting. After the sprayed cast is allowed to dry for at least 5 minutes, the addition of the blockout wax can begin.

Blockout technique

Blockout wax can be purchased as a commercially prepared product or it can be compounded to the technician's personal preference by using a combination of common dental waxes. One sheet of soft baseplate wax with one stick of green inlay wax will yield a compound that is neither too brittle nor too soft. The wax is normally kept fluid in an electrically heated pot during the working day. It is placed on the master cast with a spatula (Fig. 11-15).

It is *absolutely critical* that the blockout wax be placed only below the height of contour and not in the area to be contacted by the clasp tip (Fig. 11-16). Any wax placed above the contour line and not completely removed during the shaping of the wax with the blockout instrument *adds* to the dimension of the refractory cast and will result in a casting that does not contact the tooth in that area. Attempts to remove wax from above the contour line with the blockout instrument run the risk of removing some of the cast surface. When the cast's surface is weak or chalky, this scraping action *subtracts* from the dimension of the cast and inevitably results in a casting that is too small to seat without reshaping. Efforts to adjust the metal are always arbitrary and require a trial-and-error approach that often abrades the master cast. Although the casting may fit the master cast, it may not fit the mouth. If this problem is encountered often, the clinician should verify the laboratory's blockout procedures.

When excess blockout wax has been placed into all undercut areas where the framework will contact the teeth (Fig. 11-17), the actual shaping of the wax can begin.

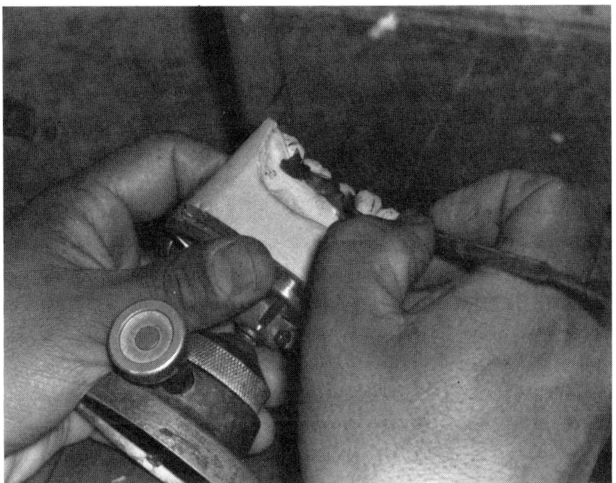

Fig. 11-15. Fluid blockout wax is placed on cast with a spatula.

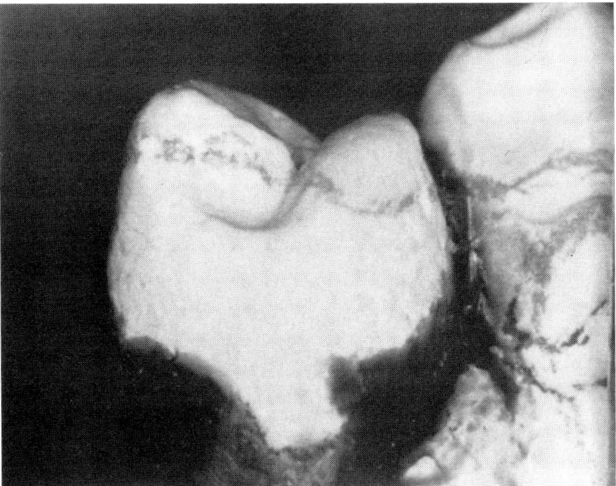

Fig. 11-16. Blockout wax must not be placed above survey line or in area to be occupied by retentive clasp tip.

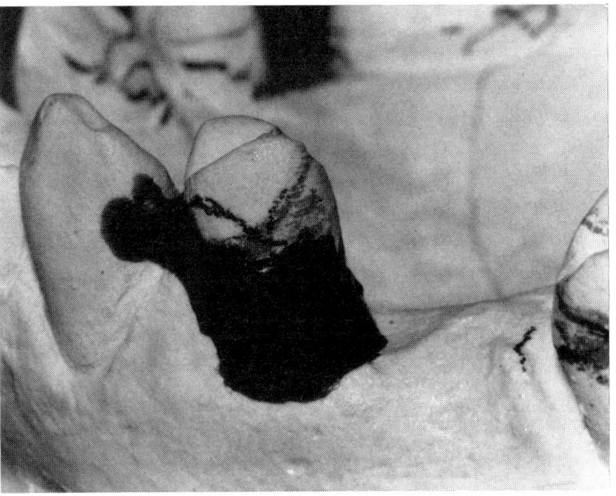

Fig. 11-17. Excess blockout wax is placed in undercut areas in preparation for shaping.

Tapered versus parallel blockout. The blockout wax is shaped by contouring it in some predetermined relation to the desired path of insertion. Excess wax is removed with a bladelike device mounted in the dental surveyor (Fig. 11-18). The blade surface will normally be perpendicular to the surveyor base. Other blades are available that offer a degree of taper from the vertical (usually 2 to 4 degrees). Large commercial laboratories often employ electrically heated shaping blades attached to long (3-foot) rods suspended at right angles to a flat base. These rods are connected to a vertical support with elastics, allowing a range of motion. They can be positioned to provide a range of taper to the wax by placing the cast on a specific area of the base.

The decision to block out the undercuts exactly parallel to the path of insertion and removal or to allow some degree of taper is a clinical one and should be included in the work authorization order. All tooth-borne partial dentures can be blocked out parallel to the path, whereas tooth-tissue-borne dentures may be given a tapered blockout to allow some freedom of movement in function before the framework binds on the abutment teeth. Personal design philosophy will determine the degree of blockout.

Wax contouring. With the blockout blade properly positioned, the excess wax is carefully removed from beneath the height of contour until the entire undercut has been shaped (Fig. 11-19). The blade can be warmed slightly by passing it over a burner flame to make the contouring easier.

When infrabulge clasp arms are to be used, soft tissue undercuts in the area of the clasp arm must be

A

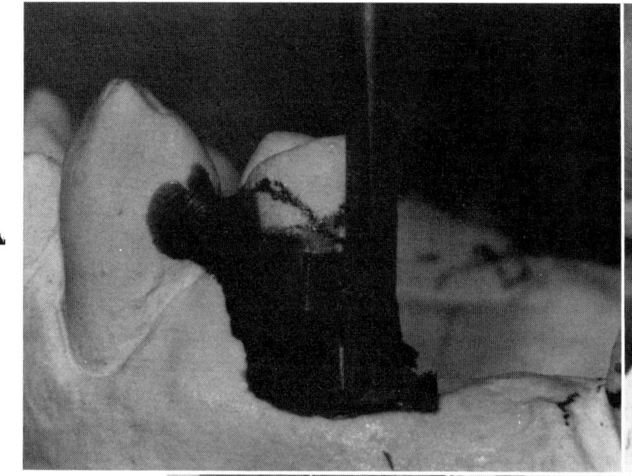

B

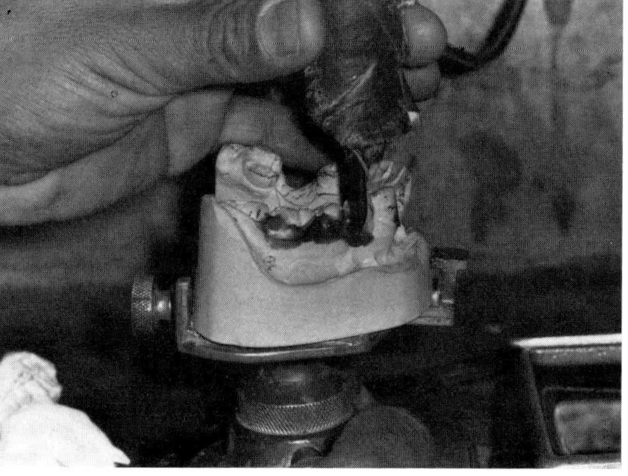

C

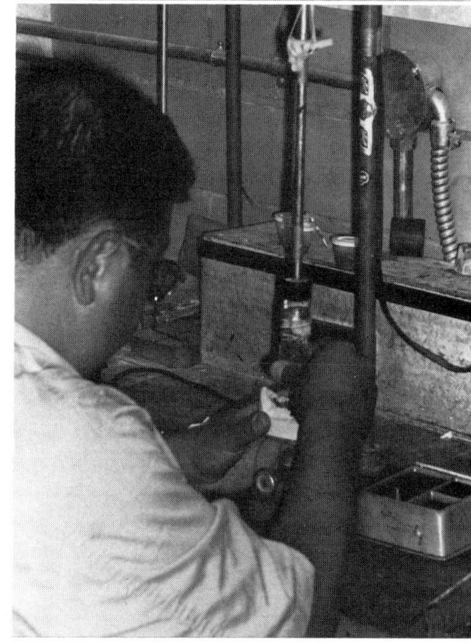

Fig. 11-18. Excess wax may be removed with a parallel wax carving blade, **A,** or a tapered blade, **B,** placed in surveyor, or with an electrically heated shaping blade, **C.**

blocked out as well (Fig. 11-20). If this phase is carefully carried out, the results will be a smooth layer of wax that eliminates all undesirable undercuts. Smooth wax will result in a uniform internal surface on the casting. The wax can be smoothed by careful flaming with the torch. (If this is overdone, undercuts can be recreated.)

The area involved with the clasp tip is critical to the success of the denture. The blockout wax can be shaped with hand instruments to provide a slight ledge just apical to the clasp tip (Fig. 11-21). This ledge guides the placement of the wax or plastic pattern to ensure that the clasp actually lies at the desired position in the undercut area.

Inadequate mouth preparation may leave undercuts in the area of the body and shoulder of the clasp arm. Since only one third to one fourth of the clasp should be placed in the undercut, these areas will require blockout. No part of the clasp arm proximal to the tip can lie in an undercut if the clasp is to function properly (Fig 11-22). It is the clinician's responsibility to evaluate tooth contours on the master cast before submission to the laboratory to ensure that the clasp can be constructed as designed.

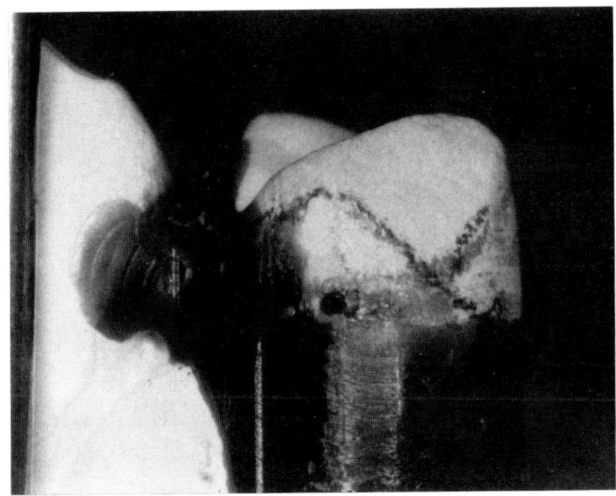

Fig. 11-19. Excess wax has been removed to shape entire undercut area.

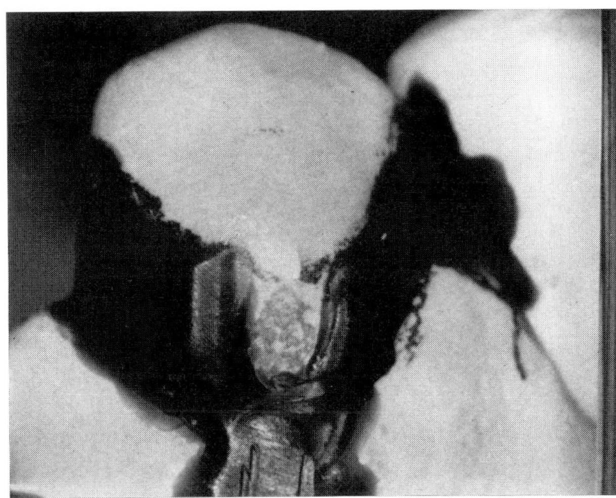

Fig. 11-20. Soft tissue undercuts are blocked out in areas to be covered by approach arm of an infrabulge clasp.

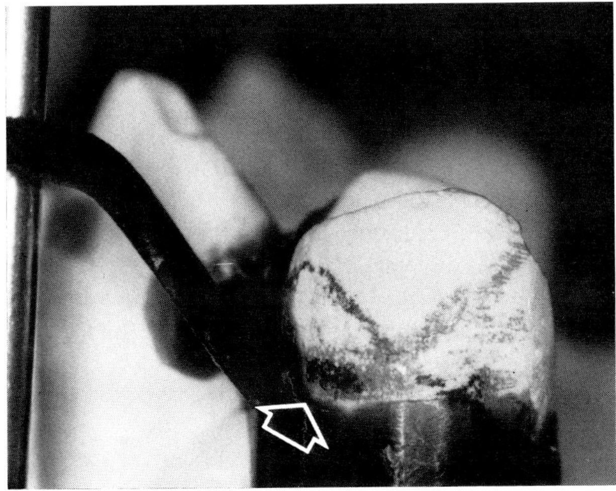

Fig. 11-21. A hand instrument is used to carve a narrow ledge of blockout wax (arrow) to help position apical margin of retentive clasp tip.

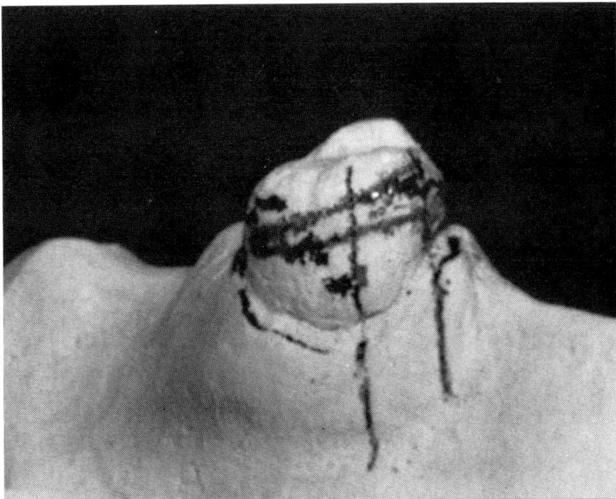

Fig. 11-22. Only the distal one third of retention clasp arm can lie in an undercut.

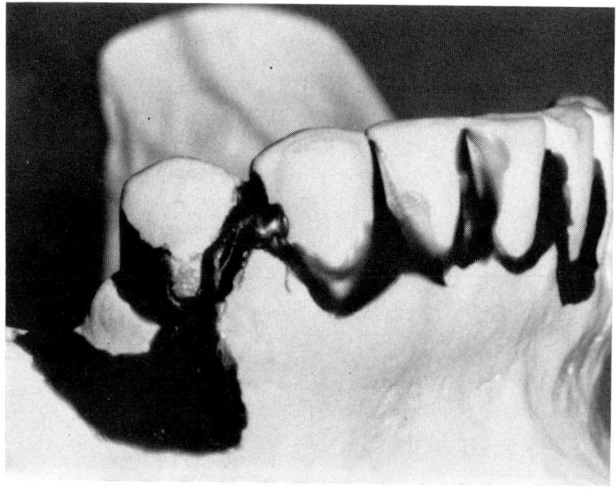

Fig. 11-23. Undercuts in areas not involved with framework are blocked out with wax.

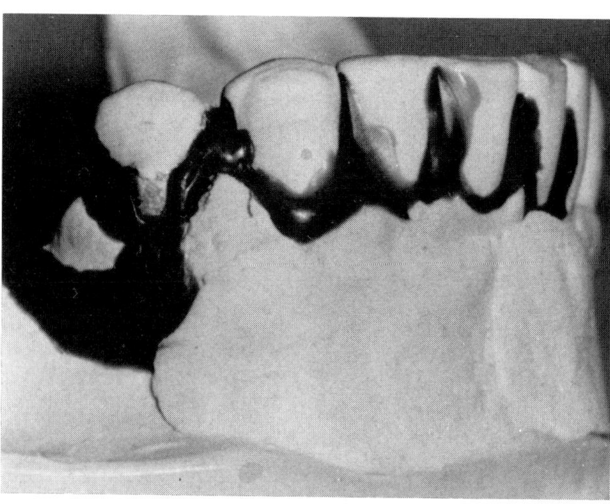

Fig. 11-24. Large undercuts in noncritical areas are arbitrarily blocked out with clay or similar material.

Arbitrary blockout. Areas of undercut not involved with the framework should also be recontoured with wax to minimize distortion during duplication (Fig. 11-23). The duplication colloids can rebound from the distortion caused by removing the cast from the mold only if there are no large undercuts present (2 to 3 mm maximum). Larger undercuts will distort or even tear the fragile colloid. This blockout is arbitrary and is *not* contoured with the blockout instrument. Areas of gross soft tissue undercuts can be arbitrarily eliminated using soft wax, clay, mortite, or similar material (Fig. 11-24).

Deep maxillary palatal clefts and irregularities in the area covered by the major connector are flushed with wax to eliminate potential sharp areas on the tissue surface of the casting (Fig. 11-25).

The same approach is taken with the mandibular cast. Since intimate soft tissue contact is not desirable because of the thin unattached tissue, a great amount of finishing time can be saved by flowing a very small amount of wax over the major connector area and smoothing the wax by flaming or polishing it with gauze or cotton batten (Fig. 11-26).

Relief

The construction of the removable partial denture requires that specific areas be deliberately relieved. The most common relief is associated with the denture base. The retentive meshwork must be raised above the edentulous area to allow resin to completely surround it. The thickness of the relief wax determines the amount of space for resin under the frame mesh. There is a common tendency to make this relief too thin. The technician knows that the higher the mesh is off the ridge, the more time and effort it will take to fit the denture teeth over the mesh. It is, however, critical to the long-term success of the denture that at least 1 mm of resin surround the tissue surface of the mesh. Thinner resin is often porous and weak and should not be in contact with soft tissue, especially at the free gingival margin of the abutment teeth.

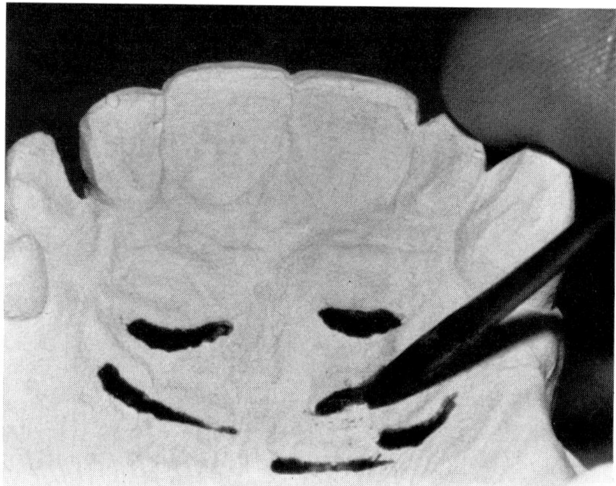

Fig. 11-25. Palatal clefts and other irregularities in areas to be covered by maxillary major connector are filled in with wax.

One margin of the relief wax forms the internal finish line of the framework. The clinician must demand that a sharp, definite internal finish line be present on every denture. The finish line must have a uniform depth of at least 1 mm and be no closer than 1.5 to 2 mm from the abutment teeth. This distance will ensure that po-

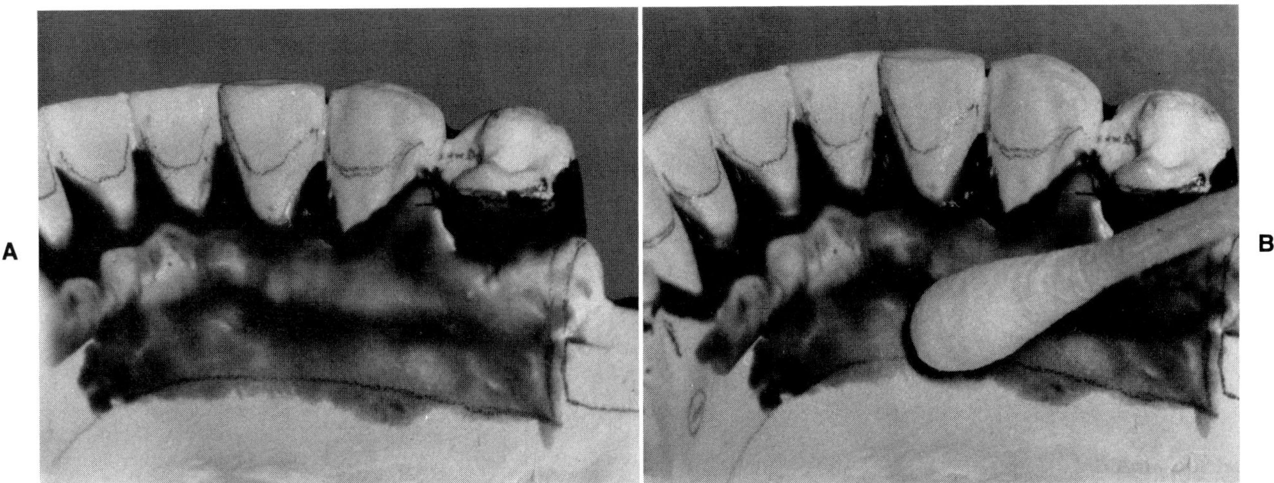

Fig. 11-26. A, Thin layer of wax is used to create a smooth surface in areas to be covered by mandibular major connector. **B,** Cotton applicator stick is used to smooth wax.

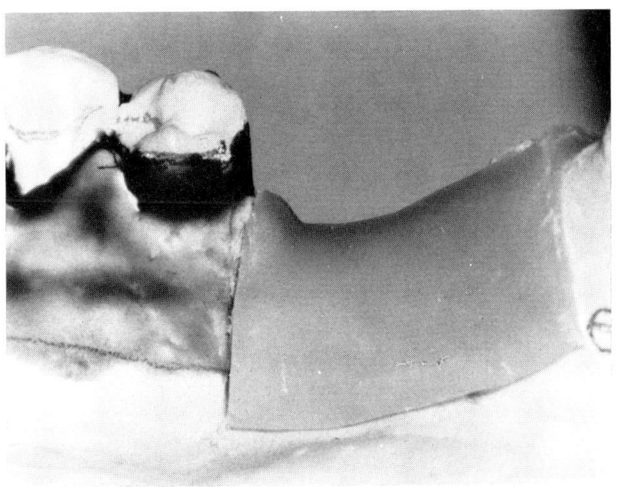

Fig. 11-27. Relief wax forming internal finish line is placed 1.5 to 2 mm from the abutment tooth.

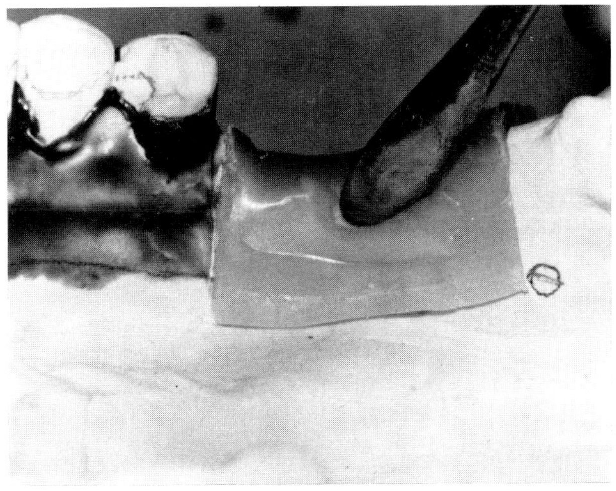

Fig. 11-28. Relief wax is luted to cast with a hot spatula.

rous resin does not come in contact with marginal gingiva (Fig. 11-27).

One thickness of baseplate wax makes an ideal mesh relief pad. The wax is softened over the flame and placed on the cast to cover the meshwork design. It must be luted to the cast with a hot spatula so that it does not separate and lift from the cast during duplication (Fig. 11-28). Special wax sheets with adhesive on one side are available to facilitate the placement of the pad.

When the wax is firmly attached to the cast, it is trimmed to the internal finish line with a sharp blade. The blade must be held at 90 degrees to the surface of the cast so that the internal finish line in the casting will be sharp and allow the metal-resin junction to be at right angles. A small square of wax must be removed at the designed tissue stop; 2 mm is sufficient for a solid tissue stop (Fig. 11-29). Again, the blade must be at 90 degrees to the cast.

There is no need to trim any other part of the mesh relief wax. The sheet need only cover the design and can end anywhere in the denture base area.

Tori, maxillary and mandibular, are often relieved with a uniform wax covering. Both the work authorization order and the diagnostic cast should carry the information to instruct the technician as to position and

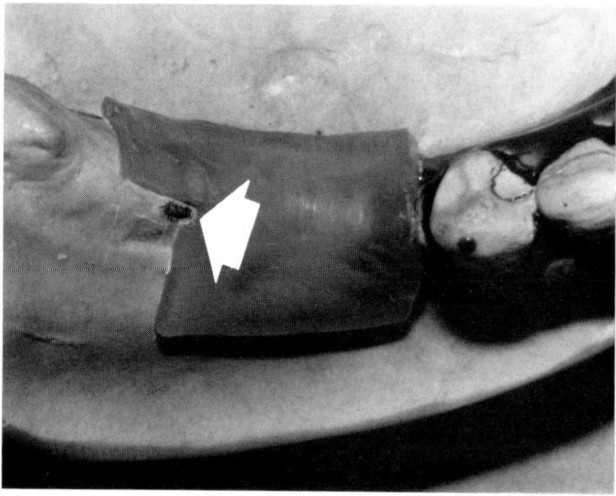

Fig. 11-29. A 2-mm square of wax (arrow) is removed to allow placement of a tissue stop.

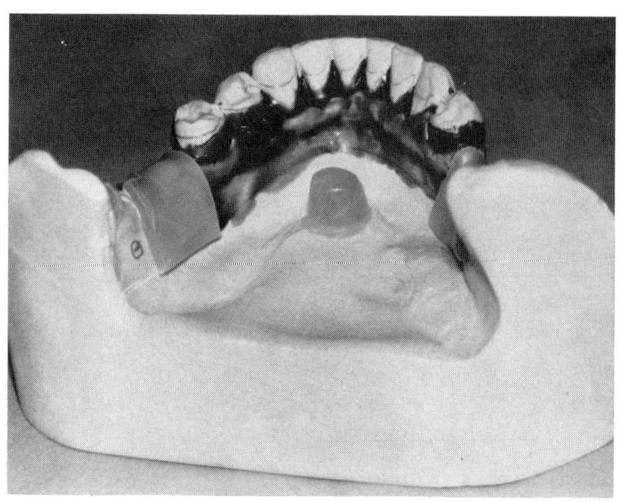

Fig. 11-30. A tapered cylinder of wax is placed on cast in position where main sprue will be placed on refractory cast.

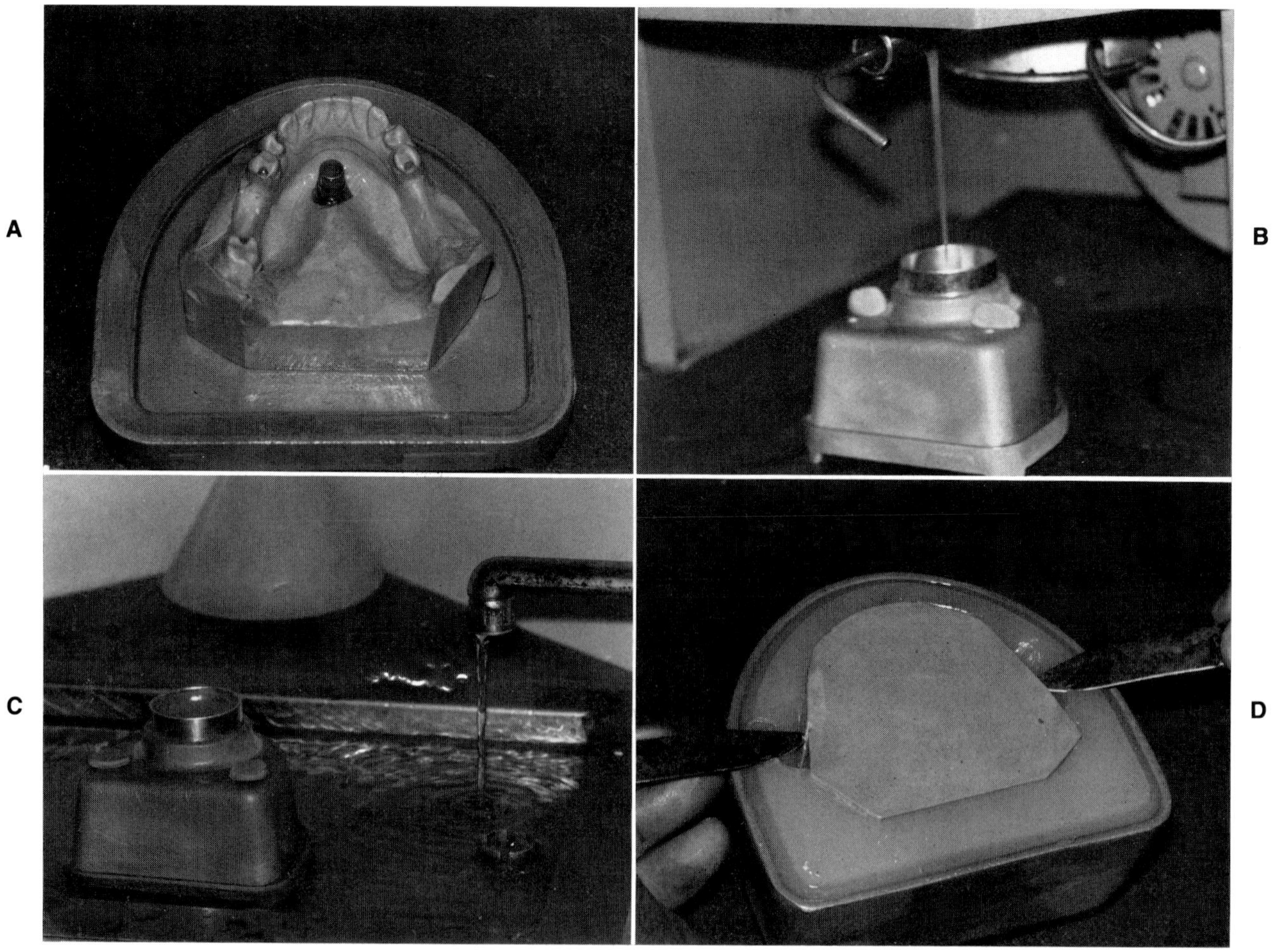

Fig. 11-31. A, Relieved and blocked out master cast is positioned on base of the duplicating flask. **B,** Duplicating flask is filled slowly with hydrocolloid material. **C,** Base of flask rests in a container of cool running water. **D,** cast is teased from hydrocolloid duplicating material.

amount. Unlike mesh relief, the borders of the wax are blended so that no sharp demarcation is found in the metal.

Sprue guide placement

Some removable partial denture alloys are sprued with an overjet. This technique requires the placement of a small metal, resin, or wax tapered cylinder on the master cast in the exact position where the main sprue will be placed on the refractory cast (Fig. 11-30). The placement of this overjet is entirely a laboratory procedure and is governed by the instructions from the company that francises the alloy.

Duplication

Regardless of the alloy system to be used, the blockout philosophy and technique will be the same. Once the duplication phase begins, techniques and materials developed for specific alloys come into play. They are critical and must be followed exactly because the dimensions and expansion of the refractory cast determine the ultimate fit of the denture. For example, low-heat alloys can use gypsum-bound investments. In these situations reversible hydrocolloid with a water base is used for the impression to create the refractory cast. High-heat alloys, on the other hand use phosphate-bound investments and glycerine-base colloids for duplication.

Impression

Many similarities exist between all duplication techniques. To make the impression (Fig. 11-31) the blocked out master cast is placed on the base of a duplicating flask. Duplicating colloid at the proper temperature is poured in a steady stream into the flask, and the flask placed in a regulated cooling tank. Up to an hour may be required to fully set the colloid. The flask is then disassembled, and the master cast carefully removed with two knife blades or a gentle blast of compressed air directed to the cast-colloid junction. The mold must then be carefully examined to detect flaws in the colloid.

Duplicating colloids are capable of being reused many times. They must be cleaned and remelted after each use. Most laboratories have special equipment to remelt the colloid and then store it at the working temperature (Fig. 11-32). It is possible, however, to prepare the duplicating material with less sophisticated means. The clean colloid can be cut in small pieces and reheated in a double boiler to a fluid consistency. It must then be reduced to a working temperature cool enough to flow easily without melting the blockout wax. A breakdown temperature of 100° C (212° F) and a working temperature of 63° C (145° F) will be suitable for most duplicating materials.

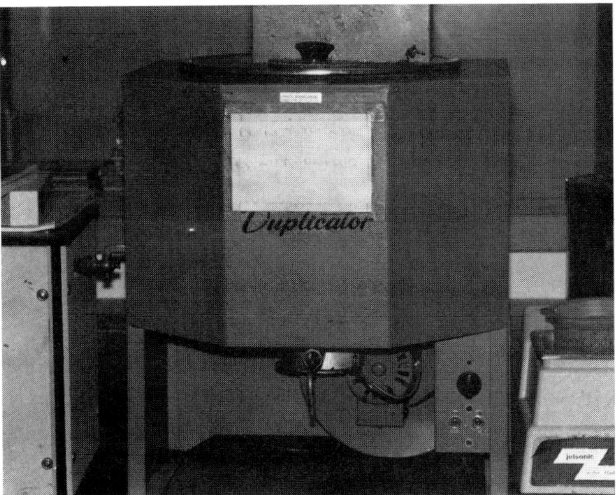

Fig. 11-32. Automatic duplicating machines prepare and store irreversible hydrocolloid.

Equipment. Flasks used in the duplication process will have a metal base on which the master cast is fixed with plastocene clay. The metal base will conduct the cooling temperature of the water bath to the colloid and cause the material to shrink toward the master cast, resulting in an accurate mold of the cast. The water in the cooling bath must be shallow so that only the base is cooled. The sides of some flasks are nonconductors to facilitate the cooling toward the base. Others are completely metal but are based on the same principle. The ideal water bath, used by large commercial laboratories, has a cooling system that circulates water at a regulated temperature. Cold tap water circulating through a sink drain will accomplish the same end, but if the temperature of the water is above 21° C (70° F) the process will take longer to completely set the colloid.

Refractory cast. Refractory, or investment, materials must be measured and mixed exactly according to the manufacturer's instructions to ensure that the expansion of the mold during burnout will match the shrinkage of the alloy.

Gypsum-bonded investments, commonly called *low-heat* investments, are used for casting Type IV partial denture gold and Ticonium. This refractory material can be burned out at 704° C (1300° F) without causing breakdown of the investment.

Investments used for Vitallium, Nobillium, Jelenko's LG, and other chrome-cobalt alloys are termed *high-heat* and are burned out at temperatures in the area of 1037° C (1900° F). These high-heat investments are phosphate bonded and usually require a special liquid to mix with the refractory material.

The colloid mold is carefully cleansed of debris and poured immediately with refractory material. The material is introduced into the mold in small amounts so

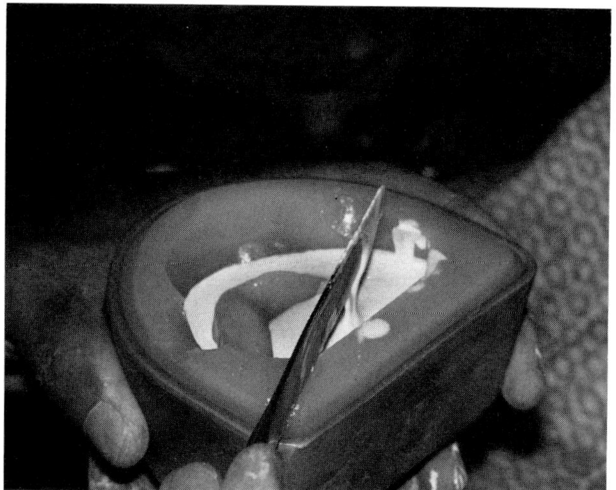

Fig. 11-33. Investment material is flowed slowly into mold.

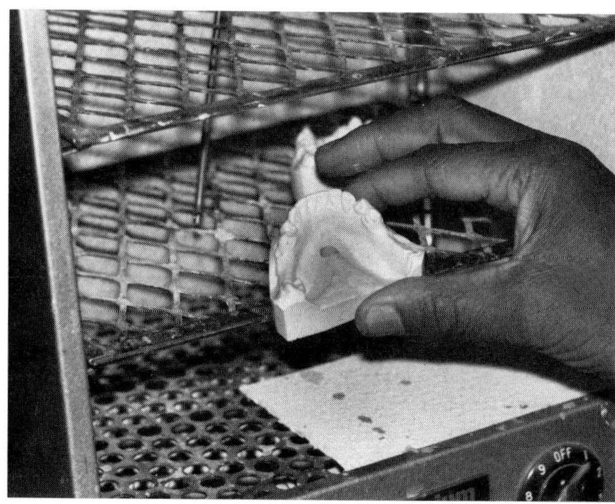

Fig. 11-34. Refractory cast is dried in oven at 93° C (200° F) for 1 hour.

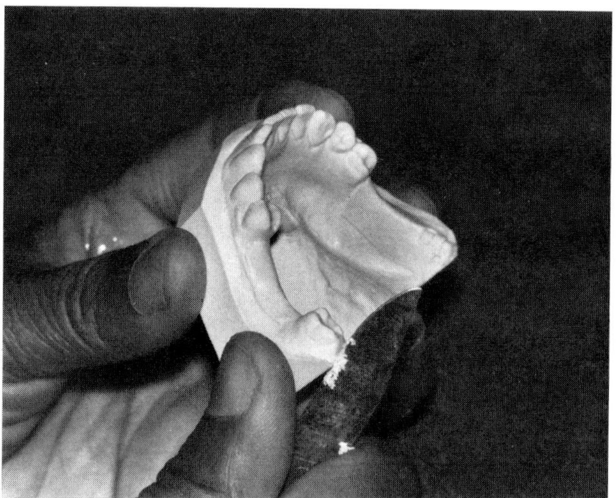

Fig. 11-35. Cast is trimmed either by hand or on model trimmer.

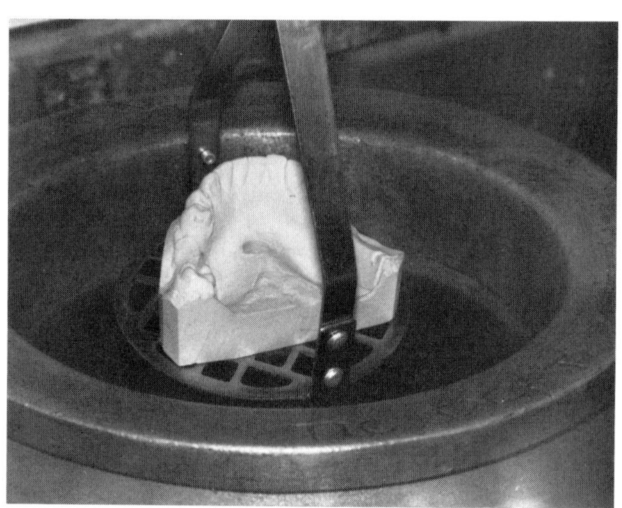

Fig. 11-36. Refractory cast is dipped in hot beeswax.

that no air will be trapped in the area of the teeth (Fig. 11-33). The remainder of the refractory material is added to the mold with a minimum of vibration, and the mold is set aside, covered with a wet towel to keep the colloid moist while the refractory material sets.

The manufacturer's instructions give the time required for complete set of the refractory material. When this stage is reached, the cast is carefully removed from the mold and placed in a drying oven at 93° C (200° F) (Fig. 11-34). When dry, the cast is trimmed to within 6 mm of the proposed design (Fig. 11-35). The trimming should be done on a dry cast trimmer to eliminate the possibility of a slurry mixture accumulating on the cast and changing its contours and dimensions.

Beeswax dip

To ensure a smooth, dense surface on the refractory cast and to eliminate the need for soaking the cast before investing, the dry refractory cast is dipped in hot beeswax (Fig. 11-36). The cast is dried in a hot air oven at 82° to 93° C (180° to 200° F) for ½ to 1 hour, dipped into beeswax at 138° to 149° C (280° to 300° F) for 15 seconds, and set immediately on end to allow all the excess wax to run off. Once the cast has cooled to room temperature, it is ready to be waxed.

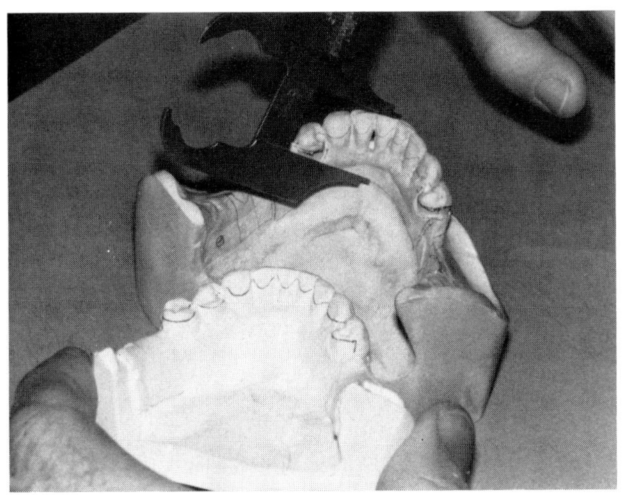

Fig. 11-37. Boley gauge is used to determine position of inferior border of major connector for accurate transfer of design to refractory cast.

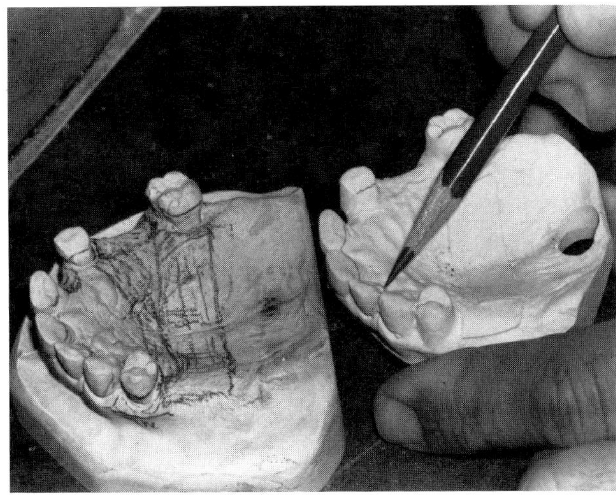

Fig. 11-38. A sharp soft-lead pencil is used to transfer the design onto refractory cast.

Waxing the framework

Design transfer

Before the actual waxing can begin, the design must once again be transferred. The master cast is evaluated and measurements made with a Boley gauge to transfer exactly the outline of the framework to the refractory cast (Fig. 11-37). A common soft lead pencil, sharpened to a point, is used. Care must be taken to draw with a minimum of pressure so that no damage to the cast surface can occur (Fig. 11-38).

The position of the clasp tips is the most critical part of the transfer. If the blockout created a ledge for the retentive clasp tip, this step is made much easier and more exact (Fig. 11-39). Other areas of the design outline are not as critical and can be accurately transferred with reasonable care.

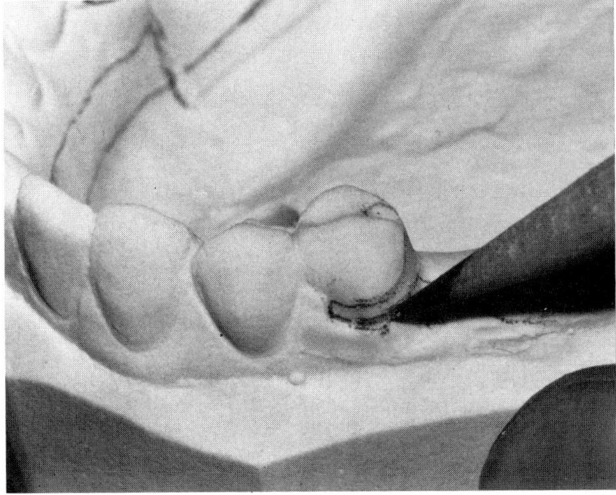

Fig. 11-39. A ledge created by blockout wax is used as a guide in positioning retentive clasp arm.

Materials

Actual waxing of the framework is a individualized operation. Care must be taken to develop an orderly sequence so that no part will be overlooked. The first decision that faces the technician is which plastic patterns to use for clasp arms, major connectors, and retentive meshwork. The plastic pattern has almost totally replaced freehand waxing of the framework. The manufacturer of the alloy system provides, as part of its franchise, a variety of patterns. Retentive clasp arms should be formed with patterns that have a width/thickness ratio approaching 2:1 if maximum flexibility is desired. Clasps that are roughly square (width/thickness ratio 1:1) will serve best as reciprocal clasps. These pattern choices are greatly influenced by clasp length. The clasp that is longer than 10 mm can be thicker than a shorter clasp and still have the same degree of flexibility. When the clasp is short (near 5 mm), it must have a width/thickness ratio near 2:1 or the forces placed on the abutment teeth will far exceed the ability of the periodontal ligament to withstand lateral movement.

Some experience is required to evaluate the rigidity of major connector patterns. In general, those having the recommendation of the manufacturer will prove sufficient for the average situation. The clinician has the responsibility to evaluate the connector and inform the laboratory if the framework is clinically flexible, which it must not be.

Waxing technique

The plastic patterns are "glued" to the refractory cast with a mixture of acetone and plastic pattern scraps mixed to a watery consistency. The tacky liquid is painted on the design outline with a fine brush and allowed to dry for just a few seconds (Fig. 11-40). The pattern can then be adapted with confidence that it will adhere to the cast. Should the pattern separate from the refractory cast—even a small amount—the accuracy of the casting will be destroyed. There is a tendency to respond to this potential problem by painting on a thicker coat of the adhesive liquid. Although this may increase the chance of a positive attachment of the pattern, the film thickness will result in increased dimension of the cast metal in the form of a flash of thin metal around the pattern. This excess metal requires careful finishing to ensure that the basic pattern form is not altered.

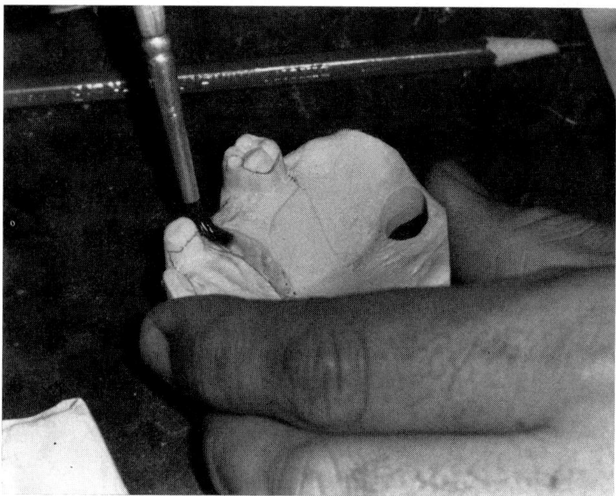

Fig. 11-40. A tacky solution of acetone and plastic is painted on area to be covered by plastic pattern.

Plastic patterns are received from the manufacturer on cards. Some care is required to remove the pattern from the card without distorting it. If the cards are kept cold, as in a standard refrigerator, it is easier to pick the patterns off with a quick snap. It is particularly important that retentive clasp patterns not be distorted. The shape of the clasps greatly affects their flexibility. The clasp pattern is cut to a length greater than that actually desired with a sharp Bard Parker blade and snapped off the card with a quick lateral motion of the blade (Fig. 11-41).

After the plastic patterns have been placed on the refractory cast, they must be adapted to the contours without distortion. A soft rubber pencil eraser shaped into a wedge is most useful in this adaptation (Fig. 11-42). The pattern is placed on the refractory cast at its tip and lightly pressed into the previously painted-on tacky liquid. The pattern is then slowly positioned along the design outline with the rubber wedge. At every step of this operation the technician must exercise extreme care not to stretch the pattern. A Bard Parker knife is used to trim the pattern extending beyond the outline drawn on the cast (Fig. 11-43). Major connector patterns are not normally distorted beyond use, but retentive clasp patterns often are. If the clinician has prepared the tooth in a manner that allows the clasp to be curved primarily in one plane, the distortion potential is greatly decreased.

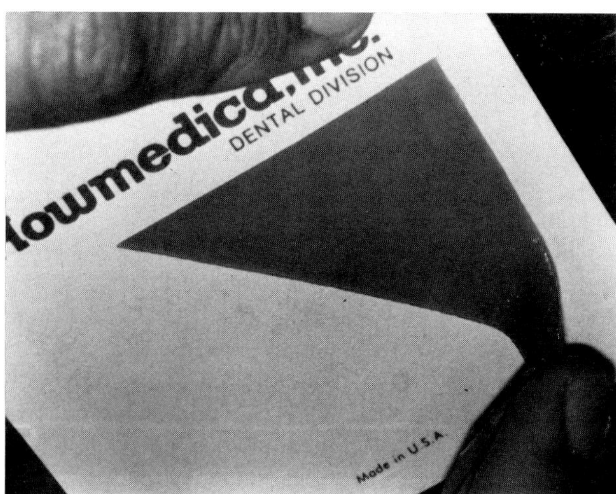

Fig. 11-41. Plastic pattern is snapped off card with a quick lateral motion to minimize distortion.

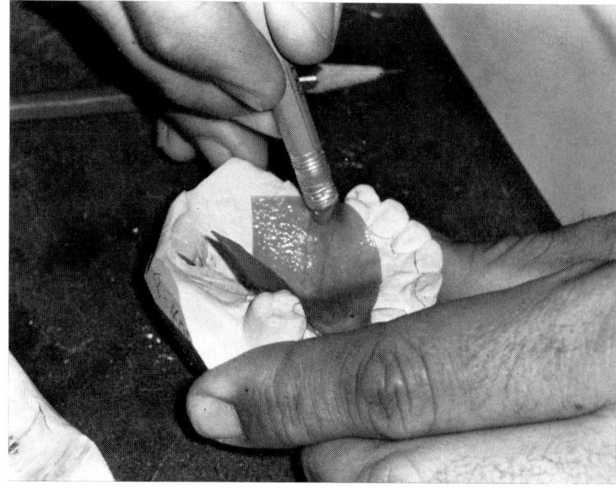

Fig. 11-42. A contoured pencil eraser is used to adapt plastic pattern to cast.

Once the plastic patterns are in place on the refractory cast, they must be joined together with wax. A wax with a formulation similar to blue inlay wax is indicated because it sets hard and polishes easily. This wax is also used to seal down the margins of the major connector and to freehand wax the minor connectors and rests (Fig. 11-44). The areas where the retentive meshwork joins the major connector must be reinforced (Fig. 11-45). The meshwork does not have as great a bulk as the connector, and thin spots in the joint can result in fracture during function.

For final contouring each technician will develop his own set of instruments. Carvers with miniature rounded blades are most apt to be used. The standard Hanau torch is too bulky and hot for partial denture wax finishing. A tiny, controlled torch made from a hypodermic needle and a piece of rubber hose attached to the Bunsen burner provides a flame that can be used to smooth even the finest details of the framework (Fig. 11-46).

Spruing the framework

Technique

The actual spruing construction depends almost entirely on the instructions provided by the manufacturer of the alloy system. Ticonium uses a single sprue ap-

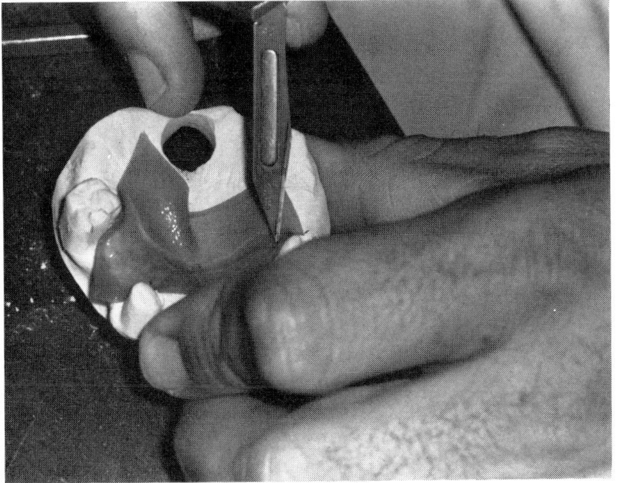

Fig. 11-43. Excess plastic pattern is trimmed with a Bard Parker knife.

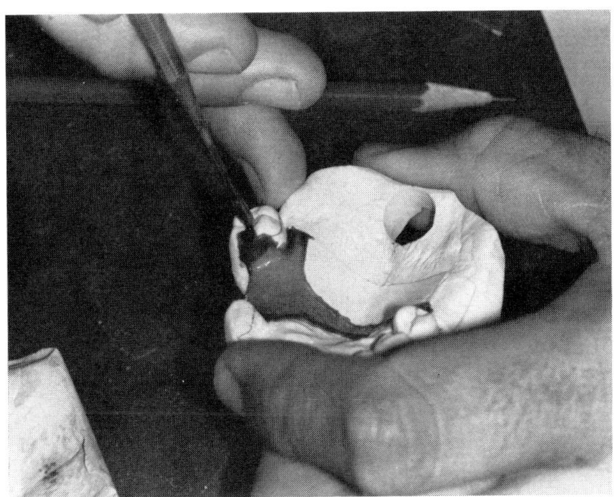

Fig. 11-44. Minor connector and occlusal rest are waxed with blue wax.

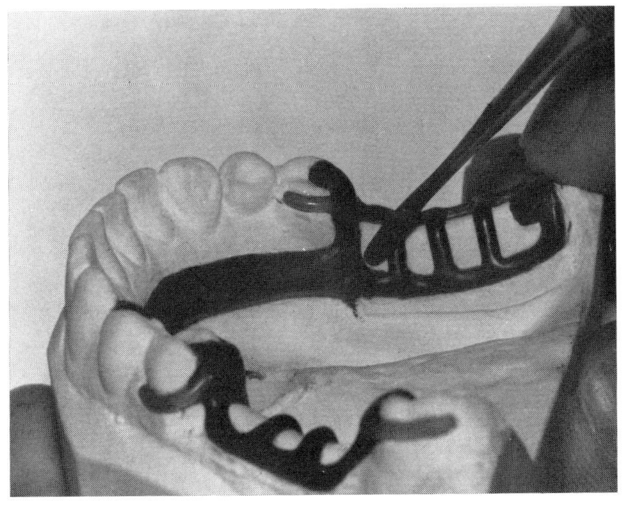

Fig. 11-45. Junction of acrylic resin retentive latticework with major connector must be reinforced with additional wax.

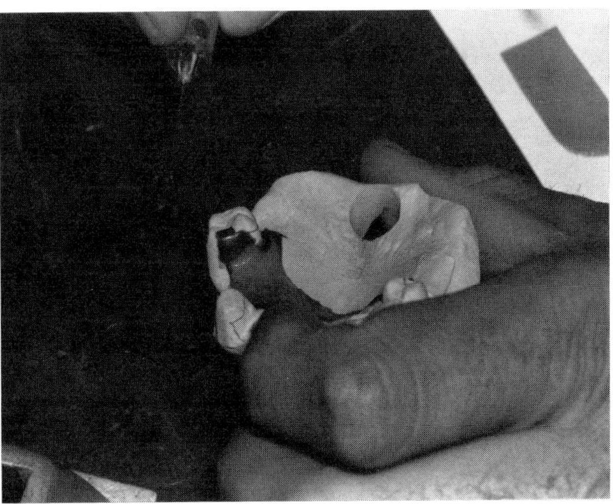

Fig. 11-46. A tiny torch made from a hypodermic needle and a piece of rubber hose is used to smooth wax.

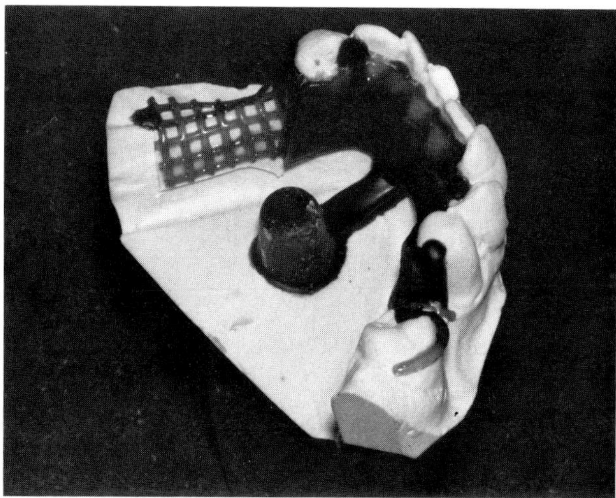

Fig. 11-47. A single sprue is traversing through base of cast to mandibular framework as recommended by the Ticonium Company.

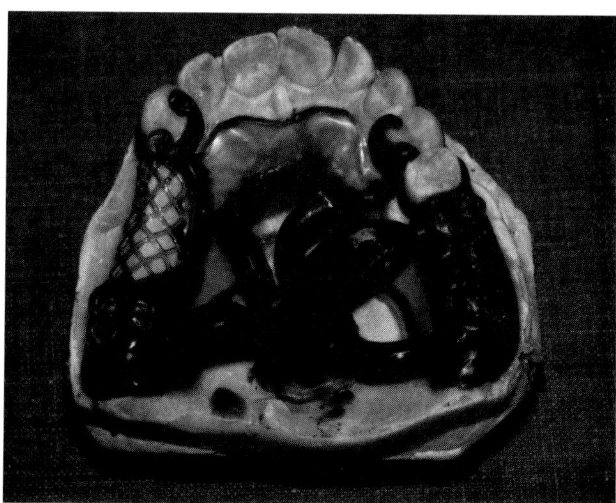

Fig. 11-48. Multiple sprues are used to cast gold and some high-heat chrome-cobalt alloys.

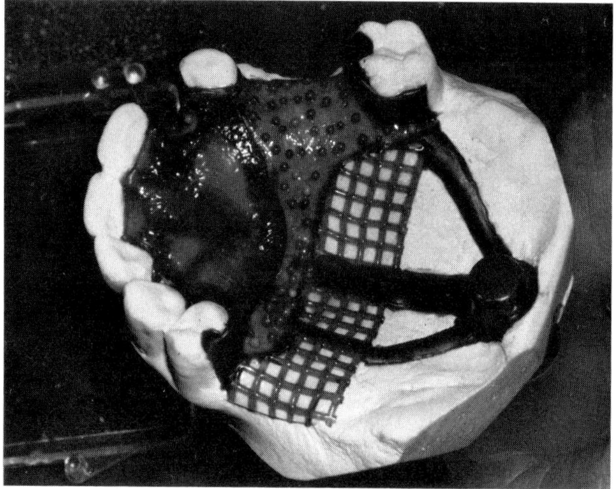

Fig. 11-49. Secondary sprues are placed to ensure flow of metal to areas separated from main sprue by thin areas of pattern.

proach through the refractory cast (Fig. 11-47). Gold castings and a number of high-heat chrome-cobalt alloys sprue the casting from above with multiple sprues (Fig. 11-48). No matter which technique is used, special care must be taken to round all sprue connections. Any sharp edges remaining in the refractory cast are apt to be broken off by the force of the molten metal cast into the mold and enveloped in the metal as inclusions that will ruin the casting.

Sprue size

Gauges of the wax used for the sprue leads are critical, and the manufacturer's directions must be followed exactly. There must be *no* constrictions in the sprue lead that would cause the molten metal to flow from a thick to a thin area and then back to a thick area. The turbulence set up by this type of sprue often results in internal mold deformation and castings that have inclusions.

Auxiliary sprues

Any area that is separated from the bulk of the framework by long spans of retentive meshwork will require a secondary sprue lead off the main lead to ensure that sufficient molten metal reaches the area (Fig. 11-49). Secondary sprues are also required to support heavy metal pontics where the molten metal might have to flow from thinner areas into the thicker metal pontics. These secondary sprues are made from round wax forms one-third to one-fourth the dimension of the major leads. The smaller leads must be connected to the main sprue in a gentle curve with no sharp angles.

The main sprue must conform to the alloy system and be large enough to ensure that the molten metal will hit the sprue and not splatter against the wall of the mold.

Investing the refractory cast

As in spruing, the investment procedures are controlled totally by the alloy manufacturer. There is little that the clinician can do to monitor this phase of removable partial denture construction.

Two-part mold

Some systems require a two-part investment, the first part being a thin (3 to 4 mm) "paint-on" layer (Fig. 11-50). This layer is literally painted on the waxed re-

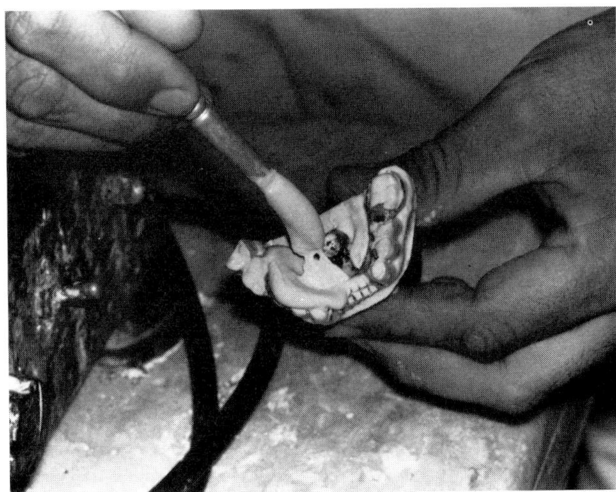

Fig. 11-50. First layer of investment is painted on pattern.

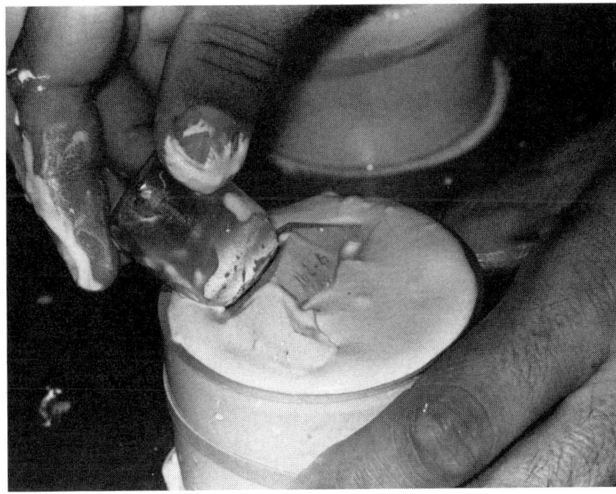

Fig. 11-51. Refractory cast is worked into soft investment in investment ring.

fractory cast slowly and carefully to ensure that no voids are present. The refractory cast must be dipped into slurry water to moisten its surface before this first layer is applied. This wetting keeps the dry refractory cast from taking up water from the paint-on layer and causing it to become sluggish as it is applied to the cast.

As soon as the first layer reaches its initial set, the second part of the investing procedure begins. An investment ring large enough to accommodate the refractory cast and its first layer is chosen according to the alloy manufacturer's directions. The refractory material is measured, mixed, and placed in the ring. The refractory cast is moistened, held by the sprue base, and worked into the mass in the ring (Fig. 11-51). Some skill is required to place the cast in the proper relation to the bottom of the ring so that an adequate thickness of investment is available to strengthen the mold and still allow for the escape of gas during casting.

Mold storage

Certain alloy systems remove the investment ring before placing the mold in the burnout furnace. Others burn out the mold with the ring in place. In either situation the sprue lead, if it is formed of metal or plastic, is removed and the entrance to the mold carefully inspected to eliminate any debris or sharp edges that might break off and be carried into the mold by the force of the molten metal. The molds are normally stored in a plastic bag to keep them from completely drying out until enough of them are available to fill the burnout furnace.

Burnout

Time and temperature

The time and temperature required to eliminate the wax and resin that were applied to the refractory cast are factors of the refractory-alloy system. This system is developed to provide thermal and/or hydroscopic expansion that closely matches the anticipated shrinkage of the alloy as it solidifies. Since the ultimate fit of the restoration depends totally on this relationship, the manufacturer's directions must be followed exactly.

Furnaces

Burnout furnaces can be either electric or gas and must be vented to allow the noxious fumes that result from the burnout to escape the work area. They vary greatly in capacity, from industrial-type gas furnaces capable of holding 25 dental casting molds to small electric furnaces with a capacity of only 1 or 2 molds (Figs. 11-52 and 11-53).

Modern furnaces are controlled electronically to permit a time/temperature relationship to be set exactly to the alloy manufacturer's specifications. The refractory molds can be placed in the furnace and the furnace set to turn itself on and have the molds at the proper temperature at the most appropriate time for casting. If the molds go into the furnace at the end of the workday, they should be placed inside a thin plastic garbage bag to keep them from drying out. When the furnace turns on in the early morning, the bag will burn completely.

Although insufficient burnout can result in many technical problems (short castings, insufficient mold expansion), there is little that the clinician can do to influence the laboratory management of these areas. Fortunately, the franchised laboratory will operate in accord with the standards set by the alloy manufacturer, and these problems should not arise.

Heating the mold beyond the intended range inevit-

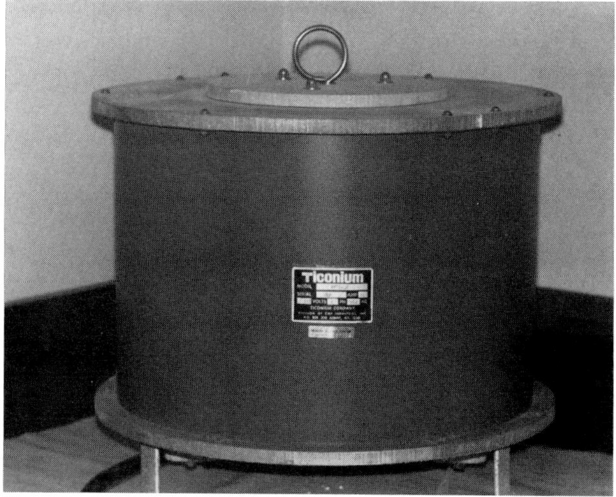

Fig. 11-52. Large electric burnout furnace.

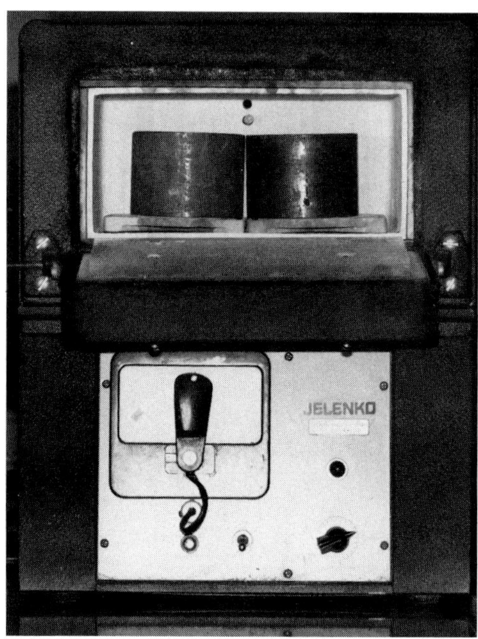

Fig. 11-53. Small burnout furnace.

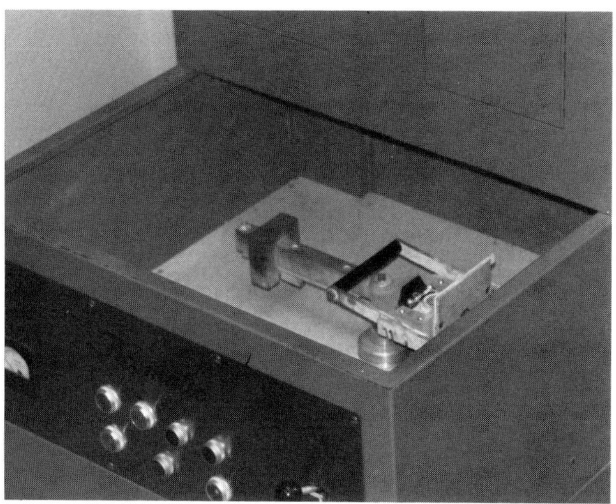

Fig. 11-54. An induction casting machine.

ably results in a breakdown of the binder material and destruction of the mold. Again, modern furnaces protect against this potential problem.

Casting

Induction casting

Induction casting of removable partial denture frameworks has become the method of choice for modern dentistry. Excellent castings can be made using gas and oxygen for alloys that melt close to 1093° C (2000° F). Oxyacetylene mixture is available for castings requiring higher heat. Torch casting requires a level of experience that is directly proportional to the melting temperature. The higher the temperature required, the more experience needed. Since removable partial denture alloys cast in the 1371° C (2500° F) range, they are particularly technique sensitive. Induction casting machines (Fig. 11-54), although expensive, allow technicians with minimum experience or training to cast these alloys successfully.

Induction casting is based on the electric currents in a metal core caused by induction from a magnetic field. A heating coil of copper tubing is shaped to fit closely around the casting crucible and is attached to an alternating current source. The alternating current in the coil sets up eddy currents of electrons in the crucible and the alloy in it. These currents, through the power generated in the magnetic field (I^2R), melt the alloy. The coil is cooled by a flowing water source running through it so that it is not permanently affected by the power dissipation.

The temperature of the melting mass is measured by an electronic eye directly above the crucible (Fig. 11-55). The sensitive optical system in the sensing eye can be set to activate the casting mechanism at any temperature selected by the operator. Some of these sensing devices are driven by the infrared wavelengths emitted by the metal and are classified as optical pyrometers.

The casting machine is set to the manufacturer's directions to include the revolutions per minute that the casting arm will spin as well as the temperature that is required to set off the machine. Most machines have the capability to revolve at up to 600 RPM.

An uncontaminated crucible with the proper amount

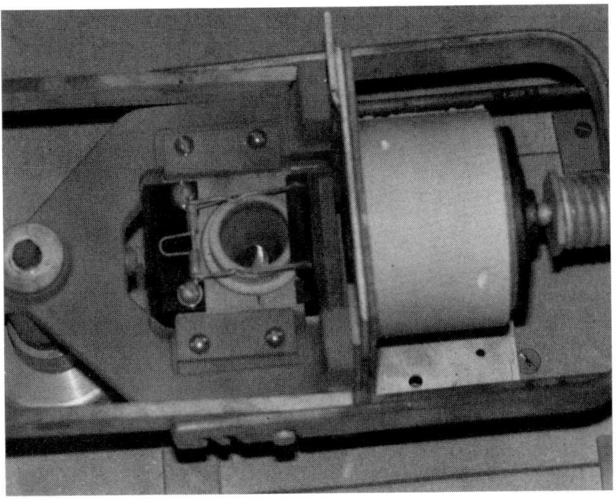

Fig. 11-55. Electronic eye measures temperature of melt and activates casting process.

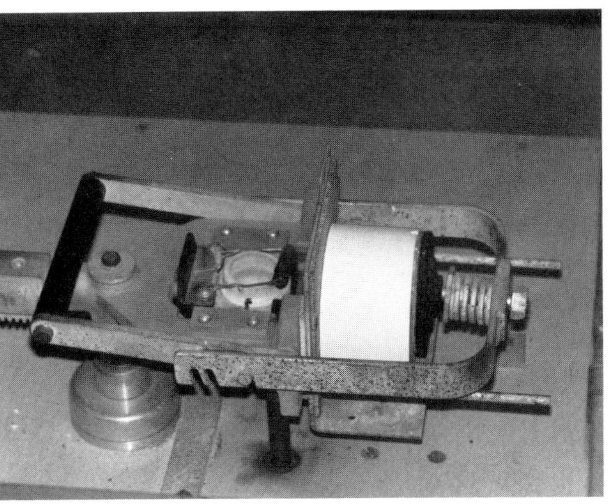

Fig. 11-56. A clean crucible loaded with alloy begins casting sequence.

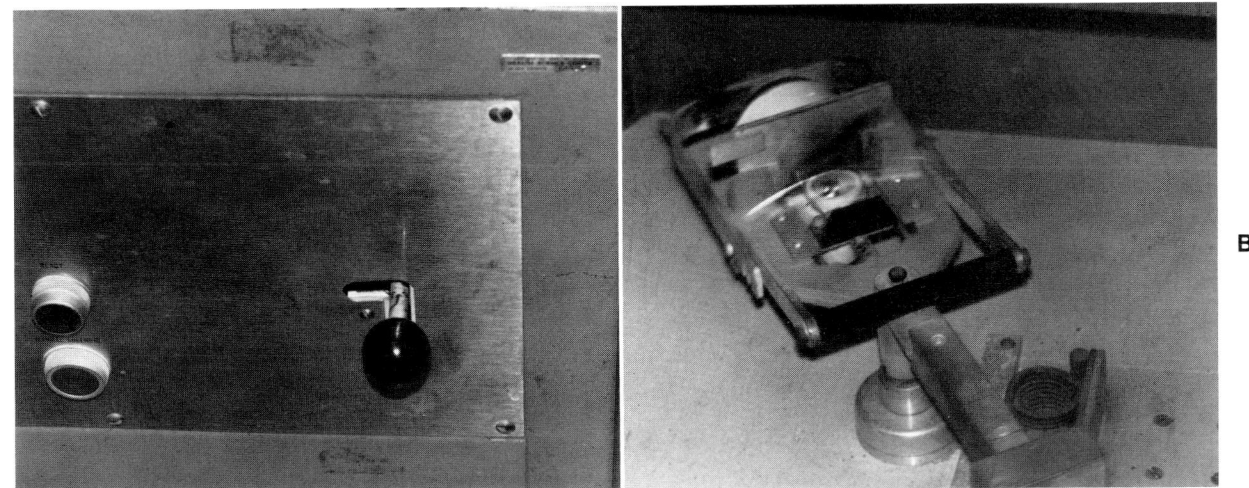

Fig. 11-57. A, Manual release for centrifugal casting machine. Lever is moved up and laterally to start machine. B, Molten metal is released by casting machine.

of clean alloy in it begins the casting sequence (Fig. 11-56).

The melt is begun by activating the alternating current; and while the alloy is heating, the mold is removed from the furnace and placed in the holding mechanism. This device varies from one casting machine to another, but every cast must be balanced to the approximate weight of the mold by placing a counterweight or counterweights on the casting arm. Balance must be obtained before the actual casting procedure begins because there is no time to carry out this step once the melt has begun.

Modern induction casting machines are normally set to cast once the desired temperature has been achieved. Some alloys require a heat soak period of up to 3 seconds during which the alloy is kept at the casting temperature by a rapid on and off of the alternating current. These machines can be set to allow the operator to determine the exact moment to cast (Fig. 11-57). To do this requires both experience and a means to view the molten metal. To look directly into the crucible is *never* recommended unless the eye is protected by a dense blue lens used by welders. Each alloy will have its own distinctive appearance under this protective lens when it is ready to cast.

Casting recovery

When the actual casting is complete, the mold is removed from the machine and allowed to cool according to the manufacturer's directions. At the appropriate time the mold is broken by tapping it with a wooden mallet to break off the outer layer of investment. The first layer of investment is then removed by sand blasting, usually in a self-contained machine especially manufactured for this purpose. The casting can now be examined for defects and the finishing and fitting procedures begun.

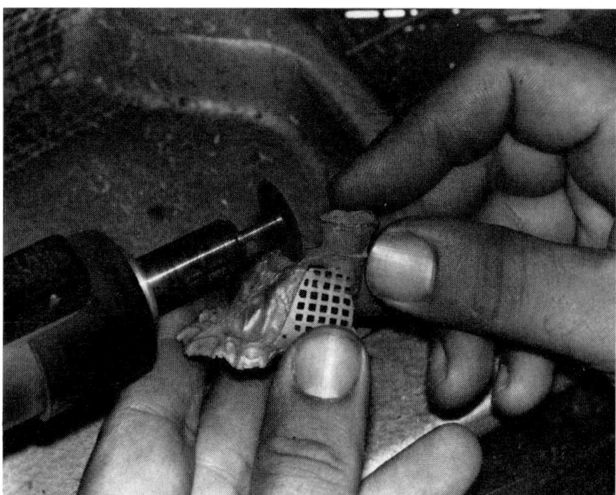

Fig. 11-58. Sprues are removed from casting with a coarse abrasive disk in a high-speed lathe.

Finishing the framework

Sprue removal

With high-speed lathes and large abrasive disks, the sprue leads are cut from the casting (Fig. 11-58).

Rough finishing and shaping

Before any fitting of the framework can begin, the casting must be shaped to its ultimate form and then rubber wheeled to a "satin" surface. Any attempt to seat the casting on the master cast before this stage is reached runs the risk of damaging the cast and reducing its value in finishing the framework. The experienced technician develops a positive plan in the finishing operation using coarser disks and stones at first and then going to a finer grade of stone (Fig. 11-59). The stones themselves must be shaped by the technician with a shaping stone (Fig. 11-60). The shaping stone creates a contour on the finishing stone that relates to the desired shape of any particular area. Until some skill is developed in this shaping operation, the technician can expect to have trouble creating smooth, flowing contours.

Areas requiring special attention (rests, retentive clasp tips, and guiding plane minor connectors) must receive an absolute minimum of finishing and polishing (Fig. 11-61). The clinician should carefully inspect these areas when the framework returns from the laboratory

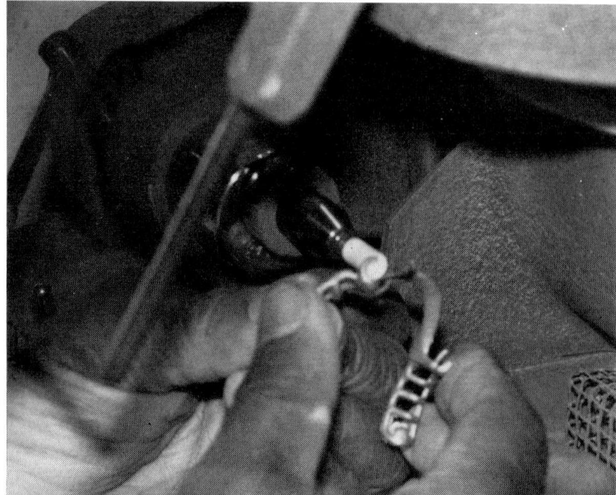

Fig. 11-59. A coarse stone, shaped to fit lingual bar, is used to start polishing procedure.

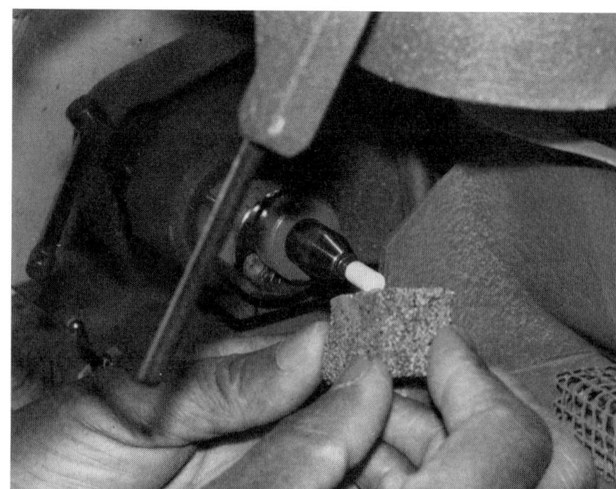

Fig. 11-60. A truing, or shaping, stone is used to shape grinding stones to desired configuration.

and has every right to complain if there is evidence of overfinishing.

When the clinician is not pleased with the treatment of his castings, he must realize that he needs to take the responsibility for the final finishing of these critical areas himself. Some additional chair time will be needed to fully seat the casting. With disclosing wax or a mixture of gold rouge and chloroform painted on the internal surface, areas that bind can be identified and then removed carefully with fine stones (Fig. 11-62).

Fitting the framework

The technician begins to fit the framework by carefully seating the casting on the master cast and attempting to identify the first spots that bind (Fig. 11-63). Special powdered sprays and liquid disclosing media are commercially available. Powdered deodorant sprays can be used equally as well. The seating and spot grinding continues until the rests completely contact the cast. Because the retentive clasp tips engage an undercut area, they will most likely be the first area that binds. The technician must carefully relieve the cast in

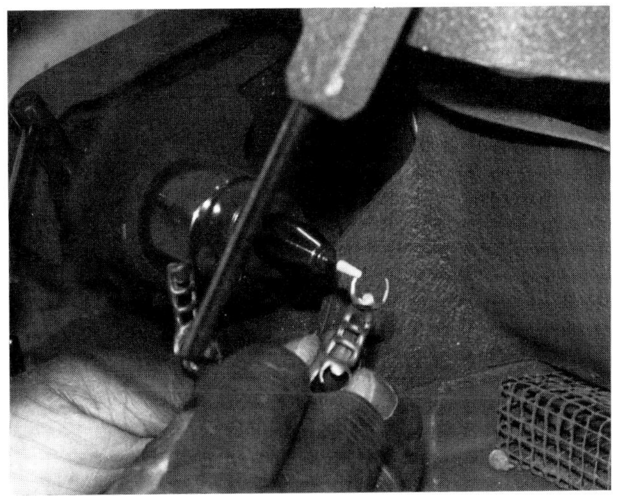

Fig. 11-61. A fine stone is used to shape such critical areas as retentive clasp tips.

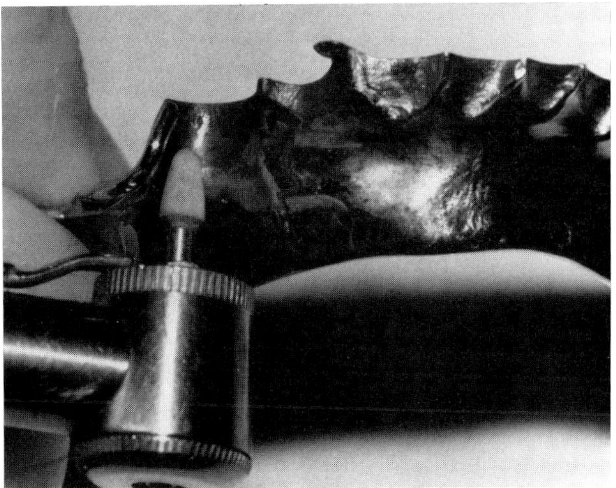

Fig. 11-62. Areas of interference to complete seating of framework are removed with a fine stone.

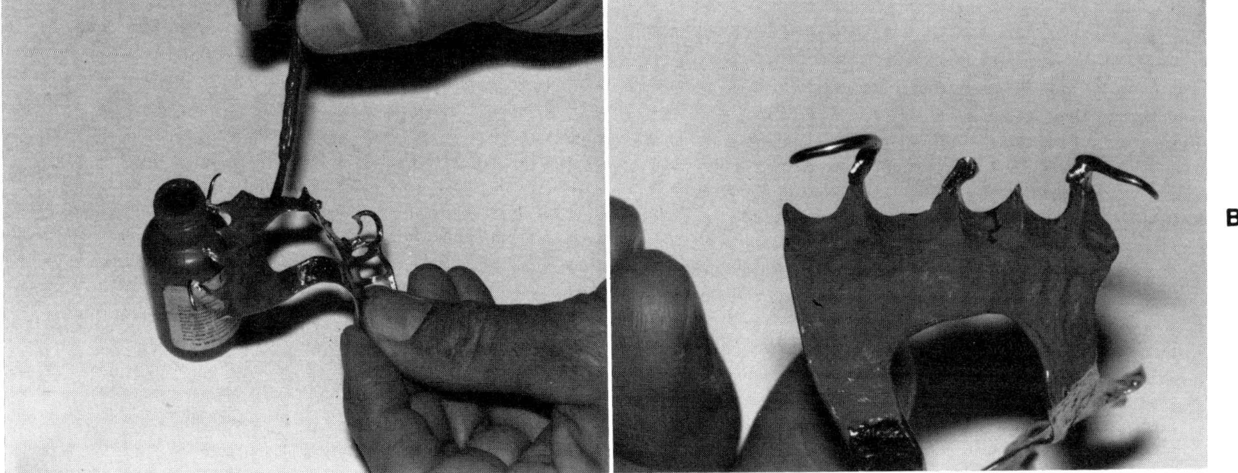

Fig. 11-63. A, Laboratory technician can improve fit of framework on cast by using a disclosing medium. Liquid is painted on metal that will contact cast and allowed to dry. **B,** Areas that are interfering with complete seating of casting are indicated by displacement of disclosing medium.

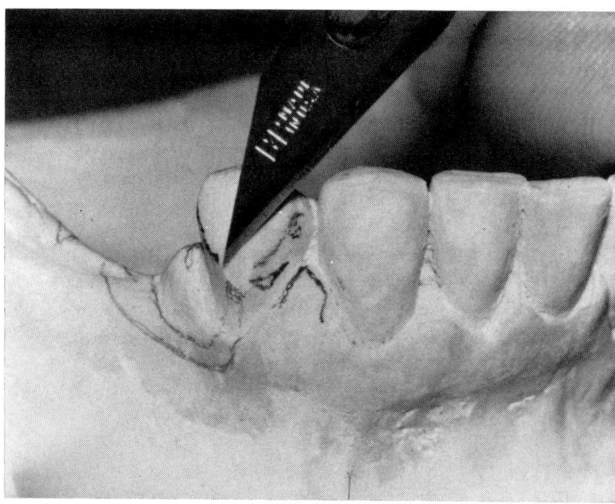

Fig. 11-64. Undercut in area of clasp tip is removed to allow framework to seat without binding on cast.

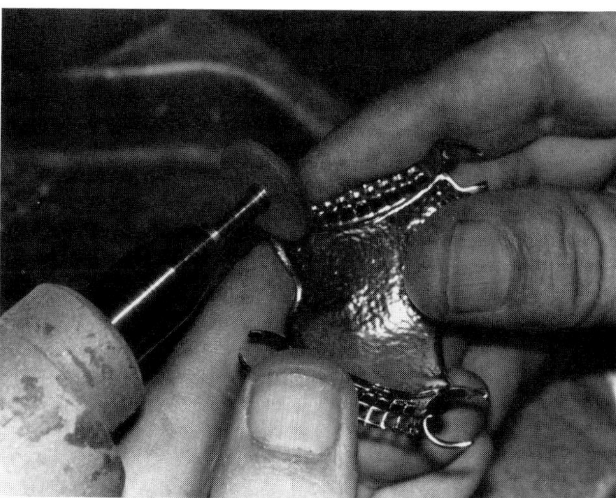

Fig. 11-65. A Carborundum-incorporated rubber wheel is used to smooth scratches and irregularities caused by finishing procedures.

the area of the clasp tip undercuts to allow the clasps to pass the height of contour (Fig. 11-64). Some technicians, to save time and preserve the master cast, bend the retentive clasp arms away from the cast and then attempt to recontour the clasp back into contact. This act requires a good deal of skill and seldom results in a truly passive clasp.

Some laboratories duplicate the master cast and then do all but the final fitting on the duplicate. This approach allows the added advantage of having an unabraded master cast available for a remake should the casting exhibit a major discrepancy.

Rubber wheeling and final polish

Once the casting seats completely on the master cast without rocking or other evidence of distortion the technician will proceed with the final rubber wheeling and polishing operation (Fig. 11-65). Each alloy manufacturer sells, as part of its franchise, a variety of polishing compounds especially suited to its alloy. Rag and felt wheels are used on the high-speed lathe to apply the final polish.

Ultrasonic cleaning is commonly used to remove all traces of the polishing materials. The framework is inspected and, if acceptable, returned to the clinician on the master cast (Fig. 11-66).

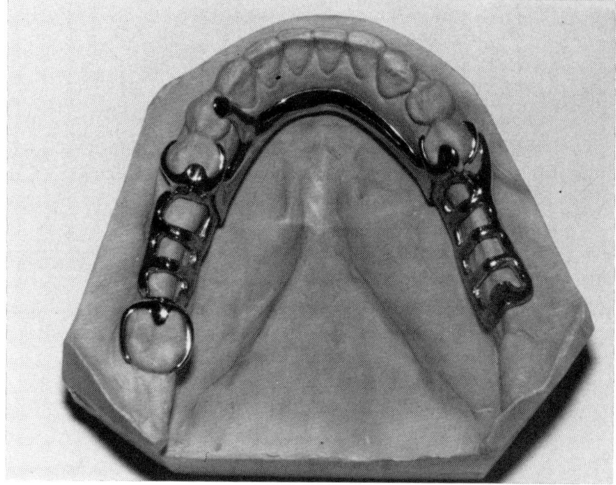

Fig. 11-66. Fitted framework is returned to clinician on master cast.

Sectioning and resoldering the framework

There are many advantages to trying in and adjusting the framework before completing the partial denture. If the clinician has verified the fit of the framework, he can then be certain that any interferences at the insertion appointment must be caused by the denture teeth or denture base. This will greatly reduce the time required for the insertion appointment and should increase patient confidence by decreasing the number of postinsertion adjustments. Should an altered cast impression be indicated for a distal extension area, the framework will be adjusted before the impression is made.

When either the clinician or the technician finds that the framework will not seat completely on all rests (usually apparent by trying to elicit a "rock"), an attempt can be made to section the casting, seat the sections, and solder them together in a new relationship. This approach is common in the construction of the fixed

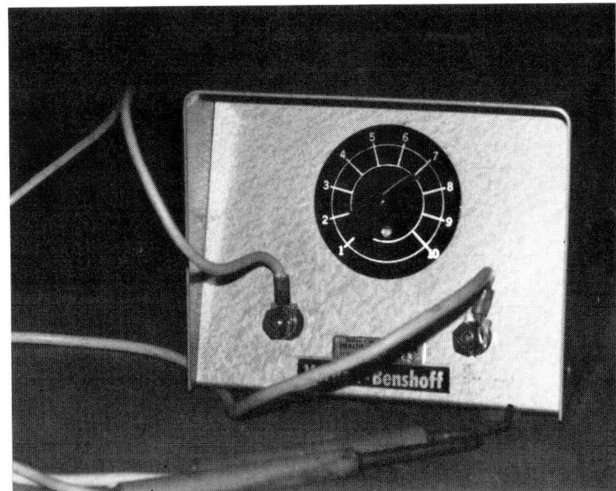

Fig. 11-67. Electrosoldering machine. Resistance of metal to be soldered to a flow of electric current provides heat necessary for soldering procedure.

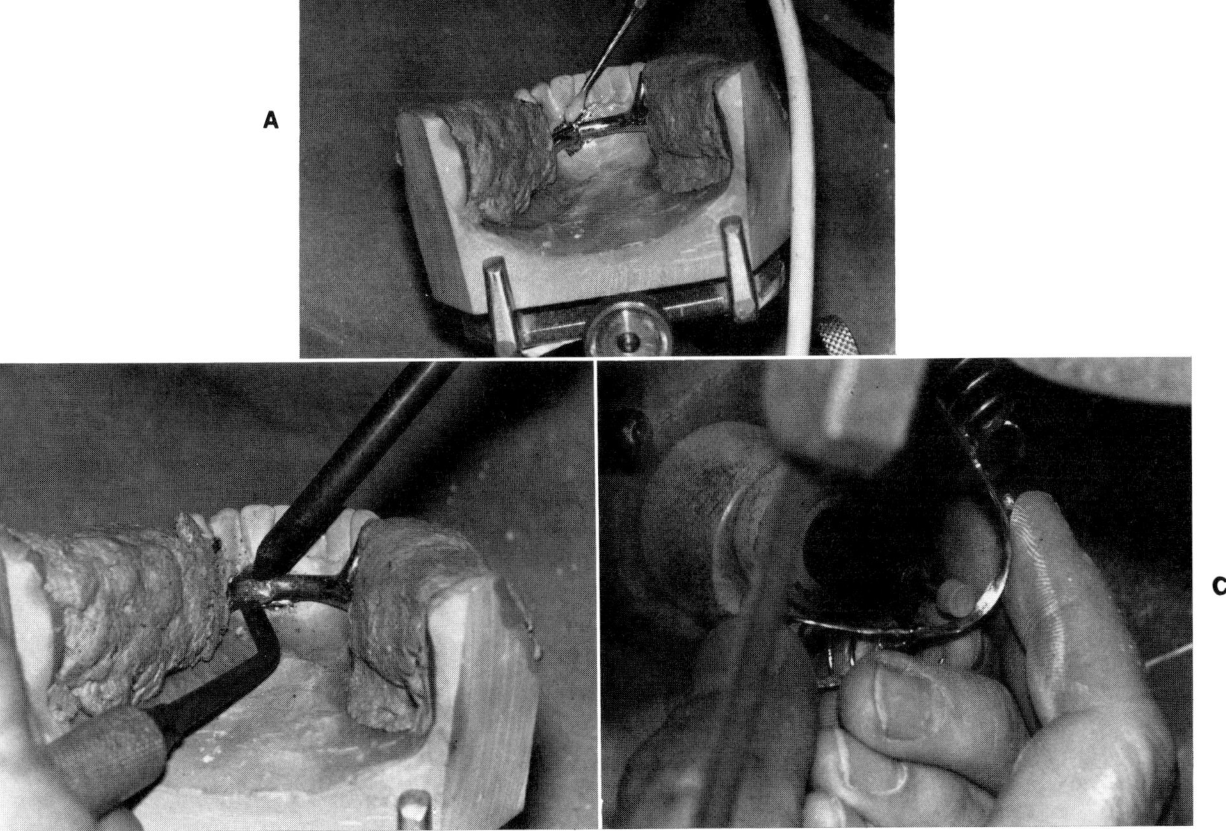

Fig. 11-68. A, Fractured lingual bar is reassembled on a soldering cast. Soldering flux is added to area of break. **B,** Electrosoldering tips are placed, one on each side of joint, and current activated. **C,** Soldering area is smoothed and polished.

partial denture, but much more difficult to accomplish in the removable partial denture because of the complexity of form. Minor connectors and some major connectors can be sectioned and soldered with either precious metal solder or nonprecious brazing alloys. This type of soldering is normally done with the electrosoldering device (Fig. 11-67), a common piece of equipment in the removable partial denture laboratory.

Sectioned segments must be satisfactorily related in the mouth and then transferred with either a plaster index or a resin matrix to the laboratory. The technician then pours a soldering cast against the casting and finally places foil over the cast in the area of the joint and completes the soldering operation (Fig. 11-68).

Adjusting occlusion

The laboratory should receive an opposing cast and suitable jaw relation records from the clinician if the clinician desires a framework that is in harmony with the existing occlusal relationship.

Occlusal and incisal rests must be waxed heavily enough to allow them to cast completely (Fig. 11-69). In many instances they must be waxed into hyperocclusion to develop this needed bulk.

Once cast, these areas are adjusted to return to the occluding vertical dimension. This obviously requires articulated casts.

Although the clinician has the responsibility to create sufficient space for the framework he designs, at times the technician finds minimum clearance for rests and embrasure clasps (less than 1.5 mm). Rather than risk weakening the metal, the interfering part of the opposing cast should be relieved and marked positively with red pencil to call the attention of the clinician to the potential problem area. This approach allows the clinician the option of doing the final adjusting himself, reducing the opposing tooth, or both, and relieves the technician of making a clinical decision.

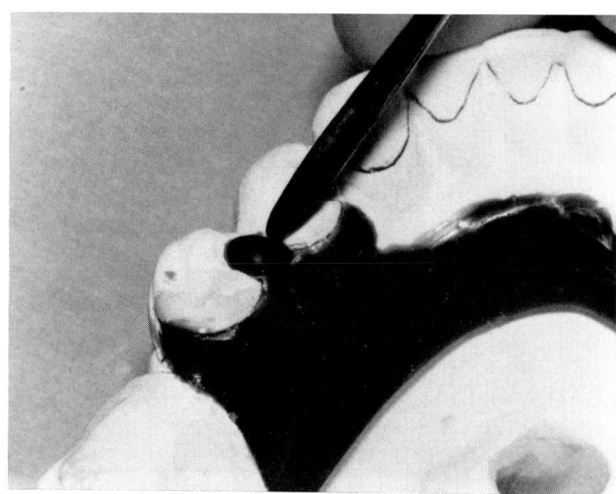

Fig. 11-69. Occlusal rest is waxed heavily to ensure that it will cast completely.

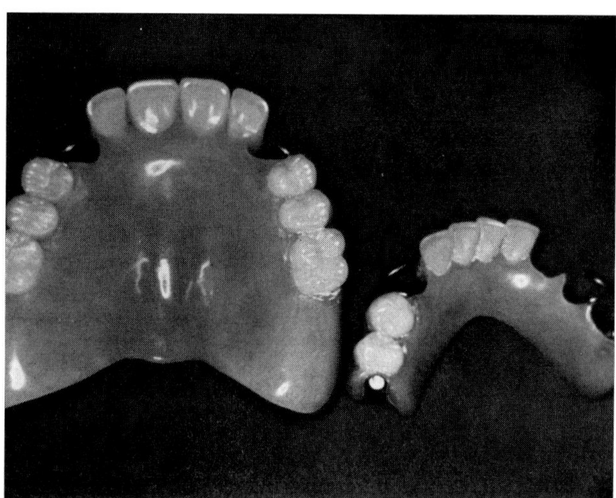

Fig. 11-70. Wrought wire clasps are used frequently in temporary prostheses.

Wrought wire retentive clasp arms

Retentive clasp arms can be constructed of wrought wire as well as cast alloy. Many clinicians prefer the wire clasp, believing that they will have a greater degree of control in adapting and adjusting the clasp. Since wrought wire is normally round, it will flex equally in all directions. This uniform flexibility is thought to be "kind" to the abutment tooth.

Wires available for removable partial dentures normally run from 17 to 20 gauge and can be made of either precious metal alloys (gold, palladium, platinum, silver) or nonprecious alloys (stainless steel, nickel-chromium, nickel-chromium-cobalt). Eighteen- and nineteen-gauge nickel-chrome-cobalt wires are currently the most popular. The high cost of precious metals has reduced the use of these wires. There is every indication that nickel-based alloys perform as well if not better than the precious metal wires.

Wrought wire clasps are almost universally used as repair additions for fractured or distorted cast clasps and on a variety of temporary and transitional prostheses as well (Fig. 11-70). It is essential that the clinician develop and maintain skill in the manipulation of the wrought wire clasp.

Wire bending skills vary greatly, with few concrete rules to guide the student. In general the best results occur when the wire is held with the pliers and bent with the fingers (Fig. 11-71). Rather than attempting to start at the clasp tip and form the entire clasp from that

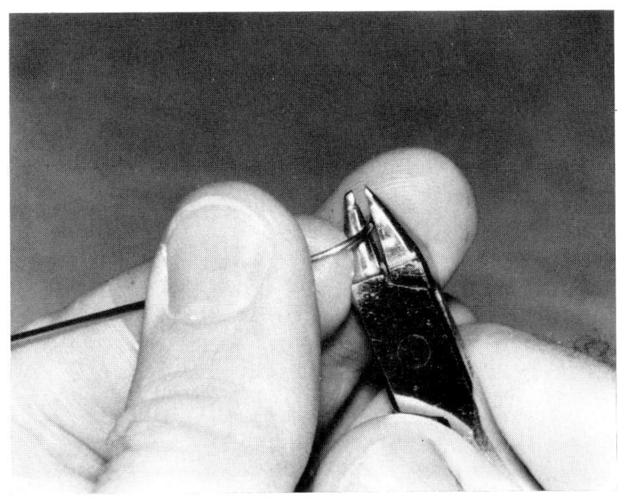

Fig. 11-71. Wire is contoured by holding wire with a pliers and bending it with finger pressure.

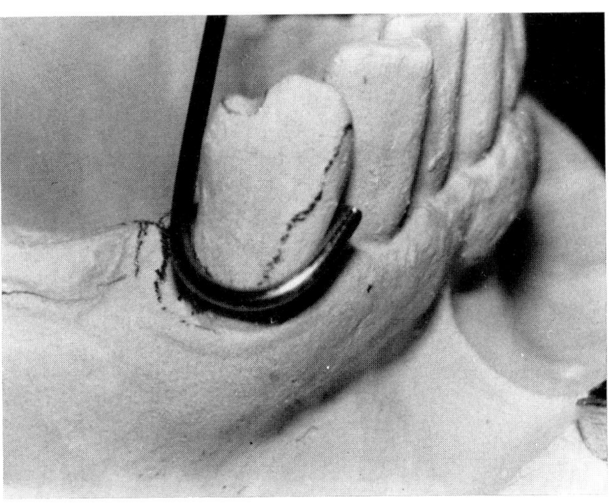

Fig. 11-72. Bent wire is positioned on cast to coincide with desired clasp position.

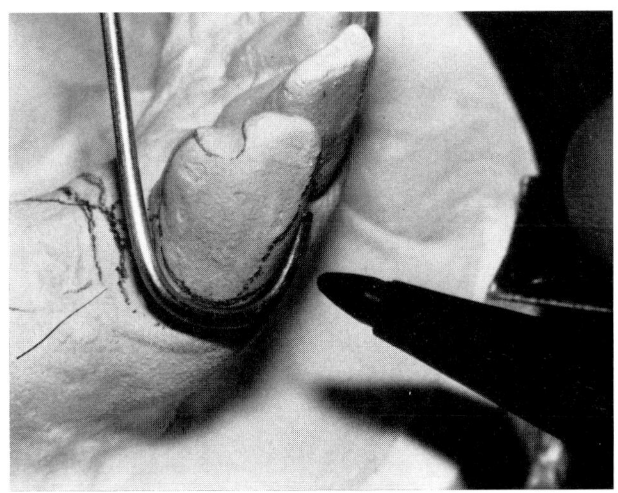

Fig. 11-73. Wire is marked with a wax pencil to indicate tip of the clasp, and excess wire is cut off.

point, the beginning student will find it much easier to estimate and then bend the wire in a basic curve that corresponds to the surface of the tooth to be clasped. The wire curve can then be moved along the tooth until it coincides with the desired clasp position (Fig. 11-72). Any part of the wire extending beyond the intended clasp tip is marked with a wax pencil and cut off (Fig. 11-73). This technique is most applicable to non precious wires because of their low cost.

The same approach is indicated for clasp forms other than circumferential.

Wire clasps can be attached to the removable partial denture in four ways. The most obvious way, and the one used primarily in repair situations, is to embed the wire in the resin of the denture base (Fig. 11-74). The wire can also be included in the wax-up of the framework and the metal cast to the wire. The joint formed here is primarily a mechanical one.

Dependable results can be achieved by contouring the wire after the framework is complete and then attaching the clasp by soldering it to the framework (Fig. 11-75). If the clasp is soldered at the rest—minor connector junction, it will be affected by the heat of the soldering operation but usually not as greatly as in the casting process. The best method of attaching the wrought wire clasp to the framework is by soldering it back on the retentive meshwork, well away from the area where it will be required to flex (Fig. 11-76). In this manner the destructive potential of the soldering operation will be limited to an area that will be covered by denture base resin.

The soldering itself is best done with an electrosoldering device and nickel-based industrial alloys (solders). Precious metal solder can be used, but it gives no particular advantage and the cost is considerably higher. The electrosoldering technique is far easier to master than torch soldering and permits the use of very high fusing alloy solders. Fluxes containing fluoride must be used in this procedure. The electrosoldering machine is basically a step-up transformer with two terminals, one copper and one carbon. When the carbon tip is placed on the solder and the copper tip on the framework a short distance from the soldering area, the electric circuit is completed through the framework and the electric energy dissipated as heat (resistance) to melt the solder.

Normally no finishing is needed on the soldered clasp if the joint is to be enclosed in the denture base resin.

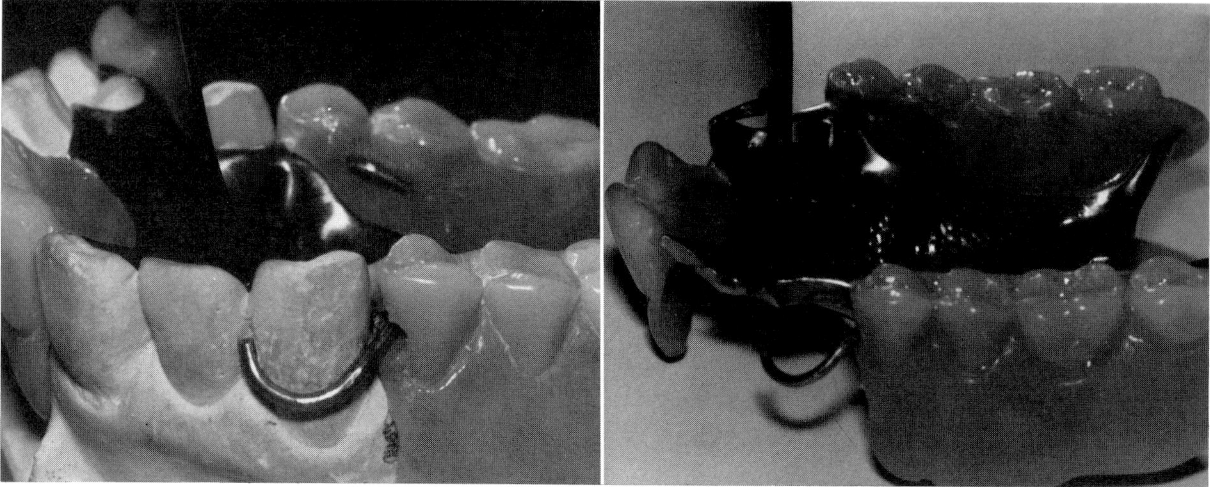

Fig. 11-74. Wrought wire clasps can be added to a prosthesis by embedding wire in acrylic resin.

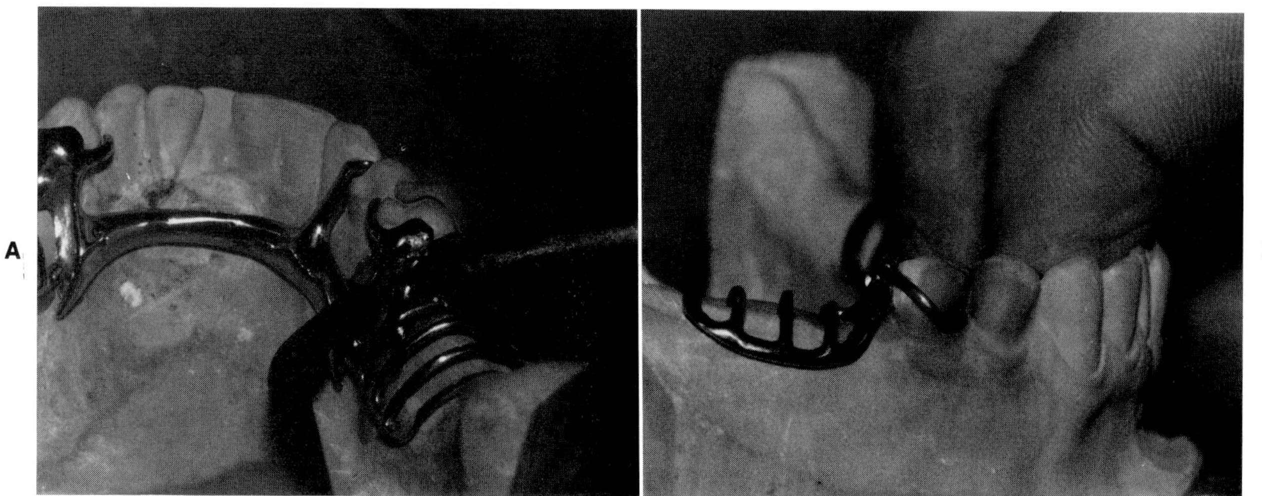

Fig. 11-75. A, A wrought wire clasp can be added to a framework by soldering wire to minor connector and rest seat. **B,** Wire can be shaped to tooth after soldering.

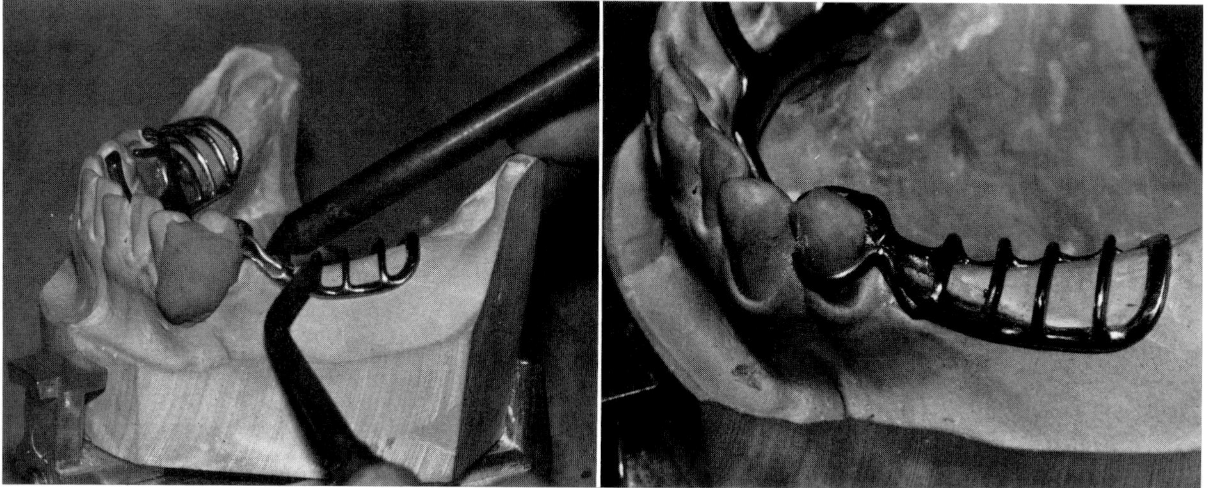

Fig. 11-76. Wire can more safely be soldered to acrylic resin retention farther from tooth.

CONCLUSIONS

Although it is certainly impractical and perhaps impossible for the clinician to be actively involved with the construction phases of the removable partial denture framework, the dentist should maintain and update basic dental school knowledge in this area.

The dentist who has the confidence to interject personally into the construction phase of the framework and establish and maintain a rational dialogue with the laboratory gains not only a better mechanical product but also the respect of the auxiliary. The information in this chapter, broad as it is, can serve as the basis for this relationship.

BIBLIOGRAPHY

Applegate, O.C.: Alloys for removable partial dentures. Factors to be considered in choosing an alloy, Dent. Clin. North Am. **4**:583-590, November 1960.

Asgar, K: A new alloy for partial dentures, J. Prosthet. Dent. **23**:36-43, 1970.

Asgar, K., and Peyton, F.A.: Casting dental alloys to embedded wires, J. Prosthet. Dent. **15**:312-321, 1965.

Beck, H.O.: Alloys for removable partial dentures, Dent. Clin. North Am. **4**:591-596, November 1960.

Blatterfein, L., and others: Minimum acceptable procedures for satisfactory removable partial denture service, J. Prosthet. Dent. **27**:84-87, 1972.

Brown, E.T.: The dentist, the laboratory technician, and the prescription law, J. Prosthet. Dent. **15**:1132-1138, 1965.

Calomeni, A.A.: Problem areas encountered by dental laboratories, J. Prosthet. Dent. **19**:523-529, 1968.

Cunningham, D.M.: Comparison of base metal alloys and Type IV gold alloys for removable partial denture frameworks, Dent. Clin. North Am. **17**:719, 1973.

Dootz, E.R., and others: Simplification of the chrome-cobalt partial denture casting procedure, J. Prosthet. Dent. **17**:464-471, 1967.

Dutton, D.A.: Standard abbreviations (and definitions) for use in dental laboratory work authorizations, J. Prosthet. Dent. **27**:94-95, 1972.

Earnshaw, R.S.: Cobalt-chromium alloys in dentistry, Br. Dent. J. **101**:67-75, 1956.

Elbert, C.A., and Ryge, G.: The effect of heat-treatment on microhardness of a cobalt-chromium alloy, J. Prosthet. Dent. **15**:873, 1965.

Fletcher, C.F.: Combatting the illegal practice of dentistry, J. Prosthet. Dent. **35**:92-96, 1976.

Gehl, D.H.: Investment in the future, J. Prosthet. Dent. **18**:190-201, 1967.

Giovanone, A.: The philosophy of cooperation of dentist and dental laboratory processing technicians, Dent. Lab. News, **25**:3-7, 1963.

Grunewold, A.H., and others: The role of the dental technician in a prosthetic service, Dent. Clin. North Am. **4**:359-370, 1960.

Henderson, D.: Writing work authorizations for removable partial dentures, J. Prosthet. Dent. **16**:696-707, 1966.

Henderson, D, and Frazier, Q.: Communicating with dental laboratory technicians, Dent. Clin. North Am. **14**:603-615, July 1970.

Hickey, J.D.: Responsibility of the dentist in removable partial dentures, J. Dent. Assoc. **17**:70-87, 1965.

Horner, S.J.: Dentistry's responsibility to the prosthetic patient, J. Prosthet. Dent. **1**:750-760, 1951.

Klein, I.J.: Danger ahead for prosthodontics, J. Prosthet Dent. **36**:122-123, 1976.

Mann, W.R., and others: Comparison of some properties of chromium alloys, J. Mich. Dent. Assoc, **23**:207, 1941.

Morris, H.F., and Asgar, K.: Physical properties and microstructure of four new commercial partial denture alloys, J. Prosthet. Dent. **33**:36-46, 1975.

Morris, H.F., and others: The influence of heat treatment on several types of base-metal removable partial denture alloys, J. Prosthet. Dent. **41**:388-395, 1979.

Payne, S.H.: The school, the practitioner, and the denturist, J. Prosthet. Dent. **12**:812-816, 1962.

Peyton, F.A., and Bush, S.H.: A comparison of tensile properties of cast gold and chrome-cobalt partial denture alloys, J. Mich. Dent. Assoc. **35**:250-252, 1953.

Pulshamp, F.E.: A comparison of the casting accuracy of base metal and gold alloys, J. Prosthet. Dent. **41**:272, 1979.

Quinn, I.: Status of the dental laboratory work authorization, J. Am. Dent. Assoc. **79**:1189-1190, 1969.

Smith, G.P.: The responsibility of the dentist toward dental laboratory procedures in fixed and removable partial denture prosthesis, J. Prosthet. Dent. **13**:295-301, 1963.

Taylor, D.F., and others: Physical properties of chromium-cobalt dental alloys, J. Am. Dent. Assoc. **56**:343-351, 1958.

Tomlin, H.R., and Osborne, J.: Cobalt-chromium partial dentures: a clinical survey, Br. Dent. J. **110**:307-310, 1961.

Walsh, Sir J.: The profession's responsibility, Int. Dent. J. **17**:75-82, 1967.

Weintraub, G.S.: The dental student as a technician: to what degree? J. Prosthet. Dent. **39**:459-465, 1978.

12 Fitting the framework

There are three phases in removable partial denture service. The first, the planning phase, takes place following the examination and diagnosis and during the survey and design of the prosthesis. The second phase is the mouth preparation and laboratory construction of the partial denture. Although both the dentist and the laboratory participate in this phase, the dentist is responsible for determining whether the result is clinically acceptable. The third phase is that of fitting the prosthesis to the patient. This chapter is concerned with the initial portion of that phase, the fitting of the framework.

No matter how much care is taken in making the final impression, in pouring an accurate master cast, and in the laboratory steps of blocking out, duplicating, waxing the framework, casting, and finishing the cast metal framework, discrepancies in the finished product will occur. The vastly improved dental materials currently available have reduced the number and size of discrepancies but have not eliminated them. Several years ago an informed panel of practitioners postulated that 105 errors can take place in removable partial denture service. Controlling these errors can be a monumental task. It is hoped that discrepancies will be held to a minimum, but errors that do take place must be corrected if the framework—and ultimately the partial denture—is to provide the health service the patient deserves.

It has been estimated that as many as 75% of removable partial dentures do not fit the mouth on the day of insertion. This may account for the fact that in the past many partial dentures either were not worn, or, if worn, produced changes in the oral structures.

During the clinical appointment described in this chapter the dentist must determine not only that the framework goes to place in the mouth, but also that all minor discrepancies in the fit are corrected and that the fit is accurate and precise. It is regrettable that the term *precision attachment* is sometimes used synonymously with internal attachment, because this implies that partial dentures with extracoronal retainers do not require precision. Nothing could be further from the truth. The effective extracoronal removable partial denture must be completely passive as it lies in the mouth. It should not exert any force on the teeth or on the underlying soft tissue and ridges. If forces are generated by the prosthesis, damage will result. Orthodontic forces may cause teeth to move to counter the force. Over time this orthodontic movement may produce passivity, but this is not the ideal way of achieving the passive state.

It should be remembered that retentive clasp tips are designed to lie passively in a specific undercut. If the retentive tip cannot reach this undercut because the partial denture is not completely seated, the tip will not be passive. Instead it will flex to cross the height of contour (see Fig. 3–29). The flexed clasp will exert a constant force against the abutment tooth, and the usual result is that the tooth becomes sore or painful. This is not uncommon with inaccurately fitted removable partial dentures.

The appointment for the try-in of the metal framework should be made as soon as practical after the framework is returned from the laboratory. This will lessen the possibility of changes taking place in the position of the teeth. Migration of the teeth is not likely to occur unless there is a long delay between the making of the final impression and the fitting of the framework. Recent periodontal therapy and recent extractions of teeth adjacent to abutment teeth increase the possibility of migration, which should be considered in planning treatment and scheduling appointments.

EXAMINATION OF FRAMEWORK

Before the patient arrives, the design cast and the master cast with the framework seated must be examined critically, preferably under magnification, and in an orderly sequence (Fig. 12-1). The importance of this examination sequence cannot be overemphasized. Although many dental schools no longer require students to perform the laboratory procedures necessary to construct a clinical, or even a preclinical (technique), partial denture, it is imperative that the student and practitioner be able to recognize deficiencies in a completed framework. The dentist must also be able to communicate instructions to a laboratory technician in an intelligent and understandable manner. Considerable emphasis should be placed on this phase of removable partial denture construction.

To expedite the examination of the completed labo-

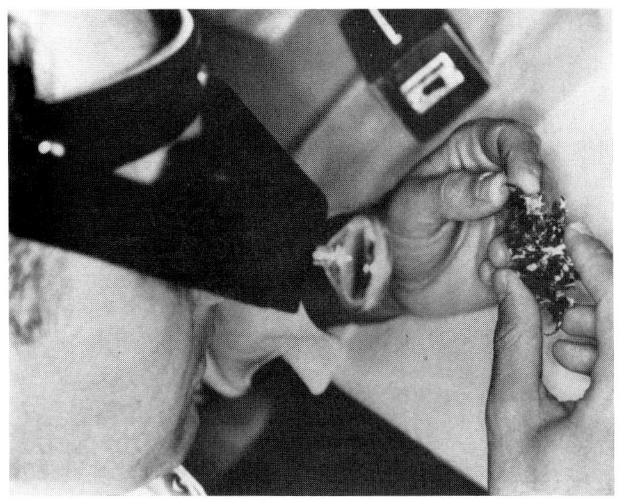

Fig. 12-1. Examination of cast framework under magnification is preferable.

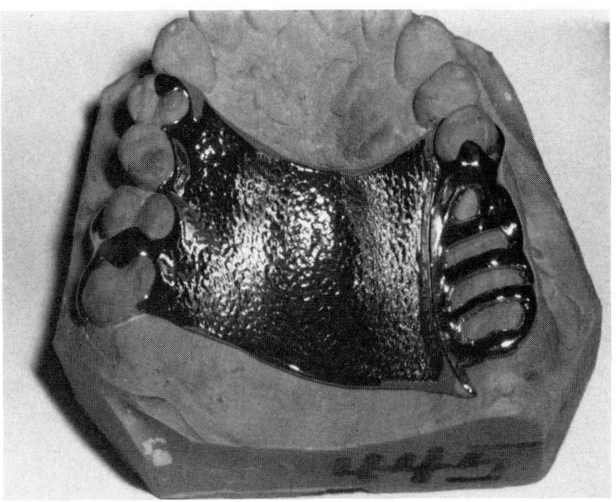

Fig. 12-2. Framework must fit cast accurately.

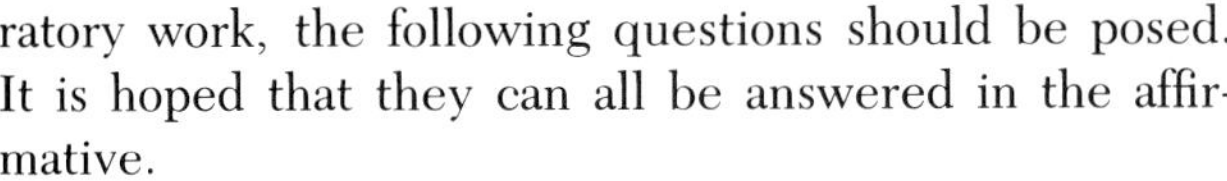

ratory work, the following questions should be posed. It is hoped that they can all be answered in the affirmative.

1. *Was the design drawn on the diagnostic cast followed?*

a. *Is the major connector positioned as requested?*

b. *Are the retentive clasp tips in the position and in the amount of undercut asked for?*

c. *Are the acrylic resin finish lines positioned correctly?*

d. *Are the indirect retainers and other rests located where desired?*

e. *Have soft tissue undercuts been handled as directed?*

The dental laboratory should never alter a design without a personal or telephone consultation with the submitting dentist. Although it is not unusual for a dentist in drawing a design to overlook some detail or to make an error, a respectable laboratory will always contact the dentist before making a change. A close rapport between the dentist and the laboratory will generally result in a higher quality of work.

If any discrepancy exists between the prescribed design and the framework returned by the laboratory, the reason for the difference should be determined before the try-in appointment.

2. *Does the framework fit the master cast accurately* (Fig. 12-2)? The framework will typically fit the cast tightly; in fact, it may be difficult to remove it because of the friction between the rough surface of the stone and the clasps. More often than not, the framework will not be nearly as retentive in the mouth. When the framework is removed from the cast, it is a good practice to cut the retentive undercuts from the stone teeth.

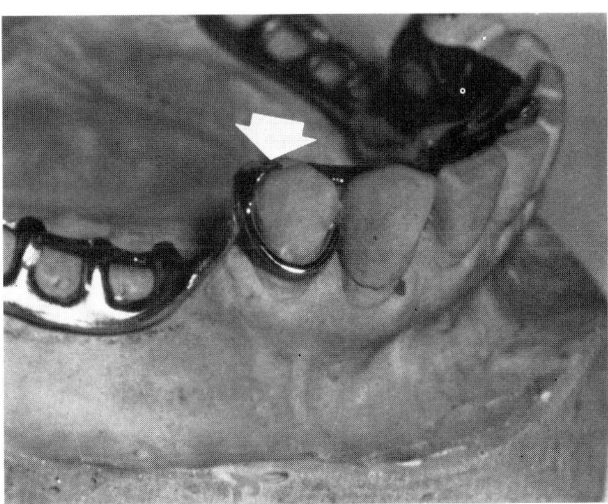

Fig. 12-3. Rest seats must be fully seated in rest seat preparations (arrow).

This will facilitate handling the framework and will not require the retentive clasp tips to flex excessively.

a. *Are the rests fully seated in their preparations* (Fig. 12-3)? If the margins of the rests are not flush with the margin of the rest seat or if evidence of incomplete seating is present, the reason for this should be determined now. The chance of a framework fitting the mouth and not fitting the master cast is extremely slim.

b. *Are reciprocal clasp arms and/or lingual plating in intimate contact with tooth surfaces?* If the blockout, waxing, and metal finishing were correctly done, there should be no space between the metal and the tooth (Fig. 12-4). Spaces that exist in these situations are damaging because debris will collect between the

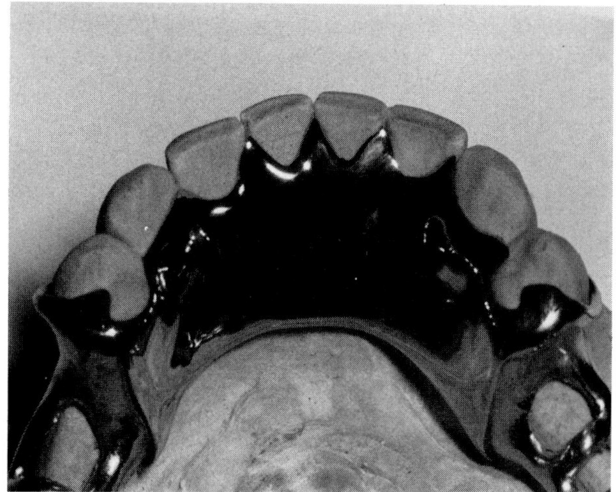

Fig. 12-4. Intimate contact between lingual plating and teeth is required to prevent damage to teeth and supporting structures.

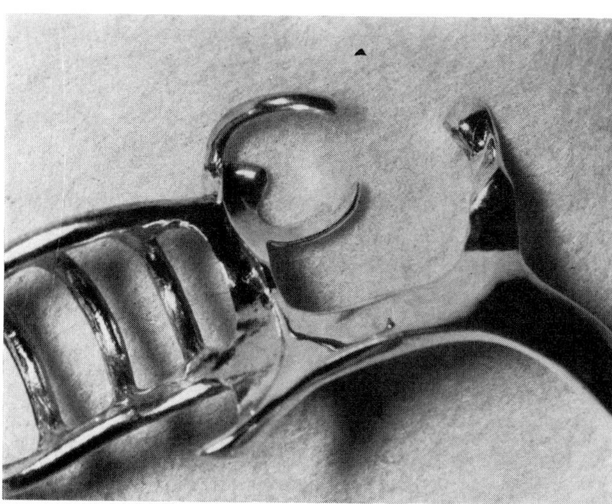

Fig. 12-5. Minor connectors, rests, and internal surfaces of clasps must be smooth and free from defects.

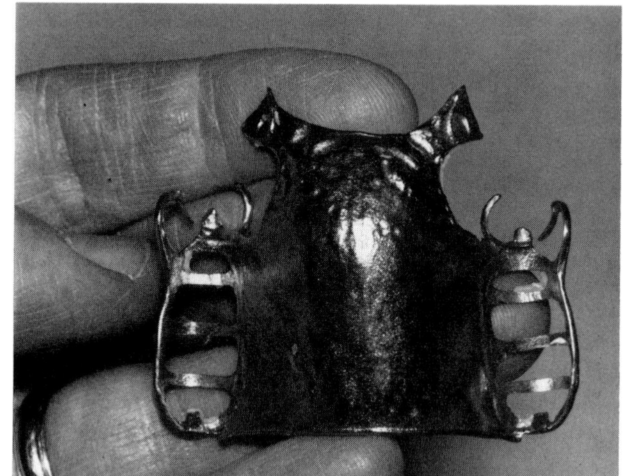

Fig. 12-6. Tissue surface of a maxillary major connector is not highly polished.

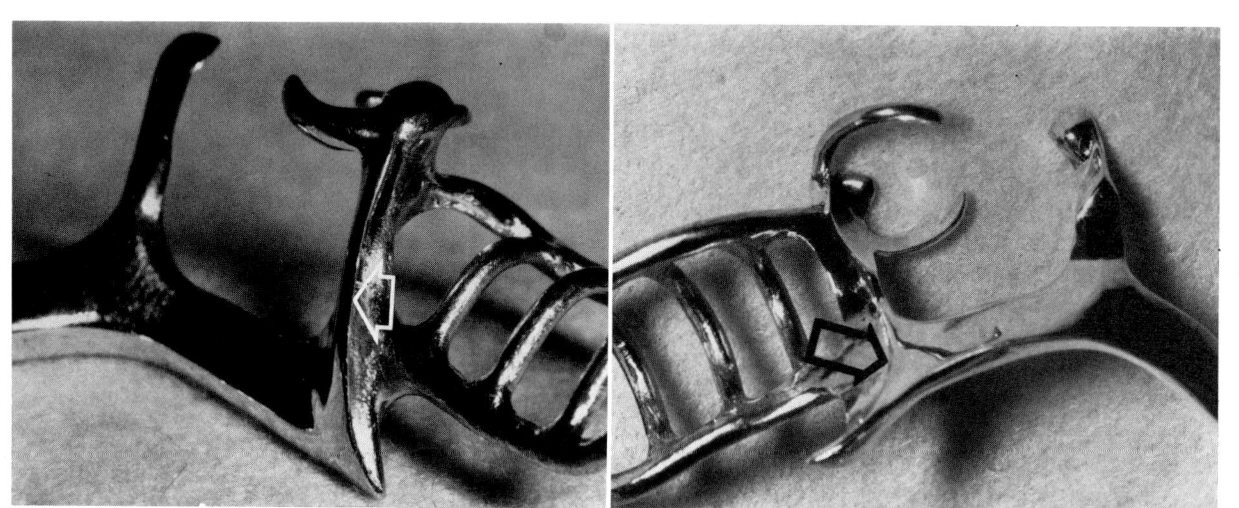

Fig. 12-7. A, An external finish line (arrow) is sharp and undercut. **B,** Internal finish line (arrow) is sharp but must not weaken framework.

framework and the tooth and cause decalcification of the hard tissue or inflammation of the soft tissue.

An especially critical location for this close adaptation of framework to tooth is in a lingual plate for the mandibular anterior teeth. If the interproximal projections of the plating do not completely close off the interproximal spaces, food will be packed between the teeth and rapid destruction of the supporting tissues may take place.

A properly designed and constructed mandibular lingual plate will be scalloped to fill the interproximal spaces and cover the cingulum of the teeth.

3. *Has the finishing and polishing of both the external and internal surfaces been carried out correctly?* The tissue side of the framework should be examined carefully for bubbles and other artifacts that might impede the smooth insertion of the framework into the mouth. A bubble of metal might not only prevent the seating of the framework, but it might also cause damage or pain to the patient.

Inner surfaces of clasps and minor connectors should be free from pits and scratches (Fig. 12-5).

The tissue surface of maxillary major connectors should not be highly polished but should be free from irregularities not caused by the impression of the soft tissue (Fig. 12-6).

Both internal and external finish lines should be sharp, definite, and slightly undercut to provide a firm mechanical lock for the acrylic resin (Fig. 12-7). A careful check should be made that the metal was not thinned excessively in providing the finish lines. This is a major cause of the entire denture base fracturing off during function.

The external surfaces of clasps and mandibular major connectors should be highly polished and free from waves, pits, and other irregularities.

The taper of clasps, particularly retentive clasps, should be uniform and free from nicks and notches.

The rigidity of the major connector should be tested with finger pressure. If the connector can be bent even slightly with light finger pressure, the framework should not be inserted. Rigidity is the first requirement of a major connector (Fig. 12-8).

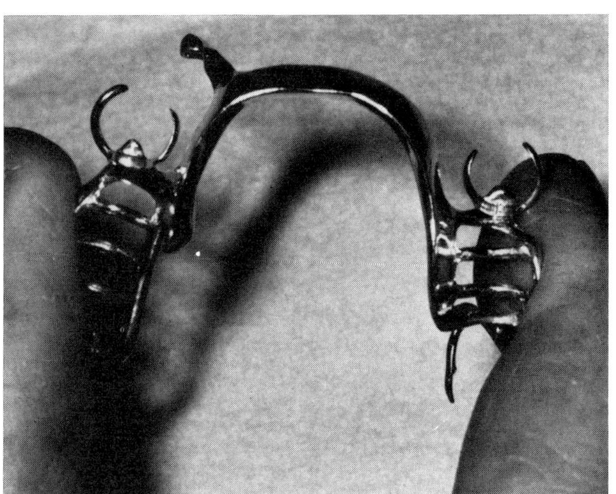

Fig. 12-8. Major connector must be rigid.

CLINICAL PROCEDURES

This appointment has two separate objectives. The first is to fit the framework to the teeth and the second is to adjust the framework to the opposing occlusion. The second should not be attempted until the first has been completed.

Fitting framework to teeth

Metal frameworks will practically always go to place and fit reasonably well with little or no adjustment. However, the fit of the framework must *not* be taken for granted. It is *always* possible to improve the fit to some degree by judicious machining of the metal. Frameworks that are close to being accurately fitted can be as damaging to the remaining oral structures as can grossly malfitted frameworks. A partial denture that is not quite seated can produce discomfort far out of proportion to its lack of accuracy.

One reason that removable partial dentures have been held in disfavor in past years was the lack of recognition that a near fit is not sufficient; an accurate fit is essential for success. The few minutes required to produce accuracy are more than compensated for in the high level of patient acceptance and the greatly decreased time needed for subsequent adjustment appointments.

Use of disclosing media

To locate small areas on the framework that are interferring with the fit, some type of disclosing medium is needed. Jeweler's rouge dissolved in chloroform and painted on the metal is an excellent pressure-indicating substance but a little more trouble to use than commercially available disclosing waxes (Figs. 12-9 and 12-10). Disclosing wax is simple to use and will give excellent results if the surface of the wax is read with caution. One must differentiate between a normal wiping away of wax during passage over a guiding plane, a showthrough of metal caused by an excessive area of pressure, and a wax tear caused by its sticking to the tooth surface. These all have different appearances, which the practitioner must learn by experience.

The greatest advantage of disclosing wax over other disclosing agents is that it is three dimensional. It will

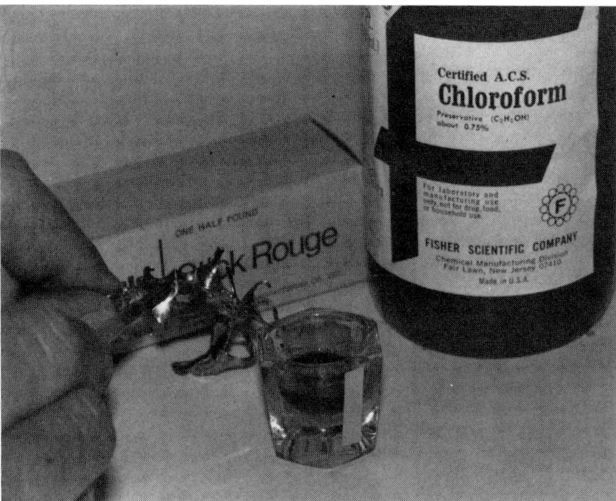

Fig. 12-9. Jeweler's rouge dissolved in chloroform and painted on internal surface of framework is one method of refining fit of prosthesis.

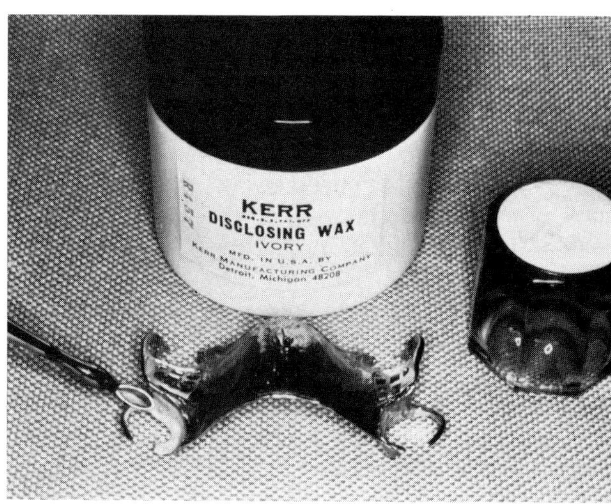

Fig. 12-10. Disclosing wax, has advantage of showing thickness when used to fit framework.

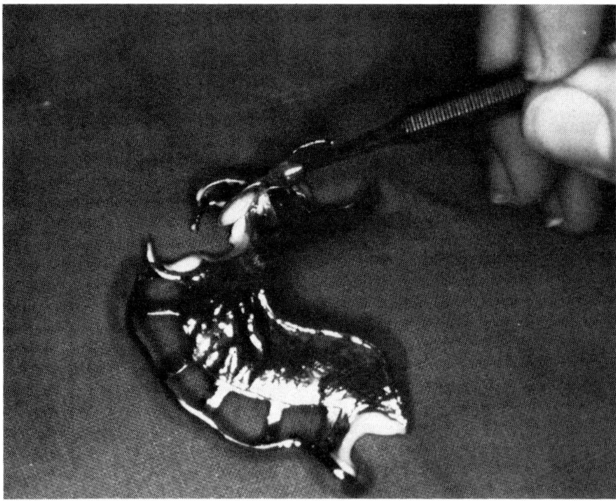

Fig. 12-11. Disclosing wax is placed on all metal surfaces that will contact tooth structure.

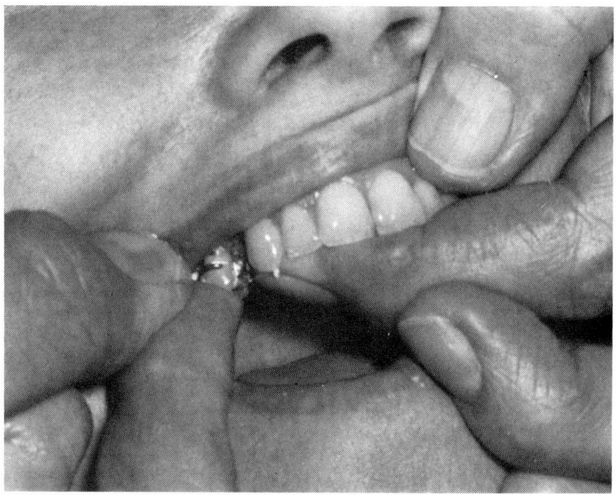

Fig. 12-12. Finger pressure alone is used to seat framework originally.

not only show whether a rest fits its rest seat and what is keeping it from being seated, but by the thickness of the remaining wax it will tell by how much the framework is not seated. Whereas a visual check may indicate that the framework fits adequately, disclosing wax may demonstrate a 1 to 2 mm space between the inner surface of the metal and the tooth surface. Correction of such errors is critical.

Melted disclosing wax is placed on all framework surfaces that will contact the teeth (Fig. 12-11). A Roach carver is the best instrument to use for this process. A thin, even coat of wax is desired.

The framework should be aligned over the abutment teeth and finger pressure applied in the direction of the planned path of insertion (Fig. 12-12). Excessive force should be avoided. If resistance to seating is great, the framework should be reexamined for distortion. Occasionally a clasp arm will have been bent, which will prevent proper seating. The surfaces of the master cast should also be examined for areas that have been abraded as the framework was seated to position and removed. These abraded areas may represent portions of the casting that are in undercuts of the teeth because of incorrect blockout.

At times it is desirable to adjust retentive clasp tips to decrease the amount of retention. This will make the insertion and removal of the framework much easier.

Particular care should be shown when circumferen-

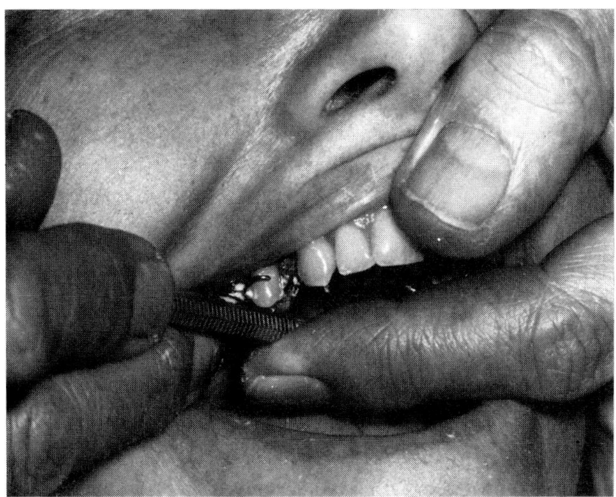

Fig. 12-13. Once framework has been seated, additional force applied via handle of instrument may be used to ensure full contact with teeth.

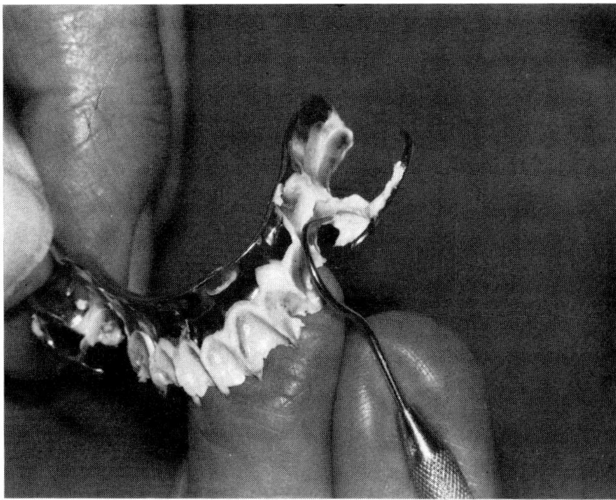

Fig. 12-14. Thickness of wax under occlusal rests can be measured.

tial or vertical projection molar clasps are present. It is easy to pinch the buccal mucosa between the clasp and the tooth, resulting in pain that can shake the patient's confidence abruptly.

When the framework is in place in the mouth, firm vertical pressure should be applied to occlusal rests or indirect retainers to seat the casting as nearly as possible. An instrument such as the mirror handle may be used to apply the seating force, but must be controlled to prevent the instrument from slipping and injuring the patient. The side of the instrument handle, not the end, should be used (Fig. 12-13).

In the case of a distal extension framework, no pressure should be applied over the distal extension area. This would cause the framework to rock and would produce misleading readings in the disclosing wax.

Correcting discrepancies

The framework should be carefully removed from the mouth to avoid damaging the surface of the disclosing wax and then examined under magnification. The thickness of wax beneath occlusal rests or indirect retainers reliably indicates the degree to which the framework fails to seat (Fig. 12-14).

The inner surface of the framework, under the disclosing wax, should be examined for "high spots," or areas of metal showthrough that prevent the seating of the casting. The most common points of showthrough that interfere with seating occur above the survey line on the teeth. As shown in Fig. 12-15, these areas generally occur *under rests*, at the *shoulder of circumferential clasps*, under *embrasure clasps*, and in *interproximal extensions* of lingual plating.

A showthrough area below the survey line on the tooth will not prevent the framework from seating. This type of showthrough is seen most frequently on posterior lingual plating and on minor connectors; it is caused when the component remains in contact with the greatest bulge of the tooth as the framework is seated. This will appear as a wipe-away of the disclosing wax, but it should not be relieved because it is beneficial. These areas are the guiding planes that guide the framework to place and prevent the tooth from being rocked each time the removable partial denture is inserted or withdrawn (Fig. 12-16).

The located areas of interference should be relieved by grinding the metal showthrough, which is most efficiently accomplished with a No. 2 round carbide bur in the high-speed handpiece (Fig. 12-17). After the areas have been relieved, the disclosing wax that has been contaminated by the metal grindings is removed completely and fresh wax is added. The contaminated wax can be removed from the framework by wiping with pledgets or, perhaps best and most efficiently, by holding the framework over a small flame just long enough to melt the low-fusing wax and then blowing the melted wax from the framework with the air syringe (Fig. 12-18). If the heat melts the wax only, the framework will not be compromised.

The entire procedure should be repeated until the framework is seated. The framework fits properly when the disclosing wax is displaced evenly, leaving a thin film of wax under rests and indirect retainers. If chrome is used for the framework, the wax will have a grayish hue from the metal's reflecting through the wax. Proper accomplishment of this procedure can do more than any

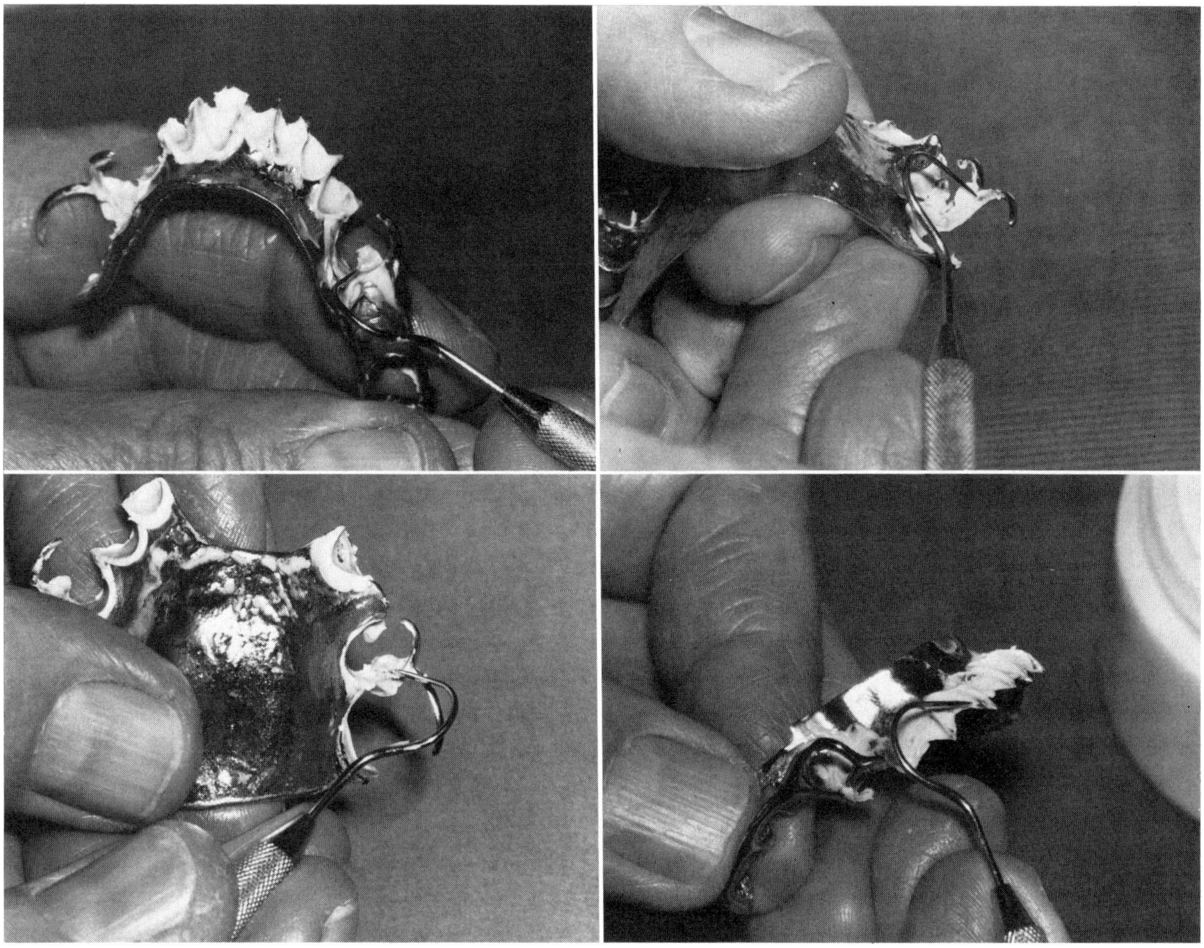

Fig. 12-15. Small metallic points of showthrough prevent framework from seating. They are most commonly seen under occlusal, incisal, or cingulum rests, **A,** at shoulders of circumferential clasps, **B,** under embrasure clasps, **C,** and in interproximal extensions of lingual platings, **D.**

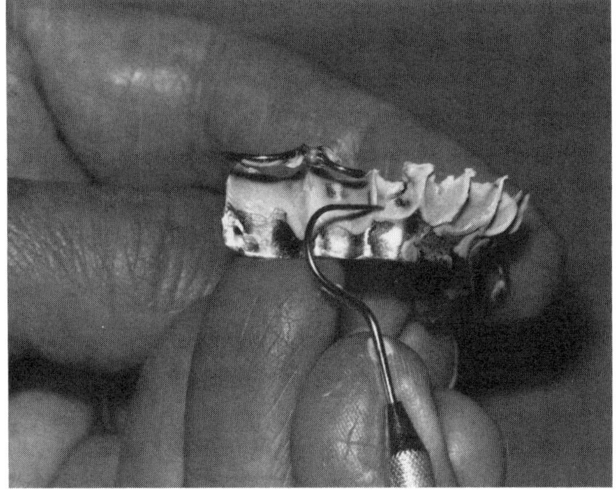

Fig. 12-16. Wipe-away of disclosing wax on guiding plane surfaces should not be interpreted as interference.

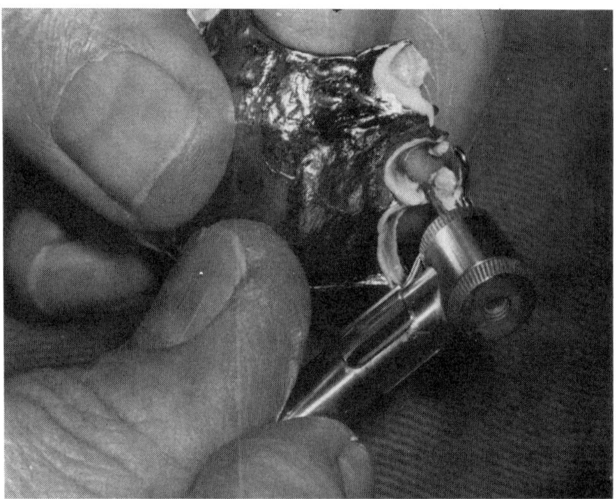

Fig. 12-17. A small round carbide bur in high-speed handpiece is used to eliminate interferences.

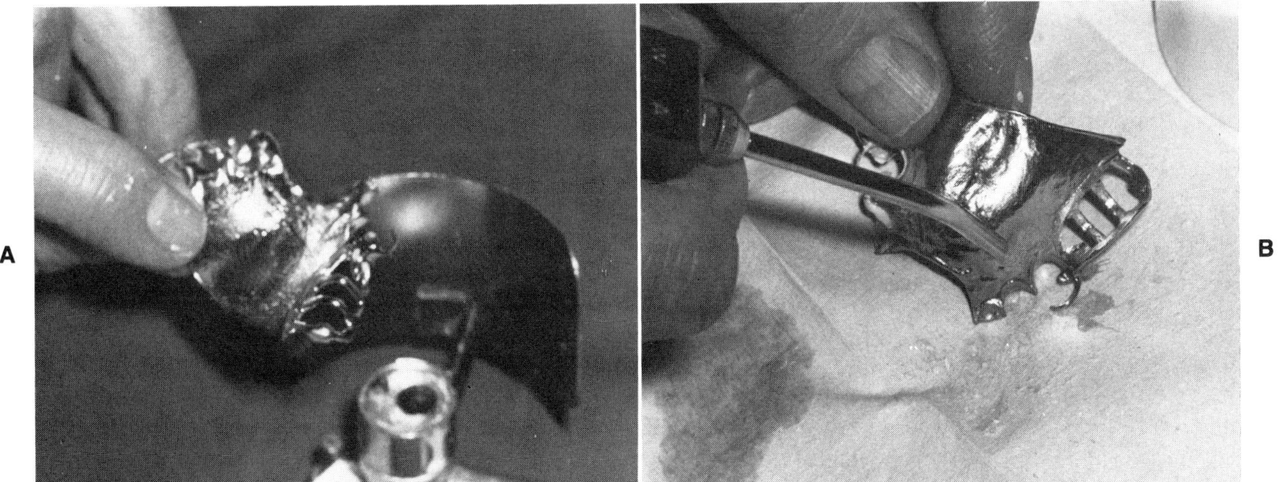

Fig. 12-18. To remove contaminated disclosing wax, framework is heated over flame, **A,** and melted wax is eliminated by air syringe, **B.**

other step in partial denture construction to ensure the success of treatment.

The time involved in this portion of the appointment varies depending on how great the error in fit is at the start of the appointment, but 15 to 20 minutes is normal. The feel of the partial denture as it goes to place changes drastically. Instead of the grating or snapping feeling that is present at the beginning of the appointment, a sliding or gliding action can be noted as the partial denture is inserted at the end of the appointment. Neutralization of some lateral forces generated by the discrepancies accounts for the decreased resistance to insertion.

One must always decide whether the discrepancies are so great that suitable correction cannot be made in the fit of a specific framework. The decision should be made as early as possible so that, if necessary, a new impression can be made for the construction of a new framework. The original master cast should not be used because in the vast majority of cases the cast represents an inaccurate reproduction of the semiedentulous arch because of an inaccurate impression. Even if the cast were accurate, its surface would be too marred to be used again.

Fitting framework to opposing occlusion

After the framework has been fit to the teeth, it must be adjusted to the opposing occlusion. It has been mentioned previously that rarely should the vertical relationship of the jaws be changed by removable partial dentures. For this reason great care must be taken to correct all occlusal discrepancies. The framework must not keep the natural teeth from making normal occlusal contacts in either centric or eccentric closures. If both

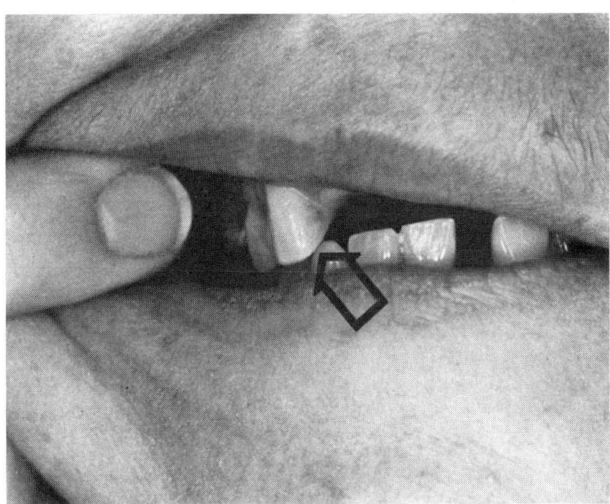

Fig. 12-19. Relationship between a maxillary and a mandibular tooth is noted with nothing in mouth.

maxillary and mandibular frameworks are being constructed, *only one at a time should be corrected.* The most reliable and simplest method of correcting occlusal errors is to have the patient close in centric occlusion with *nothing* in the mouth. In this position the relation of a maxillary natural tooth to a mandibular natural tooth can be noted. Most patients have at least one point of interocclusal contact between natural teeth that can be observed (Fig. 12-19). The same interocclusal relationship between those two natural teeth should exist when both frameworks are in the mouth.

One framework is positioned in the mouth, and the patient guided to closure in centric occlusion. The amount of occlusal interference will be evidenced by

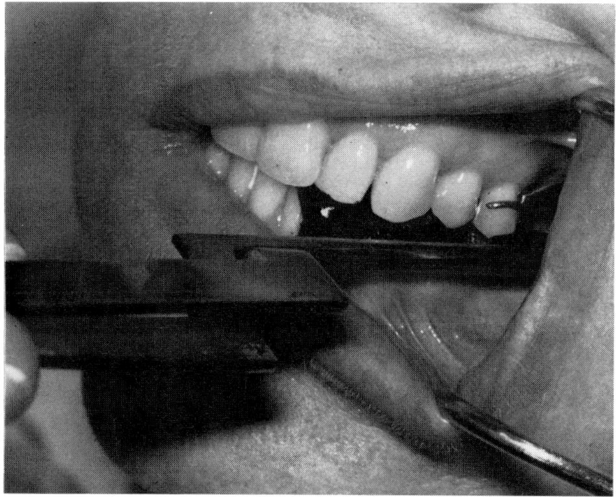

Fig. 12-20. Thin articulating paper or ribbon is used to check for premature occlusal contacts against metal.

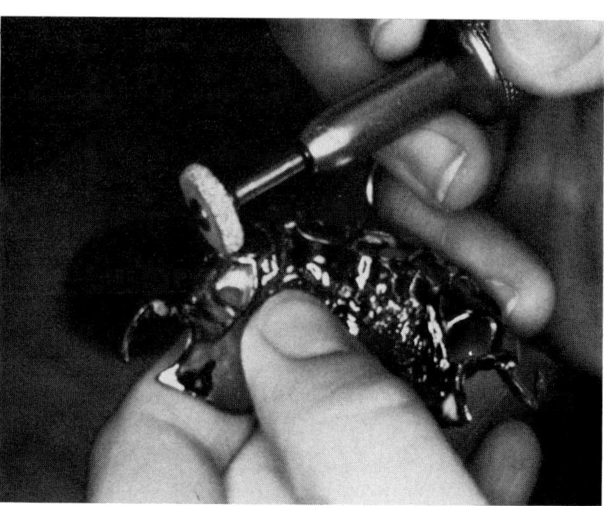

Fig. 12-21. Reduction of occlusal prematurities on metal is made with framework out of mouth.

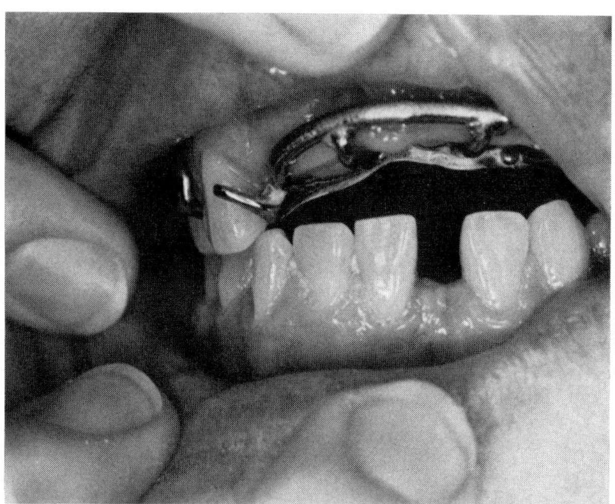

Fig. 12-22. Checks for occlusal interference must also be made in eccentric jaw positions.

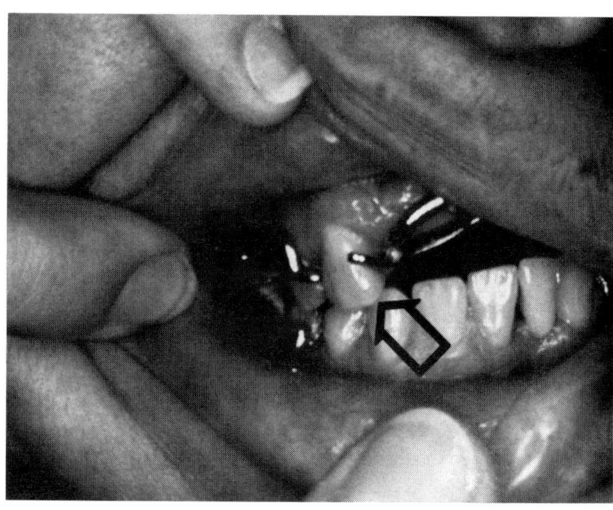

Fig. 12-23. Natural tooth-to-tooth contact (arrow) must be restored with both frameworks in place.

the observed amount of space between the natural teeth. Thin articulating paper, held in forceps, is placed over the teeth on one side of the arch (Fig. 12-20). The patient is asked to tap the teeth together with light vertical force. This movement should then be repeated with the articulating paper held on the opposite side of the arch. The tapping movement will transfer ink from the articulating paper to the area of metal that is causing the interference. Reduction or correction of the discrepancy should be made with the framework out of the mouth because most patients object to the sensation produced by grinding on this very hard metal in the mouth (Fig. 12-21). Heatless stones or diamond instruments in the high-speed handpiece are used to reduce the interferences.

Once centric occlusion has been reestablished as witnessed by the visual contact between the natural teeth, the patient should be guided into eccentric positions, both lateral and protrusive, with the articulating paper in place to locate interferences in these positions (Fig. 12-22). The eccentric interferences are corrected the same way as in centric occlusion. Each framework should be cleared in this manner individually. Then, they should be tried in the mouth together. Any inter-

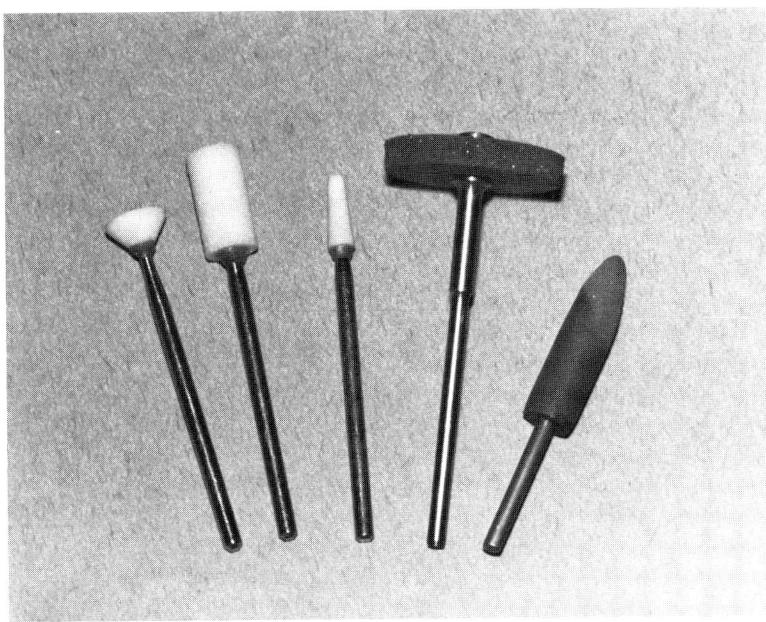

Fig. 12-24. Chrome finishing stones and Carborundum-impregnated points and wheels are used to restore smooth finish to all surfaces of framework, both internal and external, that were ground in fitting procedure.

ference noted now will be *between the metal of the opposing frameworks.* A final correction should be made using articulating paper to locate the points of interference (Fig. 12-23).

Correcting discrepancies

When occlusal discrepancies on the framework are corrected, care must be used not to cut excessively and thus weaken the important elements of the partial denture. If an occlusal rest is removed by overcutting, important support of the denture will be lost. This would have to be repaired before the partial denture could be inserted. Too much relief on a clasp may also weaken it so that it may break after insertion. The problem of obtaining sufficient interocclusal space should have been solved during design planning and mouth preparation. Unfortunately, however, occlusal clearance is often insufficient. It is almost a prosthodontic maxim that sufficient mouth preparation is never accomplished. In preference to weakening the framework by too much metal reduction, the opposing tooth surfaces or restorations may be judiciously relieved to obtain the necessary clearance.

Finishing and polishing ground surfaces

After the framework has been fit and occlusal adjustments have been made, the surfaces of the metal and the teeth that have been ground or reshaped must be finished and polished (Fig. 12-24). Special care must be observed not to destroy the accurate fit of clasps, minor connectors, and guiding planes. Adequate thickness of metal must also be preserved to avoid breakage during function.

Depending on the degree of correction of fit and of occlusal adjustment required, the experienced practitioner should require 30 to 45 minutes for this appointment. The beginning student will normally need 2 to 3 hours.

NEXT APPOINTMENT

Determination of what the next appointment will consist of should be made before the patient is dismissed. At this point in treatment it is possible to follow several different directions, depending on the type of partially edentulous patient being treated. The possible courses for the next appointment follow:

1. *Corrected or altered cast.* This appointment is required for all mandibular distal extension patients, for some long-span maxillary distal extension patients, and for some long-span anterior replacement patients.
2. *Jaw relation.* This is the next appointment if an altered cast impression is not needed and if the casts cannot be accurately hand articulated. This may be accomplished during the framework adjustment appointment if time is available.
3. *Esthetic try-in.* This appointment will be next if a corrected cast is not needed, a jaw relation record is not required, and missing anterior teeth are to be replaced with denture teeth on a denture base. If facings

or tube teeth were designed, they would have been tried in before framework construction.

4. *Insertion.* If none of the above appointments are needed, the removable partial denture may be completed and inserted at the next appointment. Generally, a try-in for the replacement of posterior teeth only is not needed. If all the posterior teeth are being replaced, a try-in may be required.

When all the replacement teeth are tube teeth, metal pontics, or facings, insertion may be accomplished during the framework-fitting appointment if time permits. If this is the case, patient instruction for care of the prosthesis and oral hygiene should be reviewed.

BIBLIOGRAPHY

Fadal, R.E.: Disclosing cast restorations—a must, G.P. Texas Acad. Gen. Dent. **7**(1):1981.

Kaiser, D.A. and Wise, H.B.: Fitting cast gold restorations with the aid of disclosing wax, J. Prosthet. Dent., **43**:227-228, 1980.

Ostlund, L.E.: Improving the marginal fit of cast restorations, J. Am. Acad. Gold Foil Oper. **17**:56, 1974.

Rudd, K.D., and Dunn, B.W.: Accurate removable partial dentures, J. Prosthet. Dent. **18**:559-570, 1967.

Shillingburg, H.T., Jr.: Cast gold restorations. In Clark, J.W., editor: Clinical dentistry, New York, 1976, Harper & Row Publishers.

Stewart, K.L., and Rudd, K.D.: Stabilizing periodontally weakened teeth with removable partial dentures, J. Pros. Dent. **19**:475-482, 1968.

13 Special impression procedures for tooth-tissue–supported removable partial dentures

PURPOSE

With removable partial dentures that are completely tooth supported (those in Class III and many Class IV partially edentulous arches), the occlusal forces transmitted to the abutment teeth are directed vertically down the long axes of the teeth through the occlusal, incisal, or lingual rests (see Fig. 4-2). The edentulous ridges will not contribute to the support of the partial denture, because the teeth absorb these forces before the forces are transmitted to the residual ridge. Since the denture base does not contribute to the support of the partial denture and since the underlying mucosa and bone are not subjected to functional forces, a tooth-supported removable partial denture can be constructed on a master cast made from a single, pressure-free impression that records the teeth and the residual ridge in their anatomic form. (The procedure for making this impression and master cast is described in Chapter 9).

A tooth-tissue–supported removable partial denture constructed on such a cast, however, will exert excess pressure on the teeth that help support the denture as the soft tissue under the denture base compresses. A dual impression technique is used to equalize as much as possible the support derived from the edentulous ridge and that received from the abutment teeth. The impression of the teeth should be made with a material that captures the teeth in anatomic form, because normally the teeth do not change position under function to any measurable degree. The impression of the soft tissue, on the other hand, must be made in such a manner as to record the tissues in a functioning form. The impression must (1) record and relate the tissues under the same loading, (2) distribute the load over as large an area as possible, and (3) delineate accurately the peripheral extent of the denture base.

FACTORS INFLUENCING SUPPORT OF DISTAL EXTENSION BASE

To determine to what extent the soft tissue supporting the denture base should be displaced during the impression procedure, a number of factors influencing the amount of tissue displacement are considered.

These factors will be considered independently, but it must be remembered that each factor will influence the other.

Quality of soft tissue covering edentulous ridge

The soft tissues covering the bony residual ridges are composed of tissues that are compressible to varying degrees. It is essential that this variability be recognized as the partial denture treatment progresses. Not only may the degree of displaceability of the soft tissue over the edentulous ridge vary from one patient to another, but differences will occur in the same patient depending on the location on the ridge being tested. The more displaceable tissue present over the edentulous ridge, the less support for the denture base can be derived from that ridge. A firm, tightly attached mucosa, several millimeters thick, will offer the greatest support (Fig. 13-1). If excessive redundant soft tissue has accumulated, particularly over maxillary tuberosities, surgical removal of this tissue may be indicated to have firm, nonmovable support for a denture base. Removal of this tissue not only improves the prospect of decreased vertical displacement of a denture base but also improves the resistance to lateral displacement.

Type of bone making up denture-bearing area

Cancellous bone, as compared with cortical bone, is less able to resist vertical forces because its irregular surface acts as an irritant to the overlying soft tissue if vertical stress occurs (Fig. 13-2). The result of the irritation is chronic inflammation, which leads not only to constant patient discomfort but eventually to resorption of the cancellous bone. The crest of the maxillary and mandibular ridge is composed mainly of cancellous bone and therefore should not be considered as the prime source of support for a distal extension denture base.

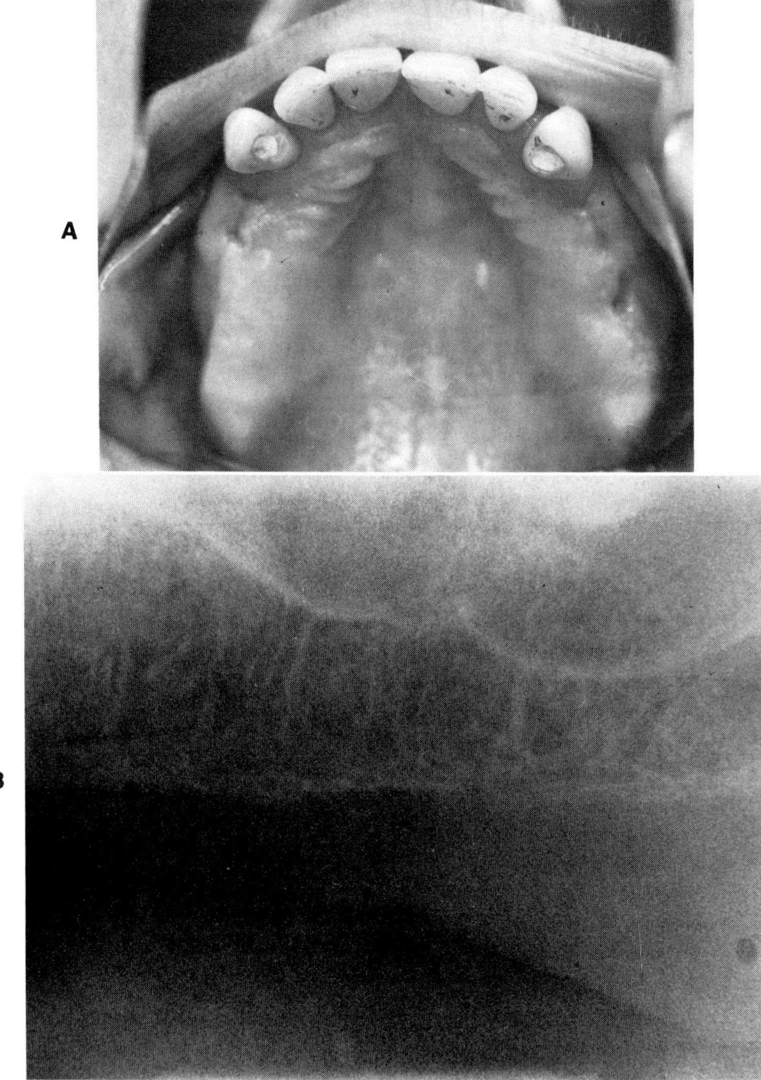

Fig. 13-1. A, Broad edentulous ridge covered by firm, nonmovable mucosa. B, Radiograph shows excessive, redundant soft tissue coverage of bone over tuberosity.

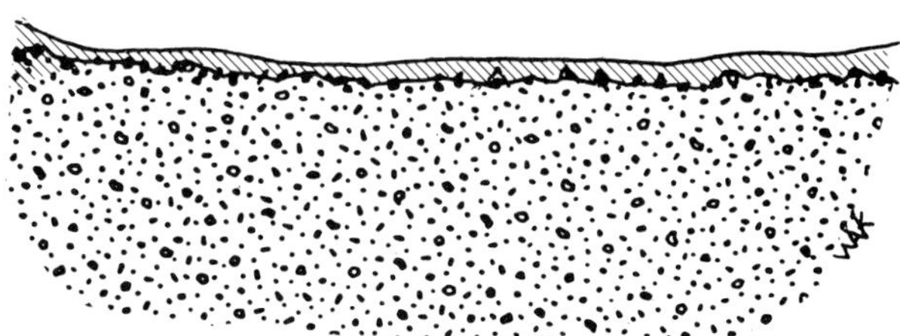

Fig. 13-2. Irregular surface of cancellous bone can irritate overlying mucosa if vertical force occurs.

Design of partial denture

Knowledge of basic mechanical principles can greatly help control functional forces occurring against the distal extension ridge (Fig. 13-3). By using additional components of the partial denture, the rotational forces taking place around the fulcrum line passing through the most distal or posterior rests can be decreased or altered. The most efficient method of controlling the rotational movement is the use of indirect retainers anterior to the fulcrum line. The indirect retainer is most often in the form of a rest attached to the major connector by a minor connector. If the distal extension denture is bilateral, two indirect retainers, one on each side of the arch, are used. If the denture is unilateral, normally only one indirect retainer is needed and is positioned anterior to the fulcrum line and on the opposite side of the arch from the distal extension ridge.

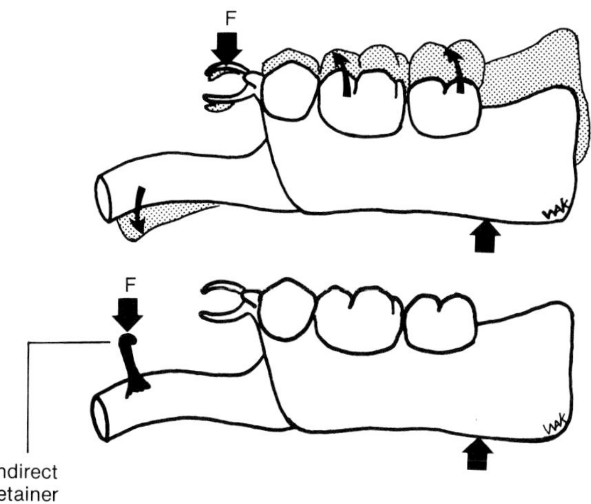

Fig. 13-3. Rest attached to major connector or anterior to fulcrum line serves as indirect retainer and helps control rotation of prosthesis away from residual ridge.

Amount of tissue coverage of denture base

To counteract the tissueward component of the rotational force, the denture base must cover the maximum amount of surface area of the edentulous ridge. The broader the coverage of the edentulous ridge, the greater will be the distribution of the load occurring against it per unit of area (Fig. 13-4). All available space must be used without encroaching on movable tissues. Not only will overextensions of the denture base cause soft tissue irritation, or ulceration, but, even worse, the lifting or dislodging forces on the base by the tissues will cause torquing of the clasped abutment teeth and possible orthodontic movement of the teeth anterior to the fulcrum line (Fig. 13-5).

Amount of occlusal force

The total amount of occlusal force applied to a denture base on a distal extension ridge influences the amount of support required to stabilize that denture base. A denture base that is opposed by a full complement of natural teeth in a young, vigorous individual with well-developed muscles of mastication requires more support than a denture base opposed by a complete denture in an elderly patient. In the first instance maximum coverage of all available ridge is an absolute necessity. In addition, narrowing the food table of the

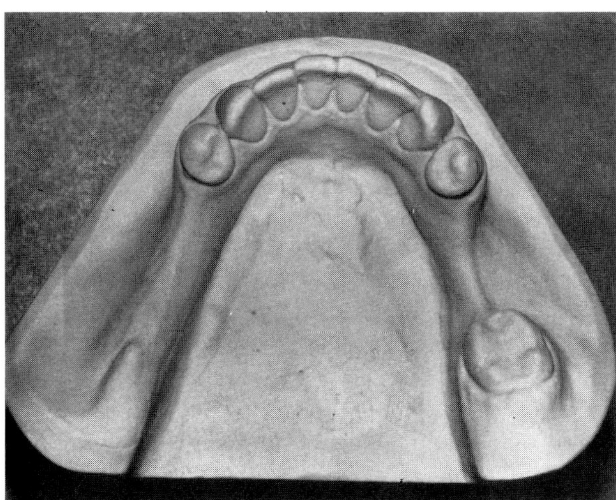

Fig. 13-4. The larger and broader the edentulous ridge the greater will be the distribution of undesirable forces.

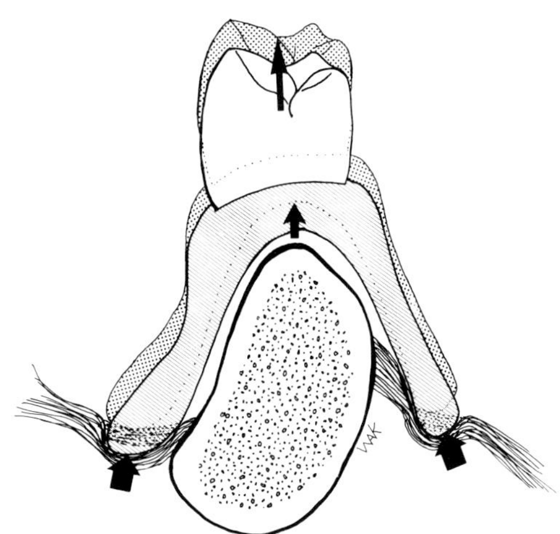

Fig. 13-5. Denture base, if overextended onto movable tissue, is lifted by that tissue, and torquing forces are transferred to abutment teeth.

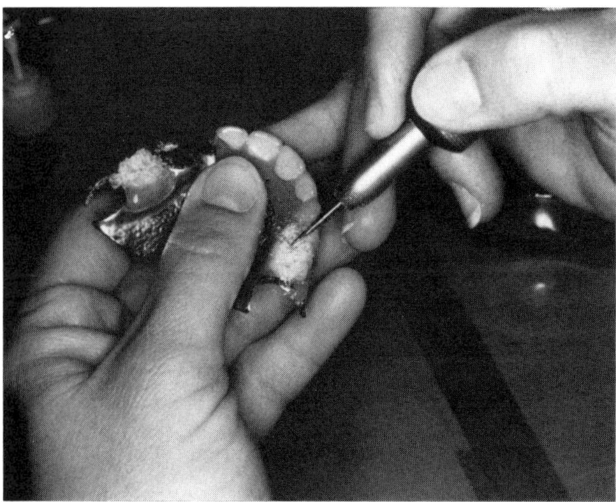

Fig. 13-6. Anatomy of denture tooth is accentuated to improve cutting efficiency.

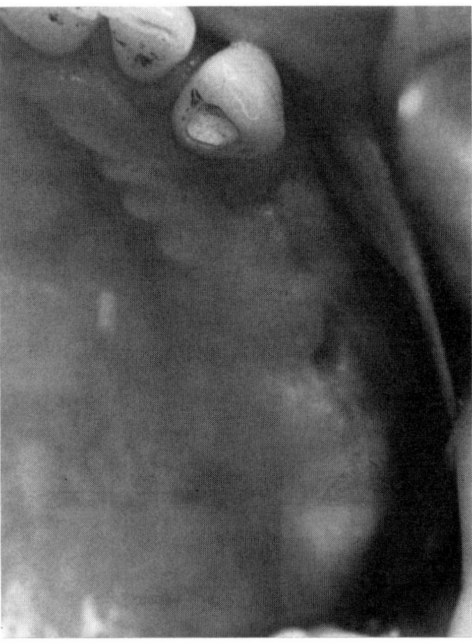

Fig. 13-7. Most vertical support for denture base in maxilla comes from ridge crest.

artificial teeth will help reduce the load transmitted to the denture base. Increasing the efficiency of the occlusal surfaces of the artificial teeth by the addition of supplemental grooves and sluiceways aids the cutting action and improves the masticatory performance of the teeth (Fig. 13-6). Improving the efficiency of the teeth will require less force in chewing, and less force will then be transmitted to the residual ridge. All these actions help improve the support for the denture base.

Denture-bearing area

To distribute the forces of occlusion to the ridge most efficiently, the majority of the force must be directed to portions of the ridge that are most capable of withstanding that force. Because the crests of both maxillary and mandibular edentulous ridges are normally composed of cancellous bone, structures other than the ridge crests must be looked to for primary support of the denture base.

Maxillary edentulous ridge

In the maxillary arch, because of its morphology, few structures other than the crest of the ridge are capable of serving as a primary support, or primary stress-bearing area. The buccal slopes of the ridge, normally covered by a layer of cortical bone, can withstand stress. Unfortunately, the buccal slope is rarely perpendicular to the vertical forces occurring against it, so it offers little resistance to them. The buccal slope will, however, resist lateral forces, reducing the total force. Some resistance to vertical displacement can be derived from the mucosa overlying the hard bony palate. If an attempt is made to use vertical support for the denture base from the palate, the mucosa over the palate must be as compressible as that over the ridge crest. If palatal mucosa is less compressible, pain may result from compression of tissue over the median raphe.

As undesirable as it may seem, the majority of denture base support for the maxillary distal extension partial denture must come from the ridge crest (Fig. 13-7). The mucosa covering the crest is usually firm, dense tissue that is capable of resisting occlusal forces to a large degree. If the crestal mucosa is not firm and dense, it should be surgically corrected to properly support a denture base.

Mandibular edentulous ridge

The crest of the mandibular ridge cannot be used as a primary stress-bearing area because it is composed of cancellous bone and often the tissue overlying the bone is less firm and dense than that in the maxilla. The very dense cortical bone forming the buccal shelf area, bordered by the external oblique line laterally and the crest of the ridge medially, makes this area an excellent primary stress-bearing site (Fig. 13-8). The soft tissue covering the cortical bone in this region is usually firm and dense. The anatomy of the buccal shelf area is normally perpendicular, or nearly so, to the vertical forces that would be occurring against it, making it well able to tolerate the stresses. The slopes of the residual ridge, both buccal and lingual, have cortical bone coverage and can contribute to resisting horizontal forces.

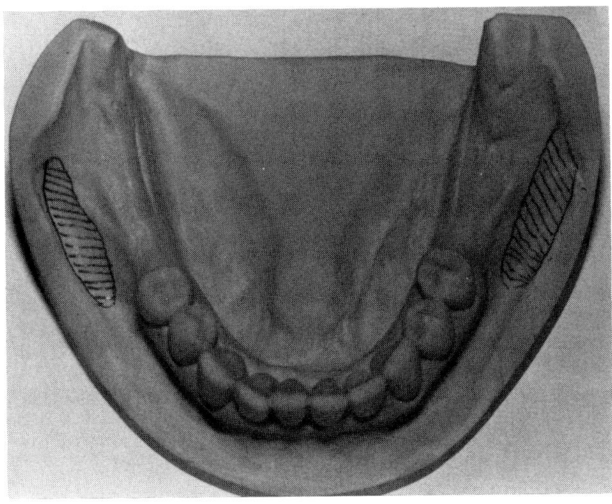

Fig. 13-8. Buccal shelf area of posterior mandibular ridge (shaded areas) can serve as primary stress-bearing area.

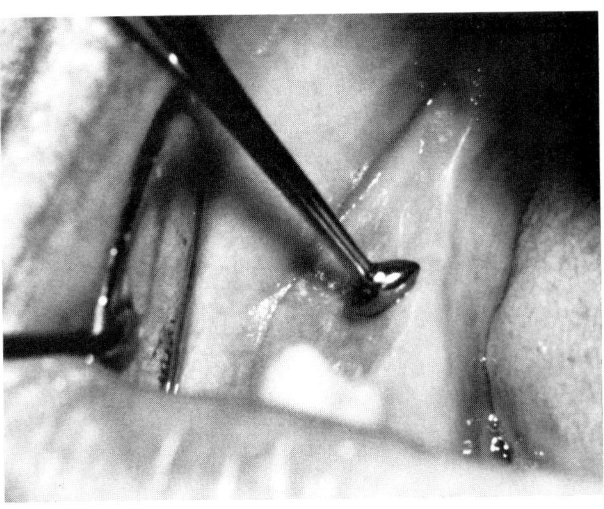

Fig. 13-9. Displaceable tissue can be measured with ball burnisher.

Fit of denture base

The denture base must be made to fit such that the areas in both arches that can serve as primary stress-bearing areas do so. The rest of this chapter discusses how best to record these areas to take advantage of the anatomic features.

INDICATIONS

In some mouths the soft tissue displacement is slight. If a thick healthy mucosal coverage is present, which is particularly apt to be true in the maxillary arch, the contour of the mucosal foundation may be virtually the same under an applied load as it is at rest.

The decision as to whether a dual impression is necessary in a given case may be determined by the following test: Acrylic resin bases are added to the framework, the framework is placed in the mouth with the attached resin bases, and finger pressure is applied to the base or bases. If the base can be depressed enough that the indirect retainers or lingual plating lifts away from the teeth, a dual impression should be made. If, however, there is no discernible movement, consideration should be given to dispensing with the dual impression technique. Other methods of measuring the displaceability of tissue such as that shown in Fig. 13-9 may be used.

It should be pointed out that dispensing with the dual impression procedure eliminates the opportunity of establishing precisely accurate and functionally formed denture borders.

The dual impression technique is most often indicated for the mandibular distal extension ridge because only a limited ridge area can be used as a stress-bearing site. In addition, obtaining the proper peripheral extension for the denture base in the mandibular arch is much more complicated than in the maxillary arch because of the movable tissues in the floor of the mouth.

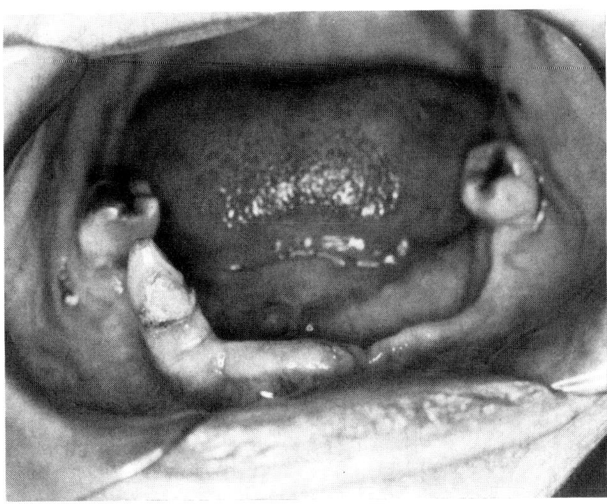

Fig. 13-10. In a long-span situation, corrected cast technique can more accurately distribute occlusal load over edentulous ridge.

Because the maxillary distal extension ridge is usually covered by a firm, dense, well-attached mucosa, or can surgically be prepared in that form, and the stress-bearing area must be the crest and buccal slope of the ridge, a dual impression does not often improve the stress distribution. The border definition is also much simpler and can be read from a single, anatomic impression.

The other indication for a dual impression is a long-span anterior edentulous ridge (normally including at least the six anterior teeth), where the ridge must supply some support for the partial denture (Fig. 13-10). Improving the accuracy of that portion of the cast with a secondary impression and defining the peripheral extension of the anterior flange can be helpful in distributing forces that will take place against a normally weaker portion of the dental arch.

IMPRESSION METHODS

There are basically two dual impression techniques.

The *physiologic, or functional, impression technique* records the ridge portion of the cast in its physiologic, or functioning, form by placing an occlusal load on the impression tray as the impression is being made. The underlying supporting tissues will be displaced because displacement will normally occur under function. Three physiologic impression techniques are discussed in this chapter: McLean's and Hindels's methods, the functional relining method, and the fluid wax method.

The *selected pressure impression technique* not only equalizes the support between the abutment teeth and the soft tissue, but has the added advantage of directing the force to the portions of the ridge that are most capable of withstanding the force. This is accomplished by providing relief in the impression tray in selected areas and permitting the impression tray to contact the ridge in other areas. Those areas where relief is provided, normally the crest of the ridge, will be the least displaced as the impression is recorded. In those areas of the tray where relief was not provided (the buccal shelf of the mandibular ridge and the buccal slope and crest of the maxillary ridge), greater displacement of the underlying mucosa will occur.

In both the fluid wax functional impression technique and the selected pressure technique an impression of the displaced edentulous ridge is made by using an impression tray attached to the framework, and the master cast is altered to accommodate the new ridge impression (Fig. 13-11). For this reason the technique is often referred to as the altered cast impression technique or the corrected cast impression technique. The procedures for making the fluid wax functional impression and the selected pressure impression will be described in the discussion of correcting the master cast.

An attempt has been made to differentiate between the amount of tissue displacement that takes place following a physiologic or selected pressure impression. Tissues are said to have been placed, rather than displaced, if after the partial denture has been inserted and worn by the patient no adverse response of the tissue in the form of inflammation, ulceration, or bony resorption has taken place. In other words, the tissue has responded favorably to the additional stresses placed on them by the prosthesis. If, on the other hand, the tissues beneath a partial denture demonstrate an inflammatory response with an accompanying resorption of bone, the tissues are said to have been displaced.

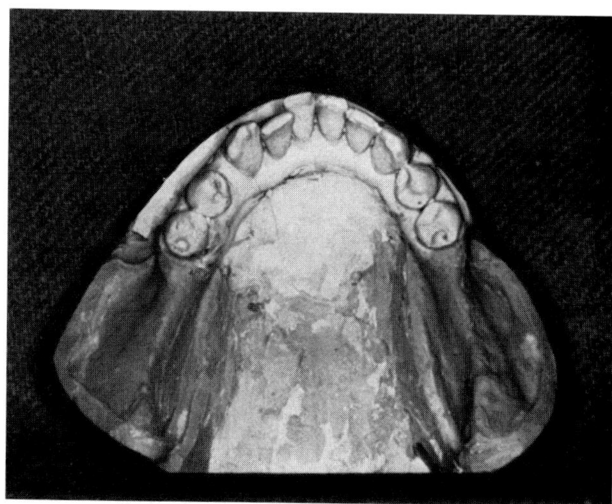

Fig. 13-11. A completed altered cast. Difference in color of dental stone indicates new edentulous ridge portion of cast that has been added.

The advantage of the difference in terminology is doubtful, and the descriptive terms *minimally displaced* to refer to the situation that has responded favorably and *excessively displaced* to that which responds unfavorably are used in this book.

McLEAN'S PHYSIOLOGIC IMPRESSION

The need for physiologic impressions was first recognized by McLean and several others a number of years ago. They realized the need of recording the tissues of the residual ridge that would eventually support a distal extension denture base in the functional, or supporting, form and then relating this functional impression to the remainder of the arch by means of a second impression.

For this dual impression a custom impression tray was constructed over a preliminary cast of the arch, a functional impression of the distal extension ridge was made, and then a hydrocolloid impression was made with the first impression held in its functional position with finger pressure (Fig. 13-12). The greatest weakness of the technique was that finger pressure could not produce the same functional displacement of the tissue that biting force produced. The apparent advantage of the technique was lost with this weakness.

Many variations of this technique have been developed and advocated, but all require some form of finger loading pressure as the second impression is made.

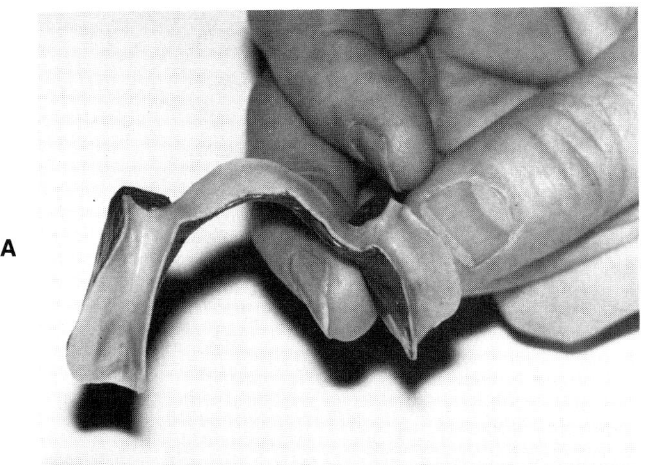

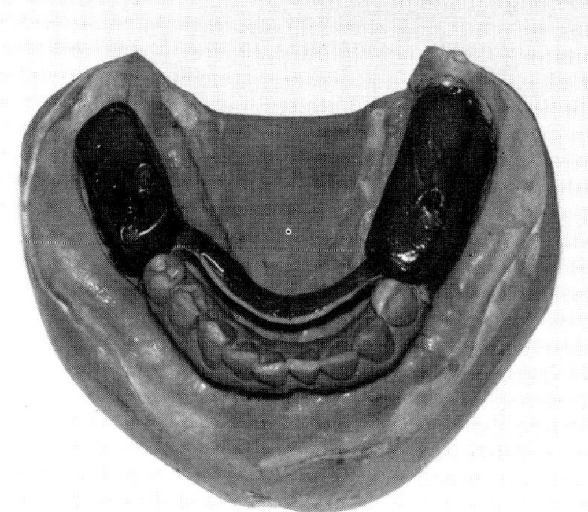

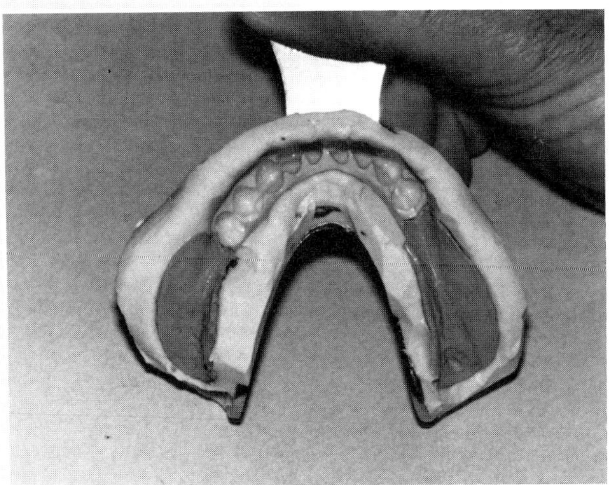

Fig. 13-12. A, Custom tray for McLean functional impression technique has modeling plastic occlusion rims. **B,** Impression paste is used to make an impression in tray over distal extension ridge only. Patient applies steady biting force to occlusion rims during procedure. **C,** Functional impression is related to remainder of arch by making alginate impression with first impression held in its functional position with finger pressure.

Hindels and others developed irreversible hydrocolloid trays for the second impression that were provided with holes so that finger pressure could be applied through the tray as the hydrocolloid impression was made (Fig. 13-13). The main change that Hindels introduced to McLean's original technique was that the impression of the edentulous ridge was not made under pressure but was an anatomic impression of the ridge at rest made with a free-flowing zinc oxide–eugenol paste. As the hydrocolloid second impression was being made, however, finger pressure was applied through the holes in the tray to the anatomic impression. The pressure had to be maintained until the alginate was completely set. The finished impression was a reproduction of the anatomic surface of the ridge and the surfaces of the teeth. The two were related to each other, however, as if masticating forces were taking place on the denture base.

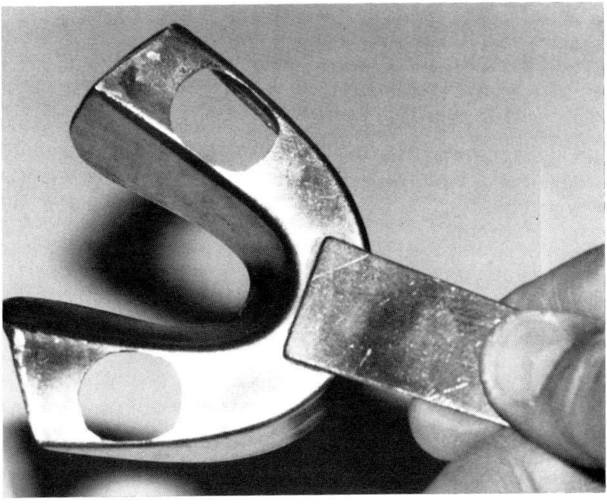

Fig. 13-13. Hindels impression tray. Holes are used by dentist to apply finger pressure to underlying impression of ridge area.

The main purpose of these techniques was to relate an impression of the edentulous ridge to the teeth under a form of functional loading.

A disadvantage of these techniques was that if the action of the retentive clasps of the partial denture is sufficient to maintain the denture base in relation to the soft tissues in the displaced or functional form, interruption of blood circulation would ensue, with possible adverse soft tissue reaction and resorption of the underlying bone.

If the action of the retentive clasps was not sufficient to maintain that functional relationship of the denture base to the soft tissue when the partial denture was in the mouth at rest, the partial denture would be slightly occlusal to the position it would assume when occlusal force was applied (see Fig. 7-41). This means that each time the patient's teeth came together, contact with the artificial teeth would occur first and the remaining natural teeth would contact only after the mucosa had been displaced to the position at which the impression was made. This early or premature contact of the artificial teeth is objectionable to many patients.

FUNCTIONAL RELINING METHOD

Most methods of obtaining a physiologic impression for support of a distal extension denture base accomplish the impression procedure before completion of the denture, usually following the construction of the framework. It is possible, however, to obtain the same results after the partial denture has been completed. The technique is referred to as a functional reline. It consists of adding a new surface to the inner, or tissue, side of the denture base. The procedure may be accomplished before the insertion of the partial denture, or it may be done at a later date if, because of bone resorption, the denture base no longer fits the ridge adequately.

Although the functional reline has many advantages, and for correcting the fit of a denture base that has been worn for a period of time is essential, it does present many difficulties. The main problems that arise are caused by failure to maintain the correct relationship between the framework and the abutment teeth during the impression procedure and failure to maintain accurate occlusal contact following the reline.

In Chapter 21 the procedures for relining and rebasing an existing removable partial denture are discussed in detail. The functional reline discussed here is that done to a completed partial denture before initial insertion for the purpose of perfecting the fit of the denture base to the residual ridge.

The partial denture is constructed on a cast made from a single impression, usually irreversible hydrocolloid. This is an anatomic impression, and no attempt is made to alter it or produce a functional impression of the edentulous ridge.

To allow room for the impression material between the denture base and the ridge, space must be provided. One of the most accurate methods of ensuring uniform space for the impression material is to adapt a soft metal spacer (Ash No. 7 metal) over the ridge on the cast before processing the denture base. After processing, the metal is removed, leaving an even space between the base and the edentulous ridge (Fig. 13-14).

The portion of the technique that introduces the greatest hazard is the making of the reline impression. The patient must maintain the mouth in a partially open position while the border molding and impression are being accomplished because (1) the border tissues, cheek, and tongue are thus best controlled and (2), the relationship between the partial denture framework and the teeth must be observed (Fig. 13-15).

The actual impression making for the functional reline consists of flowing low-fusing modeling plastic over the tissue surface of the denture base, tempering the modeling plastic in a water bath, and seating it in the patient's mouth. The heating, tempering, and reseating must be accomplished several times until an accurate impression of the ridge is made (Fig. 13-16). The border extensions are determined by limiting the application of heat to the borders and manipulating the cheek and tongue. (The technique of manipulating the border tissues is described later in this chapter in the discussion of border molding for correcting the master cast.)

After the application of modeling plastic is complete, the final impression can be made. To provide space for the impression material, the entire surface of the modeling plastic may be scraped to a depth of approximately 1 mm, or the entire thickness of the modeling plastic may be removed over the crest of the ridge (Fig. 13-17). Either method will prevent the distortion or displacement of the underlying tissue.

The final impression is made with a free-flowing zinc oxide–eugenol paste. If undercuts are present on the ridge, light-bodied polysulfide or silicone rubber may be used.

In the functional reline procedure, as in all reline procedures, occlusal discrepancies must be corrected after the new denture base has been processed. Since the open mouth impression technique must be used, it is impossible to maintain previously established occlusal contacts. If errors in occlusion after the denture has been processed are slight, the correction may be accomplished in the mouth. However, in a majority of cases it will be necessary to remount the partial denture on an articulator to correct and refine the occlusion. (The technique for remounting a partial denture to correct occlusal discrepancies is described in Chapter 16.)

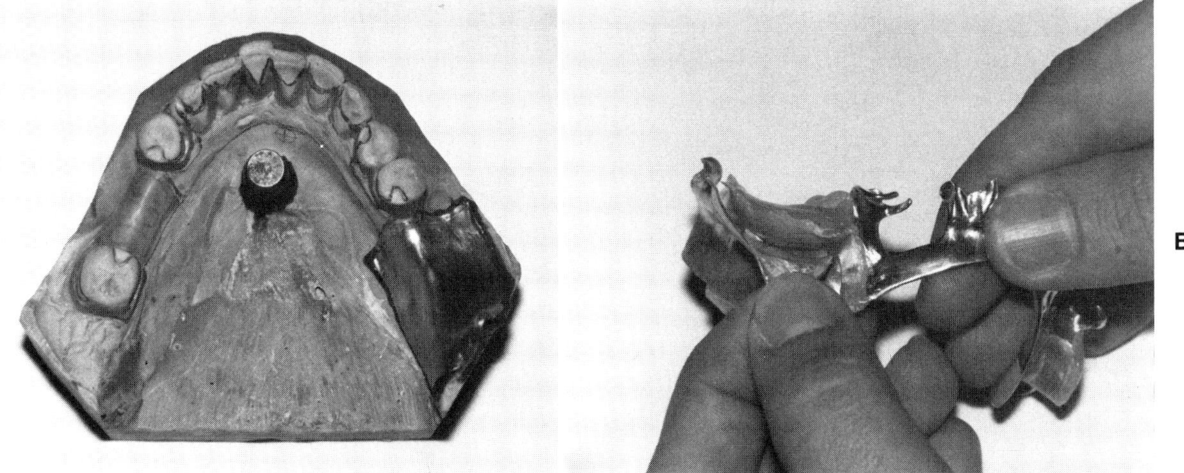

Fig. 13-14. A, Metal spacer in position on cast to provide space for functional reline. **B,** After denture base has been processed, metal spacer is removed.

Fig. 13-15. To reline a partial denture, there must be at least three points of contact between metal of framework and teeth. These contacts are usually in form of occlusal, incisal, or lingual rests or lingual plating. Occlusal rests supporting metal pontic replacing left first molar, indirect retainer resting on left first premolar, and occlusal rest on right first premolar form three points of contact here.

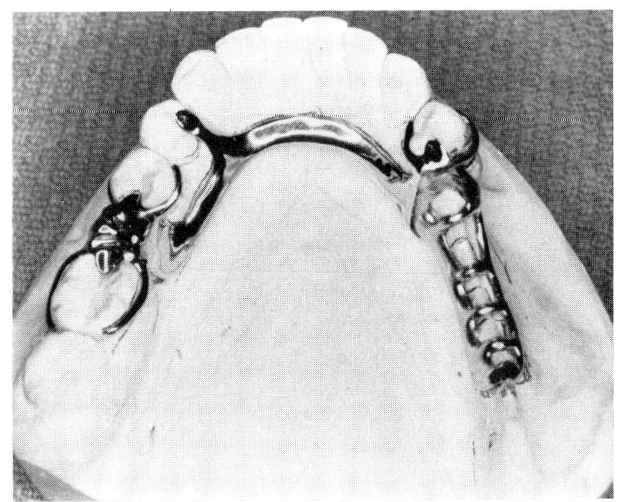

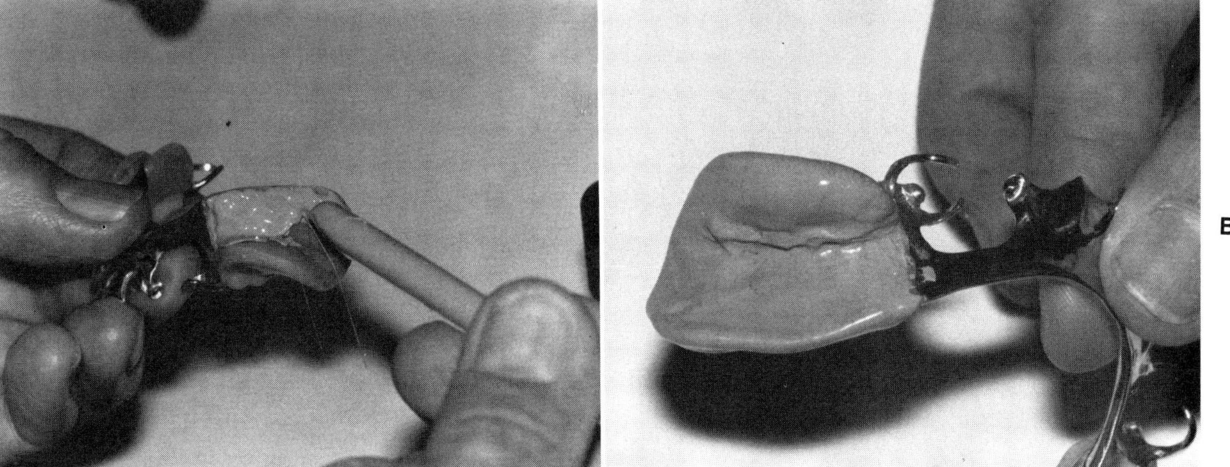

Fig. 13-16. A, Modeling plastic is put on tissue surface of the denture base. **B,** Modeling plastic impression is completed.

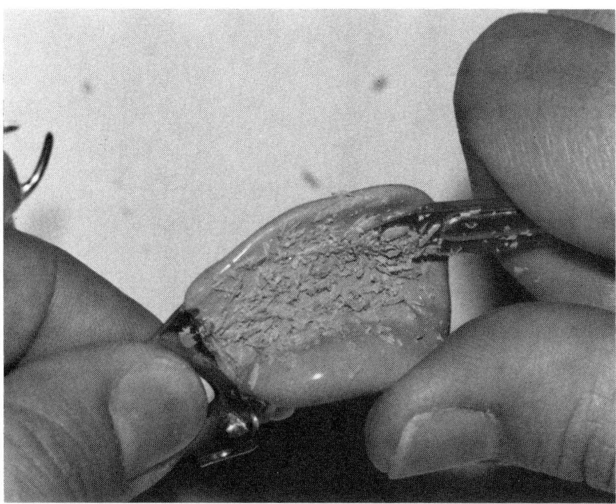

Fig. 13-17. Modeling plastic over ridge is relieved before final impression is made.

The functional reline method of improving the fit of the denture base to the residual ridge, although fraught with potential danger, has the advantage that the amount of soft tissue displacement can be controlled by the amount of relief given to the modeling plastic before the final impression is made. The greater the relief, the less will be the tissue displacement.

CORRECTING MASTER CAST

Making impression tray

Preparation for the corrected cast impression appointment requires the construction of an impression tray attached to the acrylic resin retention minor connector of the framework as shown in Fig. 13-18. This can be accomplished before the appointment if a separate appointment has been made for the purpose of making the altered cast impression.

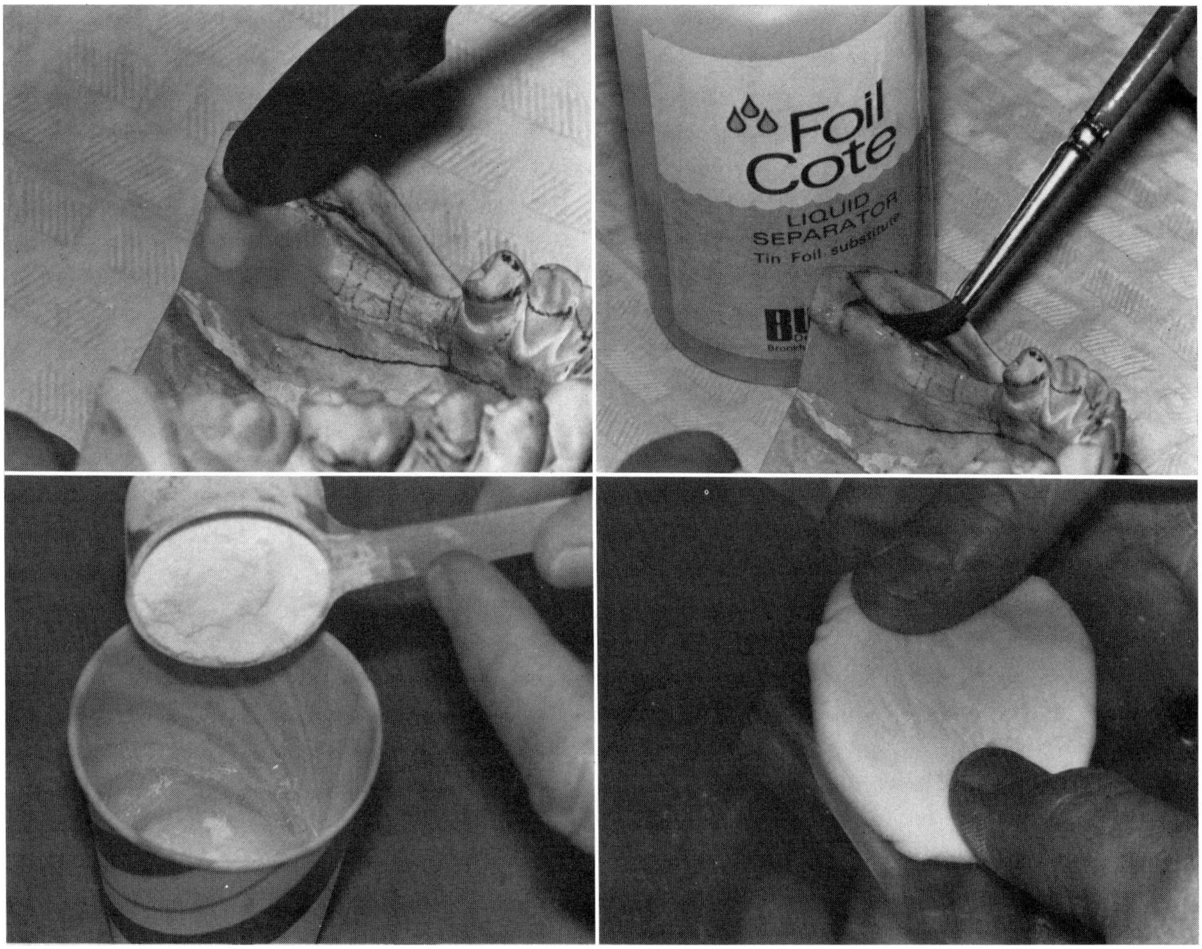

Fig. 13-18. A, Undercuts on cast that would interfere with removal of tray are eliminated with baseplate wax. **B,** Several coats of tinfoil substitute are painted on cast after undercuts are relieved to prevent acrylic resin tray material from adhering to cast. Acrylic resin tray material is mixed according to manufacturer's directions in disposable cup, **C,** and formed into patty approximately size of edentulous ridge to be covered, **D.**

There will be times when the fitting of the framework and the correction of the opposing occlusion have proceeded without complications and time may permit the impression to be made at the same appointment. If this can be done, it will decrease the overall treatment time.

It is not good practice to adapt the acrylic resin impression tray to the framework before attempting to verify and improve the fit of the casting. The presence of the impression tray greatly complicates the try-in of the framework.

Before the tray is constructed, the master cast must be examined critically. Occasionally the lingual extension of a mandibular ridge will have been obliterated in the original impression by the floor of the mouth and sublingual gland being trapped within the impression tray. (One reason for modifying the impression tray with modeling plastic is to prevent this from happening). This lack of lingual ridge should be corrected before constructing the tray by carving with a knife or large bur an approximation of the lingual extension on the master cast (Fig. 13-19). The extension of the tray will be corrected in the mouth.

The tray should be contoured and smoothed with arbor bands. The tissue surface should not be relieved at this time.

Correcting peripheral extensions of tray

The framework with the tray attached is seated in the mouth.

NOTE: From this point until the framework is recovered from the corrected cast, every time the framework is seated on the cast or is seated in the mouth, visual verification of the correct position of the framework must be made.

This description is primarily concerned with adjusting the extensions for a mandibular distal extension impression, but manipulating border tissues to arrive at the proper tray contour applies to any other situation.

The buccal extension of the tray should be observed as the cheek is moved downward, outward, and upward. This is the same movement that will be used

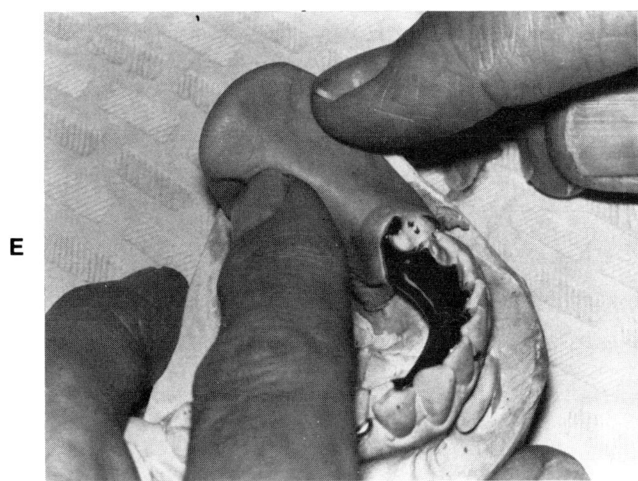

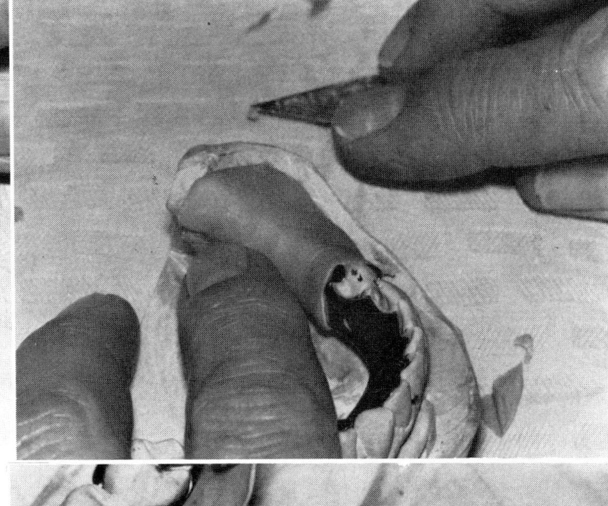

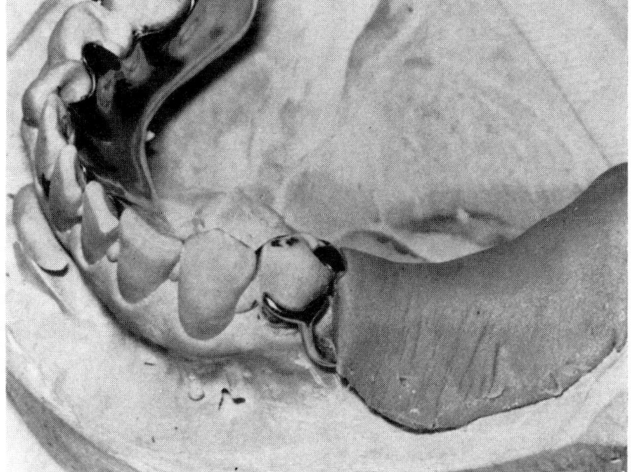

Fig. 13-18, cont'd. E, Patty is molded over acrylic resin retentive minor connector and edentulous ridge with finger pressure. **F,** Excess material is trimmed while still soft. **G,** Final peripheral extensions will be determined in mouth.

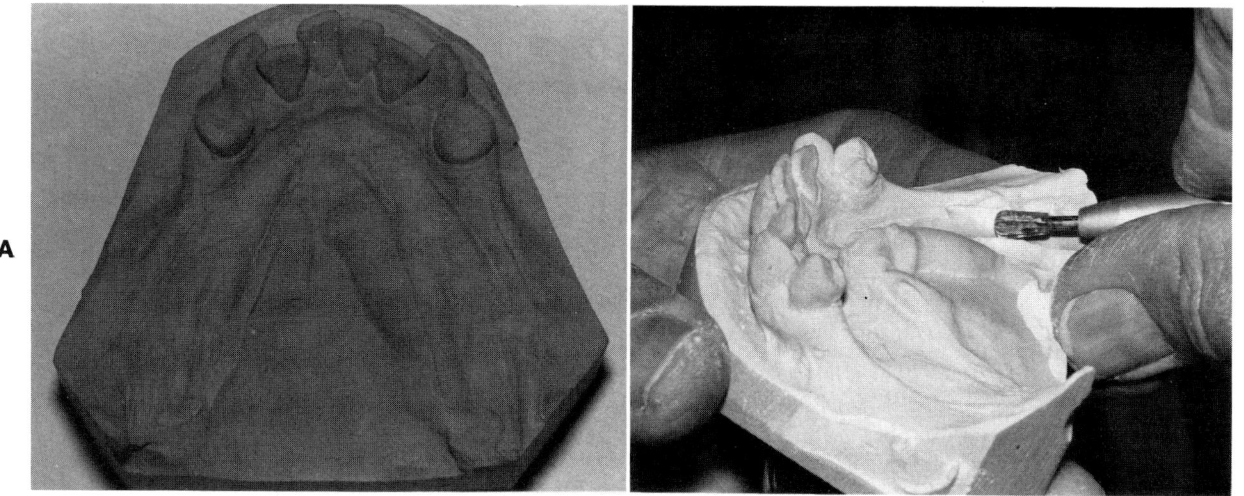

Fig. 13-19. If lingual extension of edentulous ridge was not adequate on master cast, **A,** cast is reshaped with vulcanite bur, **B.**

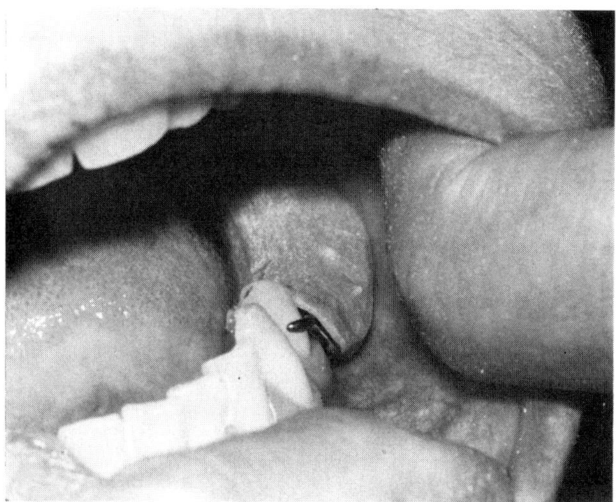

Fig. 13-20. Movable tissue should not be observed under margins of impression tray.

eventually to border mold the softened modeling plastic. As this movement is taking place, the edge of the tray should be just shy (1 or 2 mm) of the movable tissue (Fig. 13-20).

The posterior extension of the tray should end at two-thirds coverage of the retromolar pad. This must be determined by direct observation.

The distal lingual tray extension is determined by the patient protruding the tongue so that the tip contacts the upper lip. The operator's fingers should rest lightly on the tray as this protrusion takes place. If the tray tends to lift, even slightly, during this movement, the distal lingual length should be shortened.

The remainder of the lingual flange extension is checked in a similar manner. With the operator's fingers resting lightly on the tray the patient moves the tongue into each cheek. This need not be a forceful move, but enough to distend the cheek slightly. If the tray moves during this movement, the lingual flange opposite the cheek toward which the tongue moved should be shortened.

When the tray extensions are correct, moderate manipulation of the border tissues, including thrusting the tongue forward and into both cheeks, should not produce any movement of the tray. An overextended tray will cause a constant force to be placed on the abutment teeth as the border tissues try to unseat the denture.

Border molding the impression tray

The mandibular distal extension tray may be border molded in two steps: (1) from the anterior extent of the buccal flange to the most posterior extent of the tray and (2) the remainder of the lingual and distal lingual flange.

The border molding is basically the same as that for complete dentures. Tissue manipulation will be as in correcting the peripheral extensions of the tray. A low-fusing modeling plastic, green or gray stick, is used for the procedure, which is illustrated in Fig. 13-21.

When the border molding is complete, the tongue and other tissues should have freedom of motion without dislodging the tray.

Relieving tray and making impression

When the acrylic resin tray material was adapted to the framework on the master cast, no relief was provided between the ridge and the tray so that the tray material would be securely attached to the latticework

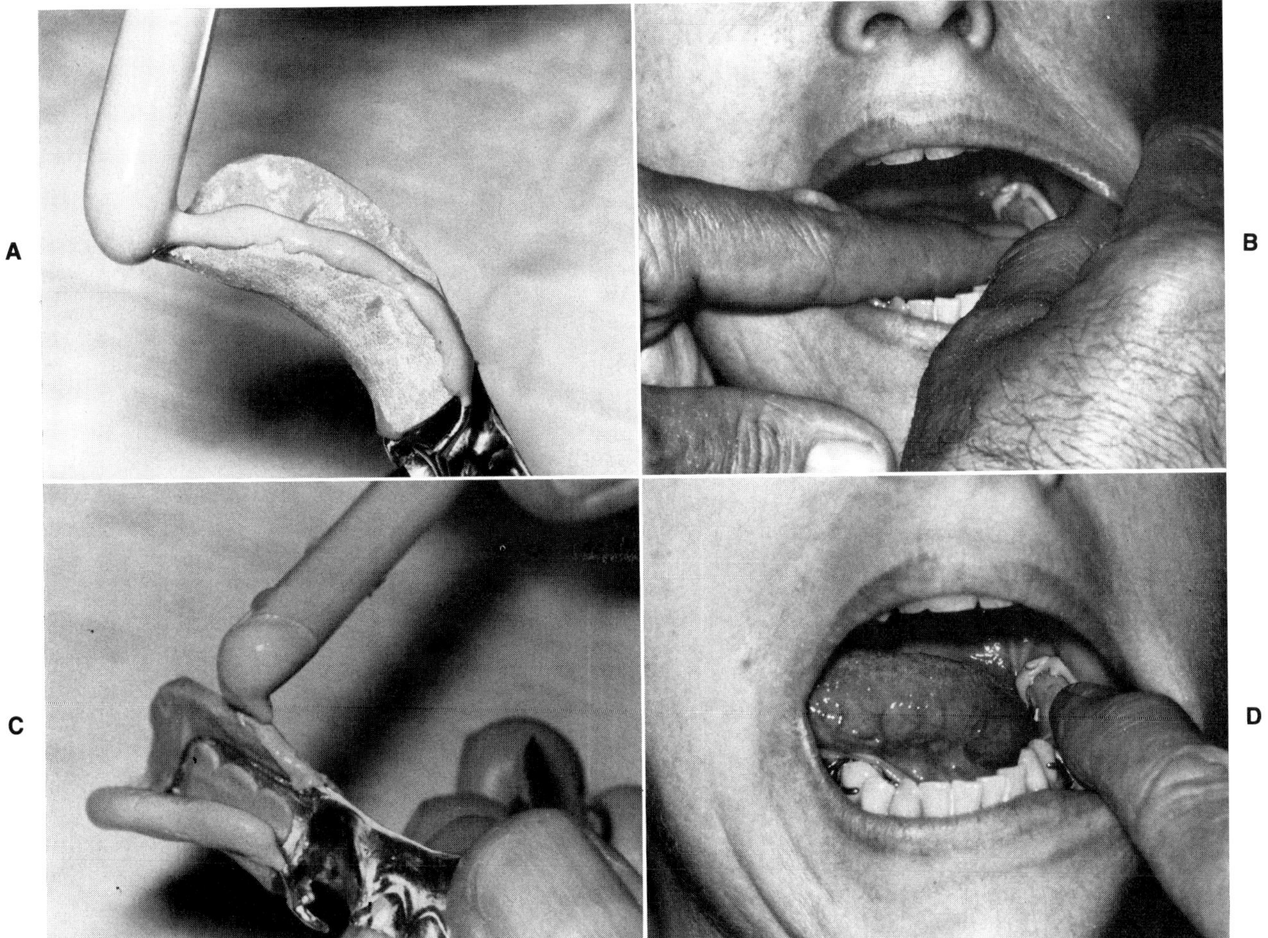

Fig. 13-21. Low-fusing modeling plastic is applied to buccal peripheral margin of impression tray, **A,** flamed with alcohol torch, tempered in water bath, and seated in mouth. **B,** Cheek is moved downward, outward, and upward while modeling plastic is still soft. Finger prevents impression tray from moving. If difficulty is encountered in developing distal buccal angle of tray, patient may bite on cotton rolls to activate masseter muscle fibers. Adding modeling plastic to correct deficiencies may be done as required. Surface must be flamed again, tempered, and border molded. Modeling plastic is added to lingual flange periphery, **C,** flamed, tempered, and seated. **D,** Patient must immediately move tongue forward and then into each cheek. This movement will usually need repeating several times. Action of mylohyoid muscle should be seen in lingual border molding and superior constrictor's action seen in distal lingual molding.

and so that the tray would be stabilized during the border molding procedure.

It is now necessary to provide relief under the tray for the impression material. It is at this point in the procedure that the technique for the fluid wax functional impression differs from that of the selected pressure impression.

Fluid wax functional impression

The fluid wax impression may be used to make a reline impression for an existing partial denture or to correct the distal extension edentulous ridge portion of the original master cast.

The objectives of the technique are to obtain maximum extension of the peripheral borders of the denture base while not interfering with the function of movable border tissues, to record the stress-bearing areas of the ridge in their functional form, and to record non-pressure-bearing areas in their anatomic form. The fluid wax impression is made with the open mouth technique so that there is less danger of overdisplacement of ridge tissue by occlusal or vertical forces.

The term *fluid wax* is used to denote waxes that are firm at room temperature and have the ability to flow at mouth temperature. The most frequently used fluid waxes are Iowa wax, developed by Dr. Smith at the

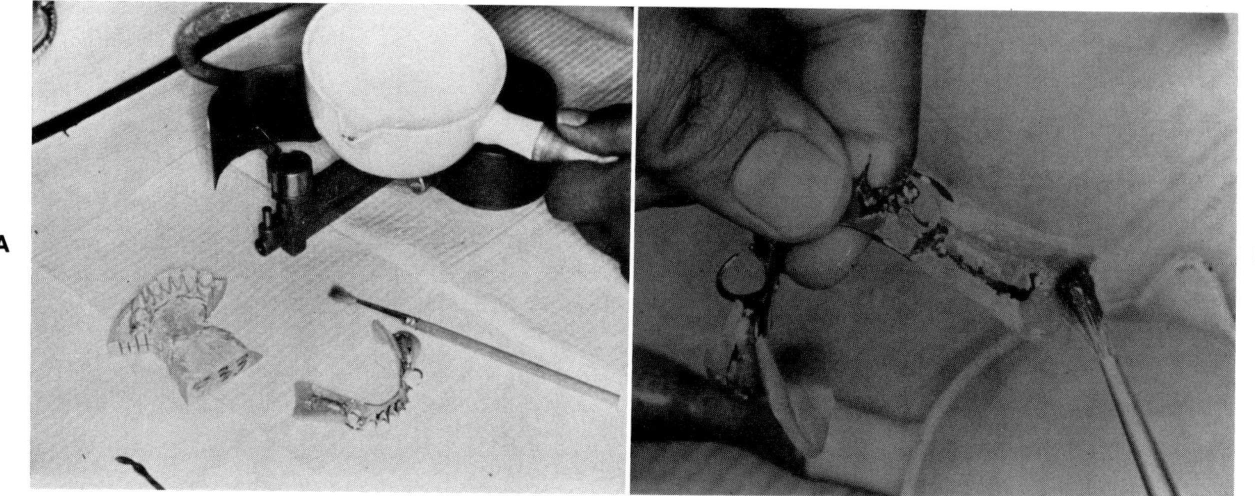

Fig. 13-22. Fluid wax is heated, **A,** preferably in temperature-controlled water bath, and painted over tissue surface of impression tray, **B.**

University of Iowa, and Korrecta wax No. 4, developed by Drs. O.C. and S.G. Applegate at the Universities of Michigan and Detroit, respectively. Korrecta wax No. 4 is slightly more fluid than Iowa wax.

The key to the use of fluid wax lies in two areas: space and time. Space refers to the amount of relief provided between the impression tray and the edentulous ridge. The impression wax flows sluggishly, and a thin layer of wax will flow less readily than a thicker layer. Relief between the tray and the ridge of 1 to 2 mm is the desired amount. Each time the tray is introduced into the mouth, it must remain in place 5 to 7 minutes to allow the wax to flow and to prevent buildup of pressure under the tray with resulting distortion or displacement of the tissue.

The clinical technique for the use of the fluid wax calls for a water bath maintained at 51° to 54°C (125° to 130° F) into which a container of the wax is placed. At this temperature the wax becomes fluid. The wax is painted on the tissue side of the impression tray with a brush (Fig. 13-22). The peripheral extension of the impression tray is critical. The borders must be short of all movable tissues, but not more than 2 mm short because the fluid wax does not have sufficient strength to support itself beyond that distance. Inaccuracies will develop if the wax is extended beyond that length. Originally a harder wax, Korrecta wax No. 1, was used to support the softer No. 4 wax if extension beyond that length was needed. The No. 1 wax, however, is no longer available.

The wax is painted on the surface of the tray to a depth slightly greater than the amount of relief provided. The tray is seated in the mouth. The patients must remain with the mouth approximately half open for about 5 minutes. The tray is removed, and the wax examined for evidence of tissue contact. Where tissue contact is present the wax surface will be glossy, and where there is no contact the surface will be dull. If needed, additional wax is painted on those areas not in contact with the tissue. The tray must remain in the mouth a minimum of 5 minutes after each addition of wax. The peripheral extensions are developed by tissue movements by the patient. For the buccal and distobuccal extension in a mandibular impression the patient must move to a wide-open-mouth position. This will activate the buccinator muscle and pterygomandibular raphe and produce the desired border anatomy. For the proper lingual extension for a mandibular impression the patient must thrust the tongue into the cheek opposite the side of the arch being border molded. The distolingual extension is obtained by having the patient press the tongue forward against the lingual surfaces of the anterior teeth.

These movements must be repeated a number of times after the impression has been in the mouth long enough for the wax to have softened sufficiently to flow.

When the impression evidences complete tissue contact and when the anatomy of the limiting border structures is evident, the impression should be replaced in the mouth for a final time. The impression should be left in the mouth for 12 minutes this final time to be certain that the wax has completely flowed and released any pressure that may be present (Fig. 13-23).

The finished impression must be handled carefully and the new cast poured as soon as possible because the wax is fragile and subject to distortion.

The fluid wax impression technique can produce an accurate impression if the technique is properly exe-

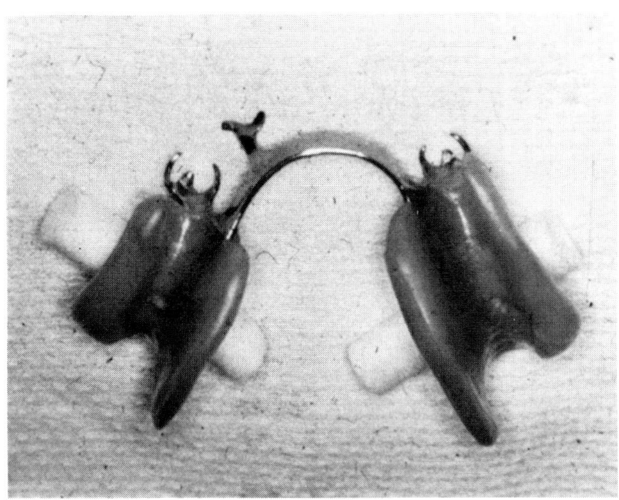

Fig. 13-23. Completed wax impression shows evidence of tissue contact.

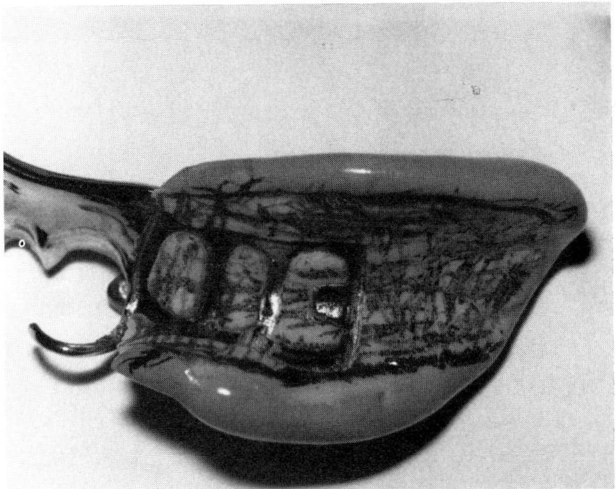

Fig.13-24. Areas of tray to be relieved are indicated by pencil marks.

cuted. The procedure is time consuming, but if the time periods are not followed accurately, an impression with excessive tissue displacement will result.

Selected pressure impression

The previous impression techniques discussed, included in the general category of physiologic impressions, produced a generalized displacement of the mucosa to a greater or lesser degree. This displacement was intended to record the tissue in the configuration it would assume when occlusal loading was applied to a partial denture in function.

The selected pressure impression attempts to direct more force to those portions of the ridge able to absorb the stress without adverse response and to protect the areas of the ridge least able to absorb force. To do this, the tissue surface of the tray is selectively relieved (Figs. 13-24 and 13-25).

For the mandibular posterior ridge, the crest of the ridge is not considered to be a pressure-bearing area, so the undersurface of the tray is relieved down to the metal retention struts. This is done with an acrylic bur. The amount of relief obtained will depend on the amount of relief the laboratory provided as the master cast was blocked out, relieved, and duplicated in producing the refractory cast. This will usually be at least 1 mm. The buccal shelf is the primary stress-bearing area, so only slight relief is provided, again with the acrylic bur. Any excess of modeling plastic that flowed onto the tissue or inner surface of the tray should be removed. The tissue contact area of the border molding should be scraped lightly with a knife.

The lingual slope of the residual ridge may furnish a little vertical support at times, but principally it resists horizontal or rotational forces. The relief provided in the tray over the lingual slope should be the same as over the buccal shelf. These tissues should be recorded by the impression in a slightly displaced form.

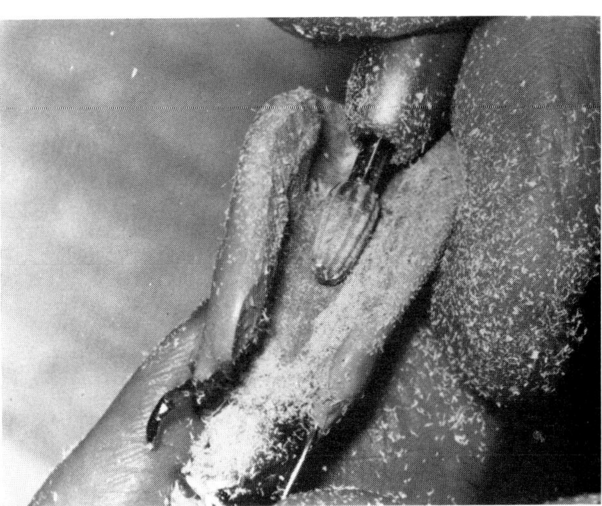

Fig. 13-25. Tissue surface of impression is relieved with acrylic bur over crest of ridge.

As the impression is made, the material over the crest of the ridge that is not closely confined will exert minimal tissueward force, and minimal tissue displacement will result. The impression material over the buccal shelf, being closely confined, will exert somewhat greater tissueward force, and a slightly greater amount of tissue displacement will occur.

The end result of this selected pressure impression is that the denture base made from this impression will be closely adapted to, and in firm contact with, the tis-

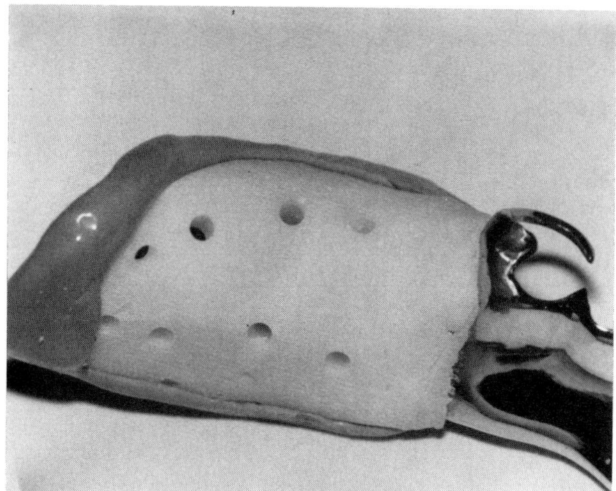

Fig. 13-26. Holes are made through tray to provide extra relief for displaceable soft tissue.

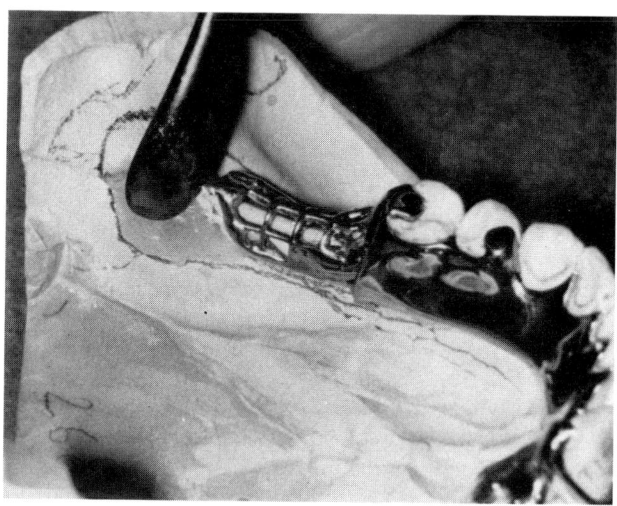

Fig. 13-27. If bony undercuts on edentulous ridge are present, as shown by placement of relief wax, polysulfide rubber impression material should be used for selected pressure impression.

sue covering the buccal shelf area of the edentulous ridge. This area is the primary stress-bearing area and is able to withstand the forces acting against it. The ridge crest, on the other hand, is lightly adapted to the tissue and the effects of occlusal loading will be less in this area.

In some patients the soft tissue covering the ridge will be softer and easily displaced. To obtain more relief and prevent excessive tissue displacement, holes may be made through the impression tray to permit the impression material to flow through and dissipate pressure that might otherwise occur, (Fig. 13-26).

Several impression materials can be used to record the selected pressure impression. The viscosity of these materials varies; and the more viscous a material is, the greater will be the tendency for compression or displacement of soft tissue. Overdisplacement of resilient tissue should be avoided, because the result may be an inflammatory reaction beneath the denture base. Displaced tissue also has a tendency to rebound to its former contour, putting additional stress on abutment teeth.

An understanding of the physical properties of the impression materials and of the manipulative techniques that are geared to those properties will result in correct border extensions and proper pressure distribution.

Zinc oxide–eugenol paste. Zinc oxide–eugenol paste is an accurate impression material of intermediate viscosity. One of its main advantages is that it requires a minimum of time. The impression must be obtained in a single insertion, so correct placement of the framework is essential. Although some authorities state that defects in an impression can be corrected by small additions of a second mix, this is not good practice. It will usually result in uneven distribution of forces and incomplete seating of the framework.

Zinc oxide–eugenol paste is generally considered to be the impression material of choice if the edentulous ridge is free from gross undercuts. It is effective when soft, flabby tissue is involved.

Rubber base materials. Both polysulfide and silicone rubber base impression materials are excellent for recording the selected pressure impression. They are only slightly more viscous than zinc oxide–eugenol paste, and this viscosity can be reduced by using a higher percentage of light-bodied material in the mix.

Slightly more time is required to make the impression because of the prolonged setting time.

Defects in an impression should not be corrected by an addition of a second mix. The entire impression must be stripped from the tray and remade.

An adhesive should be used to paint the tissue surface of the tray to ensure that the rubber adheres to the resin and to the modeling plastic.

Rubber base impression material is particularly indicated for those patients with bony undercuts in the edentulous ridge (Fig. 13-27).

To help prevent the slightly more viscous material from displacing soft tissue, several holes, the size of a No. 8 round bur, may be drilled through the tray over the crest of the ridge. This will eliminate the possibility of excess pressure from the confined material. The holes will also help prevent air from being trapped in the tray. This may be especially helpful when the impression is being made of a long edentulous ridge.

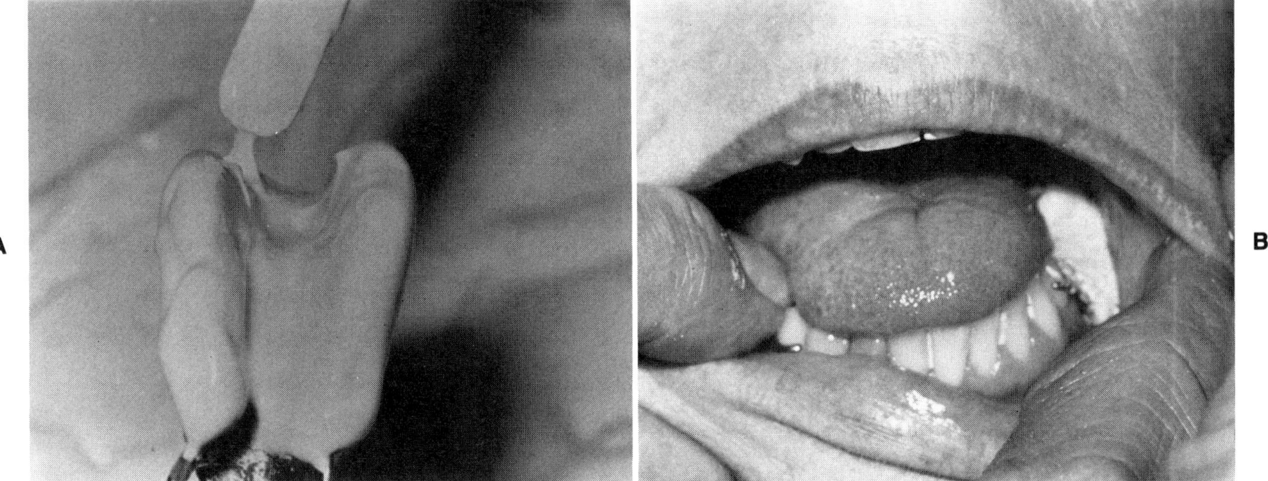

Fig. 13-28. A, An even thickness of impression material is placed over entire tissue surface of tray. **B,** Patient protrudes tongue when impression is completely seated.

Impression technique. The area of the mouth that is to be involved in the impression should be dried and isolated with gauze packs before the impression material is mixed. The 2 × 2 inch gauze packs should be unfolded and placed both buccally and lingually to the ridge or ridges of which the impression will be made.

The material should be mixed according to the manufacturer's directions and painted evenly over the tissue surface of the tray *and the peripheries.* Overloading the tray complicates the impression technique. The material should not be allowed to flow onto the inner surface of the minor connector or under the occlusal rest.

The framework should be seated on the teeth after the gauze pads are removed. The buccal tissues should be cleared as previously described by moving the cheek downward, outward, and upward as the tray is being seated.

The patient must keep the tongue relaxed as the tray is seated and then should protrude the tongue so the tip is just anterior to the incisal edges of the teeth (Fig. 13-28).

The critical point is for the operator to determine visually that all rests and indirect retainers are completely seated while the impression material is still fluid. Pressure should be applied to occlusal rests until the material has reached its final set. Care must be taken to avoid applying any downward pressure on the impression tray. This could cause the partial denture to rotate around the occlusal rests, lifting the indirect retainers from their seats and producing an inaccurate impression.

The patient's mouth must remain open and the tongue protruded until the final set of the material. The tendency on the part of most patients is to allow the tongue to fall back in the mouth and to allow the mouth to close partway. These positions will cause inaccurracies in the impression. The operator must remind the patient from time to time of the correct position.

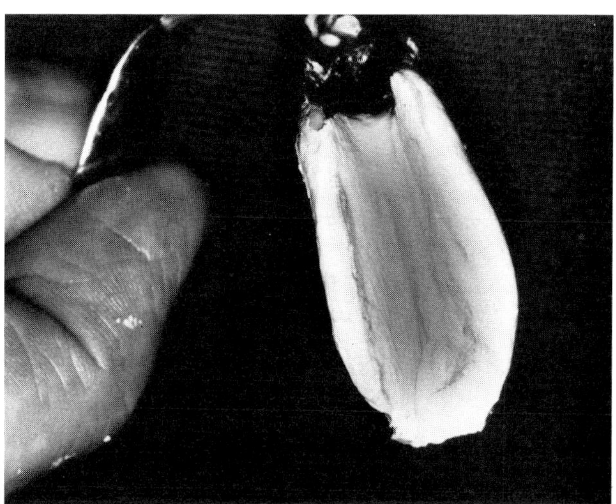

Fig. 13-29. Any void in impression such as that seen at anterior extent of lingual flange must be assessed as to its significance on final denture flange. This one would be acceptable.

Examining impression

Causes for rejection of the impression will be similar to any impression with several additions. A void on the tissue surface or periphery (Fig. 13-29) or an obvious underextension should not be accepted. In addition, any evidence that the framework was not seated com-

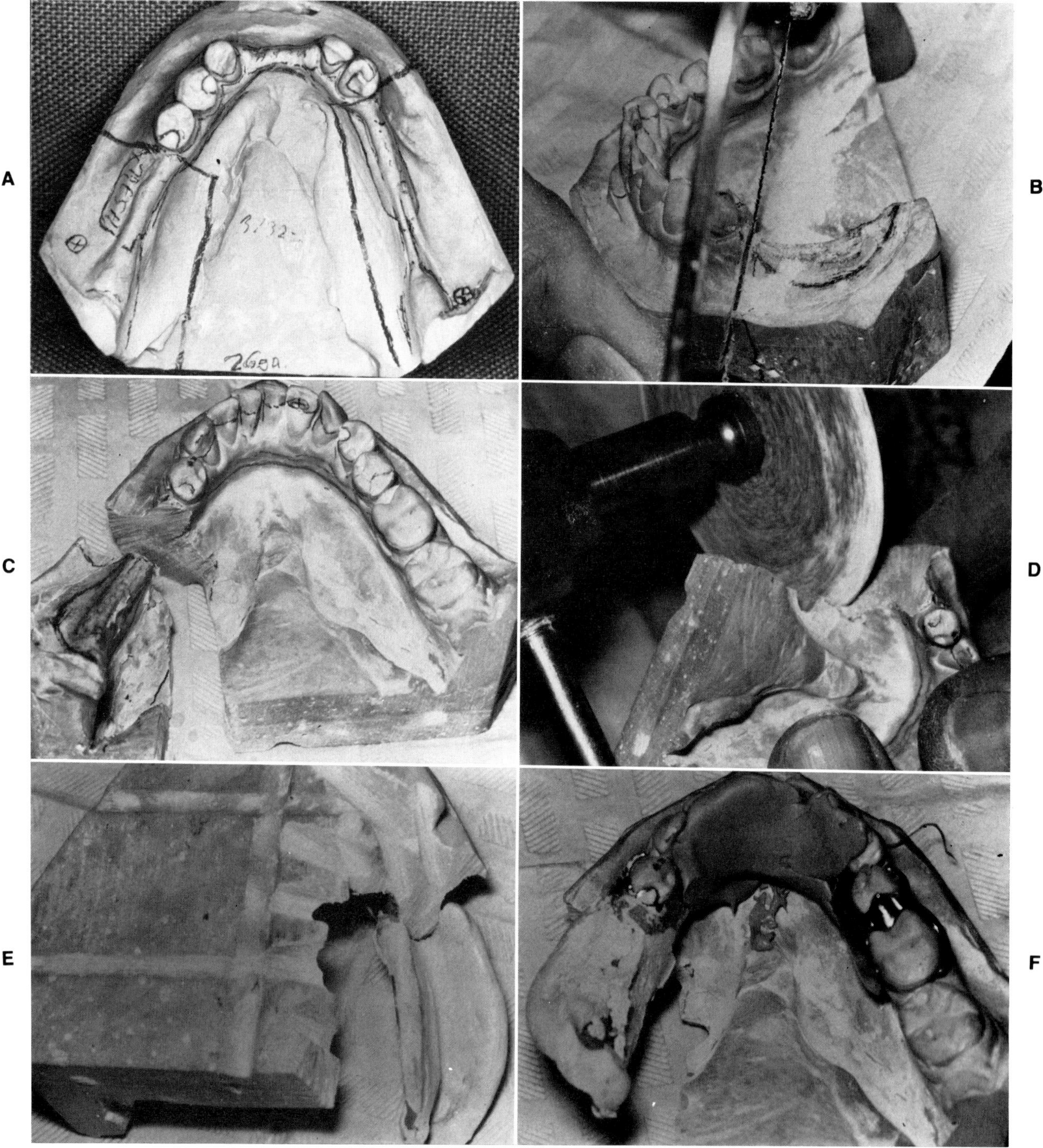

Fig. 13-30. A, Area of cast that will be replaced by corrected cast impression is outlined. Line is drawn 1 mm posterior to distal abutment tooth at right angles to long axis of ridge down both sides of ridge and down side of cast. Second line is drawn at right angles to first, beginning medial to lingual sulcus and proceeding posteriorly to end of cast while staying just medial to reflection of tissue in lingual sulcus. **B** and **C,** Outlined area of cast is removed with handsaw. **D,** Knife-edged stone on lathe is used to make longitudinal retention grooves on cut surface of cast to provide mechanical retention for new portion of cast to be poured. **E,** Framework is seated on sectioned cast. Impression must not contact cast. **F,** Framework is sealed to cast with softened modeling plastic.

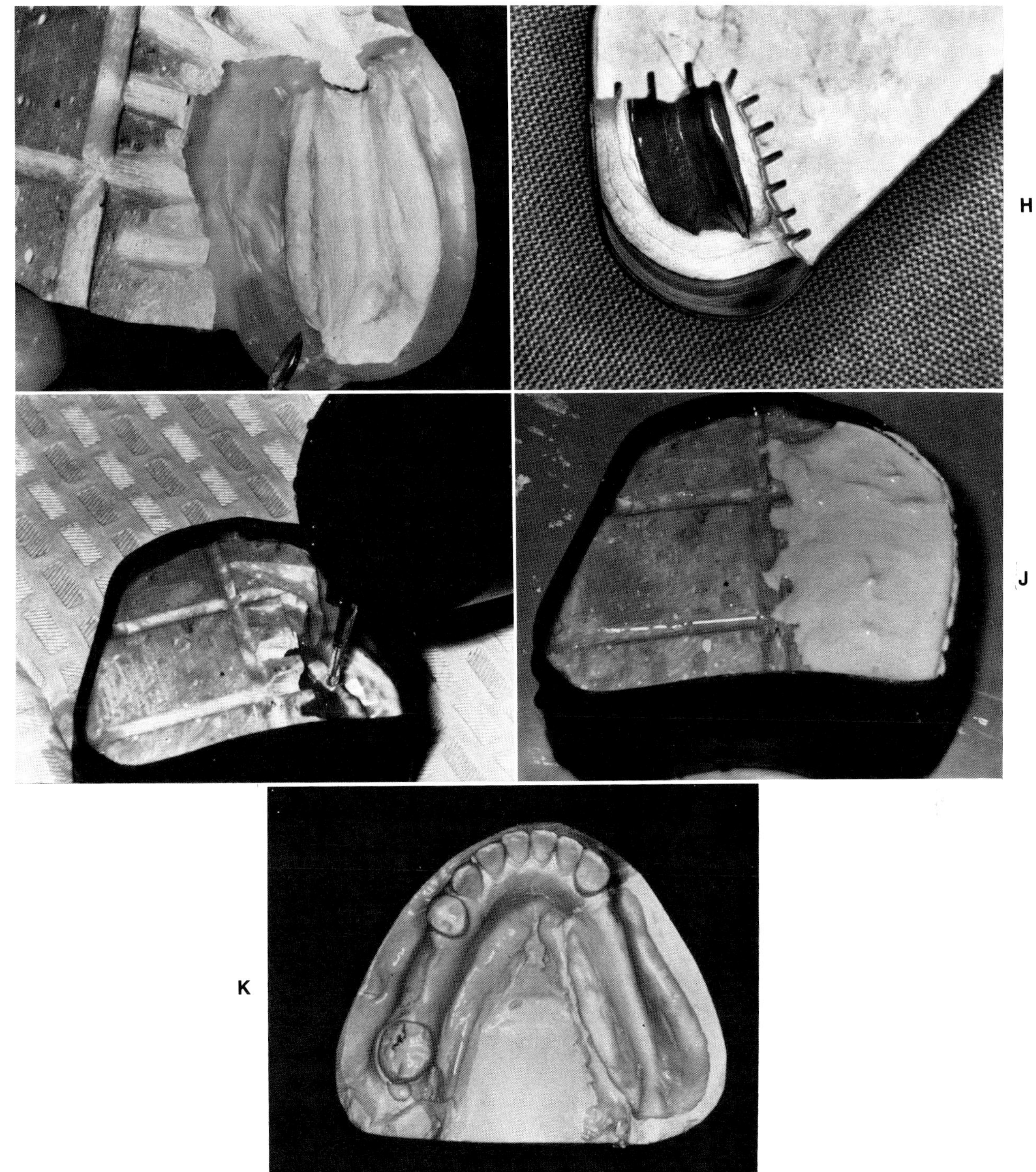

Fig. 13-30, cont'd. G, Utility wax is used to bead impression. Land area, 2 to 3 mm below peripheral margins of impression and extending outward 3 to 4 mm from impression, is developed. **H,** Boxing wax is added around beading wax to confine dental stone. **I,** Original cast is soaked in slurry water for 10 minutes. **J,** Minimal expansion dendrite stone is used to pour altered cast. Vibration should be used cautiously to prevent dislodging framework and impression. **K,** After final set, boxing is removed and cast is trimmed. Corrected cast is used to complete partial denture.

pletely, such as the presence of impression material beneath rests, is reason to remake the impression. If any doubt exists, the impression must not be accepted.

Preparing original cast and pouring corrected cast

Fig. 13-30 shows the procedure for producing an altered cast for a mandibular distal extension edentulous condition. The steps can be applied to any other situation.

Length of appointment

The experienced clinician should accomplish the corrected cast impression in 20 to 30 minutes. The dental student will usually require about 2 hours.

BIBLOGRAPHY

Applegate, O.C.: An evaluation of the support for the removable partial denture, J. Prosthet. Dent. **10**:112-123, 1960.

Applegate, O.C.: The partial denture base, J. Prosthet. Dent. **5**:636-648, 1955.

Applegate, O.C.: Essentials of removable partial denture prosthesis, ed. 2, Philadelphia, 1960, W.B. Saunders Co.

Beckett, L.S.: Partial denture. The rebasing of tissue borne saddles; theory and practice, Aust. Dent. J. **16**:340-346, 1971.

Craig, R.G.: Dental materials, St. Louis, 1978, C.V. Mosby Co.

Cummer, W.E.: Impression in partial denture service, D. Cosmos. **70**:72, 278, 1928.

DeVan, M.M.: Basic principles of impression making, J. Prosthet. Dent. **2**:26-35, 1952.

Everett, G.E.: Impression taking with a fluid wax compound, J. Aust. Dent. Soc. **2**:294, 1922.

Hindels, G.W.: Load distribution in extension saddle partial dentures, J. Prosthet. Dent. **2**:92, 1952.

Hindels, G.W.: Stress analysis in distal extension partial dentures, J. Prosthet. Dent. **7**:197-205, 1957.

Holmes, J.B.: Influence of impression procedures and occlusal loading on partial denture movement, J. Prosthet. Dent. **15**:474-481, 1965.

Leupold, R.J.: A comparative study of impression procedures for distal extension removable partial dentures, J. Prosthet. Dent. **16**:708, 1966.

Leupold, R.J., and Kratochvil, F.J.: An altered cast procedure to improve tissue support for removable partial dentures, J. Prosthet. Dent. **15**:672, 1965.

Lytle, R.B.: Soft tissue displacement beneath removable partial and complete dentures, J. Prosthet. Dent. **12**:34-43, 1962.

McCracken, W.L.: A comparison of tooth-borne and tooth-tissue–borne removable partial dentures, J. Prosthet. Dent. **3**:375-381, 1953.

McLean, D.W.: The partial denture as a vehicle for function, J. Am. Dent. Assoc. **23**:1271-1278, 1936.

Melty, A.C.: Obtaining efficient soft tissue support for the denture base, J. Am. Dent. Assoc. **56**:679, 1958.

Rapuano, J.A.: Single-tray dual-impression technique for distal extension partial dentures, J. Prosthet. Dent. **24**:41-46, 1970.

Vahidi, F.: Vertical displacement of distal-extension ridges by different impression techniques, J. Prosthet. Dent. **40**:374-377, 1978.

Walter, J.D.: Composite impression procedures, J. Prosthet. Dent. **30**:385-389, 1973.

Weinnann, J.P., and Sicher, H.: Bone and bones, ed. 2, St. Louis, 1955, The C.V. Mosby Co.

Wilson, J.H.: Partial dentures–relining the saddle supported by the mucosa and alveolar bone, J. Prosthet. Dent. **3**:807-813, 1953.

14 Establishing occlusal relationships

The clinical appointment for establishing the final jaw relation in order to position the artificial teeth is frequently neglected in partial denture construction. This appointment is necessary if the opposing casts cannot be accurately hand articulated or if the denture is being constructed at the centric jaw relation position. The appointment is most often needed following the corrected cast impression procedure, because the lack of posterior occlusion in Class I and II partially edentulous arches precludes the possibility of accurately hand articulating the master casts.

The desired occlusion for a removable partial denture will vary from closely resembling the occlusion needed for a complete denture (bilaterally balanced occlusion) to that of a fixed partial denture (complete disclusion in eccentric jaw positions). The number, position, and condition of the remaining teeth as well as the type of opposing occlusion will dictate the form of the occlusion to be established.

The goal in developing an occlusal scheme for the partial denture is the same as that for any restoration in the oral cavity: to establish and maintain a harmonious relationship with all oral structures and to provide a masticatory apparatus that is efficient and esthetically acceptable. For the tooth-tissue–borne partial denture it is necessary also to ensure that the effects of occlusal loading be distributed as evenly as possible to all supporting structures capable of receiving the forces. By developing a harmonious occlusion, the undesirable effects of rotational or torquing forces on the prosthesis can best be controlled.

Occlusal harmony must be present in centric relation, centric occlusion, and all eccentric positions the jaw may assume during the chewing cycle. Deflective contacts in any position, over time, will produce pathologic changes in the supporting structure of the teeth or in the neuromuscular mechanism that controls mandibular movement.

When occlusal relationships are established to position the artificial teeth correctly, the vertical and horizontal components of the jaw relation are equally important.

VERTICAL JAW RELATION

Vertical dimension, as the term is used in prosthodontics, refers to a vertical measurement of the face between two arbitrary points: one below the mouth, usually on the chin, and the other above the mouth, generally on the nose.

Two vertical dimensions are recognized for each patient: the vertical dimension of rest (Fig. 14-1) and the vertical dimension of occlusion (Fig. 14-2). The first is taken when the patient is in an upright position and is completely at rest. The mandibular position depends on a balance among the muscles of mastication, the postcervical muscle group, and the infrahyoid and suprahyoid muscle groups. If the patient being measured has natural dentition, the teeth will not be touching. The space between the teeth when the mandible is in its resting state is referred to as the free-way space.

If the patient with natural dentition elevates the mandible from the rest position so that the teeth contact in the maximum intercuspal relationship and the vertical dimension is again measured, this measurement will be the vertical dimension of occlusion.

It is obvious that the vertical dimension of rest will always be greater than the vertical dimension of occlusion. The difference in these measurements for most patients will be between 2 and 4 mm.

Niswonger measured the free-way space in 200 patients with natural teeth, and found that 83% of the patients had a free-way space of $^{4}/_{32}$ inch, or approximately 3 mm. Of the patients studied, none displayed less than $^{1}/_{32}$ inch, slightly less than 1 mm, and none more than $^{7}/_{32}$ inch, about 6 mm, of this interocclusal space.

Altering the existing vertical dimension of occlusion

For most patients requiring removable partial dentures, measurement of the vertical dimension is not necessary. If natural teeth in opposing arches contact in centric occlusion, this vertical separation of the jaws should be considered the vertical dimension of occlusion for that patient and the prosthesis should be con-

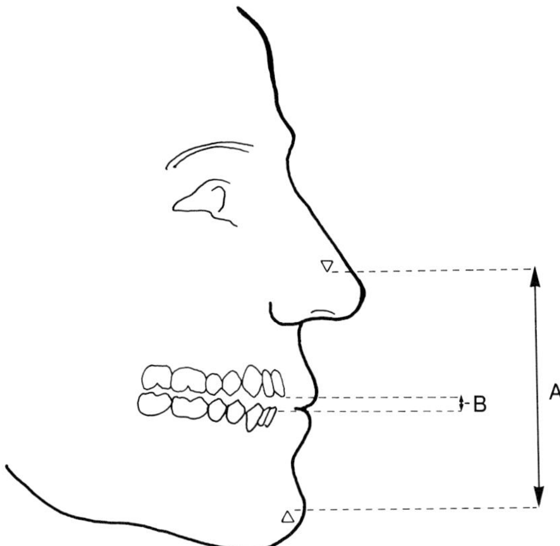

Fig. 14-1. Vertical relationship of mandible to maxillae is one part of jaw relation. *A,* Vertical dimension of rest, or physiologic rest position. Patient must be in nose-to-chin upright position and completely at rest for measurement to be correct. *B,* Free-way space.

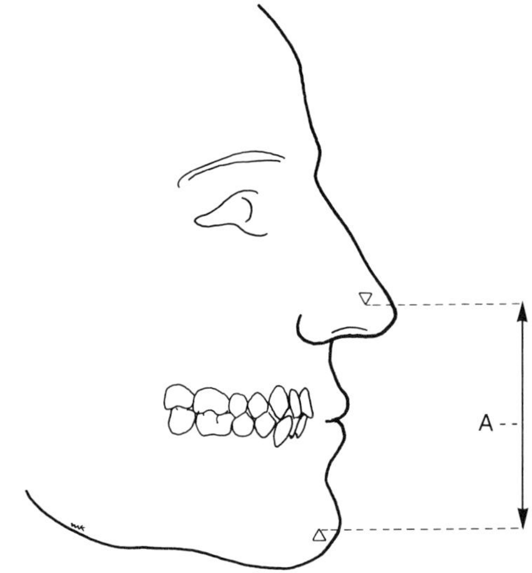

Fig. 14-2. With mandible elevated so that teeth contact, chin-to-nose distance, *A,* is vertical dimension of occlusion.

structed at that vertical dimension (Fig. 14-3). Changing this vertical dimension of occlusion should be considered only if the patient displays symptoms that suggest the vertical dimension of occlusion has been diminished, such as tired aching muscles, unexplained pain in the head or neck, or an appearance of premature aging caused by a shortened nose-chin distance (Fig. 14-4). The most significant sign of overclosure, however, is excessive free-way space (difference between the vertical dimension of rest and the vertical dimension of occlusion). The fact that the occlusal surfaces of the teeth have been worn excessively does not in itself warrant the assumption that the vertical dimension of occlusion is lessened because a compensating eruption of the teeth usually maintains the proper vertical dimension.

Another clinical sign that has often been misinterpreted because of the erroneous belief that the bite has collapsed is an extreme anterior vertical overlap in which the mandibular teeth actually strike the soft tissue of the palate (Fig. 14-5). This condition may or may not indicate a decrease in the vertical dimension of occlusion; no treatment should be instituted without more definite proof that a loss of vertical dimension has occurred.

Confirmation of loss of vertical dimension requires history of physical discomfort related to overclosure, cephalometric examination confirming migration of the condyles, and greater than 4 mm of free-way space.

If these signs and symptoms are present, a temporary increase in the existing vertical dimension can be considered. The increase in interocclusal height must be accomplished with a temporary removable appliance. The appliance should be in the form of an acrylic resin occlusal overlay (Fig. 14-6). If at all possible only one arch should be overlaid. It is normally more convenient to construct the appliance to cover the maxillary teeth because less interference with tongue movement is encountered. The most important consideration is that *all*

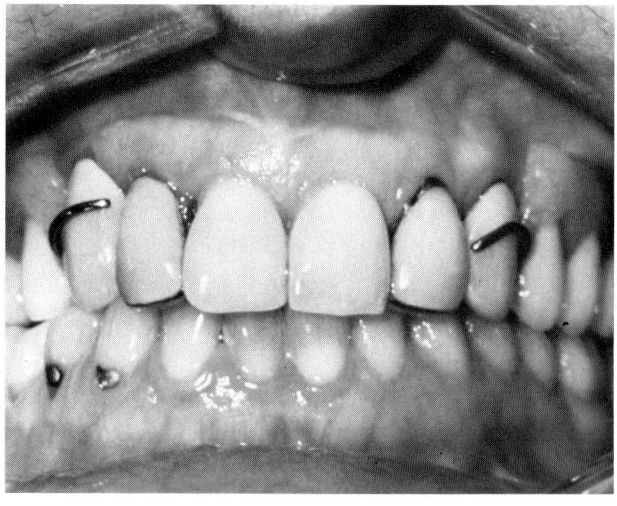

Fig. 14-3. Natural teeth are present in opposing arches and contact in centric occlusion. This vertical position of jaws is vertical dimension of occlusion.

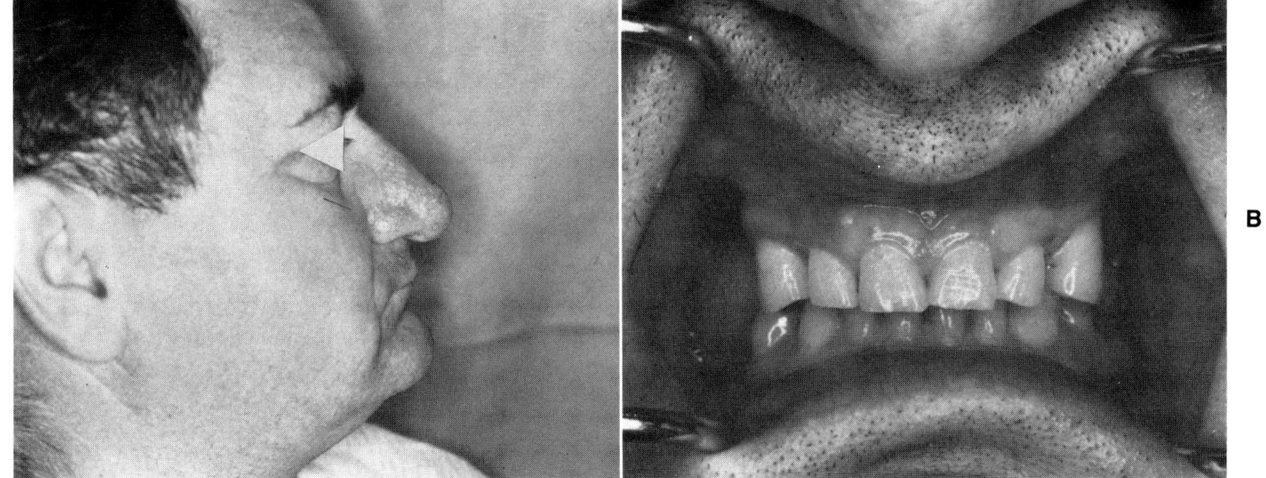

Fig. 14-4. A, Appearance of premature aging because of loss of nose-to-chin distance may indicate loss of vertical dimension of occlusion. **B,** Wear of occlusal surfaces or incisal edges does not necessarily mean that vertical dimension of occlusion has been reduced.

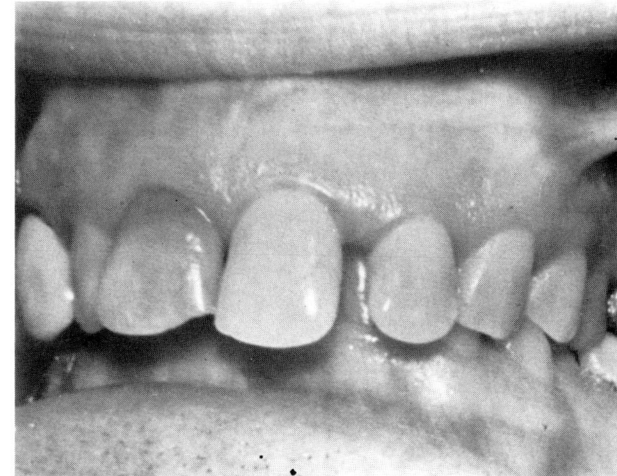

Fig. 14-5. Extreme anterior vertical overlap does not always indicate loss of vertical dimension of occlusion.

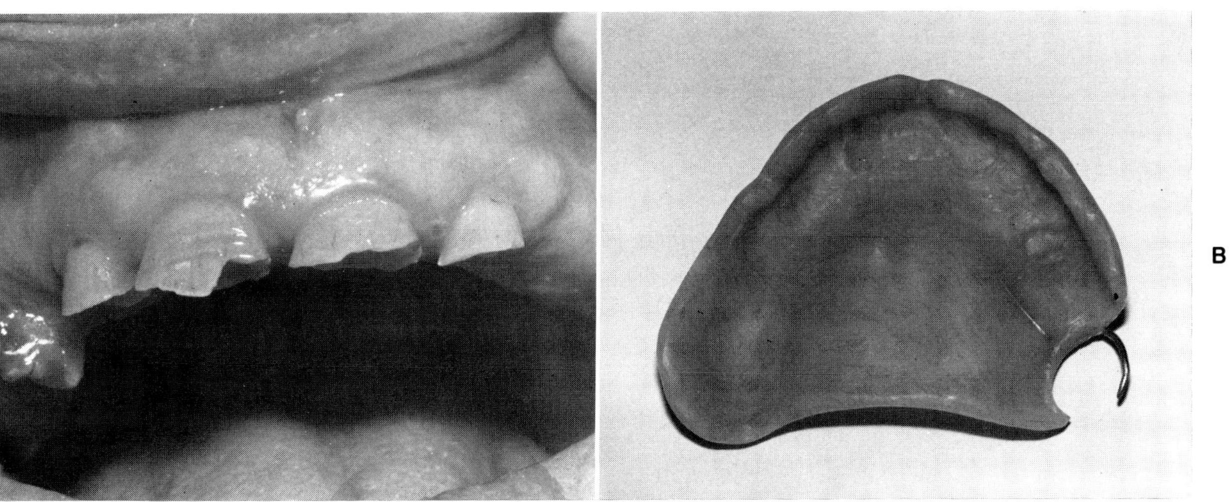

Fig. 14-6. A, Severely abraded teeth should not be restored until proof has been obtained that vertical dimension is decreased. **B,** Acrylic resin temporary prosthesis should be used to overlay remaining teeth. Note imprints of remaining teeth in resin.

remaining teeth in both arches must be contacted by the prosthesis (Fig. 14-7). Otherwise, (1) teeth not contacted by the appliance will tend to erupt to reestablish functional contact, or (2) if a sufficient number of remaining teeth are not used to support the appliance, the supporting teeth will be submerged or depressed to an infraocclusal position (Fig. 14-8). The latter result was commonly observed three to four decades ago when all unexplained maladies of the head, neck, and oral cavity were treated with "bite-opening" appliances. It is an absolute maxim that when the free-way space between the mandibular and maxillary teeth is encroached on, the physiologic rest position required for the maintenance of health will somehow be restored. The person may refuse to wear a removable appliance (which is a positive reaction), or may wear the appliance, producing ultimately either the depressing of the supporting teeth to reestablish the correct free-way space or the destruction of the supporting alveolar bone with loss of teeth.

If, however, the physiologic response of the patient to this temporary appliance is positive (cessation of muscular and neurologic discomfort of the head and neck, and a general feeling of improved health by the patient) for several months, permanent correction can be instituted. Caution should be used in evaluating an early favorable patient response. This is normally to be expected because in most patients any treatment will decrease undesirable symptoms. This condition often does not last long, and the symptoms that caused the treatment to be instituted return.

When permanent treatment is begun, it must be planned so that all occlusal-dimension–restoring prostheses, fixed and removable, are inserted at the same time. Crowns and fixed partial dentures should never be inserted before the construction of the removable partial denture. It is usually advisable to insert the fixed replacements temporarily for observation before final cementation is accomplished. Cementing a single or even several fixed units and allowing them to maintain the vertical dimension of occlusion for even a few days can result in the destruction of the supporting tissues of those teeth.

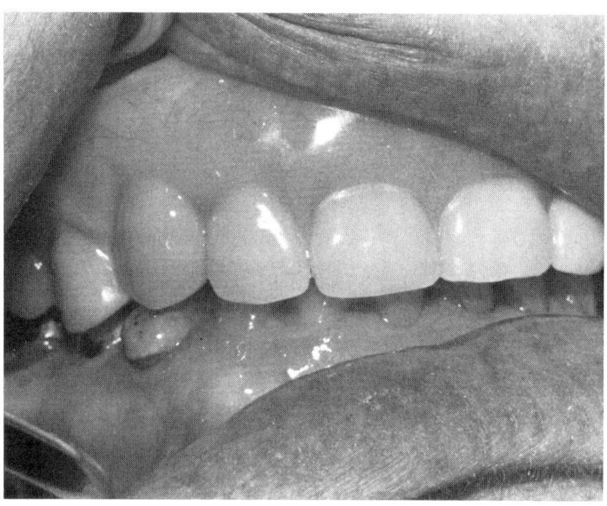

Fig. 14-7. All remaining teeth must contact temporary prosthesis.

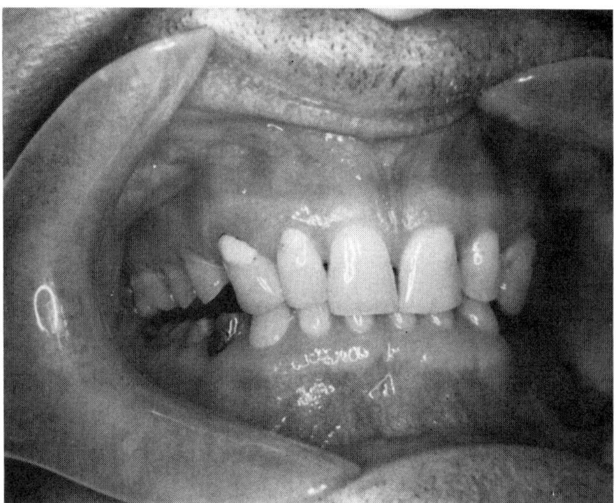

Fig. 14-8. Result of prosthesis covering only posterior teeth. Prosthesis exceeded vertical dimension of occlusion, and posterior teeth have been depressed.

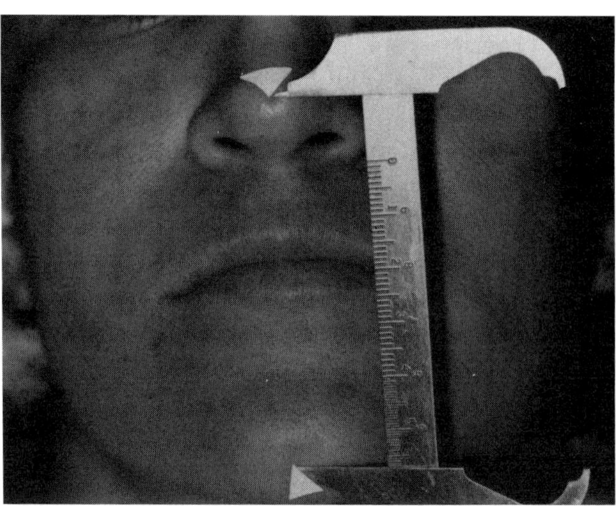

Fig. 14-9. Vertical dimension of rest is distance between points on nose and chin with mandible in physiologic rest position. Patient must be standing or sitting upright with no head support. Mandible will be in correct position immediately after patient swallows sip of water or immediately after he stops making *m* sound. A number of measurements should be made until repeatable results are obtained.

Establishing vertical dimension of occlusion

Only a small percentage of partial denture patients (those for whom a complete denture will oppose a partial denture and those who have lost all the posterior teeth in one or both arches and for whom contact of the anterior teeth cannot be relied on to provide an accurate measurement) need to have the vertical dimension of occlusion established by measurement. This is done by measuring the vertical dimension of rest (Fig. 14-9) and then subtracting 3 mm (the average amount of free-way space). It is at this figure the prosthesis will be constructed. Since the calculation is based on the average free-way space for a large group of patients, vertical dimension of occlusion must be verified for each individual patient when the partial dentures are tried in the mouth before completion.

HORIZONTAL JAW RELATION

Two horizontal relationships of the mandible to the maxilla are of importance in the occlusion for partial dentures (Fig. 14-10).

The first of these relationships is centric relation, the most retruded, unstrained position of the mandible in relation to the maxillae at a given vertical dimension from which lateral movements can be made. Many authorities now feel that the latter portion of the definition "from which lateral movements can be made" is not applicable, because lateral movements are possible from practically all mandibular positions. In any event the position of centric relation remains constant, or nearly so, throughout life, except in the event of injury or disease of the temporomandibular joint. Centric relation is a bone-to-bone relation of the mandible to the maxillae, and cuspal relation of the teeth is not considered. The mandible can be returned to this position repeatedly, so it is considered to be a reference point in developing the occlusion for a patient.

The second horizontal relation of the mandible to the maxillae is centric occlusion, the relationship of the teeth in one jaw to the teeth in the opposing jaw where there is maximum intercuspation (Fig. 14-11). This is a tooth-to-tooth relationship, and there is no mention of jaw position. This is not a terminal or end position of the mandible but takes place usually somewhere within the border limits of the chewing cycle. It is a position of learned, conscious, habitual closure. Even though a patient returns to this position constantly during function, it is not thought to be repeatable, and doubt remains as to whether it can be considered a reference point in the development of an occlusal scheme for a patient.

In more than 90% of all persons, centric relation and centric occlusion do not coincide. When different, centric occlusion will always be anterior (the position of the

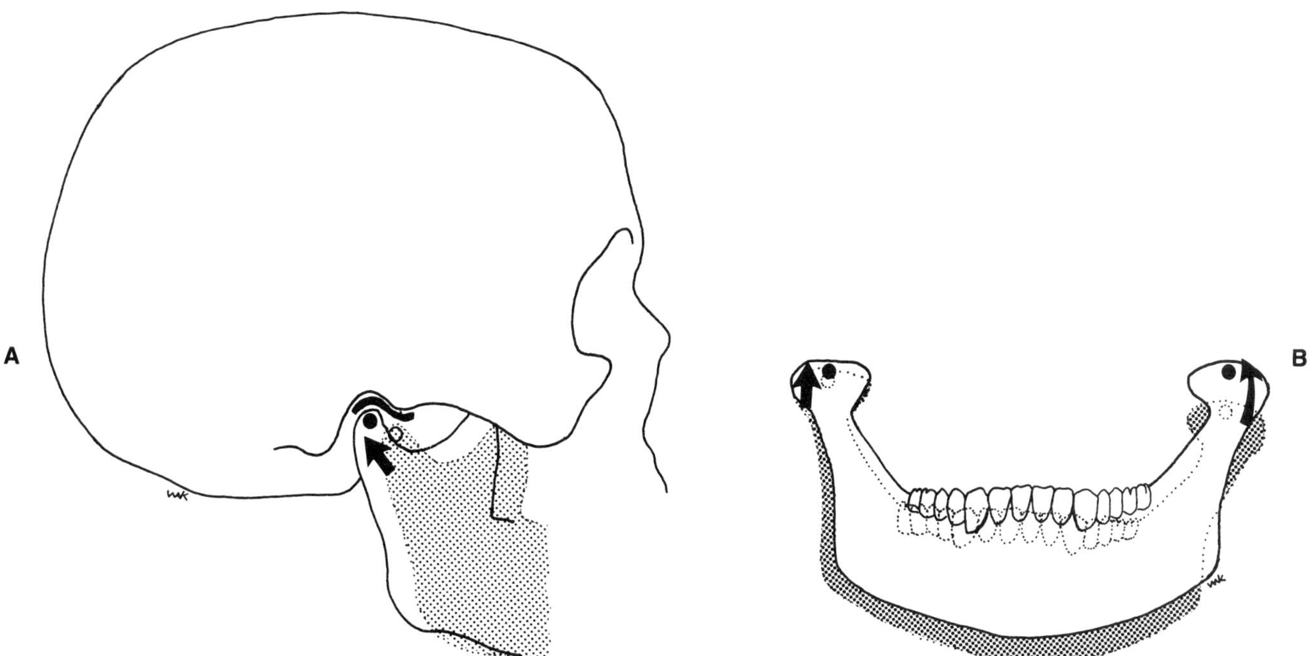

Fig. 14-10. A, Anteroposterior relationship of mandible to maxillae is one component of horizontal jaw relation. Mandible (shaded) must be moved upward and backward to reach centric relation. **B,** Lateral relation is other component of horizontal jaw relation. Both condyles must be elevated and retruded evenly.

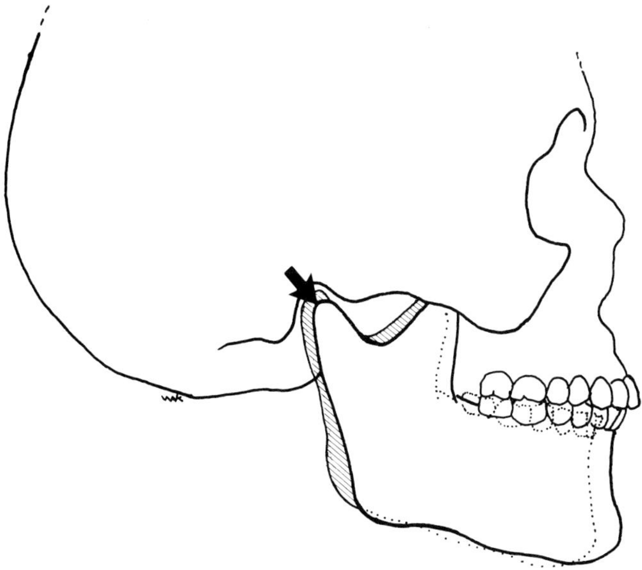

Fig. 14-11. Centric occlusion is position of maximum intercuspation. Jaw position is not a consideration. Mandible moves forward and downward slightly.

mandible in relation to the maxillae) to centric relation. The difference can range from tenths of a millimeter to 5 mm or more, but 1 to 2 mm is most frequent. Regardless of the position selected from which to develop the occlusal scheme for a prosthesis, harmony between these two positions must be maintained. Even though centric occlusion is not thought to be a repeatable position, a patient with partial dentures who has cusps on remaining natural teeth can be guided back to that position by the remaining teeth. Patients will always function in these two positions and in the intervening space, so deflective occlusal contacts in either position must be avoided.

FACTORS INFLUENCING DEVELOPMENT OF OCCLUSION

Several factors influence the final occlusal scheme for the partial denture patient.

Rudolph L. Hanau, a number of years ago, postulated his laws of articulation. These were nine purely physical laws that he thought had to be obeyed to produce balanced articulation (a continuous change from

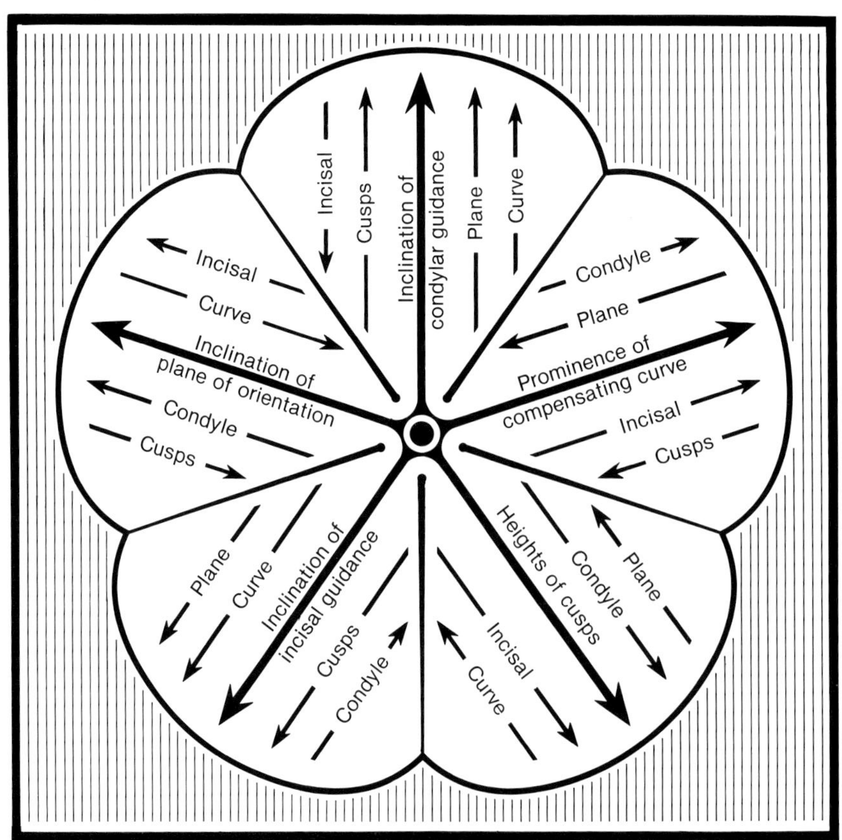

Fig. 14-12. Hanau Articulation Quint. Arrow pointing away from center indicates *increase of;* arrow pointing toward center indicates *decrease of.* (Courtesy Teledyne Hanau.)

one balanced occlusion into another for all occluded mandibular excursions). Today this concept is accepted mainly in the practice of complete denture prosthodontics.

Of the nine factors Hanau originally proposed, five, known as the Hanau Quint (Fig. 14-12), have come to be recognized as important in the field of prosthodontic restorations:

1. The inclination of the condylar guidance (Fig. 14-13)
2. The prominence of the compensating curve (Fig. 14-14)
3. The inclination of the plane of orientation (Fig. 14-15)
4. The inclination of the incisal guidance (Fig. 14-16)
5. The heights of the cusps (Fig. 14-17)

In complete denture prosthodontics the compensating curve, the plane of orientation, the incisal guidance, and the heights of the cusps may be changed to satisfy the needs of each patient. The one factor that cannot

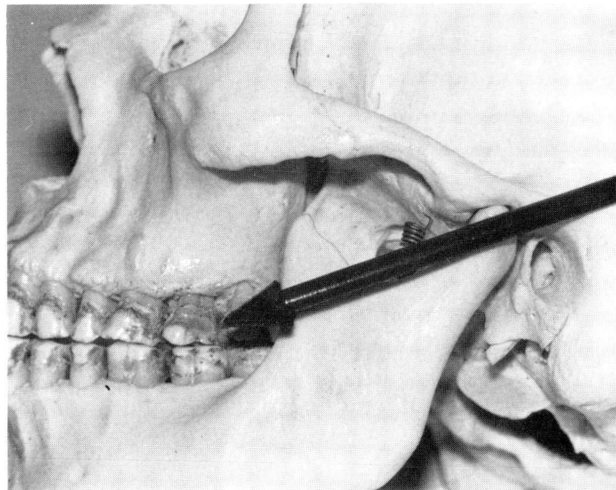

Fig. 14-13. Inclination of condylar guidance is a definite anatomic feature that depends on inclination of floor of glenoid fossa (indicated by shaft of arrow). Dentist cannot alter this inclination.

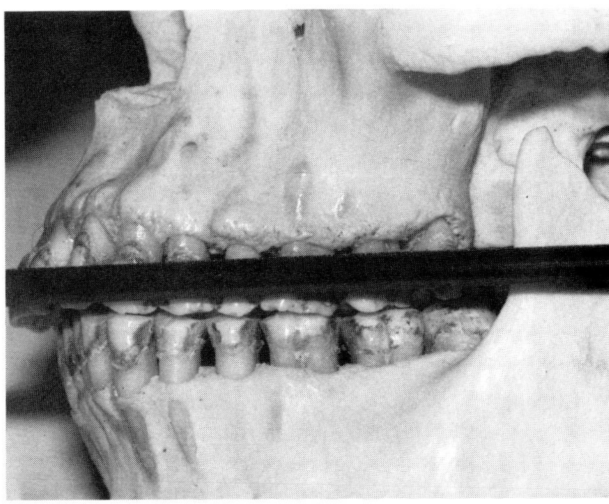

Fig. 14-14. Compensating curve (degree of anteroposterior concavity formed by mandibular posterior teeth) in this specimen has been worn relatively flat.

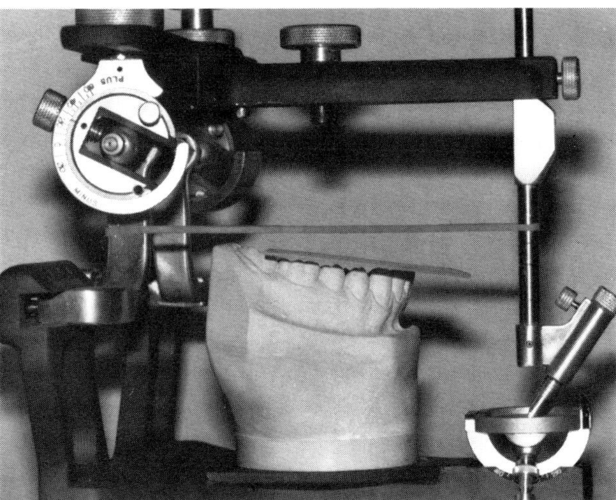

Fig. 14-15. Plane of orientation is plane that passes through contact point of central incisors and tips of mesiobuccal cusps of last molars. Inclination of plane is angle formed posteriorly with horizontal plane of articulator.

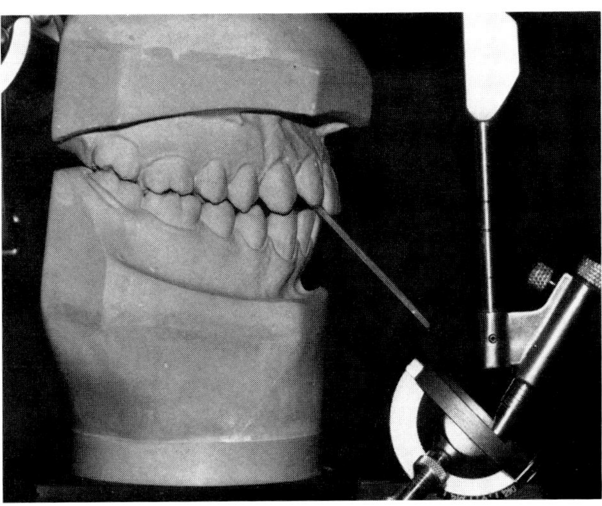

Fig. 14-16. Incisal guidance is determined by relationship of mandibular anterior teeth to lingual surfaces of maxillary anterior teeth. Inclination of incisal guidance is angle formed by lingual surfaces of incisor teeth and horizontal plane of articulator.

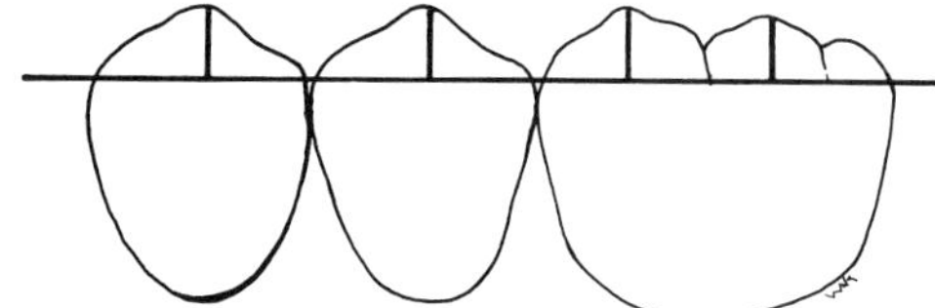

Fig. 14-17. Cusp height is distance of vertical projection from imaginary cusp base to cusp tip.

be altered for a complete denture patient is the condylar guidance. The ability to change four factors of articulation makes the development of an occlusal scheme relatively easy for a patient with complete dentures.

In a patient who has partial dentures, however, the factors governing the occlusal patterns are already determined. The presence of some natural teeth means that the prominence of the compensating curve has been determined, the plane of orientation is present, the incisal guidance is determined by the presence of anterior teeth, and the height of the cusps is known. This means that in partial denture construction the remaining natural teeth will dictate the form and position of the artificial teeth. The only exceptions are (1) when the removable partial denture is opposed by a complete denture and occlusal harmony can be obtained and (2) when only anterior teeth remain in both arches and the incisal relationship is noninterfering.

METHODS OF ESTABLISHING OCCLUSION

There are basically two methods of establishing the occlusion for a removable partial denture: (1) the functionally generated path technique and (2) the articulator, or static, technique.

Functionally generated path technique

The theory on which the functionally generated path technique is based is that when the pathways each tooth opposed to the edentulous space makes throughout all functional movements of the mandible are recorded, the artificial tooth may thus be positioned and formed so that it will remain in harmonious contact with its antagonist at all times.

The pathways are created by the patient in a wax occlusion rim. The patient performs all functional excursions while the opposing teeth contact the surface of the occlusion rim. The recording produced in the wax is actually a negative record of the movement of each opposing tooth as the mandible executes the functional movements (Fig. 14-18).

The pathways so generated are poured in hard improved stone to produce a cast against which the artificial teeth are set. Each ridge or groove in the resulting

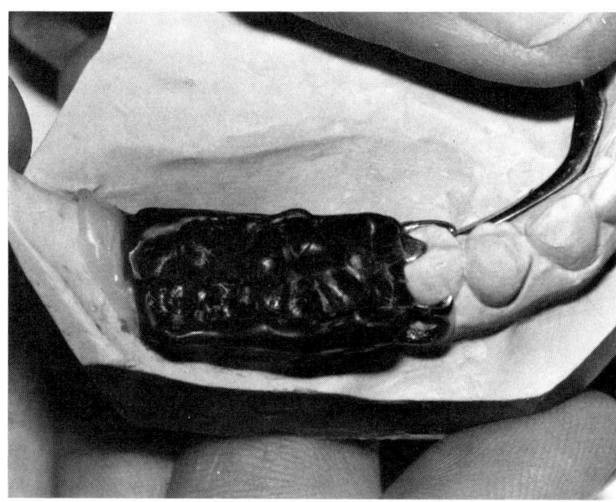

Fig. 14-18. Functionally generated pathway is dynamic record of movement of opposing tooth surfaces.

stone cast represents the path of a cusp. Setting the teeth in contact with the paths should result in a completely functional and harmonious occlusion.

Clinical procedure

An acrylic resin denture base is attached to the framework in a manner similar to that used for the record base. On the acrylic resin base is constructed a specially compounded hard wax occlusion rim. Many subscribers to the method of recording the occlusal pathways use a hard inlay wax (purple) because they believe that the purple color makes reading of the facets cut in the wax easier.

There are two methods of having the patient grind the occlusal pathways.

The first method is to have the patient take the framework with the denture base and occlusion rim attached home and to wear it continuously for 24 hours except when eating and when drinking hot or chilled drinks.

The occlusion rim is constructed so that when first inserted it is slightly high in occlusal contacts and will keep the remaining natural teeth apart from 0.5 to 0.75 mm. The extra height is necessary to develop the full range of motion. The occlusion rim should be made several millimeters wider than the buccolingual width of the tooth opposing the rim. The extra width is necessary to record the full range of functional motion (Fig. 14-19).

Ideally there should be occlusal contact between at least two opposing natural teeth so that the original vertical dimension of occlusion can be maintained. If such contact is not present, careful vertical measurements at

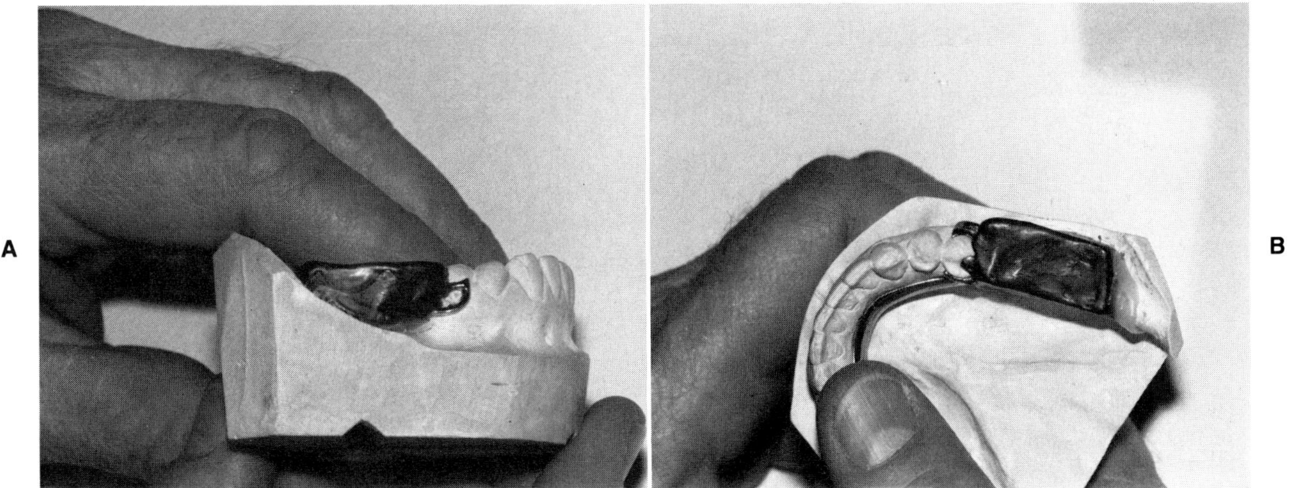

Fig. 14–19. A, Occlusion rim for functionally generated path technique is constructed slightly higher than occlusal plane. **B,** Buccolingual width of rim is several millimeters greater than that of opposing teeth.

the vertical dimension of occlusion (3 mm less than the vertical dimension of rest) must be made and recorded between two recognizable landmarks in the opposing arches. These measurements may be made by using dividers. The gingival crevicular margins of opposing teeth are frequently helpful and usable landmarks.

The patient who wears the prosthesis overnight must be reminded to intermittently close the jaws together firmly and to grind against the wax in all possible jaw positions. The patients must be taught to retrude the mandible before the prosthesis is worn.

The value of the patient's wearing the denture while sleeping is that involuntary or bruxing contacts will be recorded. The resulting pathway will be a record of all possible jaw movements and tooth contacts even though some of the contacts may be undesirable.

The completed wax pattern will resemble a slightly larger version, buccolingually, of the teeth that originally occupied the edentulous space. The occlusal size is increased because the pattern represents the extreme of the lateral and protrusive positions of the tooth-to-wax contacts.

This wax pattern is boxed and poured in improved dental stone to provide a permanent record of the generated pathways. The stone record is mounted on an articulator, and the artificial teeth of the partial denture are fitted to contact the record (Fig. 14-20).

The second method of generating the functional path is for the patient to create the pathway in the dental office directly under the supervision of the dentist. This obviously has the advantage of the dentist's being able to observe and correct the movement the patient is making. The disadvantage is that normally a patient will require at least 30 minutes of active movement to complete a pathway. The record should be removed and examined every few minutes. The wax will exhibit a glossy surface where tooth-wax contact is occurring. Those areas not in contact will appear dull. Wax may be melted and added to those areas to ensure complete and even contact. The record is boxed and poured the same as for the overnight record.

Artificial teeth set to the generated path. The incisal guide pin is opened 1 mm before the artificial teeth are positioned. This increase in vertical dimension will be returned to normal by selectively grinding the denture teeth. The selective grinding also develops the occlusal anatomy of the denture tooth to conform to the functionally generated stone path.

The denture teeth are positioned over the framework in the correct anteroposterior and buccolingual position. Care should be used not to position mandibular posterior teeth too far buccally because when the height of the tooth is reduced by selective grinding it will appear to have a more buccal position because of the contour of the tooth.

After the teeth are set in correct alignment, the incisal guide pin is returned to correct vertical dimension of occlusion. A water-soluble Prussian blue dye is painted on the surface of the generated path. The articulator is locked in centric relation, and opening and closing tapping movements are made of the stone path against the denture teeth.

The spots of dye transferred from the stone pathway to the denture teeth indicate the areas of contact and are reduced by grinding.

Selective grinding is continued until the incisal pin

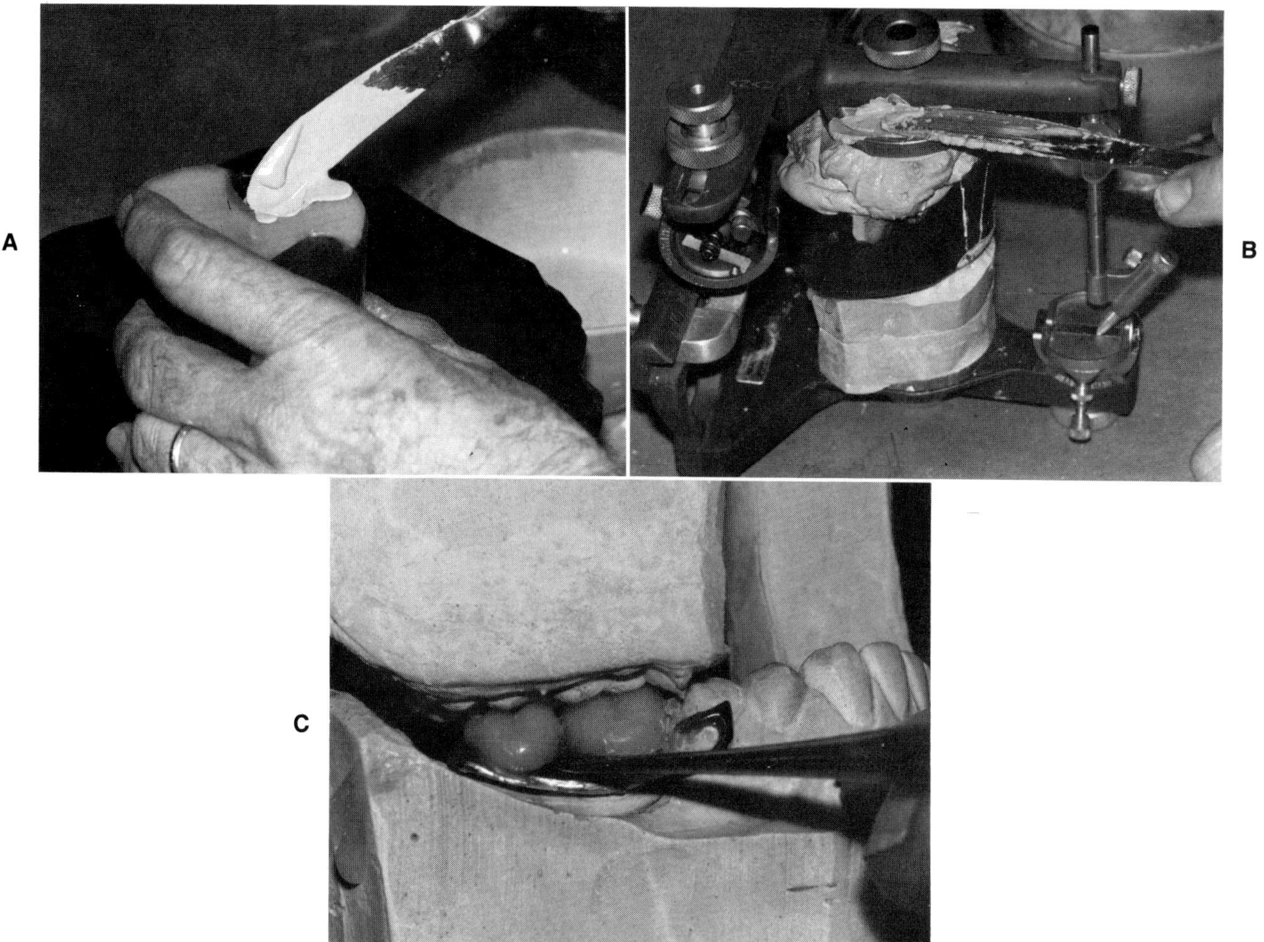

Fig. 14-20. A, Completed pathway is boxed and poured in dense stone. **B,** Stone record is mounted on articulator. **C,** Artifical teeth are fitted to record.

again contacts the incisal table. At this time, intimate contact should be present between the artificial teeth and the stone pathway. The articulator is not moved into protrusive and lateral excursions because these positions are incorporated in the pathway.

Advantages and disadvantages

Possibly the greatest advantage of the functionally generated path technique is that it eliminates the need for adjusting an articulator with interocclusal records or a tracing device. Advocates of this approach in developing the occlusion claim that a far greater potential for error lies in attempting to adjust an articulator to follow jaw movements precisely than in generating a functional pathway. This method also eliminates the need to make a face-bow transfer, because all the information derived from a face-bow transfer is contained in the pathway.

There are limitations to the use of the generated path. The occlusion in one of the arches must be complete before a generated path can be developed. If opposing partial dentures are required, one of the partial dentures must be completed before the other can be made.

This method also does not lend itself well to developing the occlusion for a partial denture opposing a complete denture. Here the solution would be to complete the partial denture by the articulator method and then to functionally generate a pathway for the complete denture.

Other disadvantages may be present also. During the generation of the path in the hard inlay wax, movement of a distal extension base carrying the occlusion rim is possible. This will produce an inaccurate pattern that will appear to be complete. Verification of a recording in the mouth is difficult. Numerous studies have also shown that the masticatory cycle differs depending on the type and texture of food being chewed. This may mean that the pattern developed in the wax is accurate for the wax only and that foodstuffs may fall inside or outside the particular chewing cycle.

Articulator technique

First, methods of establishing occlusal relationships by using record bases and occlusal rims attached to the framework are discussed. The use of this jaw relation record is essential to the articulator, or static, method of establishing an occlusal pattern for partial dentures if the casts cannot be hand articulated and if the position of centric occlusion has been selected as the proper jaw relation.

Direct apposition of casts (hand articulation)

Hand articulation may be used in place of making a jaw relation record when sufficient opposing teeth remain in contact to make the existing jaw relationship obvious (Fig. 14-21). It should be used when only a few teeth are to be replaced.

The occluded casts are secured together with wooden sticks and sticky wax and mounted arbitrarily on an articulator (Fig. 14-22). A face-bow mounting is generally not indicated.

There are limitations to using this method, yet it is better than using an inaccurate wax record, a so-called sandwich bite or mush bite, between the remaining natural teeth.

The principal danger in this technique is that it perpetuates the existing vertical dimension and any existing occlusal disharmony.

If this method is used, a clinical appointment for establishing occlusal relationships will not be necessary.

Jaw relation record made by using the framework

In the first jaw relation record made to complete the diagnostic mounting procedure, baseplates were used to transport occlusion rims and recording media. The baseplates were constructed of either gutta-percha or autopolymerizing acrylic resin. For the final jaw relation record the framework should be used to support the occlusion rim and recording medium. The fit of the framework has already been verified at the framework try-in appointment, and any occlusal interferences have been corrected or eliminated at that same appointment. This means that the framework will be a stable and accurate base on which to record the jaw relationship.

If this appointment follows the construction of an altered or corrected cast, as it usually will, the framework with the corrected cast impression should be recovered from the boxed impression. Care must be exercised in removing the framework and impression not to damage the stone teeth on the cast or the new edentulous ridge that has been poured.

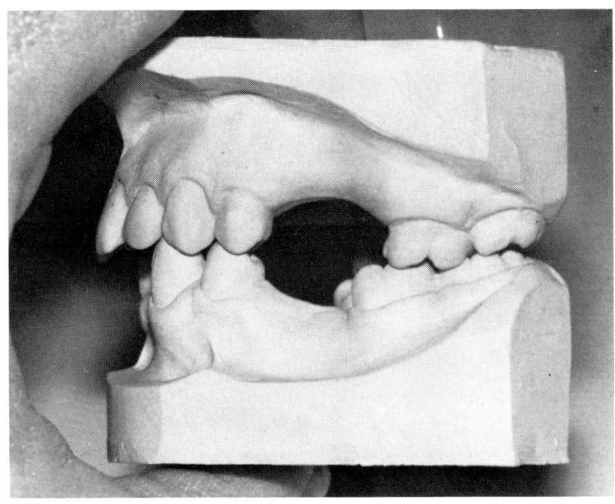

Fig. 14-21. Hand articulation. Casts must unmistakeably occlude to use this technique.

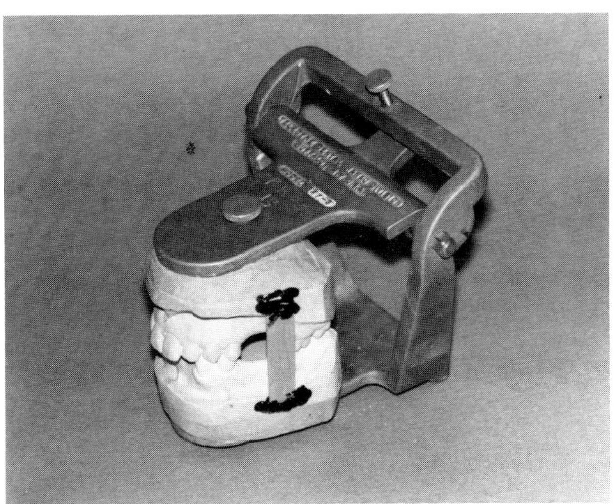

Fig. 14-22. Hand-articulated casts mounted on Hanau LTD hinge articulator.

It is advisable before removing the framework to examine the relationship of the framework to the teeth on the cast to be certain that the occlusal rests and other components of the framework did not move during the pouring of the cast (Fig. 14-23). If any change in position of the framework is evident, the corrected impression procedure must be repeated.

The acrylic resin tray that was used to make the impression must be removed from the framework. This can best be accomplished by heating the tray material over a burner until it starts to smoke and then pulling it free from the acrylic resin retention minor connector with pliers (Fig. 14-24). The impression should not be used as a recording base for the jaw relation record be-

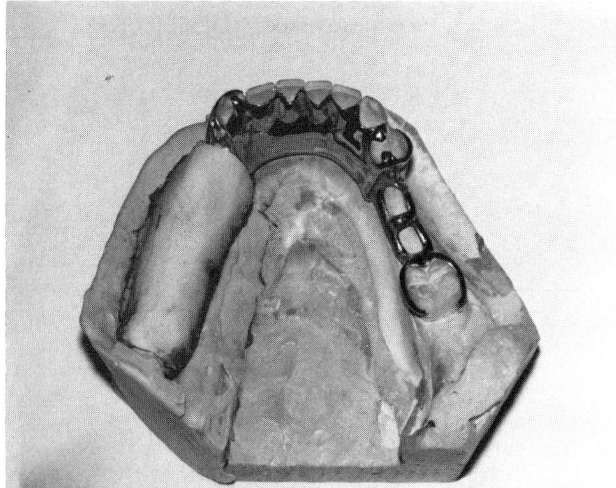

Fig. 14-23. Relationship of metal framework to stone is examined before impression is removed.

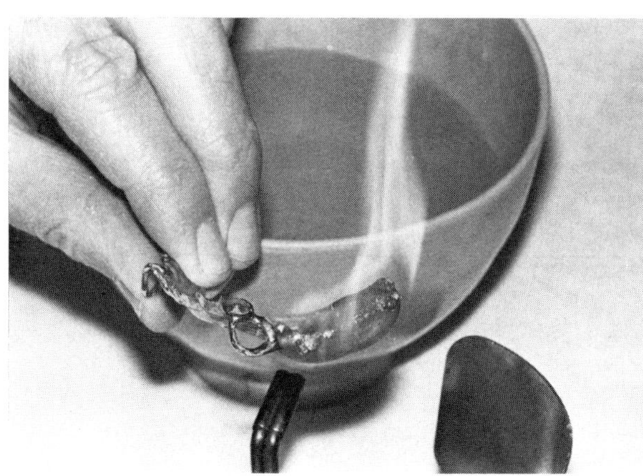

Fig. 14-24. Impression and tray are removed from framework by heating over open flame.

cause the impression generally is distorted as it is removed from the cast.

Making the record base. A new record base must be constructed on the framework to support the jaw relation record. If the edentulous space is not too long, hard baseplate wax may be formed over the acrylic resin retention metal in contact with the edentulous ridge. This will usually be strong enough if normal precautions are used in handling the framework. The jaw relation record itself will be made with a pressure-free media, so the record base will not be subjected to an occlusal pressure. The greatest danger in a baseplate wax record base is not using it to mount the casts on an articulator immediately. Allowing the wax to sit unused for any time causes distortion. On top of the wax record base an occlusion rim can be built to support the zinc oxide–eugenol impression paste that will be used to record this pressure-free jaw relationship.

Autopolymerizing acrylic resin (sprinkle-on method) or acrylic resin tray material such as that used to form the impression tray for the corrected cast impression (finger-molding technique) should be used to construct the record base if the edentulous ridge is long or if the interarch space is restricted. The former will be more accurate and slightly stronger, but the danger of damaging the master cast is also slightly greater.

Regardless of the material used to construct the record base, soft tissue undercuts on the edentulous ridge must be eliminated with baseplate wax before the separating medium is applied (Fig. 14-25). Failure to eliminate these undercuts completely can result in damage to the master cast.

Two coats of an alginate separating medium should be painted over the edentulous ridge before the framework is seated.

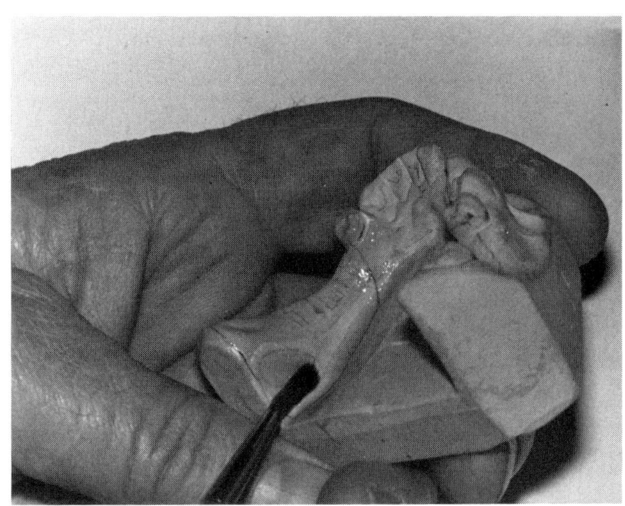

Fig. 14-25. Undercuts on edentulous ridge are eliminated with baseplate wax, and tinfoil substitute is painted over area.

When the separating medium is dry, baseplate wax or acrylic resin tray material can be adapted over the acrylic resin retention struts. It must be adapted closely enough to the ridge to offer vertical stability to the framework and closely enough to the metal to prevent movement of the base. After the base material is hard, it should be trimmed and smoothed (Fig. 14-26).

A WORD OF CAUTION: The tissue stop at the terminal end of the acrylic resin retention minor connector that contacted the edentulous ridge of the original master cast is now no longer in contact with the new ridge made from the corrected cast impression. This is primarily the result of the soft tissue's being captured in a different form by the second impression. As the wax or

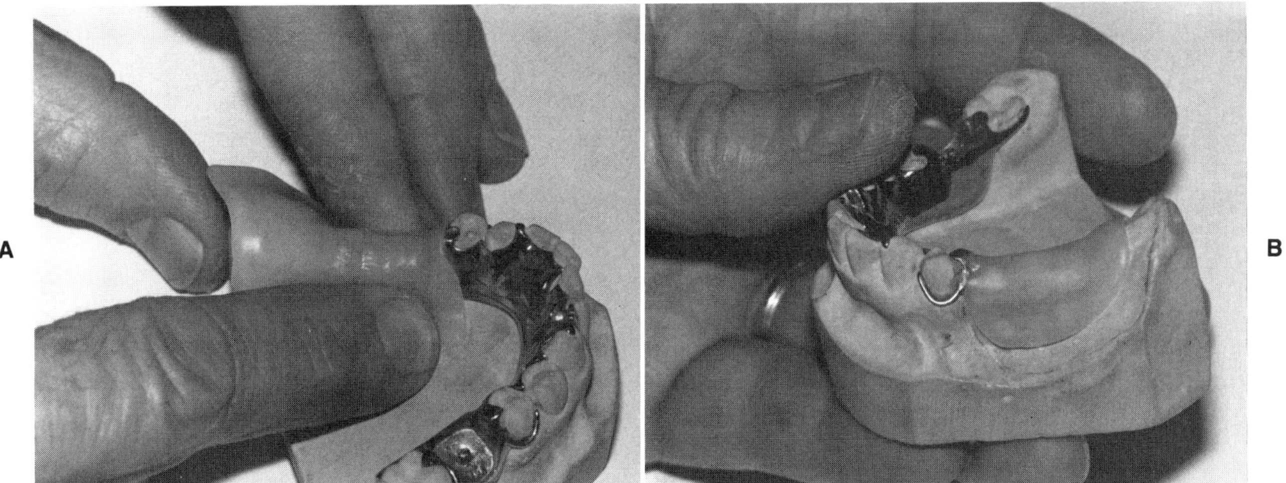

Fig. 14-26. A, Baseplate wax is adapted by finger pressure over acrylic resin retention minor connector. **B,** Wax is trimmed slightly short of final peripheral extension of denture base.

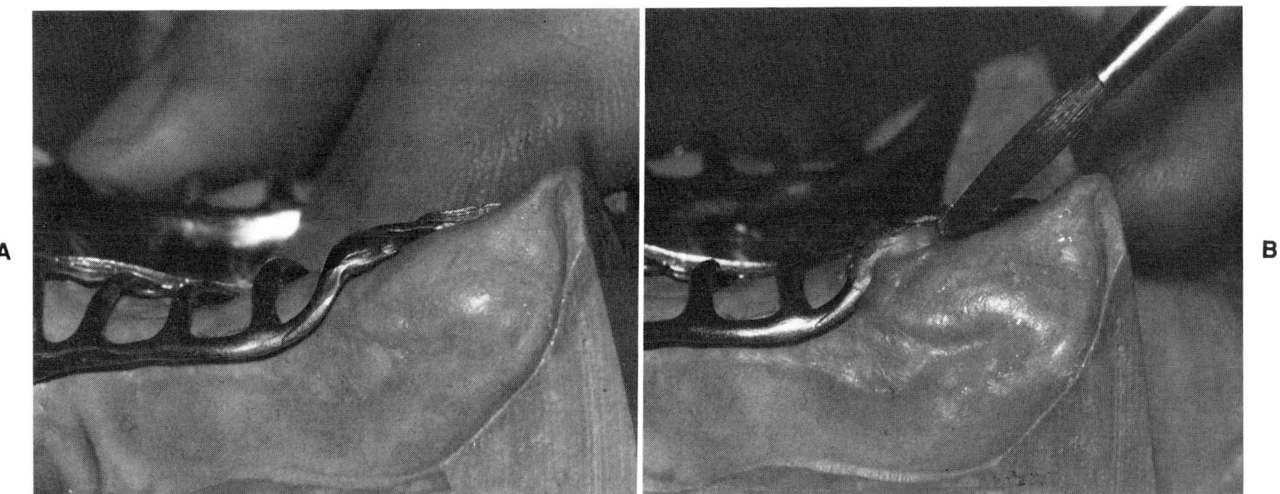

Fig. 14-27. A, Tissue stop under acrylic resin retention minor connector will not contact cast following making of altered cast. **B,** To prevent framework from being moved during record base construction or during packing of denture base, bead of autopolymerizing resin is placed between tissue stop and stone ridge.

acrylic resin tray material is adapted, care must be taken not to dislodge the framework by excessive downward force. To prevent this from happening, a bead of autopolymerizing resin can be placed between the tissue stop and the stone ridge and allowed to set before the record base is adapted (Fig. 14-27).

If an acrylic resin sprinkle-on base is to be used (the most accurate method), a peripheral border may be constructed around the edentulous space to contain the acrylic resin while it is semifluid. This peripheral border is placed after the separating medium has been applied and the framework seated. After the resin is set, it should be trimmed and smoothed but not polished (Fig. 14-28).

Occlusion rim. An occlusion rim of medium baseplate wax is added to the record base. At this time the position of the occlusion rim must be approximated but it should be centered over the crest of the edentulous ridge (Fig. 14-29). The mandibular distal extension occlusion rim may be constructed so that the height will be even with the cusps of the adjacent abutment tooth anteriorly and posteriorly to two-thirds the height of the retromolar or pear-shaped pad. The final shaping of the rim will be accomplished with the patient present.

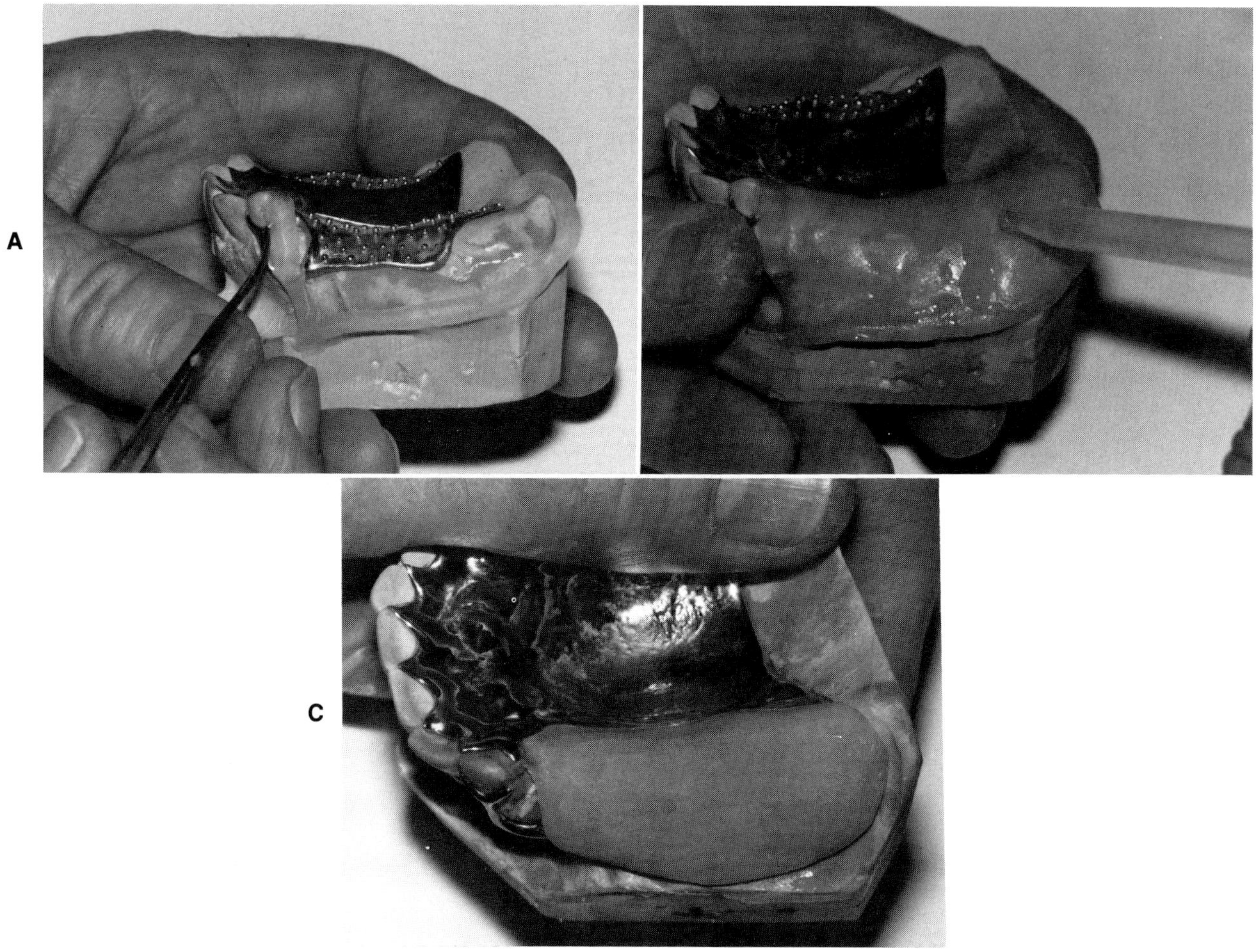

A

B

C

Fig. 14-28. A, If acrylic resin sprinkle-on record base is to be made, reservoir is made to contain semifluid resin as it is added. Reservoir is strip of utility wax attached around periphery of record base. It is joined at one end to external finish line of major connector and at other end to minor connector to which occlusal rest and clasp are attached. **B,** Record base is constructed by sprinking on dry polymer and wetting it with monomer from dropper. **C,** Completed record base is smoothed but not polished.

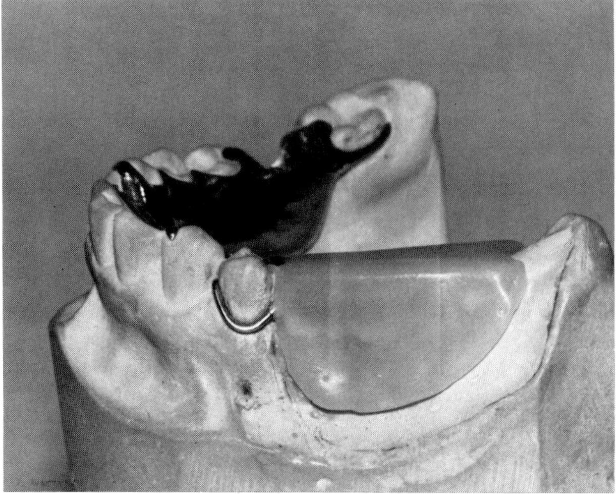

Fig. 14-29. Medium baseplate wax is used to form occlusion rim. Rim is centered over crest of ridge.

Recording media. *Zinc oxide–eugenol impression paste* is perhaps the first choice as a recording medium. It can be mixed to form a free-flowing, practically pressure-free material. Most brands have a reasonably fast setting time or can be made so by the addition of a drop of water or alcohol at the start of the mix. The material produces a record that is firm and not liable to damage. The record can be kept for an extended time, if needed, without fear of distortion.

Concentrated slurry solution mixed with Hydrocal, which is mentioned in the discussion of mounting casts on an articulator, produces a record that is hard and accurate. The mix of the material can be made so that it is free flowing and yet will set rapidly. The record can be kept for an indefinite period without fear of distortion.

If *modeling plastic* is used, it should be softened in a water bath to ensure smooth, even heating. The use of modeling plastic as the recording medium is hazardous at best, and usually should be limited to the experienced operator. It is hardly a pressure-free material and the accuracy of the record should always be verified. Once chilled, the record is hard, but it is still susceptible to distortion. It should be used to mount the casts immediately.

Baseplate wax should be used with caution to record the jaw relation. It is difficult to soften it evenly to obtain an accurate record. Waxes that contain metallic particles (such as Aluwax) can be uniformly softened, but even after this type of wax is chilled, it remains pliable and can be distorted. Merely positioning the opposing cast into the record can damage it. If this weakness is recognized and special care is taken in handling the record, accurate results can be obtained.

Clinical procedures. The framework with the record base and occlusion rim attached is tried in the patient's mouth. If the record is to be made at the centric relation position, the patient's mandible should be guided to the most retruded position and allowed to close. If the centric occlusion position is to be used, the patient should close in that position. In either case the height of the occlusion rims must be adjusted so that no contact takes place between the opposing teeth and the rim. A space of approximately 1 mm is desired (Fig. 14-30).

In the event that opposing occlusion rims are to be used, one of these should be adjusted to establish an ideal occlusal plane and the opposing rim adjusted to be short of contact. The mandibular rim is usually used to establish the ideal occlusal plane because of the landmarks that are normally present. The posterior height of the rim is established at $^{2}/_{3}$ the height of the retromolar pad and anterior to the height of the remaining teeth.

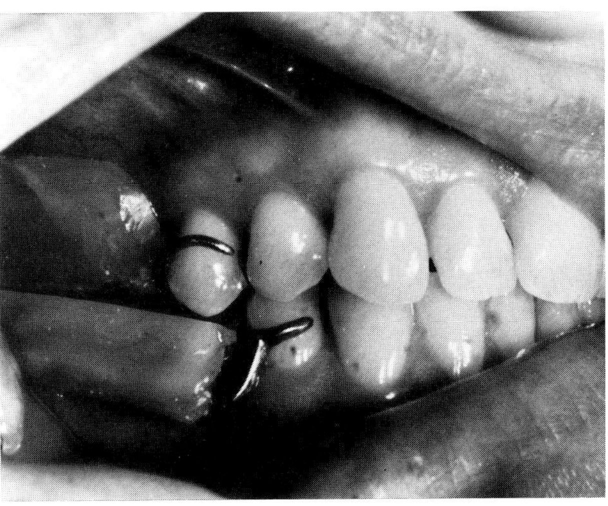

Fig. 14-30. There should be no contact between opposing occlusion rims or between occlusion rims and opposing teeth.

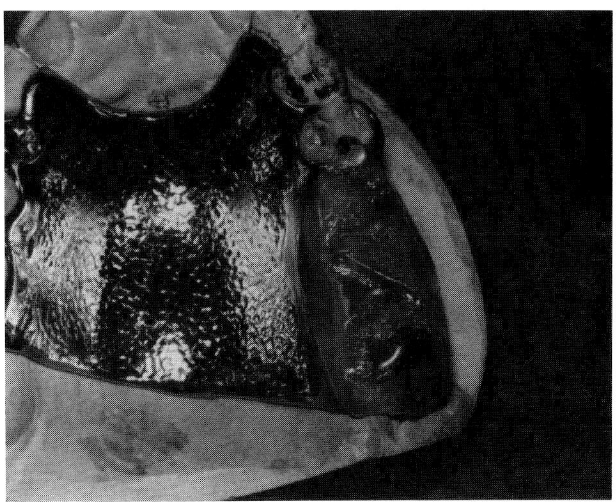

Fig. 14-31. One of the opposing occlusion rims, usually the maxillary, is indexed with several V-shaped notches.

If opposing occlusion rims are to be used, the recording medium is normally placed on the mandibular rim for convenience. The maxillary rim should be indexed with several V-shaped notches (Fig. 14-31). A separating medium, petrolatum, should also be used over the surface of the maxillary rim.

The surface of the occlusion rim that is to support the recording medium should be roughened to ensure that the record will remain attached to it. A series of scratches or small pits is sufficient for this purpose.

The patient should be instructed as to the procedure to be accomplished. An informed patient is generally more cooperative. The procedure should be rehearsed

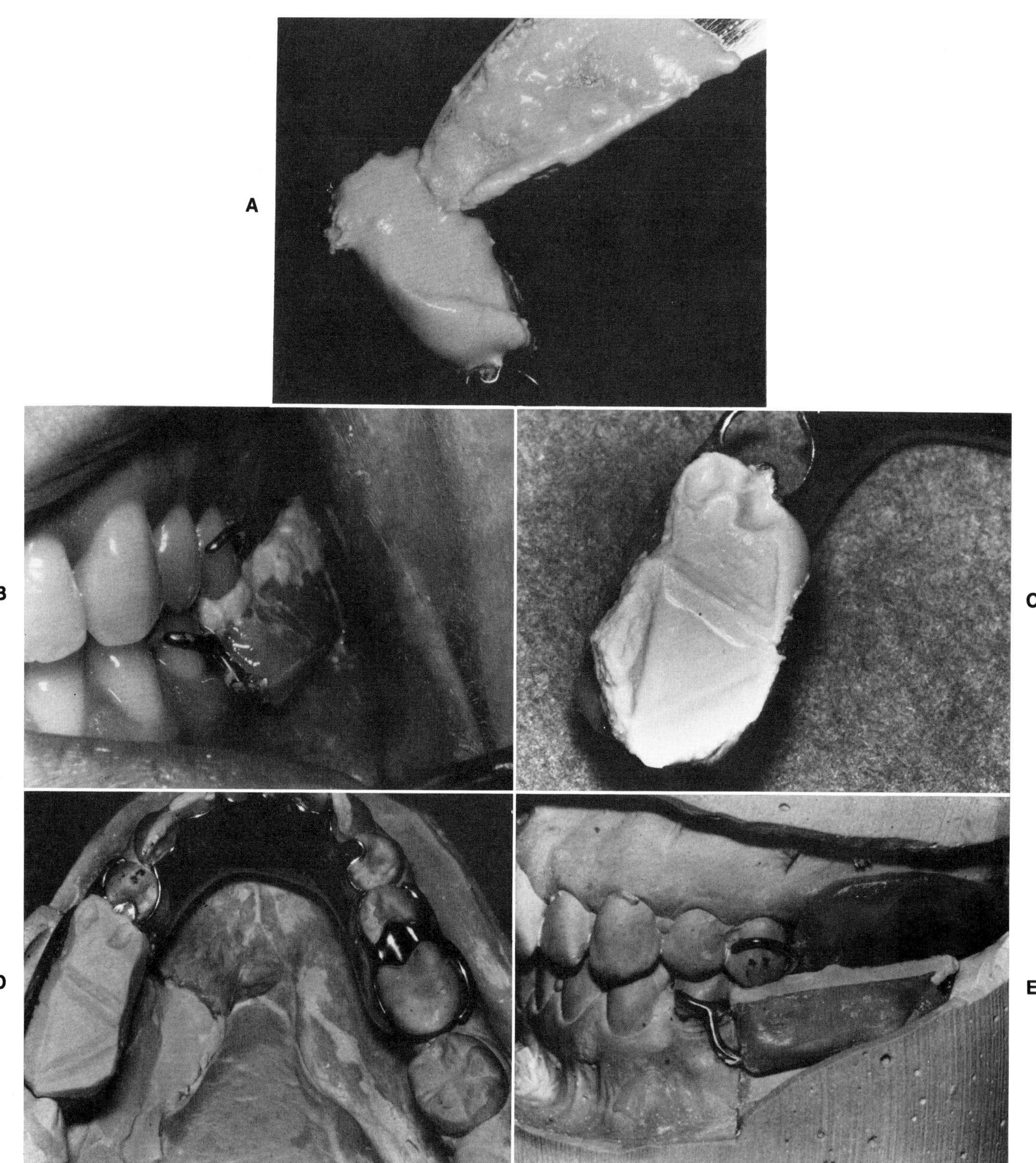

Fig. 14-32. Making jaw relation. **A,** Recording media (shown is concentrated slurry solution and Hydrocal) is mixed and located on occlusion rim. **B,** Patient is guided to correct closing position and remains in that position until material sets. **C,** Completed record is examined for evidence of showthrough. **D,** Record is trimmed so that only cusp tips and indices remain. **E,** Casts are hand articulated, and relationship of teeth on casts is compared with that in mouth. If any difference is noted, jaw relation record should be remade.

several times before the record is actually made. Fig. 14-32 illustrates the procedure.

The greatest cause of incorrect jaw relation records is pressure. If any force occurs on the occlusion rims, the distal extension record base will depress the soft tissue beneath the base. This is enough to cause an incorrect jaw relation record. If any portion of the wax occlusion rim shows through the recording medium, that portion of the occlusion rim should be relieved and the record made again.

If the jaw relation record is accurate, the casts may be mounted on the articulator and the artificial teeth selected and set.

Face-bow transfer

The casts must be mounted accurately on an articulator following determination of the vertical dimension of occlusion and the centric jaw relationship. To maintain accuracy, the length of the arc of closure of the casts should also be determined. The arc of closure is the distance from the head of the condyle to the mesial tip of the lower central incisors. Variations in the arc can have a profound influence on the position and height of the cusps on the artificial teeth. This measurement is obtained by the use of a face-bow transfer.

The use and the purpose of the face-bow (Fig. 14-33) are discussed in Chapter 6. When most or all of the posterior teeth are to be replaced in one or both arches, the use of the face-bow is essential in eliminating unnecessary problems in developing the occlusion. To properly relate artificial teeth on opposing maxillary and mandibular casts on an articulator, the casts must be related to one another in three planes: the horizontal, the frontal, and the sagittal. If the teeth were to remain in static relationship to one another, these spatial relationships would be sufficient. However, the tooth relationships do not remain static, but undergo opening, closing, and lateral movements. The mandible opens and closes on a definite arc (Fig. 14-34). The length of this arc is measured from the center of the condyle, in the sagittal plane, to the teeth. The length of the arc or the distance from the center of rotation will have a definite influence on the development of the occlusion.

It is possible to relate the occlusal plane as it is present in the mouth of a patient with the head erect to the Frankfort or horizontal plane of the skull by selecting a third point of reference anterior to the two artibrary condylar locations (Fig. 14-35). The third point normally used is the orbitale, the lowest margin of the bony orbit. When the three points of reference are used, the relation of the occlusal plane to the Frankfort plane (orbitale to tragion) is transferred accurately to the articulator. The advantage of having casts mounted on the articulator at the exact angulation that the jaws are in the mouth is that the position of the artificial teeth being placed on the cast can better be visualized as the teeth will actually appear in the patient. This is especially important when anterior teeth are being replaced or when complete dentures are being constructed.

A second major advantage of mounting the maxillary cast using the third point of reference is that any time in the future, casts of that patient can be related to the condylar elements of the articulator at the same horizontal and lateral condylar settings. Changing the horizontal and lateral angles will not materially affect cuspal position in centric relation or protrusive relationships but can produce interferences when lateral excursions are attempted.

The use of the face-bow makes the mounting of the maxillary cast on the articulator more convenient and more accurate. More frequent use of the face-bow should be encouraged.

Types of articulators

Many practitioners believe that the patient's mouth is the most accurate and usable articulator available and should be used as much as possible in preference to a mechanical equivalent. There is no doubt that the mouth is the most accurate, but many patients lack the muscular coordination and nerve perception to carry out the jaw movements required to perfect an occlusal scheme in the mouth. If the potential hazards of working directly with the patient are recognized and respected, many of the finer details in adjusting the occlusion in the mouth can be accomplished. The actions that mechanical articulators can perform range from simple open and closing movements around a fixed axis to precisely duplicating or simulating mandibular movement through all ranges of motion. The simplest and most easily understood classification system refers to the degree to which the articulator can be adjusted to conform to the jaw movements of the patient. The system consists of three categories: nonadjustable, semiadjustable, and fully adjustable. Some instruments may be completely adjustable in certain phases of jaw movements (lateral and horizontal condylar inclinations for example) yet lack the total adjustability required to accommodate the Bennett movement. An instrument of this type would be classed as semiadjustable.

Nonadjustable articulators. Nonadjustable articulators (Fig. 14-36) can open and close around a fixed horizontal axis. The condylar ball, if one is present, is normally attached to the upper member of the articulator and rotates in a groove or slot in the lower member. A few representatives of this class have a fixed condylar path along which the condylar ball can be pushed to

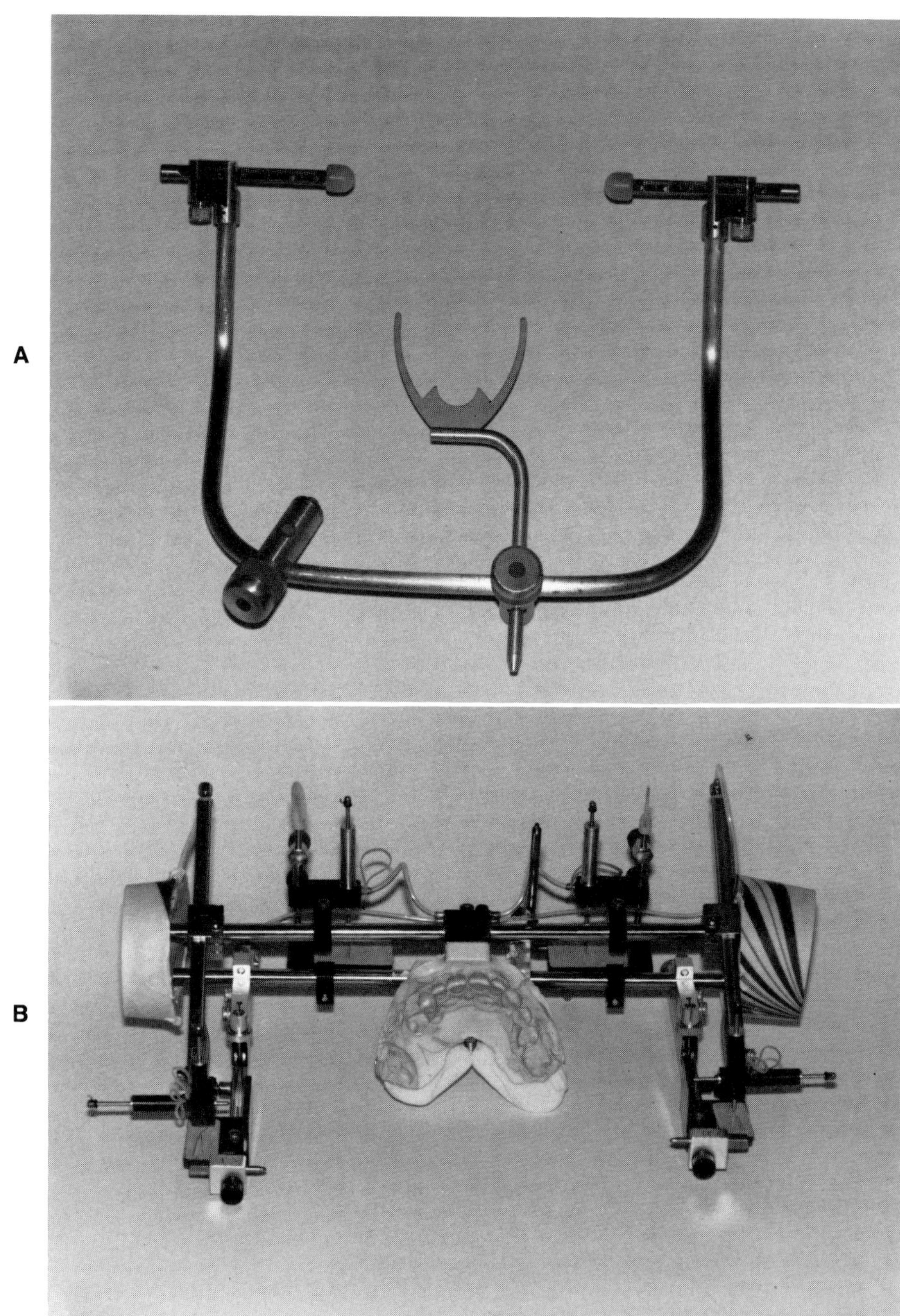

Fig. 14-33. **A,** Arbitrary face-bow. External auditory meatus is used as arbitrary hinge-axis position. **B,** Kinematic face-bow is used to locate true hinge axis on patient.

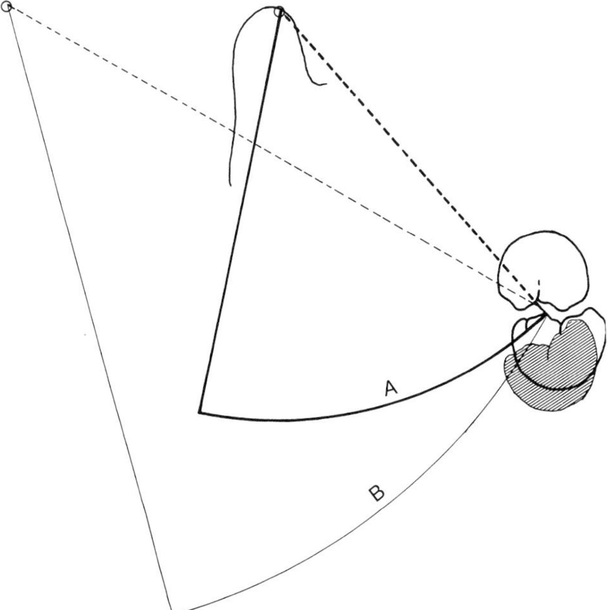

Fig. 14-34. The distance from center of rotation (head of condyle) to tooth cusps influences development of cusp. Curvature of arc *A* is more pronounced than that of arc *B*. To be harmonious, cusps developed for arc *A* would be higher than those to satisfy flatter arc *B*.

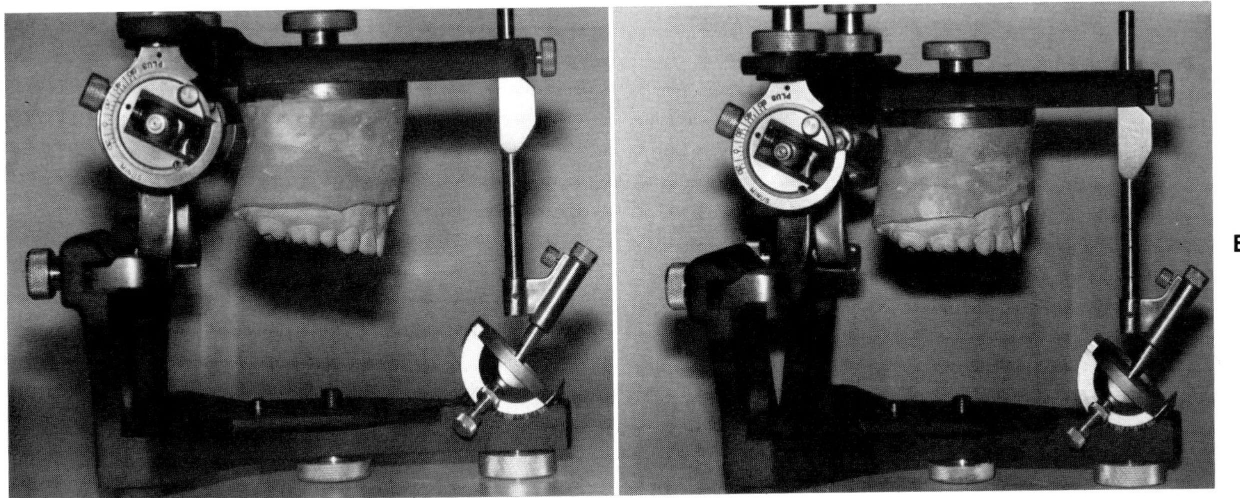

Fig. 14-35. A, Third point of reference positions cast on articulator with same orientation of occlusal plane that is present in mouth. **B,** Without third point of reference, inclination of plane of occlusion is generally flatter.

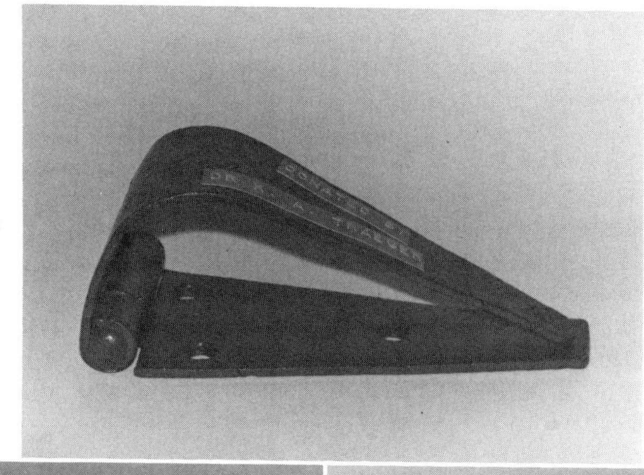

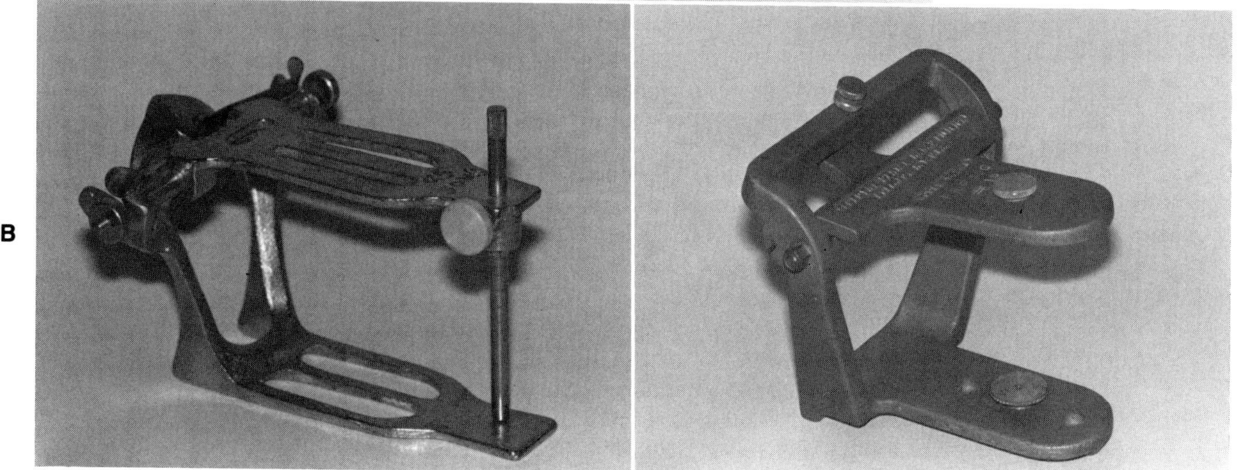

Fig. 14-36. A, True hinge that functions only in opening and closing movement. **B,** Hinge articulator with fixed condylar guidance and incisal guide pin. **C,** Hanau LTD articulator with fixed condylar guidance but without incisal guide pin. (**A** courtesy Dr. Kimball Traeger, University of Texas Health Science Center at San Antonio.)

simulate lateral and protrusive jaw movement. The condylar path is set at a fixed angle and cannot be adjusted, so the instrument is still considered to be nonadjustable. Some of these instruments also may have incisal guide pins that ride on an inclined plate. The inclination is normally fixed, and the instruments are still considered nonadjustable. The incisal guide pin or other devices designed to hold the articulator open at a definite position are an advantage in that the teeth on the mounted casts are protected against accidental closure.

Articulators representative of this group are the series of Stephens instruments and the Hanau 147-3. There are many other instruments available, but basically all perform the same functions.

The simple hinge or nonadjustable articulator is always indicated when a functionally generated pathway is used to arrange the occlusal pattern. All jaw movements have been incorporated within the pathway, and no movement of the articulator is needed or desired. An instrument used in this technique must be capable of maintaining a fixed vertical opening because slight changes in the vertical separation of the casts may be necessary as the occlusal scheme is refined.

The nonadjustable articulator may also be used for many Class III partially edentulous cases where only a few posterior teeth are being replaced and where canine or mutually protected occlusion by the anterior teeth exists. If the cusp height and cuspal angulation of the artificial teeth can be made to simulate that of the remaining natural teeth, interferences in the occlusion can be minimized. It should not be inferred that the use of a more sophisticated or adjustable articulator could not produce a more harmonious occlusal scheme—it probably would—but the time required to set the adjustments of the instrument will often be greater than the time spent refining the occlusion in the patient's mouth.

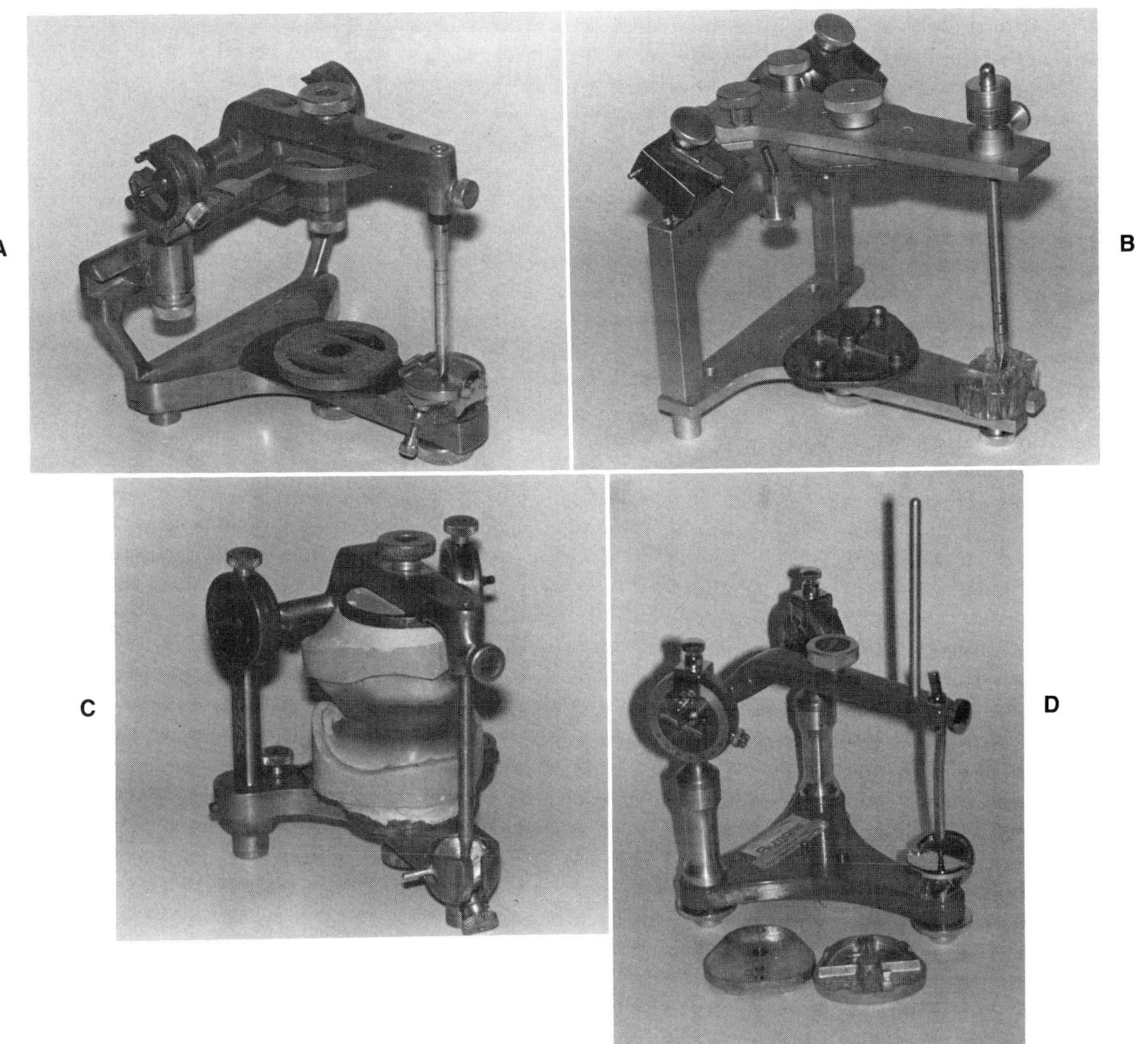

Fig. 14-37. A, Semiadjustable Hanau, University series, an arcon instrument. **B,** Whip-Mix articulator, an arcon instrument with three-position intercondylar width adjustment. **C,** Hanau H_2 articulator, a nonarcon, nonintercondylar width adjustment articulator. **D,** Dentatus articulator, a nonarcon semiadjustable instrument.

The greatest requirement for the simple hinge articulator is that it be rigid. Flexing of the upper and lower members or lateral movement of the joint between the two members can lead to errors in the occlusion. The instrument must be capable of being locked positively in the centric relation or centric occlusal position.

Semiadjustable articulators. The semiadjustable articulators (Fig. 14-37) make up the largest group in this basic system of classifying articulators according to the degree to which they may be adjusted. All these instruments have adjustable horizontal condylar paths, adjustable lateral condylar paths, and adjustable incisal guide tables. The degree and ease of these adjustments vary, but the purpose of the adjustments is to follow the mandibular movements of the individual patient closely.

Certain instruments in this class also have adjustable intercondylar distances. The condylar supports on these instruments may be moved either medially or laterally to equal the measured distance between the heads of the condyle of a particular patient. This adjustment controls the length of the radius of the arc that the mandible makes in lateral movements, permitting more accurate placement of working and nonworking cusps to eliminate cuspal interferences in lateral jaw movements.

It should not be inferred that the semiadjustable instruments are capable of following mandibular movements in their entirety. These articulators offer a close approximation of actual mandibular position, not a truly accurate one. These instruments are set principally from positional jaw relation records. The Hanau series of articulators are set or adjusted through the use of a protrusive jaw relation record. The protrusive relationship determines the angle of the horizontal condylar path. The actual setting of the angle is done through trial and error by observing the fit of the cusps of the maxillary teeth into the protrusive record. The angle selected is the one that appears to have maximal cuspal contact. The lateral condylar setting is calculated from a mathematical formula derived by Hanau: $L = \frac{H}{8} + 12$ where L is the lateral condylar inclination in degrees and H is the horizontal condylar inclination in degrees as established by the protrusive jaw relation record. Hanau's logic in using this formula of averages for all patients was that the formula compensates for a wide range of lateral condylar angles and prevents interferences in lateral movements. He also suggests that final occlusal correction in the mouth or the use of static lateral jaw relation records to mount the opposing casts in lateral positions will eliminate all possible interferences. These assumptions may be more hopeful than actual.

Other semiadjustable articulators, notably the Whip-Mix, are set through the use of lateral jaw relation records. The patient's mandible must be guided into a true lateral position and maintained in that position until the recording medium sets. This is a difficult procedure for many patients, and a series of trials or a period of rehearsing the procedure is frequently required. To set the instrument, the lateral record is positioned between the teeth of the casts as the articulator is moved to that lateral position. The condylar adjustments, both lateral and horizontal, are moved until the teeth fit the record accurately. It should be remembered that when lateral and protrusive records are used to adjust an instrument of this class, the settings will be accurate for only those positions at which the records were made. What happens between the position of centric relation and the position of the record remains unknown. The position will be accurate, but the pathways between these positions will not be. The Whip-Mix instruments also has limited (three-position) adjustment of the intercondylar width (Fig. 14-38). This increases the range of motion the articulator can simulate. The Hanau H series is not capable of accepting lateral jaw relation records.

Some semiadjustable articulators (for example, the Hanau H series, the Dentatus, and the Gysi) have the condyles attached to the upper member of the instrument, whereas others have the condyle attached to the lower member as occurs in nature. The latter instruments are referred to as *arcon* articulators. (The term *arcon* was derived by Bergström from the words *ar*ticulator and *con*dyle.) The main advantage of an arcon articulator is that after the maxillary cast is mounted on the instrument with an axis orbital face-bow mounting, the relationship of the maxillary cast to the axis orbital plane remains constant when the opposing casts are separated. As soon as opposing casts on nonarcon instruments are separated, the relationship of the casts to the axis-orbital plane is lost and true interpretation of the relation of the plane of occlusion to the horizontal plane is not possible. Articulators representative of the

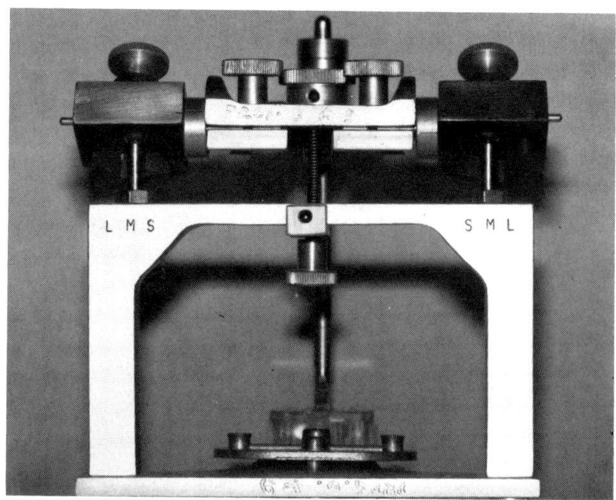

Fig. 14-38. Whip-Mix articulator with three-position intercondylar adjustment—small, medium, and large. Width is determined by face-bow measurement.

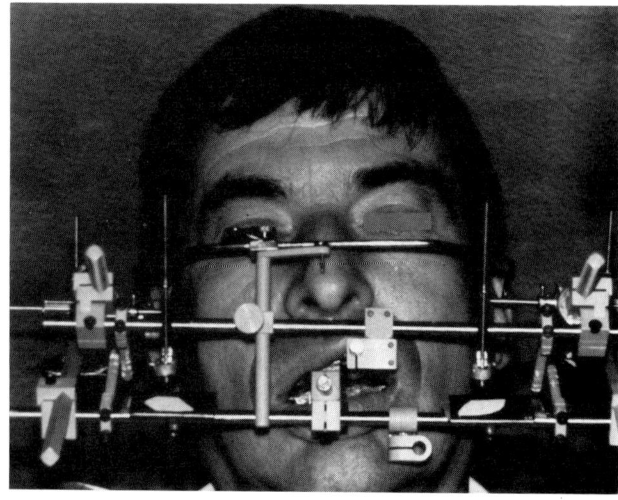

Fig. 14-39. Pantograph tracing device. Mandibular pathway is recorded in all three planes of motion: frontal, sagittal, and horizontal.

arcon semiadjustable class are the Hanau University series and the Whip-Mix instrument.

Fully adjustable articulators. Fully adjustable articulators are capable of being adjusted to follow the mandibular movement through all excursions. In contrast to the semiadjustable instruments that are capable of being adjusted to follow points along the mandibular pathway, fully adjustable articulators can follow the entire length of the mandibular pathway. To set or adjust the instrument, it is necessary to have a tracing of the mandibular pathway in all three planes of motion (Figs. 14-39 and 14-40). The tracings are accomplished by a pantographic tracing device. The actual hinge axis points on the patient's face must be located with a kinematic face-bow. Excellent sources are available that describe the technique of recording the mandibular

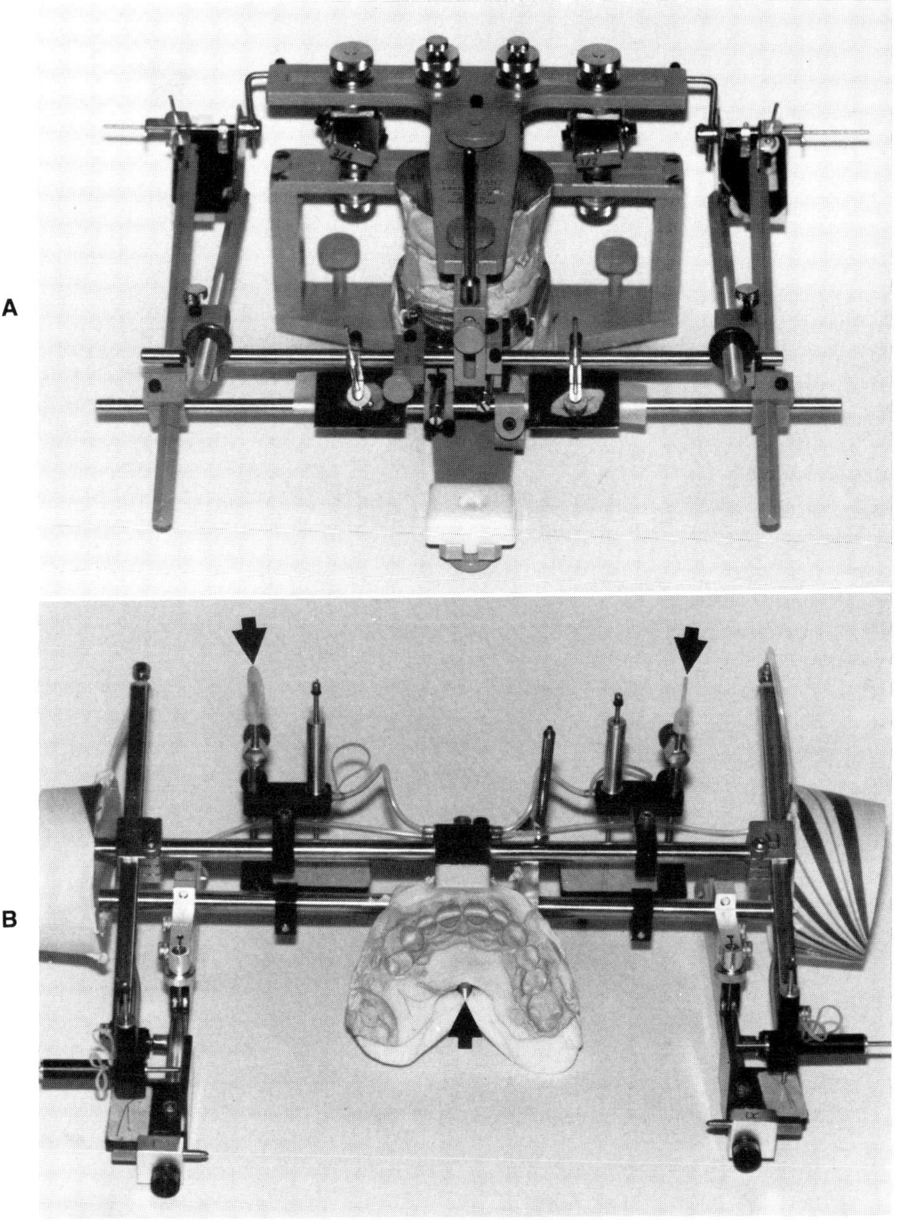

Fig. 14-40. Transfer of Stuart pantograph to Stuart articulator. **A,** Metal maxillary and mandibular clutches that support recording assemblies are luted to instrument with minimal expansion stone. **B,** Denar pantograph with acrylic resin clutches lined with zinc oxide–eugenol impression paste. Centric relationship of recording assemblies is determined by left and right centric pins and central bearing screw (arrows). Note partial cups of slurry activated stone to help maintain relationship of anterior cross bars. *Continued.*

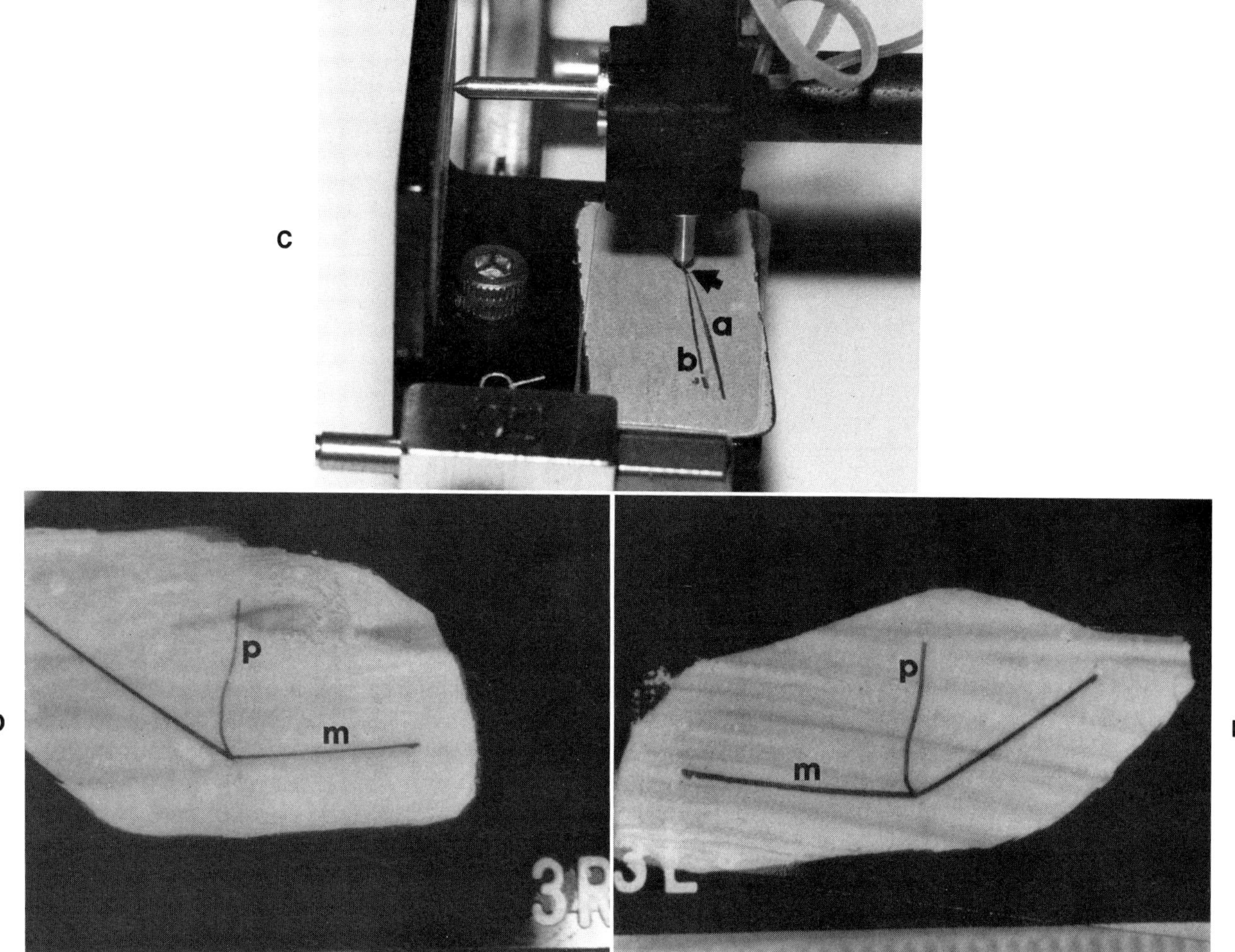

Fig. 14-40, cont'd. C, Close-up view of right posterior horizontal recording table with styli manually depressed to confirm centric relationship (arrow). Outer line, *a,* indicates timing of any immediate side shift and progressive side shift as patient makes left lateral excursion. Inner line, *b,* indicates protrusive path of mandible on horizontal plane. **D** and **E,** Anterior gothic arch tracings left and right. Tracking of anterior styli over medial tracing lines, *m,* will serve to adjust vertical axes on respective sides. Middle tracing line, *p,* indicates protrusive movement on horizontal plane.

pathways and of setting the articulator to follow the pathways, so this book does not go into detail concerning these procedures. If an articulator can be set to follow a curving tortuous motion that the mandible may take, the condylar paths must be individually carved to accommodate the moving condyles (Fig. 14-41).

In considering the use of a fully adjustable articulator, particularly in the field of removable partial dentures, the time required to accomplish the diagnostic procedures, locating the kinematic hinge axis, developing the pantographic tracing, and setting the articulator to accept the tracings must be weighed against the advantages that may be gained by the more sophisticated instrument. As a general rule, unless the entire occlusal scheme is to be rebuilt as a single unit, the more complex approach is generally not indicated. The inherent stability of most removable partial dentures makes the refining of the occlusion intraorally a practical possibility, thus erasing the necessity of involved instrumentation.

Articulators of the fully adjustable type include the Stuart instrument, the Gnatholator, and the Dena D5A (Fig. 14-42). H.O. Beck and coworkers have developed an experimental articulator that takes the factor of time into account by correlating the time of movement in each of the three planes of the skull.

Selection of articulator. A guide that should be followed for selecting the proper articulator is that the simplest instrument to accomplish the desired purposes should be used. As the complexity of the articulator in-

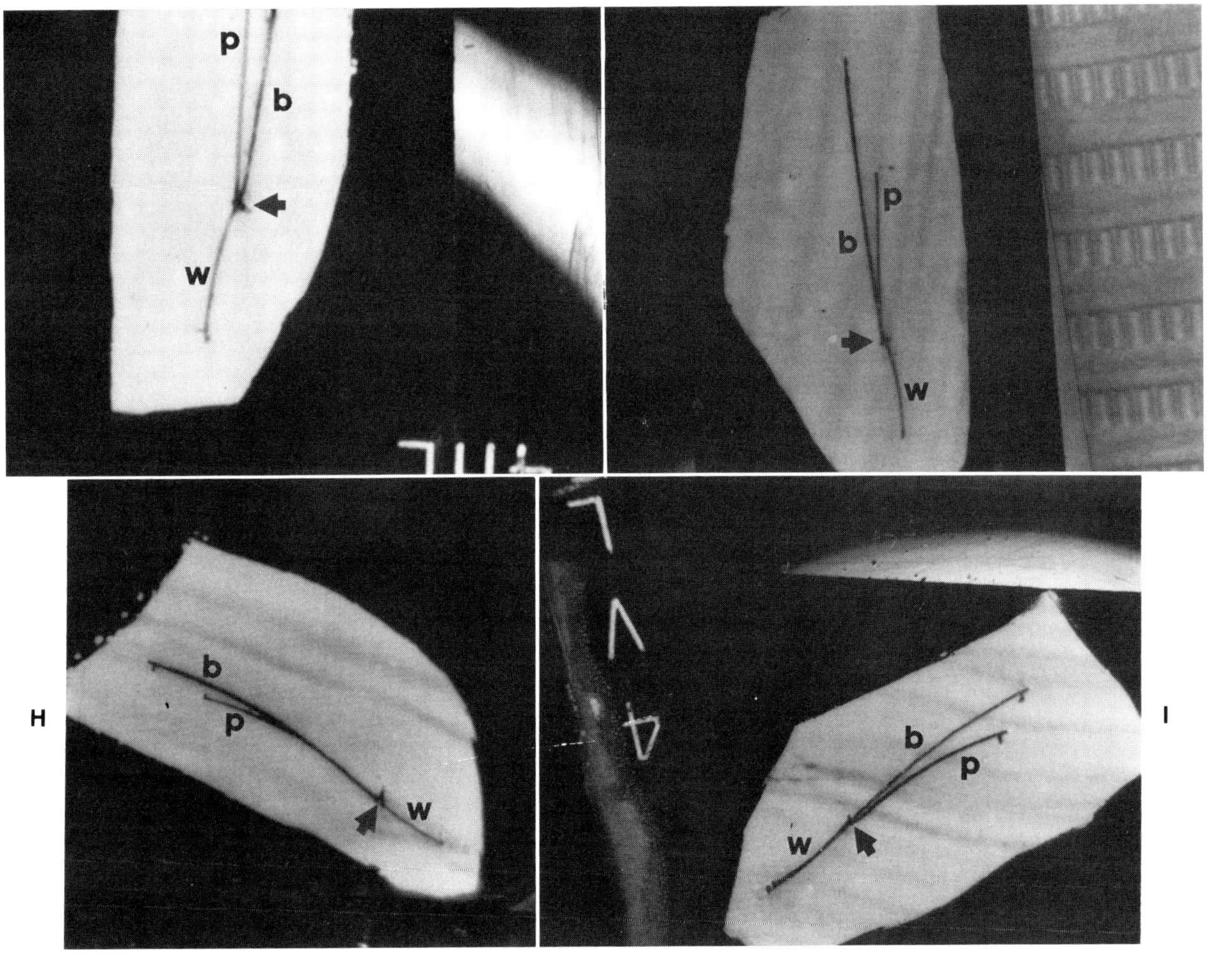

Fig. 14-40, cont'd. F and **G,** Posterior horizontal record table tracings of condylar paths of movement according to patient's temporomandibular joint characteristics. Projected paths are protrusive, *p,* balancing, *b,* and working, *w,* and junction of all three paths is centric relation (arrow). **H** and **I,** Posterior vertical record table tracings. Superior line is balancing, *b,* path; inferior line is protrusive, *p,* path. Line anterior to centric relation (arrow) is working, *w,* path of condyle.

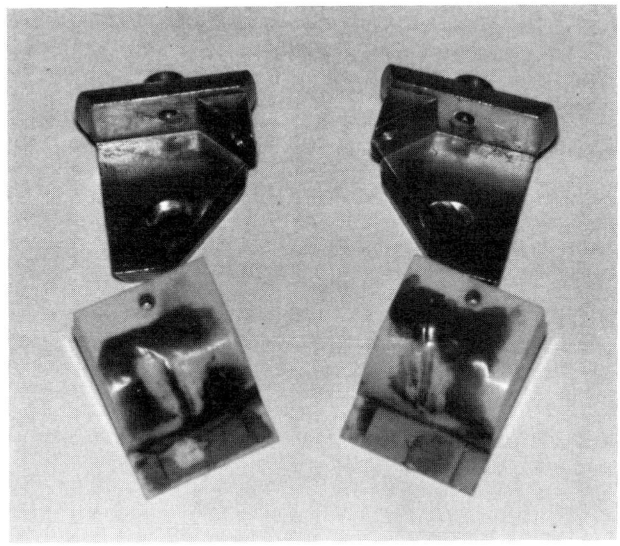

Fig. 14-41. Condylar paths, lower plastic inserts, are individually carved so that condyles will follow tracings in all three planes obtained with pantographic device. (Courtesy Col. Tom Huff, Wilford Hall, USAF Medical Center at San Antonio.)

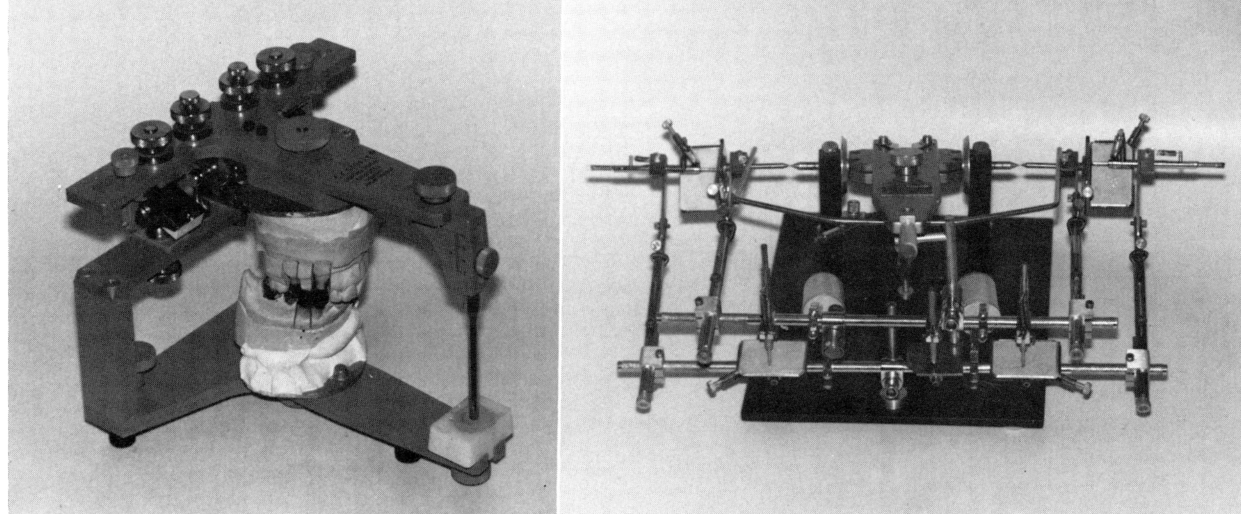

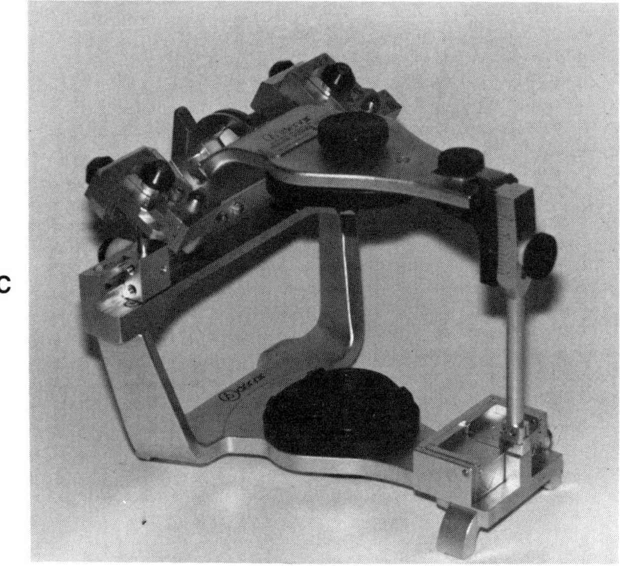

Fig. 14-42. A, Fully adjustable Stuart instrument. **B,** Gnatholator, developed by Dr. E. Granger and others, with pantograph in position. **C** Fully adjustable Denar D5A. (Courtesy Col. Tom Huff, Wilford Hall, USAF Medical Center at San Antonio.)

creases, so also do the chances of creating errors. An articulator per se is not capable of treating a patient, only of assisting the operator. A complex instrument in the hands of a partially trained individual can lead to disaster. A simple hinge or a nonadjustable articulator is frequently indicated for Class III partially edentulous patients. For most Class I and II partial dentures and for a complete denture opposing a partial denture, a semiadjustable instrument is most often indicated. The fully adjustable articulator is usually limited to those patients needing a removable partial denture and where the entire occlusal scheme is to be developed at one time by the wax additive technique (Fig. 14-43).

Selection and arrangement of artificial teeth

The various types of artificial teeth are discussed in Chapter 3.

Anterior denture teeth. As a general rule the most difficult part of selecting and arranging artificial anterior teeth is the diminished space mesiodistally. Unless anterior teeth are replaced immediately following their loss, the natural teeth adjacent to the space will either drift toward or tilt into the space. The drifting or tilting causes a loss of the original space occupied by the natural teeth and forces the selection of an artificial tooth or teeth that are narrower than the natural tooth or teeth. This will inevitably produce an artificial appear-

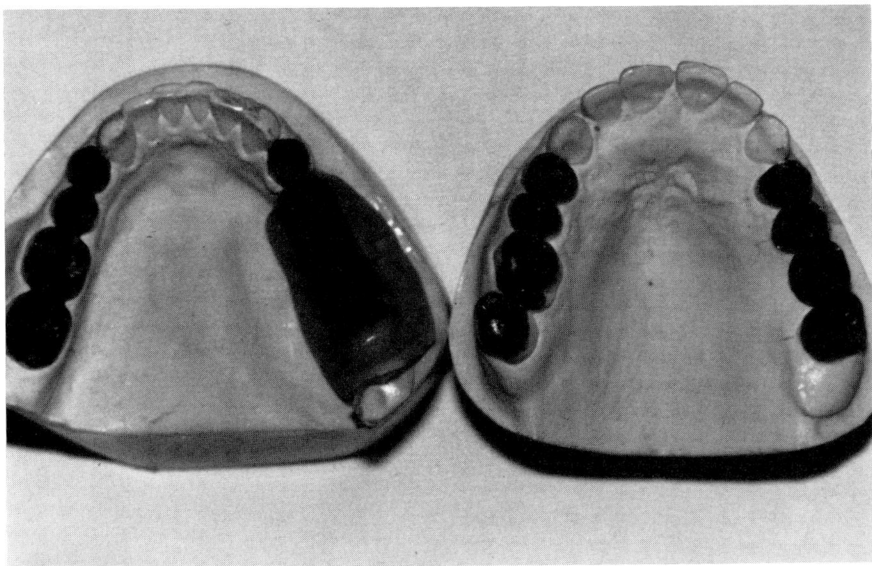

Fig. 14-43. Fully adjustable instrument is indicated where removable partial denture is being constructed as part of restoration of entire occlusal scheme. Wax additive technique is used to develop occlusal anatomy of teeth.

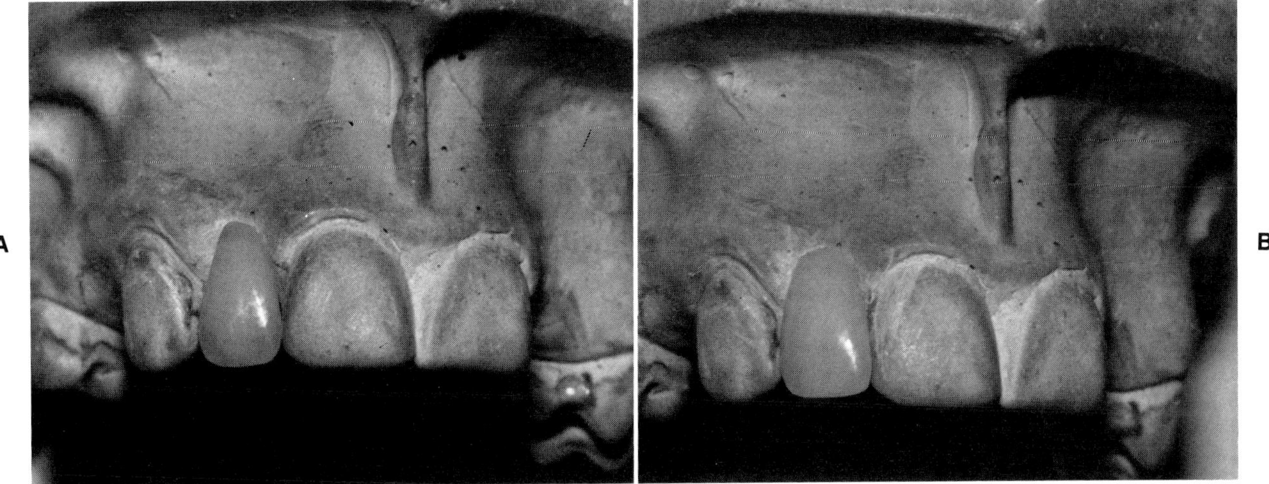

Fig. 14-44. A, Loss of mesiodistal space because of tooth drifting may cause replacement tooth to be smaller than natural tooth. This can appear artificial in mouth. **B,** Reshaping proximal surfaces of teeth adjacent to space can permit replacement tooth of normal size.

ance in the patient's mouth (Fig. 14-44). During the mouth preparation appointment an attempt should have been made to regain the original width of the space by reshaping the proximal surfaces of the adjacent teeth. If the entire width cannot be recovered, consideration should be given to overlapping the artificial teeth so that a normal-sized tooth may be used to harmonize with the patient's face and remaining teeth.

A try-in appointment should always be scheduled to obtain approval by the patient of the esthetic arrangement of anterior replacement teeth. (The try-in for anterior tube teeth, facings or RAP should have been accomplished before the framework construction; see Chapter 10.)

Denture teeth (Fig. 14-45), properly arranged, are by far the most esthetic anterior replacement. The use of the denture tooth, supported by a denture base, allows the dentist a wider choice of tooth *position,* probably the most critical factor in esthetics, than any other tooth replacement method.

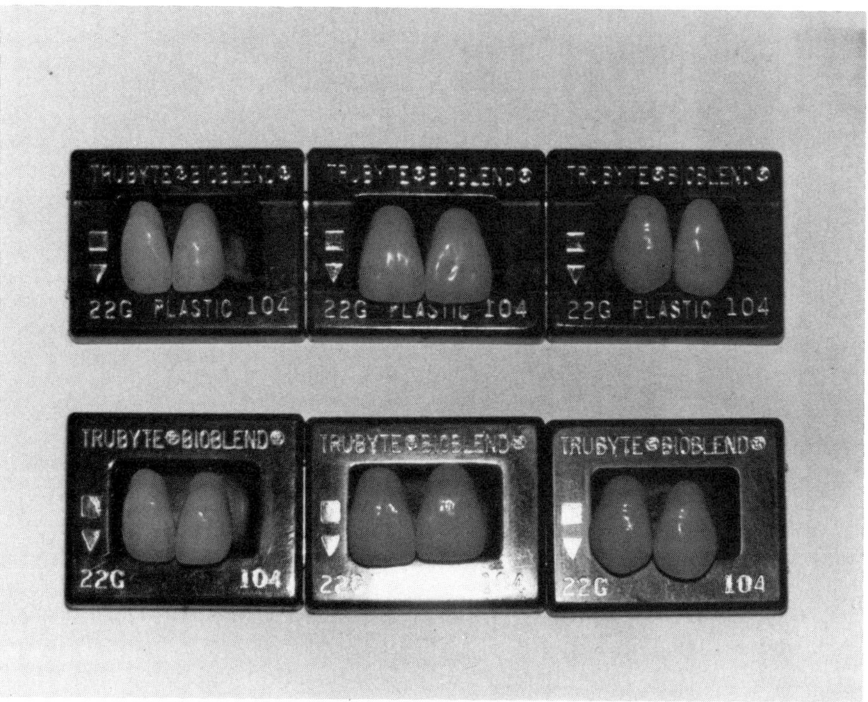

Fig. 14-45. Plastic (top) and porcelain (bottom) anterior teeth are available in identical molds and shades.

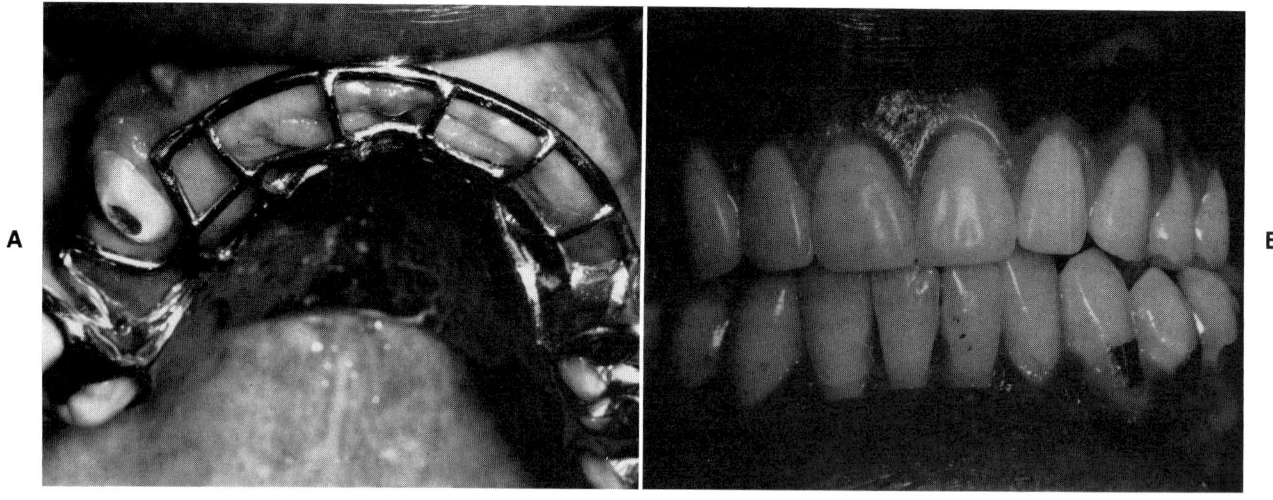

Fig. 14-46. A, Where bone loss of edentulous ridge has occurred, acrylic resin flange is used to restore lost contour. **B,** Flange allows teeth to be positioned where natural teeth had been.

The denture tooth is available in almost any shade, size, or contour that may be needed. It also may be individualized by characterizing and staining.

One of its biggest advantages is the fact that where there has been excessive loss of the residual ridge in the anterior region, the acrylic resin flange may be built to any thickness desired to support the teeth in their natural position and to restore symmetry and contour to the lips (Fig. 14-46). If, on the other hand, the ridge is full and large, the denture teeth may be butted directly to the ridge to achieve the desired effect without unnecessarily plumping the lips (Fig. 14-47).

Because of their greater ease of placement, acceptable esthetic appearance, and decreased danger of fracture, acrylic resin denture teeth are more commonly used in removable partial denture service than are porcelin teeth.

The instance in which the denture tooth is seldom

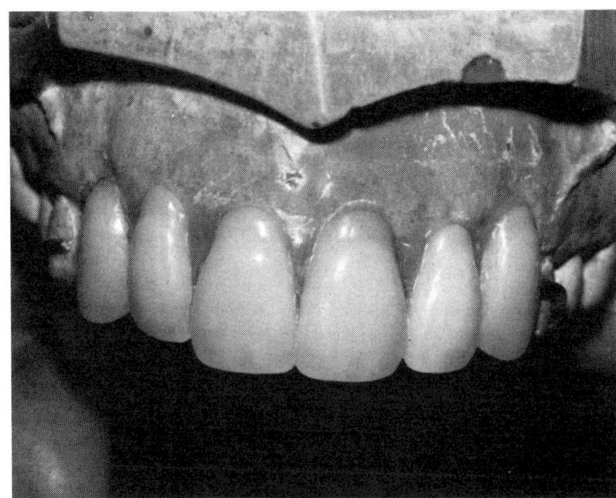

Fig. 14-47. On ridges where minimal bone loss has occurred, necks of denture teeth are butted directly against edentulous ridge.

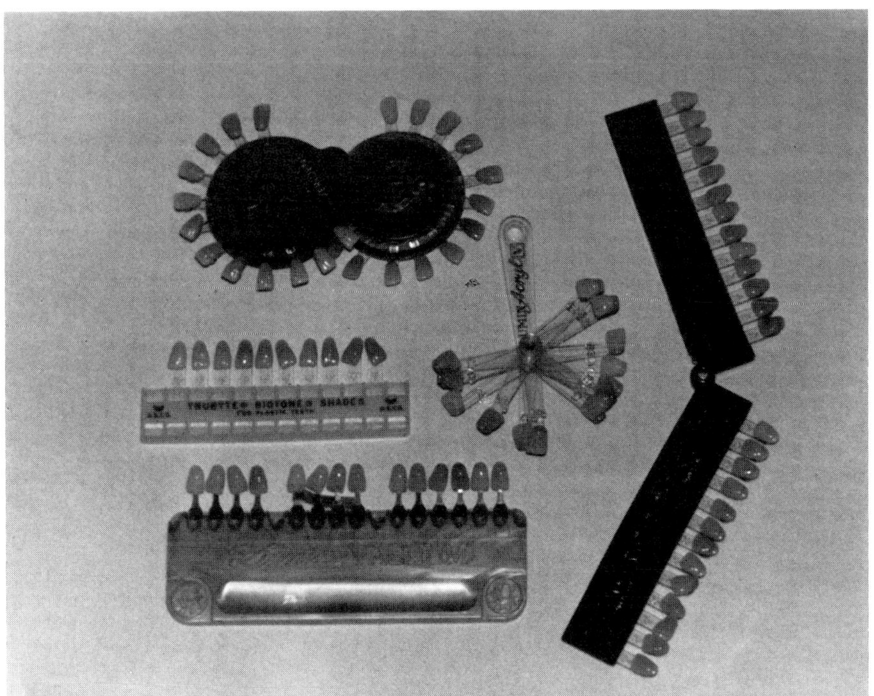

Fig. 14-48. Shade guides may differ widely. Shade guide should be same as manufacturer of teeth to be used.

indicated is for a single tooth replacement. The incising action of occlusion usually produces an excessive shearing type of stress that results in frequent breakage.

Mold and shade selection. The shade guide used should be one from the same manufacturer whose teeth will be used (Fig. 14-48). The shade guide tooth should be moistened, and the selection made in natural light if possible. If some natural anterior teeth are present, an attempt to match them as closely as possible should be made. It is not uncommon to have the remaining teeth vary in shade. If this occurs, a selection should be made that best blends with the teeth adjacent to the edentulous space.

The shade should be taken as quickly as possible. The first impression will generally be the most accurate because the ability to discriminate between shades is lost rapidly as the eye fatigues.

If single teeth are being replaced or if the losses are on one side of the midline, the remaining natural tooth on the opposite side should be used as a guide to select

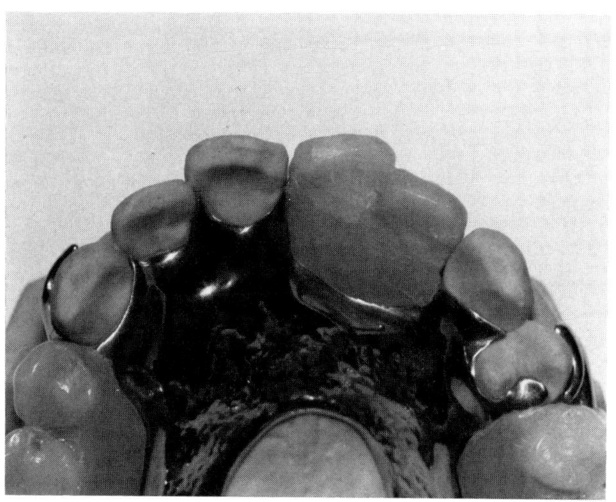

Fig. 14-49. Teeth to be replaced on one side of midline should match natural teeth on opposite side.

the proper mold (Fig. 14-49). A mold as close to the natural tooth may be chosen and then modified to match by selective grinding.

If all anterior teeth are being replaced, guides similar to those used to select teeth for complete denture patients should be followed. Teeth selected should harmonize with the patient's features. The House technique may be used to determine the proper size of the maxillary central incisors. This technique coordinates the size of the central incisor with the size of the patient's face (Fig. 14-50). It should be remembered that the calculation is based on average figures; it cannot be depended on to satisfy all patients but can be used as a starting point in tooth selection.

Preparing cast and setting anterior teeth. If acrylic resin denture bases were constructed on the framework to record the jaw relation at the previous appointment, these bases must be removed *before* the teeth are set.

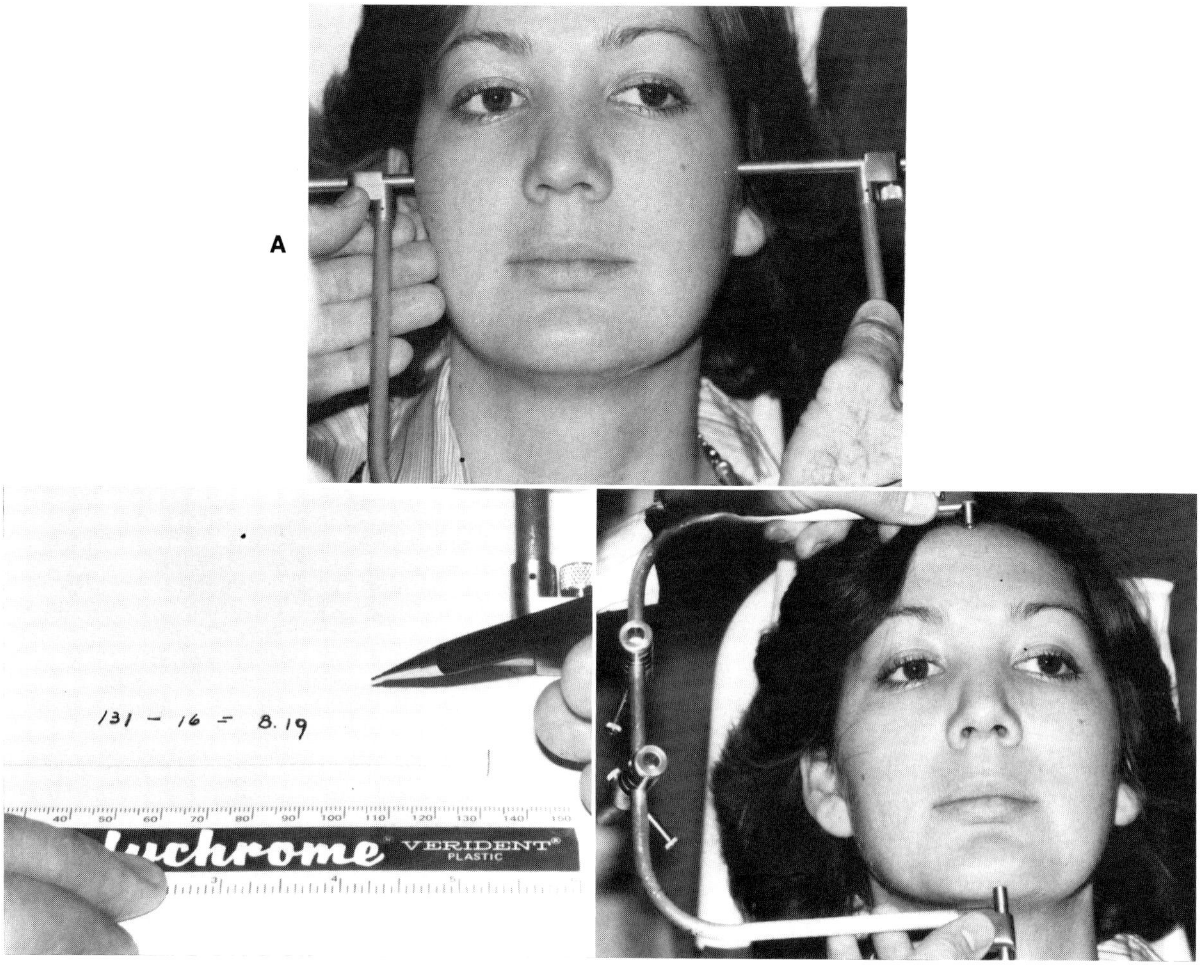

A

B

C

Fig. 14-50. Mathematic determination of maxillary central incisor size by House technique. **A,** Bizygomatic distance measured with face-bow. **B,** Bizygomatic width is divided by 16 to determine width of central incisor. **C,** Length of maxillary central incisor is determined by dividing hairline-to-chin distance by 16.

It is extremely difficult to remove these acrylic resin bases once the dentures are flasked. Baseplate wax is strong enough to support the teeth during the try-in appointment.

If teeth are missing across the midline, it is essential that the central incisors be set first to reestablish the midline at the center of the face. One of the most distracting errors in denture set-up occurs when the midline is either displaced to one side or deviates from the vertical. The proper midline should be established at either the jaw relation appointment or at the framework try-in appointment. An anterior wax occlusion rim can be adapted to the acrylic resin retention struts and shaped for proper fullness and length to support the lip naturally. The position of the nose and the philtrum of the nose will help establish the vertical mark of the midline on the wax occlusion rim. The established midline should be viewed from several angles with the patient standing and the lip raised in a smiling position (Fig. 14-51).

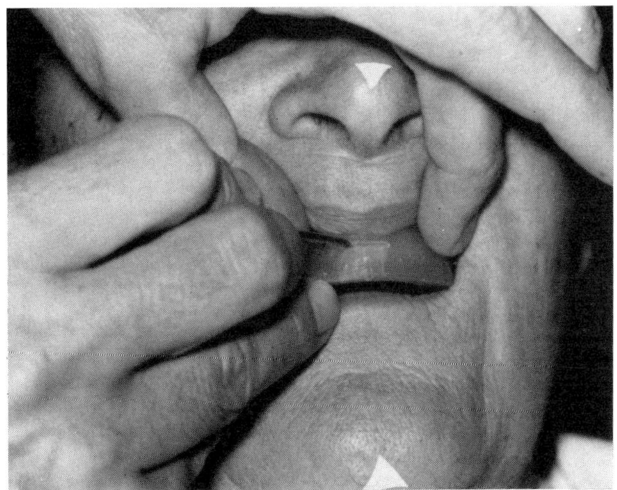

Fig. 14-51. If teeth are missing across midline, occlusion rim should be used to indicate midline and smiling or high lip line.

It will almost always be necessary to reshape the ridge-lap portion of an artificial tooth to position it over the acrylic resin retentive minor connector (Fig. 14-52). Care should be taken not to shorten the clinical crown of the denture tooth; the collar or neck should be maintained. An anterior denture tooth should be positioned as nearly as possible where the original natural tooth was located. (The biggest advantage of denture teeth on a denture base is that the tooth may be positioned ideally without concern for the location of the residual ridge. This is not true for the tube tooth or RAP. These replacements must be butted against the edentulous ridge, and if ridge resorption has taken place, an unnatural appearance will result.)

As an anterior denture tooth is positioned against a natural tooth, the proximal surface of the artificial tooth may be recontoured for better and closer adaptation to the natural tooth (Fig. 14-53). The natural morphology of the crown of the tooth should not be lost, however. The incisal angles should be maintained in a normal rounded form.

The teeth should be set before the try-in appointment to conserve as much chair time as possible. Final positioning and contouring of the teeth are done with the patient present.

The denture base flanges should be contoured and smoothed to give a natural pleasing appearance. Excess wax should be removed from the cast and framework

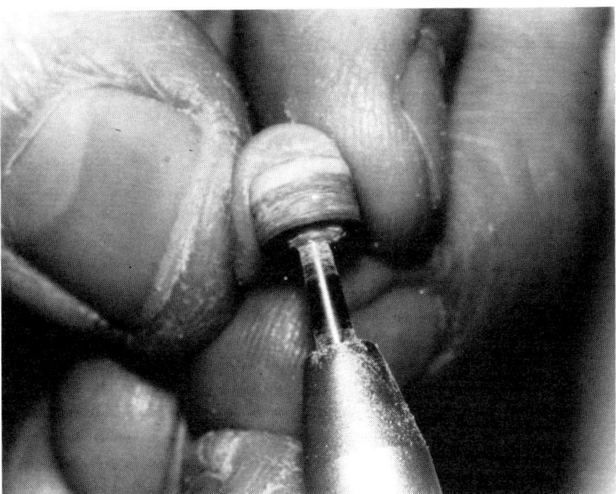

Fig. 14-52. Ridge lap portion of acrylic resin denture tooth can be shaped in order to position it over components of partial denture.

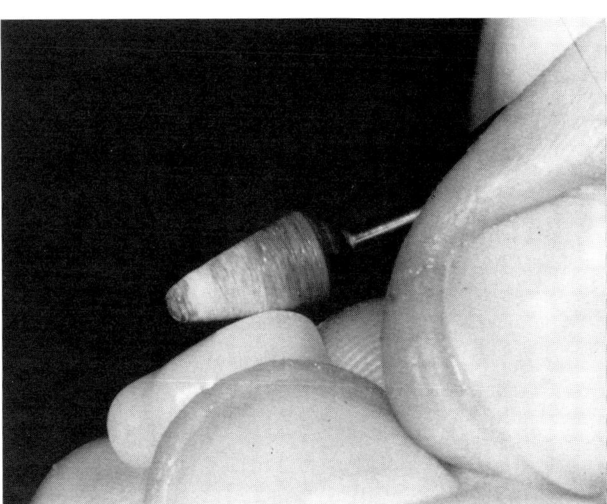

Fig. 14-53. Proximal surfaces of denture teeth are reshaped to gain better adaptation to natural teeth.

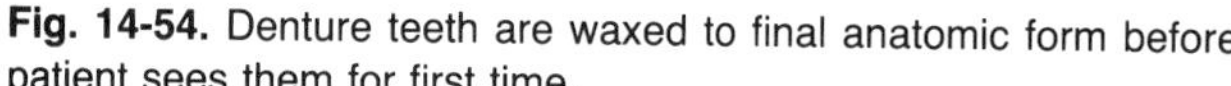

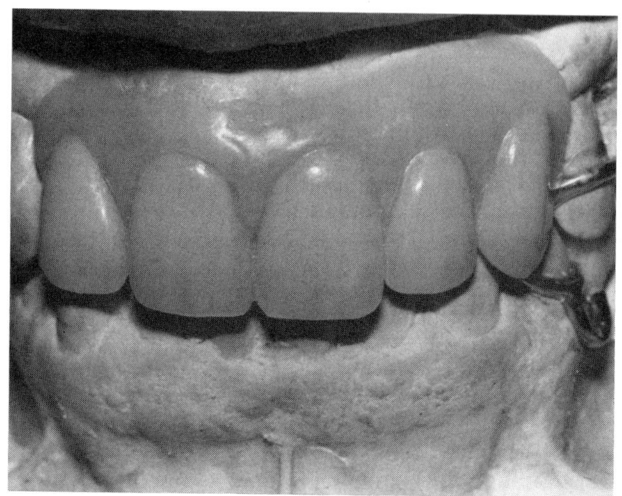

Fig. 14-54. Denture teeth are waxed to final anatomic form before patient sees them for first time.

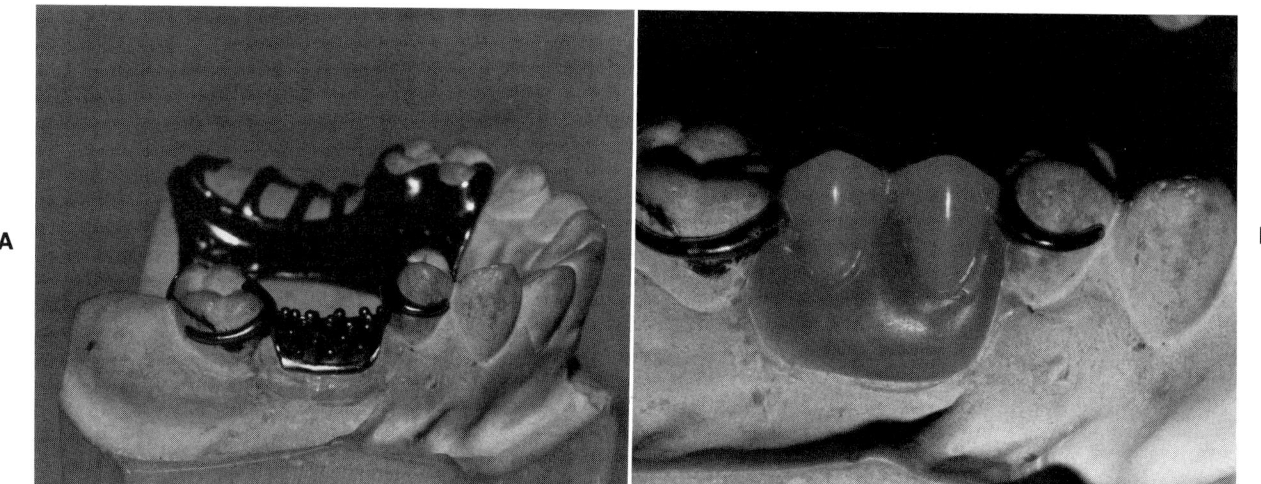

Fig. 14-55. A, Missing teeth on tooth-supported side are second premolar and first molar. **B,** Because of mesial drifting of second molar, space is available for only two premolars.

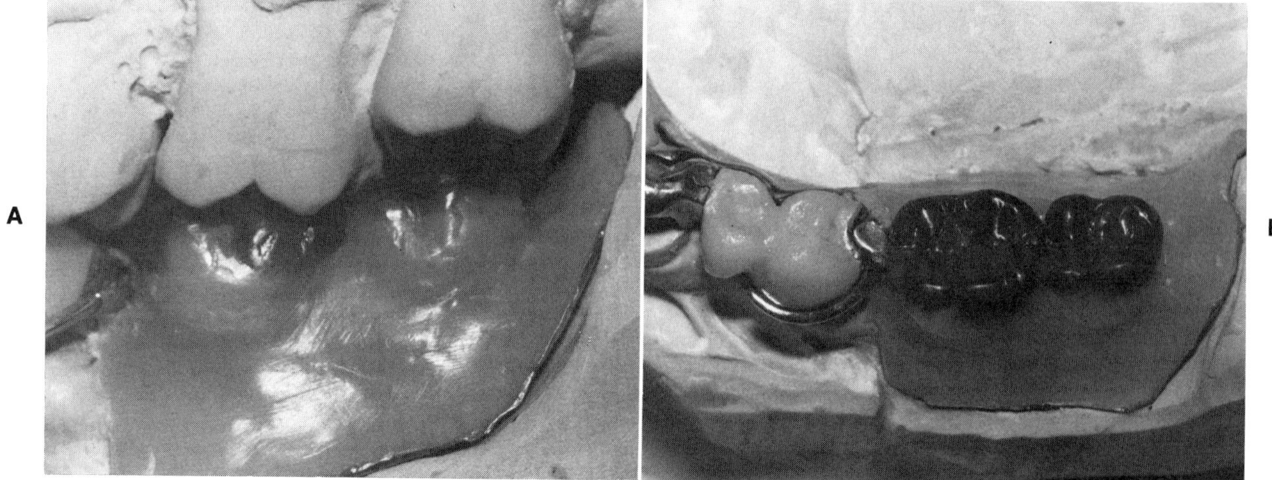

Fig. 14-56. A, Denture teeth are being developed in wax, opposing natural teeth. **B,** Occlusal surface is carved in inlay wax.

before the patient's arrival. This will be the first time the patient sees the prosthesis in its final form, and the first impression should be a pleasant one (Fig. 14-54).

Posterior denture teeth. Posterior replacement teeth must not only fit into the available edentulous spaces, but also be harmonious in composition, size, and *occlusal anatomy* with the teeth they are to oppose, whether artificial or natural.

The dentist should not be overly concerned with replacing the exact number and type of teeth that are missing. For example, the edentulous space may have been occupied by the second premolar and first molar, but, because of drifting of the remaining teeth, the most suitable replacement teeth may well be two premolars (Fig. 14-55).

For the same reasons that acrylic resin denture teeth are usually selected for anterior tooth replacement, the resin tooth is commonly indicated for posterior replacements. The shape and occlusal anatomy can be altered easily without dangerously weakening the tooth. The resin tooth may also oppose enamel or gold occlusal surfaces without abrading them.

Porcelain teeth are indicated only in the partial denture opposing a complete denture with porcelain teeth.

Construction of gold occlusal surfaces on denture teeth. The material of choice for occlusal surfaces of artificial teeth that will function against enamel surfaces or against gold surfaces such as inlays, onlays, or crowns is cast gold. The technique of producing gold occlusal surfaces for dentures is not difficult and will prevent unnecessary wear on opposing occlusal surfaces.

The construction of gold occlusal surfaces is especially indicated when the removable partial denture is to oppose a reconstructed dental arch of gold occlusal surfaces, when a functionally generated path concept is being used and considerable modifications of the denture teeth are necessary to produce occlusal harmony, and when special wax additive techniques are used on a fully adjustable articulator to produce a functional occlusion.

Gold occlusal surfaces on denture teeth have as an advantage, in addition to the physical properties of the metal: the ability to adapt to unusual occlusal problems. Disadvantages include the increased cost and, in some instances, a compromise of the esthetic result.

The occlusal surfaces to be duplicated in gold may be reproductions of the occlusal surfaces of denture teeth—always acrylic resin—that have been set on the partial denture, and the occlusion has been refined. The occlusal surfaces may also be developed in wax opposing a stone core as in the functionally generated path technique.

The technique described (advocated by Koehne and Morrow and adapted from Wallace) is that of developing wax occlusal surfaces opposing a stone pathway of opposing natural (Fig. 14-56) or artificial teeth. The method remains basically the same. The main difference is that after the occlusal surfaces of the denture teeth have been duplicated, the occlusal surfaces of the teeth have to be reduced so that the cast occlusal surfaces can be attached to the remainder of the tooth crowns.

TECHNIQUE

1. Acrylic resin denture teeth are set for the partial denture in correct buccolingual alignment against the functionally generated path or the opposing occlusion. The occlusion established should be corrected to the proper vertical dimension. The completed setup should be tried in the patient's mouth to verify correct centric relation and vertical dimension of occlusion before the gold occlusal surfaces are constructed. The partial denture is returned to the articulator, and the occlusal surfaces of the denture teeth are ground off (Fig. 14-57). Sufficient resin must be removed to provide adequate thickness for wax and subsequently for gold.
2. A lubricating medium is applied to the stone path, opposing denture teeth, or an opposing cast (Fig. 14-58).
3. Inlay wax is added to the ground denture teeth, and while it is still soft the articulator is closed to record the cusp heights and sulci depths of the opposing occlusion (Fig. 14-59). Several closures are usually necessary to reestablish the recorded vertical dimension of occlusion. The wax surface must be warmed between closures to displace the hard inlay wax. Where evidence of lack of contact between the wax and opposing occlusion is noted, additional wax can be pooled to provide contact.
4. The wax is contoured to establish the outline form of the crowns of the individual teeth. The more detailed occlusal anatomy in the form of supplemental grooves and secondary details is carved in the wax (Fig. 14-60).
5. A final check on occlusal contacts should be made to ensure maximum occlusal efficiency.
6. A mix of investment material compatible with the alloy to be cast is made and painted on the occlusal surfaces with care taken not to trap air and to ensure an accurate reproduction of the carved occlusal anatomy. A layer of investment material thick enough to provide adequate strength when handled is added to the painted-on investment (Fig. 14-61).
7. After the investment has set, it should be carefully removed and trimmed to reduce the occlu-

sogingival depth of the formed mold (Fig. 14-62). This is done to provide the desired thickness of the gold castings.

8. Inlay wax is flowed into the mold. A 12-gauge length of half-round wax shape is sealed to the exposed surface of the wax in the mold for added strength. The gold occlusal castings will eventually be processed to newly formed acrylic resin denture teeth. To ensure positive attachment to these denture teeth, the remaining inferior surface, of what is now a wax pattern of the occlusal surfaces, is painted with nail polish, and beads of acrylic resin polymer are added (Fig. 14-63).
9. The pattern is sprued and, still in the investment mold, invested, burned out, and cast following the technique suitable to the alloy being used (Fig. 14-64).
10. The castings are cleaned, and the sprues and nodules removed. The castings are checked for accuracy by positioning them against the opposing occlusal surfaces that were used during the carving procedures (Fig. 14-65). The articulator bearing the partial denture and the ground denture teeth is closed. It may be necessary to reduce the height of the denture teeth further to accommodate the retentive beads and reinforcing 12-gauge half-round bar that were added to the inferior border of the castings.
11. The gold occlusal surfaces should be polished, and an opaque resin applied to the inferior surfaces. The castings are once again placed on the opposing cast and sealed in position with sticky wax.
12. The articulator is closed, and ivory casting wax is flowed between the gold occlusal surfaces and resin denture teeth. The sticky wax is removed, and the articulator opened. Deficient areas are corrected by adding ivory wax, and proper anatomy of the crowns is restored by contouring the wax, (Fig. 14-66).
13. The baseplate wax of the denture base is removed from around the necks of the denture teeth, and the teeth with the gold occlusal surfaces attached are removed in a block.
14. The blocks of teeth are flasked with the buccal surfaces facing upward and the occlusal surfaces slightly depressed to help pack the mold later (Fig. 14-67).
15. The wax is boiled out, and all the remains of the plastic teeth are removed. A tinfoil substitute is painted on the stone mold (Fig. 14-68).
16. A mix of heat-cured resin of the correct shade is made and packed in the mold. Trial packing may be accomplished to eliminate excess resin and to ensure that the denture teeth will be as dense as possible. Characterization of the teeth may be accomplished at this time.
17. The teeth are processed with the recommended curing cycle, deflasked, and polished.
18. The blocks of teeth with the gold occlusal surfaces are once again positioned on the opposing occlusal surfaces, the articulator is closed, and the teeth are waxed to the denture base (Fig. 14-69). A try-in of the partial denture should be accomplished before the prosthesis is completed.

Text continued on p. 440.

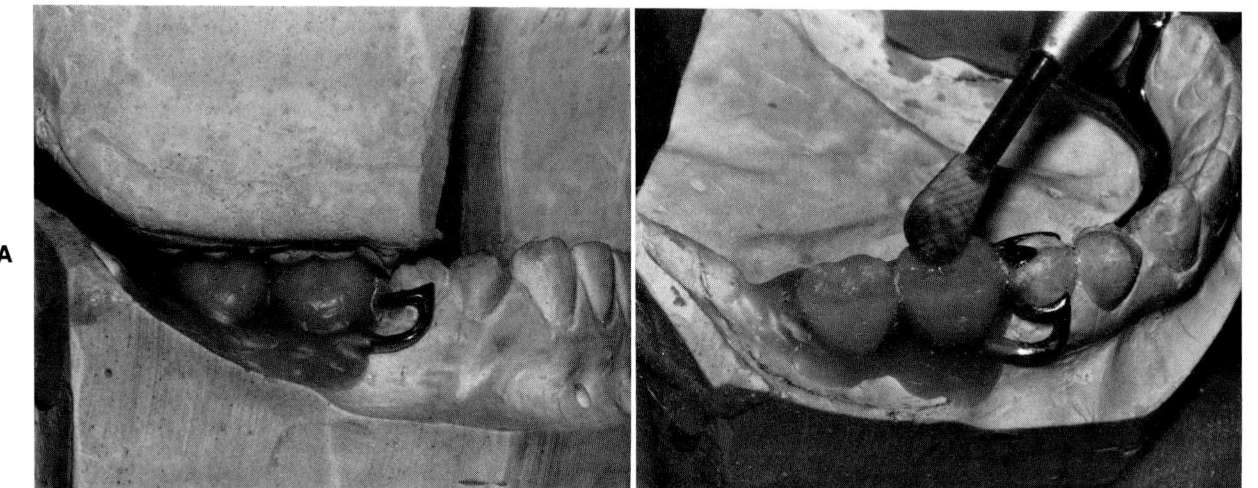

Fig. 14-57. A, Denture teeth are set against functionally generated pathway in stone. **B,** Occlusal surfaces of denture are ground away.

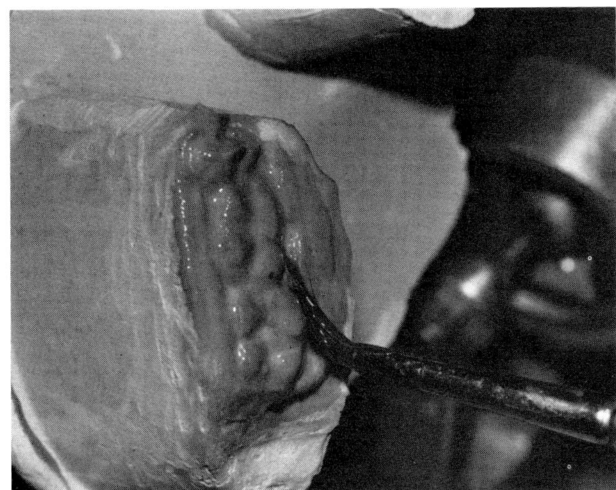

Fig. 14-58. Lubricating medium is applied to surface of stone pathway.

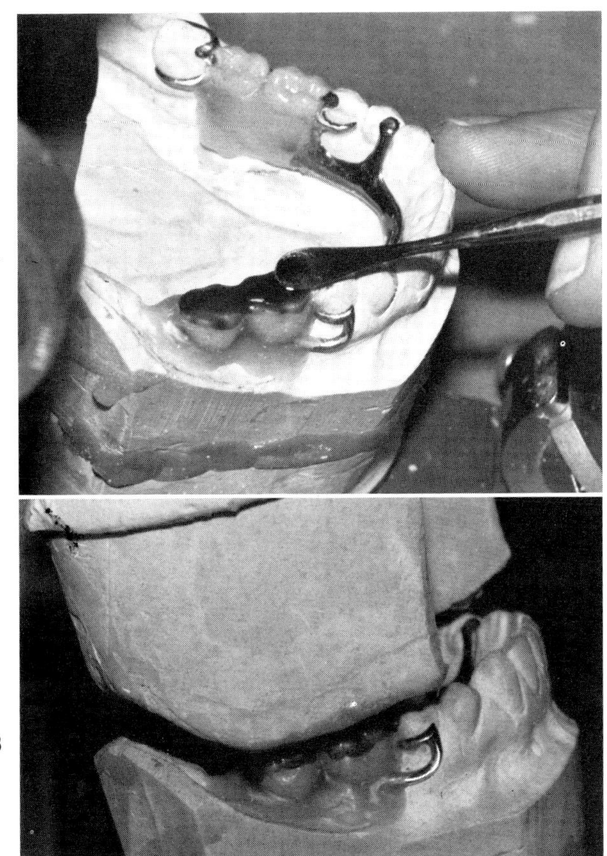

Fig. 14-59. A, Inlay wax is puddled on surfaces of denture teeth. **B,** Articulator is closed, transferring anatomy of stone pathway to softened wax. This step may need repeating several times.

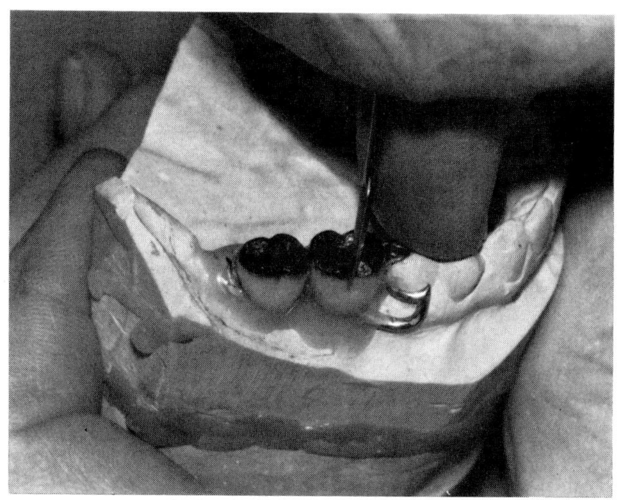

Fig. 14-60. Inlay wax is contoured to outline form of teeth, and occlusal anatomy is refined in greater detail.

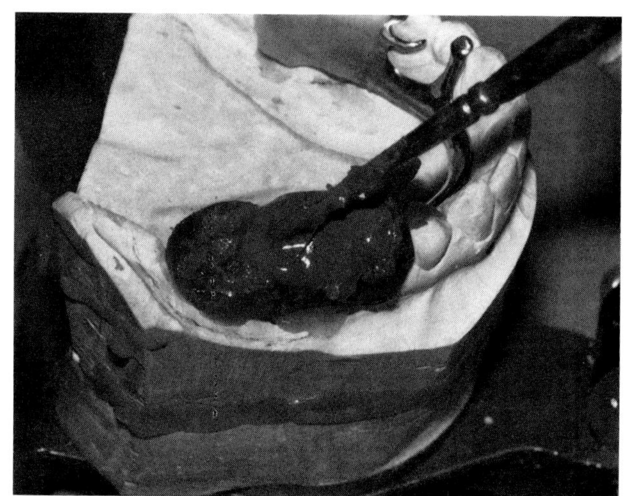

Fig. 14-61. Mix of investment material is painted on carved occlusal surfaces. Layer of investment must be thick enough to be handled safely.

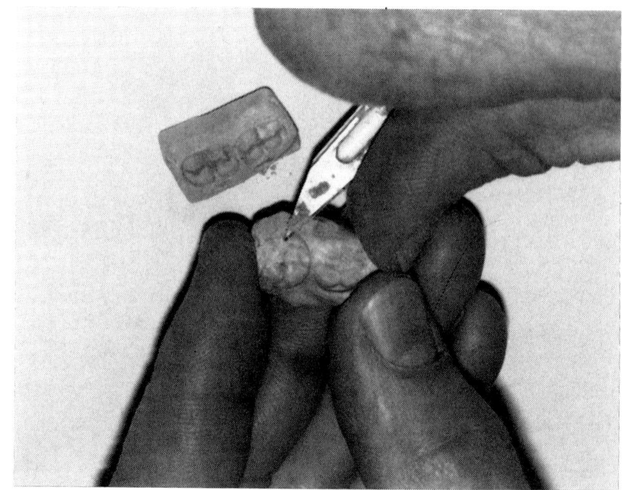

Fig. 14-62. Set investment is trimmed to reduce occlusogingival height of mold.

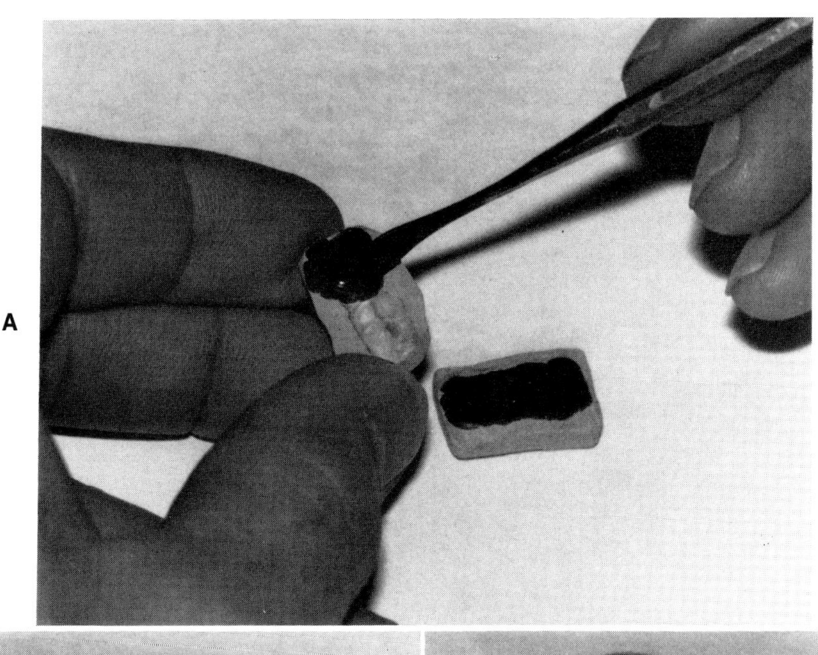

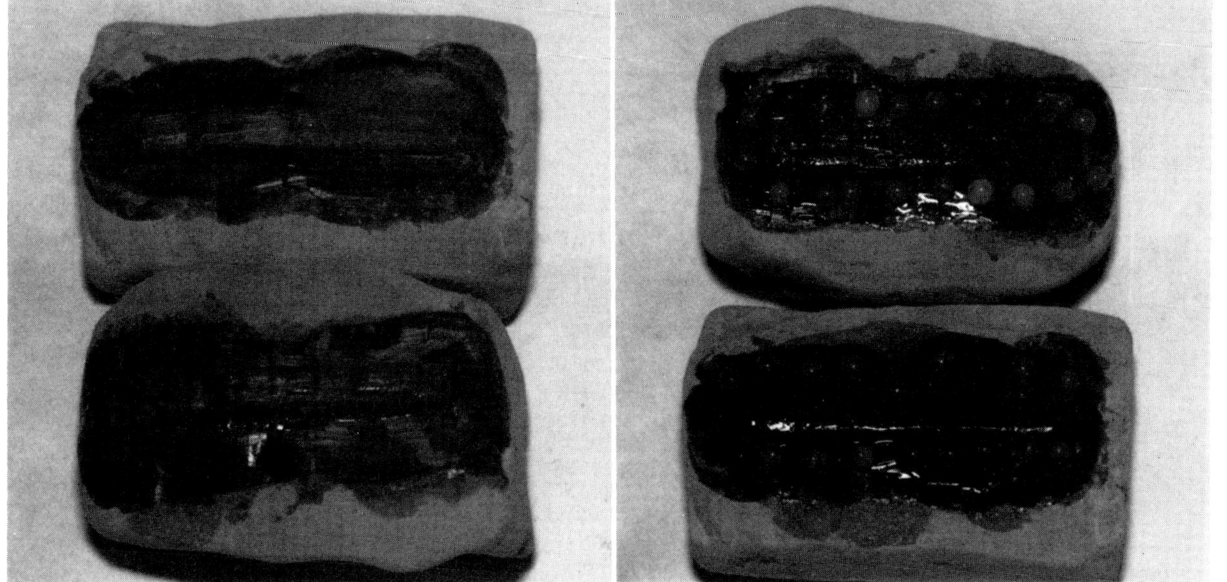

Fig. 14-63. **A,** Inlay wax is flowed to fill mold. **B,** Length of 12-gauge half-round wax shape is sealed to surface of wax. **C,** Beads of acrylic resin polymer are added to surface of wax for retention.

Fig. 14-64. Occlusal surfaces are sprued, invested, and cast.

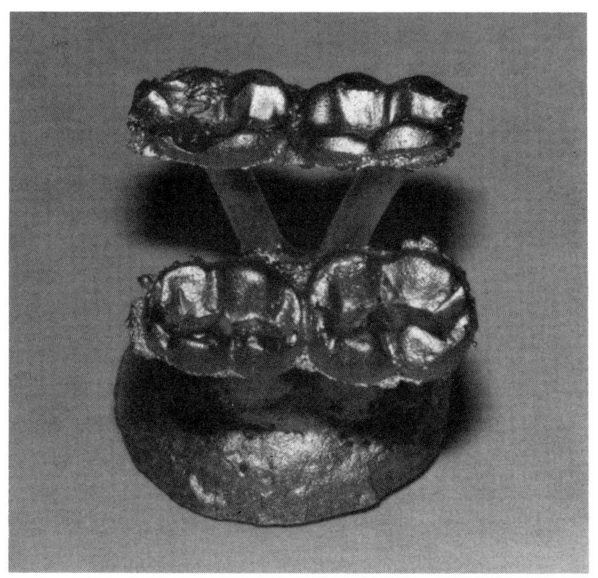

A

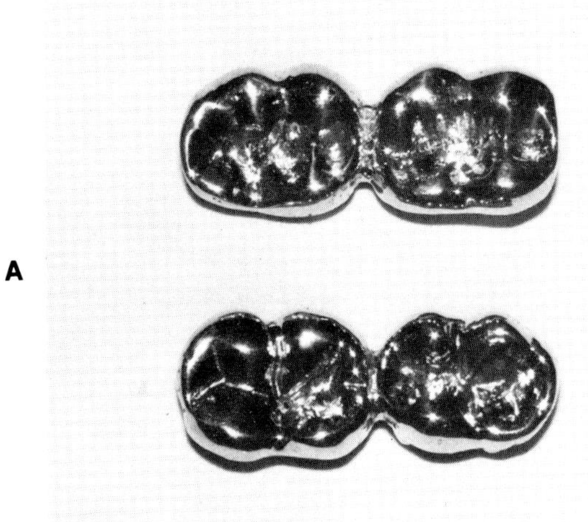

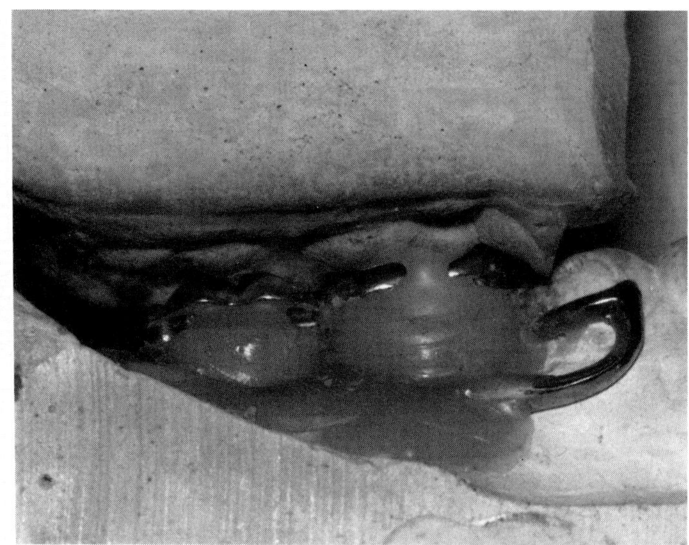

B

Fig. 14-65. A, Castings are cleaned and positioned against opposing occlusal surfaces used to carve them, either generated path or opposing teeth. **B,** Articulator is closed, and occlusal surfaces are reattached to ground denture teeth.

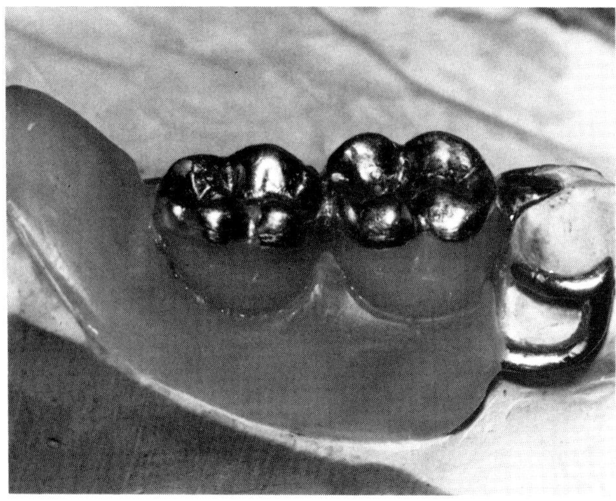

Fig. 14-66. Ivory wax is used to develop proper anatomy of crowns.

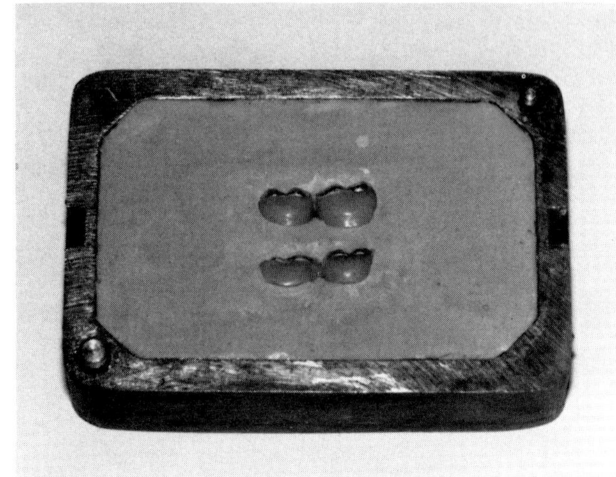

Fig. 14-67. Crowns of teeth are flasked with buccal surfaces facing upward.

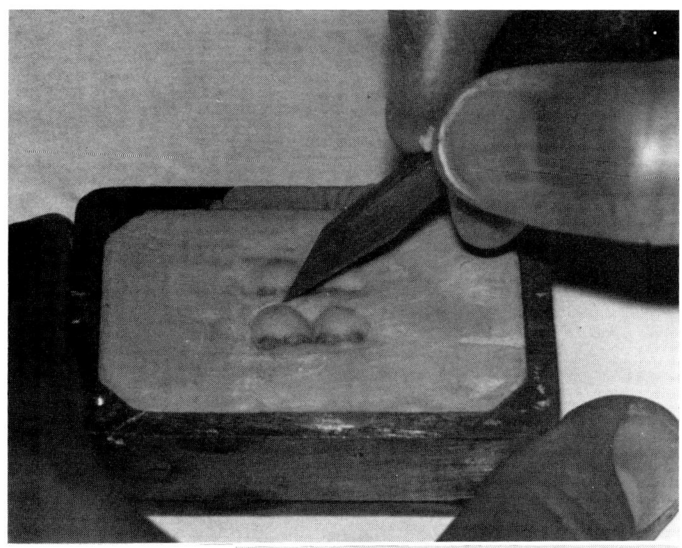

B

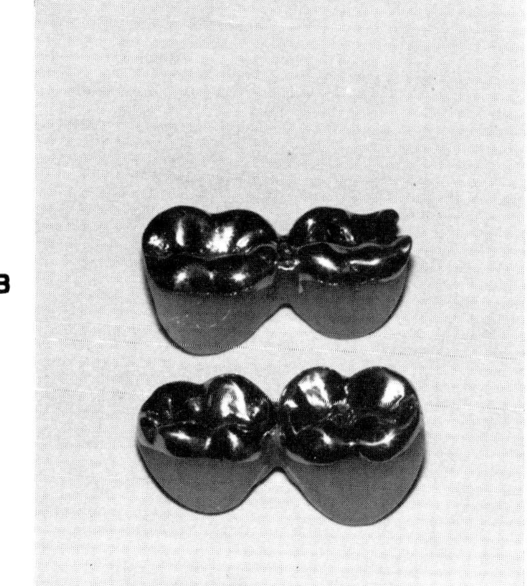

Fig. 14-68. A, Flask is boiled and opened, and wax and remnants of plastic teeth removed. Mold is cleaned, and tinfoil substitute painted on surface. Mold is packed with heat-cured tooth-colored acrylic resin. **B,** Crowns are deflasked and polished.

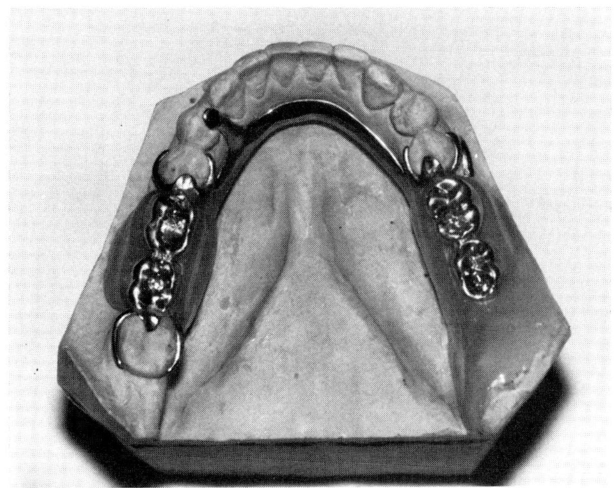

Fig. 14-69. Blocks of teeth are repositioned on framework using opposing teeth as guide. Denture should be tried in patient's mouth before it is completed.

Mold selection. The tooth size, or mold, is generally dictated by the size of the edentulous space, but certain guidelines may be followed.

For patients missing all posterior teeth a measurement may be made from the distal surface of the natural canine to the upward incline of the ramus of the mandible or to the mesial aspect of the maxillary tuberosity. This distance will normally be between 28 and 32 mm. Selection may then be made from sets of posterior teeth that correspond to the measured distance (Fig. 14-70).

A frequently overlooked measurement that must be considered is the occlusogingival height of the replacement tooth. An unfavorable esthetic arrangement results if a short artificial tooth is placed adjacent to the long clinical crown of a natural tooth, particularly in the maxillary premolar area (Fig. 14-71). At times it will be necessary to contour the ridge lap portion of the tooth so that only a thin veneer of plastic at the gingival margin remains to be butted against the edentulous ridge. This will improve the appearance of the denture, preventing a great disparity in the harmony of the cervical lines (Fig. 14-72).

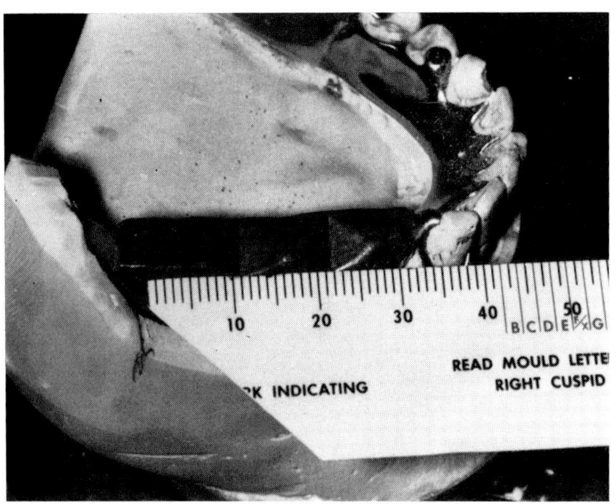

Fig. 14-70. Posterior denture teeth are selected on basis of measurement from distal surface of canine to beginning of upward incline of ramus of mandible.

Setting posterior teeth. As a general rule the classic pattern of intercuspation of maxillary and mandibular teeth should be strived for but, unfortunately, cannot always be accomplished. It is fortunate, however, that this relationship is not essential for good function. For those patients where the entire posterior occlusal scheme is being restored by partial dentures or by a complete denture opposing a partial denture, the ideal intercuspation of teeth should be achieved.

It was mentioned previously that one of the goals in establishing the occlusal pattern is to duplicate as nearly as possible the occlusal anatomy of the remaining natural teeth. In order to accomplish this, it is necessary to set the teeth originally slightly higher than will eventually be desired. This is necessary so that after the teeth have been positioned correctly, buccolingually and anteroposteriorly, the excessive occlusal height will be corrected by selective grinding of the occlusal surfaces to produce an occlusal anatomy in harmony with the remaining teeth. To obtain this slight increase of the occlusal plane, the incisal guide pin or the device that controls the vertical position of the upper member of the articulator should be increased or opened by 0.5 mm (Fig. 14-73). After the teeth are set,

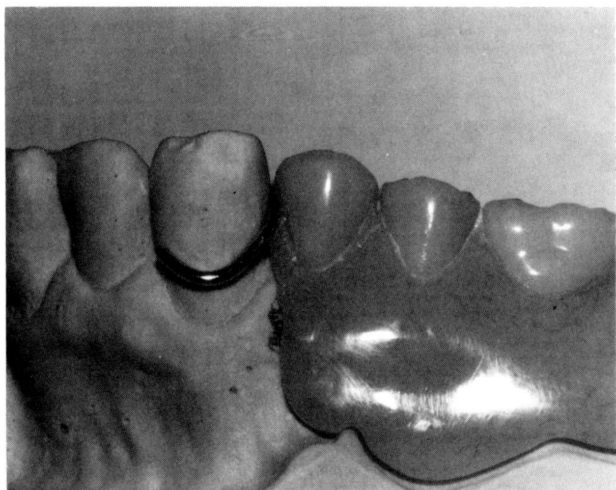

Fig. 14-71. Disparity between length of natural tooth and length of denture tooth contributes to artificial appearance.

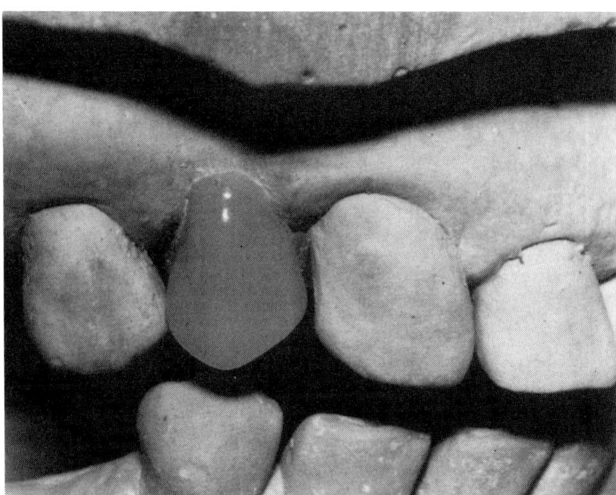

Fig. 14-72. Ridge lap of denture tooth should be trimmed so that thin buccal veneer of tooth is retained to maintain natural crown length.

the pin opening is returned to the correct position. Occlusal surfaces that contact prematurely (identified by articulating paper or tape) are reduced until the remaining stone teeth on the mounted casts are once more in contact. Following this reestablishing of the vertical dimension of occlusion, the occlusal surfaces of the artificial teeth should have grooves and sluiceways established to improve the masticating efficiency. As the occlusal surfaces are reshaped, caution must be used not to lose the occlusal contacts that have been developed. This is best done by leaving the markings of the articulating paper on the tooth surface as the supplemental grooves are added. Cuts must not be made through these marks.

Positioning tooth adjacent to clasp. The most difficult tooth to position is one that is adjacent to an abutment tooth bearing a clasp or a minor connector. The denture tooth must not only be adapted to function against the opposing occlusion but must also be adapted to conform to the clasp and minor connector, to the residual ridge, and to the denture base retention struts.

To minimize the amount of tooth reshaping or contouring that must be done at any one time, the procedure for adapting the tooth can be simplified by first removing the framework and fitting the tooth to the residual ridge and opposing occlusion (Fig. 14-74).

The ridge lap area of the tooth should be reduced by grinding mainly on the lingual and central aspect of the ridge lap in order to maintain the buccal length of the crown as much as possible. For some edentulous ridges where considerable absorption of the ridge has taken place, little or no reduction in crown height will be required. As far as occlusal contact position is concerned,

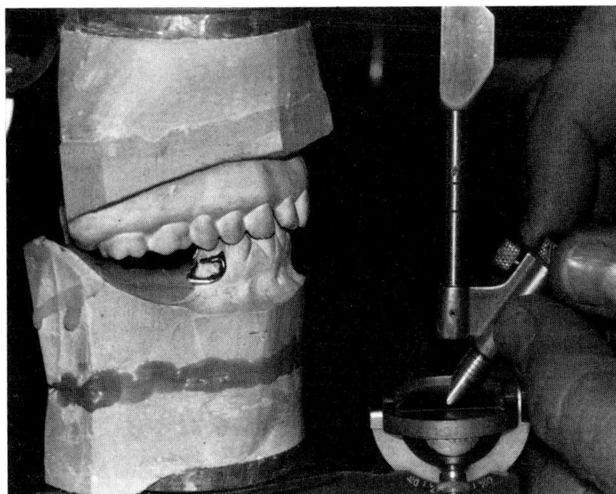

Fig. 14-73. Incisal guide is opened 0.5 mm before teeth are set. This slight increase will permit reshaping of occlusal surfaces of denture teeth to harmonize with natural teeth.

the tooth should be aligned buccolingually to provide the most ideal cusp-to-fossa relationship that is obtainable. This could require leaving a space between the artificial tooth and the abutment tooth. A space 2 mm or less in the mesiodistal direction can accommodate the minor connector on the proximal surface of the abutment tooth, but a wider space can lead to a definitely artificial appearance (Fig. 14-75). It may be necessary to reduce the mesial or distal contour of the artificial tooth that contacts the proximal surface of the abutment tooth so that more ideal intercuspation can take place. It should be realized that the amount of tooth reduction is limited in order not to produce a denture tooth width that is not compatible with the adjacent teeth. If ideal intercuspation cannot be obtained by moving the tooth mesially or distally, the occlusal surface of the denture tooth can be reshaped to harmonize with the opposing occlusion. Once correct adaptation to the opposing occlusion, to the residual ridge, and to the abutment tooth has been established (with the incisal guide pin raised 0.5 mm) the framework should be repositioned on the cast and the artificial tooth readjusted to accommodate it. The recontouring that will be required will be to the ridge lap portion of the tooth to fit the acrylic resin retention minor connector and the proximal portion of the tooth to fit the clasp and minor connector of the abutment tooth. A method of determining the areas of the denture tooth that need reshaping is shown in Fig. 14-76. It is not the purpose of adapting the ridge lap of the denture tooth to the acrylic resin minor connector to gain intimate contact between tooth and metal. Rather the purpose is only to be certain that enough space is available to position the tooth correctly in relation to the abutment tooth and the opposing teeth. There should be a space between the ridge lap of the tooth and the metal in order for the acrylic resin material of the denture base to adequately lock the artificial tooth in place. Soft utility wax may be used to hold the tooth in place while the tooth is being reshaped. Once the tooth is properly positioned, a harder baseplate wax should be used to secure the tooth firmly as final occlusal adjustments are made.

Setting the remaining posterior teeth. Any tooth that is to be set adjacent to remaining natural teeth is handled as previously described. A tooth that is to be set with natural teeth both anterior and posterior to it must have both proximal surfaces contoured to fit against the minor connector and clasp assemblies of both natural teeth.

Other posterior teeth that will be set adjacent to artificial teeth are positioned in the most favorable relationship to the opposing occlusal surfaces. Slight spacing between posterior teeth to achieve the most

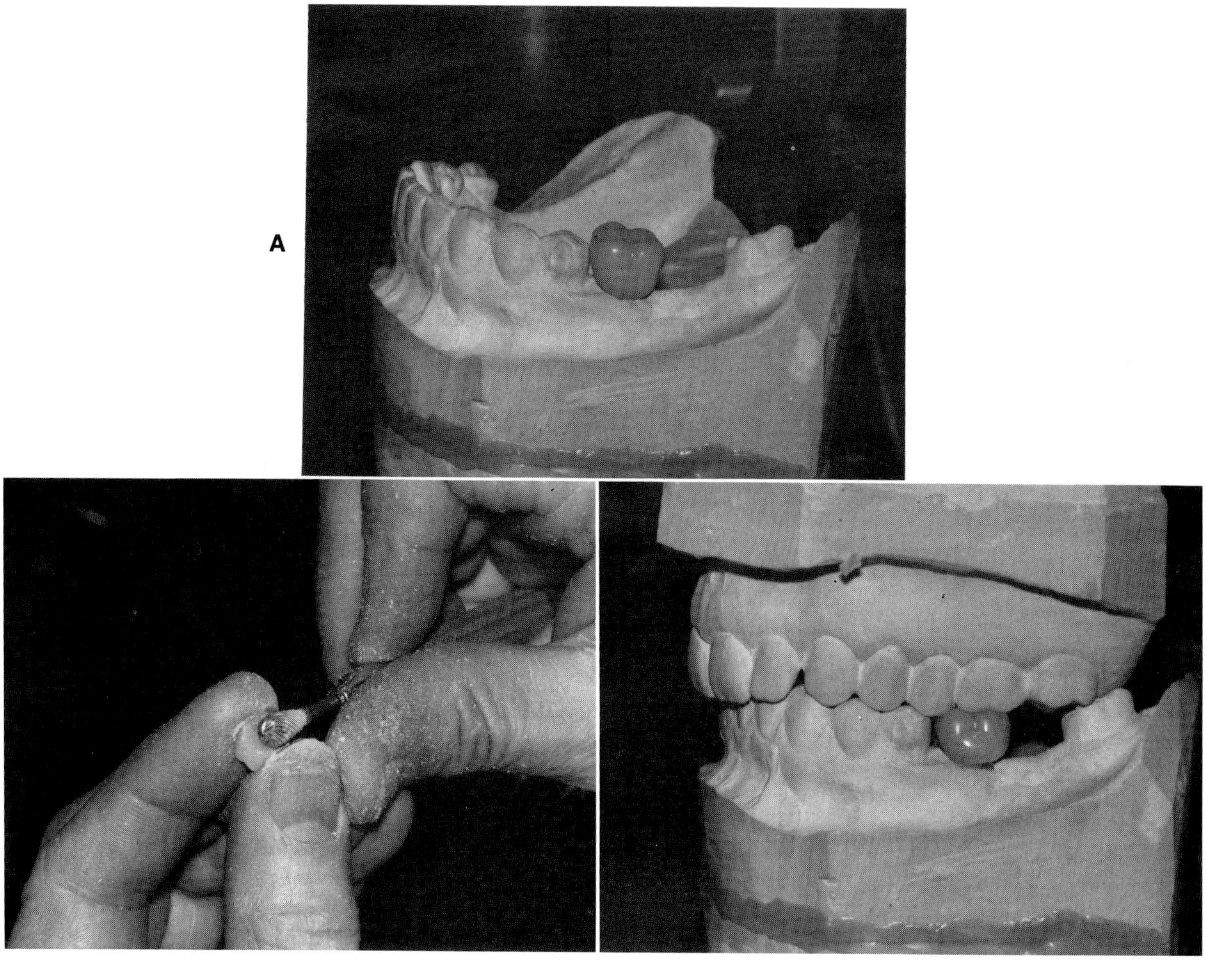

Fig. 14-74. A, Denture tooth is placed in position without framework in place to start with. Amount and location of tooth reduction necessary to provide proper alignment and occlusion can be envisioned. **B,** Ridge lap and proximal surface of denture tooth are reduced with acrylic burs. **C,** Reduction of tooth is continued until correct position is achieved.

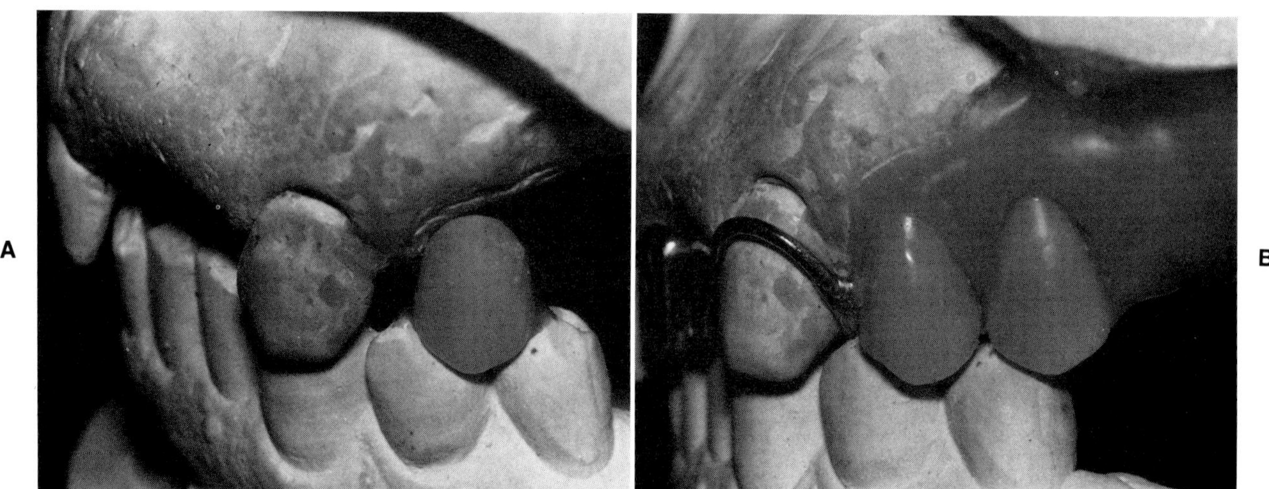

Fig. 14-75. A, Small space (2 mm) may be left between denture tooth and abutment tooth. **B,** Minor connector supporting clasp arm will occupy space. Spaces greater than this should be avoided.

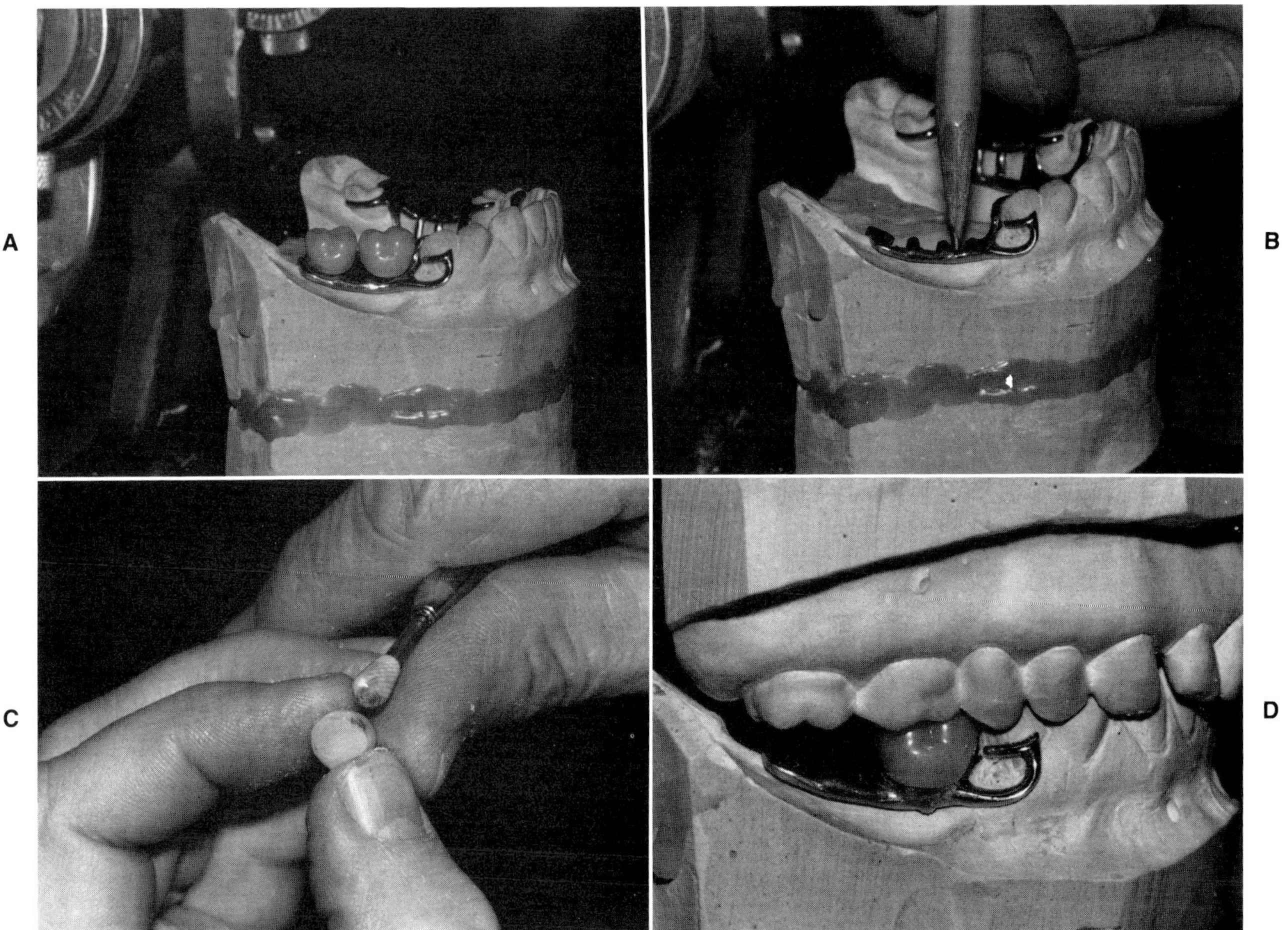

Fig. 14-76. A, Denture tooth is now shaped to fit framework. Tooth, trimmed to fit edentulous ridge, will be high when it is placed in position on framework. **B,** Coating of pencil lead is placed on framework. **C,** Denture tooth is pressed into position over framework. Pencil lead is transferred to areas of interference on tooth. Such surfaces are relieved with lathe or handpiece. **D,** Procedure is repeated until tooth is in correct position.

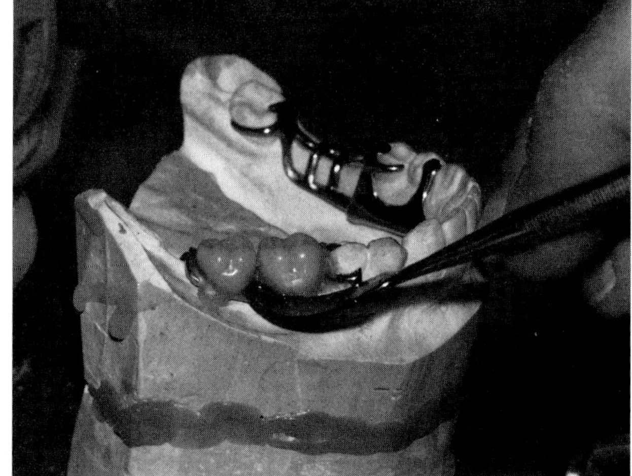

Fig. 14-77. Other denture teeth are reshaped until correct occlusion is developed. Baseplate wax is added to maintain this position.

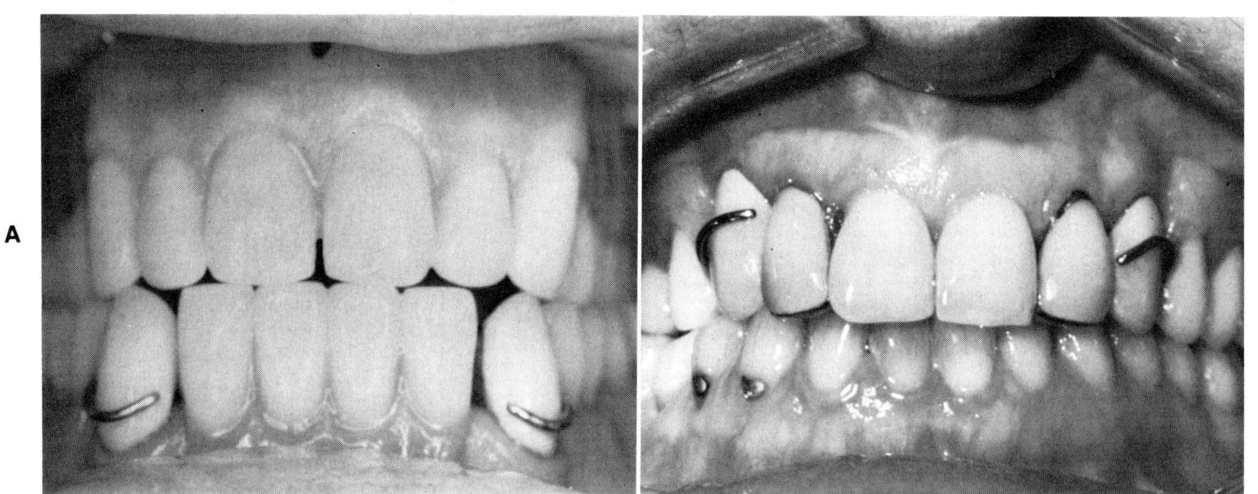

Fig. 14-78. A, Nonanatomic posterior teeth may be used in partial dentures if little or no vertical overlap is present. Occlusal problems are more easily controlled if opposing dentition is complete denture. **B,** Deep anterior overlap makes use of nonanatomic posterior teeth difficult. Balanced occlusion cannot be obtained.

desirable intercuspation is acceptable, but excessive spacing should be avoided. Recontouring of occlusal surfaces is often necessary to produce good functional occlusion without resorting to poor tooth position (Fig. 14-77).

Missing mandibular posterior teeth should always be replaced so that the central grooves of the teeth are over the crest of the mandibular ridge.

The use of nonanatomic, or zero-degree, teeth should normally be avoided in partial denture construction except when the partial denture is opposing a complete denture or where all posterior teeth, both maxillary and mandibular, are being replaced and a deep anterior vertical overlap is not present. The deep vertical overlap precludes the possibility of obtaining a balanced occlusion with nonanatomic teeth or of developing a simultaneous working side contact between natural and artificial teeth (Fig. 14-78).

Following the correct placement of the artificial posterior teeth, the teeth should be waxed securely in position with hard baseplate wax. At this time the incisal guide pin is readjusted to its correct vertical position and the occlusal surfaces of the teeth are selectively ground to reestablish the vertical dimension of occlusion (Fig. 14-79).

If an adjustable or semiadjustable articulator is being

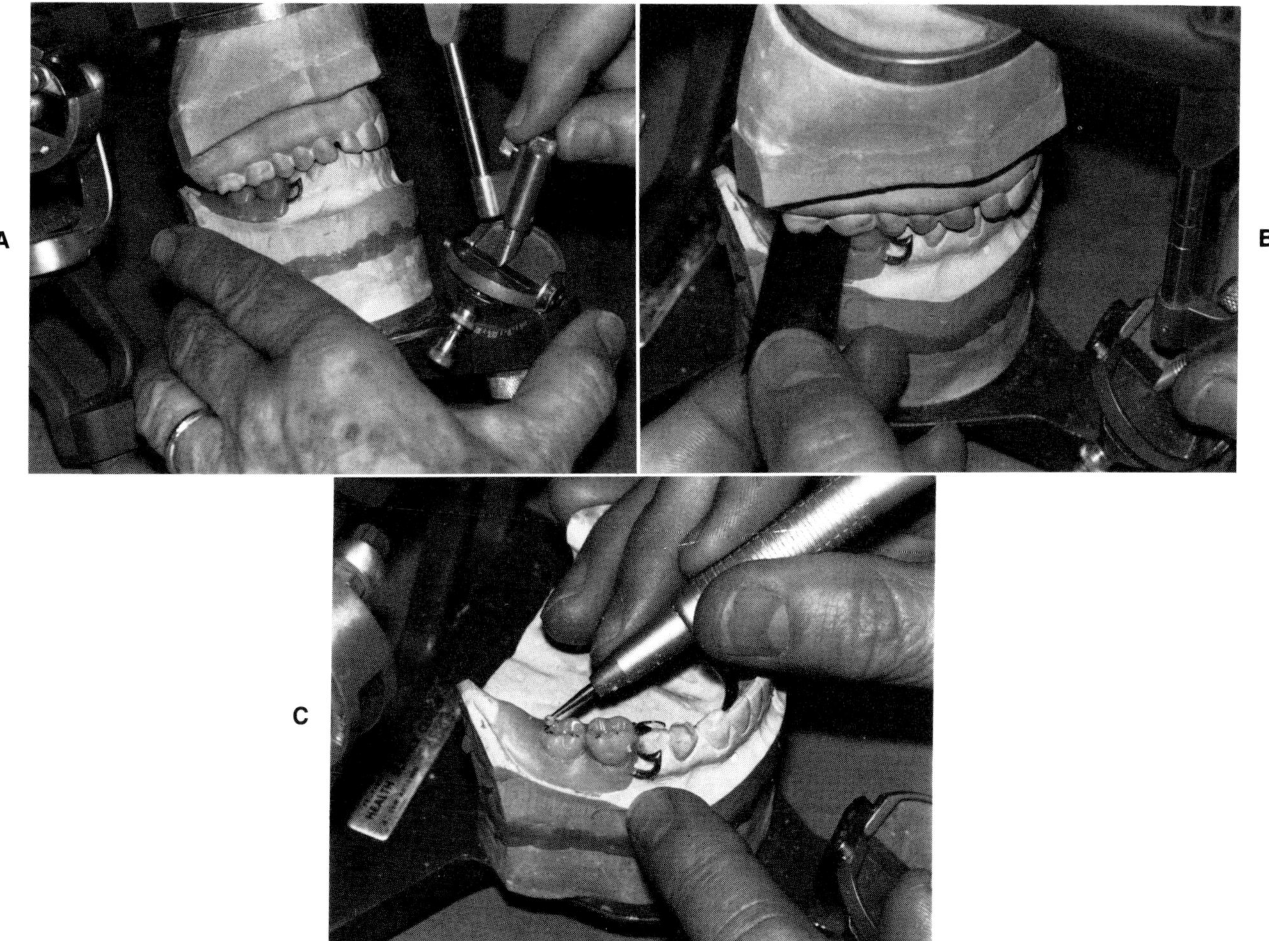

Fig. 14-79. A, When denture teeth have been waxed securely in position, incisal guide table is adjusted to protect teeth from movement or from wear of stone teeth. **B,** Articulating paper is held between denture teeth as articulator is moved to lateral position. **C,** Interferences in lateral movements, both working and balancing sides, are removed with burs.

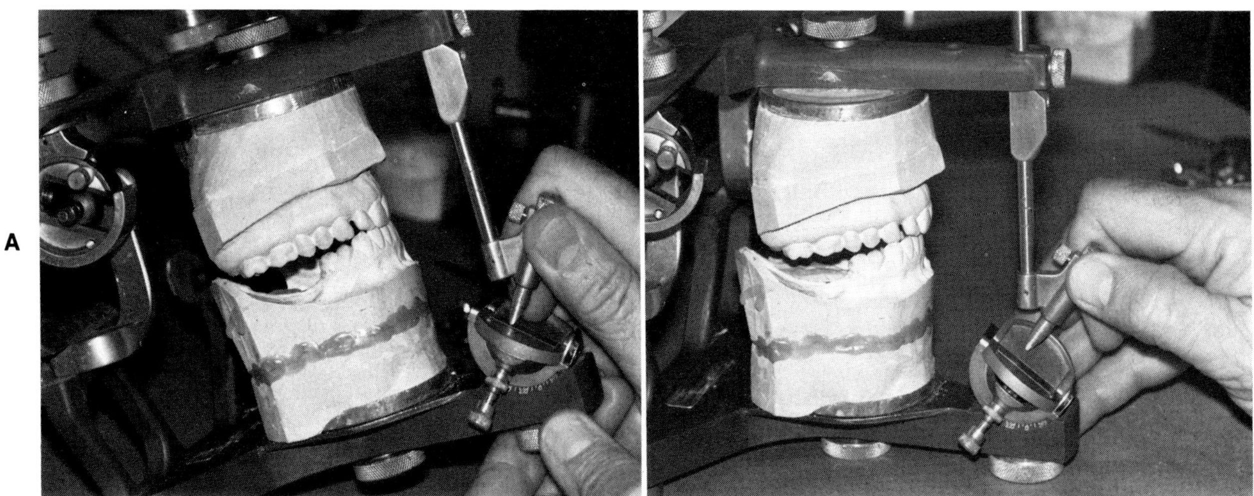

Fig. 14-80. A, Incisal guide table is adjusted to protect stone teeth in protrusive movement. With anterior teeth held in edge-to-edge relationship, guide table is tipped in anteror-posterior direction until table contacts incisal guide pin. **B,** Lateral wings of guide table are adjusted to contact incisal guide pin as stone teeth on cast are moved to right and left lateral working relationship.

used and has been set to proper condylar and incisal guidance, articulation in lateral and protrusive movements should also be adjusted. If the instrument has an adjustable anterior and lateral incisal guide table, this table and/or lateral wings must be adjusted to protect the stone teeth on the casts from being broken or abraded as the instrument is moved through the various excursions (Fig. 14-80).

The desired occlusal contacts for artificial teeth for removable partial dentures vary according to the class of partially edentulous arch being treated. The following is a summation of the various occlusal contacts desired.

1. Simultaneous bilateral occlusal contact of opposing posterior teeth in centric occlusion or centric relation is a goal of all forms of restorative dentistry (Fig. 14-81). Simultaneous contact must occur between artificial teeth, between natural and artificial teeth, and between natural teeth. A prosthesis must not hold natural teeth apart, or some form of destruction will occur.
2. For all tooth-borne partial denture (Class III) the occlusion should be similar to a harmonious natural dentition. In a high percentage of these patients a canine-protected or mutually protected occlusion where all anterior teeth act together will be the goal (Fig. 14-82). In these patients, as the mandible moves into protrusive or lateral relationship, the posterior teeth disclude, or separate, because of the lifting action of the canines or anterior teeth. This is a normal occlusal scheme and should be retained for the Class III patient. The group function concept, in which anterior and posterior contacts occur simultaneously in mandibular excursions, should not be followed except when it can be demonstrated that this concept was present in the patient's mouth before the loss of teeth and that the group function did not contribute to the loss of teeth.
3. For a removable partial denture opposing a complete denture, bilateral balanced occlusion in eccentric jaw position is desirable (Fig. 14-83). To provide stabilization for the complete denture, bilateral contacts in the working and balancing positions as well as in protrusive relationships are desired. The inability to achieve this bilateral balance will result in an unstable complete denture and premature loss of bone from the residual ridge.
4. For mandibular distal extension partial dentures, working side contact of natural and denture teeth on that side should occur (Fig. 14-84). One of the purposes of partial denture construction is to distribute the occlusal load or occlusal forces over as wide an area as possible to prevent overloading of any individual tooth or area. This can best be accomplished in the posteriorly unsupported partial denture by incorporating both natural and artificial teeth in function.
5. Maxillary bilateral distal extension dentures should have simultaneous balancing and working contacts. This is one relationship that must be most frequently compromised because of steep vertical overlap of the natural anterior teeth. This

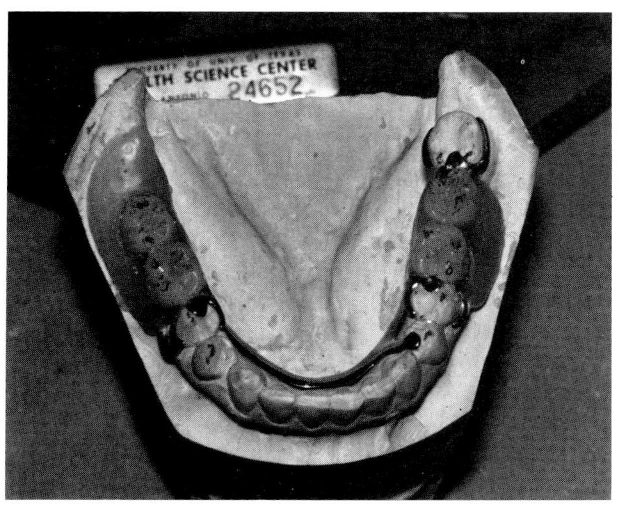

Fig. 14-81. Bilateral simultaneous contact of denture teeth and natural teeth is evidenced by articulating ribbon marking.

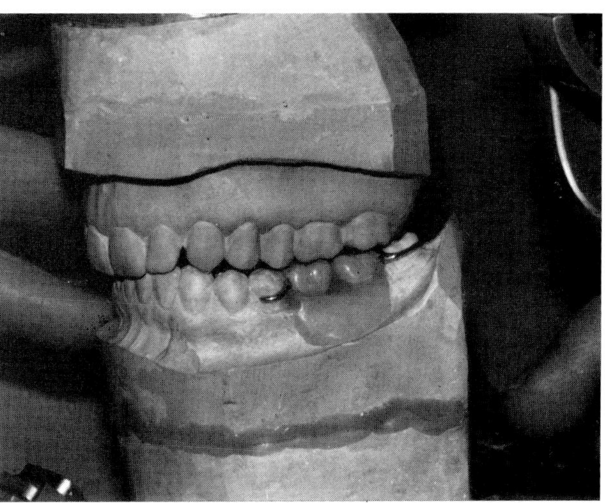

Fig. 14-82. For majority of Class III patients disclusion, or separation, of posterior teeth in lateral excursion is desirable.

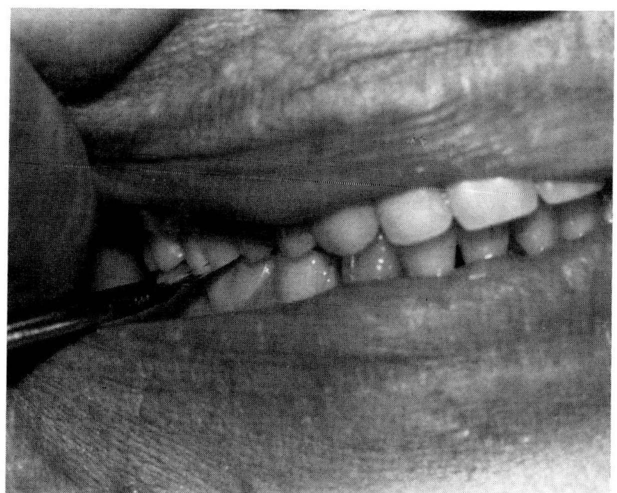

Fig. 14-83. When partial denture opposes complete denture, bilateral balanced occlusion is desirable. Bilateral contacts in working and balancing positions stablize complete denture and preserve edentulous ridge.

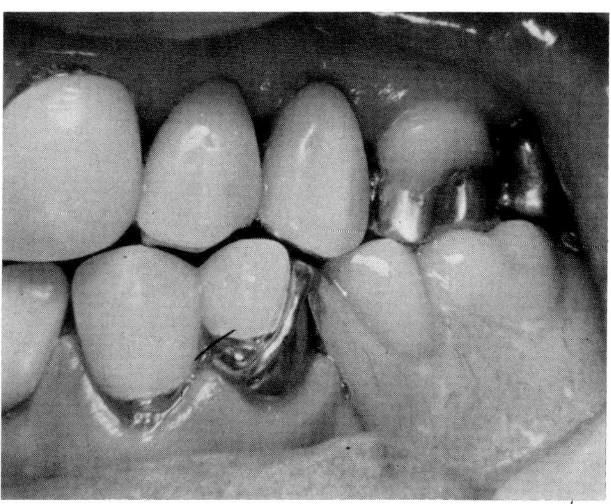

Fig. 14-84. For mandibular Class I or Class II patient simultaneous working side contact of natural and denture teeth on edentulous side is desired.

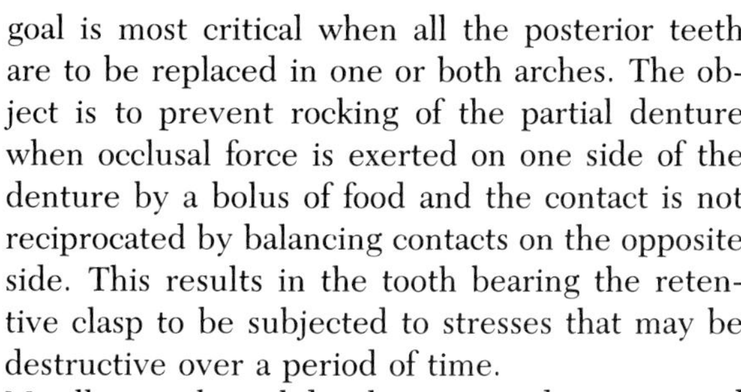

goal is most critical when all the posterior teeth are to be replaced in one or both arches. The object is to prevent rocking of the partial denture when occlusal force is exerted on one side of the denture by a bolus of food and the contact is not reciprocated by balancing contacts on the opposite side. This results in the tooth bearing the retentive clasp to be subjected to stresses that may be destructive over a period of time.

6. Maxillary unilateral distal extension dentures need only have working side contacts, because the opposite side is tooth supported. In this case forces occurring on the dentulous side are not transmitted to the denture, and forces tending to unseat the denture are distributed over several teeth and the hard palate and can be dissipated satisfactorily.
7. In Class IV situations it is desirable to have light or minimal contact with the opposing natural teeth in centric occlusion to prevent eruption of the natural incisor teeth, but contact of the anterior teeth in eccentric position is not desirable (Fig. 14-85). In situations where a deep anterior overlap is present and the maxillary anterior teeth are being replaced, the lower anterior teeth

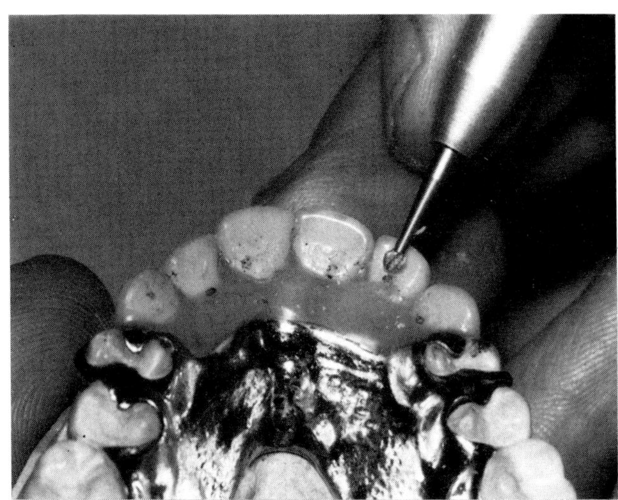

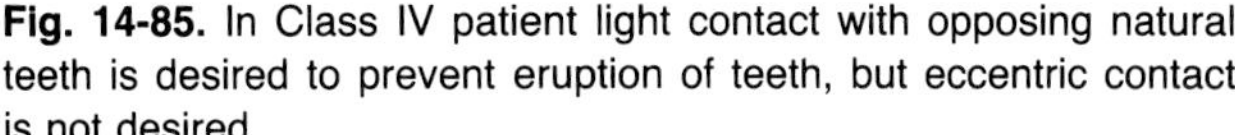

Fig. 14-85. In Class IV patient light contact with opposing natural teeth is desired to prevent eruption of teeth, but eccentric contact is not desired.

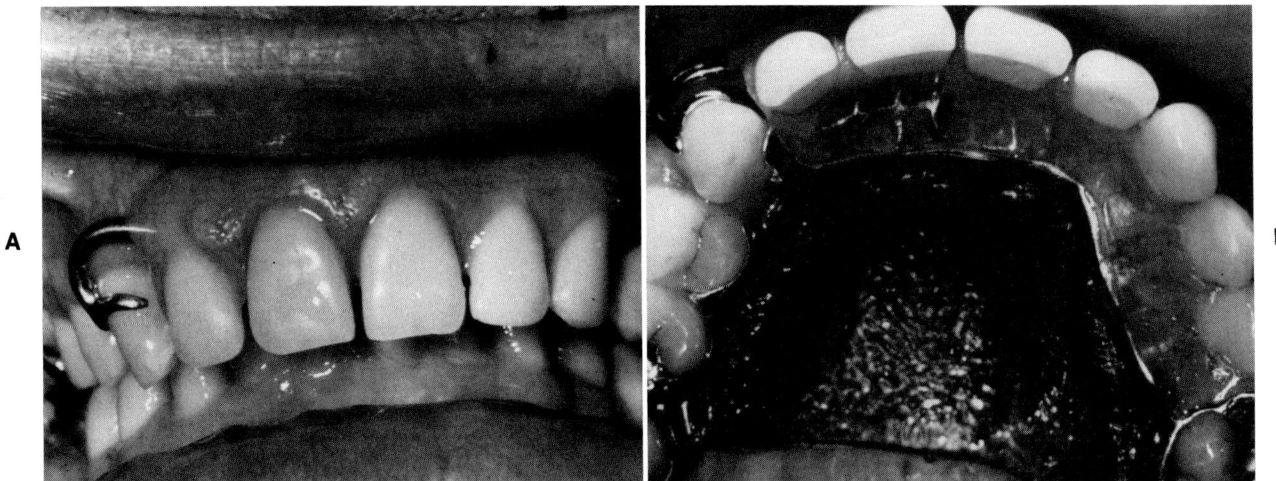

Fig. 14-86. In Class IV patient when a deep vertical overlap is present, **A,** table of acrylic resin is constructed lingual to maxillary incisor teeth, **B,** so that lower anterior teeth can contact it. This prevents over-eruption of opposing teeth.

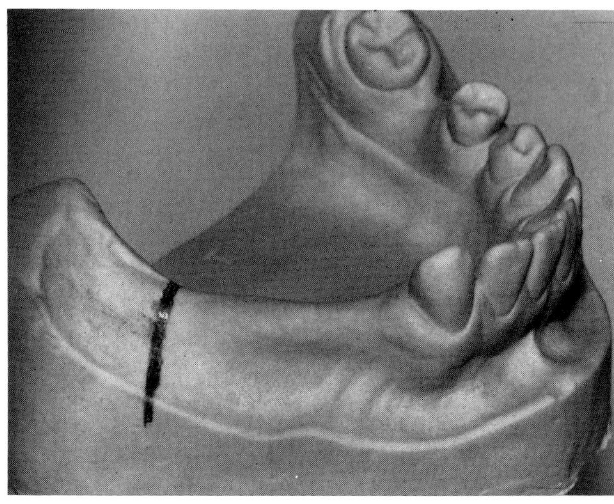

Fig. 14-87. Posterior teeth should not be positioned on upward incline of mandibular ridge.

should contact an acrylic resin table, not metal, lingual to the artificial teeth to prevent overeruption (Fig. 14-86).

8. Contact of opposing posterior teeth in straight protrusive movement is not desirable except when the partial denture opposes a complete denture.
9. Posterior teeth should not be positioned farther back than the beginning of the upward incline of the residual mandibular ridge (Fig. 14-87).

LENGTH OF APPOINTMENT

For an experienced dentist this jaw relation appointment is brief; normally 15 minutes is sufficient. For the less experienced student 45 to 60 minutes is usually required.

BIBLIOGRAPHY

Applegate, O.C.: The partial denture base, J. Prosthet. Dent. **5**:636-648, 1955.

Baraban, D.J.: Establishing centric relation and vertical dimension in occlusal rehabilitation, J. Prosthet. Dent. **12**:1157-1165, 1962.

Beck, H.O.: A clinical evaluation of the Arcon concept of articulation, J. Prosthet. Dent. **9**:409-421, 1959.

Beck, H.O.: Selection of an articulator and jaw registration, J. Prosthet. Dent. **10**:878-886, 1960.

Beck, H.O.: Choosing the articulator, J. Am. Dent. Assoc. **64**:468-475, 1962.

Beckett, L.S.: Accurate occlusal relations in partial denture construction, J. Prosthet. Dent. **4**:487-495, 1954.

Beyron, H.L.: Occlusal relationship, Int. Dent. J. **2**:467-496, 1952.

Block, L.S.: Preparing and conditioning the patient for intermaxillary relations, J. Prosthet. Dent. **2**:599-603, 1952.

Boos, R.H.: Maxillomandibular relations, occlusion and the tempromandibular joint, Dent. Clin. North Am. **6**:19-35, March 1962.

Borg, I., and Posselt, U.: Hinge axis registration: experiments on the articulator, J. Prosthet. Dent. **8**:35-40, 1958.

Boucher, C.O.: Occlusion in prosthodontics, J. Prosthet. Dent. **3**:633-656, 1953.

Brown, S.W.: Disharmony between centric relation and centric occlusion as a factor in producing improper tooth wear and trauma, Dent. Digest **52**:434-440, 1946.

Christensen, P.B.: Accurate casts and positional relation records, J. Prosthet. Dent. **8**:475-482, 1958.

Colman, A.J.: Occlusal requirements for removable partial dentures, J. Prosthet. Dent. **17**:155-162, 1967.

Craddock, F.W.: The accuracy and practical value of records and condyle path inclination, J. Am. Dent. Assoc. **38**:697-710, 1949.

D'Amico, A.: Functional occlusion of the natural teeth of man, J. Prosthet. Dent., **11**:899-915, 1961.

Emmert, J.H.: A method of registering occlusion in semiedentulous mouths, J. Prosthet. Dent. **8**:94-99, 1958.

Fedi, P.F.: Cardinal differences in occlusion of natural teeth and that of artificial teeth, J. Am. Dent. Assoc. **62**:482-483, 1962.

Fountain, H.W.: Seating the condyles for centric relation records, J. Prosthet. Dent. **11**:1050-1058, 1961.

Granger, E.R.: The articulator and the patient, Dent. Clin. North Am., **4**:527-539, 1960.

Hall, W.A.: Variations in registering interarch transfers in removable partial denture construction, J. Pros. Dent. **30**:548-553, 1973.

Hanau, R.L.: Full denture prosthesis: intraoral technique, ed. 4, Buffalo, 1930, Thorner-Sidney Press.

Henderson, D.: Occlusion in removable partial prosthodontics, J. Prosthet. Dent. **27**:151-159, 1972.

Hindels, G.W.: Occlusion in removable partial denture prosthesis, Dent. Clin. North Am. **6**:137-146, March 1962.

Jaffe, V.N.: The functionally generated path in full denture construction J. Prosthet. Dent. **4**:214-221, 1954.

Jeffreys, F.E., and Platner, R.L.: Occlusion in removable partial dentures, J. Prosthet. Dent., **10**:912-920, 1960.

Koehne, C.L., and Morrow, R.M.: Construction of denture teeth with gold occlusal surfaces, J. Prosthet. Dent. **23**:449-455, 1970.

Lucia, V.O.: Centric relation; theory and practice, J. Prosthet. Dent. **10**:849-956, 1960.

Mann, A.W., and Pankey, L.D.: The P.M. philosophy of occlusal rehabilitation, Dent. Clin. North Am. **7**:621-636, November 1963.

McCollum, B.B.: The mandibular hinge axis and a method of locating it, J. Prosthet. Dent. **10**:428-435, 1960.

McCracken, W.L.: Functional occlusion in removable partial contruction, J. Prosthet. Dent. **8**:955-963, 1958.

Mehta, J.D., and Joglekar, A.P.: Vertical jaw relation as a factor in partial dentures, J. Prosthet. Dent. **21**:618-625, 1969.

Meyer, F.S.: The generated path technique in reconstruction dentistry I and II, J. Prosthet. Dent. **9**:354-366, 432-440, 1959.

Niswonger, M.E.: The rest position of the mandible, J. Am. Dent. Assoc. **21**:1572-1582, 1934.

Nuttell, E.B.: Establishing posterior functional occlusion for fixed partial dentures, J. Am. Dent. Assoc. **66**:341-348, 1963.

O'Leary, T.J., and others: Tooth mobility in cuspid-protected and group-function occlusion, J. Prosthet. Dent. **27**:21-25, 1972.

Perry, C.K.: Transfer base for removable partial dentures, J. Prosthet. Dent. **31**:582-584, 1974.

Robinson, M.J.: Centric position, J. Prosthet. Dent. **1**:384-386, 1951.

Roedema, W.H.: Relationship between the width of the occlusal table and pressures under dentures during function, J. Prosthet. Dent. **36**:24-34, 1976.

Schuyler, C.H.: Fundamental principles in the correction of occlusal disharmony; natural and artificial (grinding), J. Am. Dent. Assoc. **22**:1193-1202, 1935.

Schuyler, C.H.: Factors contributing to traumatic occlusion, J. Prosthet. Dent. **11**:708-715, 1961.

Sears, V.C.: Occlusion: the common meeting ground in dentistry, J. Prosthet. Dent. **2**:15-21, 1952.

Shanahan, T.E.J., and Leff, A.: Interocclusal records, J. Prosthet. Dent. **10**:842-848, 1960.

Silverman, M.M.: Centric occlusion and jaw relation and fallacies of current concepts, J. Prosthet. Dent. **7**:750-769, 1957.

Silverman, M.M.: Determination of vertical dimension by phonetics, J. Prosthet. Dent. **6**:465-471, 1956.

Stuart, C.E.: Accuracy in measuring functional dimension and relation in oral prosthesis, J. Prosthet. Dent. **9**:220-236, 1959.

Teteruck, W.R., and Lundeen, H.C.: The accuracy of an ear facebow, J. Prosthet. Dent. **16**:1039-1046, 1966.

Thompson, J.R., and Brodie, A.G.: Factors in the position of the mandible, J. Am. Dent. Assoc. **29**:925-941, 1942.

Weinberg, L.A.: The transverse hinge axis: real or imaginary, J. Prosthet. Dent. **9**:775-787, 1959.

Weinberg, L.A.: An evaluation of basic articulators and their concepts, I and II, J. Prosthet. Dent. **13**:662-663, 1963.

Wilson, J.H.: The use of partial dentures in the restoration of occlusal standards, Aust. Dent. J. **1**:93-101, 1956.

Woodward, J.D., and Gattozzi, J.G.: Simplified gold occlusal technique for removable restorations, J. Prothet. Dent. **27**:447-450, 1972.

15 Try-in and completion of the partial denture

INDICATIONS FOR CLINICAL APPOINTMENT

The clinical appointment at which the patient first views the esthetic arrangement of anterior teeth that are being replaced by a removable partial denture is critical. However much a patient may state that restoration of function is the overwhelming desire, a sense of vanity always remains. An unhappy patient is seldom satisfied with a prosthesis even if it meets all mechanical and biologic requirements. Thus if anterior teeth are being replaced by denture teeth on a denture base, an esthetic try-in is essential before the denture is completed. At this stage, correction in tooth size, tooth position, or tooth shade can be accomplished easily, whereas correction after the denture is completed is a major undertaking.

The second indication for the appointment is to verify the jaw relation records that were made at the previous appointment if there is any doubt as to the accuracy of the articulator mounting. The appointment is indicated generally when all posterior teeth in one or both arches are being replaced or when the partial denture opposes a complete denture.

ESTHETIC TRY-IN

The patient should be seated in a pleasant, quiet treatment room to alleviate unnecessary tension that may develop as the patient views the replacement teeth for the first time.

Many patients object to seeing the partial denture in an articulator. The feeling of artificiality is emphasized in this situation. The denture base need not be waxed to the complete extent that it ultimately will have but should have sufficient body to support the artificial teeth and should have a neat anatomic appearance (Fig. 15-1). The patient should be cautioned against applying any biting force to the denture at this time.

The dentist should insert the partial denture carefully, making certain that it is completely seated. The patient may then close lightly to make sure there are no interferences present. The patient should be encouraged to relax. When the patient is at ease and comfortable, the teeth may be evaluated. It is better if the dentist examines the teeth in the mouth before the patient has an opportunity to observe them. In the event a gross malarrangement of the teeth has occurred, corrections can be made without upsetting the mental attitude of the patient.

Attention should be given to the anteroposterior position of the anterior teeth, particularly concerning adequate lip support. There is a definite tendency to position the artificial teeth lingual to the position occupied by the original natural teeth. Many patients, particularly if anterior teeth have been missing for any length of time, will complain of a sensation of abnormal fullness to the upper lip when the partial denture is first inserted (Fig. 15-2). Usually a thorough explanation of what is causing the sensation of fullness and the passage of a little time will eliminate this problem.

Tooth length in relation to lip length and length of the remaining natural teeth must be evaluated. If all anterior teeth are being replaced and the upper lip is of normal length, the tips of the central incisors should be visible when the lip is relaxed (Fig. 15-3). When the lip is drawn upward or in an exaggerated smile, the gingival contour of the denture base should just be evident (Fig. 15-4). There may be times when this will be difficult to accomplish because of a short upper lip or a prominent anterior edentulous ridge.

If the anterior edentulous space has been decreased by mesial drifting of the teeth, attempts should be made to rotate or overlap the denture teeth in order to restore normal or close-to-normal mesiodistal width of the replacement teeth (Fig. 15-4). An abnormal appearance usually results if fewer than the number of missing anterior teeth are replaced. This should be avoided if at all possible. If the anterior edentulous space is increased, the use of diastemas or spacing of the anterior teeth may be attempted if the patient will accept it (Fig. 15-5). Some people have difficulty adapting to the flow of air between the teeth, and speech problems can develop.

Attention should be paid to the horizontal and vertical overlap of the anterior teeth (Fig. 15-6). If some natural anterior teeth remain, the overlap should be duplicated. If no natural teeth remain, care must be taken not to create excessive vertical overlap without

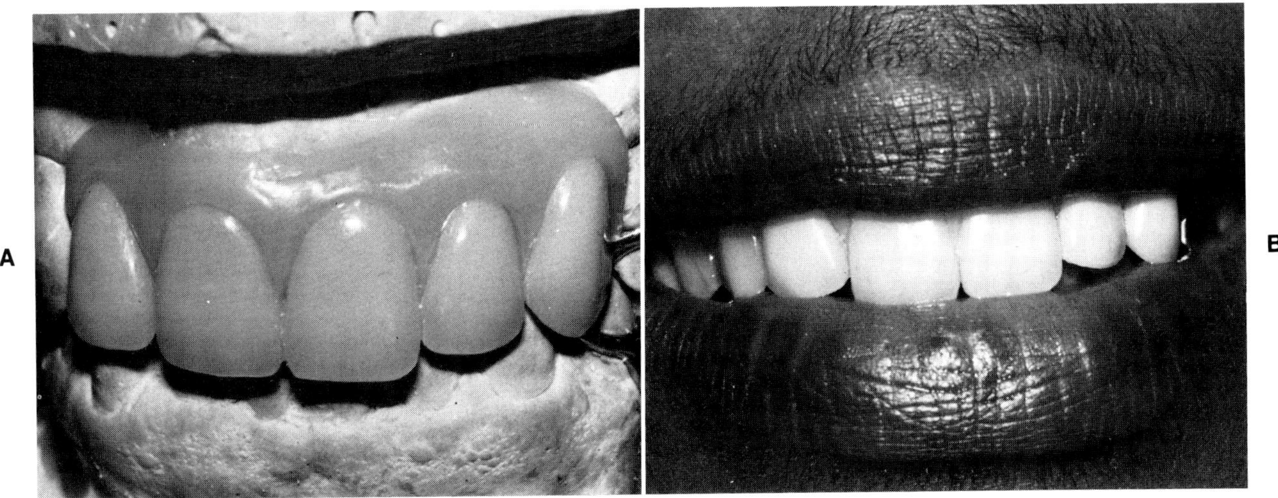

Fig. 15-1. A, Denture base is waxed to neat anatomic appearance. B, With exception of color of wax, trial denture should have same esthetic quality as completed prosthesis.

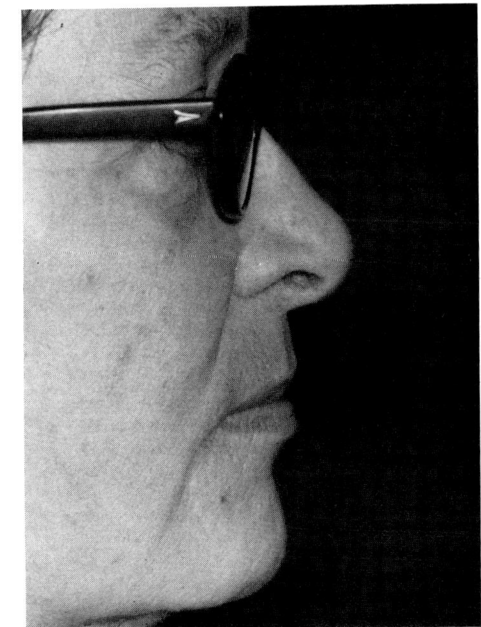

Fig. 15-2. Anterior teeth must be positioned to provide adequate support for lip and a natural appearance in profile.

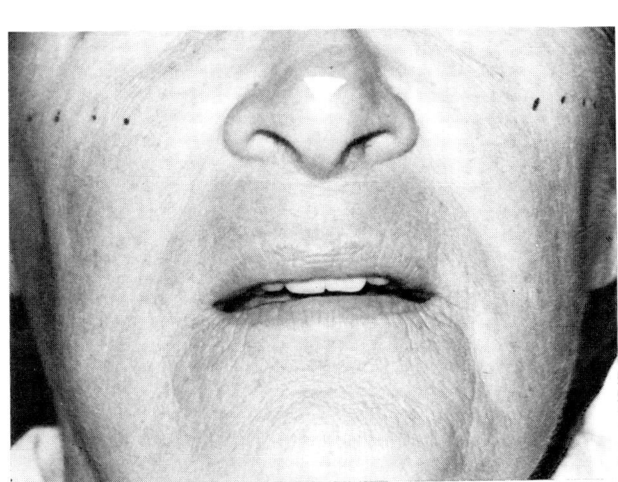

Fig. 15-3. For patient with average lip length, incisal edges of central incisors should be visible when lip is relaxed.

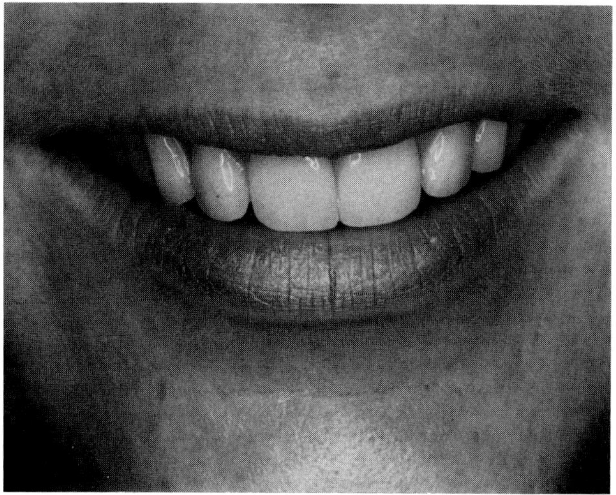

Fig. 15-4. When upper lip is in smiling position, gingival portion of denture base should just be seen. Note that slight rotation or overlapping of anterior teeth has permitted use of more normal-sized teeth in this patient, who has lost mesio-distal space because of anterior migration of remaining natural teeth.

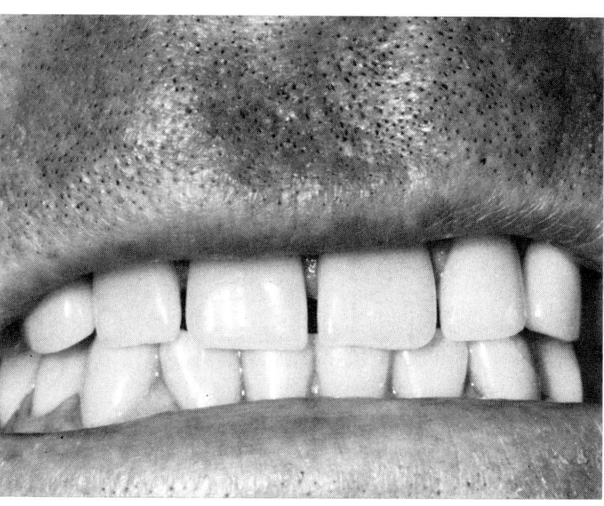

Fig. 15-5. Spacing between anterior teeth may produce natural appearance but may also cause speech problems because of air escaping between teeth.

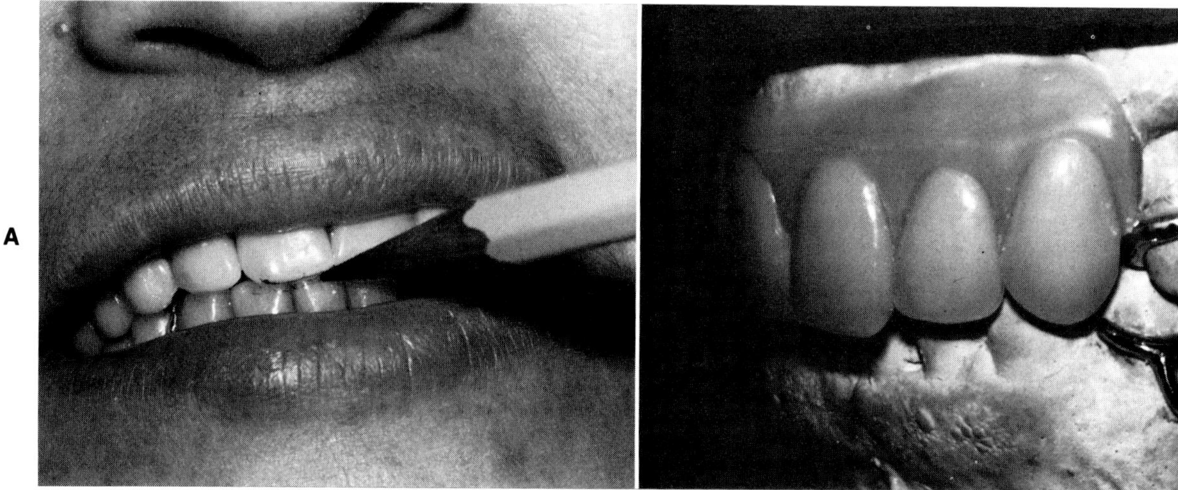

Fig. 15-6. Vertical overlap of anterior teeth, shown as measured in mouth, **A,** must be counterbalanced with sufficient horizontal overlap, as shown on articulator, **B,** to prevent undesirable tipping forçes from being transmitted to edentulous ridge.

adequate horizontal overlap. This condition could cause undesirable forces to occur on the artificial teeth and the residual ridge.

The vertical alignment of the teeth should be evaluated. A slight deviation from the vertical can produce a normal-appearing esthetic result, but a deviation of any consequence can look artificial. The midline in particular must be examined both for its vertical alignment and for its midface position (Fig. 15-7). An error in position of the midline can be extremely distracting.

As the esthetic quality of a partial denture is evaluated, the maxillary first premolar should be considered an anterior tooth because it occupies a prominent position in the arch for most patients. If the residual ridge is not resorbed excessively, the neck of the premolar tooth should be butted directly against the tissue without showing the denture base (Fig. 15-8).

Verification of the shade should be accomplished simultaneously with the evaluation of the other esthetic factors. The acceptability of the shade should be ana-

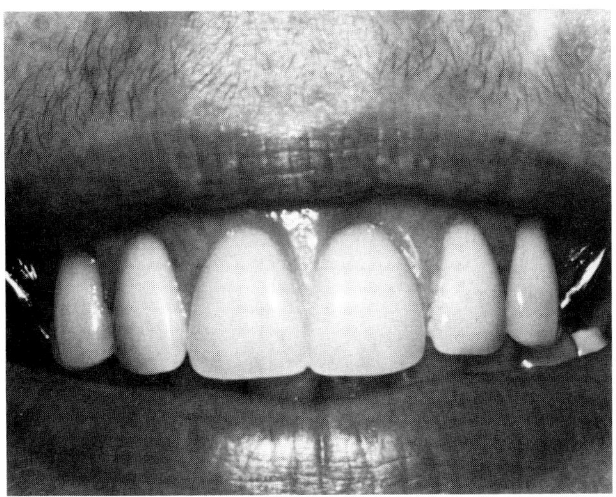

Fig. 15-7. Midline, formed by proximal surfaces of central incisors, must be in harmony with midline of face.

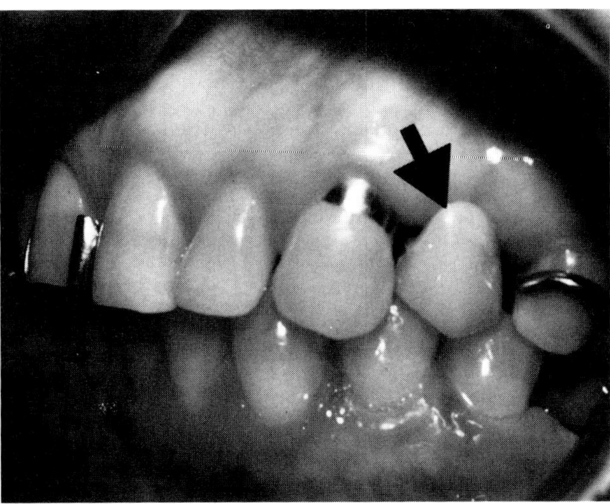

Fig. 15-8. Maxillary first premolar is considered an anterior tooth for esthetic purposes. Neck of tooth is butted directly against edentulous ridge.

lyzed in a variety of light sources. The presence of natural teeth makes the selection and approval of the shade critical and difficult.

Once the technical and mechanical requirements are satisfied, the patient should be allowed to view and comment on the results. The patient should stand several feet from a wall mirror to examine the teeth critically (Fig. 15-9). The use of a hand mirror should be discouraged because the patient's attention will be focused on individual teeth and not on the overall effect of the prosthesis. The patient's remarks should be noted carefully, and changes made in the tooth arrangement as indicated. The final satisfaction with the denture and the acceptance of the appearance must rest with the patient. Arrival at mutual acceptance by the patient and dentist frequently demands a high level of communicative skill combined with an understanding, psychologic insight.

Treatment should not proceed beyond this point until patient approval has been gained. Many practitioners insist on written patient approval.

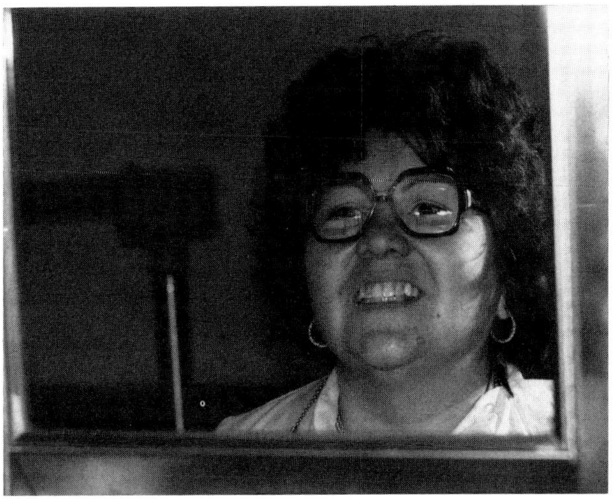

Fig. 15-9. Patient should view esthetic quality of prosthesis while standing in front of wall mirror.

VERIFICATION OF JAW RELATION

The jaw relation need be verified only in certain limited cases:

1. If, as the final jaw relation was recorded, problems were encountered handling the patient and doubt exists as to whether the recorded jaw relationship is accurate
2. If the partial denture is opposed by a complete denture
3. If all posterior teeth in both arches are being replaced
4. If there are no opposing natural teeth in contact and verification of the vertical dimension of occlusion is necessary

A dentist should never complete a prosthesis without confidence in the accuracy of the jaw relation records made to mount the casts and to set the artificial teeth. A considerable amount of unnecessary work in making corrections can be avoided if this word of caution is followed.

The procedure for verifying the jaw relation for a partial denture opposing a complete denture is included in

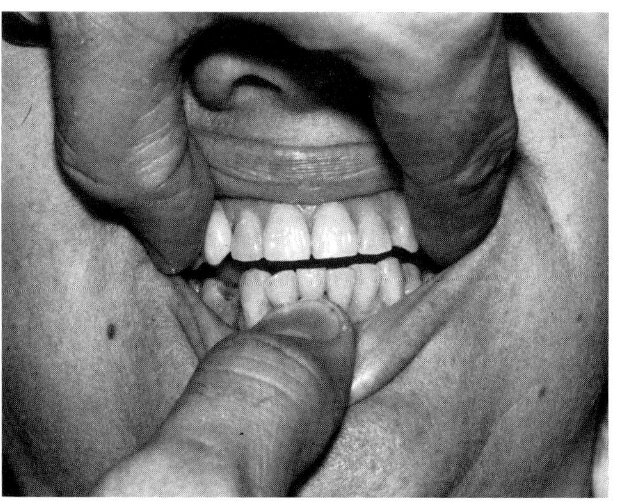

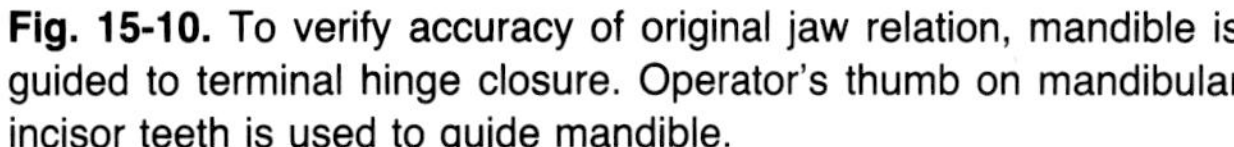

Fig. 15-10. To verify accuracy of original jaw relation, mandible is guided to terminal hinge closure. Operator's thumb on mandibular incisor teeth is used to guide mandible.

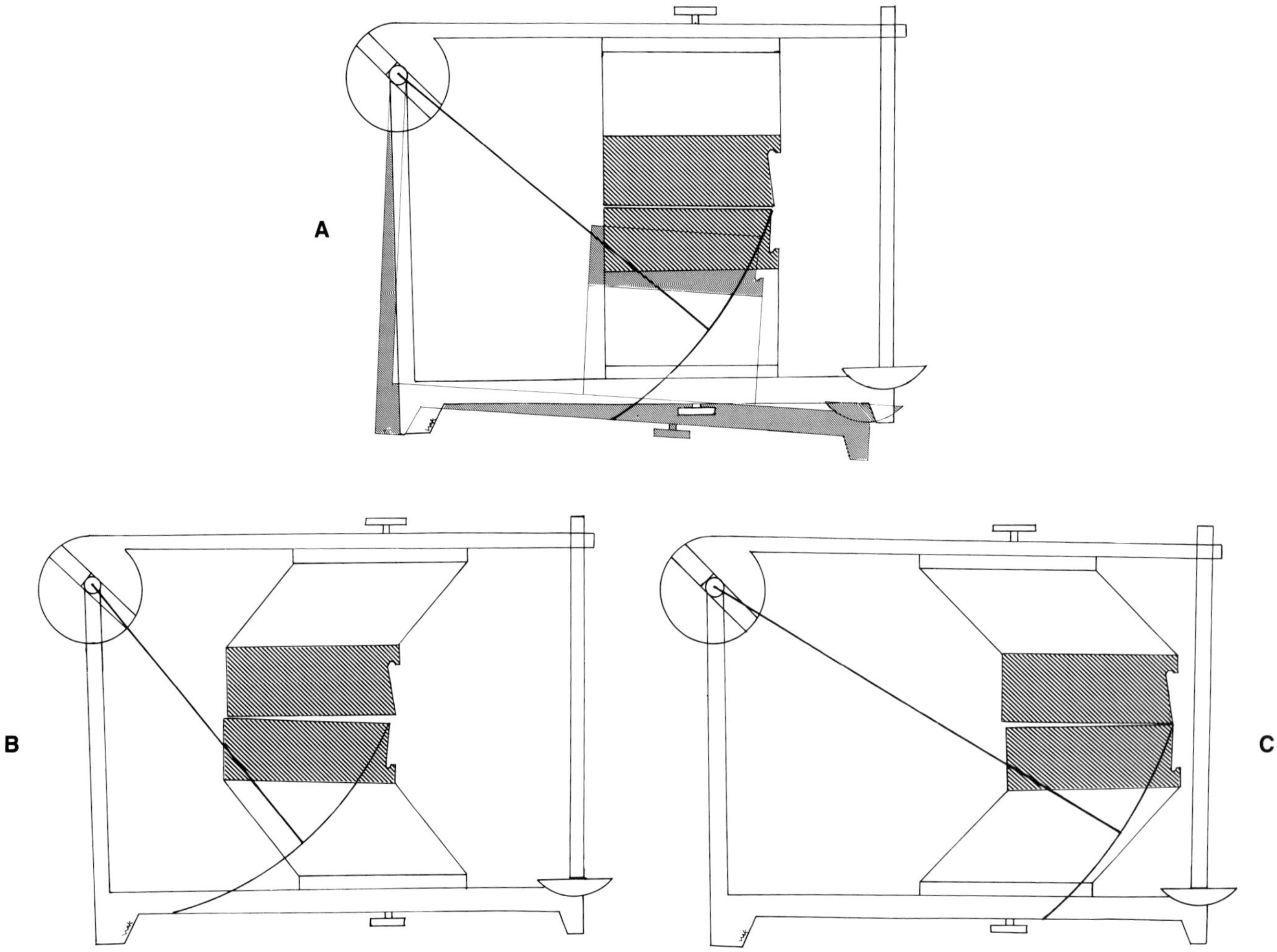

A

B

C

Fig. 15-11. A, Casts must be mounted on articulator same distance from condylar elements as jaws are from condyle in patient in order for teeth to contact correctly. **B,** If distance from condylar elements to casts is less, posterior teeth would contact first in mouth. **C,** If the distance is greater, the anterior teeth would contact first in mouth.

Chapter 19. The procedure for other partial dentures is described here.

For patients with which management difficulties were encountered during the original recording of the jaw relation either through nervousness or because of a lack of muscular control, the presence of teeth on the partial denture instead of the more cumbersome occlusion rims frequently makes the procedure less difficult. The nervous patient will tend to relax when the tongue is not encroached on, and the patient who lacks muscular coordination will often have fewer problems with the decreased bulk of the prosthesis.

Visual verification by an experienced dentist may be sufficient in some cases, but for the less experienced or to be absolutely confident in obtaining the accuracy required, verification by additional jaw relation records is essential (Fig. 15-10). Verification of centric relation is based on the premise that it is possible to transfer centric jaw relation records to an articulator, to maintain the accuracy of these records during construction of the prosthesis, and to be able to make additional centric jaw relation records that the articulator will accept accurately at a later date.

To verify the jaw relation by means other than the visual or tactile sense of the dentist, the maxillary cast must have been mounted on the articulator by means of a facebow transfer because the radius of the closing arc of the articulator must be the same as the radius of the closing arc of the patient's mandible. Otherwise the articulator will not accept a jaw relation record even though it may be completely accurate (Fig. 15-11).

The mandibular cast must also have been mounted on the articulator in centric relation. If for some reason the cast was mounted in centric occlusion, verification records cannot be made, because the position is not constantly intentionally repeatable. This is the principal reason that centric relation mountings must be used if most of the posterior occlusion is being restored.

The verification record will be made on the occlusal surfaces of the artificial teeth at a slightly increased vertical dimension of occlusion. As long as the maxillary cast is mounted correctly in relation to the condylar elements of the articulator and as long as the mandible is rotated on the terminal hinge axis in the closing movement, the increase in vertical dimension is not significant. The mandible is capable of maintaining this nontranslating rotation over an arc of 10 to 20 mm (Fig. 15-12).

Contact between opposing occlusal surfaces, either natural or artificial, must not take place. Any tooth con-

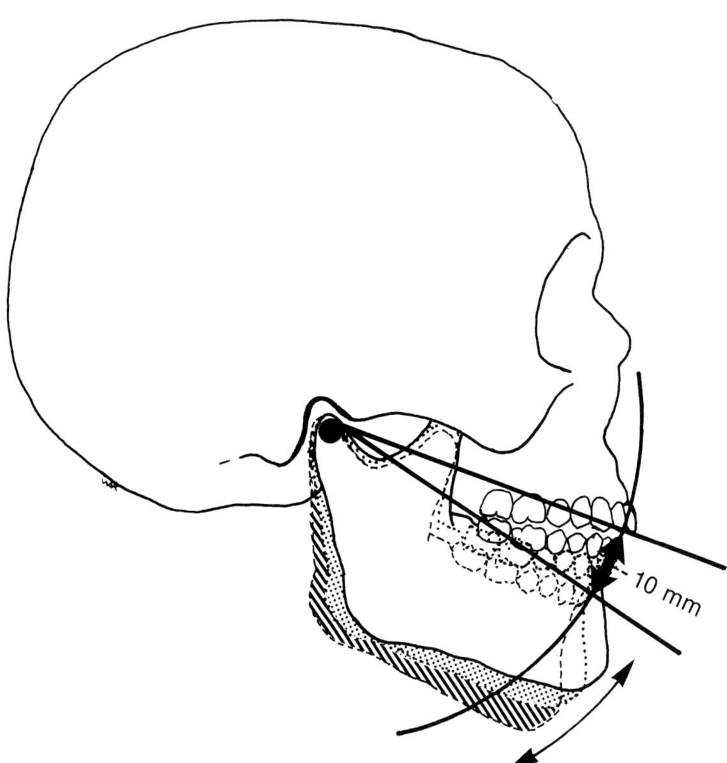

Fig. 15-12. Mandible is capable of making pure rotational movements through arc of 10 to 20 mm.

tact will result in some deviation of the mandible either by sliding on the contact or by muscular reaction to the proprioceptive mechanism in the periodontal ligament of one of the teeth involved.

Materials

The recording medium must be as pressure free as possible. Ideally the medium would be in the form of a liquid that would set to form a hard record in a short time. Obviously, confining a material such as this would be a major problem.

Materials that come closest to answering the ideal properties are zinc oxide–eugenol impression paste or Hydrocal mixed with concentrated slurry solution. Both have been described previously and the properties enumerated. They can be mixed to form a soft but firm mix that can be handled and positioned on the surfaces of the teeth without difficulty. The setting action of both is fairly fast, approximately 2 minutes, and can be accelerated if desired by adding a drop of water or alcohol at the start of the mix of the impression paste or increasing the concentration of the slurry solution. Both materials form a hard record that will resist distortion over a long period. However, a high degree of dexterity is required in using these materials. The patient must be guided to the proper mandibular position and held in that position until the material sets. The patient's mandible cannot be braced against the soft medium, and unless the patient exhibits extremely well-developed muscular coordination this technique may be beyond the ability of the patient to cooperate. The ability of the dentist may also be taxed. The mix of the material must be such that it has sufficient body not to flow uncontrollably, yet not be so thick as to offer excessive resistance. The dentist must also be capable of guiding the mandible to the terminal hinge position and maintaining that position without allowing the teeth to contact.

The use of wax to make the verification record is acceptable if all the shortcomings of the material are recognized and the deficiencies respected. Baseplace wax is difficult to soften uniformly. A temperature-controlled water bath at 63° C (145° F) (the temperature will vary some according to the hardness of the wax being used) is essential to ensure uniform softness.

Waxes containing metal particles (Aluwax containing aluminum and Cuprex containing copper) are easier to control as far as uniform softness is concerned. The metal particles make the transfer of heat quicker and smoother. This same property, however, may be a detriment because the wax remains softer and therefore is more easily distorted.

Any wax record should be used as soon as possible after it is made because wax tends to return to its original shape.

The use of modeling plastic (stick compound) as a recording medium has the same basic potential fault as wax. It is difficult to maintain thorough softness and thus be certain that pressure does not occur as the record is being made. Pressure virtually guarantees an incorrect recording.

Clinical procedure

The patient should be seated, and the partial denture tried in the mouth. Visual observation of occlusal contacts should first be made to ascertain whether gross errors are present. The patient should be permitted to wear the prosthesis for at least several minutes. Encouraging the patient to speak will hasten the time required to become accustomed to what is often a strange sensation that takes place as the denture is inserted for the first time.

Normally, if two prostheses are being constructed, the recording medium is placed on the surfaces of the mandibular teeth for convenience. However, if an insufficient number of mandibular teeth are being replaced to support a jaw relation record with enough length to stabilize the opposing cast when it is placed on the record for mounting on the articulator, the medium is placed on the maxillary prosthesis. The medium has to be slightly heavier to resist the gravitational tendency to flow.

Making wax verification record

If wax is used for the verification record, it may be in either the form of a wafer shaped to fit all the maxillary teeth or the form of narrow strips adapted to the artificial posterior teeth.

If the full-arch wafer is used (Fig. 15-13), it must be reinforced to prevent distortion. The metal-impregnated wax is available in preformed wafers with a sheet of linen incorporated on one surface of the wafer. If two of these preformed wafers are joined together with the linen surfaces contacting, the record will be well supported. If the linen-reinforced wax is not used, a double thickness of wax should be shaped to the maxillary arch and strengthened by the addition of a strip of soft metal (Ashes No. 7 metal). The strip of metal is folded over the posterior margin of the wax wafer and should extend approximately 1 inch anteriorly on both the superior and inferior surfaces of the wax.

After the wafer is formed, it is placed in a water bath for uniform softening. The metal-impregnated wax softens rapidly in 49° C (120° F) water. A baseplate wax wafer requires water at approximately 63° C (145° F) for several minutes.

After softening, the wax wafer is adapted gently to the maxillary teeth. When positioned, the wafer is supported by the thumb and index finger on each side of the arch at the premolar region. The opposite thumb is

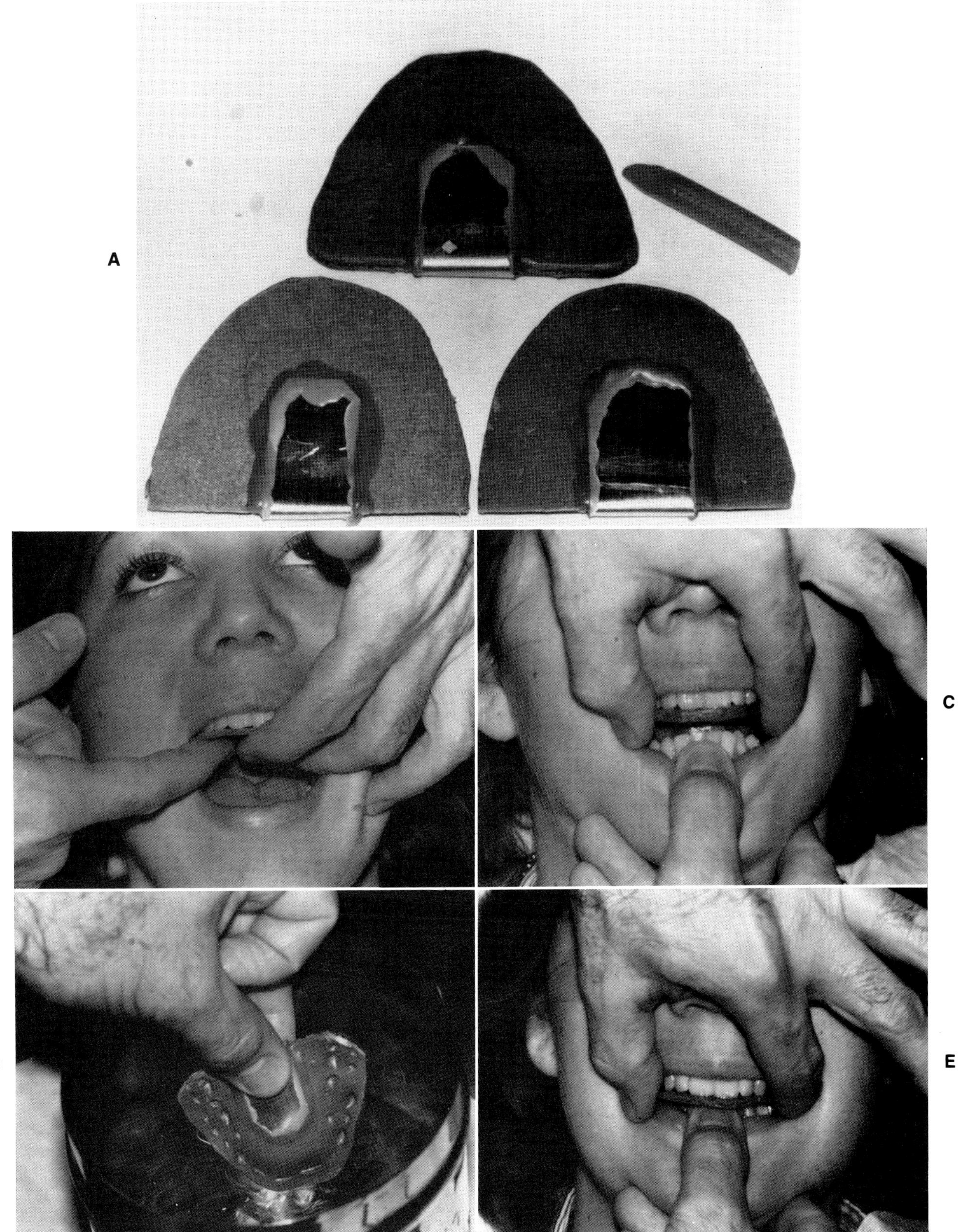

Fig. 15-13. A, Two thicknesses of Aluwax are reinforced with Ashes No. 7 metal attached to Aluwax with sticky wax. Three records are normally used for each jaw relation recording. **B,** Jaw relation record, softened in water bath, is adapted to maxillary teeth. **C,** Wax record is supported by thumb and index finger of one hand as mandible is guided to its most posterior position with other hand. **D,** Record is removed and cooled in ice water. **E,** Record is returned to mouth, and mandible guided to repeated closures. This eliminates any distortion and also verifies accuracy of record.

positioned over the gingival tissue below the mandibular central incisors and, with a firm downward and backward pressure, the mandible is retruded to its most posterior position. This movement should be rehearsed with the patient before attempting to make the verifying record. A well-prepared patient should be sufficiently relaxed to allow the operator to swing the mandible in arcing movements in the terminal hinge position. A jiggling or up-and-down movement by the operator should produce the short arcing motions. The teeth should not be allowed to contact during rehearsal and should not penetrate the wax as the recording is made.

The patient should not intentionally close the mandible; the operator must swing the mandible upward to contact the recording media.

After mandibular tooth contact with the wax wafer is made, the position should be held until the wax cools. The record should be removed and examined for sharpness of cuspal outlines. Evidence of skidding movement on the wax surface is reason to discard and reaccomplish the record.

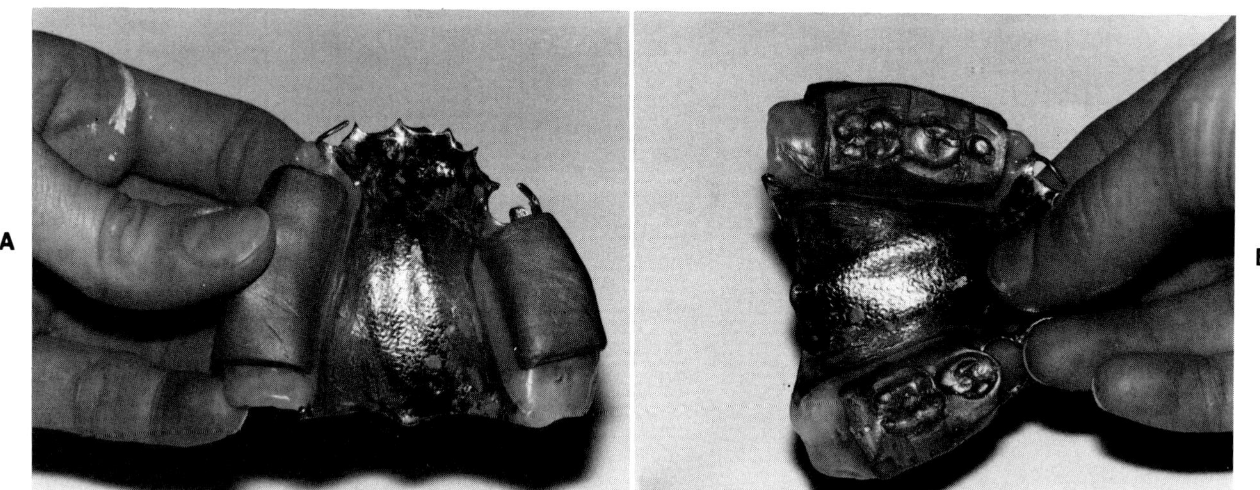

Fig. 15-14. A, Double thicknesses of Aluwax are attached over denture teeth and softened. **B,** Mandible is guided to terminal closure. Penetration of teeth through wax must not occur.

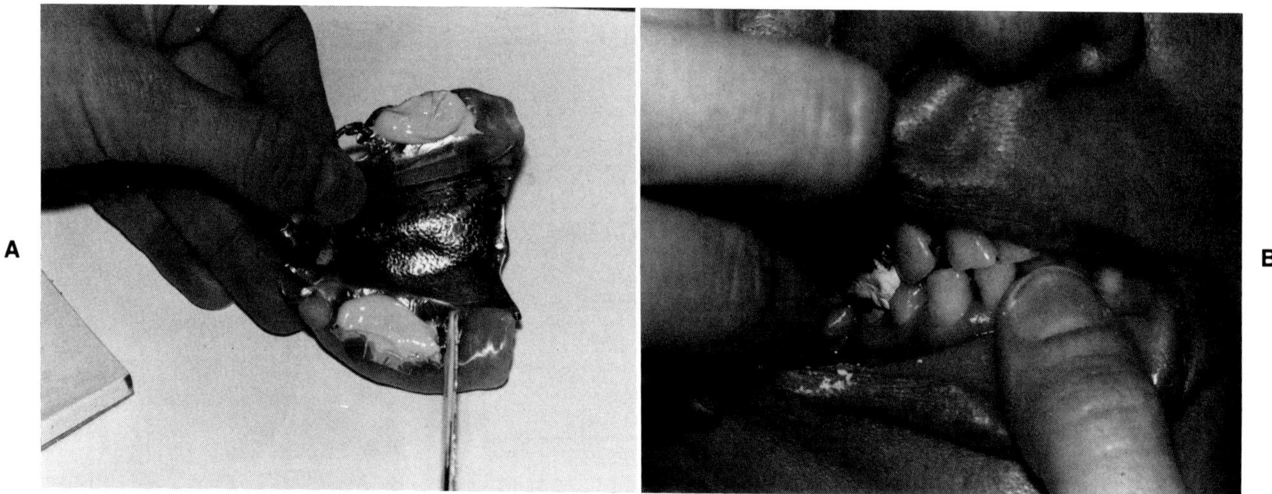

Fig. 15-15. A, Single layer of tinfoil is adapted over denture teeth. Mix of zinc oxide–eugenol paste is spread over tinfoil. **B,** Mandible is guided to its most retruded position without tooth contact occurring.

If acceptable, the record is cooled under tap water and readapted to the maxillary teeth. The mandible is again swung into contact with the record repeatedly to eliminate or correct any distortion that probably occurred as the record was removed and cooled originally. The repeated tapping of the mandibular teeth into the wafer should take place in the cuspal depressions that were made at the first closure. Multiple or varying points of contact are reason to make new records.

If narrow strips of wax adapted to the occlusal surfaces of the artificial posterior teeth are to be used instead of a wax wafer (Fig. 15-14), the partial denture should be removed from the mouth. A double thickness of wax, approximately 2 mm thick, cut in strips slightly wider buccolingually than the artificial teeth and long enough to cover all the artificial teeth anteroposteriorly is softened in the water bath.

The softened wax is quickly adapted over the occlusal surfaces of the teeth. To ensure that the wax will remain attached to the teeth, the wax should be pinched into the interproximal spaces. The partial denture must be seated quickly and the mandible guided to its terminal position and light closure of the mandibular teeth accomplished. Closure is maintained until the wax has cooled.

The partial denture with the record attached is removed and cooled under tap water. Examination of the record should be made for evidence of tooth contact through the record. If contact has been made, the record must be reaccomplished. If the record is acceptable, it may be reinserted and visually verified that the teeth are repeatedly closing into the cuspal imprints.

Making impression paste or Hydrocal verification record

If zinc oxide–eugenol impression paste is to be used, a single thickness of tinfoil should be adapted over the teeth that will support the paste (Fig. 15-15). The occlusal surfaces of the opposing teeth should be coated lightly with a separating medium such as petrolatum. If hydrocal and concentrated slurry solution are used, separating medium is not needed. Moisture from the saliva will be sufficient.

The partial denture is removed from the mouth. A mix of the material is made, and a layer of the material 3 to 4 mm high is placed over the occlusal surfaces of the artificial teeth. The partial denture is reseated quickly, and the mandible guided to the retruded position. Constant pressure must be maintained by the operator to keep the mandible in the correct position while the medium is setting. There will be a tendency on the part of the patient to close the teeth together. This must be avoided.

After the material has set, the mandible should be swung downward to break contact between the teeth and the record. The mandible should be opened still on the terminal arc to prevent damaging the record.

The partial denture should be removed and excess material trimmed from the record. The surface of the record should be carefully trimmed with a sharp knife so that only the cusp tips are shown on the record (Fig. 15-16).

The partial denture with record attached can be inserted in the patient's mouth and the record visually verified for accuracy. Evidence of opposing cusp tips sliding as the cuspal indentations in the record are ap-

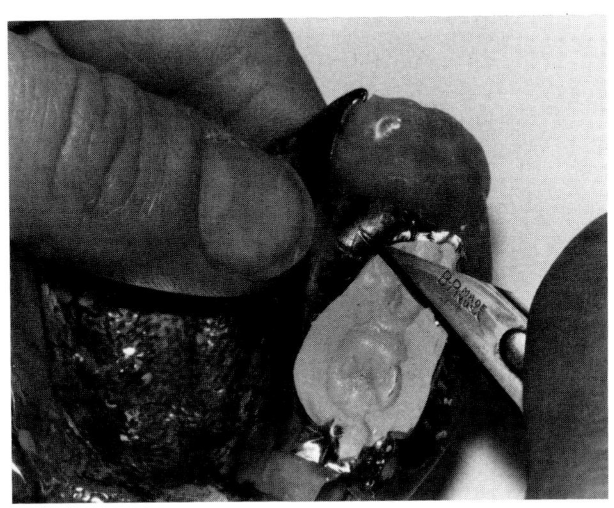

Fig. 15-16. Record is trimmed to show indentations of cusp tips only.

proached indicates that the record should be reaccomplished.

Verifying accuracy of articulator mounting

There are two commonly accepted methods of verifying the accuracy of the articulator mounting: by observing the position of the condyle balls on the articulator in relation to the condyle stops or by the split cast technique. The procedures are illustrated in Figs. 15-17 to 15-19.

The basic idea of the two techniques is the same; the variance is the point at which the accuracy is checked.

The split cast technique is more precise. For this reason it should be selected for those patients exhibiting a high degree of muscular coordination and mental cooperation.

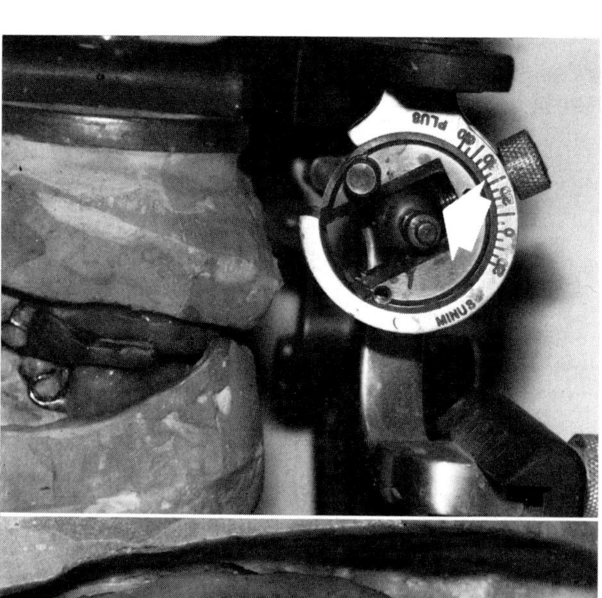

A

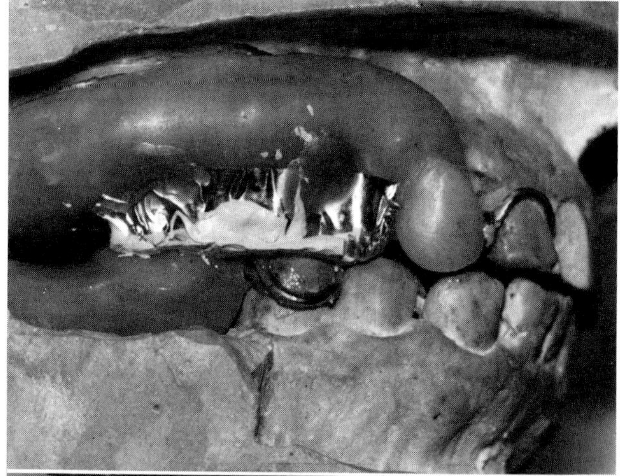

B

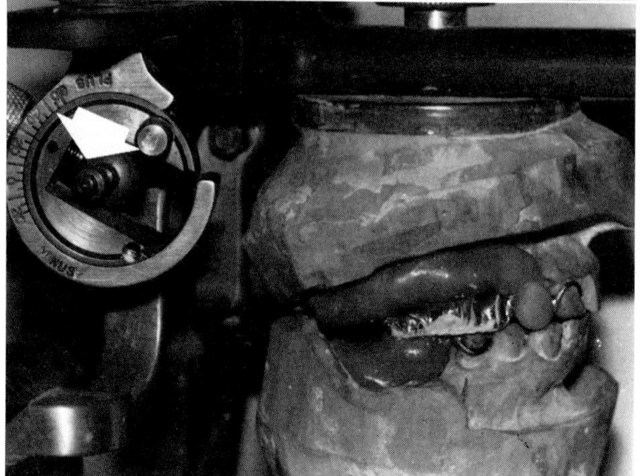

C

Fig. 15-17. Verification of articulator mounting by condylar ball position. **A,** Condyle locks on articulator are loosened so that condyle ball is free to move in condyle slot. **B,** Opposing denture teeth and stone teeth on cast are seated firmly in record. **C,** Positions of both condyle balls are noted. If one or both balls are not in contact with condyle stops, articulator mounting is not verified as being correct. If both condyle balls are contacting condyle stops, original articulator mounting is verified as being correct.

If the original mounting is not verified as being correct, another jaw relation record must be made. If this new record verifies the original mounting, the first verification record was inaccurate and the original mounting was correct. The occlusion may now be refined on the articulator and the partial denture completed.

If, however, the second record does not verify the original mounting, it must be assumed that the original mounting was incorrect. In this case the second record is used to remount the mandibular cast in a new centric relation position.

This new position must not be presumed to be correct until it has been verified by an additional record. Refinement of the occlusion and completion of the prosthesis should not be undertaken until verification is complete regardless of the number of remounts required.

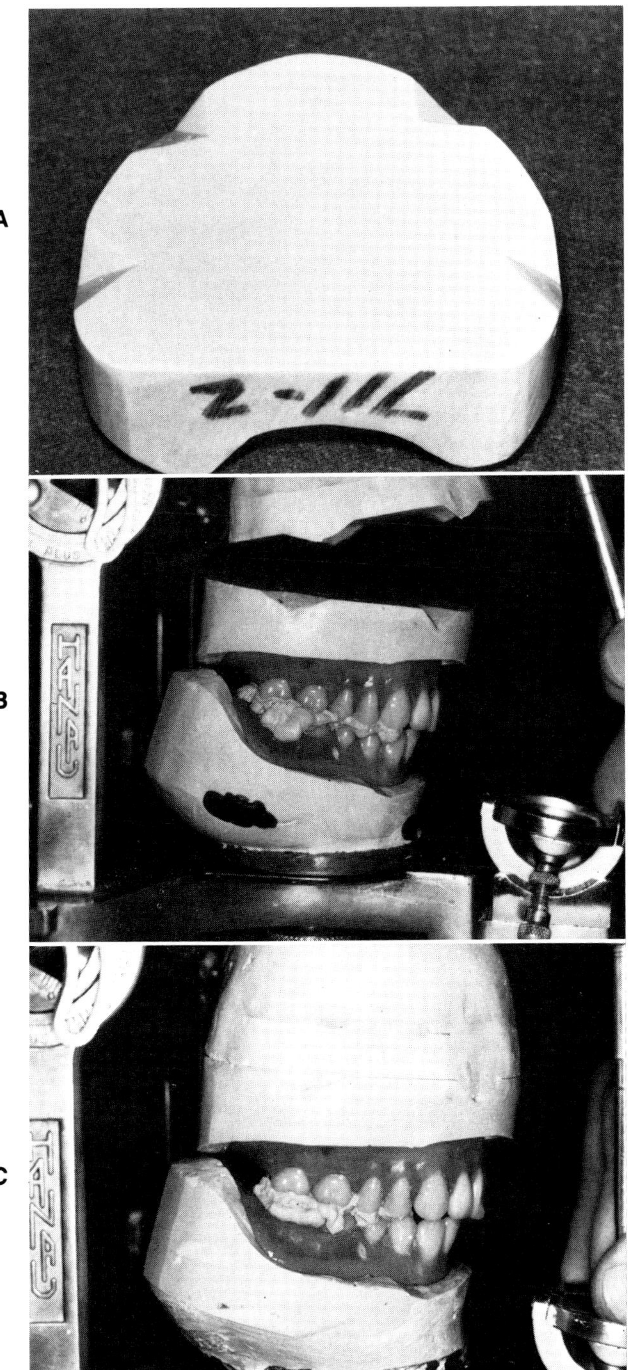

Fig. 15-18. Split cast technique with V-shaped grooves. **A,** Several V-shaped notches are made in base of maxillary master cast before mounting on articulator. Separating medium is painted over base of cast. **B,** Cast is separated from its mounting stone and jaw relation record made. **C,** With maxillary denture seated in jaw relation record, V-shaped projections of mounting stone fit accurately into notches on base of cast. This verifies original mounting as being correct.

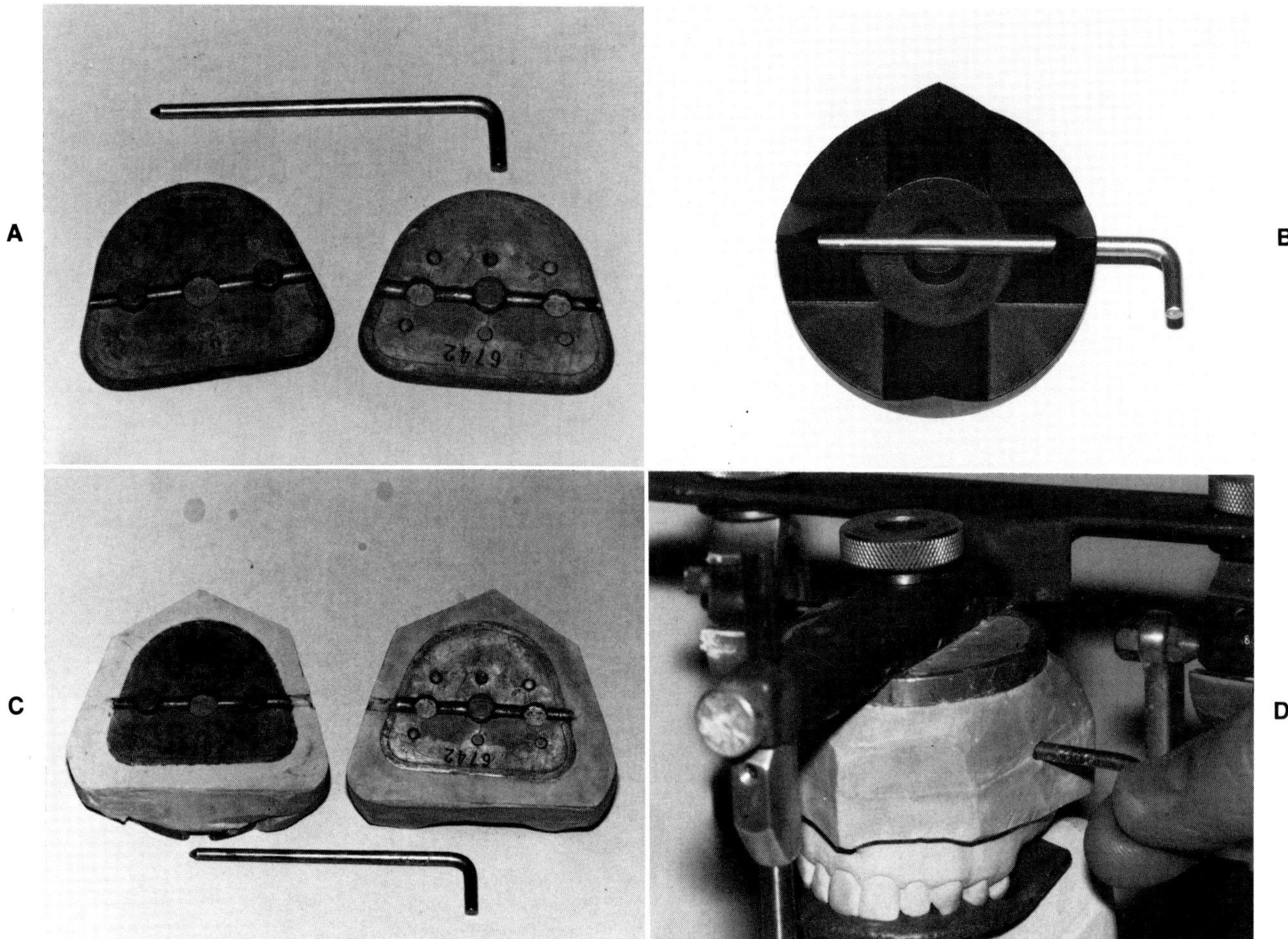

Fig. 15-19. Split cast technique with metal mounting plates. **A,** Metal mounting plates for split cast mounting technique. **B,** Pin slides through groove, locking plates together. **C,** One plate is embedded in base of cast when cast is poured. Other plate is embedded in mounting stone on articulator. **D,** Verification of original mounting is made when maxillary cast is seated on jaw relation record, articulator closed, and pin slides through its groove, engaging the two mounting plates.

Length of appointment

Depending on the difficulty encountered, the experienced practitioner should accomplish the clinical procedures in approximately 15 minutes. The dental student will usually require 45 minutes.

LABORATORY PROCEDURES REQUIRED TO COMPLETE THE REMOVABLE PARTIAL DENTURE

Waxing the denture base contour

The contour of the denture base should be such that it will add, not detract from, the retentive quality of the prosthesis. Excessive bulk of acrylic resin or overextension of denture flanges contributes to the lack of stability or retention of the partial denture. An improperly formed denture base adds to the undesirable forces on abutment teeth.

If a corrected cast impression has been made of the edentulous ridge, the proper peripheral extensions have been determined and the possibility of overextension of the denture flange is lessened (Fig. 15-20).

In general, the contour of the denture base for a partial denture is the same as for a complete denture. The main difference lies in waxing to and around parts of the metal framework. The advisability of having established definite finish lines in the metal becomes obvious as the wax is butted against the metal (Fig. 15-21).

If finish lines are not sharp, definite, and slightly undercut, the metal-to-plastic joint will be difficult to locate. Acrylic resin should never be finished to a fine edge because it lacks strength, and over a period of time will separate from the metal with resulting seepage of oral fluids and discoloration of the plastic in that area (Fig. 15-22).

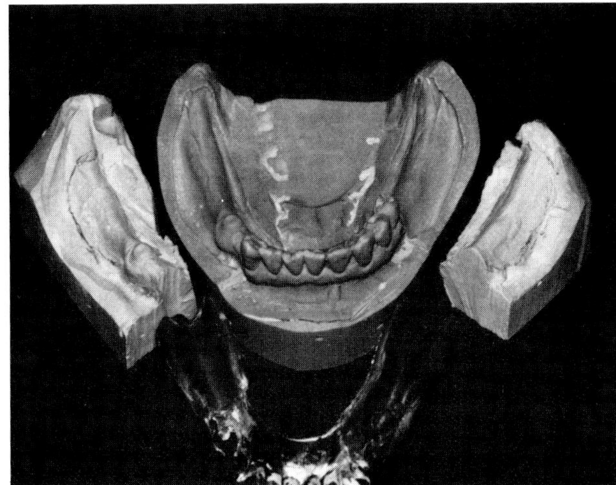

Fig. 15-20. Corrected cast impression reduces possibility of denture base flange overextension.

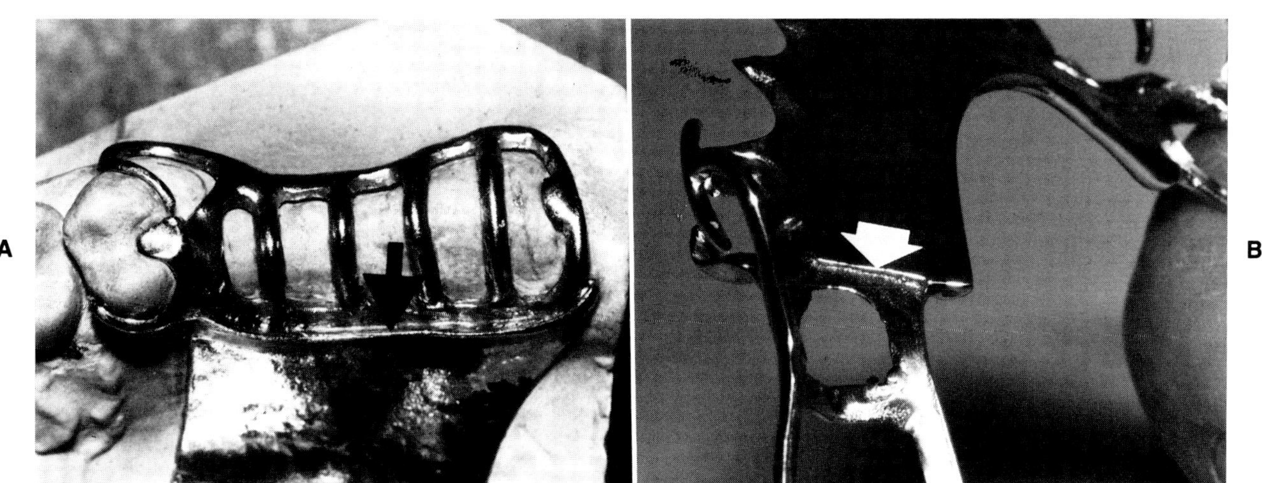

Fig. 15-21. Denture base is waxed to definite lines that were created in metal framework: external finish line, **A,** and the internal line, **B.**

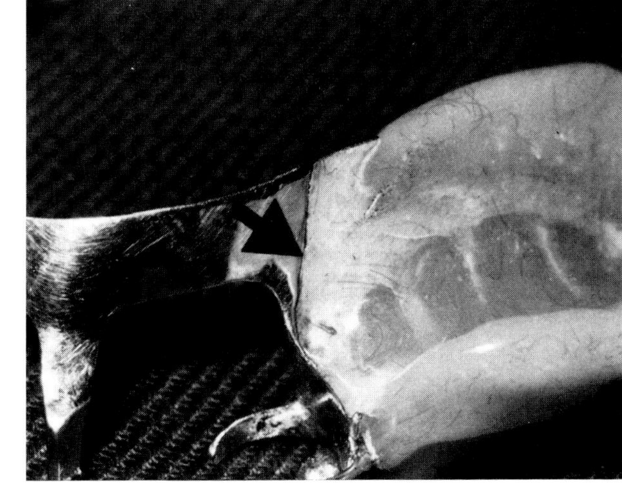

Fig. 15-22. If definite finish lines are not provided in metal, margins of acrylic resin may be too thin for adequate strength.

As one waxes to external finish lines, the wax should be left with sufficient bulk to allow for the loss of resin that will take place during the finishing and polishing phases. The height of the resin should never be below the height of the metal (Fig. 15-23).

On metal parts not having a finish line, such as minor connectors and the approach arm of vertical projection clasps, the wax should be left thick enough so that the resin will have sufficient bulk to avoid separation and seepage. Slightly roughening the metal that will be covered by resin may enhance mechanical retention of the resin (Fig. 15-24).

Gingival contour should be waxed in accordance with anatomic concepts and with the purpose of providing self-cleansing properties. The majority of prosthodontic patients will be in the middle to older age groups and as such should exhibit the normal degree of gingival recession that is expected of that age. One of the most frequent errors in waxing the gingival form around the artificial teeth is failing to keep the height of the gingival contour compatible with that of adjacent natural teeth (Figs. 15-25 and 15-26). This is particularly critical for anterior and premolar teeth. Frush and Fisher (1955) have offered several rules for determining the height of the gingival contour at various positions. For the central incisors the gingival height should be slightly below the high lip line. For the lateral incisors it should be slightly lower than the central incisors, and at the canine it should be higher than either of the incisors. At the premolars the gingival height should be lower than the canine, and it should be variable for the remaining premolars and molars.

Directly below the gingival contour of the posterior teeth a slight bulge should be waxed to act as a secondary food table to help the tongue control the bolus of food (Fig. 15-27).

Between the gingival bulge and the periphery of the denture base, a slight concavity should be provided for the soft tissues of the cheek and fibers of the buccinator muscle to fold into and prevent dislodging action from taking place.

The width of the peripheral roll should be maintained if it was developed by a secondary impression. If a secondary impression was not made, the border should be approximately 2 mm thick. If the limit of the border flange is not obvious, as in a tooth-supported segment, it is better to overwax in both length and thickness of the flange (Fig. 15-28). The final adjust-

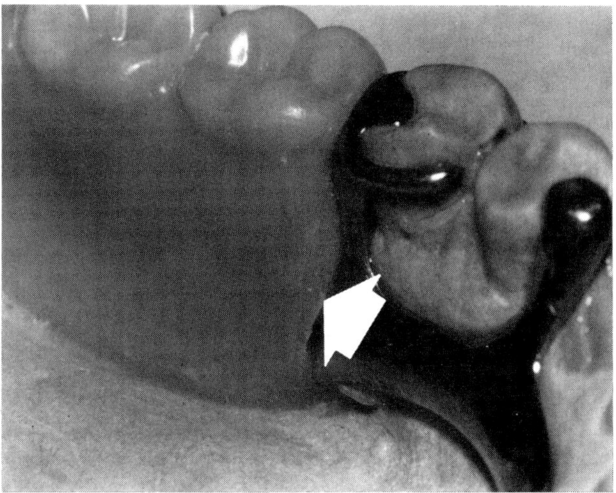

Fig. 15-23. At external finish line, wax is left slightly above height of metal. This provides for slight loss of acrylic resin that will take place during polishing procedure.

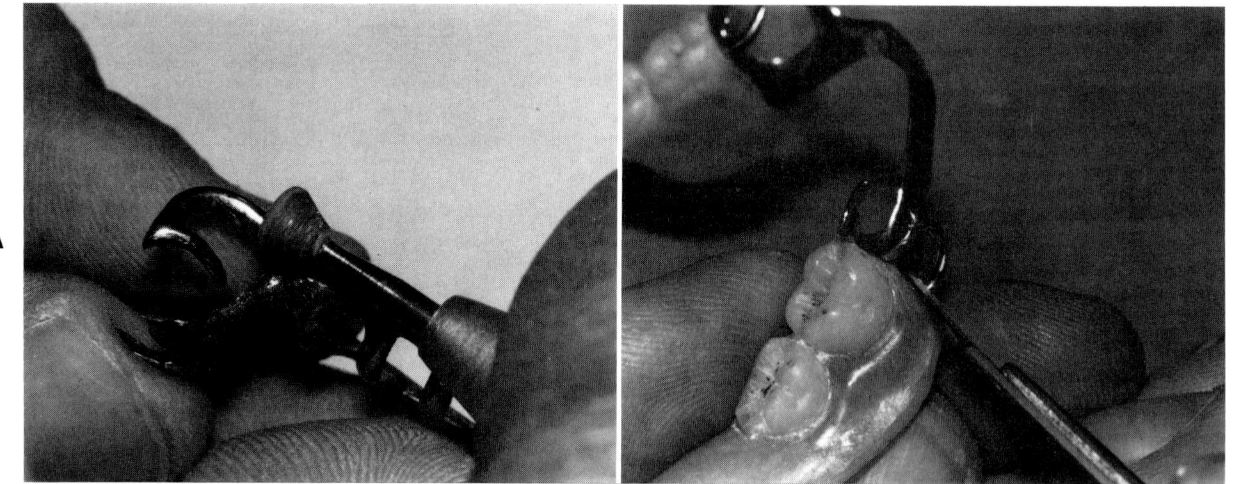

Fig. 15-24. A, Metal of approach arm for vertical projection clasp is roughened slightly with mounted point to aid in retention of acrylic resin. **B,** Resin is finished to sharp margin against approach arm.

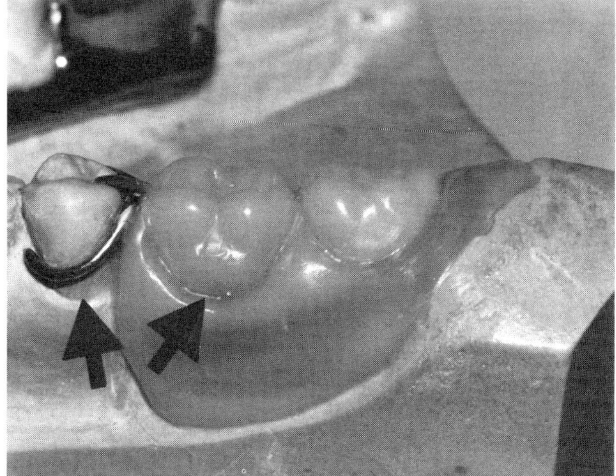

Fig. 15-25. Gingival height of artificial teeth should be compatible with that of natural teeth.

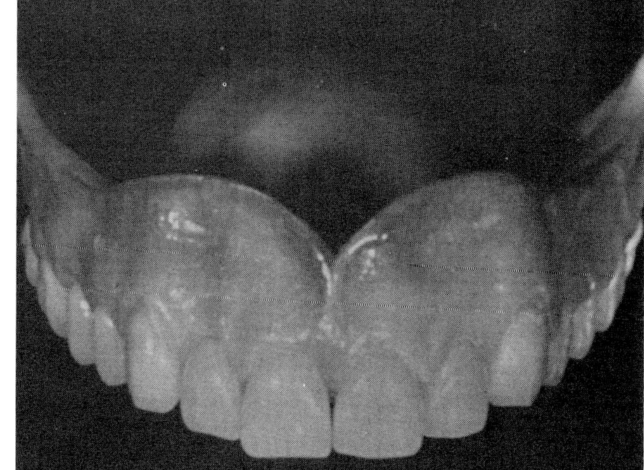

Fig. 15-26. Height of gingival contour of anterior teeth varies from central incisors, to lateral incisors, to canines.

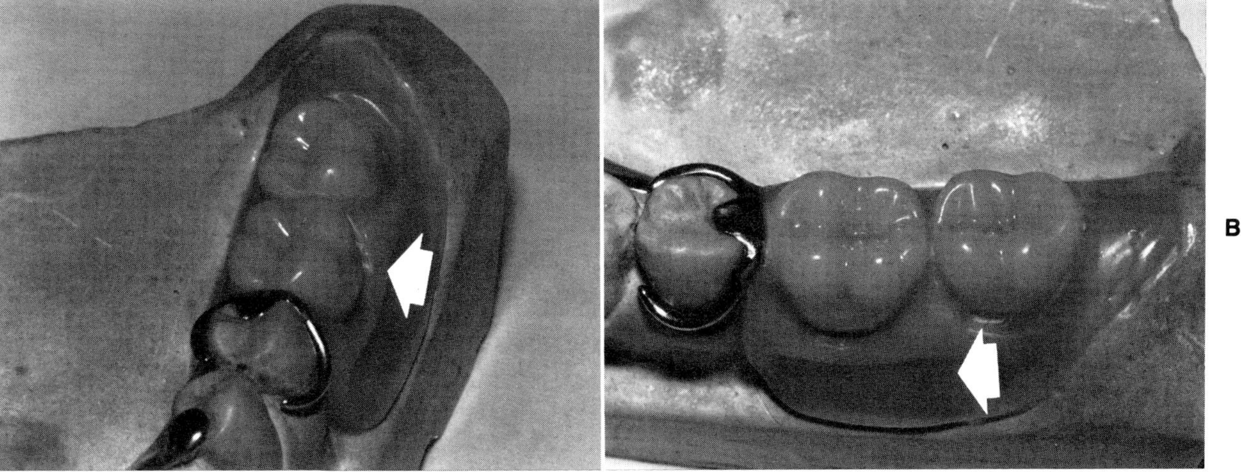

Fig. 15-27. A, A slight bulge, or convexity, is waxed below gingival contour to act as secondary food table. **B,** A concavity is carved below bulge to accommodate fibers of buccinator muscle.

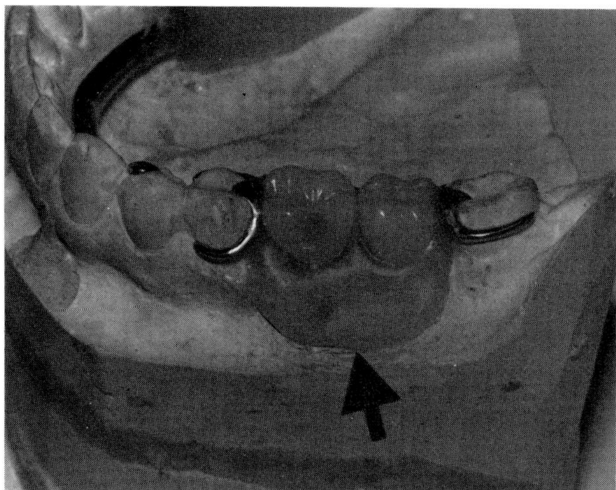

Fig. 15-28. For tooth-supported segment, denture base flange is waxed just short of reflection of soft tissue.

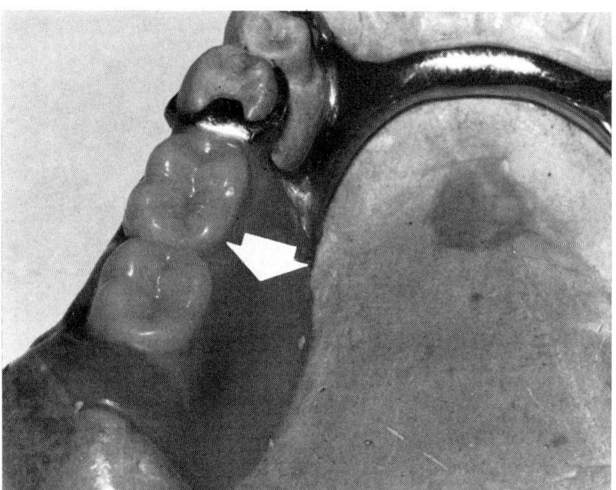

Fig. 15-29. A slight concavity is waxed in posterior lingual flange of mandibular denture base.

ments may be made at the time of insertion of the prosthesis.

Mandibular lingual posterior flanges should be waxed with a definite lingual concavity (Fig. 15-29). This will allow more space for the tongue and will contribute to retention of the denture by avoiding crowding of the tongue.

The waxing of the partial denture base should be refined to as high degree as possible to avoid the necessity of lengthy and complicated finishing and polishing procedures. The possibility of damaging the framework is always present when cloth and brush wheels are used on the lathe during polishing procedures, which might not be needed if the waxing is done properly.

Two areas of the denture base will need modifying by the dentist at the time of final polishing: the distobuccal flanges of an upper denture base (to avoid interferences with the coronoid process of the mandible) and the distolingual extension of the lower denture base (to provide more room for tongue movement).

Procedure for contouring denture base

1. Make certain the artificial teeth are firmly waxed in position.
2. Soften small pieces of baseplate wax over the Bunsen burner and mold them in position around the teeth and over the edentulous ridge (Fig. 15-30). Make certain they are well adapted to exposed portions of the framework. This technique of finger molding or sculpturing the denture base has several advantages.
   a. It decreases the time required for adding wax to the denture base.
   b. Better control can be maintained over the wax than if it is melted and flowed on.
   c. As the wax is added it is also positioned, which reduces the time required for carving it to form.
   d. If wax is melted and flowed on the cast, the chances of the artificial teeth being moved increases. This movement of teeth caused by adding hot wax is the most frequent cause of occlusal interferences in the finished partial denture.
3. On the distal extension edentulous ridge be sure that a minimum thickness of 2 mm is maintained at the periphery of the denture base. The periphery should be finished to a definite rolled margin.
4. Establish the buccal extension of the base of a tooth-supported segment arbitrarily approximately 5 mm below the gingival margin of the artificial tooth. The final shaping of this flange is normally accomplished at the insertion appointment.
5. Carve gingival contour in harmony with the adjacent natural teeth. Special care in finishing the wax around the teeth should be taken because it is *much more difficult* to finish and polish the denture base *around plastic teeth* than it is around porcelain teeth.
6. Accomplish final contouring and smoothing of the buccal and lingual flanges with emphasis on developing a slight concavity, particularly of the lingual flange.
7. When finishing and polishing of the wax is complete, return the master cast to the articulator and make a final check of the occlusion. Be certain that none of the teeth moved during the waxing procedure.

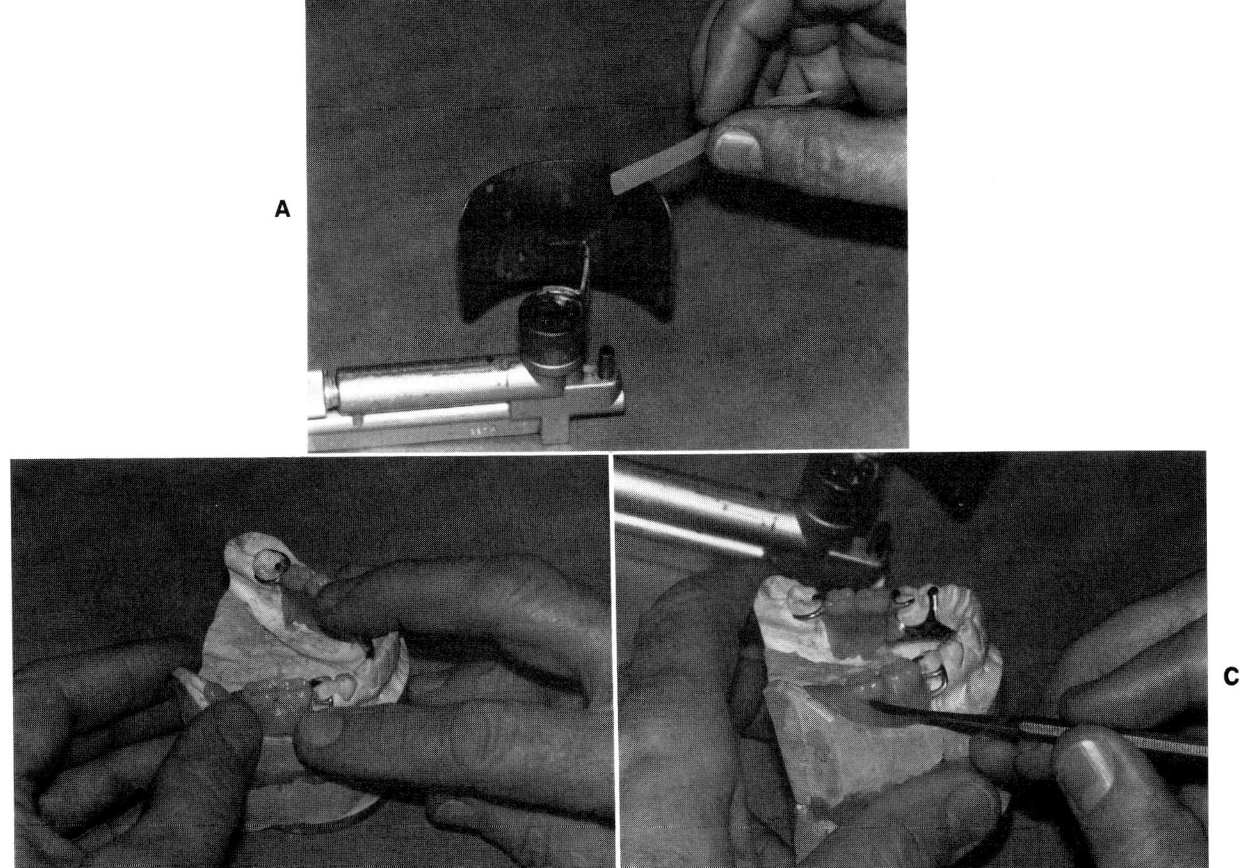

Fig. 15-30. Small pieces of baseplate wax are softened over burner, **A,** and finger molded to form denture base, **B. C,** Final shaping of wax is accomplished with wax instruments.

Investing the partial denture

There are currently several methods of investing a partial denture in preparation for processing the acrylic resin denture bases.

Single-step investing

There are single-step investments, both hydrocolloid and solid material, in which the denture may be invested. The cast with the partial denture is recovered by splitting the investment and eliminating the wax. The cast with the framework and artificial teeth are replaced in the mold and the mold reassembled. Liquid resin is flowed into the mold through previously established sprue holes. The resin used is normally autopolymerizing, and the processing is usually accomplished under warm water and air pressure.

Processing dentures with this technique offers several advantages. First, considerable time is saved as opposed to the conventional method of flasking with Hydrocal; the recovery time is lessened markedly, and little or no finishing is required. In addition, little processing error in the form of increasing the vertical dimension of occlusion, which occurs routinely with conventional processing, is noted.

The reason that this single-pour investing and processing technique has not received wider acceptance is probably that the resin in use when the procedure was first introduced was not reliable. The impact strength of the resin was low, and denture breakage a much too frequent occurrence. A persistent problem was also present in the fact that the denture teeth were often depressed below the original plane of occlusion in the finished denture.

These problems have for the most part been solved with the advent of new resin and improvement in the investment materials. It seems logical that wider acceptance of the technique should follow.

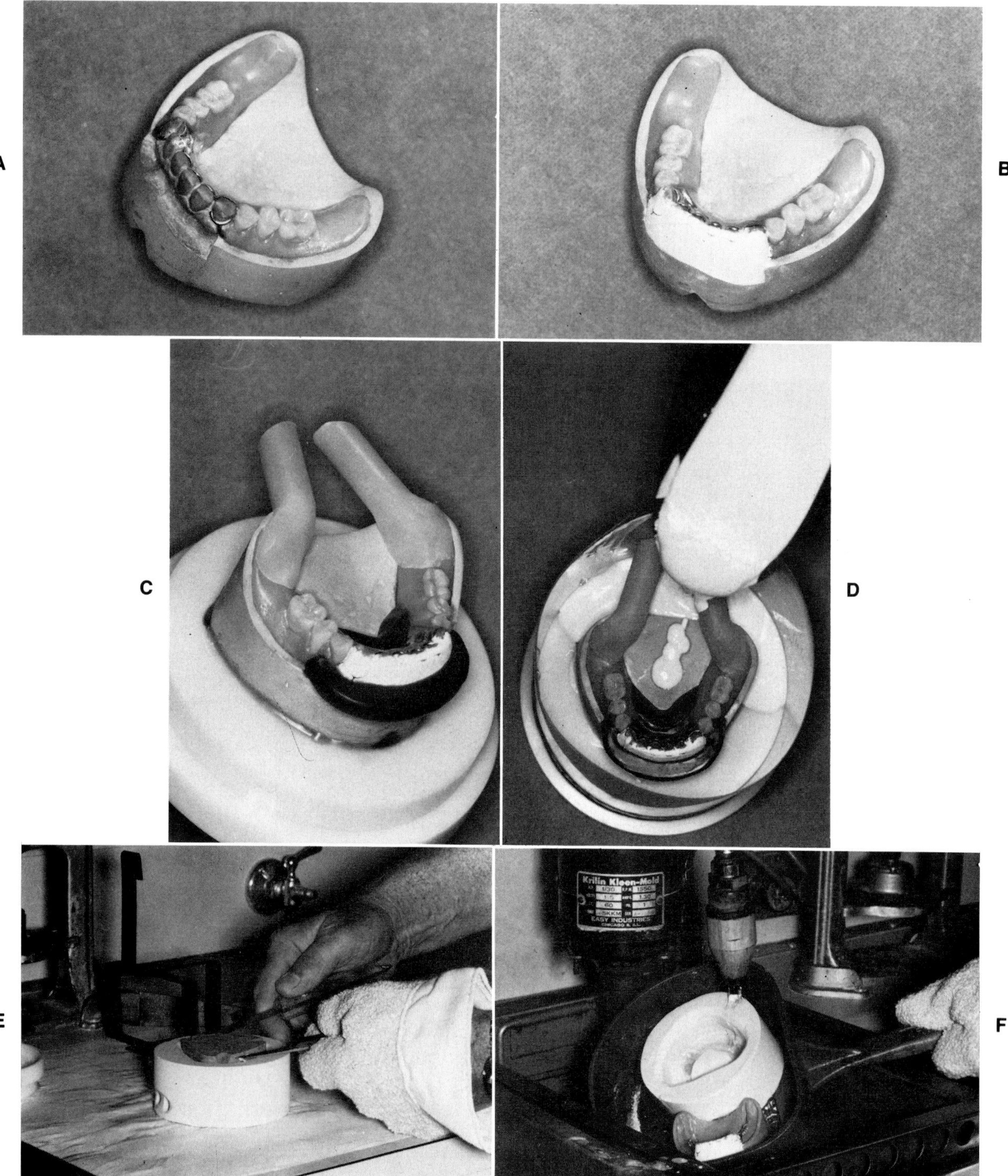

Fig. 15-31. Processing a removable partial denture in rigid mold with popular fluid resin system (Dentsply Maxum Fluid Resin System, Dentsply International Inc., 500 West College Avenue, York, Pa. 17405). **A,** Bilateral distal extension removable partial denture has been waxed for processing. **B,** Anterior undercuts are blocked out with plaster. **C,** Wax sprues have been attached. **D,** Sprued denture is invested in plastic "flask" with modified gypsum investing material. **E,** After investment has set, mold is heated in boiling water. Cast is then carefully removed. **F,** Wax is flushed from rigid mold by conventional procedures. (Courtesy Richard A. Smith, D.D.S., Director, Professional Research, Dentsply Inter., Inc., York, Pa.)

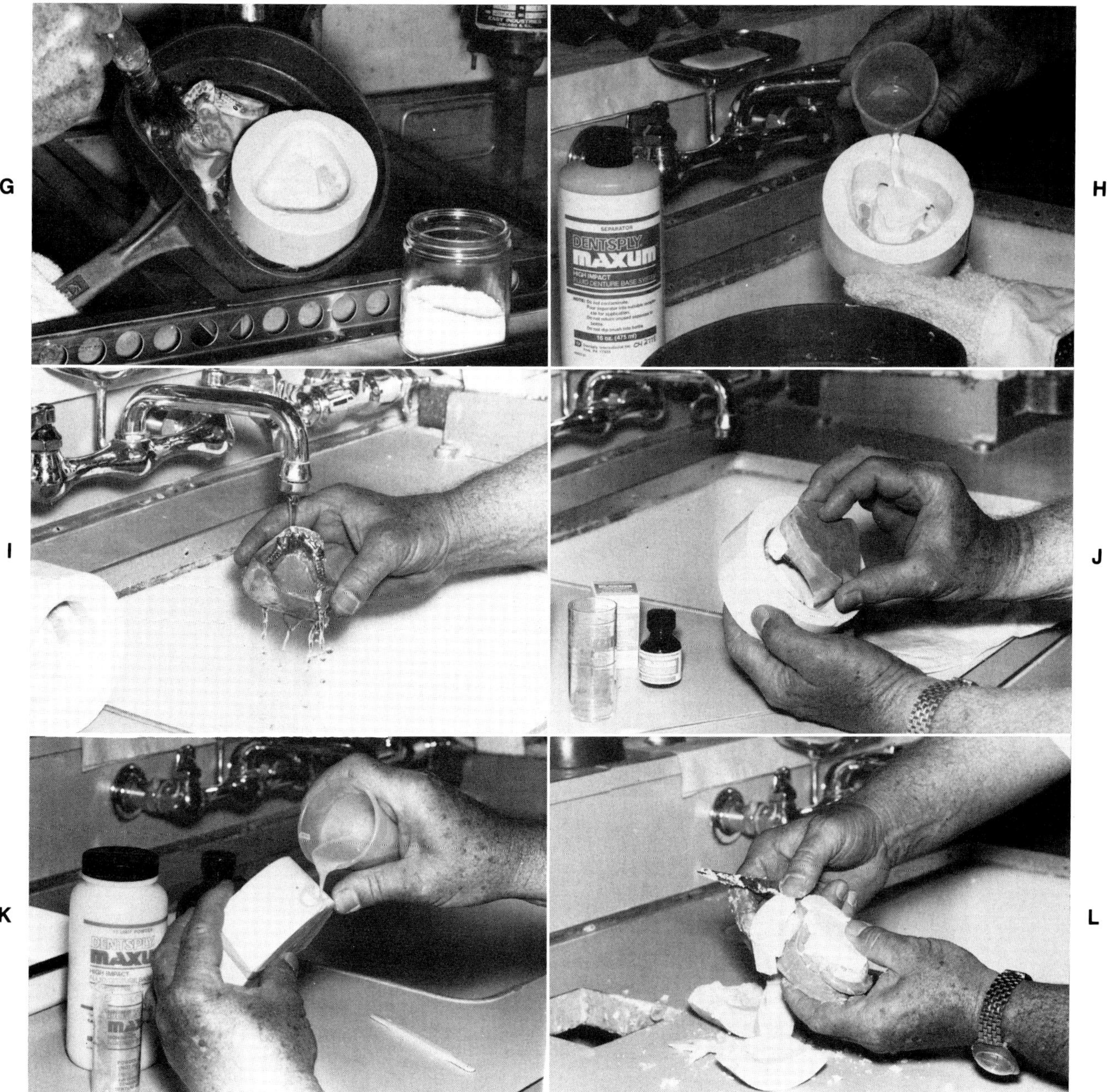

Fig. 15-31, cont'd. G, Mold, cast, teeth, and so on are scrubbed with powdered soap and water, then rinsed with clean, hot water to ensure cleanliness. **H,** Separating medium is applied. **I,** Separator is carefully rinsed from both mold and cast. **J,** Following draining and drying of separator, and a short water bath to rehydrate and cool mold, cast is repositioned in mold. **K,** Fluid resin is mixed as per manufacturer's instructions, and poured into mold. **L,** After processing, partial denture is readily recovered from "soft stone" mold.

Continued.

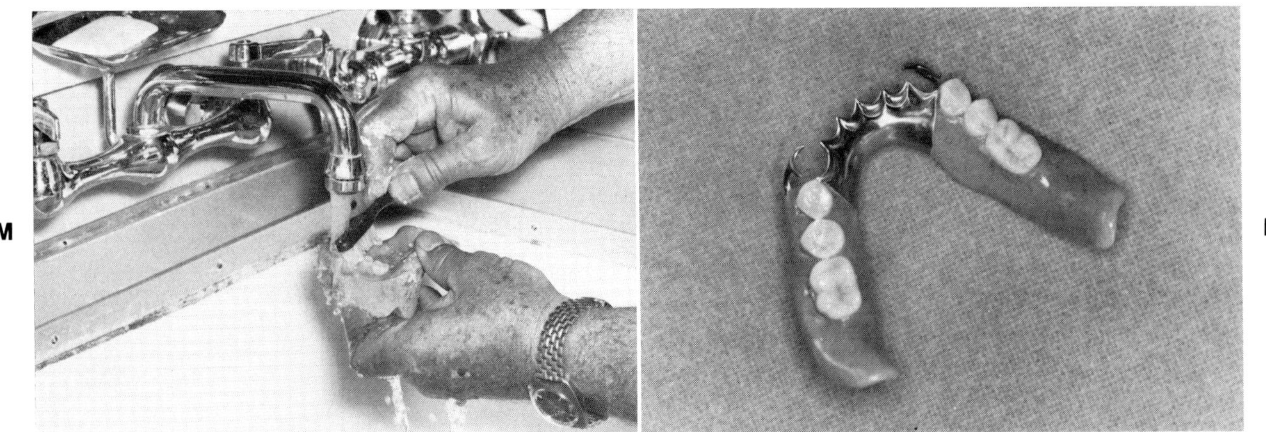

Fig. 15-31, cont'd. M, Remaining investment is easily removed with a toothbrush and water. **N,** After sprues are removed, finishing requires little more than removal of "flash" from the periphery and polishing.

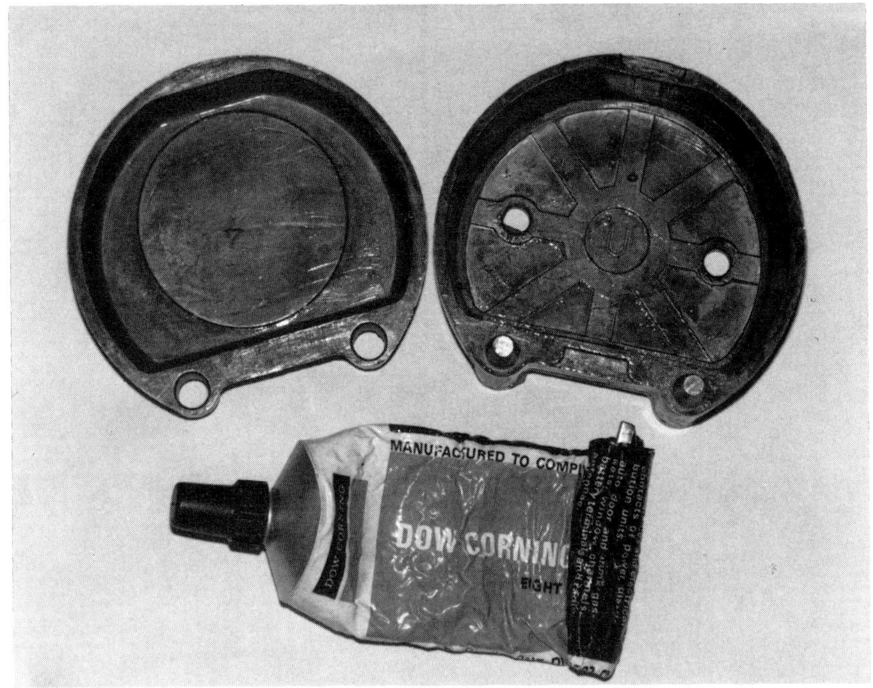

Fig. 15-32. Hanau denture-processing flasks. To prevent oxidation of the metal, a light coat of silicone ointment is applied.

Each manufacturer provides instructions for using these single-step investments (Fig. 15-31).

Split-mold investing

The purpose of investing the master cast and partial denture in Hydrocal is to provide a smooth, dense mold in which the acrylic resin may be forced under high pressure to accurately reproduce the refined wax contour of the denture base. Because of the amount of pressure used to force the resin into place, less dense investment material such as plaster of paris or a mixture of plaster of paris and Hydrocal should not be substituted. As the resin is processed after being packed in the mold, some dimensional change in the resin will occur. Using a less dense gypsum material as the investing medium will multiply the amount of processing error and may lead to errors that cannot be corrected. Commercial laboratories at times invest with plaster of paris on the mistaken belief that the denture can be recovered easier. However, if the correct investment procedure is followed, recovering the partial denture from the investment mold is not a difficult process.

As the term *split-mold* implies, the investment flask, after it is opened, will contain the master cast with the framework in place in the lower half of the flask and the artificial teeth in the upper half. Although this method of investing requires special care when the resin is packed, it is safer than transferring the framework and the teeth to the upper half of the flask. The latter method is fraught with possibilities of damaging the framework.

Preparing flasks. The flasks used for investing the denture must be kept in good condition (Fig. 15-32). The assembled empty flask should not rock when alternating forces are applied to the upper half of the flask. Unless there is solid metal-to-metal contact between the two halves, the force applied to compress the resin will not be distributed evenly and portions of the denture base may be compressed excessively and portions undercompressed.

The flasks should be coated lightly with a lubricant, silicone ointment or petrolatum, between uses to prevent oxidation, which would eventually alter the fit of the components.

First investment layer. Investing the partial denture for processing an acrylic resin denture base is done in four steps. The first step, or pour (Fig. 15-33), is the same as that for investing a complete denture. The base of the master cast to be invested should be examined for roughness, irregularities, and voids. It should be perfectly smooth if it was formed and trimmed correctly except for the intersecting V-shaped grooves. After processing, it is necessary to recover the master cast intact so that it may be returned to the articulator to correct the processing errors in occlusion that will take place. If there are bubbles or voids present on the base of the cast that would interfere with recovering the cast because the investing Hydrocal becomes locked in the discrepancies, baseplate wax may be used to eliminate these defects. It is also possible to adapt a sheet of tinfoil to the base of the cast to ensure that it will be released from the investment. If tinfoil is not used, a gypsum separating medium must be painted on the base and sides of the cast. Caution must be shown in applying the gypsum separating medium. Certain brands of the solution, if allowed to contact the wax or the teeth, will produce a discoloration of the acrylic resin. A heavy soap solution may be used in place of the gypsum separating medium, but lubricants such as petrolatum that actually occupy space should be avoided. As pressure is applied to the flask during the packing process, the cast or other layers of investment may be compressed in the space and result in changes in the position of the teeth.

The master cast with the partial denture in place should be seated in the bottom half of the flask. It is very important that there be at least 15 mm clearance between the occlusal surfaces of the teeth and the top of the upper half of the flask. This is an important reason why it is necessary to control the thickness of the cast at the time it is poured. If the cast is so thick that it must be trimmed in order to fit the flask, the indices on the base of the cast will be lost, and the cast cannot be remounted for the correction of occlusal errors after processing.

A mix of 150 g Hydrocal and 45 ml water is correct for the first investment layer. Measuring the water/powder ratio accurately will ensure an investment of consistent density. The mix is made and puddled into the lower half of the flask. The lower half is filled two thirds full, and the master cast gently teased into the mix until the land area of the cast is level with or slightly below the rim of the flask. The stone mix should be even with the land area of the cast and above the rim of the flask. The stone should be left untouched until the initial set has started. A sharp laboratory knife is used to trim the stone smoothly from the land area of the cast to the inner edge of the flask rim. The practice of smoothing the surface of the stone with tap water before the set is complete should be discouraged. The addition of water to the partially set stone produces a soft, powdery surface that, when subjected to high compression forces during the packing process, will itself be compressed and produce distortion in the contour of the denture base and in the position of the artificial teeth.

After the final set of the first investment layer, a gypsum separating medium is painted over the surface of the stone and the entire surface of the master cast. Once again, the separating medium should not contact the surface of the wax or the artificial teeth because staining of the denture base or teeth will result. Soap solution may safely be used in its place. The flask should be soaked in slurry water before the second pour is made. If gypsum separating medium is used, it may be applied before the flask is soaked. If soap is used, it should be applied after the slurry water soak.

Second investment layer. The second mix should be the same as the first, 150 g Hydrocal to 45 ml water. The mix will be formed or molded over the master cast and metal framework, covering everything but the waxed denture base and the denture teeth (Fig. 15-34). The critical point about this second mix is that it be contoured so that there are no undercuts when it is viewed from a vertical direction. This is essential so that, after the boilout, the flasks may be separated clearly between the second and third investment lay-

Fig. 15-33. First investment layer. **A,** The base of the cast is painted with a tinfoil substitute separating medium. **B,** Tinfoil may be adapted to the cast instead of using the substitute. **C,** There must be a clearance of 15 mm between the teeth and the top of the flask. **D,** The cast is pressed gently into the first mix of stone in the bottom half of the flask. **E,** The first mix is trimmed even with the land area of the cast and the edge of the lower half of the flask. **F,** Separating medium is painted on the stone surface and **G,** The flask is soaked in slurry water.

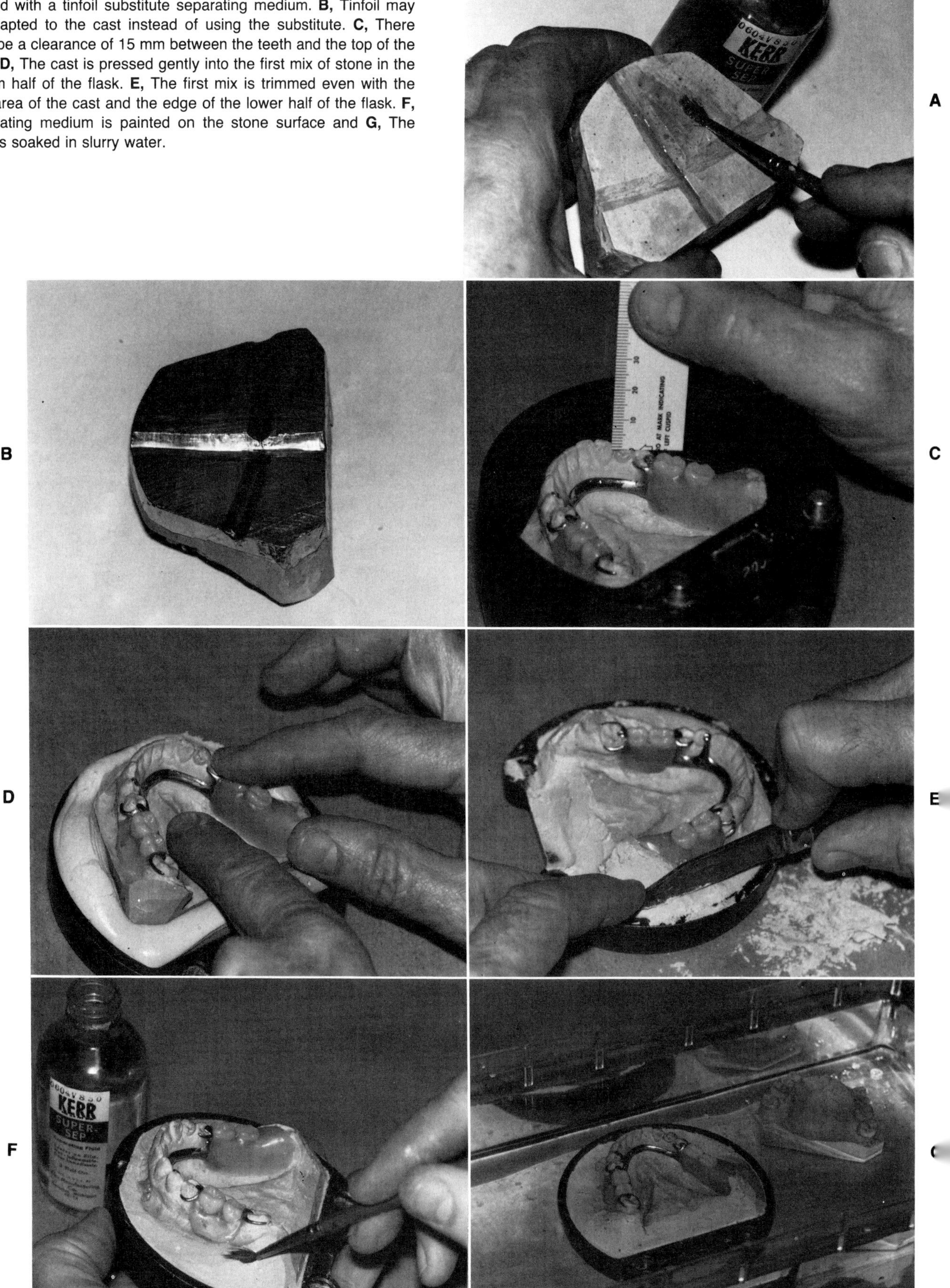

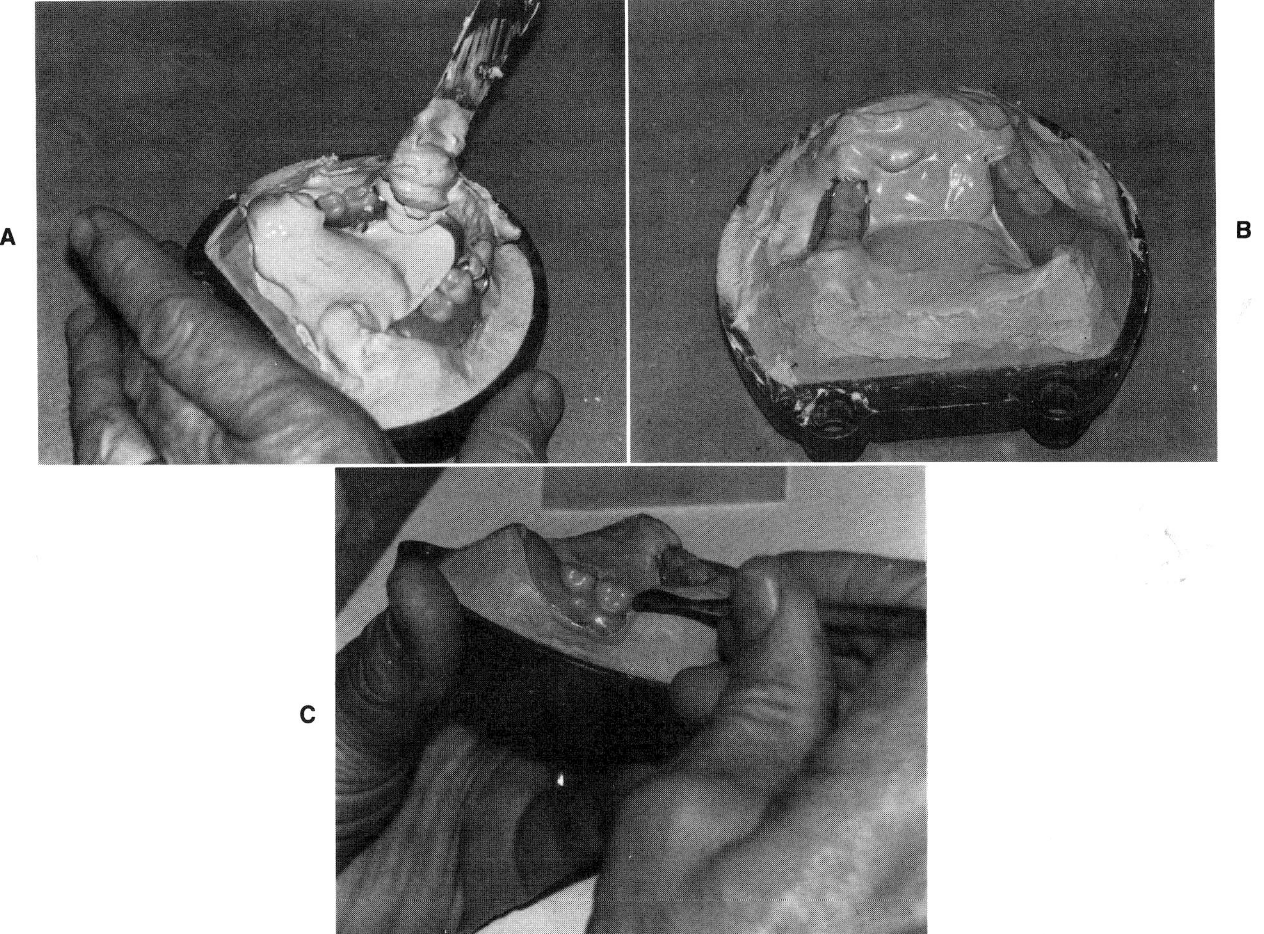

Fig. 15-34. A, Second layer of investment is added. **B,** Entire surface of cast and first investment is covered by second layer. Only artificial teeth and wax denture base are exposed. **C,** Second layer is trimmed to eliminate all undercuts and sharp projections.

ers. Any undercut in the second layer would prevent this and could greatly complicate the packing and finishing procedures. Sharp angles in the second layer should be avoided. It should be visualized that when the third pour, or cope, is made there will be no thin projections of stone that could fracture during the boil-out procedure. There should be at least 7 mm clearance between the top of the second mix and the top of the upper half of the flask. The outer edge of the second layer should end even with the rim of the lower half of the flask.

The more experienced dentist or technician can accomplish the purposes of the first and second layer in a single mix. The single mix, however, makes the deflasking procedure more difficult and hazardous.

After the second mix is set, the surface of the exposed stone must again be painted with a separating medium and soaked in slurry water. A surface-tension–reducing agent is painted on the surface of the wax to permit the next layer of investment to adapt more closely to the wax.

Third and fourth investment layers. The third investment layer, 150 g Hydrocal to 50 ml water, is accomplished in the same way as the second layer in complete denture investing (Fig. 15-35). With a fairly stiff paint brush small portions of the mix are adapted intimately against the wax of the denture base and the artificial teeth. Care should be used not to trap air bubbles in or around the necks of the teeth. Stippling should be accurately reproduced in the walls of the mold that is being formed. The more care used at this point, the more time will be saved during finishing and polishing procedures.

The upper half of the flask is positioned and the mix of stone is vibrated into the flask to within 7 mm from the top. The occlusal surfaces of the denture teeth are

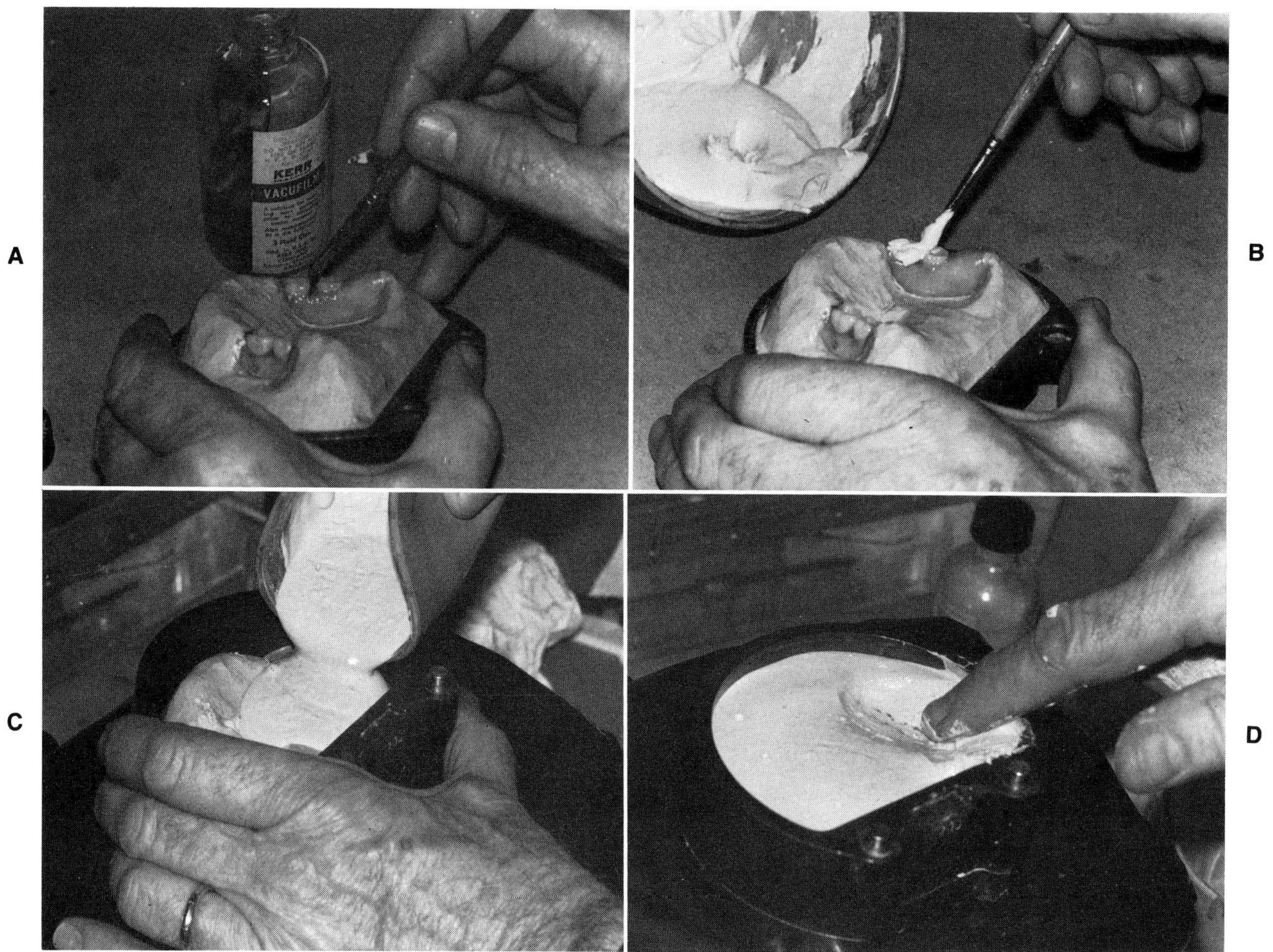

Fig. 15-35. Third investment layer. **A,** Wax denture base is painted with surface tension reducer. **B,** After second layer has been painted with separating medium and soaked in slurry water, third layer is added. Stiff brush is used to paint stone around artificial teeth and over surface of wax. **C,** Remainder of mix is vibrated into upper half of flask to about 7 mm from top of flask. **D,** Occlusal surfaces of artificial teeth are cleaned with finger, and third mix is shaped to form concavity.

uncovered with the index finger, and the soft stone is shaped to form a concavity into which the fourth or final mix will be poured. The main purpose of the fourth mix is to facilitate deflasking. Some technicians believe that this third mix can safely be made using plaster of paris or a softer investment, and the fourth mix made of Hydrocal. This last mix would then support the artificial teeth from being depressed into the softer investment and prevent an excessive amount of change in the vertical dimension of occlusion after processing. The time saved in following this technique is not worth the potential trouble that can be encountered.

The fourth investment layer, or lid, is applied into the concavity formed by the third layer. A separating medium should have been applied and the flask soaked several minutes in slurry water. The top of the flask is pressed to place immediately after the pour is complete.

The flask should set undisturbed for a minimum of 1 hour, but preferably overnight, before wax elimination is begun.

Denture release material. In the past few years a silicone rubber material has been introduced that has proven to be useful in the denture processing procedure (Fig. 15-36). The material, in the form of a paste, is applied or painted over the wax surfaces and artificial teeth immediately before the third pour of investment is made. As the name implies, after the denture has been processed, the denture base is released easily and cleanly from the silicone rubber material. Particles of investment do not adhere to the resin as often happens in conventional investing procedures. This makes the

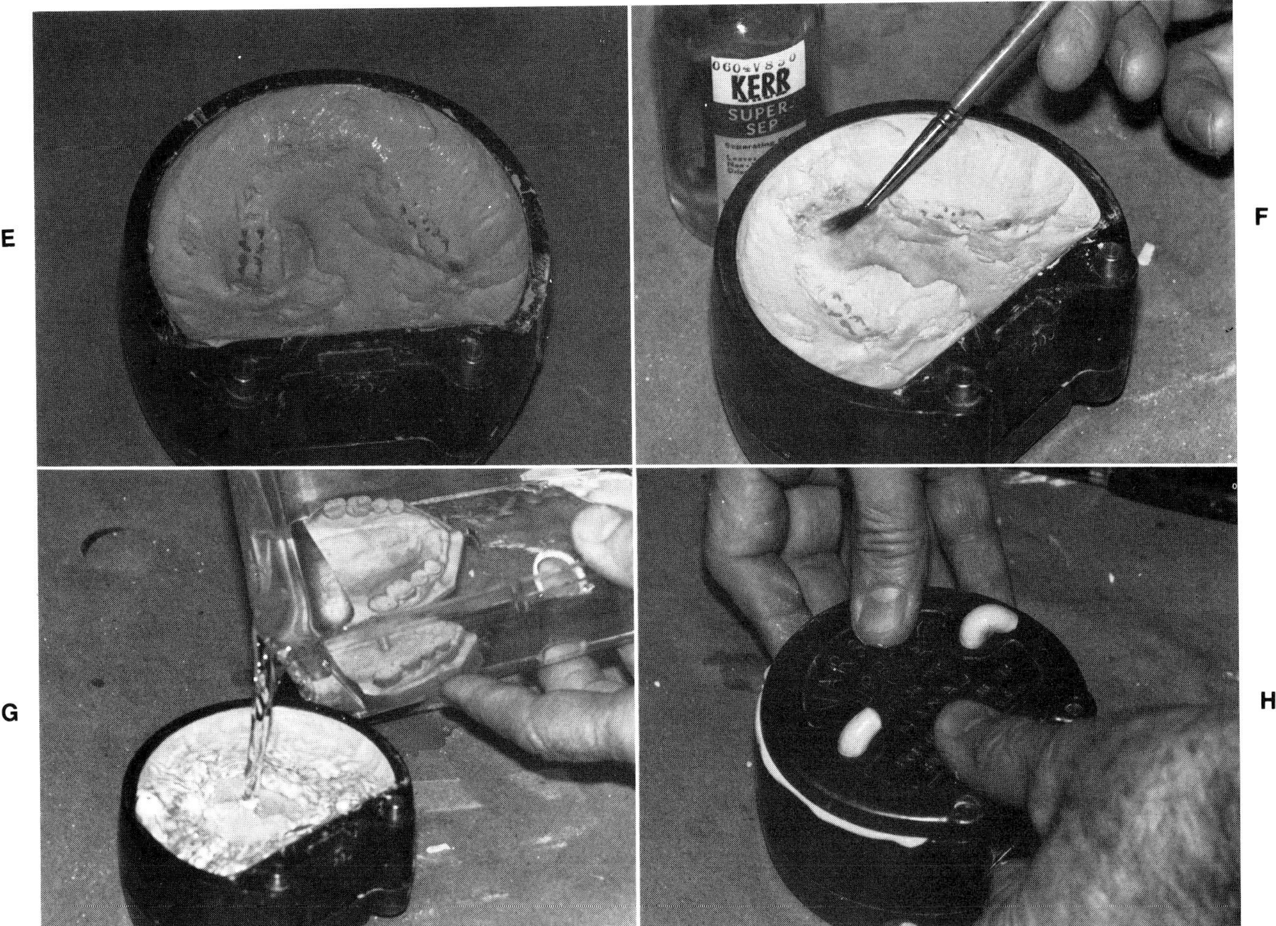

Fig. 15-35, cont'd. E, Surface of third layer is left slightly rough to secure fourth layer firmly in place. Surface of stone is painted with separating medium, **F,** and slurry water is poured into concavity to soak stone, **G. H,** After concavity is filled with fourth mix, lid is pressed to place.

finishing and polishing of the denture much faster and easier. Studies have shown tooth position in the completed denture not to be affected by the use of this soft material.

To use the denture release material, the first two investment layers are accomplished the same as for conventional flasking. A gypsum separating material is applied to all exposed stone surfaces.

The denture release material is normally supplied as a base paste in a tube and a liquid catalyst in a bottle. For most partial dentures a portion of base 1 inch in diameter is sufficient. Three to five drops of the catalyst are added, and the material mixed for 30 seconds.

Immediately after being mixed, the paste is applied to the wax surface, gingival crevice areas, and interproximal extensions with a small spatula or by finger. The paste should be approximately 1 mm thick.

While the denture release material is still tacky, the third pour of investment must be added. The same technique of uncovering the occlusal surface of the teeth and forming a concavity while the stone is still soft should be followed.

The main difference in technique that is required in the remainder of the processing procedure is that after the wax has been eliminated from the mold, detergent or other chemical wax solvents should not be used. The mold should be flushed only with absolutely clean, boiling water.

Wax elimination

If the flask has set on the bench overnight, it should be soaked at least 1 hour before the boilout procedure is started. Stone that is allowed to dry thoroughly becomes extremely hard, and breakage during flask separation following boilout is common.

The flask is placed in *boiling* water for 5 minutes. This time period is critical because the wax will become liquid and may penetrate into the investment if the

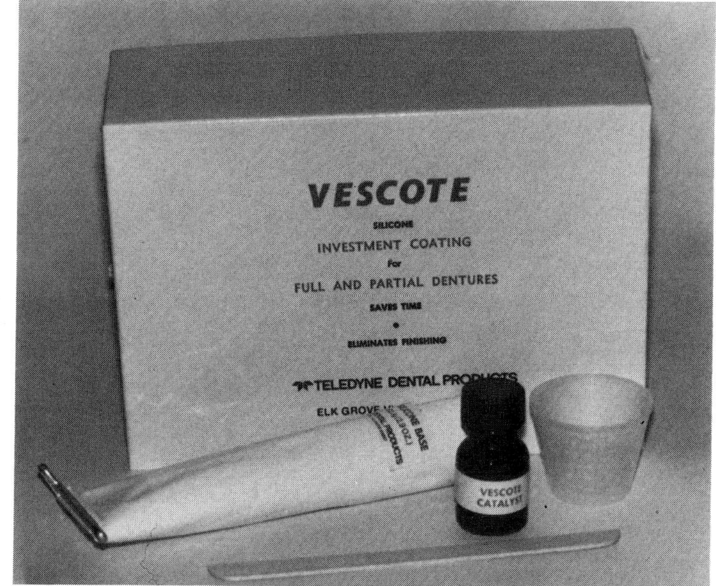

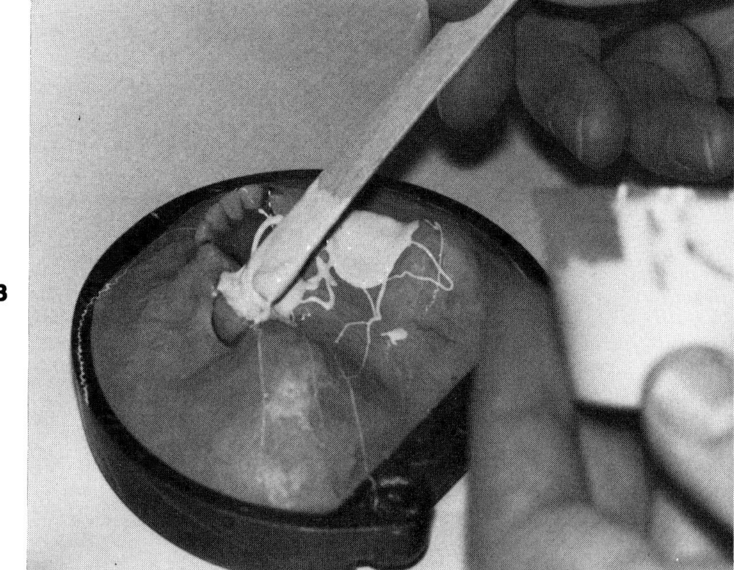

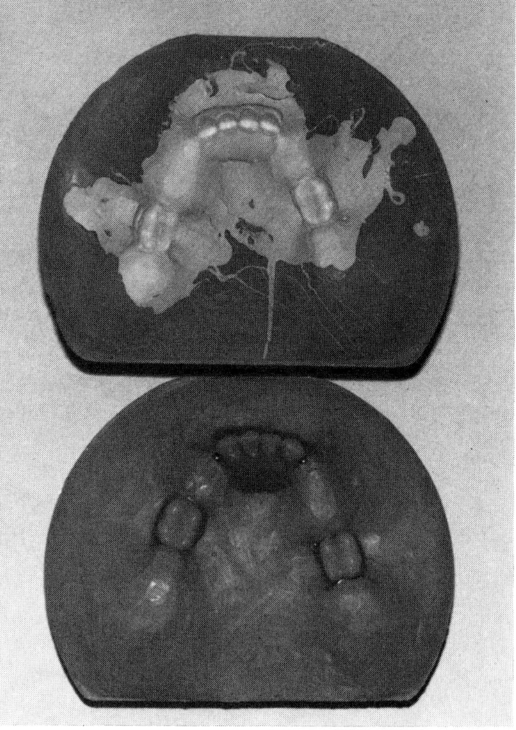

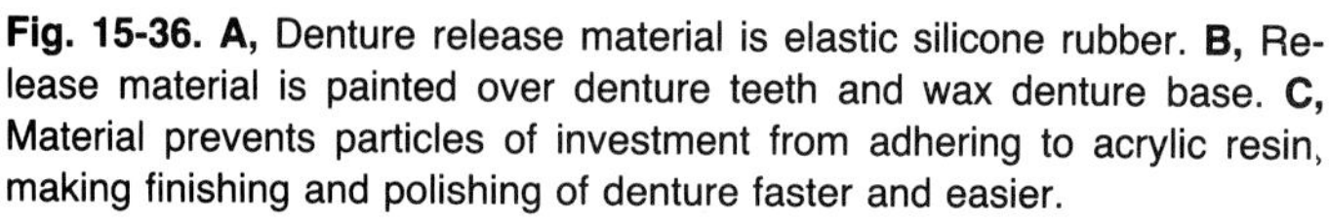
Fig. 15-36. **A,** Denture release material is elastic silicone rubber. **B,** Release material is painted over denture teeth and wax denture base. **C,** Material prevents particles of investment from adhering to acrylic resin, making finishing and polishing of denture faster and easier.

time is exceeded. If not enough time is allowed or if the water is not boiling, the wax is not softened sufficiently, and separating the two halves of the flask is difficult.

After the boilout the halves of the flask are separated carefully and the molds are prepared for packing with acrylic resin as illustrated in Fig. 15-37.

Cleansing of the stone surfaces, the areas under the acrylic resin retention struts, and the area around the denture teeth in the half of the flask opposite the framework is particularly important. Any wax that is not removed will interfere with the separating medium that must be used between the acrylic resin and the Hydrocal, producing contamination of the resin by the stone. If the separating medium does not spread evenly on the stone surface or if it tends to "ball up" in certain areas, that is evidence that wax elimination was not complete. Further detergent applications and rinsing of the surfaces a second time is warranted.

Certain precautions should be observed when paint-

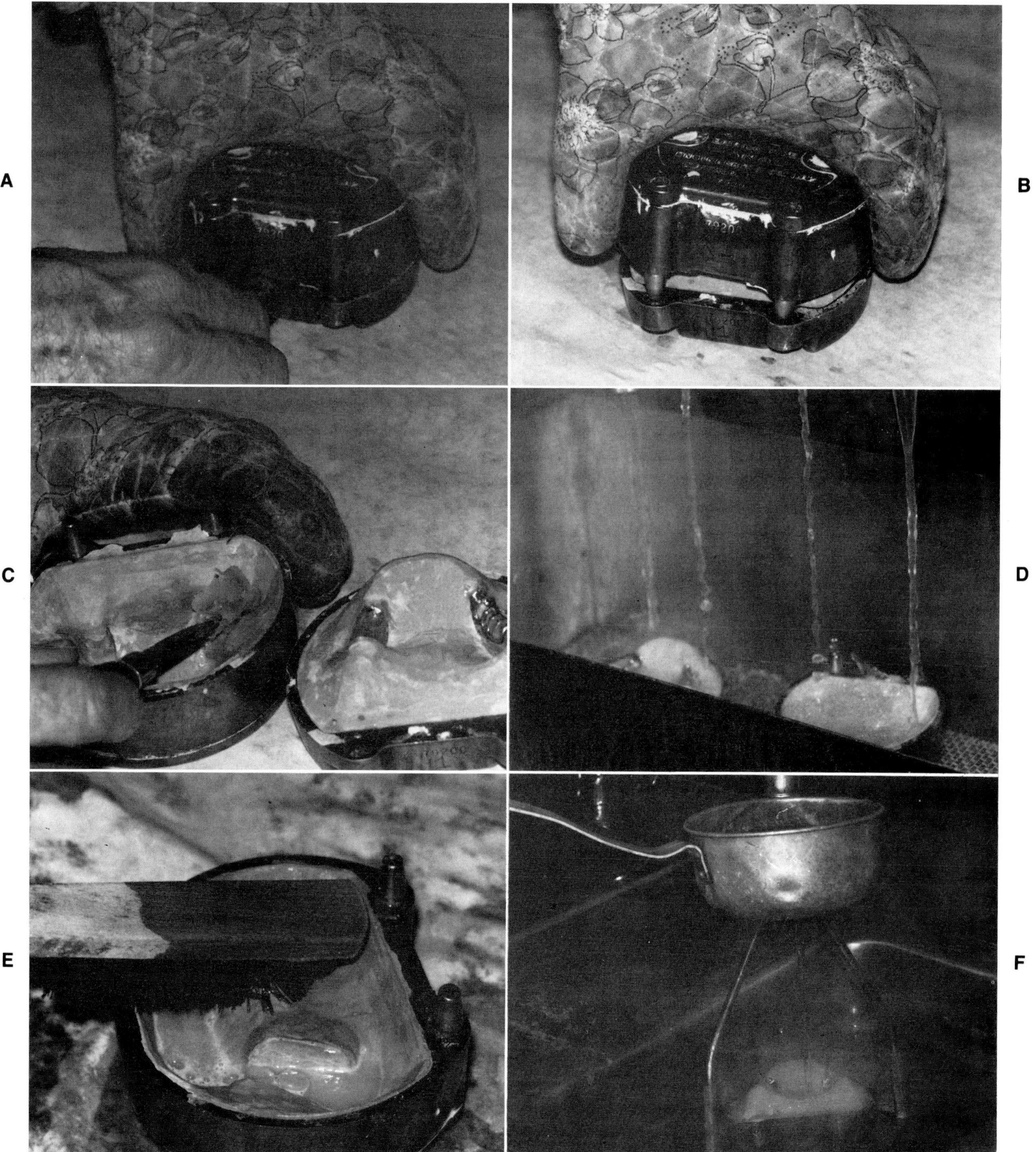

Fig. 15-37. **A,** After boilout, flask is pried open with stiff blade inserted in grooves in side of flask. **B,** Upper half is lifted as vertically as possible to avoid fracturing projections of third investment layer that may be present around contour of second layer. **C,** Bulk of molten wax is scraped from mold. **D,** Remainder of wax is flushed from mold with boiling slurry water. **E,** Detergent solution and soft brush are used to clean wax residue from mold. **F,** Finally, clean boiling slurry water is used to flush mold.

Continued.

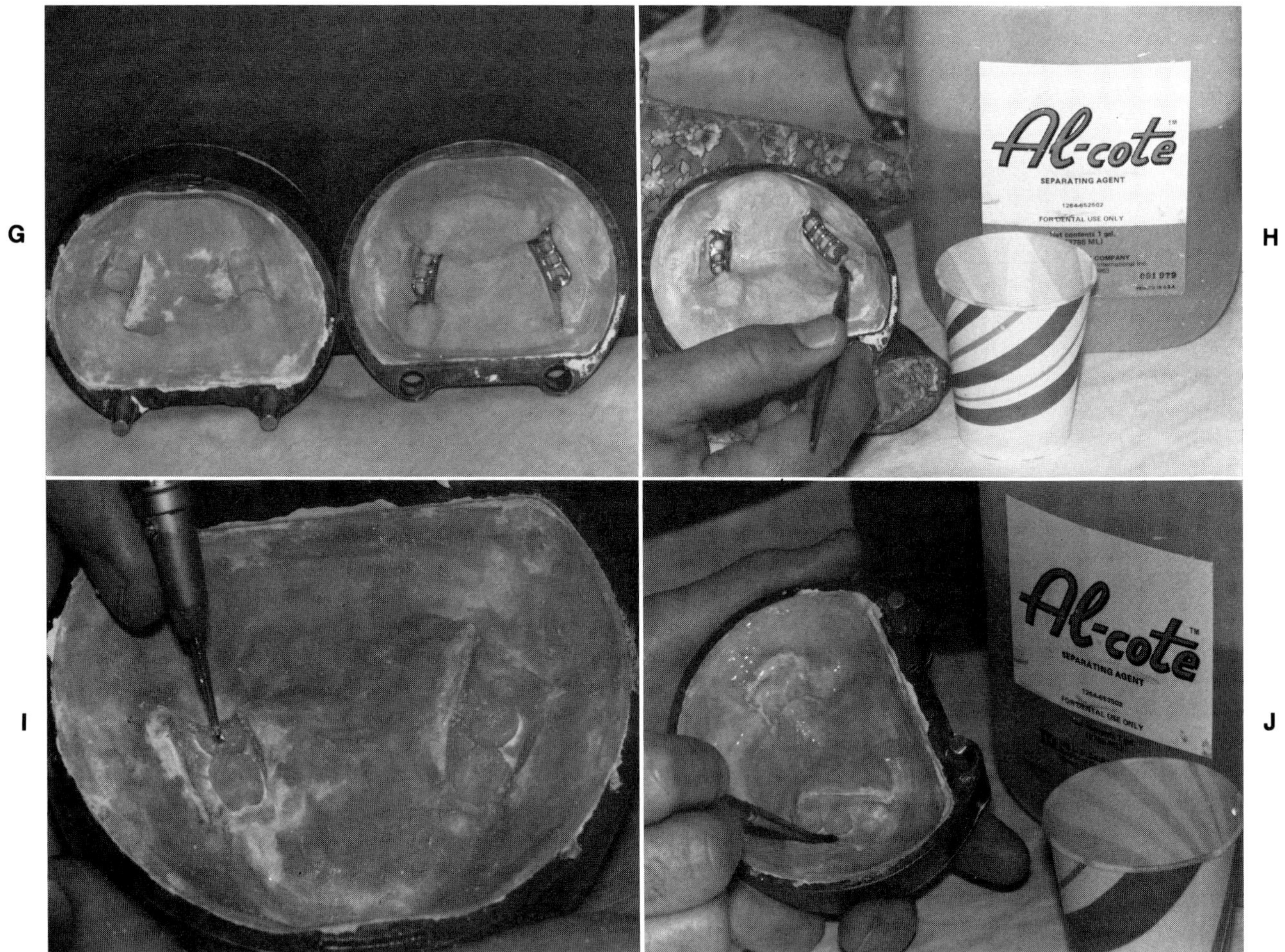

Fig. 15-37, cont'd. G, Clean flasks are stood on heels for several minutes to allow water to drain. **H,** While flasks are still warm, thorough coat of alginate separating medium is applied. **I,** Retention holes, or diatorics, are cut in denture teeth with a No. 6 round bur to ensure that artificial teeth and denture base will be locked together securely. Hole should not be too deep, or pink denture base may show through tooth. **J,** Another coat of alginate separating medium is painted on stone surfaces.

ing the stone surfaces with alginate separating medium. It is essential that a smooth and solid coating of the material be applied to prevent the stone from adhering to the resin after processing. However, the ridge lap areas of the artificial teeth should not be painted because this could prevent the acrylic resin denture base from attaching securely to the teeth.

Packing the acrylic resin denture base

If it is desired to characterize or stain the denture flanges, it is accomplished before the acrylic resin is prepared for the denture base (Fig. 15-38). Characterizing the denture base should be done for most anterior flanges, particularly if the patient has a fair or a dark complexion. Resins with stains are available in a variety of shades. The polymer, which contains the stain, is sprinkled on the outer surface of the mold in the position desired. Only a thin layer of the stain need be applied. The polymer is wet with heat-curing monomer from a dropper. The amount of monomer used must be controlled so that the stain will not flow from the location where it was placed. After the characterization is complete, the flask should be closed to prevent excess evaporation of the monomer while the acrylic resin for the denture base is being prepared.

If individual free-hand characterization is not desired, there are a number of commercial denture base resins available that are supplied with the stain incorporated in the polymer. The stains usually are identified as light, medium, or dark and can be selected to harmonize with the patient's complexion. The resin may or may not contain fibers to simulate minor blood

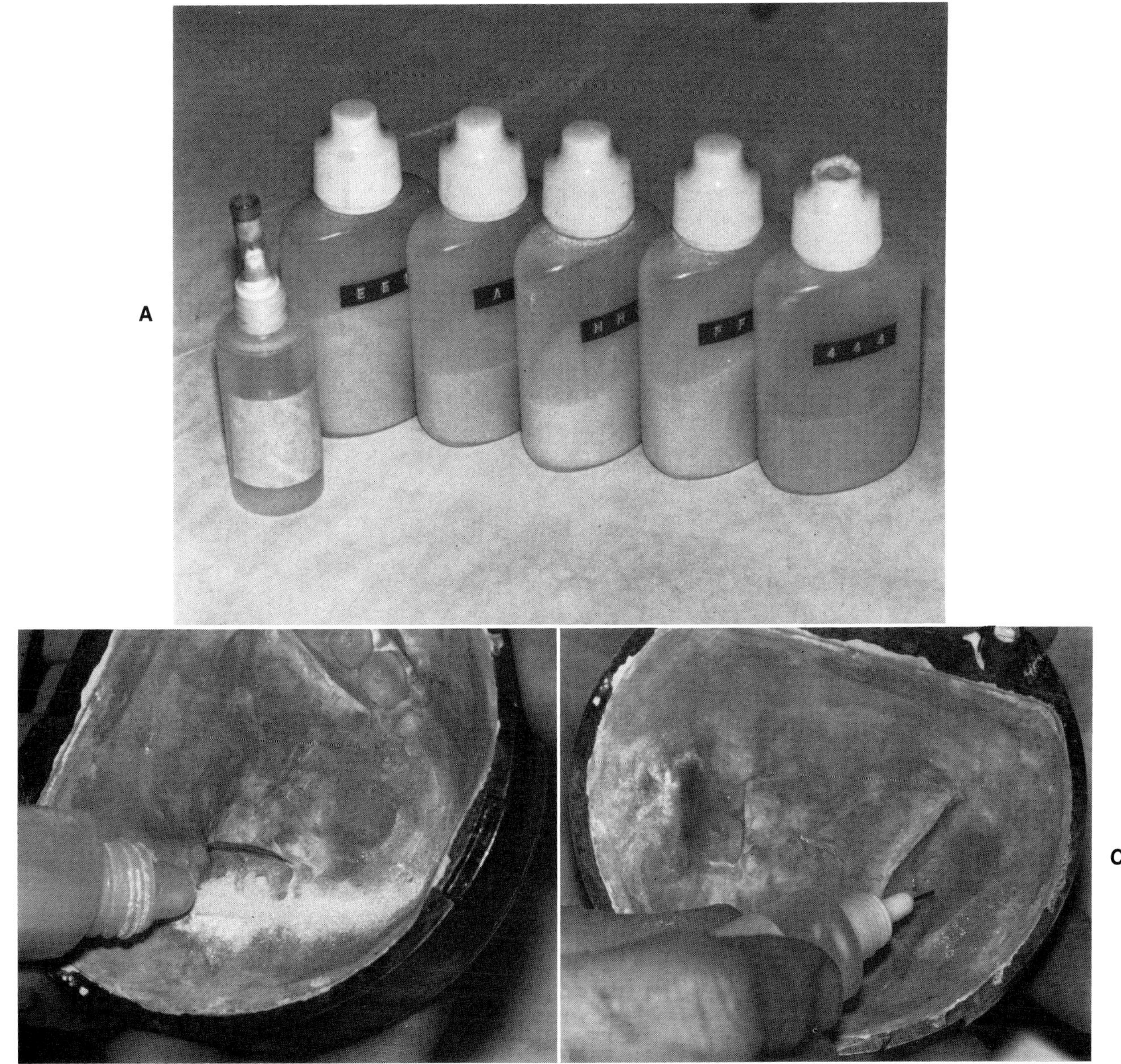

Fig. 15-38. A, Denture base can be characterized with denture base stains. **B,** Dry polymer containing stain is sprinkled on surface of mold. **C,** Polymer is wet with heat-cure monomer.

vessels in the gingival tissue. These denture resins are certainly acceptable and a definite improvement over a bland uniformly pink resin. They do lack the individuality that can be created by free-hand characterization.

An important point to be observed before packing the acrylic resin is the tissue stop at the end of the retentive latticework of a distal extension ridge. This tissue stop was waxed onto the latticework originally to support the framework on the master cast if downward force was placed against the framework. If an altered cast was made, the tissue stop will usually not be in contact with the underlying edentulous ridge of the master cast. The closing pressure of the packing procedure may distort or depress the unsupported extension of the framework. To prevent this, a small amount of autopolymerizing resin should be sprinkled on or painted under the distal end of the latticework and allowed to set before the denture resin is packed (Fig. 15-39).

The acrylic resin is mixed using 5 ml of monomer to 15 ml of polymer. The mixing jar should have a lid that can be closed tightly to prevent evaporation of the

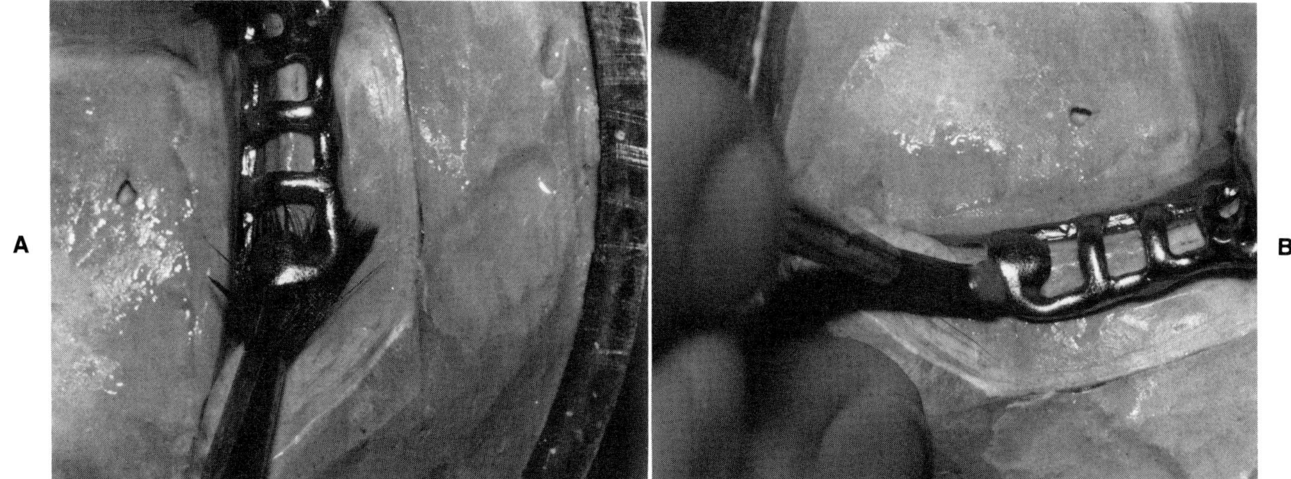

Fig. 15-39. A, Tissue stop may not contact edentulous ridge on cast. **B,** To prevent framework from being depressed or distorted during packing process, small portion of autopolymerizing resin is placed between tissue stop area of framework and stone ridge.

monomer during polymerization. The polymer and monomer are mixed for 30 seconds, or until the polymer is thoroughly wet with the monomer. The jar is closed tightly and allowed to set untouched until the mix reaches the doughy stage. This stage is characterized by separating cleanly from the sides of the jar when pulled by a spatula.

The resin should not be handled with bare fingers during either the mixing or packing phases because oil from the skin will be transferred to the resin and will influence the degree of dimensional change that the resin will undergo on processing. In addition, allergic dermatologic responses may occur if preventive measures are not observed. These allergic reactions may be severe, limiting the dentist to little or no contact with acrylic resin. This could limit the type of clinical practice a dentist could pursue markedly. Disposable plastic gloves should normally be worn during the packing process. If gloves are not available, the material should be handled between plastic sheets that will be used during the trial packing.

When the resin in the mixing jar has reached the doughy stage, packing should be accomplished as quickly as possible. The procedure is illustrated in Fig. 15-40.

A split-packing technique must be followed for the partial denture. With the framework retained in the lower half of the flask and the teeth in the upper half, some modification in the packing procedure is required. If the conventional packing procedure used for complete dentures were followed (where the resin is packed against the artificial teeth, a separating plastic sheet is used to cover the resin, and the flask halves are closed, pressed, and then opened to remove the excess resin) the chances of dislodging the framework or the artificial teeth would be great.

If sufficient resin is used in each half of the flask, there should be a flash around all margins of the denture base in both sides of the flask. One of the most frequent errors in split-packing is to assume that if an abundance of flash is present around the denture base in one half of the flask, there is sufficient resin to fill both sides of the mold. This is not true, and if the denture base is processed under the conditions described, porosity of a portion of the denture base is certain to occur as a result of underpacking. If flash is not present around all the margins, a small portion of resin should be added to the deficient area before the next trial closure. The flash that is present should be trimmed to the margin of the denture base with an instrument. Care should be taken not to loosen particles of investment onto the resin. The plastic sheet should be replaced between the halves of the flask, and the trial closure repeated.

Trial packing should be repeated until a minimal amount of flash is present. Under normal circumstances at least three trial closures should be accomplished; at times six or more may be required. The working time of different manufacturers' acrylic resin will vary considerably. The beginning student should select a brand that has the longest working time. In any event, trial closures should be accomplished as rapidly as possible while avoiding the application of pressure too quickly to the flask. Enough time must be allowed to permit the resin to flow.

After final closure has been made, the flask should be

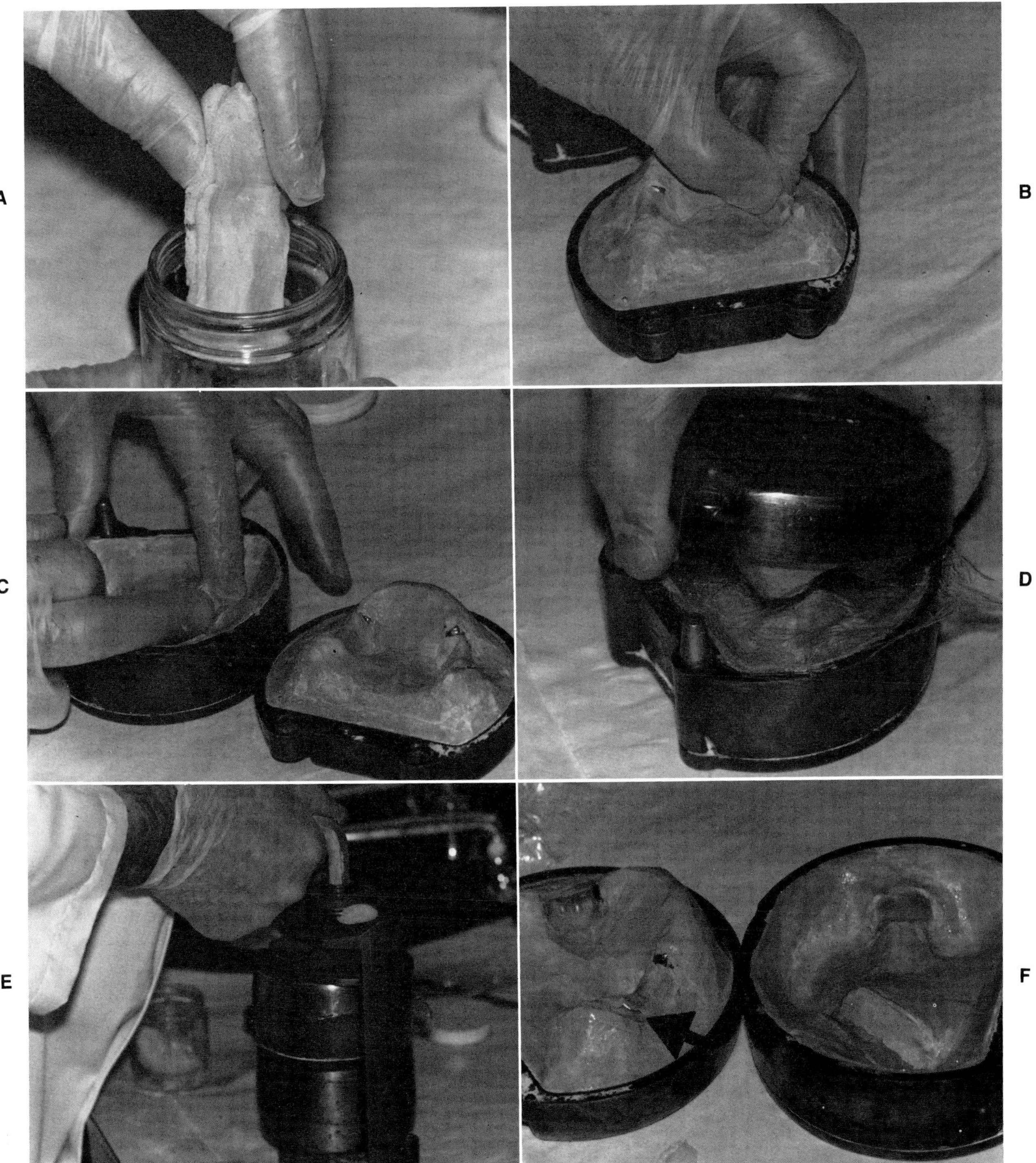

Fig. 15-40. **A,** Mix of acrylic resin separates cleanly from mixing jar when consistency is correct. Note that operator is wearing plastic gloves. **B** and **C,** Small portions of mix are pressed in and around teeth in one half of flask and in and around framework in other half of flask. **D,** Cellophane or plastic sheet is placed between flask halves as flask is closed. **E,** Flask is placed in flask press and pressure is applied slowly to force resin into intimate contact with framework, teeth, and walls of mold. Alternatively, pressure may be applied hydraulically. When considerable resistance to closing flask is encountered, press is released, flask is opened, and flash around margins of denture base is trimmed. **F,** There is no flash along one border (arrow).

Continued.

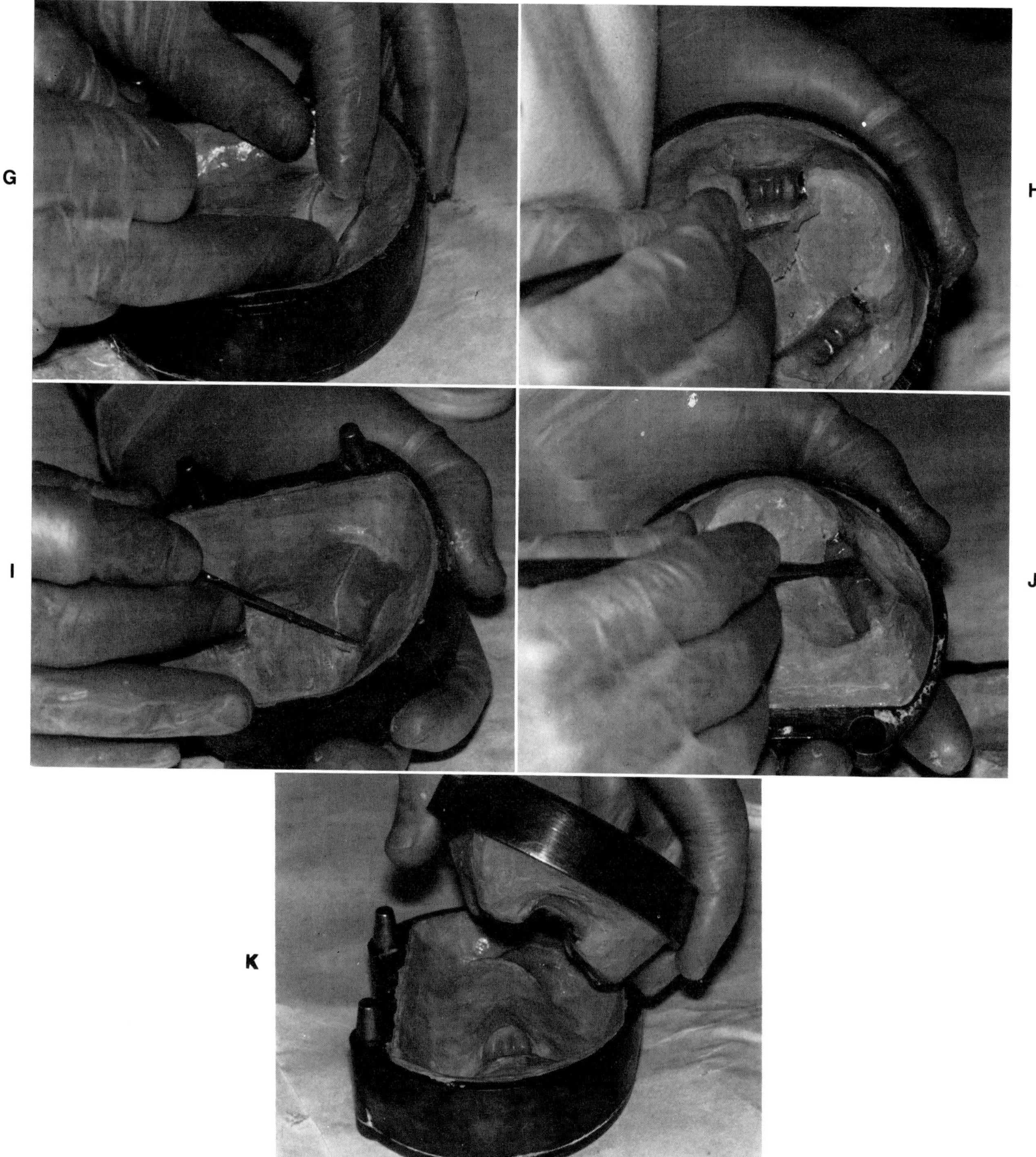

Fig. 15-40, cont'd. G, Portion of acrylic resin mix is added to deficient area, and another trial is accomplished. **H,** Flash is now present around area that was deficient. **I,** After a number of trial packs, very little flash is present. Final closure can now be made. **J,** Opposing surfaces of acrylic resin are painted with monomer. **K,** Flasks are closed without plastic sheet and placed in flask press. If press has spring compression, pressure should be reduced slightly to allow for dimensional change that will occur as heat is applied to flask.

permitted to bench cure for 1 hour before processing is started.

Processing the partial denture

After being bench cured for 1 hour, the flask and press are placed in a curing unit. If an electric curing unit is not available, the processing can be accomplished in any large metal container holding water. There must be enough water to completely cover the flask press to make certain that heat is being applied to the flask evenly. Processing can be accomplished satisfactorily using improvised equipment if the temperature of the water in the container is monitored carefully.

Heat-cured acrylic resin is processed at 71° C (160° F). Lower temperatures will not activate the resin to produce the polymerization reaction; higher temperatures will cause polymerization to proceed too rapidly and will bring about a rapid elevation of the internal temperature of the resin. This rapid rise in temperature may result in boiling of the monomer, which is one cause of porosity in the denture base. Thicker portions of the denture base should have the temperature rise to the processing temperature more slowly to avoid this dangerous internal rise in temperature. Conversely, a thinner portion of the denture base will process more slowly, since there will be less rise in internal temperature because of less bulk.

Long-cure cycle

For heat-cured acrylic resin there are two curing cycles that may be used. The most widely used is referred to as the long-cure cycle. In this cycle the flask is placed in the curing tank with room temperature water. The temperature is raised slowly to reach 71° C (160° F) in 1 hour. This temperature is maintained for an additional 7 hours. At the end of the total of 8 hours the tank is brought to a boil and maintained for 30 minutes. To use this curing cycle without an electronic control is difficult. The most widely used curing tank is the Hanau curing unit, which can accommodate six flask presses at one time (Fig. 15-41).

This curing cycle is the safest and should normally be used. If the electric curing unit is available, the processing is usually accomplished at night and the denture will be ready for deflasking the next morning.

Short-cure cycle

There may be instances where not enough time is available for a long cure. In these cases it is possible to use a short cure. The short cure consists of holding the curing tank temperature at 71° C (160° F) for $1\frac{1}{2}$ hours

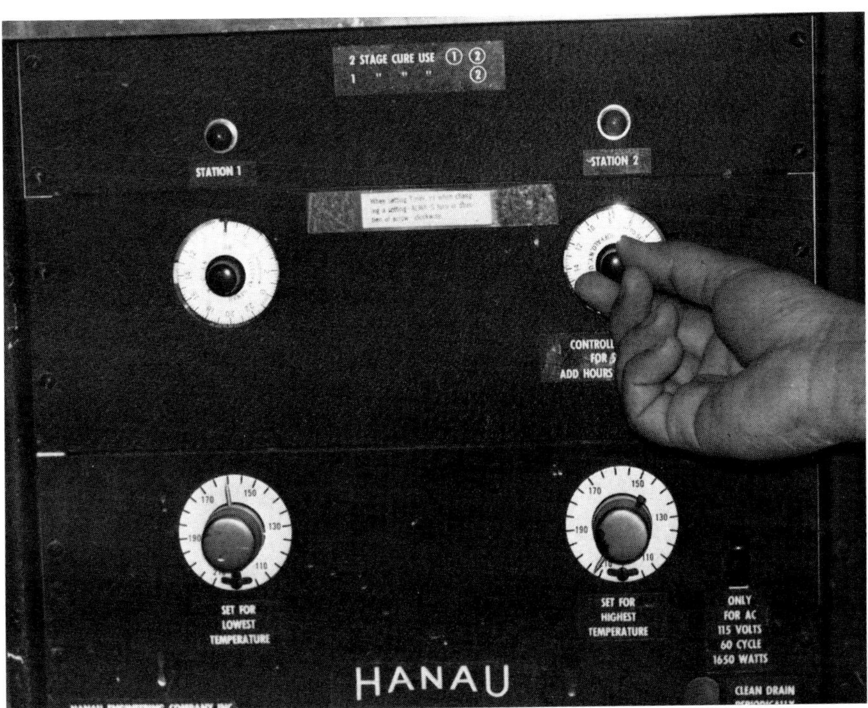

Fig. 15-41. Hanau curing unit. Station 1 is set for 8 hours at 160° F, and station 2 is set for $8\frac{1}{2}$ hours at 212° F for the long cure cycle.

followed by boiling for $^{1}/_{2}$ hour. This procedure involves a certain element of risk, usually in the form of incomplete polymerization with a high residual of free monomer remaining in the resin. Porosity in the resin is also a distinct possibility.

If deflasking cannot be done immediately after processing, the investment should not be allowed to dry. The flask should be kept covered with room temperature water until deflasking can be accomplished.

Deflasking the partial denture

The flask and the four layers of investment are removed one by one as shown in Figs. 15-42 to 15-45.

Correcting processing errors

Before the partial denture is removed from the cast, it must be remounted on the articulator for correction of any errors in the occlusion that may have taken place as a result of the processing procedure. The base of the cast must fit the mounting stone on the articulator precisely before the occlusal corrections are made.

At the present time methyl methacrylate resin remains by far the most widely used denture base material in complete and removable partial prosthodontics. Even with improvements that are constantly being made in the material, it is still one in which sizable dimensional change takes place during the polymerization process. This dimensional change coupled with the dimensional instability of the wax in which the teeth are set is sufficient to produce measurable errors in occlusal contacts of the artificial teeth. To correct the major part of this processing error, the partial denture, still mounted on the master cast, must be returned to the articulator on which the teeth were originally ar-

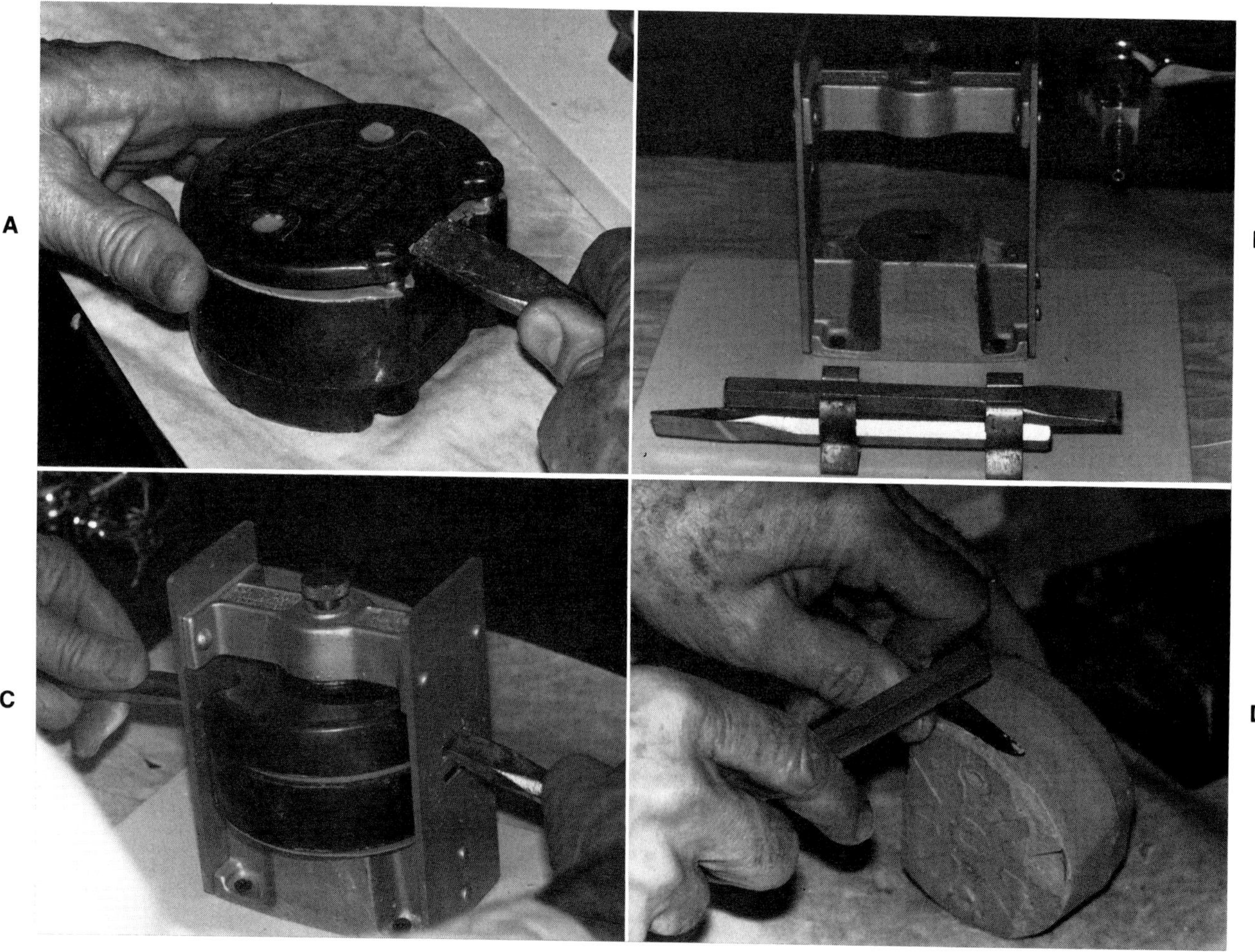

Fig. 15-42. A, Top of flask is removed by prying with chisel. **B,** Flask ejector such as this Hanau flask ejector and chisels must be used to remove remainder of flask. **C,** Flask is positioned in ejector upside down. Top knob is turned down to contact knock-out plate in base of flask. Chisels are inserted through holes in ejector and engage slots between halves of flask. Vigorous up-and-down force is applied with chisels. **D,** Knife edge is held at junction of third and fourth layers. Light tap will remove lid, or fourth layer.

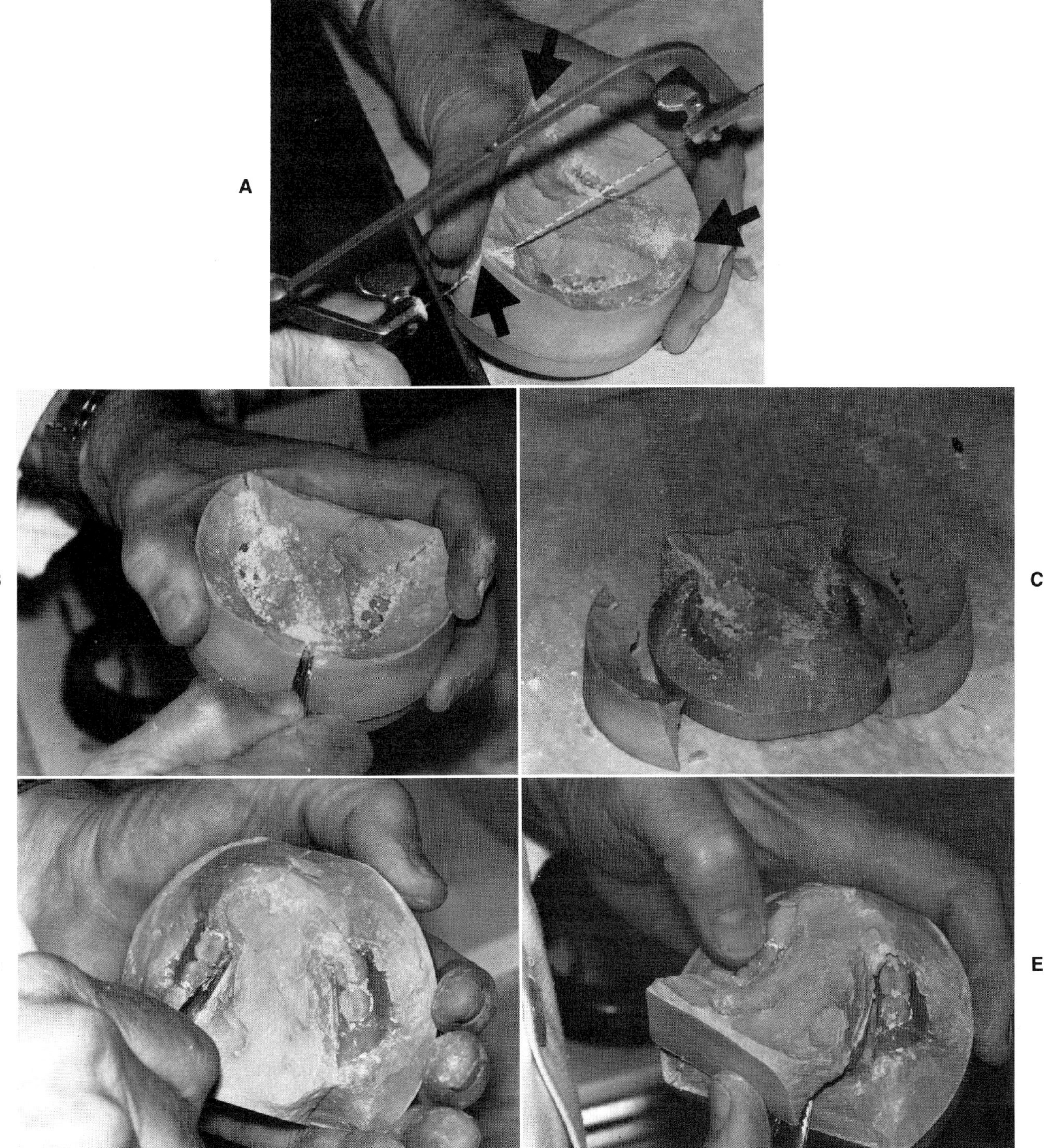

Fig. 15-43. A, Plaster saw is used to make three cuts at points indicated. Anterior cut must be deep enough to provide purchase point for knife blade but not so deep as to damage master cast. Posterior cuts should reach but not damage master cast. **B,** Knife blade is inserted into anterior cut, and twisting force applied. **C,** Sides of third investment layer separate cleanly. **D,** Lingual surfaces of denture teeth are exposed with laboratory knife. **E,** Lingual portion of third investment layer is gently pried loose.

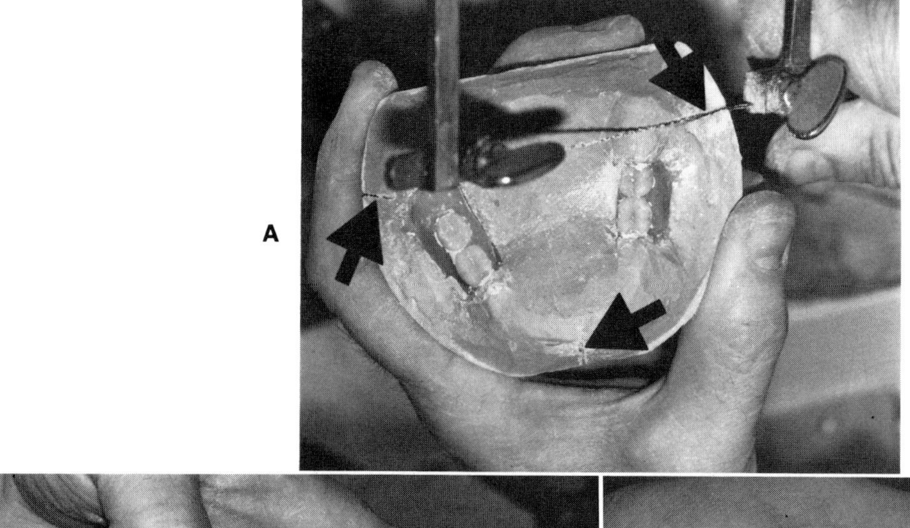

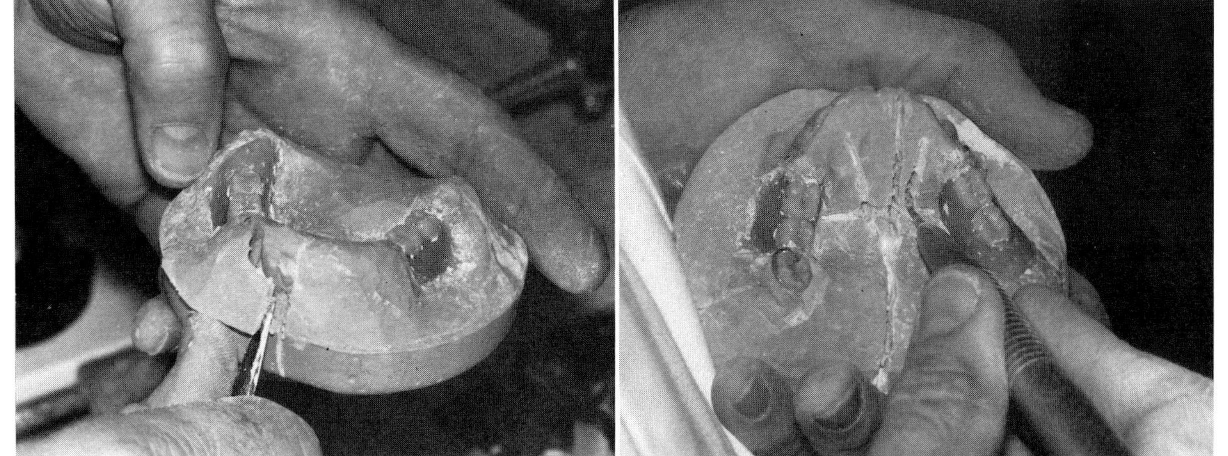

Fig. 15-44. A, Plaster saw is used again to make three cuts in second investment layer as indicated. **B,** Knife blade is inserted in saw cuts and twisted to remove sides of second layer. **C,** Fissure bur is used to section remaining lingual portion of second layer. Care must be taken not to distort or damage lingual bar or reciprocal clasp arms of denture.

ranged and the occlusion corrected by selective grinding.

Some practitioners think that the processing error can be corrected in the mouth. When only a few teeth are being replaced and the prosthesis is tooth supported, this probably can be accomplished quite accurately. However, as the number of teeth being replaced increases and when a Class I or Class II partially edentulous arch is being treated, the stability, or lack of it, of the denture bases, the accessibility of the occlusion, and the ability of the patient to perform the necessary jaw movements limit the possibility of the operator correcting the errors accurately. The procedure may involve excessive chair time and may not produce a totally acceptable result.

The articulator used may not be capable of correcting all discrepancies that have occurred in the occlusion in lateral or eccentric jaw positions, but if the occlusion can be corrected and returned to the position of centric relation or centric occlusion at which the teeth were arranged, a savings of time and energy can result. The eccentric occlusal defects may be corrected in the mouth, if necessary, or by making eccentric jaw relation records from the patient and remounting the casts on the articulator in those positions. The occlusion can be refined to a greater degree of accuracy with this technique. The procedure of remounting the partial dentures from the patient back to the articulator is an extremely valuable clinical tool and is discussed in Chapter 16.

To correct the processing error, the master cast with the partial denture still in place after being recovered from the investment is positioned on the mounting stone on the articulator. The fit of the base of the cast

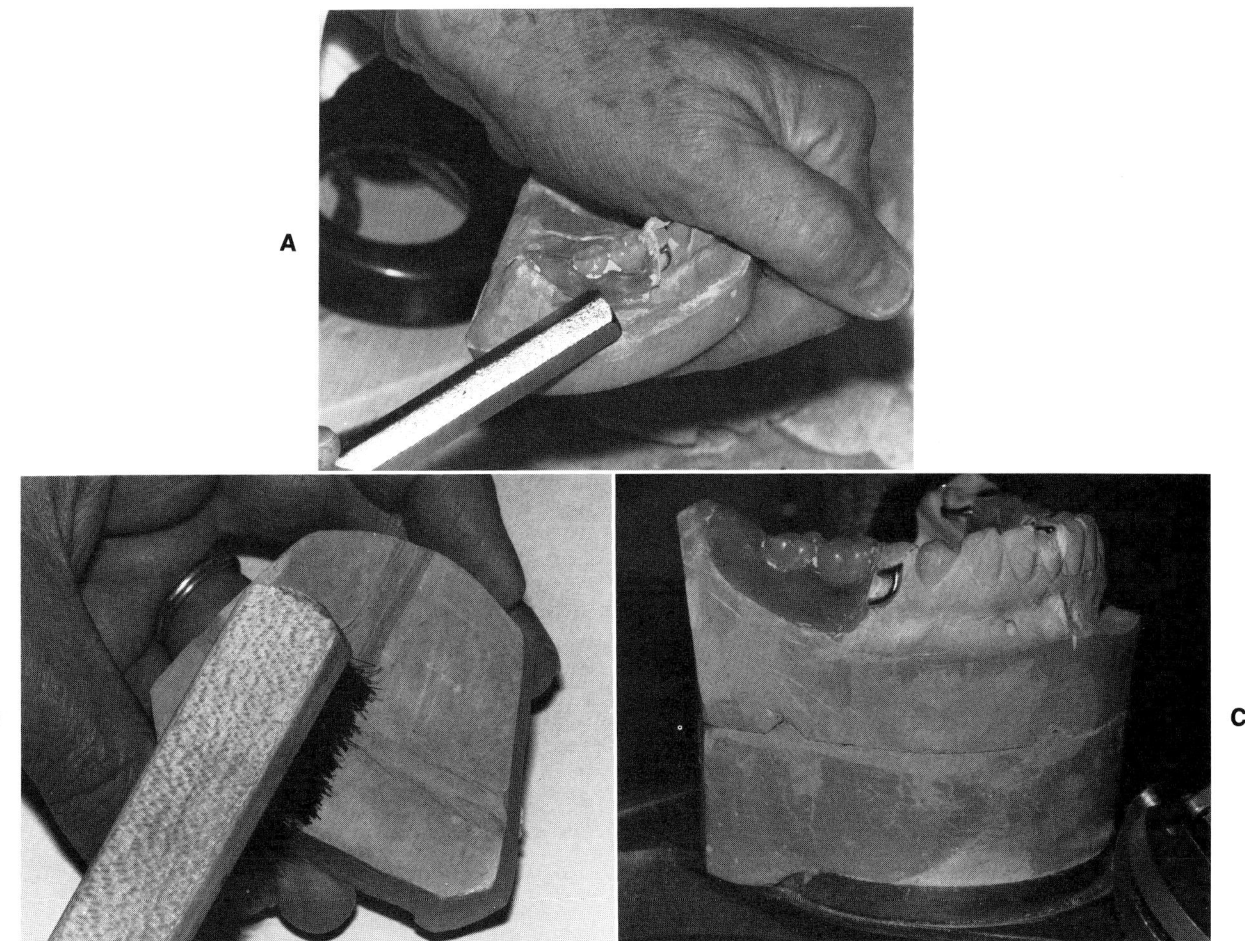

Fig. 15-45. A, First investment layer is removed by tapping with chisel or knife handle. **B,** Particles of investment are cleaned from base of cast and indices. **C,** Cast is reseated on mounting stone on articulator.

to the mount must be verified as being accurate. Even a small error in the adaptation of the cast to the mount can result in an incorrect interpretation of the occlusion. The master cast should be sealed to the mount with wax or modeling plastic to hold the cast securely while the occlusal adjustment is being accomplished.

The articulator should be closed, and the amount of opening of the incisal guide pin from the incisal table observed. If there is 1 mm or less of pin opening, the technique used in investing and processing was acceptable. If more than 1 mm of pin opening is present, some errors occurred during the investing procedure. If an excessive amount of pin opening occurs, the anatomy of the teeth may be destroyed in reestablishing the proper occlusal relationship and the masticatory efficiency of the denture may be impaired.

The condylar controls of the articulator should be locked in the centric relation position. The errors that occurred during processing can be located by tapping the teeth on the articulator together lightly while holding a piece of articulating paper between the teeth. The paper should be as thin as possible to prevent false occlusal markings. The paper should be held crosswise between the teeth rather than lengthwise. False markings on the most posterior teeth can occur when the articulating paper is held lengthwise.

The occlusion is adjusted so that opposing stone teeth on the casts are returned to equal contact (Fig. 15-46). Some practitioners believe that the artificial teeth should be left slightly high (0.5 mm) at this time and the final refinement accomplished in the mouth. This course can be followed but with the realization that extra chair time will be required when the partial denture is delivered to the patient.

In correcting for the pin opening, the tip of the cusps alone should not be removed. The occlusal surfaces of the teeth should be reshaped to provide inclines, grooves, and escapeways or sluiceways (Fig. 15-47). At

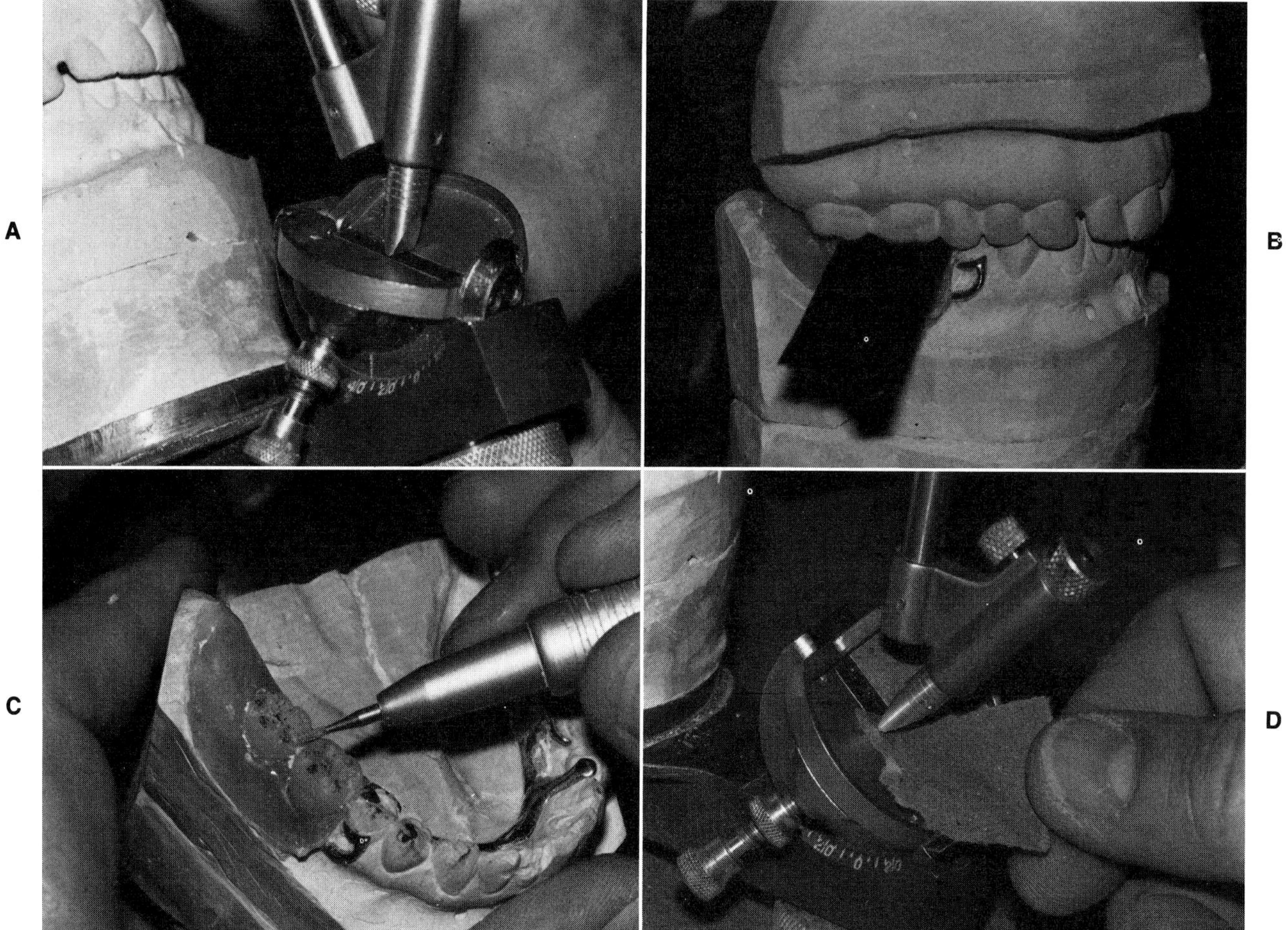

Fig. 15-46. A, Amount of incisal pin opening indicates amount of processing error that has occurred. **B,** Articulating paper is used to locate interferences. **C,** Interferences are corrected with burs. **D,** Occlusal correction is continued until incisal pin contacts incisal table.

this stage the anatomy of the occlusal surfaces of the artificial teeth should resemble quite closely the anatomy of the remaining natural teeth particularly as far as cusp height is concerned. Any disparity between the natural and artificial teeth will result in a lack of occlusal harmony.

Thin tissue paper, such as is found in the rolls of articulating paper, or Mylar tape is used to check contact between opposing teeth. It is desired to have an equal amount of resistance to pulling the paper between the opposing teeth in all positions. This judgment does require some laboratory experience.

When the vertical dimension of occlusion has been restored, the relationship of the teeth in working and balancing occlusion should be studied. The artificial teeth should never keep the natural, or the stone, teeth from contacting in any of the eccentric positions. Balancing contacts in particular must be carefully checked and, if present, eliminated by selective grinding of the artificial teeth.

Finally, the anatomy of the occlusal surfaces must be restored (Fig. 15-48). This should include the establishment of sluiceways and the breaking up of flat areas on occlusal surfaces with additional grooves. If flat surfaces are allowed to contact, excessive frictional forces can be generated, placing unnecessary stress on the abutment teeth.

Following the restoration of anatomy, a final occlusal check should be made to determine that centric occlusion has not been destroyed during the occlusal carving.

Decasting the partial denture

After processing errors have been corrected, the master cast is no longer of any value. Even if the partial denture could be recovered from the cast and the cast

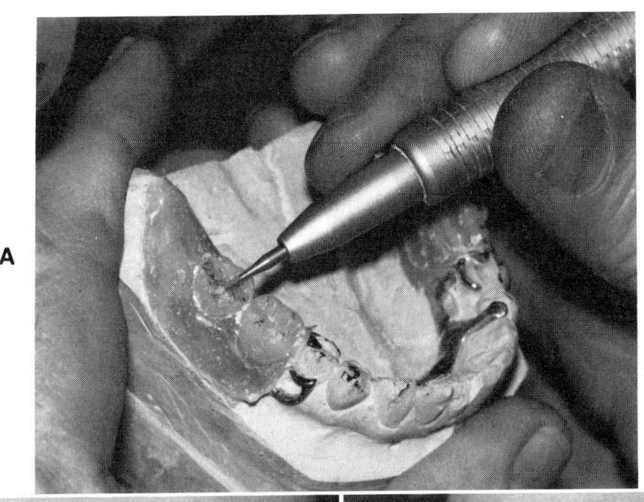

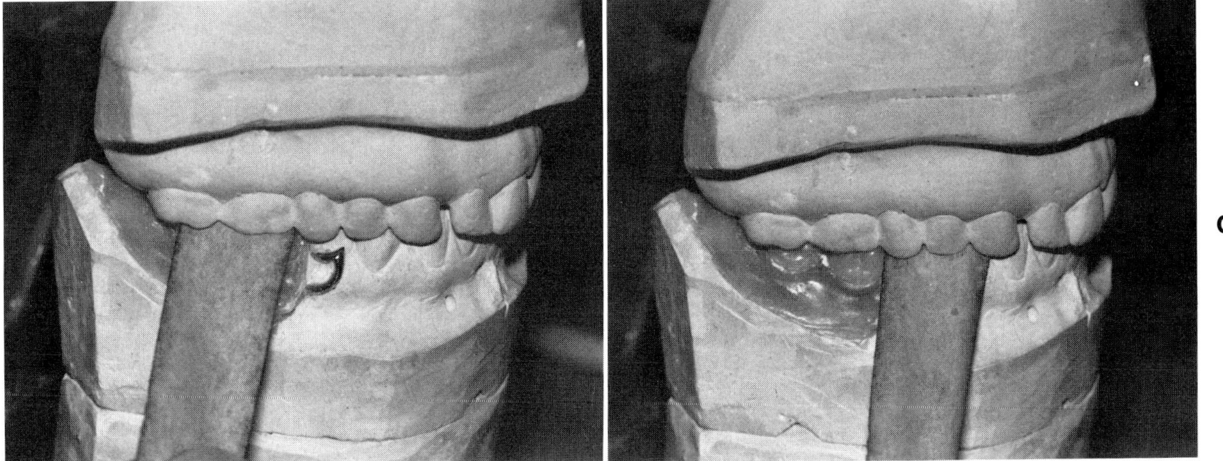

Fig. 15-47. A, Occlusal anatomy is restored to denture teeth. Occlusal contact marks left on occlusal surfaces of teeth should not be removed as anatomy is developed. Tissue paper is held firmly between artificial and natural teeth, **B,** at same time it is held firmly between natural teeth, **C,** on articulator.

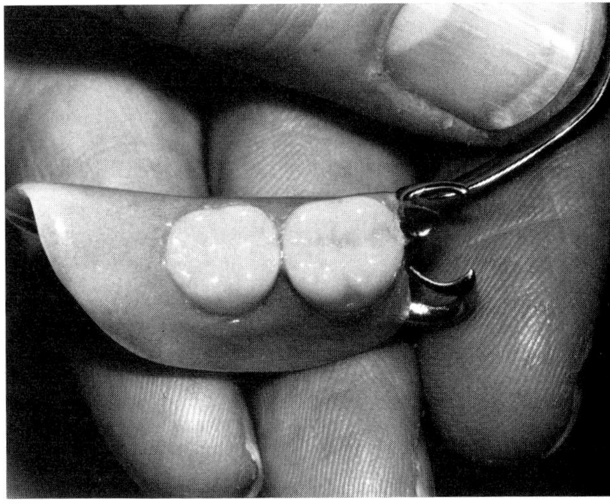

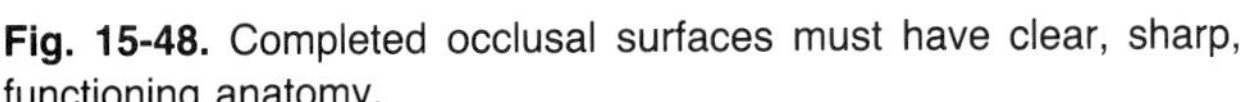
Fig. 15-48. Completed occlusal surfaces must have clear, sharp, functioning anatomy.

left intact, it should not be used as a remount cast during the insertion appointment. As the acrylic resin denture bases are released from the cast, a resultant release of stresses takes place within the resin and a dimensional change occurs in the denture base. As a result, the base will no longer fit the master cast accurately. Errors may be built into the final occlusal correction if this is attempted.

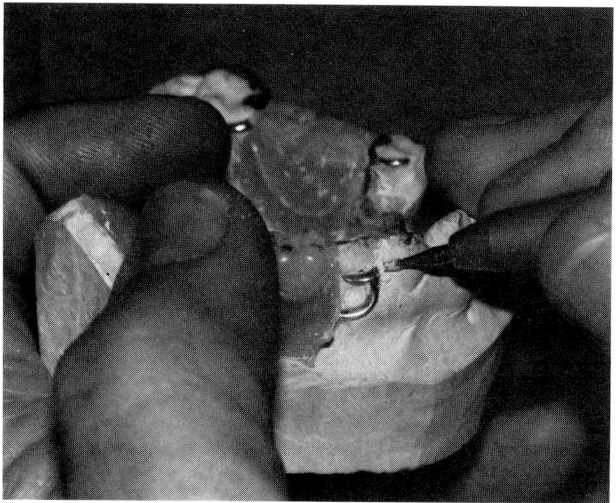

Fig. 15-49. Abutment teeth are cut from master cast with fissure bur.

The abutment teeth are cut from the master cast with a plaster saw or a fissure bur in a straight handpiece (Fig. 15-49). Care must be taken not to scratch or cut the metal or resin of the denture. Generally, when the abutment teeth have been removed, the partial denture can be carefully teased from the remainder of the cast. If, however, undercuts are present under the denture base, the master cast must be sectioned and removed piece by piece. The sectioning is done by either a plaster saw or a fissure bur in the straight handpiece. The sections should be cut starting at the perimeter of the cast and proceeding inward (Fig. 15-50). This will prevent the major connector from having to support unnecessary weight and prevent distortion of the metal. After the major part of the cast has been removed, increasingly smaller sections should be cut to avoid damaging the prosthesis.

Finishing and polishing the partial denture

When the partial denture has been recovered, particles of investment should be removed from around the teeth and from the resin-to-metal joints. This is best accomplished with small hand instruments (Fig. 15-51).

There are three areas to be primarily concerned with in finishing and polishing the partial denture: (1) the external surfaces of the denture base, (2) the periphery or borders of the denture base, and (3) the finish lines

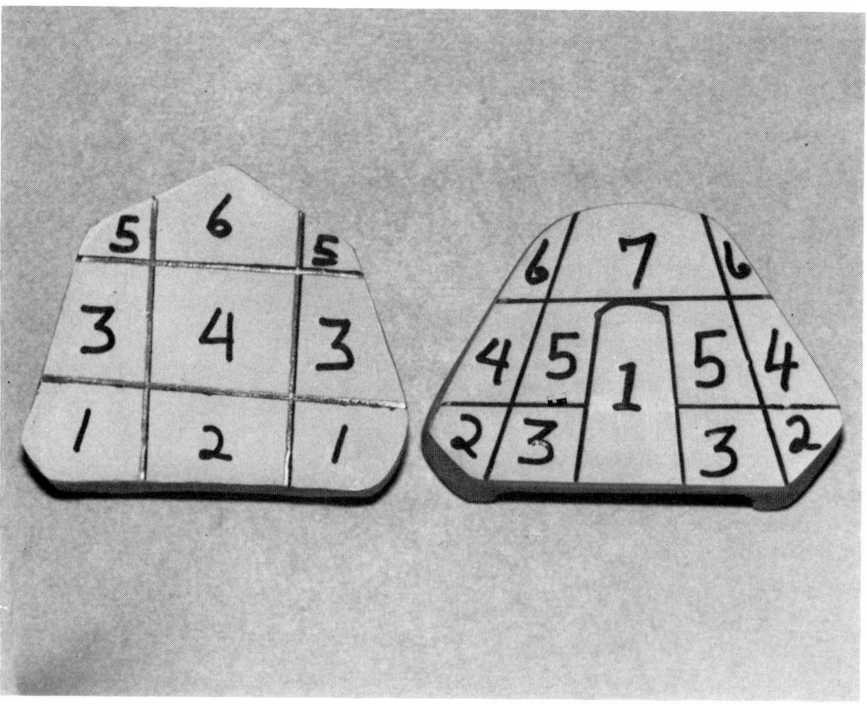

Fig. 15-50. To remove processed denture from master cast, it is occasionally necessary to section cast. Sequence of sectioning cuts is shown on base of maxillary cast, left, and mandibular cast, right.

or contact areas between denture base and metal and the base adjacent to the teeth.

The use of pumice to reduce the scratches or defects in the surface of acrylic resin must be done with caution. Pumice can rapidly reduce the surface of resin. Coarse pumice has little or no indication in smoothing the surface of a denture base. If the surface is so rough that coarse pumice is needed to correct the irregularities, the waxing technique used to produce the denture base should be reviewed.

The whole procedure used in polishing, either the resin denture base or the metal framework, is based on the philosophy of making little scratches out of big scratches. Each progressive step in polishing is designed with that concept in mind. The fineness of the finishing or polishing instrment increases as the polishing process progresses. The final polish is always attained with the most minute abrasive surface available.

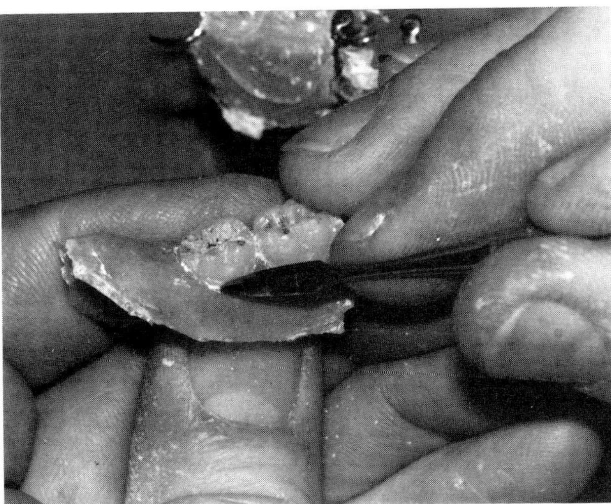

Fig. 15-51. Small hand instruments are used to remove investment from around teeth.

External surfaces

The external surfaces of the denture base should have been developed in the waxing phase to the point that only minimum finishing will be required. The gingival bulge below the gingival contour of the teeth should be maintained (Fig. 15-52). It will act as a secondary food table, enabling the tongue to be a more positive factor in denture retention. Concavities in the denture base below the gingival bulge on the facial surface and in the lingual flanges of the mandibular distal extension partial denture help provide space for the buccal tissues and for the tongue and prevent the dislodging forces these tissues can contribute if the contour is incorrect.

If the waxing was done correctly, the use of vulcanite burs or finishing burs should not be necessary. The lingual flanges should be brought to a high polish by using flour of pumice or fine pumice on a wet cloth wheel (Fig. 15-53) that has been prepared as shown in Fig. 15-54. Then the use of a resin-polishing compound on a dry cloth wheel should produce a high gloss to the resin surface.

The facial surface of the denture base, particularly on anterior flange, should not be brought to a high polish but should be smoothed. A high finish on the facial surface can produce an artificial appearance. Light stippling on the facial surface with an off-center round bur followed by light buffing with fine pumice will produce an egg-shell finish that does not reflect light and will appear more natural (Fig. 15-55).

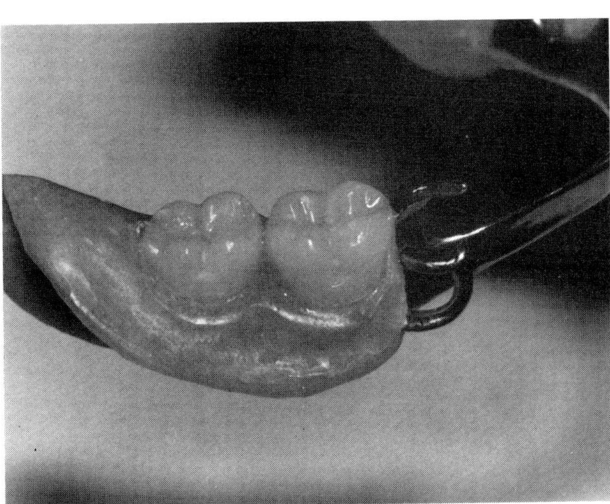

Fig. 15-52. Secondary food table and facial concavity are reproduced in acrylic resin denture base.

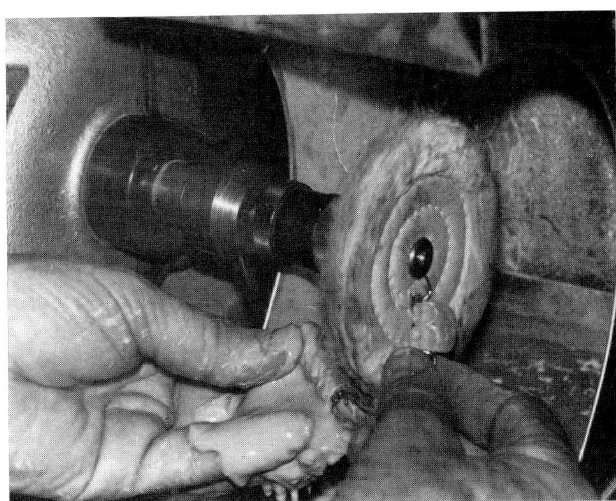

Fig. 15-53. Denture base is smoothed with wet flour of pumice on wet cloth wheel.

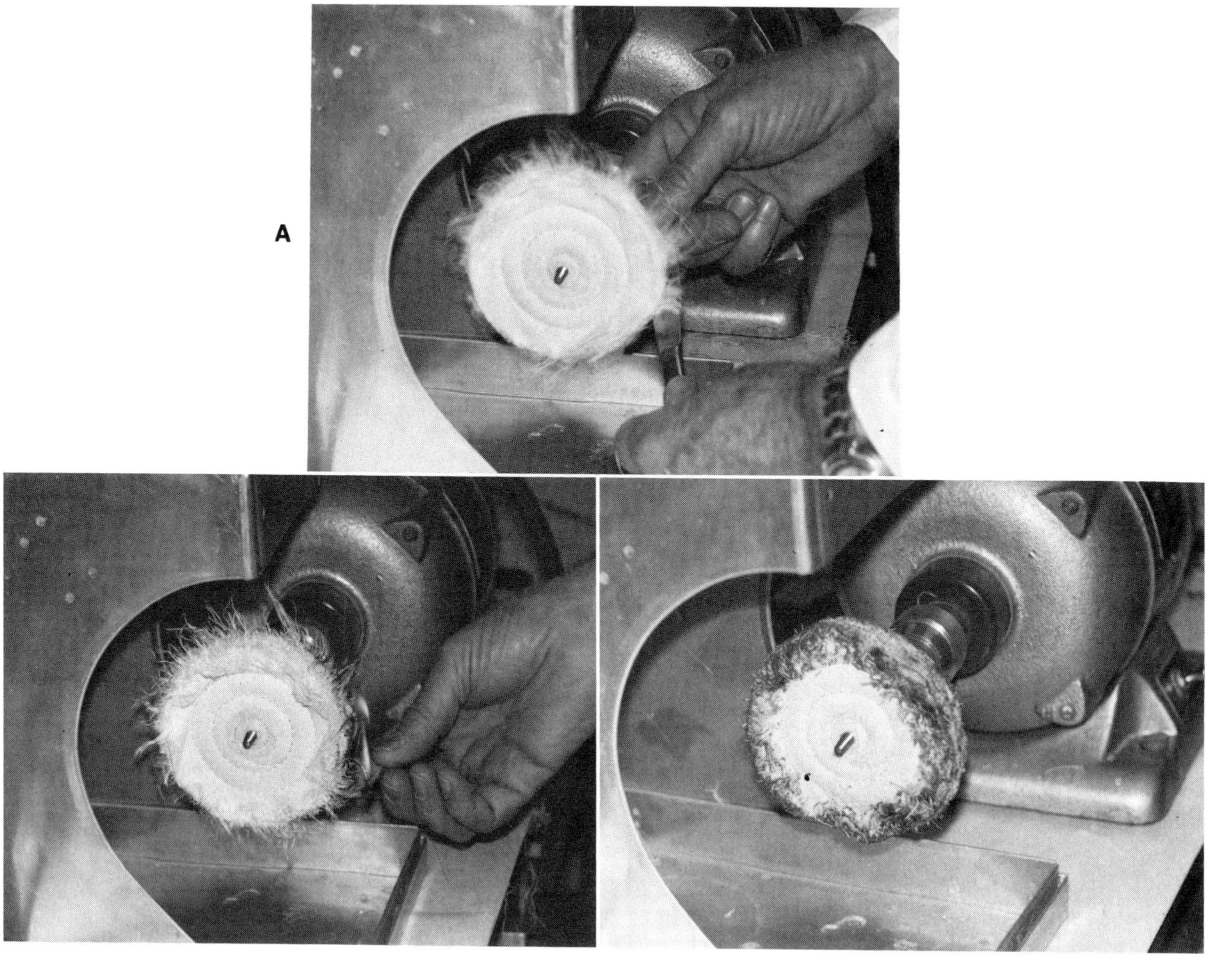

Fig. 15-54. New cloth wheel is prepared for use by running wheel on lathe against dull side of knife blade, **A,** to loosen fibers of cloth and burn loose fibers off wheel, **B. C,** Prepared cloth wheel has smooth, soft surface.

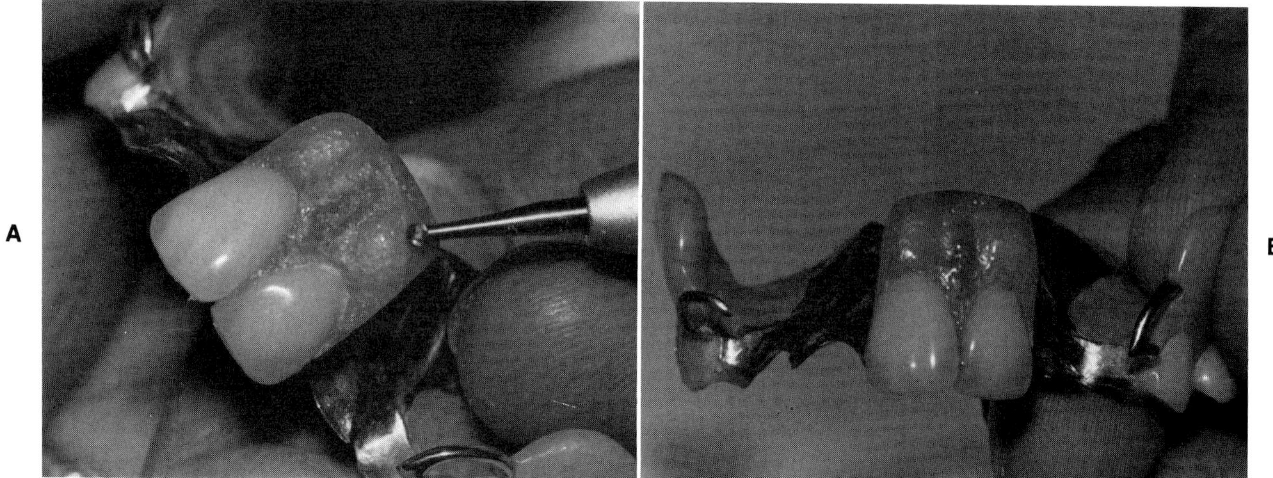

Fig. 15-55. A, Labial flange of denture base is stippled with off-center round bur. **B,** Stippling reduces light reflection and appears more natural.

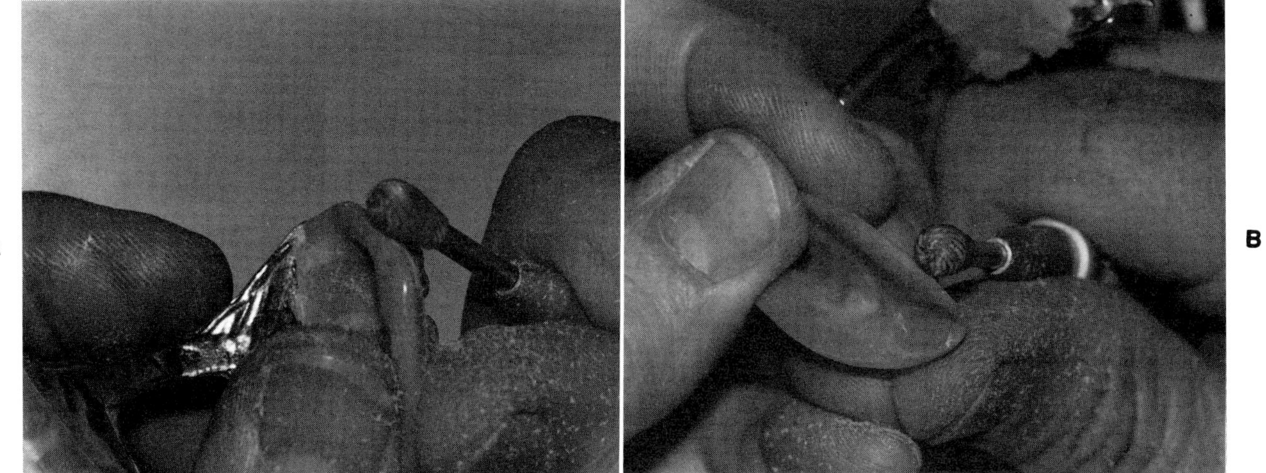

Fig. 15-56. **A,** Distobuccal extension of maxillary distal extension partial denture must be thinned to permit movement of coronoid process of mandible. **B,** Distolingual extension of mandibular free-end denture base is also thinned arbitrarily.

As mentioned previously, two areas of partial dentures must be shaped arbitrarily by the dentist (Fig. 15-56). This is best accomplished during the finishing process. The distobuccal extension of the maxillary distal extension partial denture must be thinned arbitrarily to permit freedom of movement of the coronoid process of the mandible, and the distolingual extension of a mandibular free-end saddle is thinned to allow as much room as possible for tongue movement. A flange thickness of 1.5 to 2 mm is normally desired.

Periphery or borders of denture base

Ideally the denture bases should be extended to the maximum length available to provide all the support and stabilization possible. For most mandibular distal extension partial dentures the extension of the border and the thickness of the border will be established by the secondary impression that is made to provide the altered cast. As the impression is boxed, the length and width of the border must be maintained so that the denture base will be precisely reproduced to those dimensions. To finish these borders, usually all that is necessary is to remove the flash that occurred as the result of trial packing with arbor bands and to polish with fine pumice on a wet cloth wheel followed by a resin-polishing compound.

For borders that are not determined by a secondary impression the extent and thickness must be finished somewhat arbitrarily at this time. The final adjustment will be made at the insertion appointment. For most maxillary partial dentures the tissue reflections can be read adequately on the cast and the denture base extension can be approximated accurately. In any event the denture border should not be finished to a thin edge. A sharp denture base border can be irritating to the movable tissues that contact it. The irritation over a long period of time can result in the development of an epulis fissuratum—a hyperplastic tissue response to chronic denture irritation. The denture borders, except for the two areas mentioned previously, should be at least 2 mm thick and must be rounded (Fig. 15-57). Special consideration must be given to the borders of an anterior flange; this is discussed in Chapter 16.

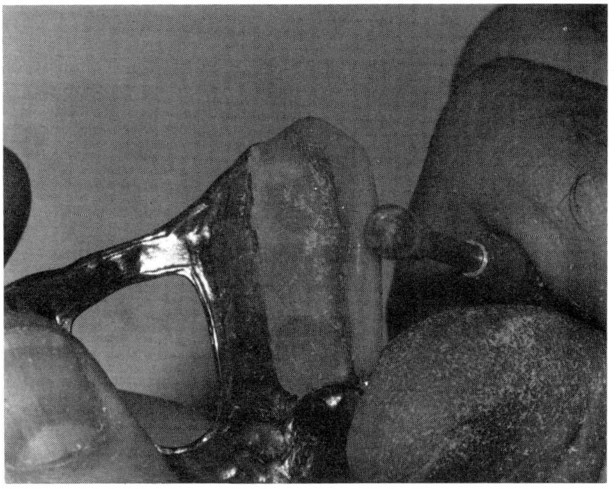

Fig. 15-57. Posterior peripheral border is finished to rounded margin 2 mm wide.

The borders of these flanges are finished and polished in the same way as the flange developed from a secondary impression. The flash is removed with arbor

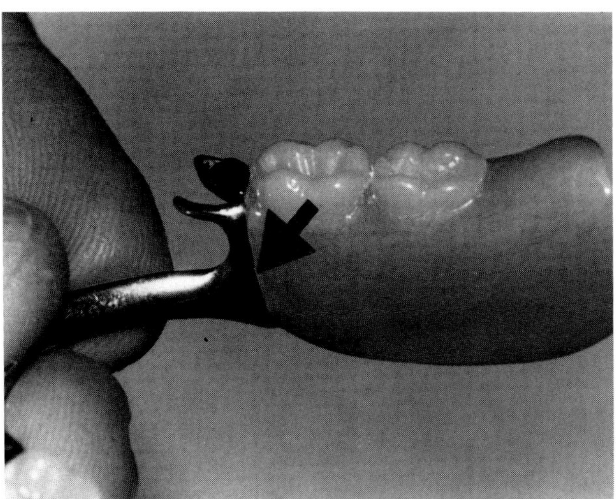

Fig. 15-58. Acrylic resin at external finish lines is left slightly above height of metal. This will be reduced during final polishing.

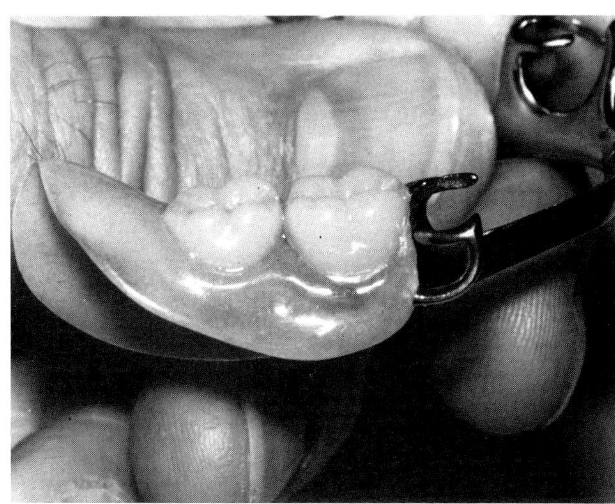

Fig. 15-59. Areas around artificial teeth and minor connector are polished with small cups and wheels to avoid destroying anatomy developed in wax-up.

bands or vulcanite burs. Smoothing is accomplished with pumice and a wet cloth wheel, and the final polish is administered with a resin-polishing compound.

Finish lines and gingival contours

The resin-to-metal junction at the internal finish lines should not be polished. If any flash is present, it must be removed and the joint between the two materials smoothed with finishing burs.

The acrylic resin at the external finish line should be trimmed smooth but left slightly elevated above the height of the metal (Fig. 15-58). This slight elevation will be removed during the final polishing. The goal in this polishing procedure is to ensure an even, flowing surface from plastic to metal. Any deviation from the surface of the plastic to metal annoys the patient's tongue.

Finishing the gingival contours, including the interproximal spaces, becomes a real challenge if acrylic resin teeth have been used, as generally is the case. If proper anatomic contour of these tissues has been established in the wax-up, any attempt to merely smooth the areas by pumicing with a brush wheel or a cloth wheel will flatten the convex surfaces and may abrade the facial surfaces of the plastic teeth. The gingival margins around the teeth are cleaned and smoothed with explorer points and small operative chisels. This cleaning operation will emphasize the value of a good wax-up. A rubber prophylaxis cup or small soft brush wheels in the dental handpiece can be used to fine pumice and polish these areas around the teeth (Fig. 15-59).

If the final polish to the partial denture—both the metal and acrylic resin portions—is done on a lathe,

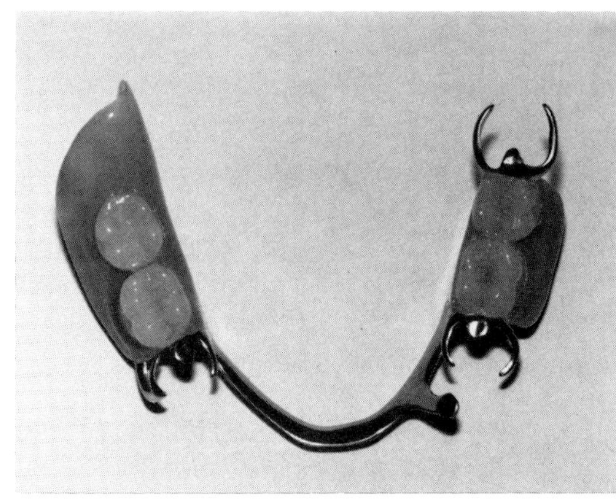

Fig. 15-60. Completed removable partial denture should be free from defects and should restore form and function to patient.

special care must be used. It is very easy for a clasp or other component to become entangled in the polishing wheel, particularly a cloth wheel. It is possible to distort a clasp arm, but more important, it is possible that the denture can be thrown with considerable force against the lathe pan. This can distort the major connector or fracture the denture base. The less experienced operator would be wise to line the lathe pan with soft towels or to keep the pan well filled with wet pumice to cushion the shock should the partial denture be thrown from the polishing wheel.

After the polishing procedures are complete, the partial denture should be washed with soap and water and a soft brush. If difficulty is encountered in removing remnants of polishing compound from the partial denture, it may be placed in an ultrasonic cleaner for a few minutes.

The partial denture should be carefully inspected, preferably under magnification, to be certain that all scratches or other minor defects have been removed (Fig. 15-60). If the inspection is satisfactory, the partial denture is ready for delivery to the patient.

REFERENCE

Frush, J.O., and Fisher, R.D.: Introduction to dentogenic restoration, J. Prosthet. Dent. **5**:568-595, 1955.

BIBLIOGRAPHY

Bolouri, A., and others: Modified flasking technique for removable partial dentures, J. Prosthet. Dent. **34**:221-223, 1975.

Clark, E.B.: Tooth color selection, J. Am. Dent. Assoc. **20**:1065-1073, 1933.

Culpepper, W.D.: A comparative study of shade matching procedures, J. Prosthet. Dent. **24**:166-173, 1970.

DeVan, M.M.: The appearance phase of denture construction, Dent. Clin. North Am. **1**:255-268, 1957.

Grunewald, A.H., and others: The effect of molding processes on some properties of denture resins, J. Am. Dent. Assoc. **44**:269-284, 1952.

Hughes, G.A.: Facial types and tooth arrangement, J. Prosthet. Dent. **1**:82-95, 1951.

Johnson, H.B.: Technique for packing and staining complete or partial denture bases, J. Prosthet. Dent. **6**:154-159, 1956.

Krajicek, D.D.: Natural appearance for the individual denture patient, J. Prosthet. Dent. **10**:205-214, 1960.

Lowe, R.D., and others: Swallowing and resting forces related to lingual flange thickness in removable partial dentures, J. Prosthet. Dent. **23**:279, 1970.

Peyton, F.A., and Anthony, D.H.: Evaluation of dentures processed by different techniques, J. Prosthet. Dent. **13**:269-281, 1963.

Pound, E.: Applying harmony in selecting and arranging teeth, Dent. Clin. North Am. **6**:241-258, March 1962.

Scandrett, F.R., and others: Layered silicone rubber technique for flasking removable partial dentures, J. Prosthet. Dent. **40**:349-350, 1978.

Smith, R.H.: Rapid removable partial denture processing with a cold-curing acrylic resin, J. Prosthet. Dent. **28**:442-444, 1972.

Sproull, R.C.: Color matching in dentistry, part I: the three dimensional nature of color, J. Prosthet. Dent. **29**:416-424, 1973.

Tillman, E.J.: Molding and staining acrylic resin anterior teeth, J. Prosthet. Dent. **5**:497-507, 1955.

Van Victor, A.: The mold guide cast—its significance in denture esthetics, J. Prosthet. Dent. **3**:165-177, 1953.

Vig, R.G.: The denture look, J. Prosthet. Dent. **11**:9-15, 1961.

Young, H.A.: Denture esthetics, J. Prosthet. Dent. **6**:748-755, 1956.

16 Delivering the removable partial denture

The climax to the long hours of intensive preparation, the apex to the sometimes lengthy clinical and laboratory sessions, is arrived at in the appointment to deliver the completed prosthesis. Throughout the many clinical appointments the clinician should be reminding and reinforcing the patient of the value of a removable partial denture. The reminder should include the fact that the principal contribution of the partial denture to oral health is not merely replacing missing teeth but providing additional support and stabilization that will help prolong the function and prognosis of the remaining oral structures.

It is imperative that these points be strongly emphasized before the prosthesis is delivered. Many patients will have a period of discomfort immediately following the placement of a removable partial denture merely because of the presence of a foreign object in the mouth. If the patient has been mentally conditioned to expect this sensation, the depression that might otherwise occur can be prevented. Even a short period of discomfort following insertion can prevent a patient from ever completely accepting a prosthesis. A significant percentage of unsuccessful partial dentures can be attributed to a lack of mental preparation of the patient by the dentist.

The objectives of the delivery or insertion appointment are (1) to fit the denture base to the edentulous ridge, (2) to correct occlusal discrepancies, (3) to adjust retentive clasps if necessary, and (4) to instruct the patient in home care and in care of the prosthesis.

The first three listed objectives should be completed in order. The occlusion should not be altered until the denture base has been completely fitted to the edentulous ridge, and clasps should not be tightened until all other adjustments have been made. Inserting and removing a partial denture numerous times as is necessary during this appointment is more easily done if the retentive clasps are not overly retentive.

CORRECTING FIT OF DENTURE BASE

Even after all the care that has been taken in securing accurate impressions of the edentulous ridge, the denture base, if constructed of heat-cured acrylic resin, will not fit the soft tissues accurately. The denture base will usually exhibit heavy contact with the lateral walls, both buccal and lingual or palatal, of the ridge and light or no contact with the ridge crest. This pattern is produced by the direction of shrinkage that takes place during polymerization of the resin. Autopolymerizing resin does not produce this shrinkage pattern. It normally requires much less adjustment than the heat-cured resin.

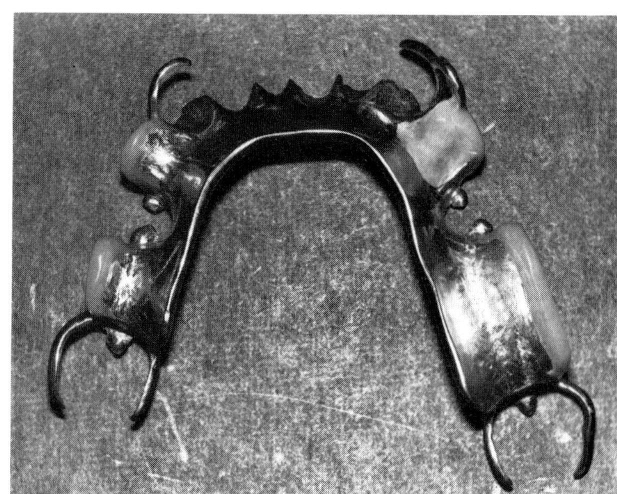

Fig. 16-1. Fit of metal denture bases is corrected or verified at framework try-in appointment. At delivery appointment it is not necessary to further adjust their adaptation.

Cast metal denture bases (often the choice for tooth-supported segments) should not require any adjustment at this time (Fig. 16-1). Any correction in the fit of the metal to the underlying tissue would have been made at the framework try-in appointment.

Pressure-indicating paste

Other than asking the patient whether the denture base feels as though it fits properly or whether there are areas that feel as though pressure from the base may be excessive, there is no way that the fit of the denture base can be verified without using a pressure-disclosing agent. The materials used to fit the metallic

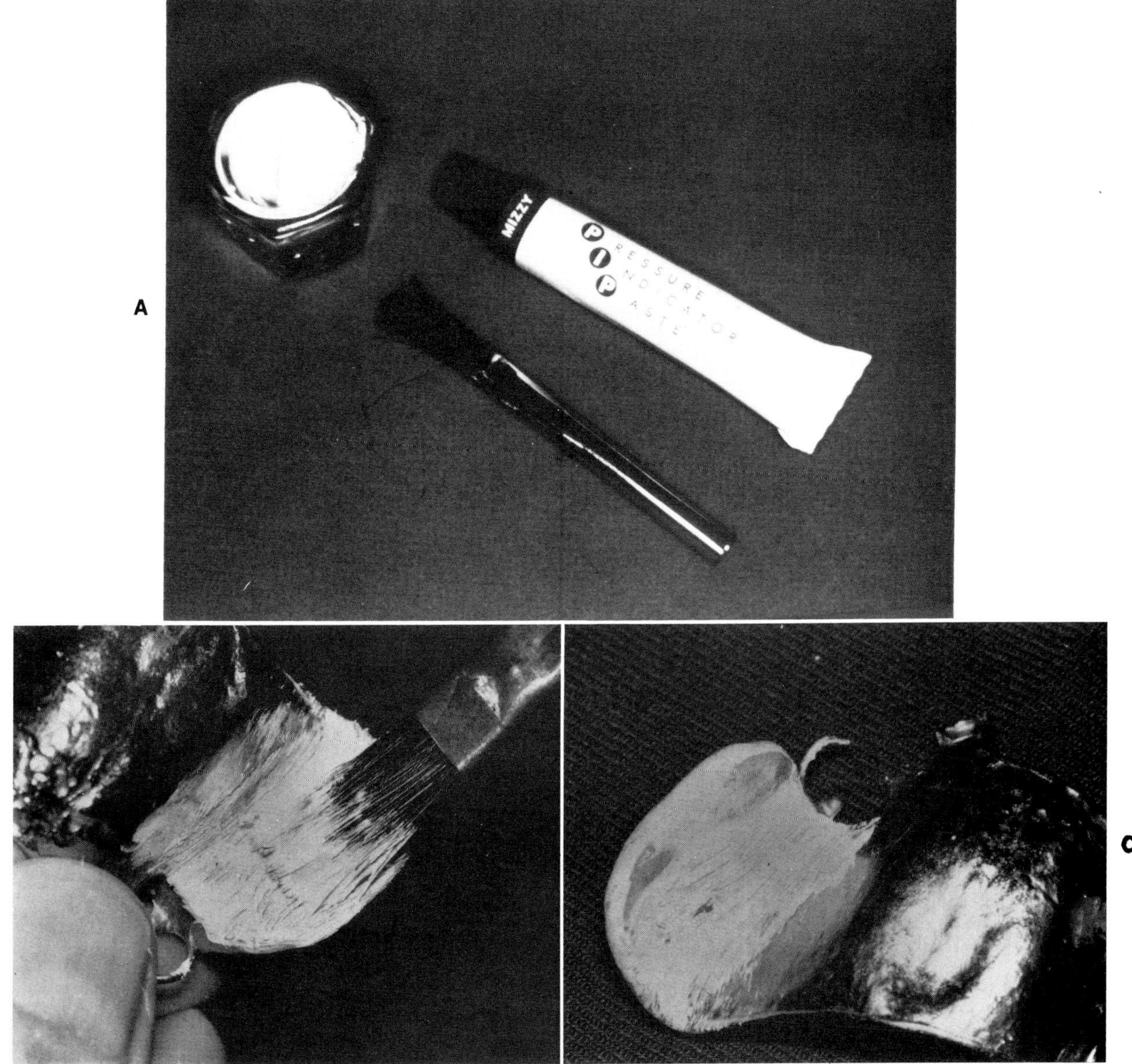

Fig. 16-2. A, Pressure-indicating paste. **B,** Paste is painted on acrylic resin denture base with stiff brush. **C,** Paste is displaced on those parts of denture base in contact with soft tissue. Brush marks remain evident when no soft tissue contact takes place.

framework to the teeth (disclosing wax or solution of jeweler's rouge dissolved in chloroform) cannot be used to locate areas of interference or pressure between the acrylic resin denture base and the soft tissue. These disclosing materials are too resistant to displacement by soft tissue under normal circumstances, and the results would not be reliable.

A softer material, more easily displaced by soft tissues, is required to check the fit of a denture base to the edentulous ridge. The various pastes available on the commercial market consist principally of zinc oxide powder combined with a medium consistency vegetable fat or shortening. Other ingredients are added to improve the odor and taste and to control the consistency. The material is referred to as pressure-indicating paste, or PIP (Fig. 16-2).

The consistency of the material should be such that it can be painted on the tissue surface of a denture base with a stiff brush. A stiff brush is preferred so that the brush marks are left on the surface of the paste. As the denture base is seated in the mouth, in those areas where the denture base and soft tissue are in intimate

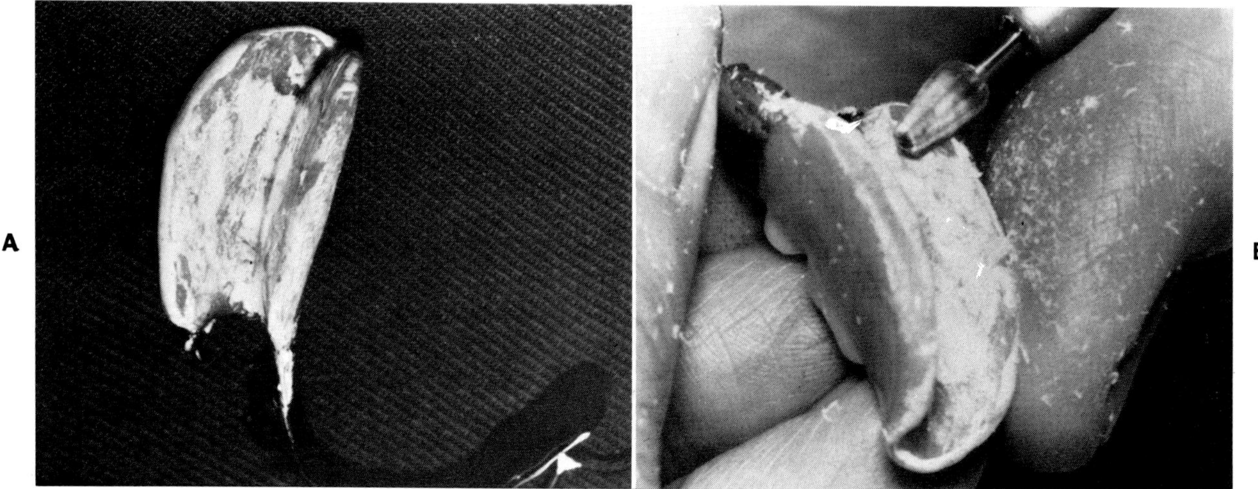

Fig. 16-3. A, Areas of interference on denture base offering resistance to seating are evident by portions of base showing through pressure-indicating paste. **B,** Areas of showthrough are relieved with vulcanite burs.

contact, the brush marks will be obliterated. When contact is not present, the marks will be obvious.

A WORD OF CAUTION: The use of a pressure-indicating material at the insertion appointment can do much to prevent unnecessary pain or discomfort several days following the insertion caused by an ill-fitting denture base. However, unnecessary or ill-advised relieving of the tissue surface of a denture base can produce a poorly fitting base that can lead to the need for early relining of the denture. This could be discouraging for a patient who was expecting longer service from the prosthesis. A certain amount of experience is necessary to differentiate between a wipe-away of paste that has occurred from normal contact with soft tissue on an edentulous ridge and the displacement of paste that occurs as the denture attempts to pass over a bony protuberance or an undercut on the ridge. The student or the beginning practitioner should always err on the side of conservation until the necessary clinical experience is developed. As with any other dental material that is used in clinical situations, if the weaknesses in the use of pressure-indicating paste are recognized and the limitations of the material respected, good results can be obtained.

Clinical use

The removable partial denture should not be tried in the patient's mouth before pressure-indicating paste is used. There are times when it will be difficult to recognize subtle undercuts that may be present on the ridge. Seating the partial denture over these undercuts can produce pain or even lacerate the soft tissue. Worse still, the exact location of the offending undercut will still not be known, and the patient will be subjected to the same procedure again, although this time with considerable apprehension.

The tissue surface of the denture base must be completely dried with air from the syringe or by wiping with a tissue. A thin coating of pressure-indicating paste is painted evenly over the entire tissue surface of the base.

When the partial denture is inserted for the first time, a very gentle seating force should be used. If resistance to the seating is encountered, the partial denture should be immediately removed and the pressure-indicating paste on the denture base examined. Any resistance met in seating the partial denture must be occurring between the acrylic resin denture base and the edentulous ridge. All other components of the partial denture have been tried in the mouth previously, and all interferences have been eliminated. The paste over the area that is preventing the partial denture from going to place will be displaced at the point of interference. This area or areas are relieved by using vulcanite burs or other rotating istruments (Fig. 16-3). It is good practice to relieve a little at a time rather than overcutting and losing all tissue contact. After each time that the acrylic resin is relieved, the denture base surface should be wiped clean of the pressure-indicating paste and the grindings of the resin and fresh paste applied. The procedure should be repeated until the denture goes to place without encountering resistance or causing patient discomfort.

The most frequently observed areas that cause problems with the seating of the denture base are undercuts buccal to the edentulous ridge in the mandibular pre-

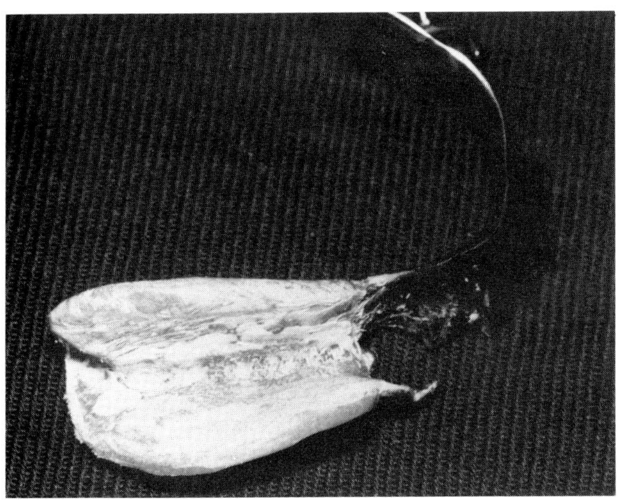

Fig. 16-4. Mylohyoid area of mandibular ridge is especially sensitive to pressure. This denture base appears to be seating properly.

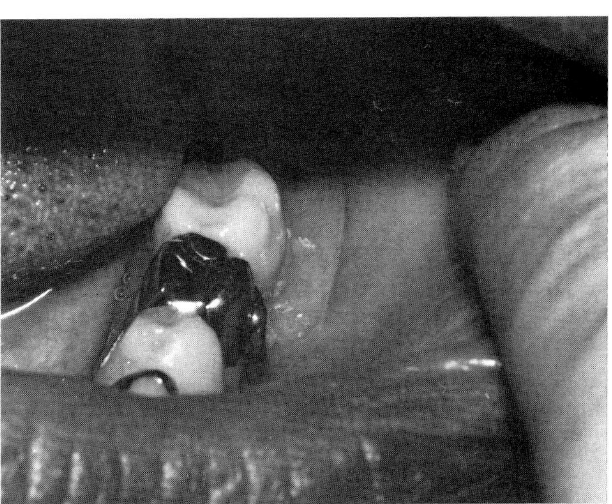

Fig. 16-5. Posterior buccal flange extensions must be checked visually. Cheek is moved downward, outward, and upward with finger. Movable tissue must not lie under denture base.

molar and maxillary tuberosity areas. Perhaps the most difficult area to correct and certainly the most sensitive to pressure against soft tissue is the mylohyoid area on the lingual surface of the mandibular posterior edentulous ridge (Fig. 16-4). Careful analysis must be made of the readings seen on the surface of the pressure-indicating paste over this area to be certain all pressure is relieved.

Modifying the peripheral extension of the denture base

The length and degree of adaptation of the denture base flanges are critical to maximum support and stabilization of the partial denture. The maximum amount of edentulous ridge must be covered so that no portion of the ridge and no abutment tooth bears a greater share of the functional forces generated by the prosthesis than it can safely accommodate.

Denture base flange length not only contributes a major share of vertical support for the partial denture but also can play an important role in offering resistance to horizontal or lateral displacement of the denture. For this reason peripheral extensions should not be arbitrarily reduced but should cover as much ridge as possible.

For practically all mandibular Class I or II partial dentures the extension of the peripheral borders will have been determined by the border-molding procedures in obtaining the corrected cast impression. A visual and digital check may be made if doubt exists as to the correct extension (Fig. 16-5). To check visually, the buccal tissues should be held between the thumb and index finger and moved downward, outward, and upward. As the movement of the tissue adjacent to the buccal border of the denture base is observed, it can be determined if any movable tissue is trapped by the denture base. Trapping or impinging of movable tissue or muscle attachments by the denture base can damage the abutment teeth. The rebound of the tissues attempting to resume the normal tissue anatomy places additional and needless stress on the abutment teeth. Hanau described this phenomenon as REALEFF—*re*silient *a*nd *l*ike *eff*ect—of tissues always attempting to return to their normal contour. This is the reason that, although maximum tissue coverage is essential, it is equally important not to extend denture borders on to movable tissues. The action of the tissues that are compromised will apply a constant unseating force to the denture, causing the abutment teeth to have to resist this unnecessary and at times destructive force.

The lingual and distolingual flange length may also be verified by tissue movement. The operator should rest the index finger on the occlusal surfaces of the artifical teeth on the distal extension denture base. The patient should then thrust the tongue straight forward and also into the cheek on the opposite side of the mouth that is being tested. The tongue thrust should be made with moderate force. If overextensions are present in the floor of the mouth or in the distolingual flange extension, the denture base will tend to rise. This movement can be felt by the operator, and necessary correction in reducing the flange length can be made.

One method of determining exactly where the overextension is located is to use disclosing wax along the denture border that is suspected of being overex-

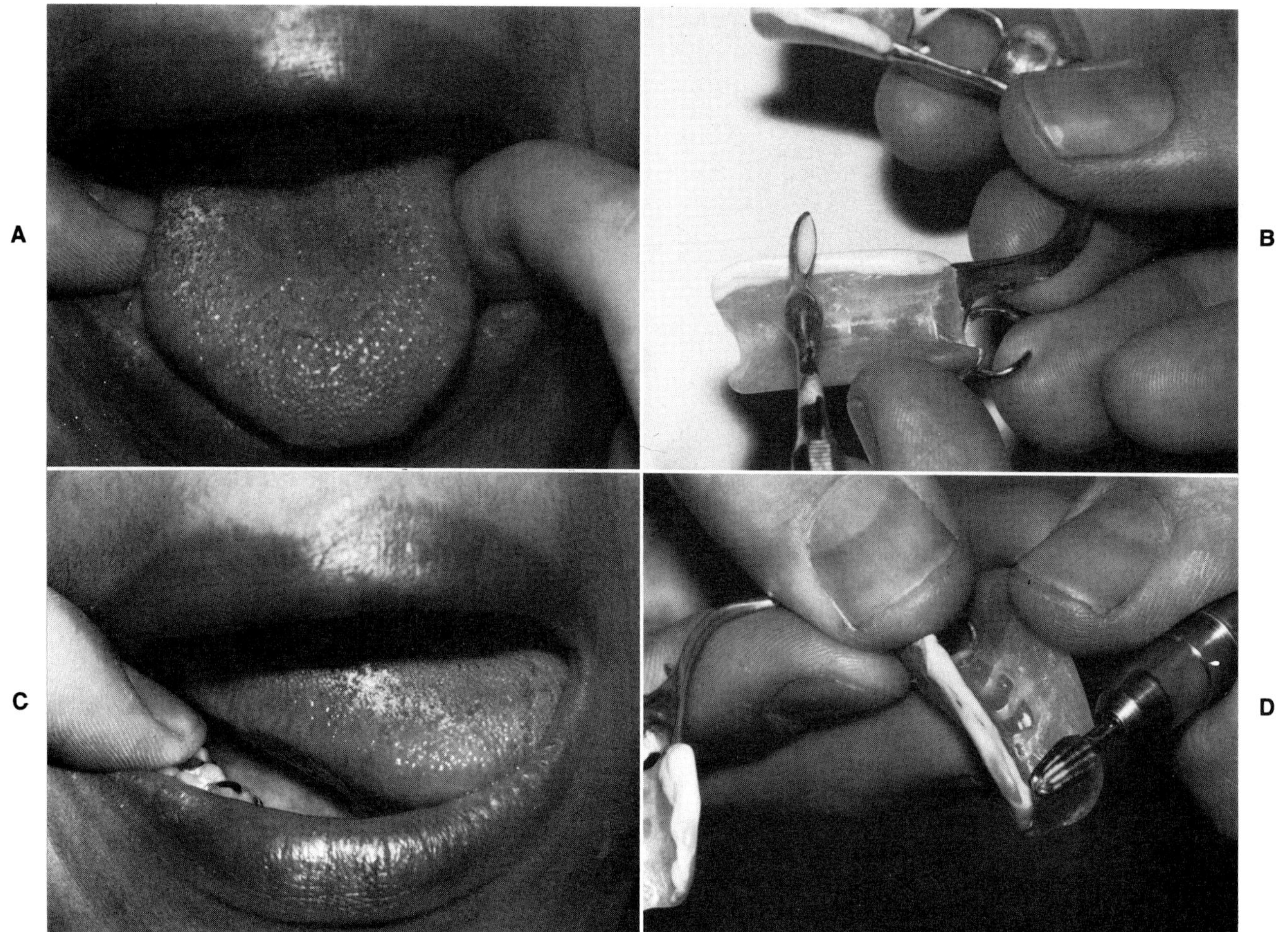

Fig. 16-6. A, Lingual flange extension of mandibular partial denture is checked by placing finger on denture teeth with patient's tongue thrust forward. Denture will lift if overextension of flange is present. **B,** To define area of overextension more accurately, disclosing wax is flowed over flange periphery. **C,** Denture is inserted carefully in order not to mar wax surface, and patient's tongue is moved into opposite cheek. **D,** Area of overextension is corrected.

tended, as shown in Fig. 16-6. The use of disclosing wax is not totally reliable and should be used only to confirm or isolate an area that is thought to be overextended as a result of other tests; it should not be used routinely in determining proper peripheral border extensions.

For maxillary Class I or II partial dentures, for which corrected cast impressions are not usually accomplished, direct visual verification of proper flange extension is the method of choice. The tissue of the cheek is lifted upward, outward, downward, and also moved anteroposteriorly. Careful observation should reveal the presence of movable tissue trapped by the denture base if an overextension is present.

In a tooth-supported partial denture—either a Class III or for a modification space of any other class—the peripheral border should extend enough to ensure tissue contact so that food impaction is prevented under the denture base. The denture base should replace the contour of the ridge by filling in the areas of missing bone as well as the missing teeth. Extending the length of the denture flance to the soft tissue reflection is normally not desired (Fig. 16-7).

All borders of the posterior denture base must be well rounded. The only areas where the flange should be reduced to less than 2 mm thick are the distolingual extension of a mandibular Class I or II denture base and the distobuccal extension over the tuberosity of a maxillary Class I or II denture base, (to provide tongue space in the mandibular arch and permit freedom of movement of the coronoid process in the maxillary arch) and the leading edge of a maxillary or mandibular posterior denture base flange (because as a patient is viewed from in front while smiling, a thick leading edge

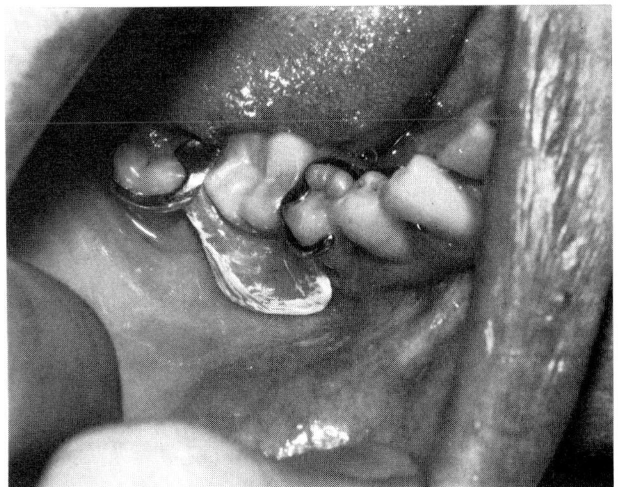

Fig. 16-7. A tooth-supported flange must not extend onto movable tissue.

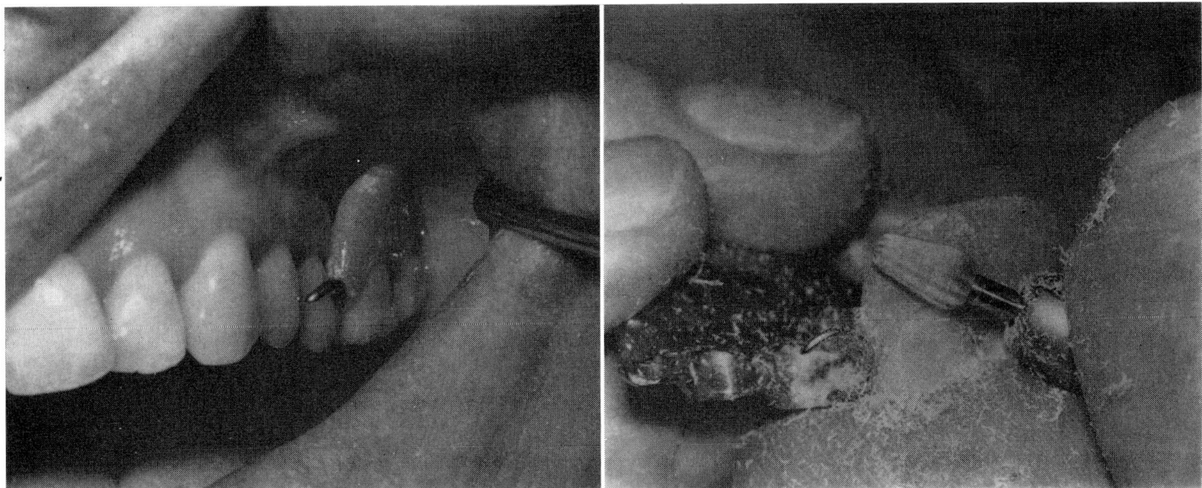

Fig. 16-8. Leading edge of posterior denture base should be thinned, but not to less than 1 to 1.5 mm, to add to esthetic quality of denture.

of the denture base detracts from the esthetic quality of the denture) (Fig. 16-8).

Contouring the anterior denture base flange

Contouring and shaping an anterior flange must be considered apart from the shaping required of a posterior flange. High priority has to be given to the esthetic requirements of the patient. Overextension of the labial flange either in length or in fullness must be prevented. Nothing can detract more from what might otherwise be a successful partial denture than a patient's lip that is plumped out of normal shape.

Pressure-indicating paste is painted on the tissue surface of the denture base and, as was done with the posterior denture base, the partial denture is positioned and seated in the mouth with gentle pressure. Nearly all maxillary anterior edentulous ridges will be undercut varying from moderately to severely. The labial flange of the denture must not be allowed to extend into an undercut area when all denture flange and tissue contact has been eliminated. This flange will do nothing but distort the shape of the lip.

As resistance to the seating of the labial flange is encountered, the partial denture is removed and the length of the flange is reduced vertically to the point of contact with the edentulous ridge (Fig. 16-9). The contaminated paste and grindings of the resin are removed, fresh paste applied, and the seating of the denture again gently attempted. If resistance is again encountered, the denture is removed and the labial flange further shortened to the point of contact as indicated on the surface of the paste. This sequence is repeated until

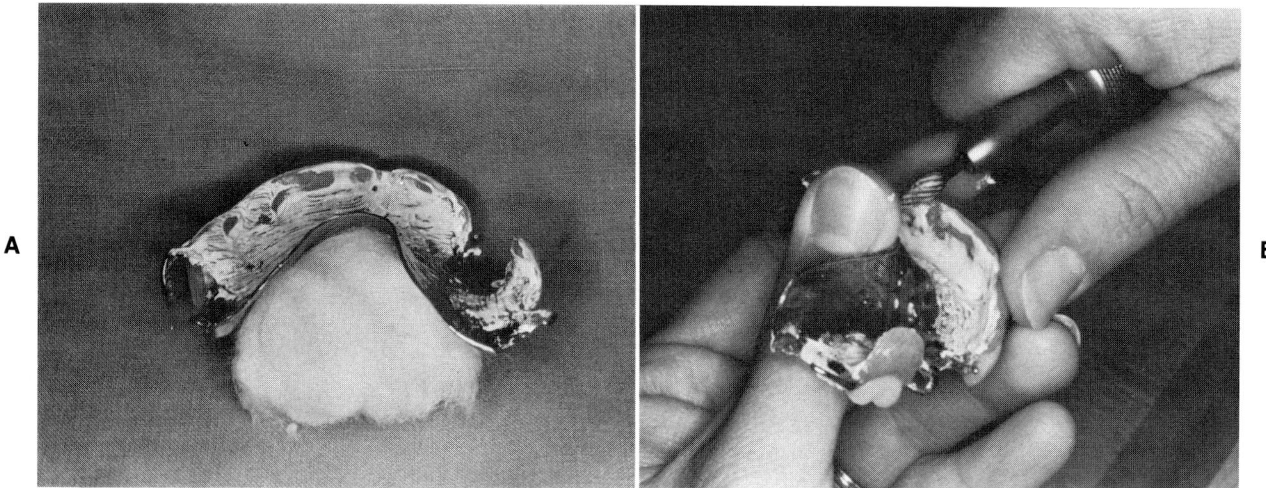

Fig. 16-9. Anterior denture flange is handled differently from posterior flange. **A,** Areas of interference preventing denture from seating are shown. **B,** Height of flange is reduced to level of interference.

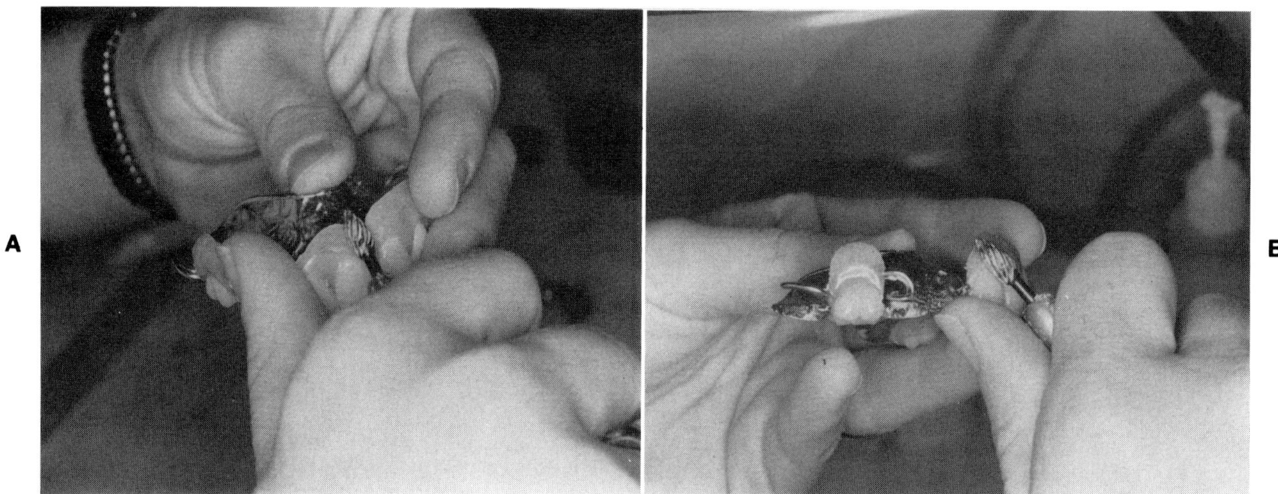

Fig. 16-10. Margins of anterior flange are beveled, both superiorly, **A,** and laterally, **B,** to blend into supporting soft tissue.

the partial denture goes to place easily without producing blanching of the soft tissues or patient discomfort.

Once completely seated, the superior and lateral margins of the denture base flange are beveled to a thin edge in order to blend into the surrounding soft tissues and to produce a natural and esthetic effect (Fig. 16-10). It must be emphasized that only anterior margins can be handled in this fashion.

It would appear to be simpler and more time saving for the dentist if the technician were to block out the undercut areas on the anterior ridge of the master cast before waxing and processing the denture base. If the denture base is formed in this fashion, the same degree of intimate contact and blending of the denture base to the mucosa will not be present. A slight resiliency of the soft tissue is necessary to produce intimate contact and disguise the presence of the denture base.

Characterizing the completed denture base

To fortify the natural appearance, particularly for those patients possessing a high degree of pigmentation in the skin and mucosa, characterization of the denture base with acrylic resin stains will greatly enhance the esthetic quality of the restoration. The staining technique is discussed in Chapter 15. Staining or characterizing the denture base may be accomplished after the partial denture is completed, but it is easier to accomplish it during the investing and processing procedure.

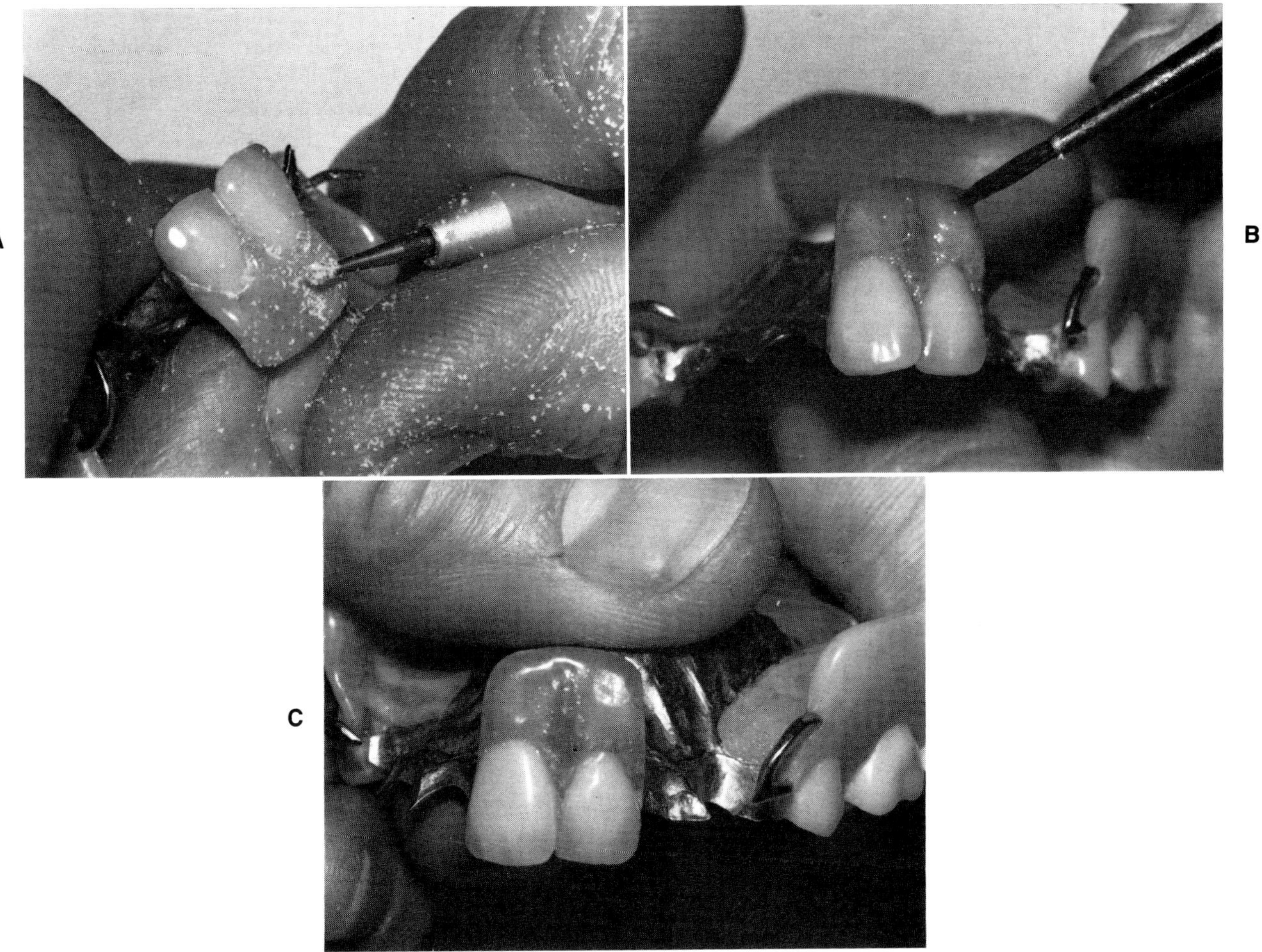

Fig. 16-11. A, To characterize completed denture base, labial surface is reduced in thickness by 1 mm. **B,** Polymer stains are sprinkled on surface of denture base and wet with monomer. Shaping or sculpturing is accomplished with brush. **C,** Completed characterized base can match tones of surrounding tissue.

The labial surface of the anterior flange must be thinned to provide space for the acrylic resin stain. A reduction of approximately 1 mm is sufficient for the stains to be added to create the desired result (Fig. 16-11).

The surface of the resin to be characterized is painted with a coat of *autopolymerizing* monomer that is compatible with the polymer stain that is being used. The stains are added by sprinkling the polymer on the surface of the denture base. The brighter or more distinctive stains are added first so that if toning down the effect is required this can be done by adding a more neutral stain over the brighter stain. The polymer is wet with the monomer by using a soft camel hair brush dipped in the monomer. The brush is also used to sculpture the soft resin to the anatomic form desired.

The characterization and sculpturing process must be carried out rapidly because the working time of the autopolymerizing resin is limited. Probably the greatest drawback of this technique is that the outer layer of the denture base, the added on stained layer, will not be as dense as the processed resin. It will tend to wear more rapidly than the rest of the denture base. To provide as dense an outer layer as possible, the final cure for the stained resin should be accomplished in an atmosphere saturated with monomer. This atmosphere can be obtained by inverting a rubber bowl or a glass jar over the partial denture on the bench top. This will decrease the amount of surface porosity caused by evaporation of the volatile monomer.

When the denture bases have been fitted and shaped to the desired contour, smoothness and polish must be restored to the surfaces involved.

CORRECTING OCCLUSAL DISCREPANCIES

The second of the four steps involved in delivering the partial denture to the patient is begun only after the denture bases have been corrected to fit the edentulous ridges. Attempting to correct occlusal errors before or during the process of fitting the denture base can not only waste time but can also damage the final occlusal scheme. Until the denture bases are seated, it is impossible to analyze occlusal contacts.

During the framework try-in appointment all interferences between opposing natural teeth and the framework and between opposing frameworks were relieved. Therefore, the only possible interferences at this appointment are between the artificial teeth in one arch and the natural teeth or artificial teeth in the opposite arch.

The basic method for correcting these discrepancies is the same as that used during the framework try-in appointment. A systematic and logical sequence to correcting occlusal errors will not only save valuable chair time but will also reduce the possibility of overlooking interferences.

The same goal that was strived for when occlusal discrepancies of the framework were being corrected is the ultimate aim for this procedure: complete occlusal harmony in all jaw positions. Included in this process must be the reestablishing of natural tooth contacts. The denture must not keep natural teeth from contacting that would otherwise normally be in contact in any jaw position. Failure to observe this maxim can account for patient's failing to accept the prosthesis. The only variation in this most important concept is when a change in the vertical dimension of occlusion is required (covered in Chapter 14).

In addition to restoring natural tooth contacts, a harmonious relationship must be developed that permits the patient to function in the most retruded position as well as the position of habitual closure, the neuromuscular position. The patient must not only be able to make equal bilateral contacts in both centric relation and centric occlusion but should be able to traverse the path between the two positions without meeting deceptive or deflective occlusal contacts.

At times in the past the patient was allowed to wear the partial denture for a short time before final occlusal correction was made so that the denture would have a chance to 'settle' in place. In light of clinical research this position is hardly justifiable.

The technique for detecting occlusal discrepancies intraorally is based on the premise that the removable partial denture or dentures being corrected are stable in the mouth. A large percentage of partial dentures fall into this category. However, in a small percentage of patients stability is a problem and intraoral detection of occlusal defects should be avoided. This group of patients includes those in whom all or nearly all the posterior occlusion is being restored and in whom the task of locating discrepancies intraorally would be difficult if not impossible. Also in this group are patients for whom a complete denture is being constructed simultaneously with a removable partial denture. For these patients in whom stability of the prosthesis is questionable or in whom so much of the occlusal scheme is being restored to contraindicate intraoral occlusal interference detection, a remount of the dentures is indicated.

Intraoral detection of occlusal discrepancies and their correction

One of the best and simplest methods of detecting occlusal discrepancies intraorally and correcting them is shown in Fig. 16-12.

If interferences are present and articulating paper is used to locate them, the point of initial contact on the artificial teeth will normally appear as a small bull's-eye. The white center of the bull's-eye is caused by the dye of the marking paper being expressed by the heavy contact of the opposing cusps. The colored ring around the center represents the accumulation of the dye in the area surrounding the heavy contact. It is necessary to differentiate between a smudge of dye or ink from the articulating paper that may be caused by near but not actual contact of opposing teeth. Before a cusp or a fossa is relieved, the operator should be certain that the articulating paper mark indicates an area of interference and not a false indication. This is best proved by holding a narrow strip of tape or tissue paper over the area in question and having the patient close. If an interference exists, the paper cannot be withdrawn.

Correction on the occlusal surfaces of the artificial teeth must not destroy the anatomy or the efficiency of the masticatory mechanism. At the time the teeth were set, the occlusal surfaces were shaped to correspond to the cusp height and cuspal inclination of the remaining natural teeth. This similarity of occlusal surfaces should not be lost by the procedures involved in eliminating occlusal interferences. As occlusal errors are corrected, the cusp tips should not be relieved arbitrarily. At times it may be necessary to shorten a cusp, but the anatomy of the cusp must be maintained. At times, by altering the incline of a cusp, interferences can be eliminated without basically changing the cusp height. Frequently a small V-shaped notch can be made on the cusp surface as indicated by the mark of the articulating paper (Fig. 16-13). The notch will not only eliminate the undesirable contact but will also add to the cutting efficiency of the cusp.

It is good practice, and one that the patient will appreciate, not to perform the occlusal correction proce-

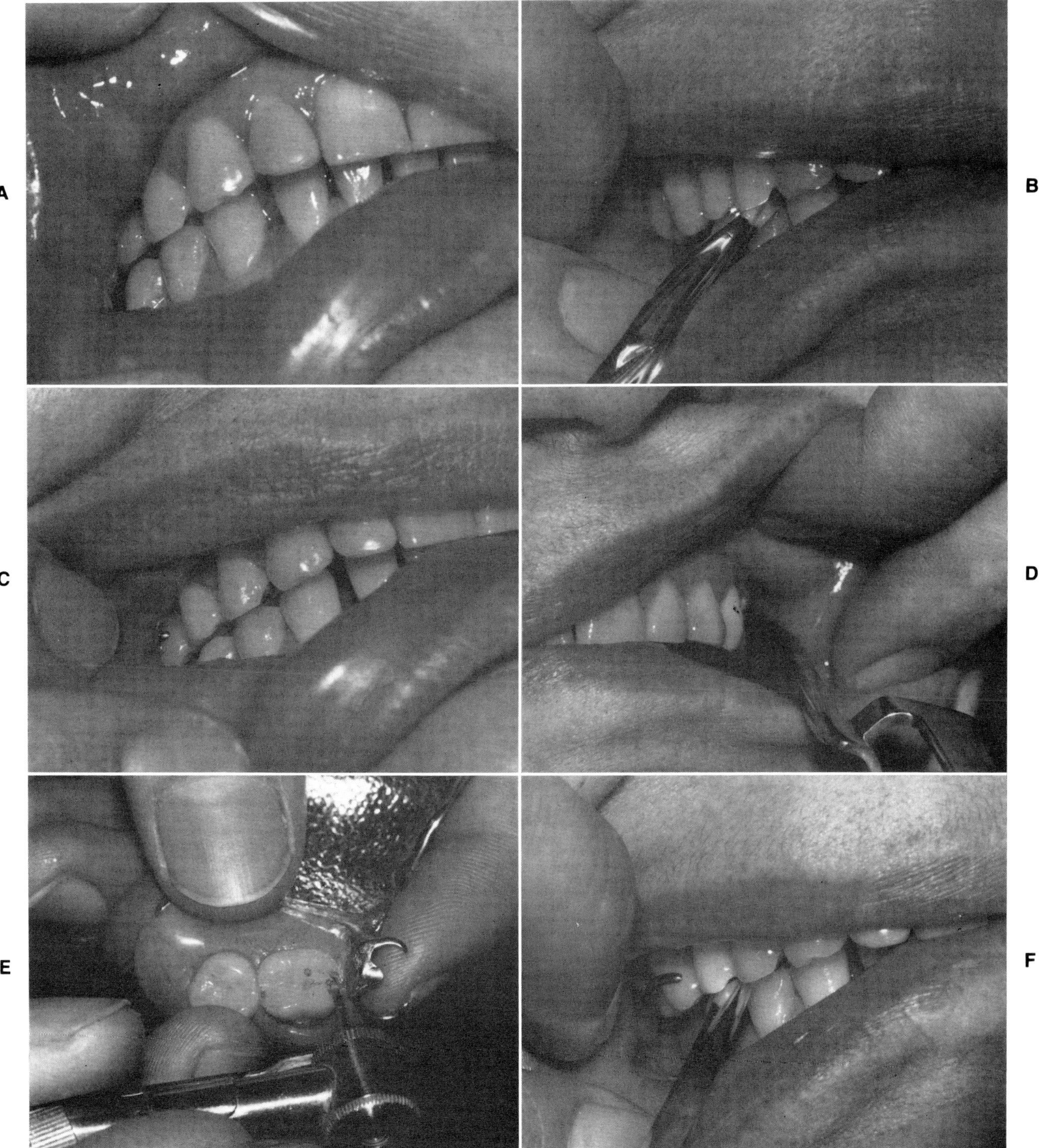

Fig. 16-12. A, With partial dentures out of mouth, two opposing natural teeth that contact when patient closes in centric occlusion are selected. **B,** The contact should be verified by using fine Mylar tape or tissue paper. **C,** With one partial denture in mouth and patient closing in centric occlusion relationship of selected index teeth is noted. **D,** If index teeth are not contacting, articulating paper or tape is used to locate interference. **E,** Interference, which must be on denture teeth, is relieved. **F,** After interferences are corrected, index teeth must be in contact. Contact must be verified by having patient close on thin strip of tissue paper or tape. There must be resistance to removing paper when teeth are together.

Continued.

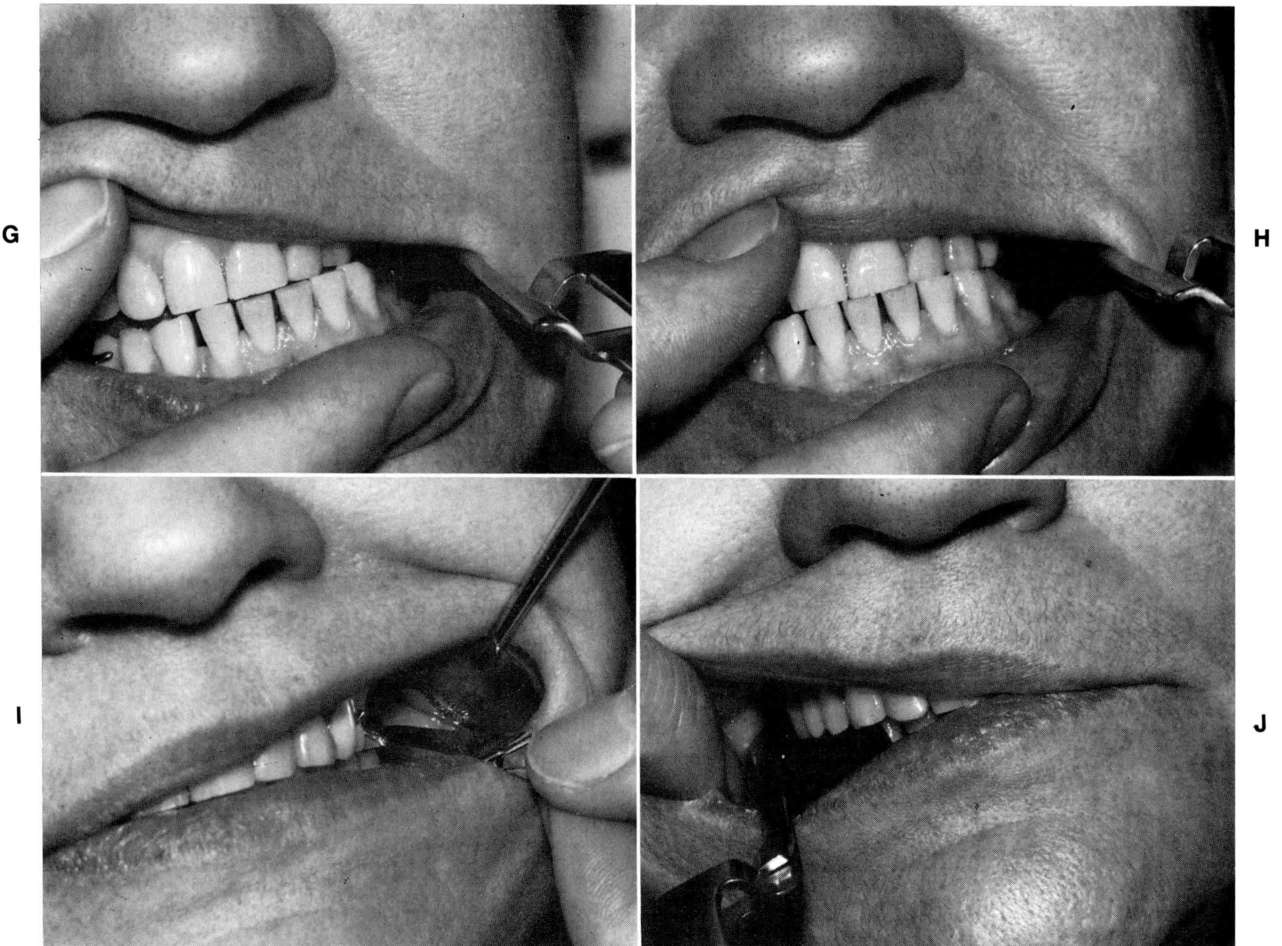

Fig. 16-12, cont'd. After interferences in centric occlusion are corrected, interferences in centric relation, in lateral excursion, **G,** and in protrusive movements, **H,** must be corrected. **I,** After all corrections have been made, fine Mylar tape is used to verify that occlusal contacts are present between natural teeth. **J,** For patient receiving two removable partial dentures, after one partial denture is cleared, same procedure is followed with opposing partial denture. After each denture has been corrected individually, final step is to correct for interferences with both dentures seated in mouth.

dure in the patient's mouth. The noise and vibration produced by the bur or mounted points are greatly magnified to the patient and can produce uncomfortable sensations. One reason for leaving the adjustment of the retentive clasps to the end of the insertion appointment is so that the partial denture can be easily inserted and withdrawn numerous times.

As a final step the occlusal anatomy of the posterior artifical teeth must be restored to reestablish the functional efficiency of the occlusion. To prevent inadvertently losing occlusal contacts while the occlusal surfaces are being restored, the marks of the contacts made by the articulating paper can be left and these points avoided as the occlusal surfaces are refined. Sluiceways and supplemental grooves should be added to occlusal surfaces to create escapeways for food and to act as cutting blades to increase the chewing efficiency. Any flat occlusal surface such as a cuspal incline should be broken up by these supplemental grooves because the friction developed when opposing flat inclines come together can greatly magnify the stresses against structures supporting the partial denture.

The use of articulating paper or cloth tape has been stressed as a means of identifying occlusal contacts. Another widely accepted method of locating occlusal interferences is the use of occlusal indicator wax (Fig. 16-14). Occlusal indicator wax may be obtained as a special item that is supplied with one surface of the wax treated with an adhesive so that it adapts firmly to the teeth being studied. Thin sheets of regular casting wax, 28- or 32-gauge, may also be used, but problems may be encountered in keeping this wax attached to the teeth.

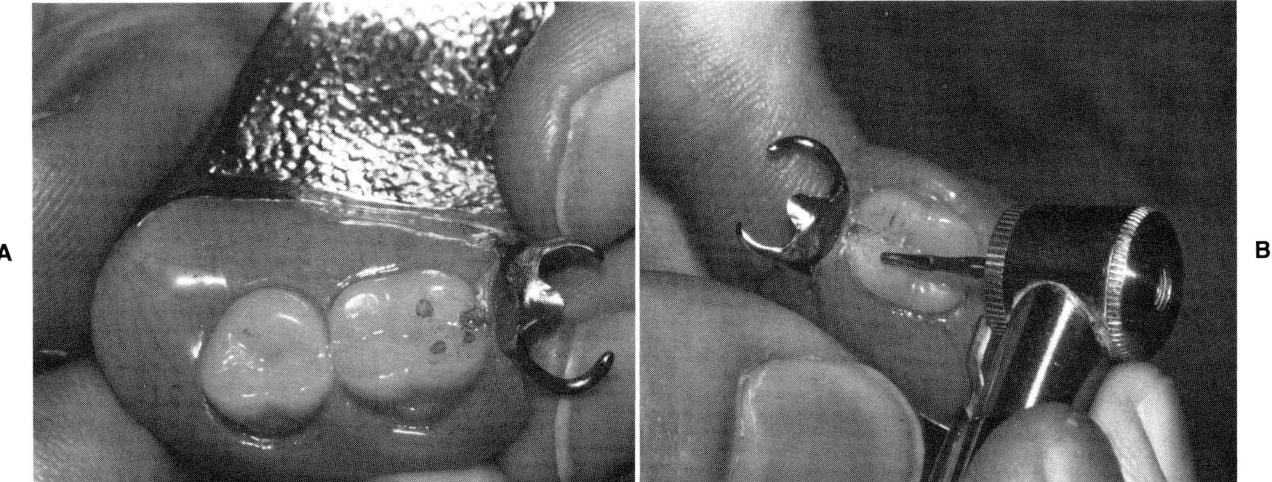

Fig. 16-13. A, Areas of interference on cuspal inclines and on marginal ridge of first molar. **B,** V-shaped cuts are made to relieve interference without destroying occlusal anatomy.

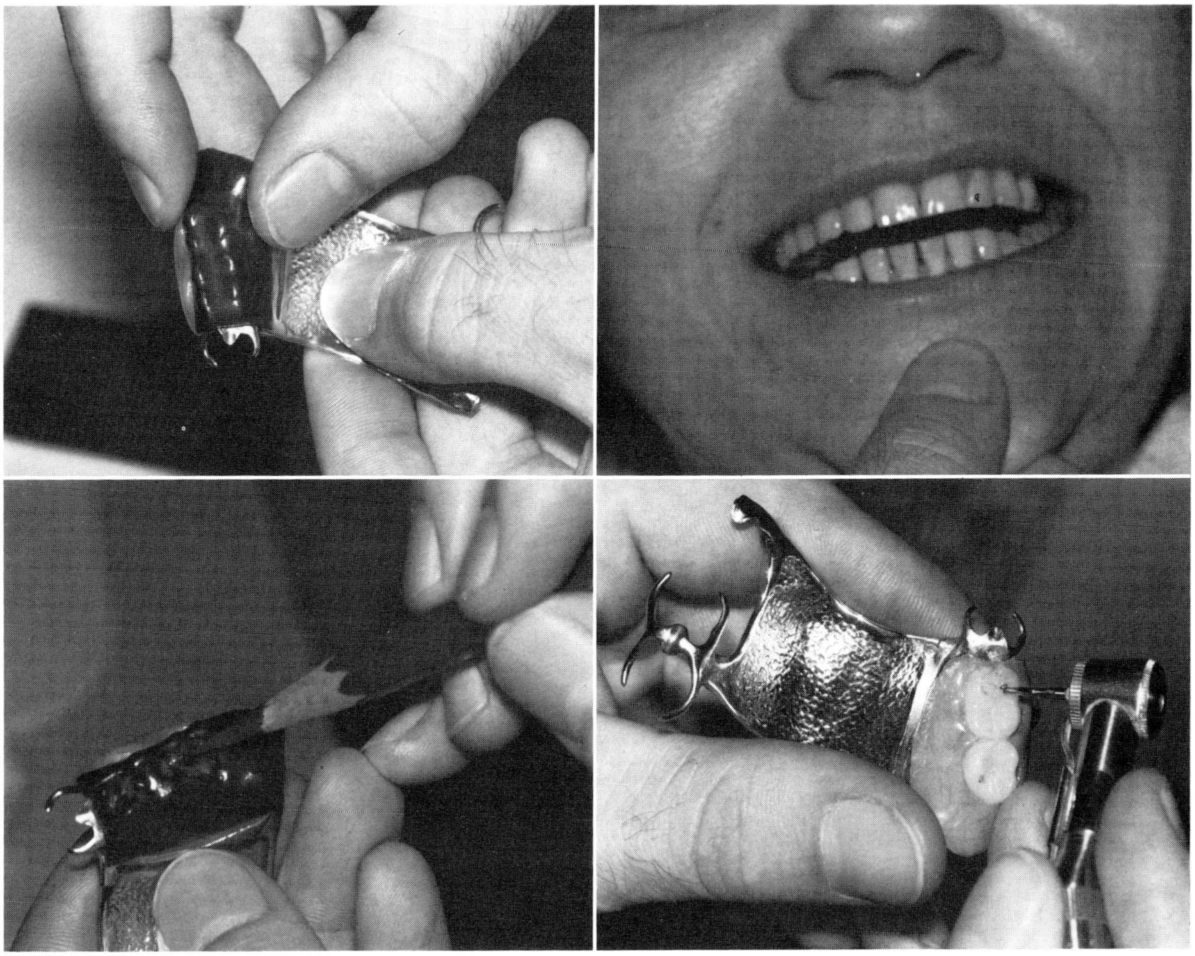

Fig. 16-14. A, Occlusal indicator wax is adapted over denture teeth. **B,** Patient is guided into repeated tapping closures at position desired. **C,** Penetrations of teeth through wax are marked with wax pencil. **D,** Penetrations or prematurities are corrected. (Alternatively, interferences may be relieved with wax still in place.)

Occlusal correction by remount procedures

Detecting occlusal errors directly in the mouth as has been described is a reliable and accurate method. It does, however, have limitations. Difficulty may be experienced in attempting to guide the mandible into the many positions of occlusal contact that are necessary to make certain that all possible areas of interference have been eliminated. In addition, if much of the posterior occlusion is being restored, the procedure becomes so difficult that its accuracy is open to question.

The alternative is to remount the completed partial denture on an articulator and perform the occlusal correction on the instrument.

The use of the articulator in developing the occlusal scheme is discussed in Chapter 14. Although access is much easier with the articulator, the shortcomings of the technique should be recognized and respected. Only the most sophisticated and fully adjustable articulators are capable of reproducing mandibular movements through a full range of motions. The most frequently used articulators, the semiadjustable instruments, are accurate only in limited positions, usually the outer limits of the envelope of motion. The pathway in between these points is not known, and the articulator can only approximate the true pathway. For this reason if occlusal corrections are made on an articulator, final intraoral refinement may still be required.

The use of the articulator to refine the occlusion of any prosthesis is based on the accepted premises that it is possible to transfer an accurate centric jaw relation to

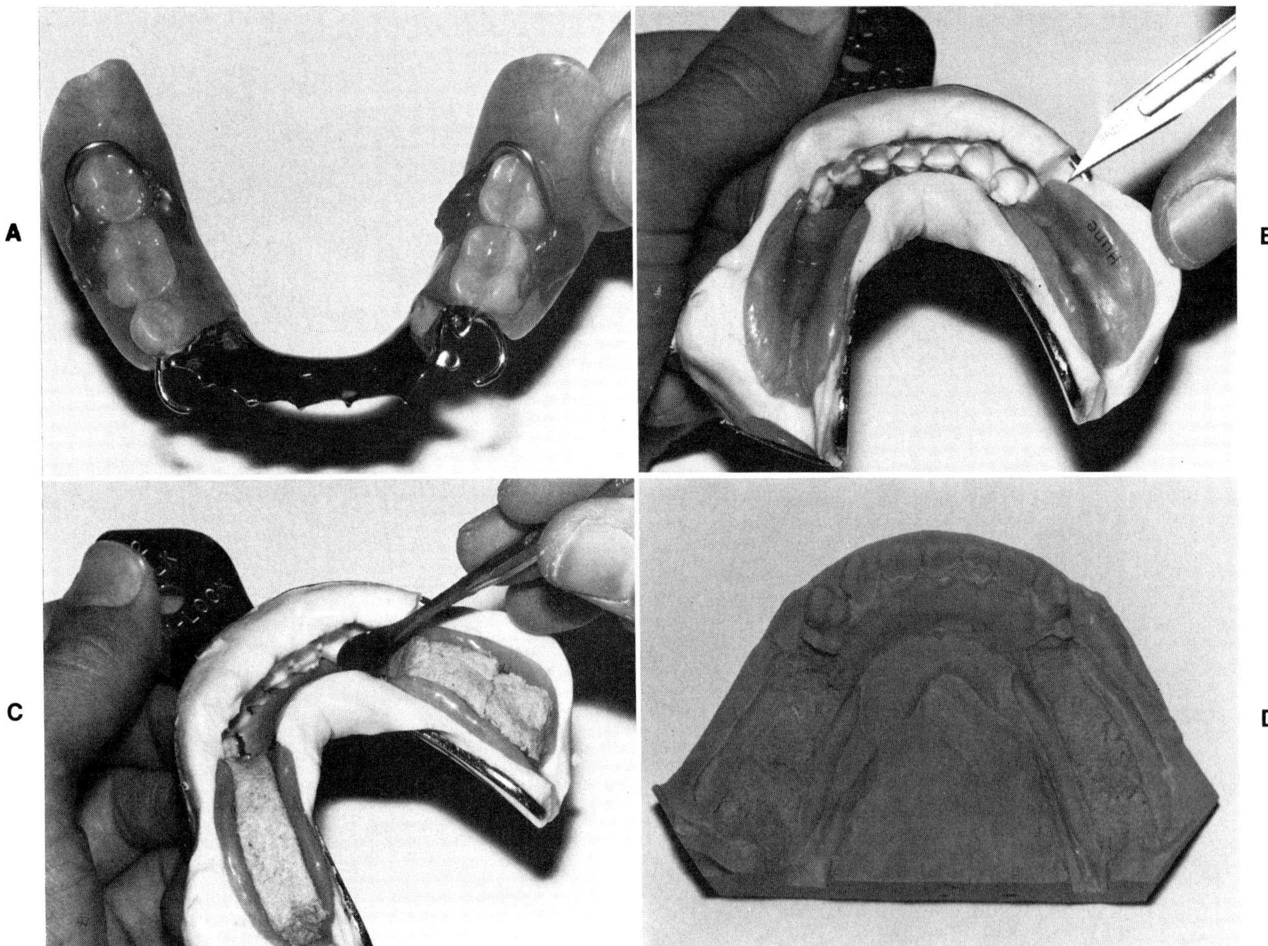

Fig. 16-15. A, To help make a pick-up impression, pieces of paper clip are attached to denture bases with sticky wax. This helps retain denture in impression. **B,** Irreversible hydrocolloid impression is made in slightly oversized impression tray over partial denture as it is seated in mouth. **C,** Undercuts in denture base are blocked out with baseplate wax, plasticine-like material, wet pumice, wet paper toweling. Enough ridge contact must remain to provide stable cast surface on which denture rests. **D,** Remount cast shows clear imprints of denture base periphery. To stabilize denture during occlusal correction, it is essential that peripheries be well defined.

an instrument and to maintain that accuracy throughout the construction of a prosthesis, and that the jaw relationship on the articulator can be verified by additional records.

To remount the partial denture on the articulator, it will be necessary to secure casts of the patient's mouth with the partial denture positioned on the casts. The casts are obtained by making an impression of the arch with the partial denture seated in position (Fig. 16-15). If the partial denture remains in the mouth as the impression is removed, it must be repositioned in the impression with great care. It is possible for a small fragment of torn alginate impression material to be lodged between the partial denture and the surface of the impression. This small displacement would be sufficient to produce errors.

The remount cast should be poured in a dense dental stone to provide as near resistant stone teeth as possible. During the occlusal correction procedure the contacting surfaces of the stone teeth will be subjected to wear and abrasion, so the teeth must be as dense and as wear resistant as possible.

If problems are anticipated in the equilibration procedure, the remaining natural teeth in the impression or an impression of the opposing occlusion may be poured in a low-fusing metal, as illustrated in Fig. 16-16.

The dimensional accuracy of this low-fusing metal is proportionate to its bismuth content. An alloy containing less than 48% bismuth will shrink during solidification. Little volumetric change occurs in alloys containing between 48% and 55% bismuth, but when more than 55% is present, the alloy expands during solidification. Most of the commonly used alloys fall into the desirable bismuth range and may be used with confidence concerning the dimensional accuracy of the cast. The teeth portion only of the impression need be poured in metal; the remainder of the cast can be poured in dental stone.

Regardless of the material with which the remount cast is poured, the maxillary cast must be mounted on the articulator with a face-bow transfer so that the arc of closure of the instrument will be identical to that of the patient. The reasons for the arc of closure being the same and the face-bow transfer technique are discussed in Chapter 14.

After the mounting of the maxillary cast on the articulator with the face-bow, jaw relation records must be obtained to mount the mandibular remount cast. The jaw relation records for the remount procedure will normally be made at centric relation because usually so much of the occlusal scheme is being replaced that the most retruded position of the mandible must be used to develop the occlusion.

The technique for securing these jaw relation records is the same as that used to verify the initial mounting after the artifical teeth were arranged in wax (discussed in Chapter 15).

After the mandibular remount cast has been mounted on the articulator following the technique described in Chapter 14, a second centric jaw relation record must be made to verify the accuracy of the mounting.

Once the remount has been verified, the occlusal correction procedures may be undertaken. Articulating paper is most easily used to locate interfering cusps and to help determine evenness of occlusal contacts. The object of the first part of the procedure is to develop even bilateral occlusal contacts in centric relation. The condylar balls of the articulator should be locked in the centric relation, posterior position, as this correction is being made. Contacts of opposing natural teeth, if they are present, must be noted. Interferences between natural teeth should have been corrected after the original diagnostic mounting procedure, but observation is necessary to make certain that these teeth contact at the same time that the artifical teeth contact. As has been noted previously, the partial denture must not prevent natural teeth from contacting if contacts are present without the partial denture in place.

Reestablishing occlusal contact in centric and eccentric positions is covered in Chapter 14 and is not repeated here. Whether group function (multiple contacts of posterior teeth in lateral movements or in working position), mutually protected occlusion (disclusion of the posterior teeth in lateral movement or protrusive movement by the lifting action of the anterior teeth working together) or canine protected occlusion (disclusion of the posterior teeth by the lifting action of the mandibular canine gliding along the lingual surface of the maxillary canine) is desired depends on the type of partial denture being delivered. The type of occlusion would have been developed as the artificial teeth were positioned before the try-in appointment, and it is the purpose of this appointment to refine the occlusion for the final time before delivering the prosthesis to the patient.

Repositioning teeth on processed denture base

Major alterations in the occlusal scheme should not be required at this time. If gross malposition of the artifical teeth has occurred (Fig. 16-17), removal of the teeth from the denture base, repositioning of new teeth in wax on the denture base, and reprocessing of the teeth on the denture base may be required.

To remove plastic teeth from the denture base, it is necessary to cut or grind the teeth from the acrylic resin denture base or to section the teeth out as a block

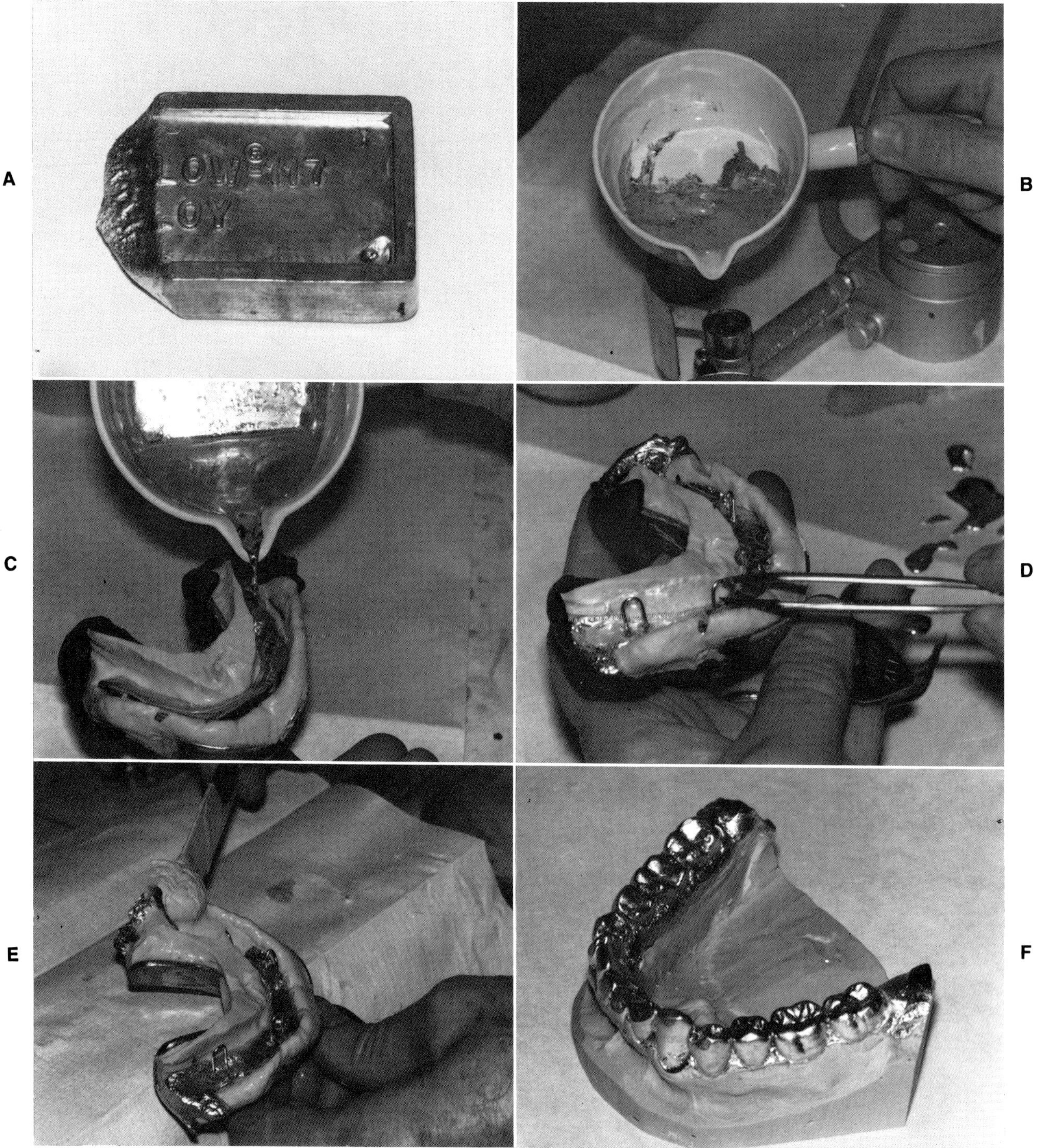

Fig. 16-16. A, Ingot of low-fusing metal, melting point 47.2° C (117° F). **B,** Metal is fused in porcelain container over open flame. **C,** As soon as it is completely liquid, molten metal is poured slowly into impression containing partial denture. **D,** After metal has solidified, pieces of paper clip are heated and buried in metal to act as retaining devices for remainder of cast. **E,** Working cast is completed by addition of dental stone. **F,** Cast, in this case an opposing cast, is used to complete occlusal correction.

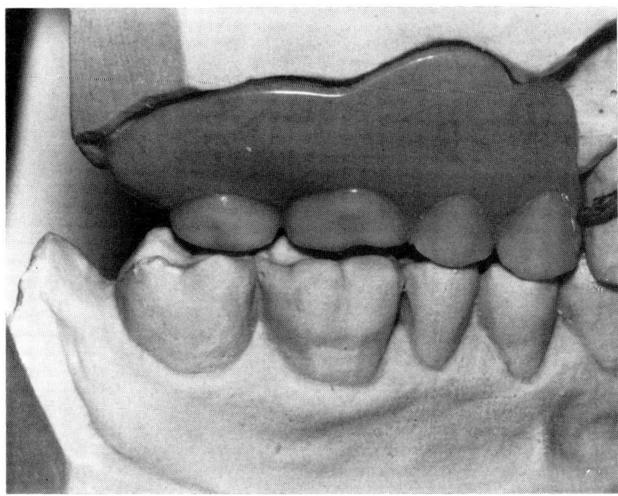

Fig. 16-17. Gross malposition of denture teeth may occur as a result of undetected errors in technique. Occlusal correction by equilibration is not possible.

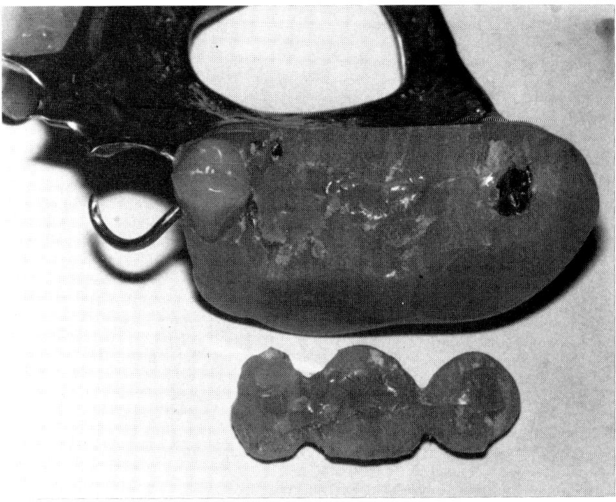

Fig. 16-18. Malpositioned teeth may be sectioned from denture in a block.

(Fig. 16-18). The latter is rarely successful because repositioning the teeth is a problem. In the event porcelain teeth were used, it is possible to apply localized heat, from an alcohol torch, to each tooth and pry the tooth free from the denture base. The application of heat is usually sufficient to soften the resin in the diatoric or around the retaining pins of anterior teeth so that the teeth may be removed intact with no distortion of the denture base.

With the casts and partial denture mounted on an articulator, the artificial teeth may be reset on the denture base in the correct position (Fig. 16-19). The denture base contour can be reestablished with baseplate wax and the teeth reprocessed to the denture base. The safest method of reattaching the teeth is by using autopolymerizing acrylic resin. Reinvesting the partial denture in the denture flask and processing the teeth in position by the heat-cured resin technique, as was done originally, may distort the base. If the heat processing procedure is followed, the temperature of the curing unit should not exceed 68° C (155° F), the long (8-hour) curing cycle should be followed, and the boiling step must be omitted.

To use the autopolymerizing technique (Fig. 16-20) to reattach the teeth to the denture base, a matrix of dental stone must be made to hold the teeth in the correct position and to contain the resin as it is flowed into place. The matrix should cover either the buccal or lingual surface, not both, because the resin will be introduced from the side of the denture not covered. Because the resin will not be contained from the side from which it is being placed, the finish or contour of that side must be accomplished freehand after the resin has polymerized. For this reason it is normally better practice to cover the buccal surface with the stone matrix and introduce the resin from the lingual surface. Finishing and contouring the lingual anatomy of the denture base around the necks of the teeth is not as critical on the lingual surface as it is on the buccal, or facial, surfaces. The major drawback to the autopolymerizing resin is that the line of demarcation between the previously processed heat-cured resin and the new self-cure resin may be noticeable. Slight surface porosity of the autopolymerizing resin is also a potential problem.

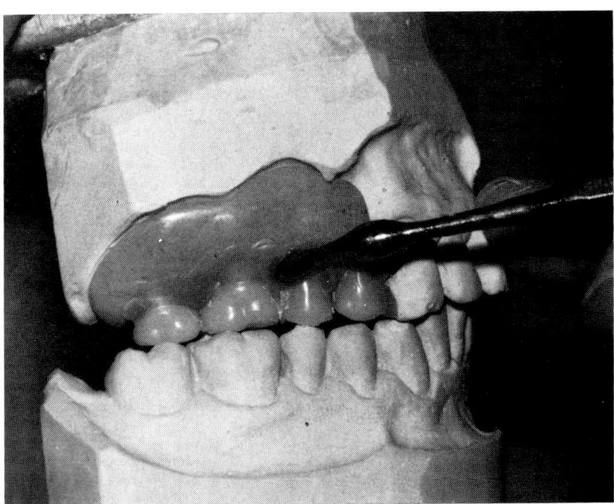

Fig. 16-19. Block of teeth is repositioned on denture base correctly and waxed to proper contour.

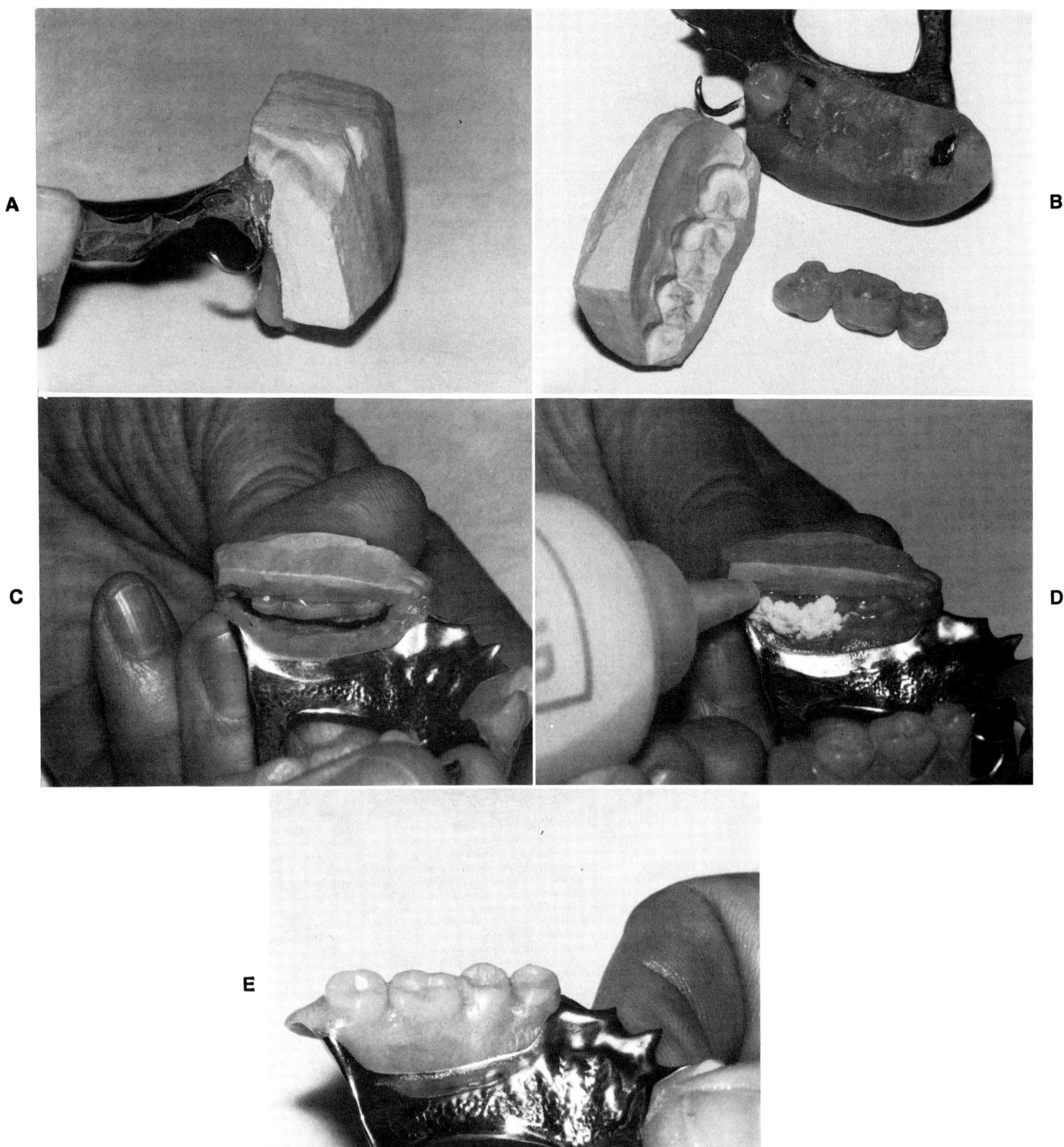

Fig. 16-20. A, Stone matrix is made of denture teeth position. Matrix covers occlusal surfaces of the teeth, buccal surfaces of teeth, and adjacent denture base that was not altered during tooth-repositioning process. **B,** Stone matrix is removed, and wax holding denture teeth is washed from denture base and teeth. **C,** Matrix, with denture teeth in position, is reassembled on denture base. **D,** Autopolymerizing acrylic resin is added by sprinkle-on method from lingual aspect of teeth. **E,** After processing, resin is finished and polished.

Reestablishment of occlusal anatomy

After the occlusion of the partial denture has been refined on the articulator, the anatomy of the occlusal surfaces should be restored. Additional sluiceways and accessory grooves should be added to increase the efficiency of the masticatory apparatus. Dull or blunt cusps can cause unnecessary forces to be transmitted to the abutment teeth and supporting structures because the patient will try to accomplish with chewing power what could otherwise be accomplished with sharp cutting and grinding surfaces.

ADJUSTING RETENTIVE CLASPS

Up to this point in patient treatment there has been no need to be concerned with the amount of retention supplied by the retentive clasps. Normally the framework will be very retentive, in fact difficult to remove, on the master cast because the friction between the surface of the stone cast and the metal clasps amplifies the retention. It is often good practice to scrape the suprabulge on the abutment teeth to decrease the retention (Fig. 16-21). This not only makes the removal of the framework from the cast much easier, but also decreases the amount of flexing the retentive clasp tip must undergo, thus decreasing the possibility of metal fatigue in the clasp and early failure of the clasp in function.

The clasp adjustment phase of the insertion appointment should make certain that unnecessary force is not being applied by the retentive clasps and yet sufficient retention is present to maintain the partial denture securely in place. As a general rule, at the time of insertion slightly less than maximum retention should be used. Many patients will have difficulty in inserting and removing the prosthesis initially, so maximum retention should be avoided.

Over the years chrome alloy developed a reputation of being difficult to adjust. The reputation for the most part was unearned. The percentage of elongation of the metal, which in actuality denotes the ease or difficulty in bending before permanent distortion occurs, is listed for most chrome alloys as 8% to 10%. This compares with a percentage of 20% for gold alloy. This means that although chrome alloy is somewhat more resistant to bending than gold, there still remains an ample margin of safety in which chrome may be adjusted.

Fracture of chrome alloy clasps during adjustment is almost always attributable to sudden quick bends or an excessive amount of bending at any one time. One philosophy of clasp adjustment to be kept in mind is never to overadjust or overbend a clasp and then have to bend or adjust it in reverse. This is a major cause for clasp breakage during adjustments. Clasps should be adjusted a small amount at a time, checked in the mouth to ascertain if the desired result has been achieved, and additional small adjustments made in the same direction if required. This technique will reduce clasp breakage to a clinically acceptable level.

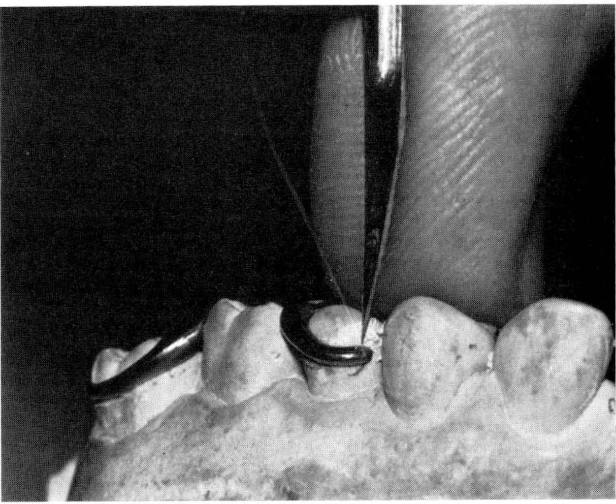

Fig. 16-21. Suprabulge of abutment teeth on cast is scraped to remove retentive undercut. This prevents clasp from deforming each time it is placed on or removed from cast.

Types of pliers

Numerous types of pliers are available for bending wires or clasps in dentistry. In the practice of orthodontics, where intricate bends may be required to direct and control the forces generated by orthodontic wires during the movement of teeth, a variety of pliers are usually required. In the practice of removable partial prosthodontics, however, where normally only gentle curving bends are needed two pliers are generally sufficient (Fig. 16-22).

A laboratory technician who bends and shapes clasps constantly in constructing partial dentures will develop or adapt a pair of pliers to best serve the technique that the technician uses. A dentist, who normally does not bend the volume of wires and does not develop specialized techniques, can function adequately with less specialized equipment.

The proper technique for bending wires or adjusting clasps is to hold the wire or clasp between the beaks of the pliers and to apply the bending force with the fingers of the hand not holding the pliers (Fig. 16-23). A bending force applied with the pliers frequently results in a bend of improper magnitude or radius. The adjustment made by the No. 200 pliers is one exception to this rule; this adjustment is made by squeezing the beaks of the pliers together. Another exception occurs when the retentive tip only of a cast circumferential clasp requires adjustment. In this instance the clasp should be grasped with the beaks of the No. 139 pliers

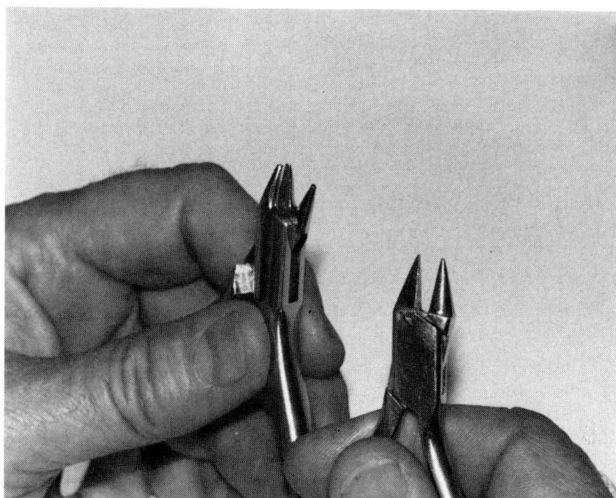

Fig. 16-22. Pliers normally used to adjust retentive clasps. Left, No. 200 pliers. If a piece of wire or clasp is held between beaks and beaks are squeezed together, crimp or sharp bend will occur where inner finger on one beak closes between two outer fingers on opposite beak. Use of these pliers is limited to adjustment of vertical projection clasps. Right, No. 139 pliers, used for most clasp adjustments. Tapered cylindric beak opposes flat surface of triangular beak.

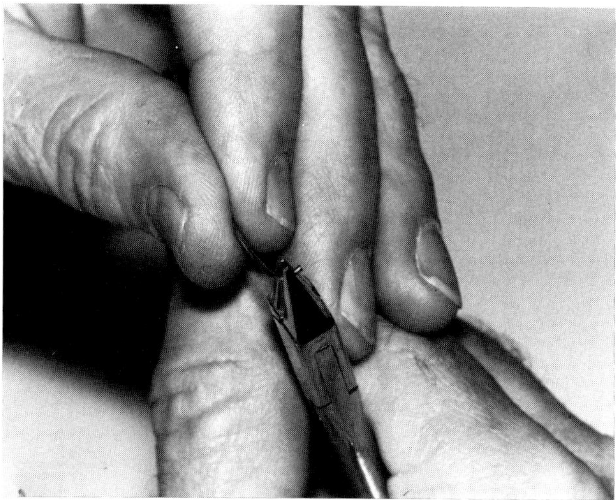

Fig. 16-23. Wire or clasp is held firmly with beaks of pliers, and bending force is applied with opposite fingers.

and a slight rotating force applied by the pliers to produce the needed result. The exact technique will be discussed under adjusting cast circumferential clasps.

Adjusting wrought wire clasps

Wrought wire clasps probably require the greatest amount of adjusting of all the varieties of clasps. The greater flexibility of the clasp can lead to abuses of the properties of the metal. Technicians tend to position the clasp in too severe a retentive undercut under the mistaken belief that lack of retention is a prime cause of patient nonacceptance of a removable partial denture. (This is a minor reason for patient rejection; most patients adapt well to minimally retentive partial dentures.) When the wrought clasp is placed in too deep an undercut, the constant flexing of the metal as the prosthesis is inserted and withdrawn from the mouth will eventually distort the metal away from the tooth. When this type of distortion is corrected, the clasp should be adjusted so that less of an undercut is engaged by the retentive tip. The clasp tip is bent upward toward the survey line as well as inward toward the tooth. (This should not be attempted for a cast clasp.) Recent research into properties of wrought wire clasps conducted in part by one of the contributors to this book, James Brudvik (1973), indicates that wrought wire clasps placed in undercuts greater than 0.015 inch will eventually fail as a result of fatigue of the metal caused by excessive flexing. The yield strength of the metal is exceeded, and permanent deformation or fracture of the wrought metal results. This fact should be kept in mind as the design for the partial denture is developed.

Another important reason for early distortion of wrought wire clasps is the manner in which the patient removes the denture from the mouth. Patients not taught the correct method tend to remove the denture by placing a fingernail under the clasp and pushing the clasp free from the tooth. It will not take long for the clasp to be distorted.

To adjust the wrought wire clasp to increase contact with the tooth, the procedure shown in Fig. 16-24 should be followed. If retention is not present once tooth-clasp contact has been reestablished, the tip is not positioned sufficiently gingival to the survey line. The round beak of the pliers will need to be placed in contact with the gingival side of the center of the length of the clasp. Force can then be applied to the denture to bend the retentive tip of the clasp in a gingival direction. When this has been accomplished, the adjusting procedure in Fig. 16-24 must be followed to adjust the clasp inward against the tooth and into a greater depth of undercut.

Small bends made by twisting or rotating the pliers should be avoided because they tend to nick or mar the smooth surface of the wrought clasp. Defects in the wire will reduce the strength of the wire. Stresses created by the flexing of the clasp will concentrate in the area that has been marred and will lead to premature fracture of the clasp. Any damage to the surface of the wire caused by pressure from the beaks of the pliers must be smoothed before the partial denture is delivered to the patient (Fig. 16-25). The smoothing can best

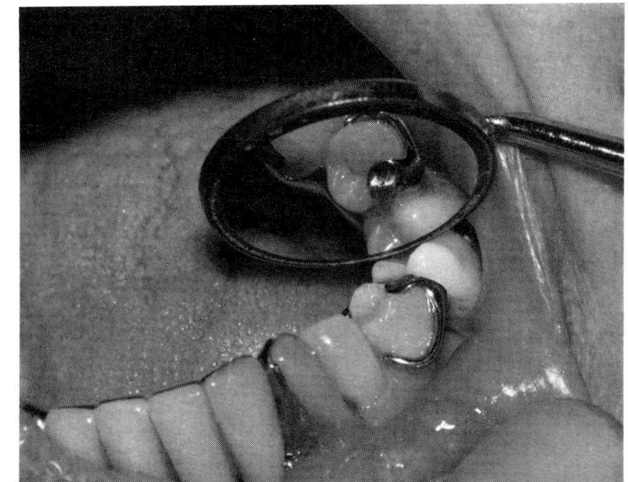

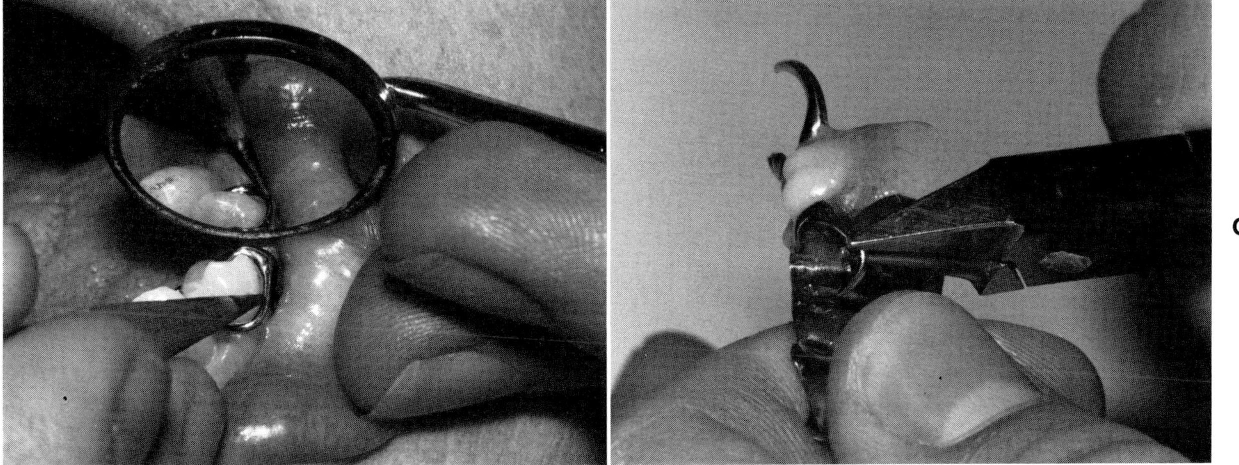

Fig. 16-24. Wrought wire clasp adjustment to increase contact with tooth. **A,** By sighting down long axis of abutment tooth in mouth mirror, contact of clasp with tooth can be observed. **B,** Point at which clasp loses contact with tooth is marked with pencil. **C,** Round beak of No. 139 plier is placed on inner aspect of clasp at point marked. Denture is rotated with opposite hand toward round beak of pliers. Only small adjustment is made, denture is returned to mouth for observation, and process is repeated until complete contact between tooth and clasp has been reestablished.

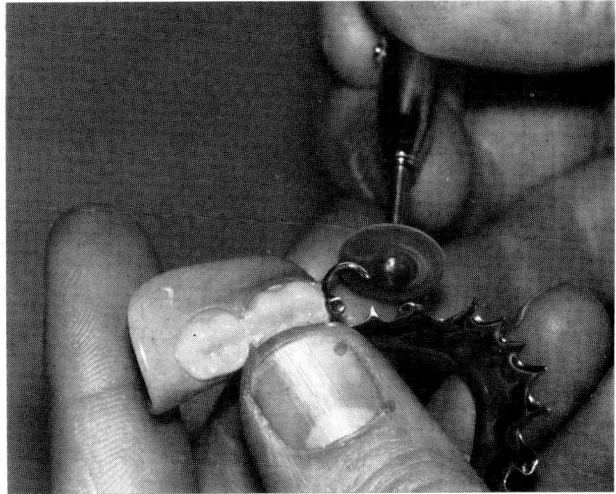

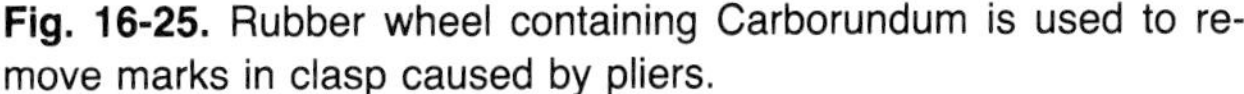
Fig. 16-25. Rubber wheel containing Carborundum is used to remove marks in clasp caused by pliers.

be accomplished by using a rubber wheel containing Carborundum. Care must be exercised not to thin the metal to the point where fracture or permanent deformation could occur.

Adjusting cast circumferential clasps

A cast circumferential clasp can be adjusted in only one plane, either inward, perpendicular to the flat surface of the clasp, or outward along the same plane. The flat, or inner, surface of the clasp represents the surface of the tooth against which the clasp was waxed. The outer surface of a well-constructed clasp will be half-round in form. Any attempt to bend the clasp in any other plane or direction will result in a twisted or distorted clasp. For this reason if the retentive tip is in too little or too great an undercut, reconstruction of the framework or the addition of a wrought wire clasp will be necessary to solve the problem.

The only set of pliers necessary to adjust the cast circumferential clasp is the No. 139. The proper technique for adjusting the clasp is similar to that of the wrought wire clasp; it is illustrated in Fig. 16-26. It must be decided at what point of the clasp arm the adjustment should be made. If the clasp is not retentive and requires adjusting inward toward the tooth, this is best done by inserting the partial denture and observing the contact of the clasp with the tooth surface with the mouth mirror and reflected light. If it is necessary to reduce the amount of retention by bending the clasp away from the tooth, the adjustment is made at the junction of the middle and terminal thirds of the clasp.

The application of force to achieve the adjustment should be made slowly and steadily. Chrome alloy is resistant to deformation or bending. Twice the amount of force is required to bend chrome-cobalt alloy as is required to bend Type IV gold alloy.

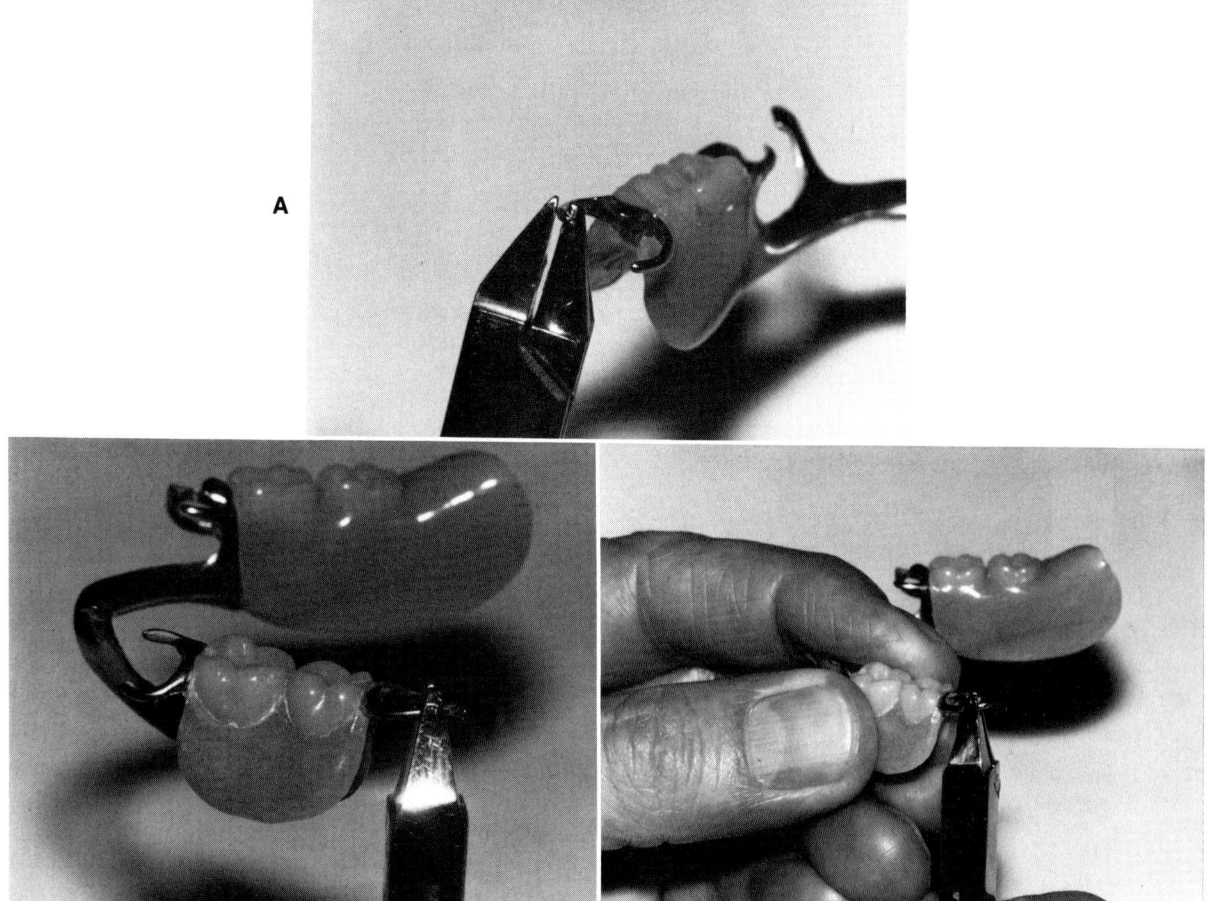

Fig. 16-26. A, Round beak of plier is placed against flat inner surface of clasp at point requiring adjustment. **B,** All support for partial denture is released. This will align flat surface of clasp with beaks of pliers. **C,** Pressure is applied with opposite hand to produce desired adjustment.

Adjusting vertical projection clasps

The vertical projection, or bar, clasp, being of cast construction, can be adjusted only inward or outward perpendicular to the flat side of the clasp. One of the most common and damaging adjustments that can be made to a bar clasp is attempting to bend or adjust the head or finger of a T or modified T clasp. Trying to adjust only the T portion of the clasp will always result in a torquing or twisting bend to the approach arm of the clasp. This will inevitably ruin the function of the clasp. A twisting bend can rarely be corrected adequately by bending in the opposite direction. A twisting bend is a complex one involving several spatial planes, and to reverse the bend in the exact dimensions as the first is virtually impossible.

If the retentive finger of a T or modified T clasp requires bending to increase retention (which is unusual because normally the entire T portion of the clasp will

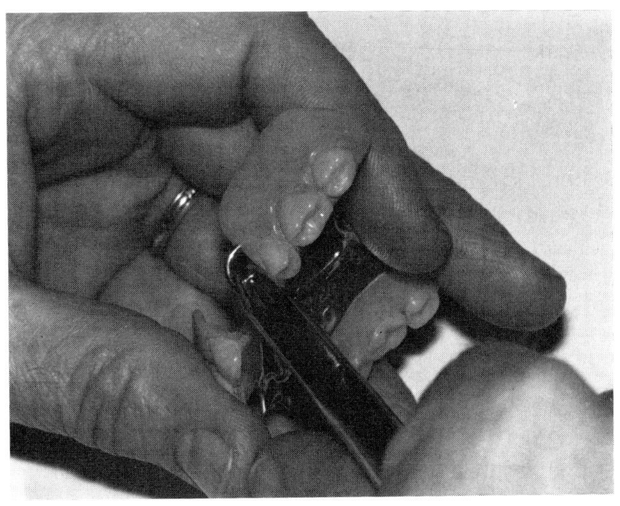

Fig. 16-27. No. 200 pliers are used to crimp retentive terminal of T clasp.

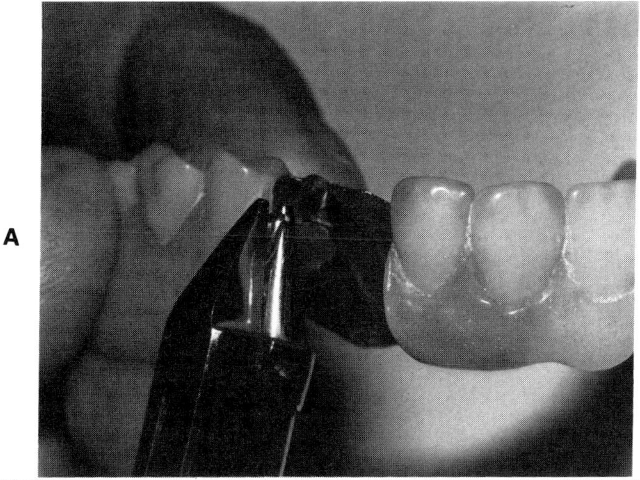

A

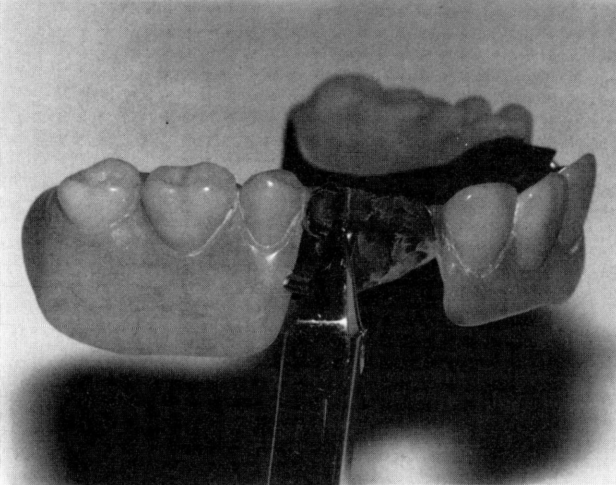

B

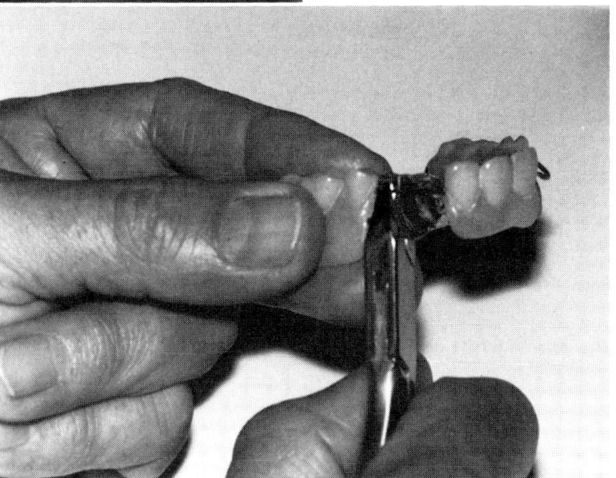

C

Fig. 16-28. Adjustment of approach arm of vertical projection clasp. **A,** Approach arm is held with beaks of No. 139 pliers down long axis, round beak on inner surface. **B,** Fingers are released from partial denture to align beaks with approach arm and prevent twisting bends from being made. **C,** Bend is made only inwardly or outwardly.

have moved away from the tooth), the No. 200 pliers must be used (Fig. 16-27). This is the only indication for the use of this set of pliers. The adjustment made in this case is not truly a bend but rather a crimp in the retentive finger of the clasp. There must be no twisting or bending force applied to the pliers. The beaks of the pliers are positioned as near the retentive tip of the clasp as possible with the single finger of the pliers on the inner surface of the clasp and the two fingers of the opposite beak on the outer surface, and squeezing force is applied. This will crimp the clasp tip and force the retentive tip toward the tooth to provide the increase in retention. This type of adjustment is considered only after other types have been considered and rejected.

The normal adjustment of a vertical projection clasp is made along the length of the approach arm as the arm approaches the tooth. Most of the time when the bar clasp loses retention it is because the clasp has moved away from the tooth. The movement may have been caused accidentally or, more probably, by the clasp's flexing on and off the tooth over a long period.

To correct for the loss of retention that has taken place or to increase or decrease retention at the time of insertion, the entire vertical portion of the approach arm must be adjusted with the No. 139 pliers (Fig. 16-28).

INSTRUCTIONS TO PATIENT

Oral hygiene

Proper instructions to the patient are extremely important. Throughout the course of patient treatment the physiologic and economic value of removable partial dentures should be stressed. Adequate home care is a prerequisite to partial denture success. No useful purpose is served when a removable partial denture is placed in an unclean mouth. This will only hasten the inevitable destruction of the remaining teeth. Thus, before this appointment the patient should have been given thorough instructions in the care and maintenance of the remaining teeth and soft tissues. Proper tooth brushing techniques and the use of dental floss should be a routine part of the patient's home care at this time. Reinforcement and reexamination of the patient must be considered a routine part of treatment. The intervals between examinations will vary depending on the condition and reaction of each patient but should not normally exceed 1 year.

The use of disclosing tablets is an excellent way to impress on the patient the need for meticulous attention in cleansing areas that are difficult to reach and to disclose areas that are susceptible to accumulation of plaque and debris (Fig. 16-29). The patient should be taught to chew the disclosing tablets with the partial denture in the mouth and then to remove the denture and examine both the inner and outer surfaces for areas of plaque. Although there will be no plaque accumulation at the insertion appointment, the technique should be demonstrated so the patient can periodically check the effectiveness of home care efforts.

Having made the point to the patient that the partial denture as well as the remaining natural teeth can become a target for plaque accumulation, the dentist should demonstrate the correct method of brushing the denture. Clasp and denture brushes should be shown to the patient (Fig. 16-30). The configuration of the brushes is such that the areas that are difficult to clean become more accessible. The material used as a cleaning agent is not as important as the physical act of brushing. Regular toothpaste may be used, but it is not any more effective than facial soap or other mild detergents. Abrasive agents such as scouring powders should be avoided because the acrylic resin denture base could be damaged, and overzealous brushing of the metal with an abrasive agent could ultimately produce a roughened surface, which may hasten the accumulation of undesirable deposits. The denture is never brushed while still in the mouth; it must always be removed for cleaning. The patient should be instructed not to hold the denture in one hand, squeezed between the fingers and the heel of the palm, while brushing. If this is done, the patient will tend to squeeze harder as the cleanser takes effect and becomes slippery, and the denture can be distorted across the midline. The preferred method of brushing is to hold one side of the denture with the fingers as the opposite side is cleansed. Another good practice for the patient to be shown is to brush the denture over a partially filled basin or bowl of water so that if the denture is dropped, little harm will be done.

Solutions in which to soak the denture overnight have received a great deal of publicity, particularly over commercial radio and television stations. It would be ideal if an all-purpose, unfailing soaking solution were available, but at this writing none are in sight. Brushing, or mechanically removing plaque and debris, still must be considered the most reliable method of ensuring cleanliness of the denture. Some commercially available solutions are helpful, however. There is currently on the market at least one overnight soaking solution (Mercene) that will actually penetrate and remove plaque. Other products contain an oxidizing agent that is only partially effective and will not attack plaque.

The patient should be cautioned against the use of any cleansing solution containing chlorine. A popular solution for soaking plastic dentures is a mixture of Clorox, Calgon, and water. This is an excellent solution for cleaning resin dentures. However, if chrome-cobalt al-

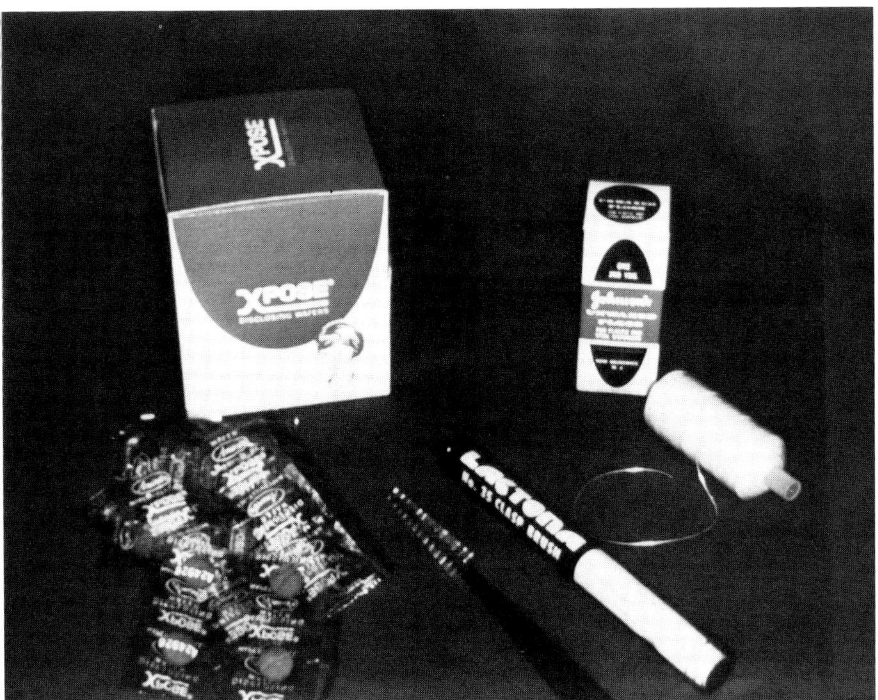

Fig. 16-29. Home care aids are shown and demonstrated to patient. Aids should include disclosing tablets and floss.

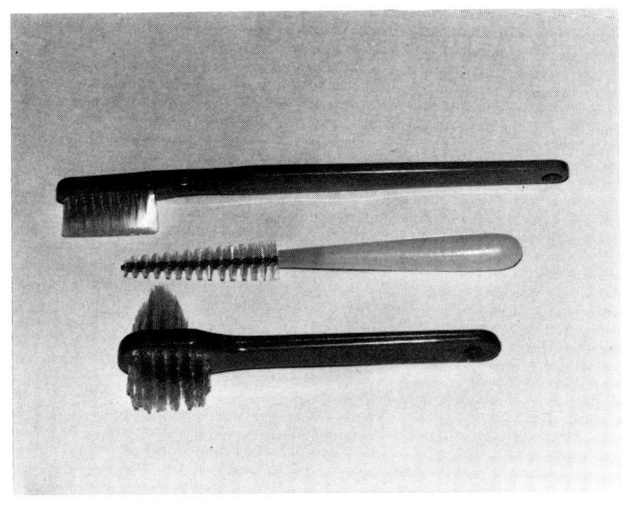

Fig. 16-30. Brushes that partial denture patient uses routinely. Top, Regular toothbrush. Center, Clasp brush for cleaning inner surface of clasps. Bottom, Denture brush for inner surfaces of denture base and minor connector.

loy has been used in the construction of the partial denture, the chlorine will attack the metal rapidly.

Patients should be reminded that a minimum of 24 hours is required for plaque to accumulate to a perceptible degree on the denture. Deposits of calculus on the partial denture should never take place if home care is exercised to even the minimum level, which consists of one thorough brushing every 24 hours. Calculus that has accumulated (Fig. 16-31) must be removed by scraping with hand instruments or by soaking the prosthesis at least 12 hours in full-strength household vinegar. This will dissolve or soften the calculus sufficiently so that it can be removed with brush wheels on a dental lathe. The denture will require polishing following the removal of the calculus deposit.

Ultrasonic cleaners for complete or partial dentures combine the chemical action of the cleansing solution with the rapid vibrating effect of the sonic unit. Tests conducted recently by the American Dental Association's Council on Dental Materials and Devices show that the action of these units is slightly more effective than that of the cleansing solution alone but that hand brushing of the denture after using the unit was still necessary to clean the denture completely. Of the solutions tested with the sonic units, none were shown to be harmful to the chrome-cobalt alloys, but each should be tested before prolonged use.

The patient should be instructed that only in rare instances should a removable partial denture be worn at night. The soft tissues covered by the denture base and the major connectors must be given the opportunity to rebound and recover from constant function. This is best done during the sleeping hours. With the reduced salivary flow that is normal during sleep, particles of food or bacteria that would normally be carried away from the teeth remain in contact with enamel surfaces and soft tissue and may ultimately produce decalcification of the hard tissue and inflammation of the soft tissue.

If a patient has only a few remaining natural teeth and is subject to bruxism, less damage may be done to the teeth if the denture is worn at night. It would, however, be a better practice in this instance to construct an occlusal night guard for the patient to wear during sleep (Fig. 16-32). The occlusal night guard can be designed to contact less soft tissue than is contacted by the regular partial denture.

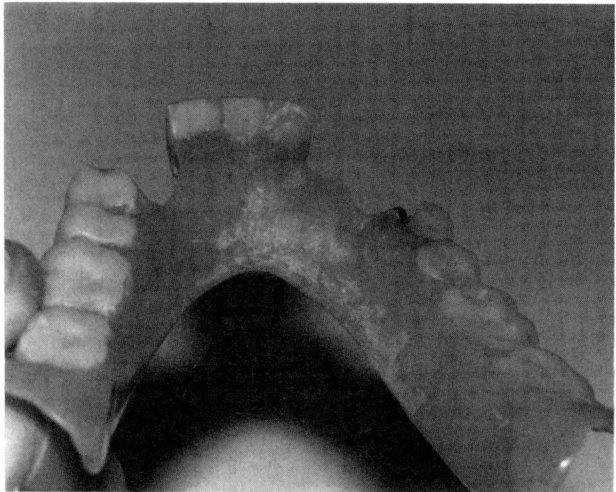

Fig. 16-31. Calculus that has been allowed to accumulate on denture can be softened by prolonged soaking in household vinegar and then removed with brush wheels on dental lathe.

In any event the removable partial denture must be left out of the patient's mouth no less than several hours each day.

Patient placement and removal

One often overlooked part of patient instruction at the time of the delivery of the partial denture is teaching the patient to insert and remove the prosthesis. The difficulty of this task depends to some extent on the muscular coordination and physical condition of the patient, the number and position of retentive clasps, and the amount of retention for each clasp.

The insertion of the partial denture is generally not a major problem. The patient should be positioned in front of a wall mirror—a hand-held mirror is not a good substitute—while the dentist inserts the denture (Fig. 16-33). The dentist should explain how the clasps must be lined up with the abutment teeth before any seating pressure is applied. The patient should be cautioned about trapping soft tissue of the cheek or tongue be-

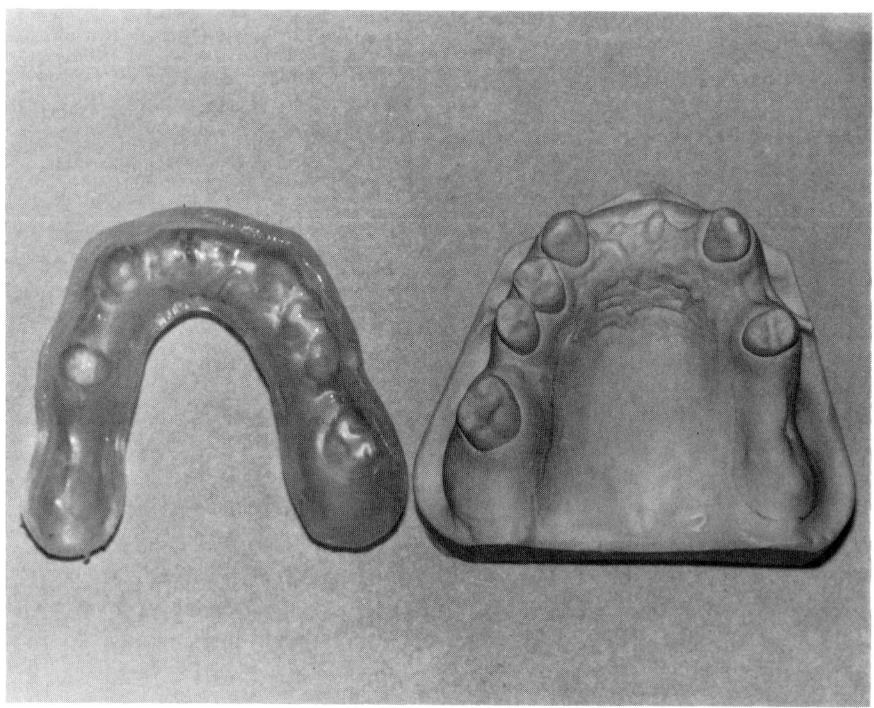

Fig. 16-32. Occlusal night guard is constructed to protect remaining teeth if bruxism by patient is a possibility.

tween a clasp and the tooth. The amount of force needed to seat the prosthesis should be demonstrated, and the patient warned that if excessive pressure seems to be needed to seat the denture, the alignment of the denture with the teeth must be incorrect. In the event that the partial denture was designed with a tilt of the surveying table, the path of insertion will be along that tilted path, at an angle to the occlusal plane. This must be explained and demonstrated to the patient. Placing the denture in the mouth and seating it with biting pressure should be discouraged because damage to the denture or the teeth and soft tissues can easily result.

After the patient has observed the placing of the partial denture, its removal must be demonstrated. The simplest way to remove the denture for most patients is to slip a fingernail or thumbnail under a buccal clasp arm on each side of the arch and to push the clasp occlusally. This method is acceptable if the clasps are cast circumferential and will not be distorted by the pressure placed against them. If, however, the clasps are constructed of wrought wire, this technique should not be used. The wrought wire clasps are easily distorted in a short period. These patients should be encouraged to grasp the saddle area on each side of the arch, if present, between the thumb and forefinger and to withdraw the partial denture in this manner (Fig. 16-34).

Patients for whom vertical projection clasps have been designed should be warned against attempting to remove the denture by the use of a fingernail under the approach arm. This not only often results in a laceration of the mucosa but also forces the retentive tip of the T clasp toward the tooth, making the removal of the partial denture even more difficult. The best method to use to remove dentures of this design is to engage the nonretentive tip of the T clasp and apply occlusal pressure. The denture should disengage easily.

The fact that the path of withdrawal of the denture is directly opposite to the path of insertion should be pointed out to the patient. Frequently this helps the patient understand the direction that the force of removal must be applied.

Postinsertion appointment

Even with all the care exercised in planning, constructing, and fitting the partial dentures, postinsertion problems should be expected and arrangements made to keep these problems to a minimum, both the severity and the number.

The types of difficulties encountered and methods of handling them are discussed in Chapter 17, but the practitioner at the delivery appointment should counsel the patient on what to expect from the prosthesis.

After the patient has been warned of the worst that may be expected, plans should be made to prevent these dire events from taking place. The partial denture must be adjusted to the patient before overt symptoms appear. There is a mistaken belief that sore teeth and/or painful soft tissue areas are an integral part of treatment with removable partial dentures. This is not the case. Teeth become tender or painful after a partial denture is inserted because the teeth are being orthodontically moved by a prosthesis that has not been adequately fitted to the teeth. Irritation, inflammation, or ulceration of the soft tissues and edentulous ridge is usually caused by denture bases that were not completely adjusted to the ridges at the delivery appointment.

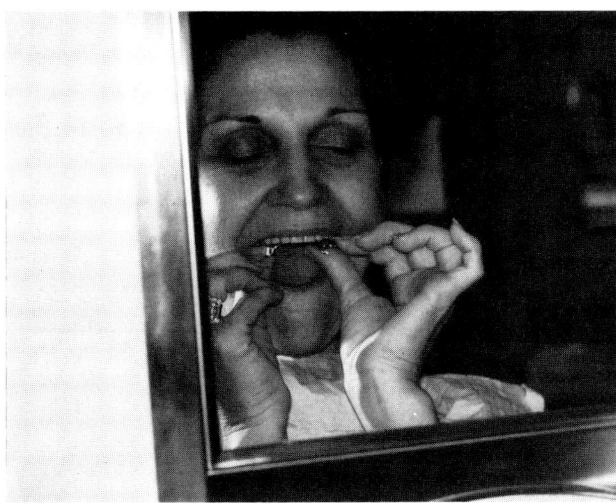

Fig. 16-33. Patient is rehearsed in inserting and removing partial denture before leaving office.

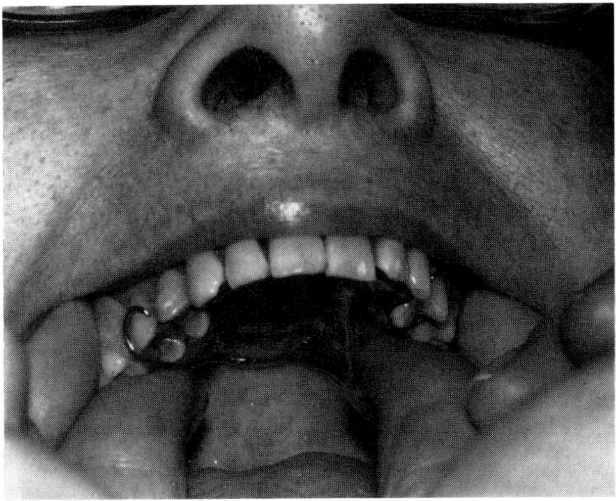

Fig. 16-34. To remove partial denture with wrought wire clasps, patient grasps saddle areas on each side of arch.

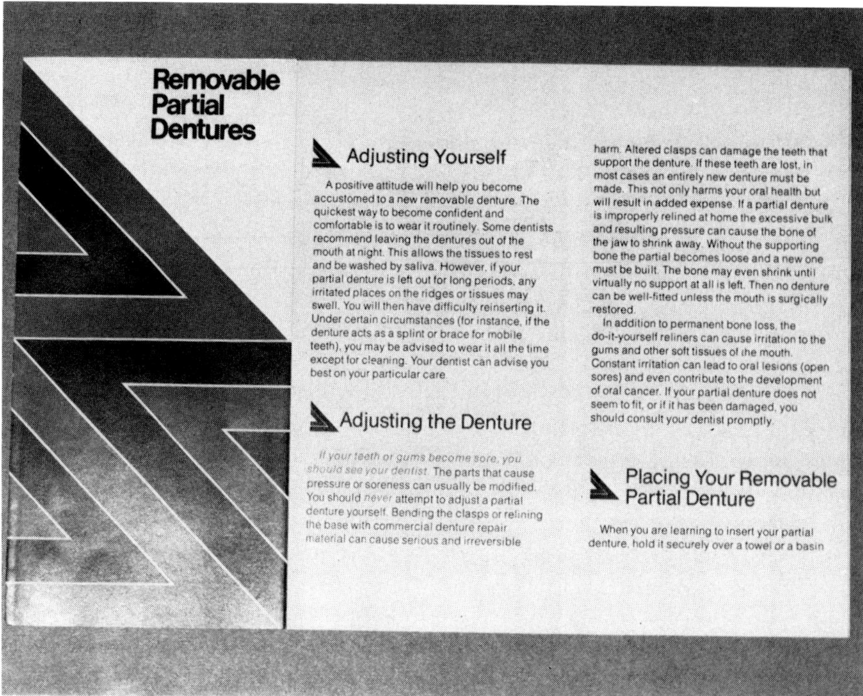

Fig. 16-35. Excellent patient education pamphlets are available. Written instructions should be discussed with and given to patient.

Adequate attention to detail during the various appointments will minimize but not totally eliminate all possible problems. To reduce patient discomfort further, a postinsertion examination within 24 hours after delivery of the prosthesis should be scheduled. Twenty-four hours is sufficient time for evidence of trouble that may be starting to be detected by the dentist but not long enough for pain or discomfort to develop to the level of patient perception. The procedures for detecting and interpreting the onset of postinsertion difficulties are discussed in the next chapter.

Written instructions

During the delivery appointment most patients are completely absorbed in attempting to adjust to and evaluate the fascinating new appliance. No patient will be able to absorb all the instructions concerned with wearing and caring for the prosthesis. For these reasons written instructions should be provided.

The written instructions may be those of the individual practitioner or one of the excellent pamphlets available from commercial sources. The American Dental Association has a very useful pamphlet for the removable partial denture patient prepared with the cooperation of the American Prosthodontic Society (Fig. 16-35).

The written instructions should cover the main points the patient must know clearly and concisely.

LENGTH OF APPOINTMENT

The experienced practitioner should accomplish the necessary procedure for this appointment in 30 to 45 minutes. The dental student will require between 3 and 4 hours.

REFERENCE

Brudvik, J.S., and Wormley, J.H.: Construction techniques for wrought wire retentive clasp arms as related to clasp flexibility; J. Prosthet. Dent. **30**:769, 1973.

BIBLIOGRAPHY

Backenstose, W.M., and Wells, J.G.: Side effects of immersion-type cleansers on metal components of dentures, J. Prosthet. Dent. **37**:615-621, 1977.

Bauman, R.: Minimizing postinsertion problems: a procedure for removable partial denture placement, J. Prosthet. Dent. **42**:381-385, 1979.

Comner, J.N.E., and others: An evaluation of an enzyme denture cleanser, J. Prosthet. Dent. **37**:147-157, 1977.

Cronas, D.: Preparation of pressure indicator paste, J. Prosthet. Dent. **37**:92-94, 1977.

Fisher A.A.: Allergic sensitization of skin and oral mucosa to acrylic resin denture materials, J. Prosthet. Dent. **6**:593-602, 1956.

Gronas, D.G: Preparation of pressure indicator paste, J. Prosthet. Dent. **37**:92, 1977.

Hanau, R.L.: Full denture prosthesis, ed. 4, Buffalo, 1930, Thorner-Sidney Press.

Jankelson, B.H.: Adjustment of dentures at time of insertion and alterations to compensate for tissue changes, J. Amer. Dent. Assoc., **64**:521-531, 1962.

Lutes, M.R., and others: Soft tissue displacement beneath removable partial and complete denture, J. Prosthet. Dent. **28**:572, 1972.

Lytle, R.B.: Complete denture construction based on a study of the deformation of the underlying soft tissues, J. Prosthet. Dent. **9**:539, 1959.

Lytle, R.B.: Soft tissue displacement beneath removable partial and complete dentures, J. Prosthet. Dent. **12**:34, 1962.

Maison, W.G: Instructions to denture patients, J. Prosthet. Dent. **9**:825-831, 1959

Means, C.R., and Flenniken, I.E.: Gagging—a problem in prosthetic dentistry, J. Prosthet. Dent. **23**:614-620, 1970.

Mehringer, E.J.: The saliva as it is related to the wearing of dentures, J. Pros. Dent., **4**:312-318, 1954.

Morden, J.F.C., and others: Effect of various cleaning solutions on chrome-cobalt alloys, Dent. Pract. Dent. Rec. **6**:304-310, 1956.

Myers, H.M., and Krol, A.J.: Effectiveness of a sonification denture cleaning program, J. Prosthet. Dent. **32**:613-618, 1974.

Neill, D.J.: A study of materials and methods employed in cleaning dentures, Br. Dent. J. **124**:107-115, 1968.

Plainfield, S.: Communication distortion: the language of patients and practitioners of dentistry, J. Prosthet. Dent. **22**:11-19, 1969.

Rodegerts, C.R.: The relationship of pressure spots in complete denture impression with mucosal irritations, J. Prosthet. Dent. **14**:1040, 1964.

Rothman, R.: Phonetic considerations in denture prosthesis, J. Prosthet. Dent. **11**:214-233, 1961.

Stevenson-Moore, P., and others: Indicator pastes: their behavior and use, J. Prosthet. Dent. **41**:258-265, 1979.

Tautin, F.S.: Should dentures be worn continuously? J. Prosthet. Dent. **39**:372-374, 1978.

Wagner, A.G.: Maintenance of the partially edentulous mouth and care of the denture, Dent. Clin. North. Am. **17**:755-768, 1973.

Wagner, A.G.: Instructions for the use and care of removable partial dentures, J. Prosthet. Dent. **26**:477-479, 1971.

Woelfel, J.B., and Paffenbarger, G.C.: Pressure indicator paste patterns in duplicate denture made by different processing techniques for the same patient, J. Am. Dent. Assoc. **70**:339, 1965.

17 Postinsertion observations

The patient should be seen within 24 hours after the insertion of any removable prosthesis, whether it be a conventional partial denture, an immediate partial denture, or a temporary partial denture. Often irritation produced by the denture will not yet be felt by the patient, but it can be detected by the dentist. If the defects are detected and corrected early, the patient may never be subjected to the pain and discomfort that might otherwise occur, and the treatment will be considerably easier.

Many practitioners believe that the partial denture should be worn continuously, except for cleaning after meals and at bedtime, for this 24-hour period. This procedure has merit, and if the patient can be made to understand that it is to be followed only on the first night, it should be recommended to the patient.

After the patient has been seated and before the mouth examination is begun, the patient should be questioned to determine whether there are specific problems and if so, the exact nature of these problems. The patient should be reassured that most problems can be solved rapidly and simply. If there are no complaints, the mouth should still be examined carefully with the prosthesis in and out of the mouth.

Complaints normally fall into three main categories: pain or discomfort arising from the soft tissue or the underlying edentulous ridge: soreness of a tooth or group of teeth: and miscellaneous items such as tongue and cheek biting, looseness of the denture, problems with phonetics, and problems with eating. Each group is discussed individually.

SOFT TISSUE IRRITATION

Laceration or ulceration

A laceration or ulceration of the soft tissue surrounding the denture base is generally produced by an overextended denture base (Fig. 17-1). The patient may not be aware of the problem at this time or may complain of soreness or irritation, in which case he can usually point to the area of soft tissue that is being compromised. In any event, careful examination of the border tissues should be made. Any area of slightly increased redness or translucency should arouse suspicion of overextension of the denture base border. The translucent appearance takes place just before actual ulceration occurs (Fig. 17-2). It may or may not be accompanied by pain.

The degree of overextension of the denture base will usually have to be determined by visual examination. With the prosthesis in position, the cheek should be manipulated in a downward, outward, upward, and anteroposterior direction. If the denture border is overextended, movement of the border tissue will be impeded. If interference with free tissue movement and a change in color of the tissue are present, the denture flange extension must be reduced.

Overextension of the denture base on the lingual aspect of the mandibular edentulous ridge may be located and confirmed by manipulation of the patient's tongue. A forward thrust or a thrust of the tongue into the cheek opposite the side being examined will usually disclose the site of overextension of the denture base.

Another method of determining denture base overextension is through the use of disclosing wax as described in Chapter 16 and illustrated in Fig. 16-6. This method must be used with caution; it is normally used to verify or to isolate an area that is under suspicion following visual observation.

The use of pressure-indicating paste for the purpose of locating areas of border overextension is generally not indicated. Because of the softness of the material it is easily wiped off and as a result is not reliable.

A dependable method of identifying an overextension is through the use of an indelible pencil (Fig. 17-3). The area of soft tissue in question is dried with a gauze sponge and marked with the indelible pencil. The prosthesis is placed in position, and the border tissues activated as described. The partial denture must not remain in the mouth very long or the indelible mark will be lost as saliva begins to flow. The area requiring relief will be outlined by the transfer of the indelible ink to the acrylic resin border.

The denture border overextension is best corrected with a vulcanite bur or an arbor band. The flange must be kept rounded as it is being shortened. The tendency is to overrelieve these areas, so it is best to err on the side of conservatism rather than to overcut the denture. Any soreness present at the time of adjustment will remain for at least 24 hours. Healing and diminishing of painful symptoms can be hastened if the patient uses a

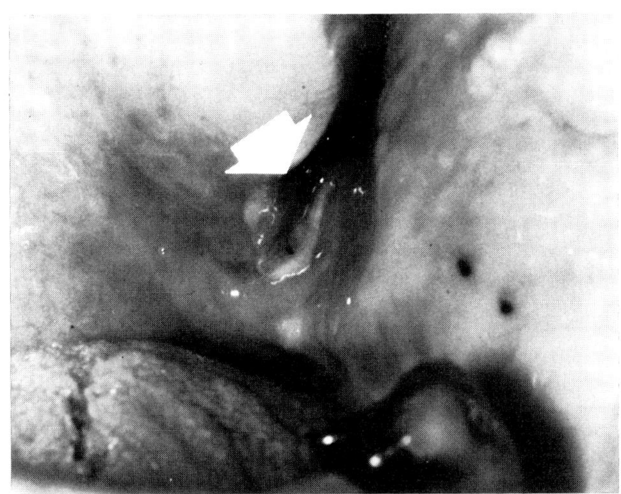

Fig. 17-1. Slight change in color, redness, indicates chronic irritation of soft tissue caused by an overextended denture base periphery.

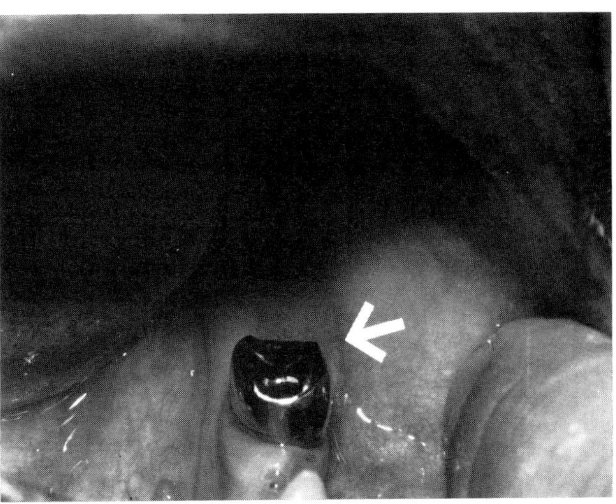

Fig. 17-2. Translucent appearance may be present along margin of slightly overextended denture base.

A

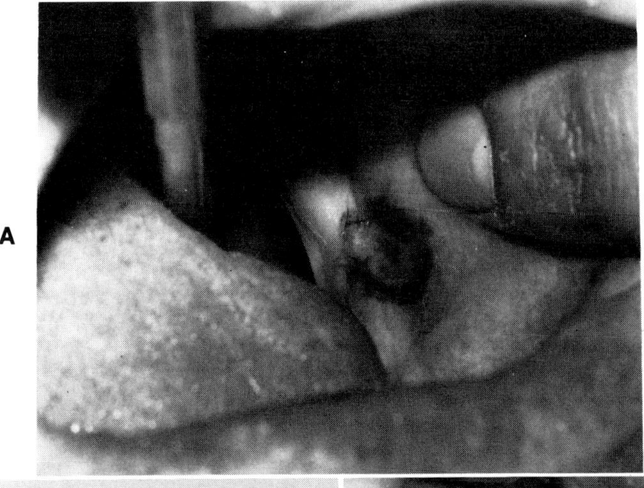

B

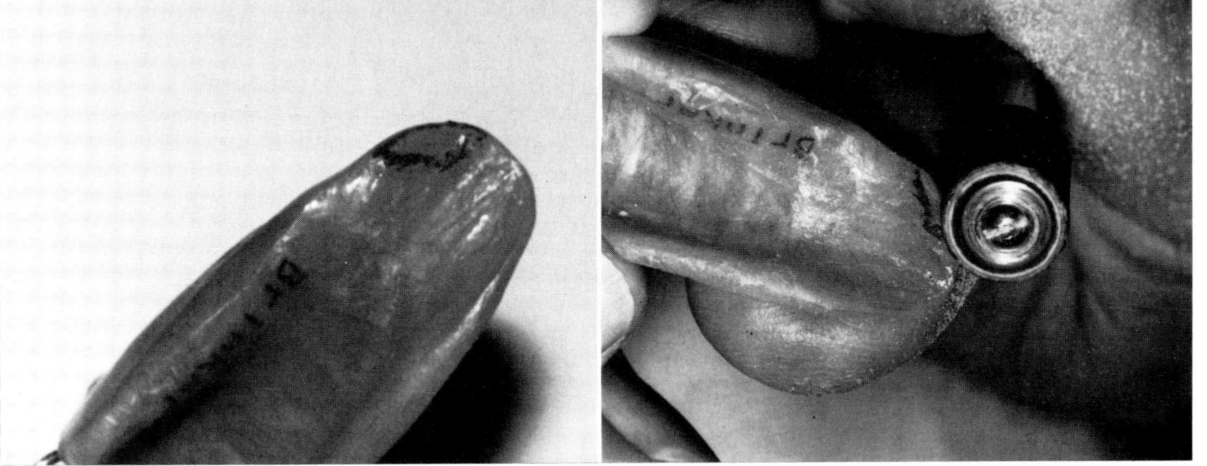

C

Fig. 17-3. A, Area of soft tissue irritation is circled with indelible pencil. B, Partial denture is seated in mouth, and pencil mark is transferred to denture base. C, Area of base causing irritation is relieved with arbor band. Margin is kept rounded.

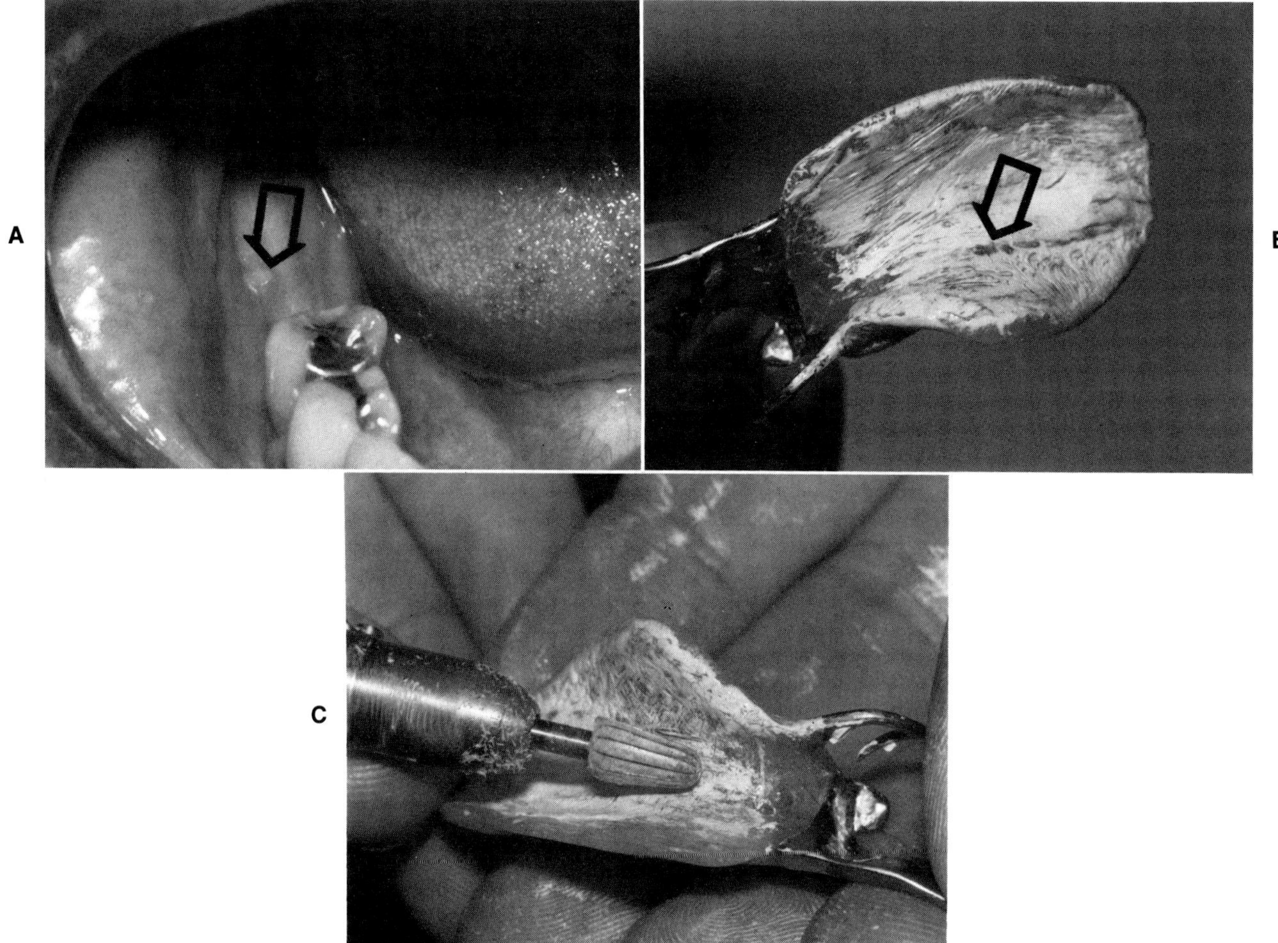

Fig. 17-4. A, Isolated area of irritation beneath denture base. **B,** Pressure-indicating paste is painted on base, and partial denture is seated. **C,** Area causing irritation, which appears as showthrough in pressure-indicating paste, is relieved.

hot saline mouthwash (1/2 teaspoon salt in a 6-ounce glass of water as hot as the patient can tolerate) at least every 4 hours. The patient should take a mouthful of the solution and hold it until the temperature of the solution drops. This is repeated until the 6 ounces is finished.

The use of topical anesthetics should not be encouraged because they will tend to mask the problem. If the patient is seen in 24 hours, there should not be pain severe enough to require this type of medication. If more time has elapsed and pain is sufficient to warrant the local application of medication, the prosthesis should not be worn until the pain has been controlled. At that time final adjustment of the prosthesis should be accomplished.

Erythema

Redness, or erythema, of the tissue covered by the denture base is generally caused either by a rough tissue surface of the denture base or by a slight rubbing movement of the denture base against the soft tissue covering the edentulous ridge during function. Roughness of the tissue side of the denture base can be corrected simply by using pressure-indicating paste to reveal the area of roughness and relieving the acrylic resin with an acrylic resin cutting stone or bur (Fig. 17-4). After the correction is made, another trial with pressure-indicating paste should be made to verify that the pressure has been relieved.

An excellent method of checking for roughness or small nodules of acrylic resin on the tissue surface that may be missed by the pressure-indicating paste is to pass the tip of a finger over the tissue surface of the resin (Fig. 17-5).

The second factor in producing this redness of the tissue underlying the denture base, and probably the more common, is the presence of occlusal discrepancies or prematurities.

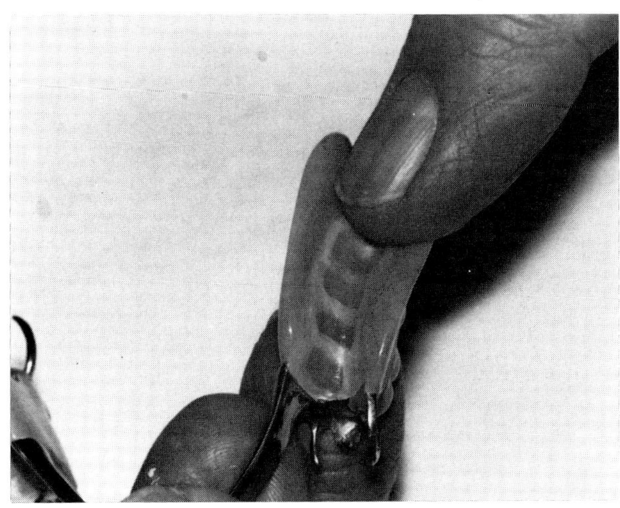

Fig. 17-5. Feeling tissue surface of denture base will often disclose nodules of resin that must be removed.

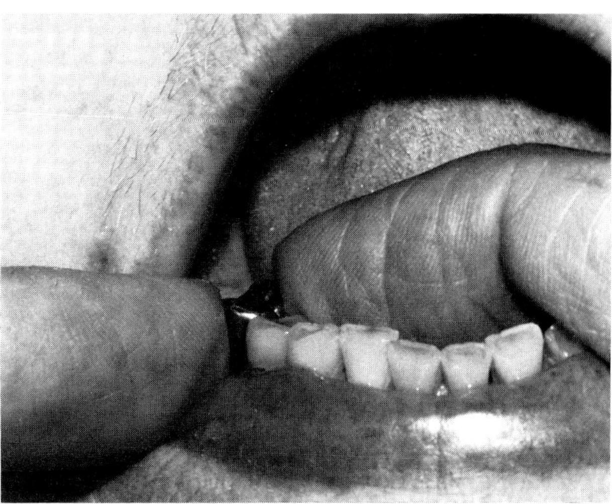

Fig. 17-6. Finger pressure is applied to each abutment tooth to detect sensitivity caused by pressure from partial denture.

This lack of occlusal harmony is by far the greatest factor in discomfort caused by removable partial dentures. Enough emphasis cannot be placed on examining the occlusion in a patient who is having problems adjusting to a partial denture. The technique for correcting the occlusal disharmony will be discussed later when the sore tooth problem is considered.

IRRITATION TO TEETH

When the soft tissue areas of irritation have been corrected, each tooth contacted by the restoration should be checked individually (Fig. 17-6). With the prosthesis out of the mouth, mesial, distal, buccal, and lingual pressure should be applied to each tooth. The pressure can best be applied by using fingers rather than an instrument because the danger of slippage is always present if an instrument or instrument handle is used. If the abutment tooth has been subjected to undesirable forces by the partial denture, a painful response to finger pressure in the direction toward which the tooth is being moved will result.

If the adjustment appointment is within 24 hours after delivery of the denture, the patient may not be conscious of pain until the tooth is pushed. If, however, a longer time has elapsed, the tooth or teeth may be so painful that it will be impossible to tell in what direction the undesirable forces are occurring and the problem will therefore be more difficult to locate and correct.

The use of disclosing wax in these instances will usually be sufficient to pinpoint the area of metal or resin that requires relieving to prevent this tooth movement. The disclosing wax should be applied to the metal or resin that contacts the tooth, and the partial denture seated in the mouth. When the denture is removed, the area that is causing the pressure will appear as a showthrough in the disclosing wax (Fig. 17-7). The showthrough will always appear on the side of the tooth opposite which the painful response was elicited by finger pressure. When carbide burs in the high-speed handpiece are used, these areas of showthrough can be removed or relieved.

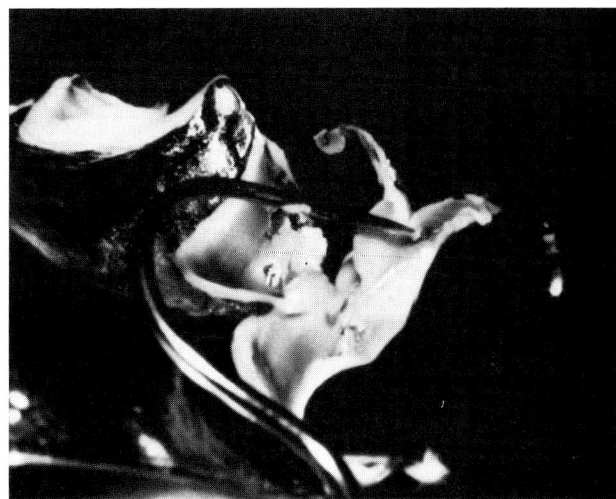

Fig. 17-7. Disclosing wax is displaced over area that is causing pressure.

If it can be demonstrated that the soreness or pain in a tooth is not caused by pressure from the partial denture, then the most logical reason for pain is occlusal interference. Failure to produce an area of showthrough in the disclosing wax is reason enough to assume that the pain is being produced by occlusal stress and not by lateral pressure from the metal or resin of the prosthesis.

One of the most common causes of pain or discomfort for a partial denture patient is occlusal interference between a natural tooth in one arch and the metal of the denture in the opposite arch. The actual tooth-to-metal contact may appear minor and may be difficult to isolate, yet the resulting discomfort can be extremely aggravating. Articulating paper or occlusal indicator wax strips must be used to locate the portion of the partial denture causing the interference (Fig. 17-8). The patient must be instructed to tap the teeth together firmly with the paper or wax in position. If articulating paper is used, the dye of the paper will be transferred to the denture where the interference is occurring. If wax strips are used, the offending cusp tip will penetrate the wax at the point of interference. Checks for occlusal prematurities in eccentric jaw positions should also be made at this time.

Premature contacts should be corrected by using heatless stones or carbide burs in the high-speed handpiece (Fig. 17-9). Diamond points may also be used, but cutting chrome alloy will reduce the life of these expensive instruments. The correction should be made with the prosthesis out of the mouth. Care must be taken not to thin the metal excessively, particularly in critical areas such as occlusal rests and retentive clasps. A particularly troublesome correction is that of the embrasure clasp (Fig. 17-10). Reduction of opposing cusps may have to be resorted to in order to prevent clasp breakage after adjustment is completed. Reduction of enamel surfaces at this stage of treatment is not

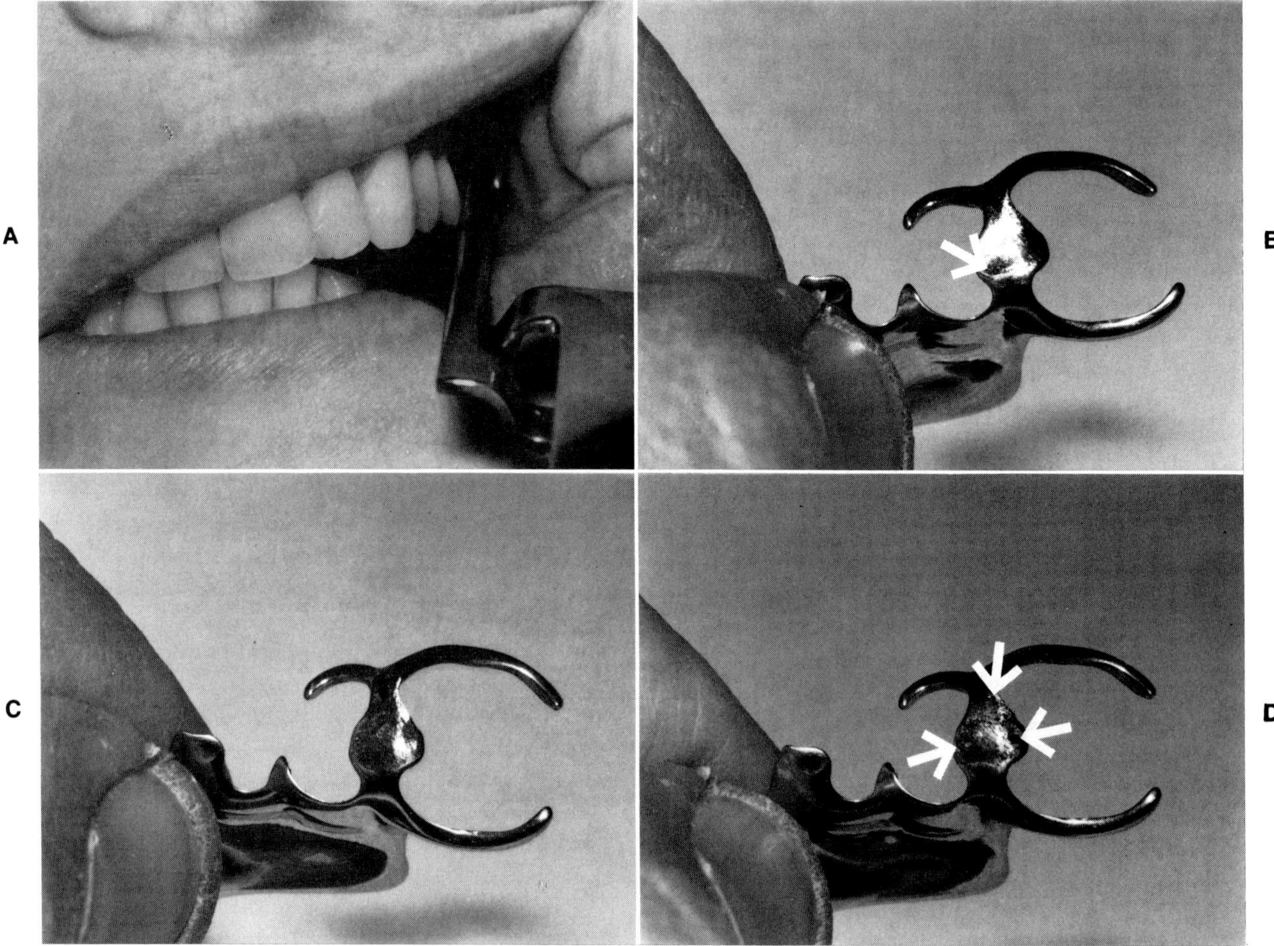

Fig. 17-8. A, Articulating paper is used to locate areas of occlusal interference. **B,** Occlusal interference is evidenced by transfer of dye from articulating paper to metal. **C,** If difficulty is encountered in transferring dye mark to polished metal surface, surface is roughened slightly with fine stone. **D,** Mark of occlusal interference is now easily read.

the method of choice. More complete planning at the survey and design stage would have prevented the problem.

An important adjunct to detecting occlusal prematurities is the patient's perception as recognized by the proprioceptive mechanism in the periodontal membrane. Perhaps fewer than 50% of patients will have this perception developed to the point where the exact spot of occlusal interference can be identified, a larger group will have the ability to recognize that an occlusal prematurity is present but cannot localize it closer than several teeth, and a smaller group will have little or no awareness of occlusal interferences. Working with complete denture patients Brill and others (1962) found that some patients could precisely locate areas of interferences as small as 0.06 mm. The presence of the periodontal membrane of the remaining teeth of a removable partial denture patient should increase the degree of perception for some patients to an even greater degree.

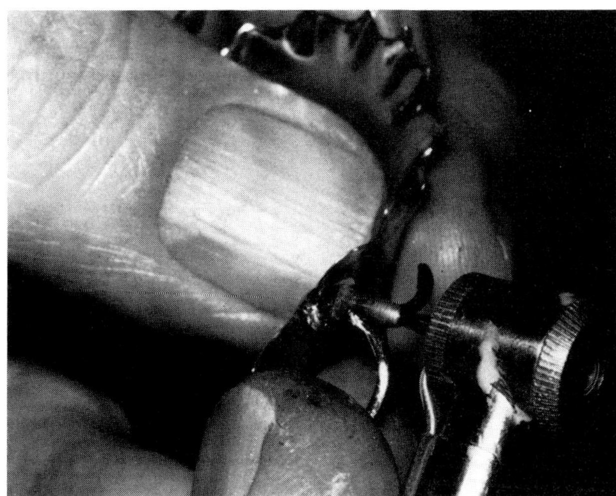

Fig. 17-9. Mounted points in high-speed handpiece are used to eliminate interferences.

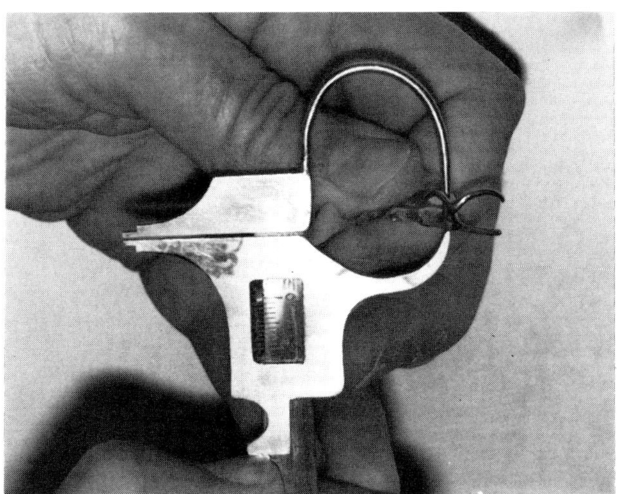

Fig. 17-10. Metal of embrasure clasp must be at least 1 mm thick.

Patients must be questioned as to the "feel" of occlusal contacts, but complete reliability cannot be accepted for all responses.

Remount procedures

A small percentage of patients will have multiple postinsertion complaints, all requiring adjustments. For the patient who cannot appear to be satisfied, a remount procedure may be indicated. Remounting the partial dentures on casts made from impressions of the patient's mouth on a semiadjustable articulator will usually reveal small discrepancies in the occlusion that were not possible to locate directly from the mouth.

Even though extra chair time is required for the procedure, it often proves to be one of the best time-saving appointments possible. The technique to be followed is described in Chapter 16. Accurate jaw relation records are essential, and the articulator mounting must be verified before any occlusal correction is attempted.

MISCELLANEOUS COMPLAINTS

Gagging

Gagging is not often a complaint of the wearer of a removable partial denture. However, if it is a complaint and if it has not been a problem up to this time, it must be resulting from a physical cause and not a psychologic one. For this reason all possible causes must be investigated rather than placing the blame on the psychologic makeup of the patient.

Gagging in the wearer of a maxillary partial denture is caused most frequently by failure of the maxillary major connector, either metal or acrylic resin, to be adapted closely enough to the hard palate. Failure to modify the impression tray to reduce the space between the tray and the palate results in the impression material slumping before the final set occurs. This produces an inaccurate cast and results in a major connector that will have a space between the tissue surface of the metal and the soft tissue of the palate. Saliva will accumulate in this space and, in some patients, produce a gagging sensation.

The remedy for this problem, if the major connector is constructed of acrylic resin, is to reline the major connector and obliterate the space. The technique for relining is discussed in Chapter 21. However, if the major connector is cast metal, a remake of the prosthesis may be necessary. (This inaccuracy of the palatal fit should have been recognized at the framework try-in appointment or at the time of delivery if correct procedures were followed.)

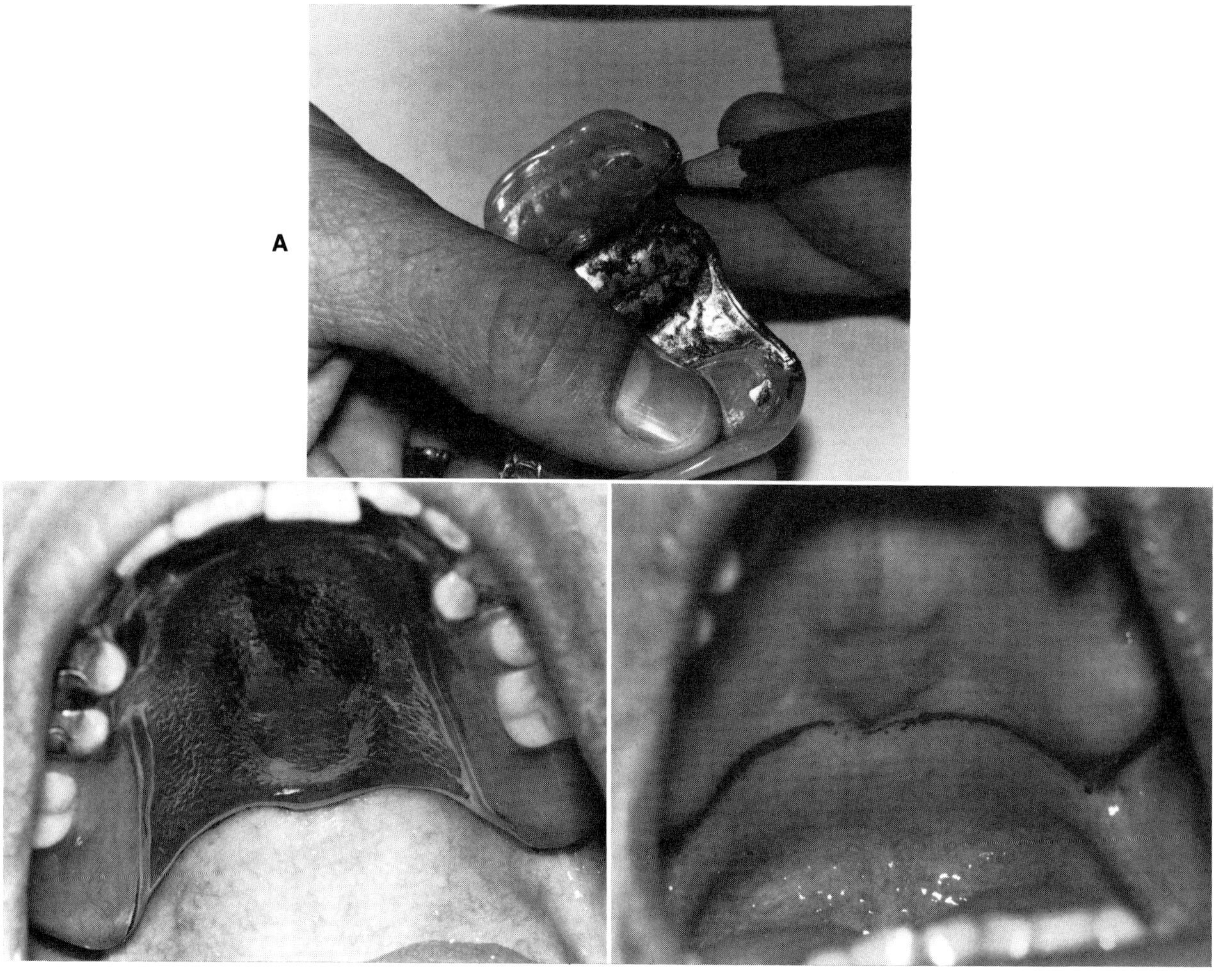

A

B

C

Fig. 17-11. A, Indelible pencil is used to mark posterior margin of major connector. **B,** Ink line is transferred to hard palate. **C,** Vibrating line is activated.

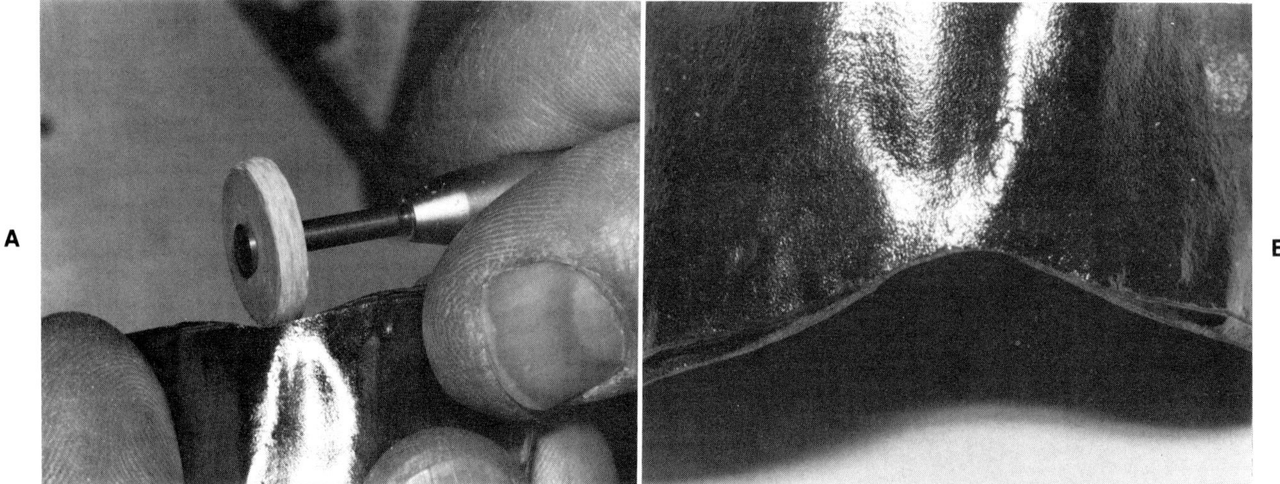

Fig. 17-12. A, Overextended major connector may be shortened by using heatless stone. **B,** Bead that prevents food debris from collecting beneath major connector is lost. This may necessitate remake of partial denture.

If the presence of a space cannot be shown for a maxillary partial denture, posterior overextension of the major connector may be causing the gagging. With the partial denture out of the mouth, an indelible pencil mark should be made along the posterior border of the partial denture. The denture is then seated and removed from the mouth. The indelible ink will be transferred in the form of a line to the soft tissue of the palate (Fig. 17-11). The relationship of this line to the soft palate can be determined by having the patient say "ahh." If any vibration of soft tissue takes place anterior to this line, the posterior border of the major connector may be extended too far on the soft palate. This overextension may result in gagging but more often will result in ulceration of the movable tissues contacting the edge of the metal. This type of overextension can be corrected by trimming the major connector (Fig. 17-12) or remaking the denture.

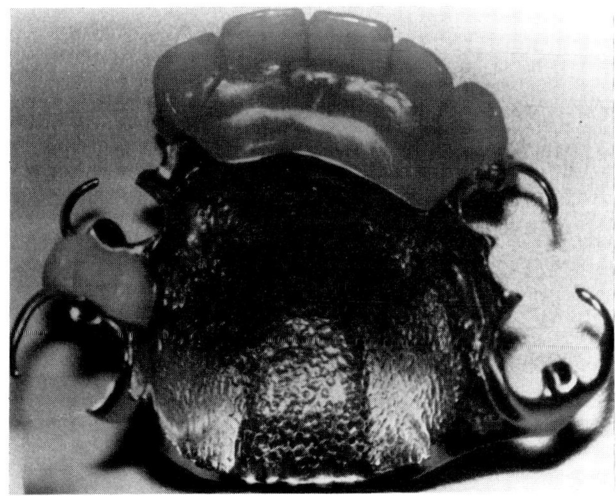

Fig. 17-13. Speech problems are encountered when maxillary anterior denture teeth are not positioned far enough anteriorly.

Gagging following the insertion of a mandibular removable partial denture may be caused by an alteration of the vertical dimension of occlusion. It was originally believed that only a decrease in the proper vertical dimension of occlusion would stimulate gagging (caused primarily by crowding of the tongue and adjacent soft tissues). More recent studies (Krol, 1963) have shown, however, that an increase in the vertical dimension of occlusion with concomitant elimination of the freeway space can also produce a prolonged gagging reaction. The exact mechanism is not well understood but is probably caused by spasms of the levator and the tensor veli palatini muscles.

Correction requires reestablishment of the proper vertical dimension of occlusion. The artificial teeth will have to be removed from the partial denture and reset to the correct vertical dimension, and adequate freeway space, on an average of 2 to 3 mm, must be maintained.

Another potential cause of gagging is the overextension, both in length and bulk, of the denture base flanges of a mandibular Class I removable partial denture. The overextension will reduce the available tongue space and produce involuntary retching or nausea. The flanges must be thinned and shortened.

Problems with phonetics

Phonetics problems are not frequently encountered with removable partial dentures. Problems that do arise are usually associated with the placement of maxillary

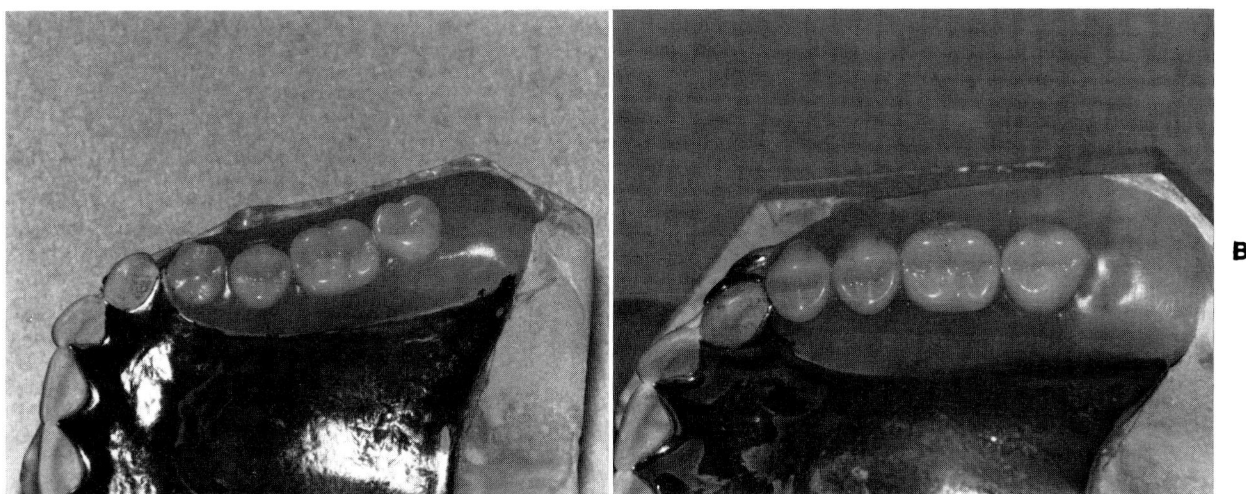

Fig. 17-14. A, Premolar teeth, if positioned too far lingually, will interfere with speech. **B,** Correcting tooth position will correct difficulty.

anterior teeth and the contour of the maxillary major connector over the rugal area.

The problem is usually attributed to a change in the contour of the speech area (the anterior part of the palate) or the anterior teeth not being positioned far enough labially (Fig. 17-13). More often than not the cause is a combination of these two factors.

The position of maxillary or mandibular premolar teeth will occasionally influence phonetics adversely (Fig. 17-14). If these teeth are positioned too far lingually, the action of the tongue is impeded and pronunciation will be changed. If these teeth are positioned too far facially, air will escape between the tongue and teeth and a whistling or slurring of the speech will be evident. If the latter error is present, soft utility wax adapted to the lingual surfaces of the premolar teeth should decrease the escape of air and the whistling or slurring effect.

For the other speech problems described the patient should be given a reasonable time (1 to 2 weeks) to adapt to the sensation and presence of the artificial teeth and to overcome the problem of articulation. Reading aloud is one of the best methods of adapting to the partial denture. If the patient fails to adapt to the denture, repositioning of the anterior teeth will have to be accomplished and consideration given to altering the contour of the palatal major connector.

Cheek or tongue biting

Cheek biting, trapping the buccal mucosa between the maxillary and mandibular posterior teeth, is usually caused by teeth positioned with insufficient horizontal

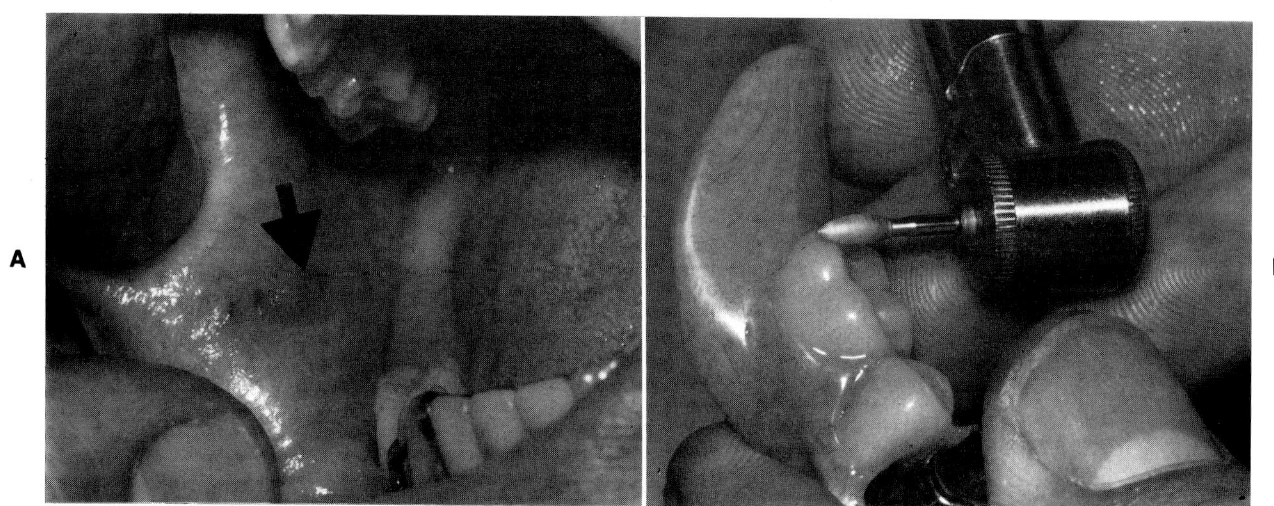

Fig. 17-15. A, Cheek biting results in line of ulcerations on buccal mucosa. **B,** Cheek biting is prevented by rounding mandibular buccal cusp tips.

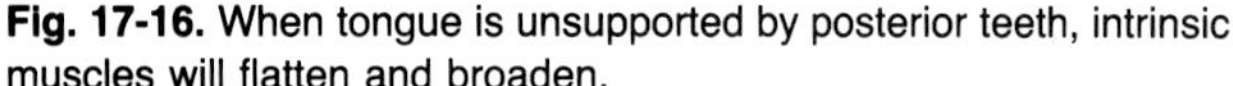

Fig. 17-16. When tongue is unsupported by posterior teeth, intrinsic muscles will flatten and broaden.

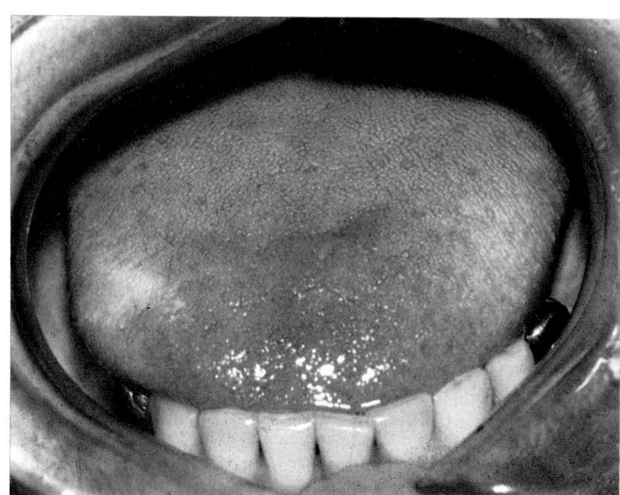

overlap. It is also possible the artificial teeth may have been set too far facially to the edentulous ridge. This may be corrected by either resetting the teeth or reducing the height of the mandibular buccal cusps by selective grinding.

Another contributing factor is when the natural posterior teeth have been missing for a long period. The buccinator muscle tends to sag into the space created by the missing teeth and may cause cheek biting. After the prosthesis is worn for a time, the muscle will regain its normal tone and resume its original position.

As a general rule, if the artificial teeth have been positioned correctly in the buccolingual relation to the edentulous ridge, the buccal cusps of the lower posterior teeth should be rounded inward to control cheek biting (Fig. 17-15).

Tongue biting frequently means that the artificial teeth have been positioned too far lingually and the tongue space has been decreased. The first attempt at correcting this condition should be recontouring the lingual surfaces of the mandibular posterior teeth by rolling in the lingual cusps of the teeth. It should be remembered that reducing the cusps of the teeth will also reduce the overall efficiency of the teeth. If tongue biting continues after the teeth have been reshaped, the artificial teeth will have to be removed and reset.

As mentioned previously, if lower posterior teeth have been missing for a long time, the intrinsic muscles of the tongue will lose tonus and will flatten or broaden considerably to fill the space once occupied by the teeth (Fig. 17-16). When the partial denture is placed, the tongue will regain its normal contour in time. The patient should be made to understand what is happening.

Difficulty in chewing

Most patients who have trouble chewing have not had posterior teeth for a number of years. The patient has lost the neuromuscular skills required to use the posterior teeth in grinding the food. The patient should be informed that a reasonable time is going to be required to relearn the masticating process. The length of time will depend to some extent on the patient's innate neuromuscular coordination and determination and on the duration of the edentulous state.

To prevent the patient from becoming discouraged, reassurance should be given that the chewing pattern will eventually be reestablished.

It is also wise to examine the occlusal surfaces of the artificial teeth. If the occlusal anatomy of acrylic resin or plastic teeth is not reestablished correctly, the result will be that the tooth is actually dull. Additional sluiceways and grooves should be added to the occlusal surface to increase the cutting efficiency (Fig. 17-17). The use of gold occlusal surfaces on the artificial teeth should also be considered, particularly if the artificial teeth oppose natural dentition.

The patient should also be advised to avoid extremely tough, stringy, or sticky food during the early period of adjustment. These foods will only add to the patient's discouragement.

Loose denture

The most common cause of a loose removable partial denture is retentive clasp tips that were not adjusted

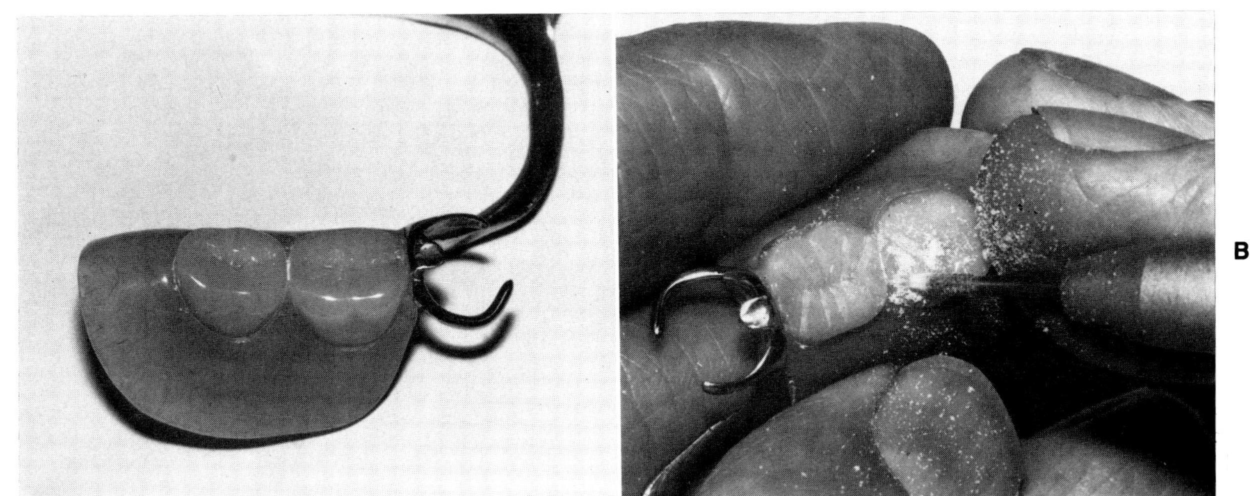

Fig. 17-17. A, Surfaces of occlusal resin artificial teeth will wear flat or can be polished flat if good technique is not followed. These teeth will function inefficiently. **B,** Additional grooves and sluiceways will improve cutting efficiency.

accurately or completely into the retentive undercuts. The technique described in Chapter 16 should be repeated to increase the retention. If adjusting the clasp does not produce the retention desired, careful analysis of the position of the retentive clasp tip on the tooth must be made. The clasp may not enter a true undercut, that is, an undercut in relation to the path of withdrawal. If this is the case, no amount of adjusting will increase the retention. A new clasp will have to be added to the denture. The method of accomplishing this is discussed in Chapter 21.

SUBSEQUENT ADJUSTMENTS

Occasionally a single postdelivery adjustment will suffice, but more frequently several additional adjustments may be required within 48 to 72 hours following the first adjustment.

A small number of patients lack confidence in wearing the removable partial denture. These patients should be seen an additional appointment or two even though they may have no specific complaints or clinical signs of difficulty. These patients should be given reassurance that they will overcome their problems and in time will adjust comfortably to the prosthesis.

A grave mistake is made by the practitioner who classifies these patients as chronic complainers and avoids continuing to work with them on postinsertion adjustments. Many dental prostheses have failed because of the dentist's reluctance to provide adequate postinsertion care.

PATIENT INSTRUCTION

The instruction given to the patient at the insertion appointment should be reinforced at the time of each adjustment. The patient's mouth should be examined carefully to observe the quality of home care that the patient has given to the partial denture and to the oral structures. The use of disclosing tablets can frequently be helpful in demonstrating to the patient areas of the prosthesis that are difficult to clean and where special care must be taken. The quality of the home care must be stressed strongly and constantly.

The patient should also be questioned about any problems encountered when inserting or withdrawing the partial denture, and the technique to insert and remove the prosthesis should be reviewed (Fig. 17-18).

Before the patient is dismissed, a reminder should be given of the necessity of continuing adequate home care and of frequent maintenance checks by the dentist. Maintenance visits should be scheduled every 3, 6, or 12 months. Seldom, if ever, should longer than 12 months elapse between appointments. The frequency of these checks will depend in part on the condition of the patient's remaining dentition. If the remaining teeth were periodontically involved or if difficulty is noted initially in controlling the rate of caries development, particularly for younger patients, the checks need to be more often.

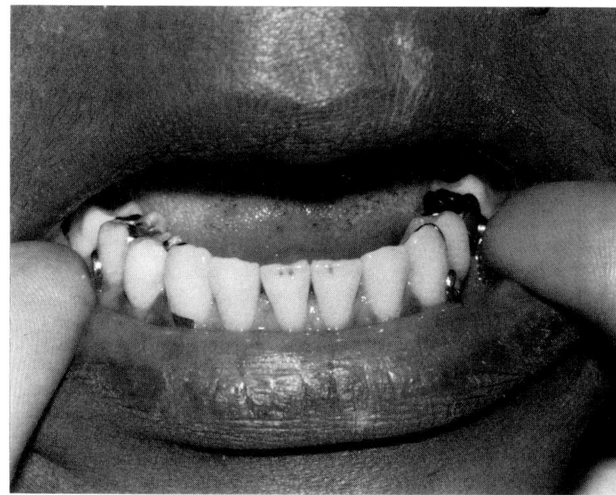

Fig. 17-18. Patient should be warned against attempting to remove partial denture by lifting against approach arm of vertical projection clasps. This distorts clasp and may abrade soft tissue.

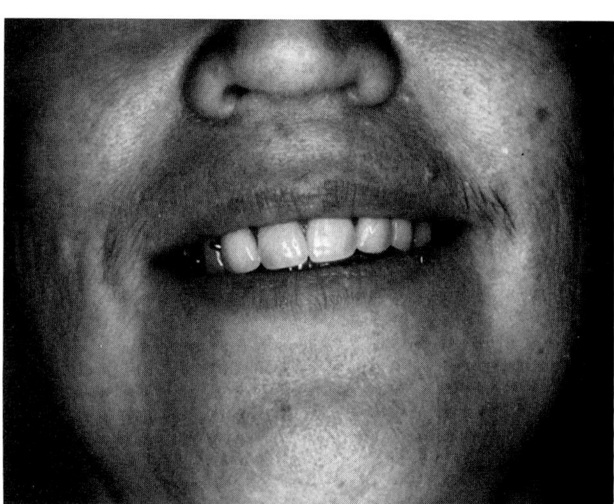

Fig. 17-19. Delivery of partial denture does not terminate treatment of patient. Postinsertion adjustments and periodic maintenance appointments are necessary part of treatment.

The insertion of a removable partial denture, or any prosthesis, does not relieve the dentist of the responsibility of providing adequate maintenance for that patient or that prosthesis (Fig. 17-19).

LENGTH OF APPOINTMENT

This appointment should be accomplished by an experienced practitioner in 15 minutes. The dental student will normally require 1 hour.

REFERENCES

Brill, N., and others: Aspects of occlusal sense in natural and artificial teeth, J. Prosthet. Dent. **12**:123, 1962.

Krol, A.J.: A new approach to the gagging problem, J. Prosthet. Dent. **13**:611, 1963

BIBLIOGRAPHY

Bauman, R.: Inflammatory papillary hyperplasia and home care instructions to denture patients, J. Prosthet. Dent. **37**:608, 1977.

Cavalaris, C.J.: Pathologic considerations associated with partial dentures, Dent. Clin. North. Am. **17**:585-600, 1973.

Derry, A., and Bertram, U.: A clinical survey of removable partial dentures after 2 years usage, Acta. Odontol. Scand. **28**:581-598, 1970.

Federation of Prosthodontic Organizations: Guidelines for evaluation of completed prosthodontic treatment for removable partial dentures, J. Prosthet. Dent. **27**:326-328, 1972.

Immekus, J.E., and Aramany, M.: Adverse effects of resilient denture liners in overlay dentures, J. Prosthet. Dent. **32**:178-181, 1974.

MacCullum, M., and others: Which cleanser? Dent. Pract. Dent. Rec. **19**:83-89, 1968.

Maison, W.G.: Instructions to denture patients, J. Prosthet. Dent. **9**:825-831, 1959.

Miller, E.L.: Clinical management of denture induced inflammations, J. Prosthet. Dent. **38**:362, 1977.

Newton, A.V.: Denture sore mouth, Br. Dent. J. **112**:357-360, 1962.

Ramsey, W.O.: The relation of emotional factors to prosthdontic service, J. Prosthet. Dent. **23**:4-10, 1970.

Rothman, R.: Phonetic considerations in denture prosthesis, J. Prosthet. Dent. **11**:214-223, 1961.

Savage, R.D., and Mac Gregor, A.R.: Behavior therapy in prosthodontics, J. Prosthet. Dent. **24**:126-132, 1970.

Schabel, R.W.: Dentist-patient communication—a major factor in treatment prognosis, J. Prosthet. Dent. **21**:3-5, 1969.

Schabel, R.W.: The psychology of aging, J. Prosthet. Dent. **27**:569-573, 1972.

Schole, M.L.: Management of the gagging patient, J. Prosthet. Dent. **9**:578-583, 1959.

Sharp, G.S.: The etiology and treatment of the sore mouth, J. Prosthet. Dent. **16**:855-860, 1966.

Sharp, G.S.: Treatment of low tolerance to dentures, J. Prosthet. Dent. **10**:47-52, 1960

Wagner, A.G.: Maintenance of the partially edentulous mouth and care of the denture, Dent. Clin. North. Am. **17**:755-768, 1973.

Webb, C.S.: Gagging: a method for positive control, Dent. Surv. **42**:54-56, 1967.

Young, H.A.: Factors contributing to success in prosthodontic practice, J. Prosthet. Dent. **5**:354-360, 1955.

18 Temporary and immediate removable partial dentures

The three types of temporary removable partial dentures—interim, transitional, and treatment—are types of temporary removable dentures, identified according to the reason for which the denture is to be used. The immediate partial denture does not make up a special variety by itself but may be a treatment approach to any of the other three. It has a great many indications and should be planned as often as possible where indicated.

INTERIM PARTIAL DENTURES

Indications

The interim partial denture is indicated when age, health, or lack of time precludes a more definitive treatment. It is indicated most often in young patients who have, usually inadvertently, suffered the loss of an anterior tooth or teeth (Fig. 18-1). In these instances the size of the pulp chambers of the adjacent teeth makes crown preparation for a fixed partial denture on the teeth hazardous at best (Fig. 18-2). The risk of mechanically exposing the pulpal tissue and performing endodontic therapy is not warranted. With the proper instructions on home care and with continuous and regular follow-up examinations, a young patient can be treated with an interim partial denture, or a series of dentures if necessary, until the teeth adjacent to the space have matured sufficiently to permit abutment preparations for a fixed partial denture. Patients have been treated in this manner successfully for periods longer than ten years.

The interim partial denture may also be indicated for the young patient who, because of accident, undetected rapid caries, or hereditary partial anodontia, has missing posterior teeth. The edentulous spaces should not be allowed to remain untreated, or a lifetime of dental ills caused by migration or overeruption of unsupported teeth can result. The dental pulp of these adjacent posterior teeth will also be large, and abutment tooth preparation for fixed prosthodontic replacement will not be possible. In some instances it will be possible to maintain the edentulous space using orthodontic means (bands and wires) (Fig. 18-3). However, if the clinical crowns of the adjacent teeth are short, as is most often

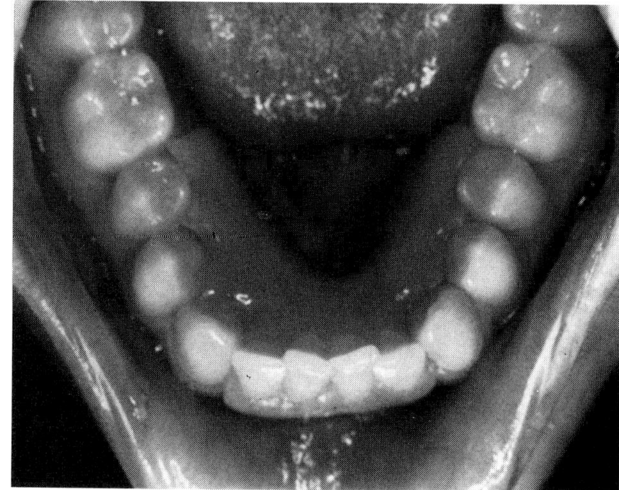

Fig. 18-1. Interim partial denture in 12-year-old patient. Clasps are not needed for retention.

the case, maintaining the bands and wires in position can be difficult. Construction of an interim removable partial denture, always bilateral in design, can solve the problems of maintaining the space adequately and restoring occlusal function at the same time (Fig. 18-4). This temporary prosthesis must never be unilateral. A unilateral partial denture offers a definite hazard, not only because the patient may swallow or aspirate the prosthesis, but also because the denture fails to distribute forces over a sufficient area of the soft tissue and remaining teeth to prevent damage to these structures.

In addition to the interim partial denture being indicated for the young patient, there are many elderly patients whose health contraindicates the lengthy and, at times, physically trying appointments needed to construct fixed replacements for missing teeth. For these patients the simple clinical procedures required to construct and insert an interim partial denture can normally be well tolerated. Health limitations are, of course, not limited to the geriatric patient but can be encountered in any age group. Many patients are reluctant to be seen without anterior teeth regardless of their medical prognosis. Often the psychologic lift pro-

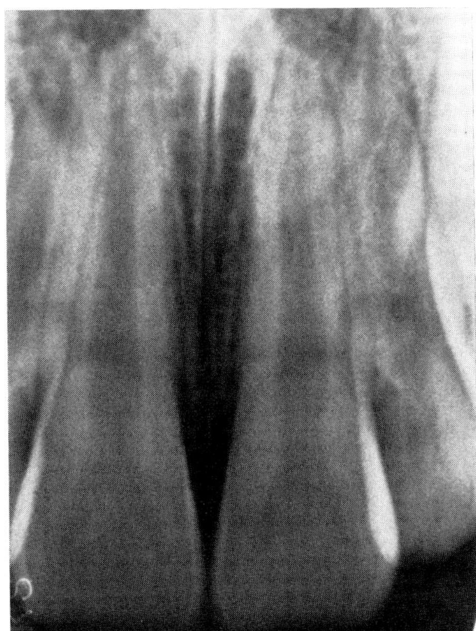

Fig. 18-2. Size of pulp chamber in young patients contraindicates crown preparation for fixed partial denture.

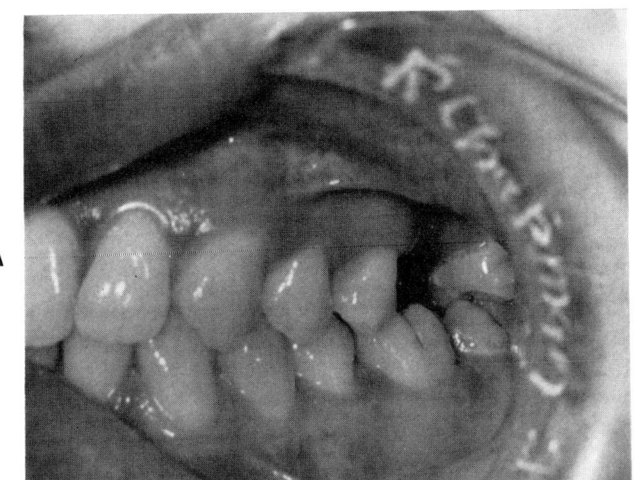

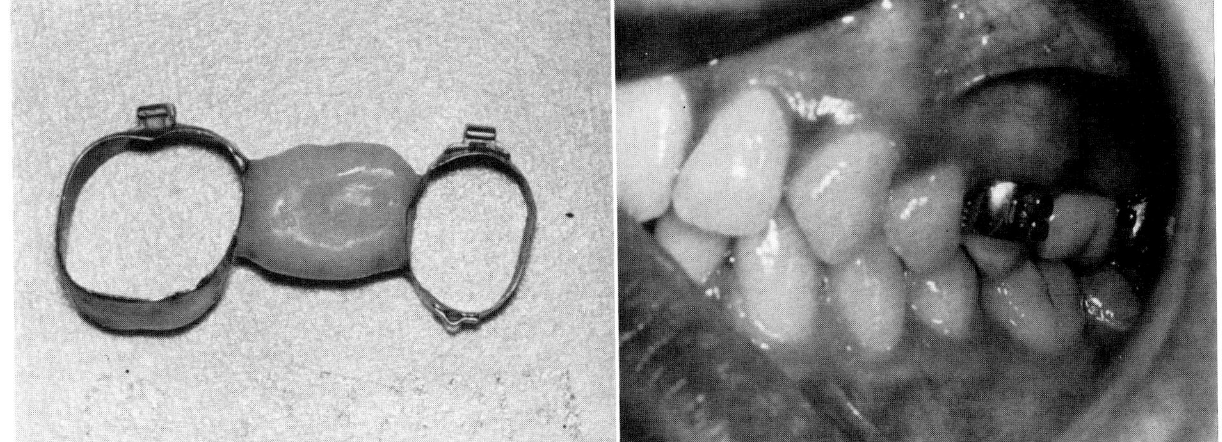

Fig. 18-3. Posterior missing tooth in young patient, **A,** may be replaced on interim basis with plastic pontic suspended between orthodontic bands, **B. C,** Bands and pontic in position. (Courtesy Department of Orthodontics, University of Texas Health Science Center at San Antonio.)

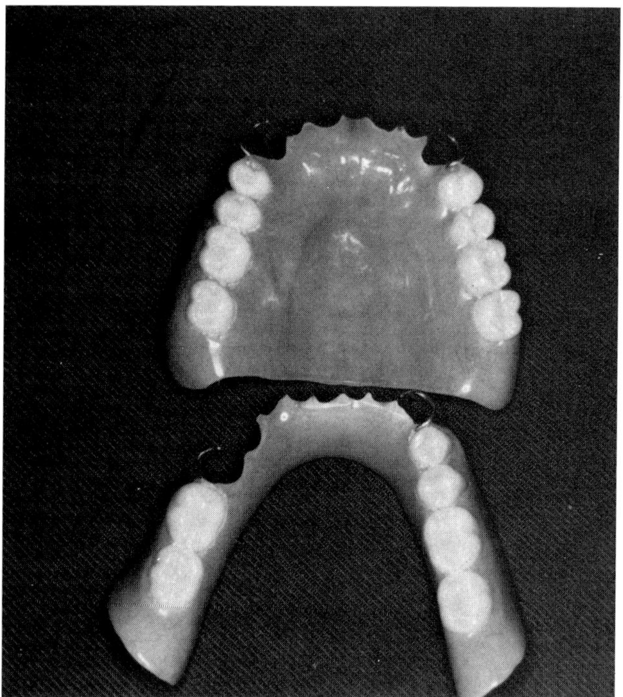

Fig. 18-4. Temporary partial dentures should be used to replace posterior teeth until definitive treatment can be carried out.

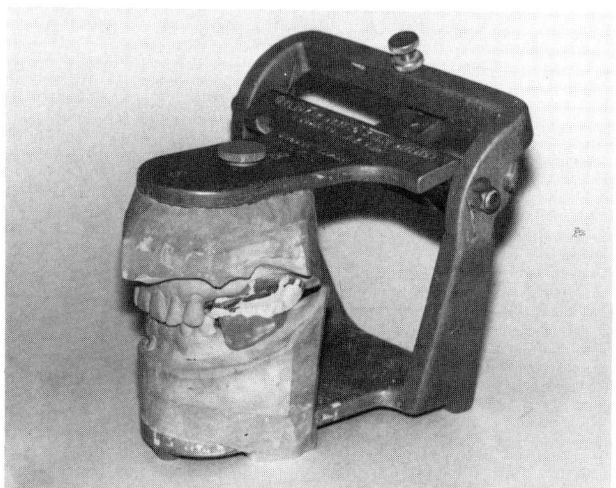

Fig. 18-5. Master casts mounted on articulator with jaw relation records made on gutta-percha baseplates.

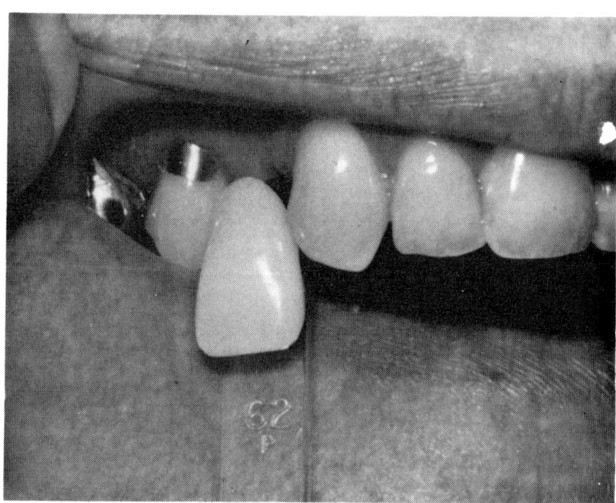

Fig. 18-6. Shade of adjacent teeth is taken with shade guide from manufacturer of artificial tooth that will be used.

vided by an interim denture greatly improves the mental outlook for these patients.

Another indication for the interim partial denture may occur in patients who have suffered a temporary financial setback. The cost of this service to the patient can be considerably less than for the definitive treatment that will be required eventually. This is not to imply that the interim partial denture should be considered as anything other than a temporary form of treatment.

Patients will often come in for treatment of an unexpected loss of a tooth or teeth and with business trips or other important engagments scheduled. The time available for the necessary dental work will not be sufficient. In this case, construction of an interim partial denture is indicated. It is far better for the health of the patient to provide an interim replacement rather than attempting to rush the permanent treatment and compromise the end result.

Clinical procedures

After the teeth have been cleaned, accurate irreversible hydrocolloid impressions are made of both arches. The impressions should be extended sufficiently to capture the peripheral roll in at least the area of the missing teeth. In the mandibular impression the tongue must be controlled to produce the anatomy of the ridge lingual to the natural and missing teeth. This is the part of the impression most often lacking in completeness.

In the maxillary impression the impression tray must be altered to obliterate excessive space between the tray and the hard palate. If this is not done, the impression material may sag, resulting in an inaccurate cast.

The impressions should be poured in a dense dental stone by the double-pour technique. This technique is discussed in Chapter 5.

If the casts can be unmistakeably hand articulated, a jaw relation record will be not be necessary. It would be a rare situation when an interim removable partial denture would be constructed at any position other than centric occlusion. If a jaw relation record is

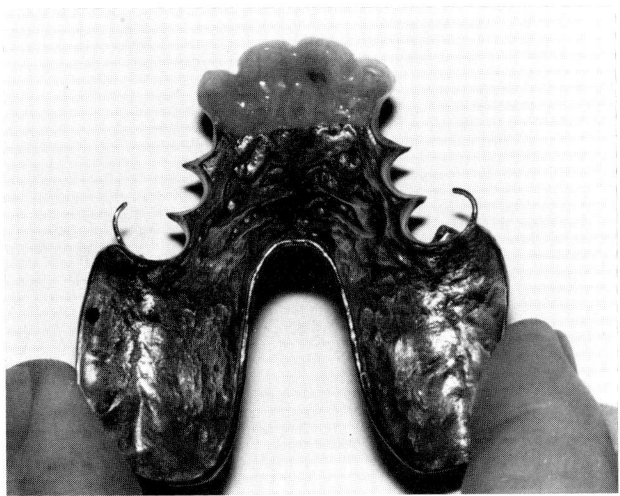

Fig. 18-7. If temporary prosthesis is to be worn for extended time, cast metal base is more hygienic than acrylic resin.

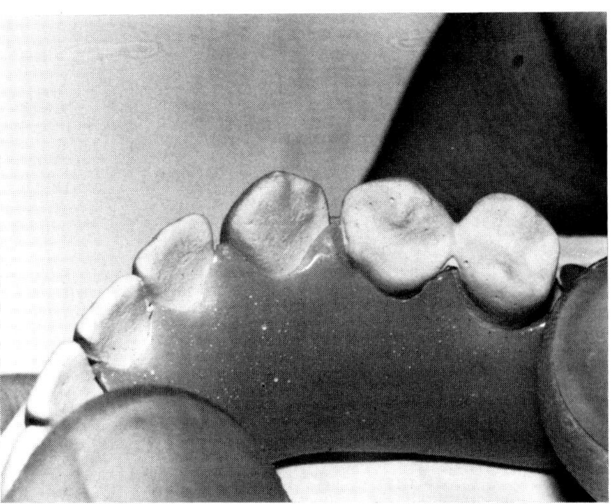

Fig. 18-8. Acrylic resin denture base extending into interproximal areas of teeth provides retention for prosthesis.

needed, it must be made on the master cast. Either a gutta-percha baseplate or sprinkle-on autopolymerizing acrylic resin may be constructed following the technique described in Chapter 9 (Fig. 18-5).

A shade of the remaining teeth must be taken with the appropriate shade guide (Fig. 18-6). This is one of the most overlooked steps in denture construction. It should be established as a routine step in all patient treatment in prosthodontics. It can be inconvenient for the dentist and also for the patient to have to schedule an additional appointment to record the shade that had been forgotten at the original appointment. The mold and size of the artificial teeth to be used can be determined from the remaining natural teeth on the master cast.

Laboratory procedures

Most temporary removable partial dentures have an acrylic resin denture base and acrylic resin artificial teeth. When it is known that a patient must wear an interim denture for a prolonged time, such as for a 10- or 12-year-old patient, consideration may be given to using a cast metal denture base (Fig. 18-7). The fit of the casting undoubtedly will be more accurate, and it will be easier to maintain oral hygiene.

The casts must be mounted on an articulator. A simple hinge articulator is normally adequate for this purpose.

Retentive clasps are optional for interim partial dentures. Most patients can accommodate easily to a partial denture that is retained by the adaptation of the denture base to the soft tissue. It is also possible for the acrylic resin contacting the lingual surfaces of the teeth to project into slight interproximal undercuts and add to the retention of the denture (Fig. 18-8). This type of retention takes advantage of the linear change in dimension that occurs as acrylic resin polymerizes. If the material did not change volumetrically this retention would not be effective.

When retentive clasps are desired, a surveyor must be used to locate areas of retentive undercuts. Minimum retention is desired. In the event undercuts are not present for a conventional clasp, a ball clasp can be used. The ball clasp consists of a ball of solder on the end of a piece of wrought wire. The wire crosses the marginal ridges between two teeth, and the ball engages the interproximal space (Fig. 18-9). This clasp can provide adequate retention without an untoward display of metal.

Wrought wire is usually used for retentive clasps. The wrought wire should be of lighter gauge than that used for a conventional removable partial denture; 0.040 inch is adequate.

When the wrought wire retentive clasps are designed, careful analysis must be made for occlusal clearance, or space between the opposing teeth to accommodate the thickness of the wire (Fig. 18-10). Reshaping of enamel surfaces should be kept to a minimum. This is not to suggest that enamel surfaces should not be altered if success or failure of the prosthesis depends on changing the tooth contour. In preference to delivering a partial denture that the patient cannot adjust to or one that may be damaging to the remaining oral structures—such as one in hyperocclusion because of misplaced wrought wire clasp—tooth altering procedures should be included in the treatment plan. The main reason that retentive clasps are not always included in the design of interim partial

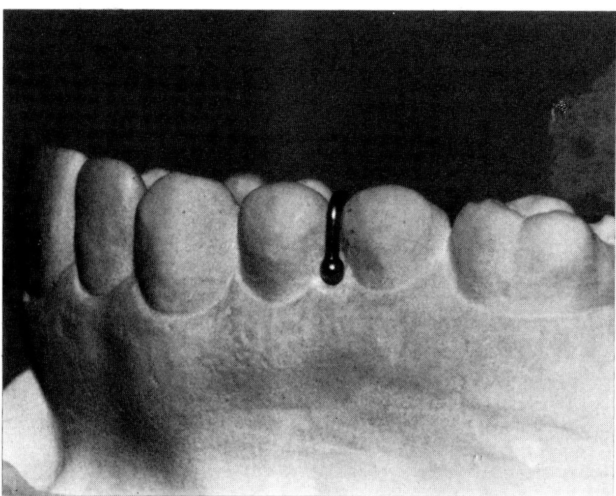

Fig. 18-9. Ball clasp fits into interproximal space buccal to posterior teeth to provide retention.

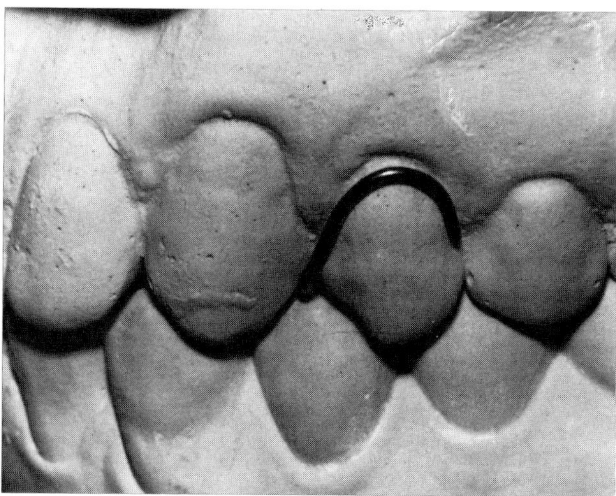

Fig. 18-10. Wrought wire clasps may be used for retention, but occlusal space must be present. Note relation of lower first premolar to clasp.

dentures is that, particularly in the younger patient, occlusal freedom for the placement of the clasps may not be present and removal of enough tooth structure to provide the needed space may require excessive tooth structure removal.

Retentive clasps, if used, will be attached to the denture base by embedding the nonretentive portion of the clasp in the denture base. After the retentive portion of the clasp is formed, the remainder of the clasp is coiled upon itself and bent so that as it rests in the position on the cast at which it will ultimately be constructed; the coiled or acrylic retention portion will be slightly out of contact with the lingual or palatal surface of the cast. This will allow the acrylic resin of the denture base to flow completely around the wrought wire and lock it securely in place.

The retentive clasps are the first component of the interim partial denture to be formed. After being formed, they should be attached to the tooth surface with sticky wax applied on the buccal surface of the tooth (Fig. 18-11, *A*).

The next component to be selected and shaped is the artificial tooth or teeth (Fig. 18-11, *B* and *C*). If little or no resorption of the edentulous ridge has taken place, the neck of the tooth should be butted directly to the cast and no labial flange of the denture base should be planned. To ensure intimate contact with the mucosa in the mouth, the crest and labial portion of the edentulous ridge should be scraped slightly. This will provide for the slight compression of the soft tissue that may have taken place during the impression procedure and guarantee intimate contact between the ridge lap portion of the replacement tooth and the tissue. This area will be further adjusted at the time of delivery to make certain excessive pressure against the tissue is not present.

In the event that resorption of the edentulous ridge has occurred, scraping the ridge will not be necessary because the denture base will cover the ridge and support the teeth in the position the natural teeth originally occupied. Shaping of the ridge lap portion of the artificial teeth in this case may be kept to a minimum, only enough to ensure that the tooth is in its correct position.

The selection of the artificial tooth will be governed by the mesiodistal and occlusogingival space available and by comparison with the same tooth on the opposite side of the midline if one is present. If all anterior teeth are being replaced, guides such as are used to select anterior teeth for complete denture patients should be followed. It is especially important to maintain the midline formed by the central incisors in harmony with the midline of the face. Any great deviation of the midline will result in an artificial appearance. The number of teeth used as replacements is also important. Every attempt should be made to restore the same number of anterior teeth that are missing. The number of posterior teeth is not important as long as occlusal harmony and function are restored. For the anterior region, overlapping of the teeth if the space is diminished, or creating diastemas if the space has increased, should be resorted to before a tooth is omitted or added.

One of the chief advantages in using plastic teeth is that reshaping the teeth is relatively simple. Contouring incisal edges can be done with sandpaper disks to match or harmonize with the natural teeth. Other forms of altering the denture tooth can be accomplished to match adjacent teeth. Materials are also available that

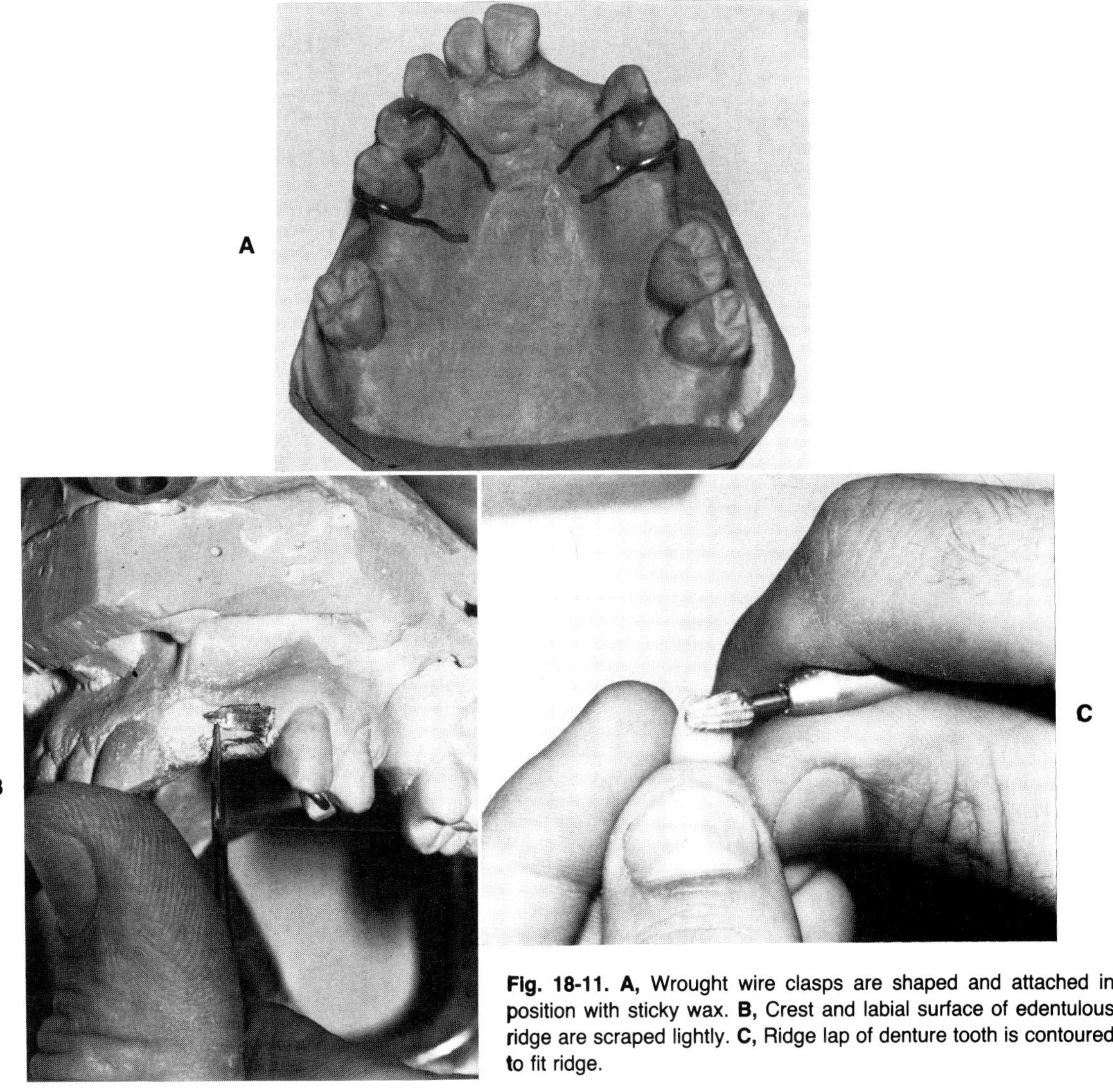

Fig. 18-11. A, Wrought wire clasps are shaped and attached in position with sticky wax. **B,** Crest and labial surface of edentulous ridge are scraped lightly. **C,** Ridge lap of denture tooth is contoured to fit ridge.

make characterizing the denture tooth a quick and simple process.

After the denture teeth have been positioned on the cast as desired (the occlusion should be developed as the teeth are positioned), a stone matrix should be made to retain the teeth as the denture base is formed. If a heat-cured denture base is to be used, the matrix will not be necessary. The denture base can be waxed and the master cast invested and processed as with complete dentures. The split packing process that was described for the conventional removable partial denture need not be followed.

Esthetic try-in of anterior teeth

If verification of the esthetic quality of anterior tooth replacements is desired, and most often it should be, the try-in should be scheduled before the formation of the stone matrix (Fig. 18-12). A try-in appointment should be used on a routine basis for interim partial dentures that are expected to be used for an extended period.

After the denture teeth have been positioned as desired, a double thickness of baseplate wax is adapted to the master cast. The wax is adapted to the lingual surfaces of the natural teeth and extended onto the palate, or to the lingual ridge of the mandibular arch, far enough to provide strength for the try-in appointment. The denture teeth are attached to the baseplate wax and the wax chilled. Obviously, care must be used in handling this temporary try-in partial denture, but if the patient is cautioned against attempting to function with the denture, an esthetic evaluation can be made.

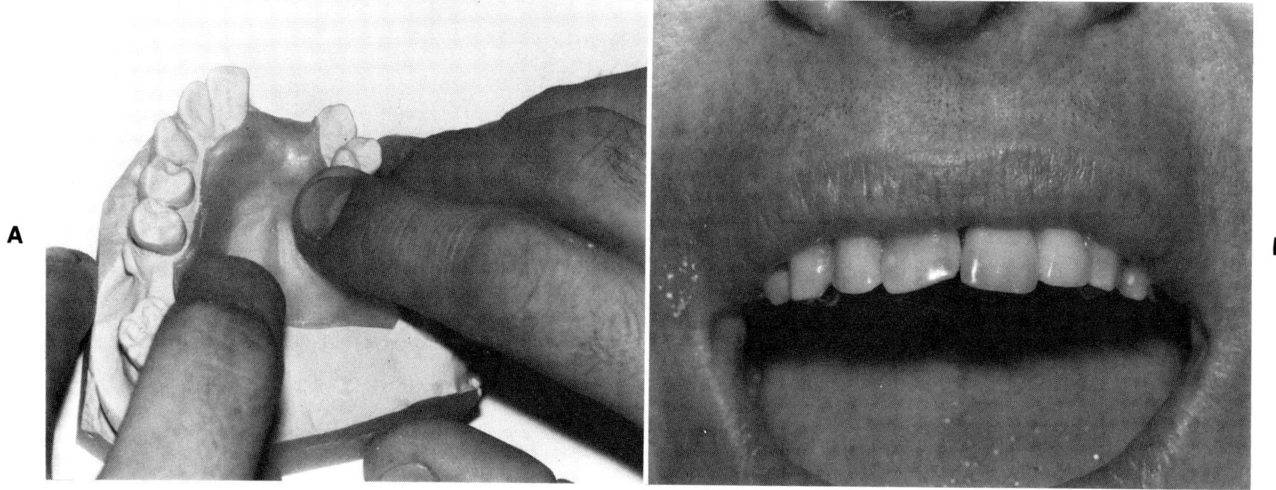

Fig. 18-12. A, Baseplate wax is softened and contoured to fit palate of cast. **B,** Denture tooth is contoured, attached to baseplate wax, and tried in patient's mouth.

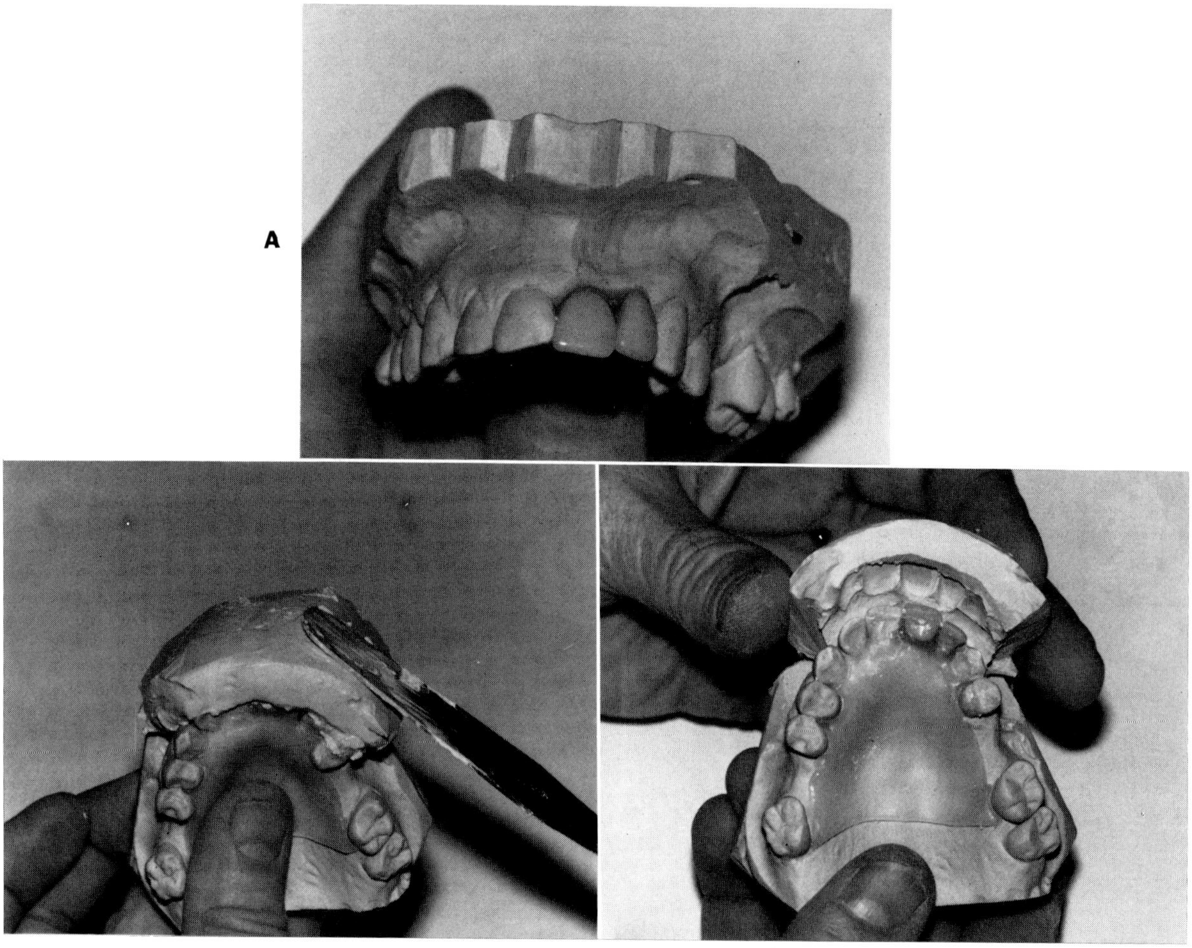

A

B

C

Fig. 18-13. A, Base of cast is notched, and cast soaked in slurry water. **B,** Thick mix of accelerated stone is formed over labial surface of cast and teeth. **C,** Stone matrix is removed after stone has set.

Any necessary changes in tooth position or shade can be made with the patient present. When both the dentist and the patient are satisfied, thc matrix can be constructed.

Completing the interim partial denture

The majority of temporary partial dentures will be constructed of autopolymerizing acrylic resin using the sprinkle-on technique. For this reason a stone matrix is necessary to maintain the position of the artificial teeth (Fig. 18-13). The master cast must be soaked thoroughly in slurry water and a gypsum separating medium painted over the stone surfaces to be contacted by the matrix. This should include the facial surfaces and incisal or occlusal edges of several teeth on each side of the artificial teeth and a portion of the soft tissue and side of the base of the cast. The side of the base of the cast may be indexed with several V-shaped notches to ensure that the matrix will be repositioned accurately.

A thick mix of dental stone, one that can be handled and sculptured with the fingers, is made using Hydrocal and concentrated slurry solution. If a facial or labial denture base flange has been planned, the flange must have been waxed to its final form before the matrix is adapted to the cast and artificial teeth. The mix of dental stone is adapted or lightly vibrated into place on the facial surface using fingers, not a mechanical vibrator because this could loosen the denture teeth. The matrix should be made of uniform thickness, between 8 to 10 mm, to provide strength adequate for supporting the denture teeth as the denture base is formed. The working time of the Hydrocal–concentrated slurry solution is limited, so the matrix must be formed rapidy.

When the final set of the matrix has occurred, it is teased off the cast and trimmed. The baseplate or utility wax that was used to support the denture teeth during construction of the matrix is removed from the denture teeth and cast with boiling slurry water (Fig. 18-14).

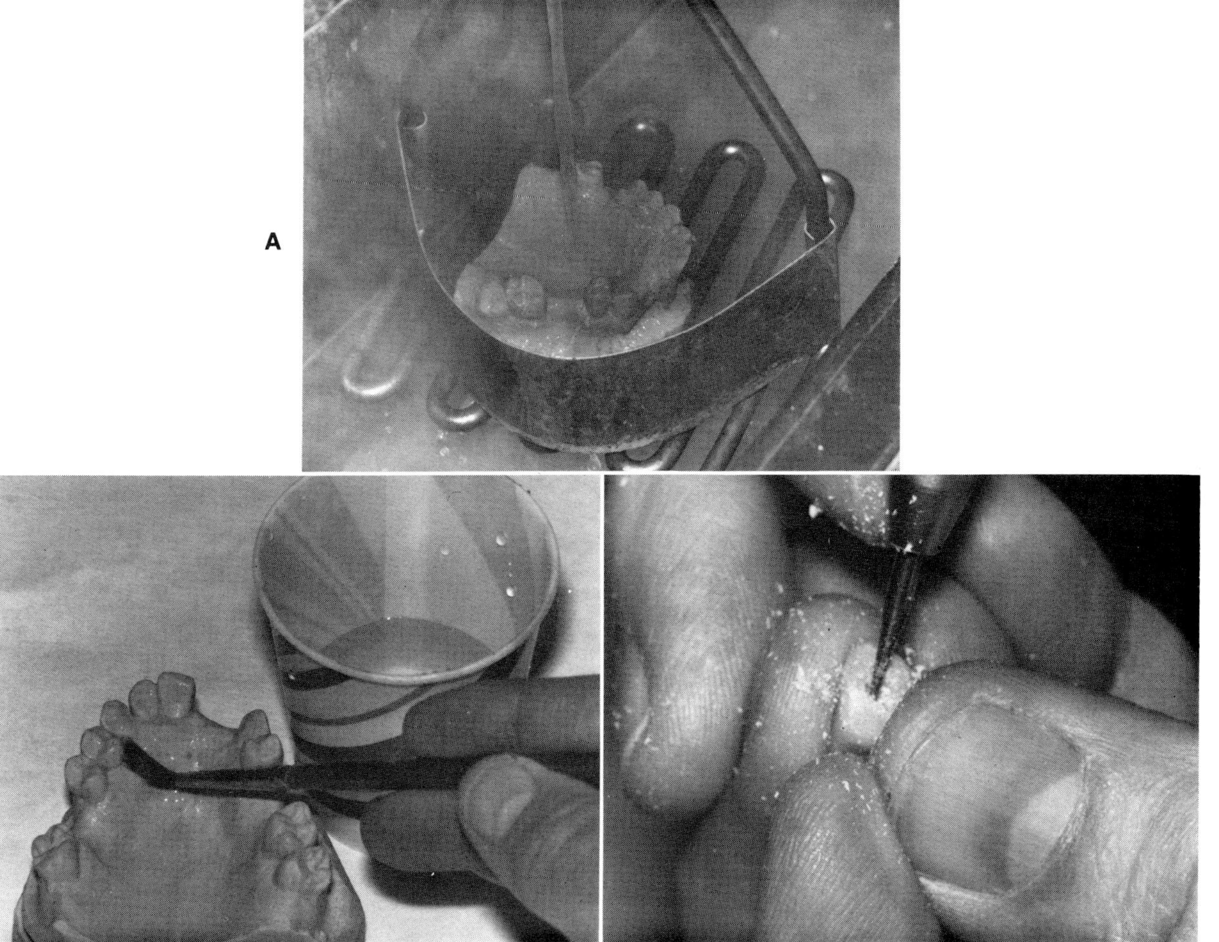

Fig. 18-14. A, Baseplate wax is flushed from cast with boiling water. **B,** Separating medium is painted on warm cast. **C,** Retention holes (diatorics) are drilled in ridge lap portion of denture tooth for acrylic resin denture base.

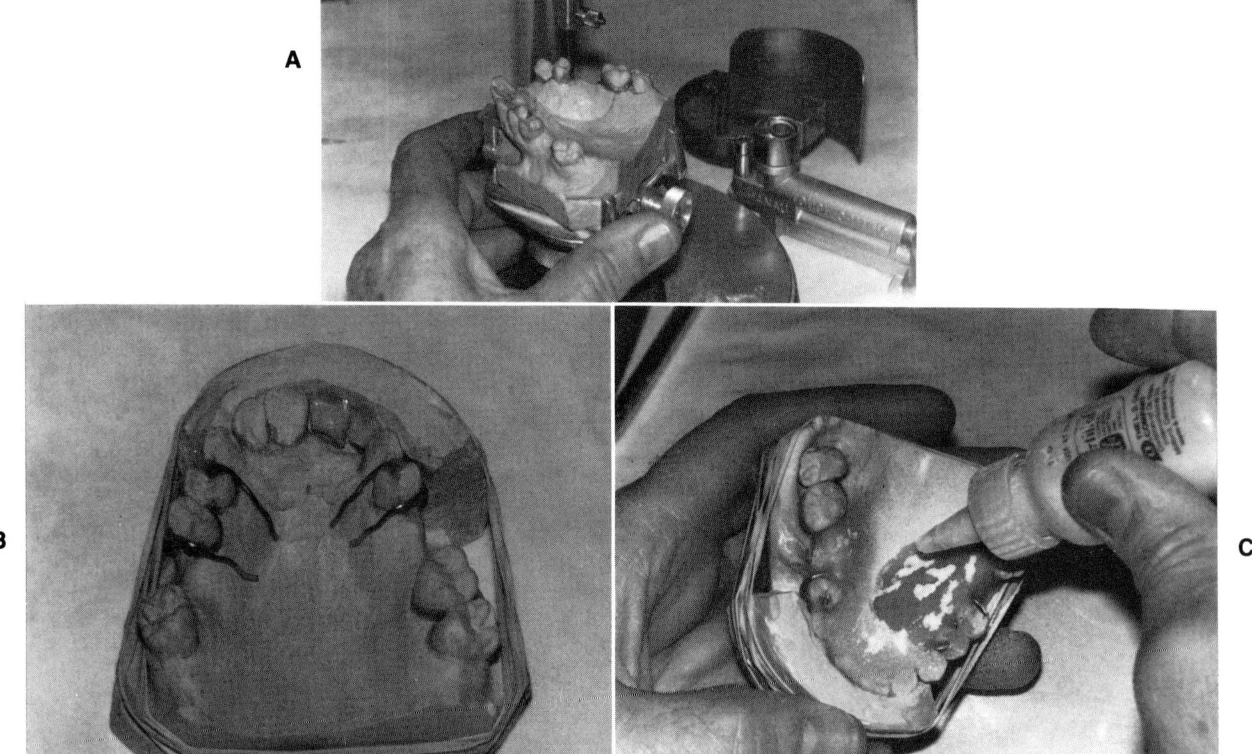

Fig. 18-15. A, Undercuts to path of insertion are blocked out with wax. **B,** Denture teeth and matrix are reassembled on master cast. Rubber bands are used to hold matrix in position. **C,** Acrylic resin is added using sprinkle-on method.

Several coats of an alginate separating medium are painted on the surface of the cast while it is still hot from the boilout procedure. To provide mechanical retention of the artificial teeth to the denture base, diatorics, or retention holes, may be drilled in the ridge lap portion of the teeth. Care should be exercised not to penetrate into the tooth so deeply to allow the shade of the denture base to alter the shade of the tooth.

Following the boilout procedure to remove all residues of wax from the master cast and teeth, the cast, denture teeth, and matrix are assembled. The teeth are positioned in the matrix and secured in place with sticky wax. The sticky wax must be placed so as not to interfere with the fit of the matrix against the cast. The surface of the matrix should also have been treated with a separating medium before the teeth are placed in position.

Before the denture base is formed, gross undercuts (greater than 0.030 inch as measured by the undercut gauge on the surveyor) on the lingual surfaces of the teeth to be contacted by the denture base should be eliminated (Fig. 18-15).

If autopolymerizing resin is to be used to form the denture base, baseplate wax or a mix of Hydrocal and concentrated slurry solution can be used to eliminate the undesirable undercuts. The analyzing rod in the surveyor is used to determine that parallel blockout has been achieved. The blockout must be accomplished with the tilt of the cast such that it will be parallel to the path of insertion of the partial denture.

Slight undercuts on the teeth need not be eliminated because a certain amount of retention can be gained from them. The slightly resilient acrylic resin will engage the undercuts and provide some resistance to displacement of the denture.

Slight undercuts of the soft tissue need not be eliminated at this time. During the delivery appointment these areas can be relieved if necessary.

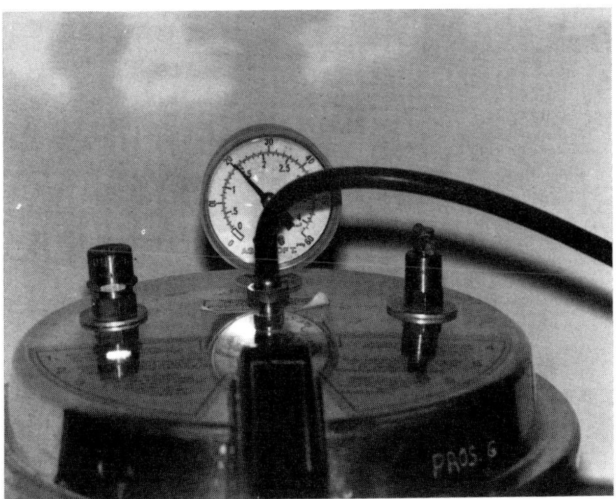

Fig. 18-16. Autopolymerizing resin is processed in pressure pot under 20 pounds of pressure for 20 minutes.

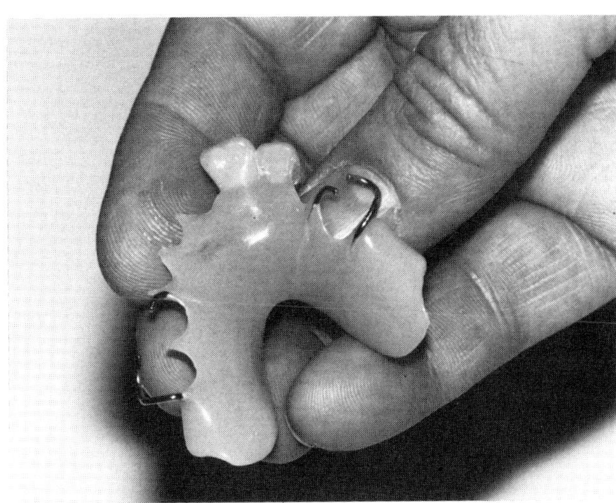

Fig. 18-17. External surface of temporary prosthesis must be highly polished.

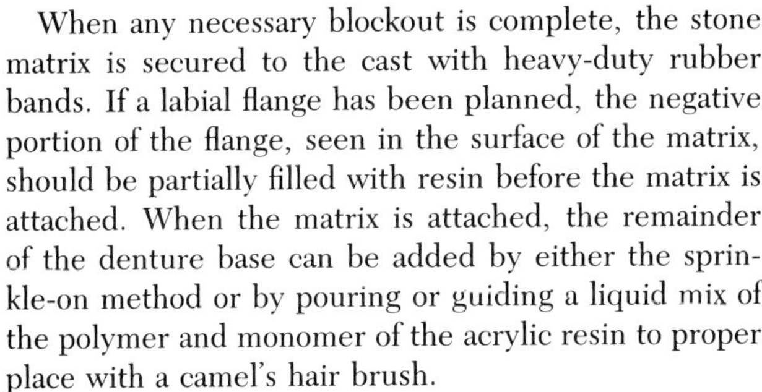

When any necessary blockout is complete, the stone matrix is secured to the cast with heavy-duty rubber bands. If a labial flange has been planned, the negative portion of the flange, seen in the surface of the matrix, should be partially filled with resin before the matrix is attached. When the matrix is attached, the remainder of the denture base can be added by either the sprinkle-on method or by pouring or guiding a liquid mix of the polymer and monomer of the acrylic resin to proper place with a camel's hair brush.

The outline of the denture base for an interim removable partial denture in the maxillary arch will normally be that of a horseshoe major connector with the acrylic resin contacting the lingual surfaces of the remaining teeth. If anterior teeth are being replaced, the posterior extension should at least include the first molar teeth. This will provide sufficient soft tissue contact to ensure adequate vertical support for the prosthesis.

For the mandibular arch the denture base will also be in the form of lingual plating and should extend inferiorly as far as possible without encroaching on the movable tissues of the floor of the mouth. Posteriorly it also should extend minimally to the distal lingual surface of the first molar if anterior teeth are being replaced. This is required not only to distribute forces generated by the presence of the partial denture but also to provide stability of the denture against anterior tipping forces.

The denture base after being formed should be allowed to cure, preferably in a pressure pot under twenty pounds of pressure, for at least 20 minutes (Fig. 18-16). If a pressure pot is not available, the polymerization should take place in an environment saturated with acrylic resin polymer (obtained by placing the cast in a closed container with a small amount of polymer or by inverting a rubber mixing bowl over the cast). The saturated environment prevents excessive loss of polymer from the denture base through evaporation and thus prevents porosity of the denture.

After the processing is complete and before the denture is removed from the cast, the cast should be returned to the articulator to correct any occlusal errors that may have developed during denture base construction. This is accomplished using articulating paper following the procedure described in Chapter 15. The interim denture is then recovered from the cast and finished and polished following the regimen used in finishing and polishing the denture bases for the conventional partial denture (Fig. 18-17).

Delivery of interim partial denture

At the delivery appointment the tissue surface of the interim partial denture should be painted with pressure-indicating paste before attempting to place the denture in position (Fig. 18-18). The paste will help show areas that may prevent the denture from seating. An interference indicated by the presence of an area that has been wiped away should be visually verified before a correction to the surface of the denture base is made. The most common areas that will interfere with the seating of the interim denture are the interproximal projections between the natural teeth and the contact areas of the artificial teeth with the proximal surfaces of the natural teeth adjacent to the edentulous space.

For the first seating little pressure should be applied after resistance to seating is encountered. It is possible for the acrylic resin, under heavy force, to spring over undercuts from the teeth and become locked in place

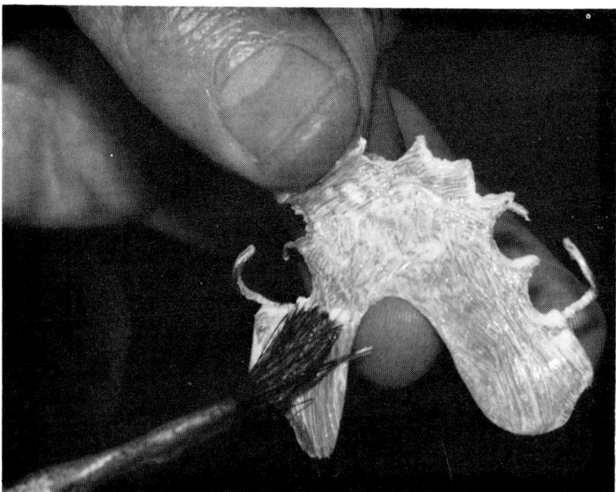

Fig. 18-18. Pressure-indicating paste is painted on tissue surface of temporary partial denture.

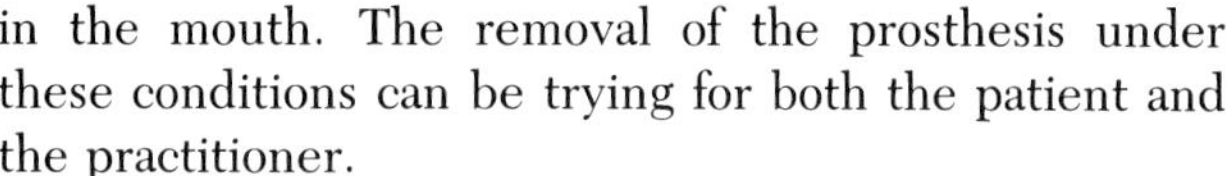

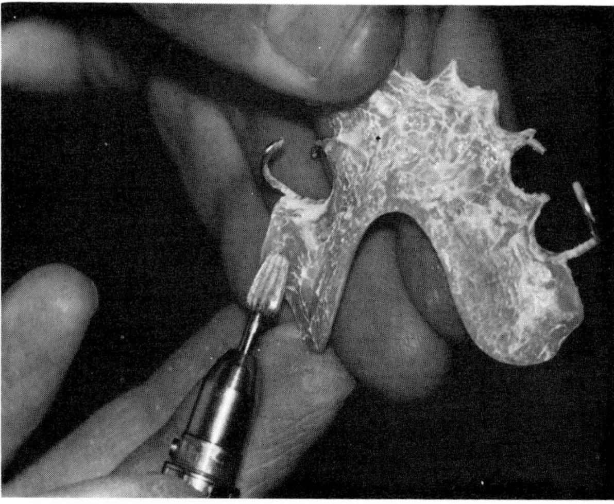

Fig. 18-19. Areas of excess pressure, as indicated by complete displacement of the paste, are relieved.

in the mouth. The removal of the prosthesis under these conditions can be trying for both the patient and the practitioner.

After visually verifying areas of the denture that are preventing the denture from seating, the areas should be carefully reshaped, not just haphazardly eliminated, with vulcanite burs or acrylic resin stones (Fig. 18-19). The alterations at each trial insertion should be kept to a minimum. If a denture base flange is present, it must also be viewed as a possible area of interference and should also be checked with pressure-indicating paste at each trial insertion. Blanching of the soft tissue under and around the flange as the denture is seated indicates interference caused by the denture base flange. Intimate contact between the edges of the denture base and the soft tissue is desired, but not to the extent that ischemia of the tissue is produced.

The number of seatings that will be required before the denture goes to place with minimal interference will be in direct proportion to the height of the clinical crowns of the remaining natural teeth. The greater the height of the crowns, the greater number of trial seatings will be required. It should also be understood that the shorter the clinical crowns, the less will be the retention.

When the interim denture is seated completely, the impression of the soft tissues will be clear on the surface of the pressure-indicating paste. There must be no excessive pressure under the denture base against the soft tissue (indicated by the obliteration of the paste in isolated areas). Any pressure spots must be relieved with appropriate burs. Ideally the pressure-indicating paste should be equally or evenly displaced over the entire tissue surface of the denture base. Once the accurate fit of the denture base has been confirmed, the occlusion must be checked.

Since the majority of interim partial dentures will be used to replace anterior teeth, the goal of the artificial tooth position is to be free from contact with opposing teeth in centric relation or centric occlusion (Fig. 18-20) and to have light contact in lateral or protrusive jaw positions. When the mandible is protruded to bring the anterior teeth into an edge-to-edge relationship, the tooth contact should offer slight resistance to a piece of tissue paper being drawn between the teeth but should not be great enough to cause displacement of the partial denture.

When posterior teeth are being replaced, light occlusal contact is again the desired goal in developing the final occlusal scheme. If multiple posterior teeth are being replaced and normal occlusal contacts are necessary to provide the patient with a functional occlusion, some method of providing vertical support for the prosthesis may be necessary to prevent damage to the underlying soft tissue and edentulous ridge. Rapid resorption of the alveolar bone can take place if occlusal overloading is present. Occlusal rests can be incorporated into the interim partial denture during construction if necessary. The simplest method of constructing occlusal rests is by bending a piece of wrought wire to engage the occlusal surfaces of at least one posterior tooth on each side of the arch (Fig. 18-21). The wire must be positioned so as not to interfere with the opposing occlusion. The opposite end of the wire is bent to form several angles. The purpose of the angles is to provide a firm attachment to the denture base because this end of the wire will be embedded in the acrylic resin. This type of occlusal rest will provide sufficient

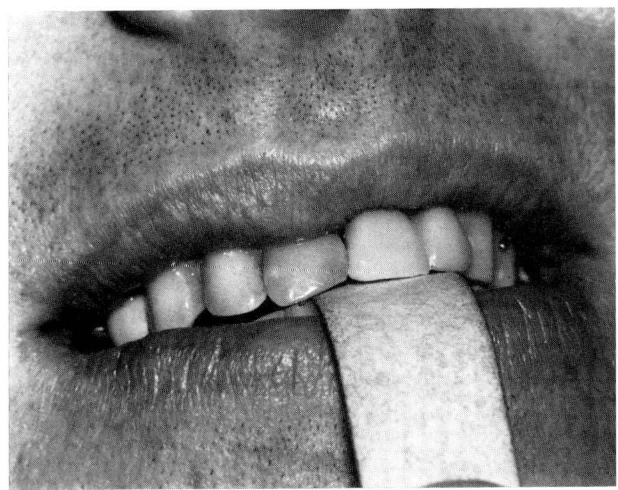

Fig. 18-20. There should be no contact between artificial anterior teeth and opposing natural teeth. Tissue paper should slide between teeth.

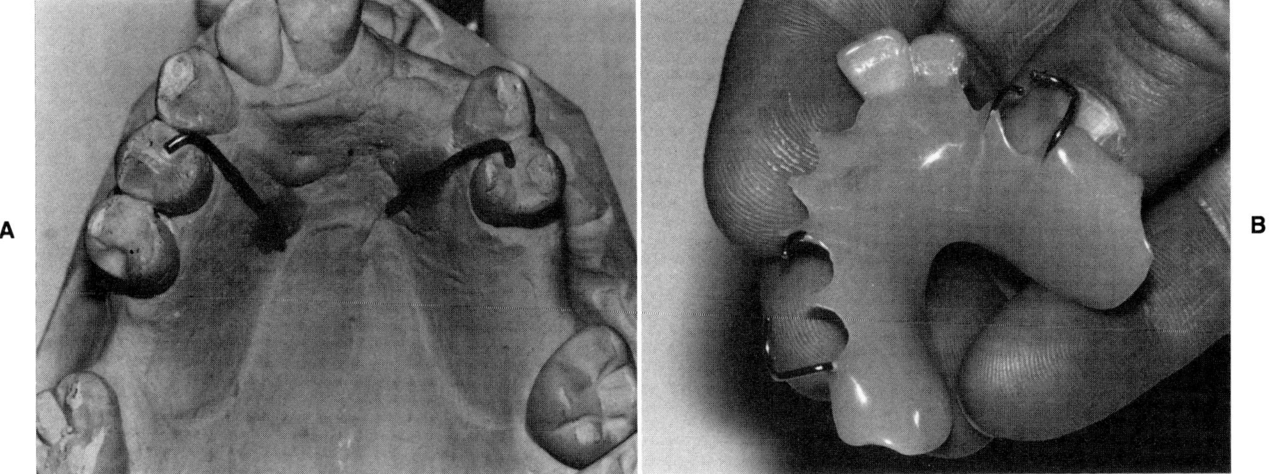

Fig. 18-21. A, Occlusal rests can be incorporated in interim prostheses. Wrought wire is adapted to nonfunctioning fossae. **B,** Occlusal rests are incorporated in denture base for support.

resistance to vertical displacement of the prosthesis during function to protect the gingival tissue and alveolar bone from excessive trauma.

When all necessary occlusal corrections have been accomplished, the patient must be thoroughly counseled in the care of the temporary partial denture and the remaining teeth and soft tissue. The prosthesis must never be worn continuously. Ideally the denture should not be worn during sleep. This is the best time to allow the soft tissues to recover the normal architecture of healthy tissues. If the patient insists on wearing the prosthesis at night, and frequently a woman will refuse to allow her husband to see her with missing anterior teeth, then for at least several hours during the day, when she is alone, she must do without the denture to allow the soft tissue to recover.

The care and cleaning of the denture will be the same as for the conventional partial denture appointment (described in Chapter 16). If no metal has been used in the construction of the denture, a chlorine-containing solution may be used safely for soaking or cleaning the denture.

The use of disclosing tablets with the partial denture in the mouth should be demonstrated to the patient. This will reveal areas of the partial denture that will require special consideration in the cleaning procedure.

Before the patient is dismissed, a program for instituting definitive care should be established. To avoid possible legal entanglements at a later date, the patient must be made to understand that the treatment rendered up to this point must be considered temporary. If a long period must elapse before permanent treat-

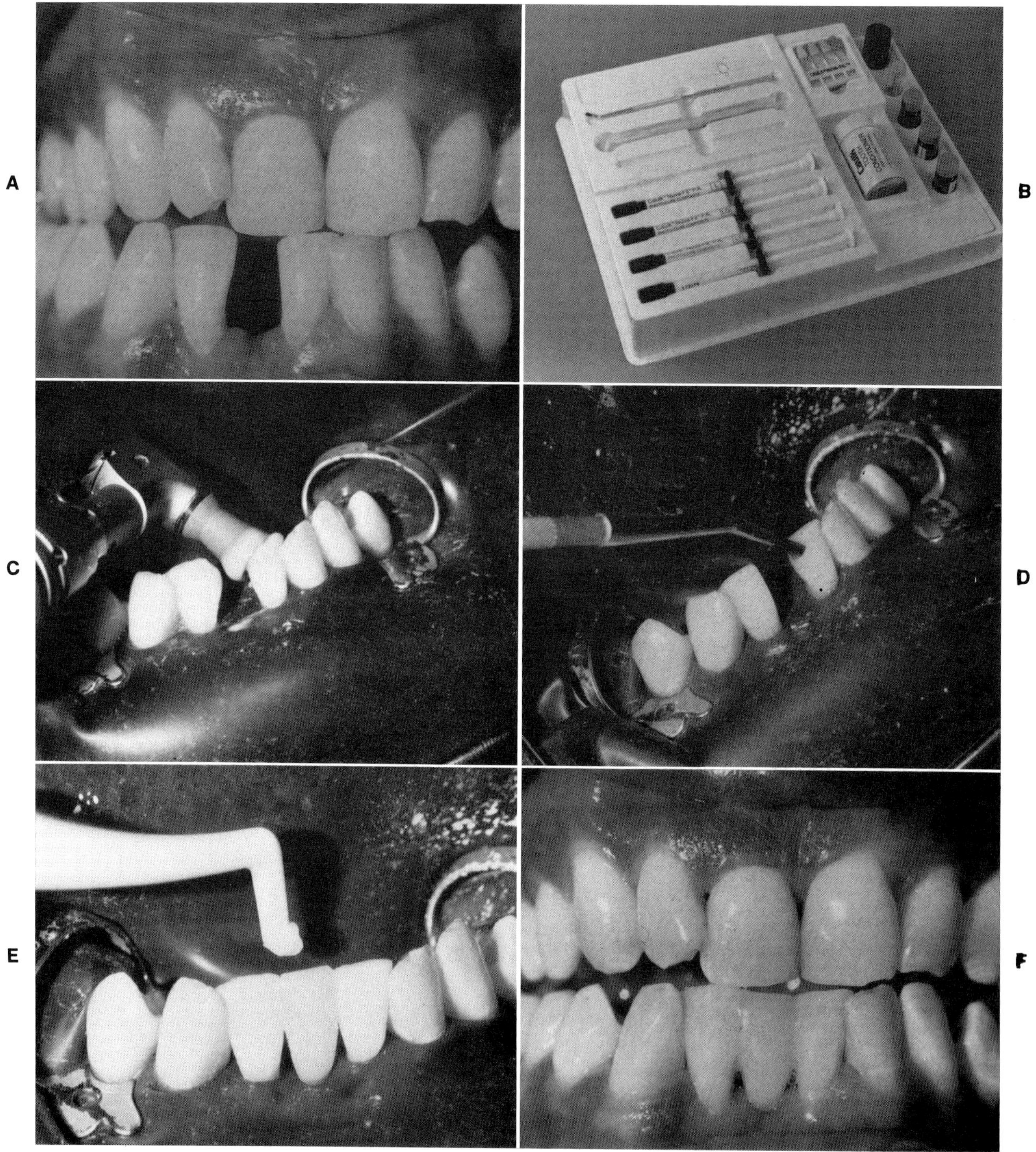

Fig. 18-22. A, Central incisor avulsed in young patient. **B,** Caulk Nuva-Fil acid etch kit (The L.D. Caulk Co., Milford, Del). **C,** Teeth isolated with rubber dam and cleaned with flour of pumice. **D,** Acid painted on proximal surfaces to etch enamel. **E,** Plastic pontic in place and photocure composite added to attach pontic to adjacent teeth. **F,** Completed restoration following cure of composite. (Courtesy Dr. Mervyn Yankelson, University of Texas Health Science Center at San Antonio.)

ment can be started, arrangements must be made for periodic examination and maintenance appointments. Insertion of a temporary partial denture should never be considered a termination to treatment.

Alternative treatment

In the past few years an alternative temporizing method has been developed. This technique consists of acid etching the enamel surfaces of the teeth adjacent to the edentulous space, usually with phosphoric acid, and attaching an acrylic resin denture tooth or a polycarboxylate crown form to these prepared surfaces with an acrylic or aromatic dimethacrylate cement (Fig. 18-22). If meticulous attention is paid to the preparation of the enamel surfaces of the natural teeth, this method of providing a temporary fixed partial denture can be used successfully over a long period. A number of excellent sources describe this technique in detail, so it is not covered in this text. The main problem encountered is the difficulty at times in obtaining a solid union between the enamel surface and the bonding or cementing material. The esthetic result obtained with this method is frequently not as pleasing as may be developed with a temporary removable partial denture. Problems may also be encountered in keeping the gingival tissue beneath the joint between the natural tooth and pontic in an acceptable state of health, particularly if a long treatment period is anticipated.

TRANSITIONAL PARTIAL DENTURES

Indications

The transitional denture is planned when some or all of the remaining teeth are beyond the point of restoration but immediate extractions are not indicated for physiologic or psychologic reasons (Fig. 18-23). The teeth will be removed over a long period of time, and the patient must be provided with a functional prosthesis during treatment.

For an elderly patient or a patient suffering from a chronic debilitating disease where multiple extractions could exacerbate the basic illness, this treatment plan can be used effectively. By removing the hopeless teeth as adverse symptoms arise, the patient may be spared a major crisis in the physical condition.

Another significant group of patients who may be served with this treatment concept are those who are psychologically unable to accept the loss of teeth. In the minds of many people the presence of teeth is related to sex appeal, youth, and happiness, whereas the loss of, or the absence of, teeth indicates the opposite—lack of appeal to the opposite sex, loss of youth, and gloom and despair. The dentist should not attempt to become an amateur psychologist in treating patients of this sort but should understand that the loss of a single tooth, especially the last one, can be a frightening emotional experience for some patients. The dentist, in the pretreatment plan interview, should attempt to gain some insight as to the value the patient places on the retention or the loss of teeth. If the patient is truly concerned over the loss of teeth but the loss is inevitable, the treatment should be carried out over as long a period as possible. During treatment the patient should be constantly reassured as to the success of treatment and prepared mentally to accept the unavoidable result. This type of problem can be lessened, if not removed entirely, if the dentist remembers at the initial patient interview, to "meet the mind of the patient before meeting the mouth" as De Van (1961) so aptly put it.

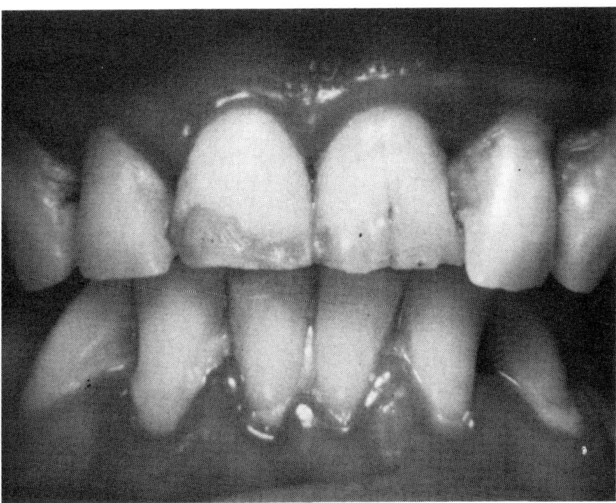

Fig. 18-23. When permanent restoration is not possible but immediate extraction is not indicated, transitional partial denture is indicated.

Clinical procedures

The clinical procedures for this and all temporary partial dentures remain basically the same, requiring accurate, well-extended irreversible hydrocolloid impressions poured with a dense Hydrocal to form an accurate cast. Jaw relation records will most often be required to mount the casts in a semiadjustable articulator in order to set the artificial teeth correctly (Fig. 18-24).

If the transitional denture is not to be an immediate partial denture (see the discussion of immediate temporary dentures at the end of this chapter), the construction of the denture will be the same as that for the interim partial denture. The denture base will normally be constructed of acrylic resin. If the denture is to serve for a long time, cast chrome metal may be used. When cast metal is planned, special design considerations must be used so that as additional teeth are lost

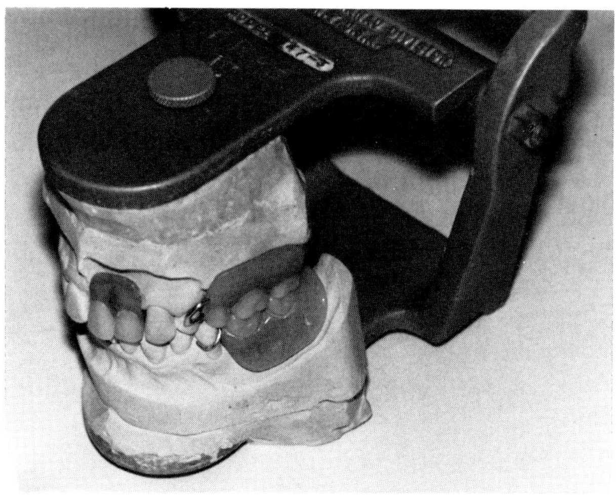

Fig. 18-24. Master casts for transitional partial dentures are mounted on articulator, and denture teeth are set.

the teeth can be added easily and economically to the metal framework. The design to be used most often to satisfy this requirement is to lingual plate, with the cast metal, the teeth that are most apt to be lost (Fig. 18-25). As the teeth are extracted, metal retention loops can be soldered to the lingual plating and artificial teeth processed to the retention loops. With this form of treatment the patient will never truly be without teeth.

This concept of partial denture design should be followed whenever a design is made for a patient who has remaining teeth with a guarded or limited prognosis. The design should be such that teeth may be added to the original framework, preventing the necessity of remaking the partial denture merely for the loss of a single or several teeth. Teeth that most often have to be given special consideration are the mandibular anterior teeth. Loss of bone supporting these teeth can be advanced, yet the decision to retain the teeth for as long

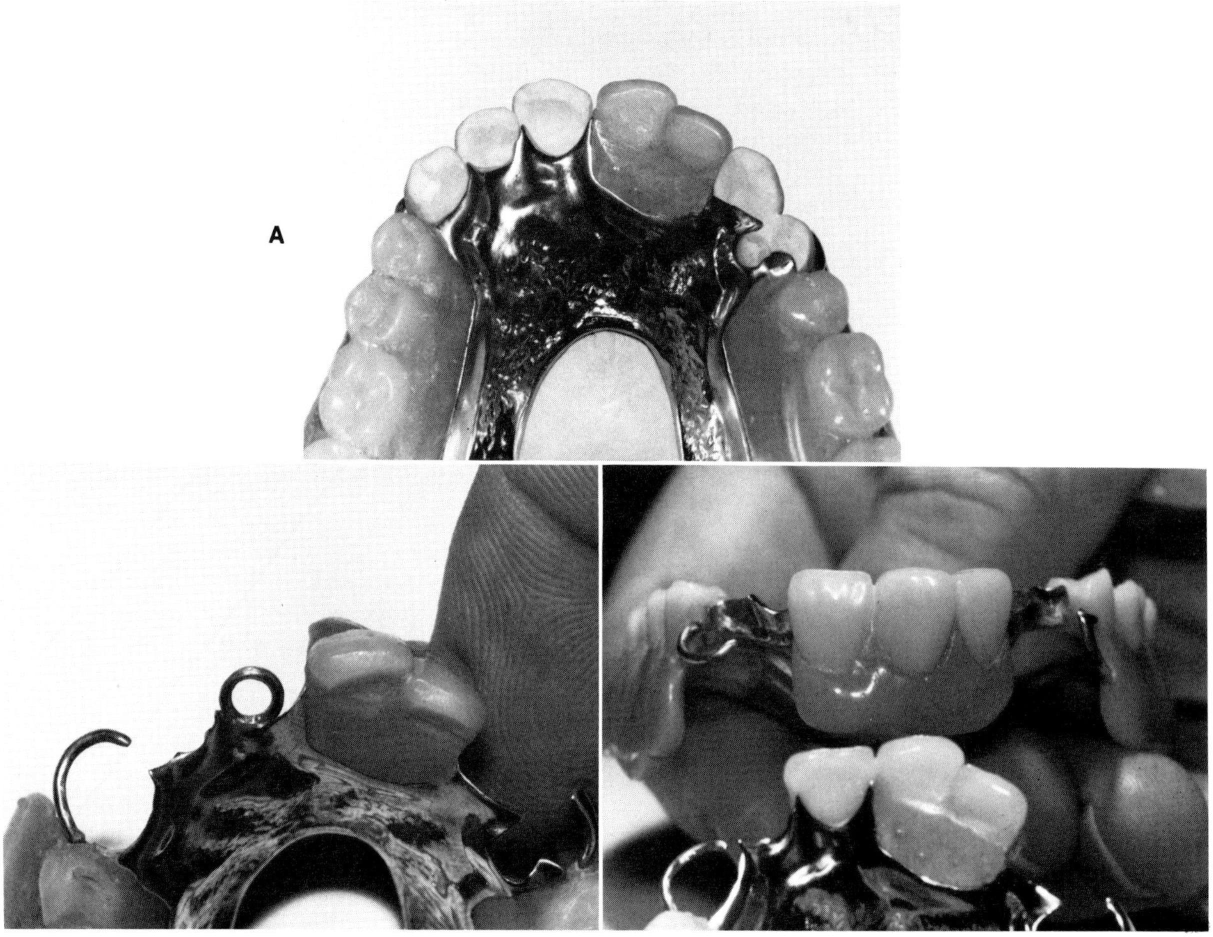

Fig. 18-25. **A,** Right central incisor is to be extracted and added to transitional partial denture. **B,** Metal retentive loop to hold new tooth is soldered to lingual plate. **C,** Mirror view shows adaptation to lingual plate and addition of labial flange.

as possible can dictate that the definitive partial denture be designed so that these anterior teeth can be added to it as required. In this case, if the mandibular major connector is designed as lingual plating of the anterior teeth, additions of artificial teeth can be made relatively easily. As mentioned previously, retention loops of wrought metal can be added to the inner surface of the lingual plating by a soldering procedure. To these retention loops can be processed, usually by tooth-colored autopolymerizing resin, denture teeth to replace the teeth that are lost. A simpler method of adding these teeth, but one that is not as reliable, is to drill holes through the lingual plating and allow these holes to serve as points of retention for the added teeth. This technique obviously will not provide the strength that soldered metal retention loops will provide.

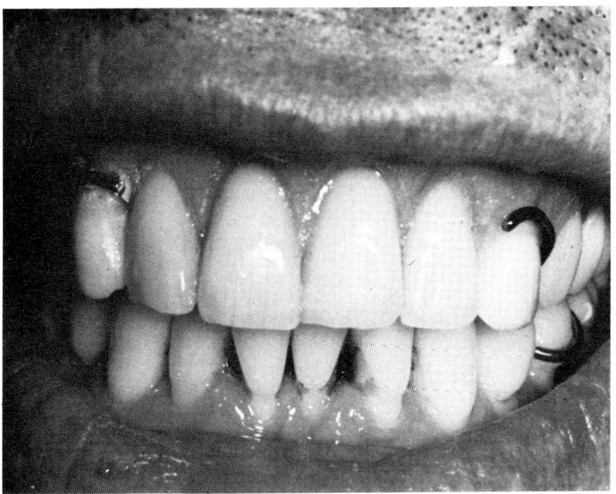

Fig. 18-26. Maxillary transitional partial denture that has been converted to temporary complete denture. Clasps have been left on denture to retain natural appearance.

The transitional partial denture concept of treatment can be used with a preexisting partial denture, provided the design is such that teeth can be added safely and conveniently. In this case the transition will usually be from the partially edentulous state to the completely edentulous condition (Fig. 18-26).

If the design of the existing partial denture is such that teeth may be added to it, the clinical procedures to add teeth to the denture are as follows. The removable partial denture is seated in the mouth. With a slightly oversized impression tray, an alginate impression is made over the denture (Fig. 18-27). In a majority of cases the partial denture will remain in the impression as it is removed from the mouth. This is desired, but close inspection must be made to be certain that the position of the denture in the impression is correct. In the event the denture does not remain in the impression as it is removed from the mouth, the denture must be repositioned in the impression. To facilitate the denture staying in the pickup impression, retentive clasps may be adjusted to reduce the amount of retention before the impression is made.

Before the working cast is poured, any area of undercut in the denture bases must be blocked out. As teeth are added to the partial denture, it will be necessary to remove it from the cast. The blockout may be accomplished with baseplate wax, modeling clay, or wet paper toweling.

After the cast is poured in a hard densite stone, the partial denture is recovered from the cast. The teeth on the cast that are to be extracted and replaced are cut

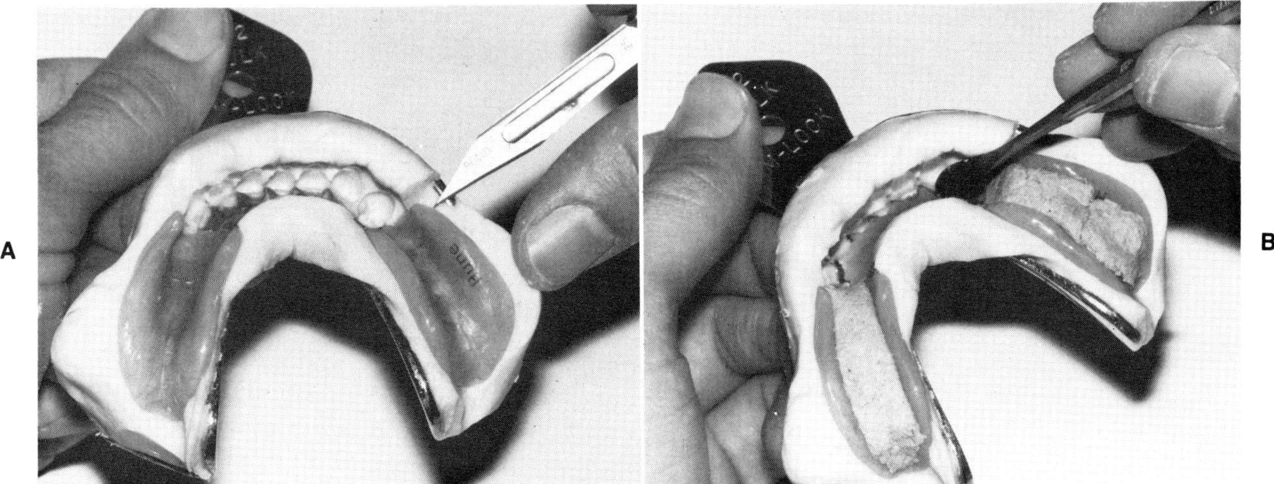

Fig. 18-27. A, Transitional denture to which teeth will be added is "picked-up" in alginate impression. **B,** Undercuts in denture base are blocked out, and thin film of wax is flowed on tissue side of lingual plate.

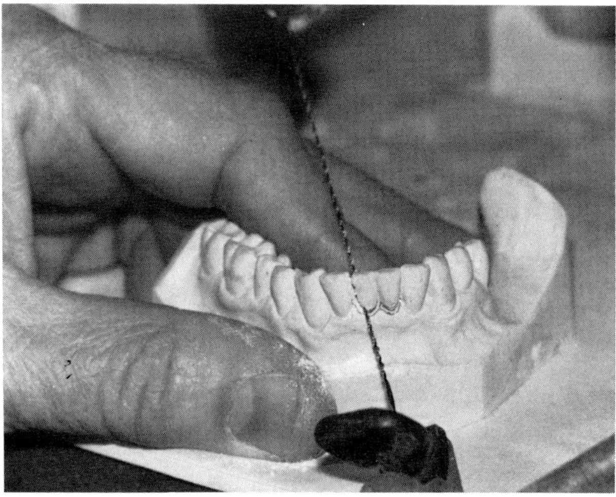

Fig. 18-28. Teeth that are to be extracted and replaced are cut from cast.

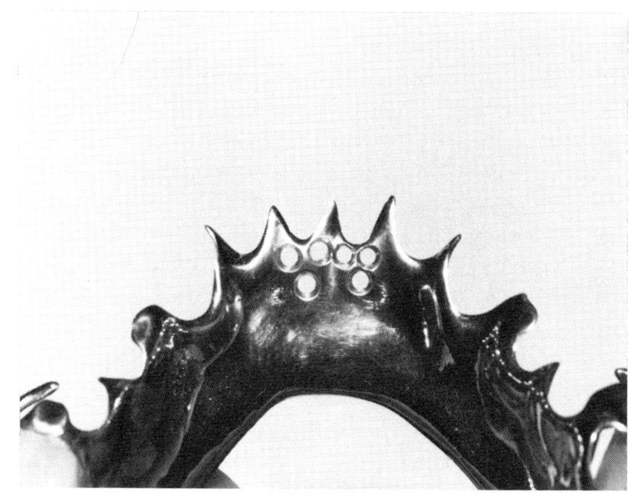

Fig. 18-29. Holes are cut in lingual plate to retain denture teeth.

A

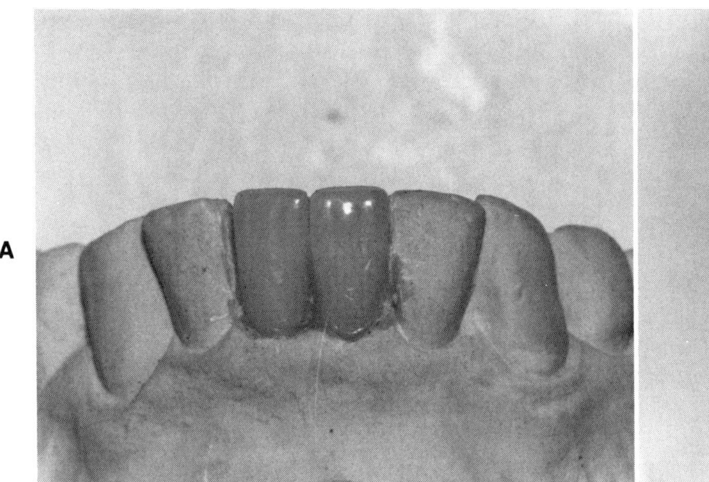

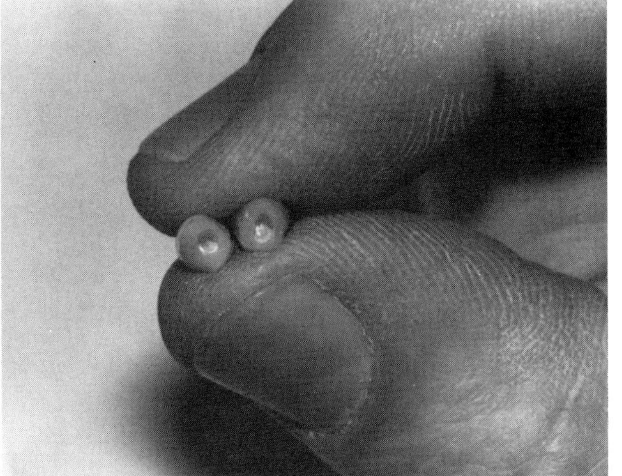

B

Fig. 18-30. A, Necks of denture teeth are contoured to butt against edentulous ridge. **B,** Diatorics, or retention holes, are cut in denture teeth for attachment to acrylic resin denture base.

from the cast. The initial cut should be even with the surrounding gingival tissue (Fig. 18-28). The tooth socket on the cast should be prepared as a slight concavity with the center 2 mm deeper than the perimeter. If an anterior tooth is being replaced, the labial surface of the socket should be scraped lightly.

Some method of retention for the teeth to be added must be developed on the framework. The retention may be in the form of wire loops soldered to lingual plating or perforations through the plating. The denture teeth can be attached to these retention areas with autopolymerizing acrylic resin (Fig. 18-29).

With the partial denture seated on the cast, denture teeth are ground to fit the trimmed cast. If a denture flange is not present or planned, the necks of the teeth should be butted to the ridge. This is the reason the labial surface of the tooth socket should be scraped lightly on the cast before the denture tooth is contoured to fit the ridge (Fig. 18-30). The light pressure of the tooth against the soft tissue in the mouth will give a more normal appearance.

Small diatorics (holes for retention) should be drilled into the ridge lap area of the tooth to provide a more positive retention between the tooth and the acrylic resin that will be used to retain the tooth.

After the teeth have been added to the partial denture, the patient is prepared for the extractions. Following the surgery, pressure-indicating paste is painted

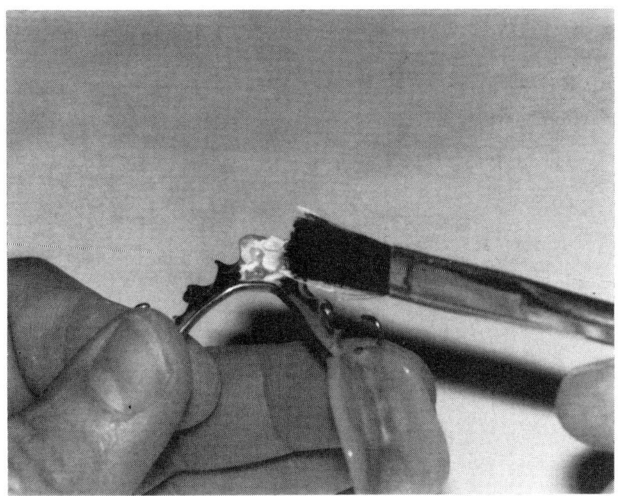

Fig. 18-31. Pressure-indicating paste is used at insertion appointment to locate areas of excess pressure.

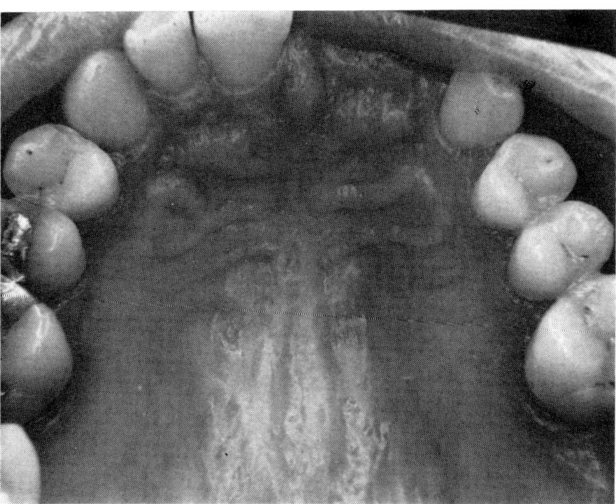

Fig. 18-32. Marginal gingivitis caused by prolonged wearing of partial denture and poor oral hygiene.

on the tissue surface (Fig. 18-31), the denture is seated in the mouth, and areas of excessive pressure (where the pressure-indicating paste is displaced) are relieved with acrylic resin burs or stones.

These patients should routinely be seen in 24 hours as a follow-up to both the surgical procedure and the insertion of the transitional partial denture. This early recall will prevent major discomfort.

Patients receiving transitional partial denture service should normally be placed on a routine recall system (at intervals not greater than 3 months) so that the questionable remaining teeth can be monitored closely. The usual cause for the inevitable loss of teeth is advanced periodontal disease. Deep periodontal pockets will frequently be present, and acute exacerbation in the form of periodontal abscesses may be expected if adequate home and office care is not practiced.

TREATMENT PARTIAL DENTURES

Indications

The treatment partial denture may be used (1) as a vehicle to carry tissue treatment material to abused oral tissues, (2) to increase or restore the vertical dimension of occlusion on a temporary basis while the results of the increase can be observed, (3) as a splint following surgical corrections in the oral cavity, and (4) as a night guard or mouth protective device to correct or control undesirable oral habits or to protect the mouth and teeth from trauma.

Vehicle for tissue treatment material

Soft tissue on which a removable prosthesis, either complete or partial, rests is subject to the normal response of soft tissue anywhere in the body. If the prosthesis causes excess force against the soft tissue, an adverse soft tissue reaction may take place. This is especially true if poor oral hygiene is also present. The reaction can be in the form of simple erythema, or reddening, of the tissue, which may be controlled by adjusting or relining the denture. The reaction may also be more severe in progressive degrees.

One of the most potentially dangerous soft tissue reactions is marginal gingivitis of the gingival crevicular tissue (Fig. 18-32). Prolonged marginal gingivitis can lead to chronic periodontal disease if enough time and contributing factors such as plaque accummulation are also present. This condition is commonly seen if temporary partial dentures are used for too long without adequate recall examination and professional hygiene care.

Soft tissue, particularly gingival tissue, will respond in one of two ways if subjected to chronic irritation. Hyperplasia may occur with abnormal enlargement of the tissue as a result, or the tissue may recede from the factor that is causing the irritation (Fig. 18-33 and 18-34). In either event the source of irritation must be identified and corrected before the result of the irritation becomes irreversible.

A frequent site of inflammatory hyperplasia is beneath the major connector of a maxillary partial denture (Fig. 18-35). The condition is referred to as papillary hyperplasia, or papillomatosis, and is most often seen in the palatal tissue beneath a complete denture. The acute infection and inflammation present in the hyperplastic tissue can be controlled by the local application of a tissue treatment material lining the existing prosthesis, but the condition is not truly reversible. Surgical intervention of stripping the palatal tissue with scalpel

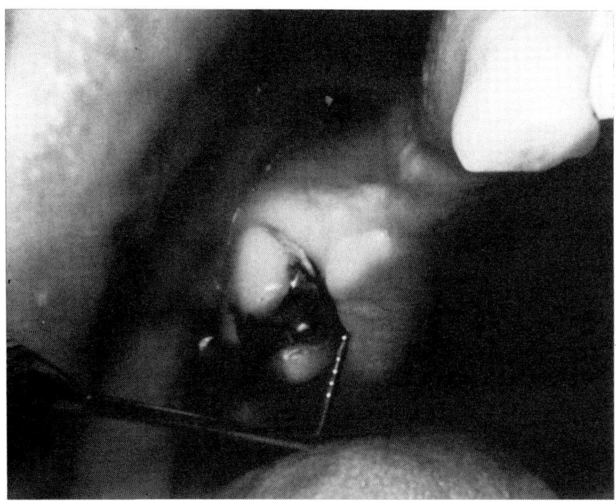

Fig. 18-33. Gingival hyperplasia caused by chronic irritation of poorly fitting removable partial denture.

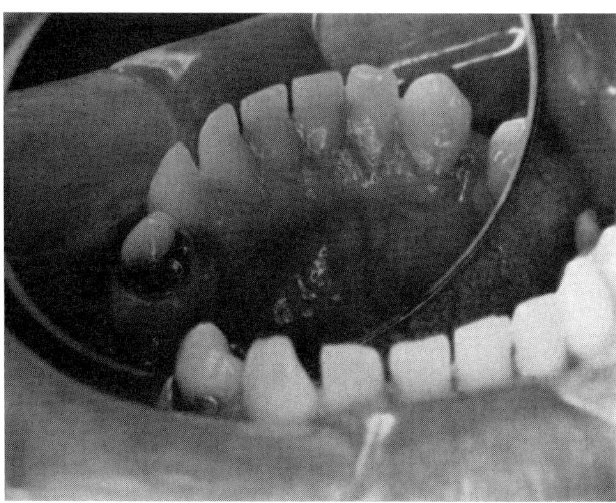

Fig. 18-34. Gingival recession lingual to anterior teeth caused by chronic irritation from partial denture.

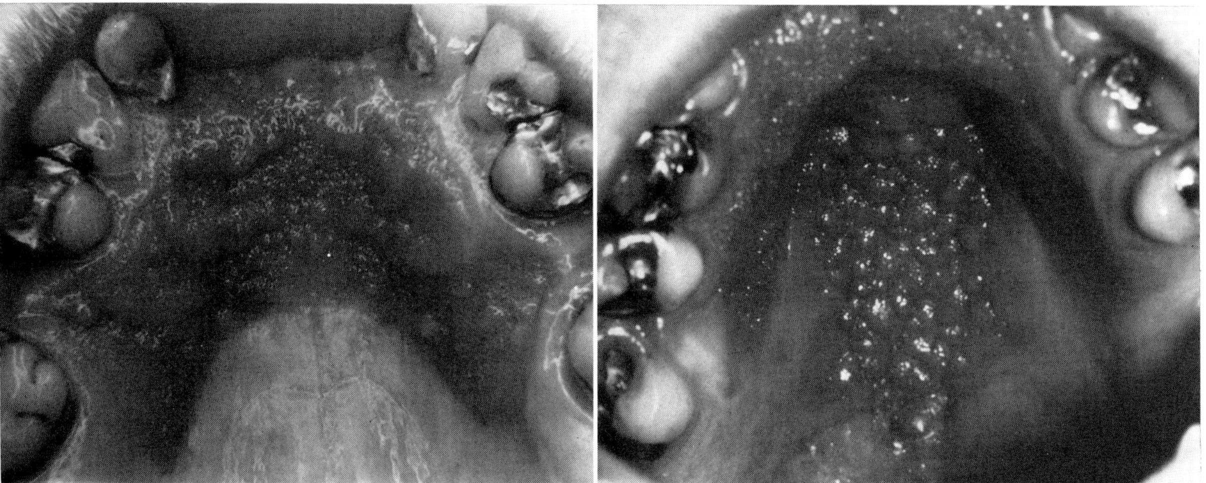

Fig. 18-35. Papillary hyperplasia, or papillomatosis of palate. Condition is seen under poorly fitting major connectors accompanied by poor oral hygiene.

or with rotating instruments is usually required (Fig. 18-36). The technique can be found in oral surgery texts.

Two common factors can almost always be found associated with an hyperplastic tissue response: (1) the patient has been wearing the prosthesis continuously, not giving the tissues a chance to recover, and (2) oral hygiene habits, including cleansing of the prosthesis, are poor if not altogether absent. Examination of the prosthesis and the mouth and questioning the patient will confirm the presence of these two factors in practically all instances, especially papillary hyperplasia.

Another abnormal tissue response that may indicate treatment partial dentures is an epulis fissuratum, a hyperplastic tissue response to an overextended periphery of a denture base (Fig. 18-37). The overextension of the denture base is not so great as to produce pain of sufficient magnitude to cause the patient to seek help but is enough to cause a proliferation of the border tissues. Simple shortening or adjusting the length of the denture base flange may, if the proliferation is not severe, result in a slow dissolution of the hyperplastic tissue. Usually, however, treatment of the area with tissue treatment material supported by a treatment partial denture will be needed to reverse the process. This treatment may be required over a period of several weeks. If the response of the tissue is not complete following use of the material, surgery may have to be re-

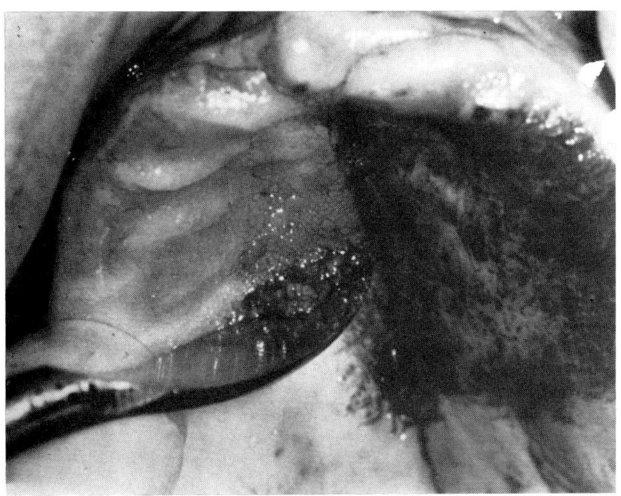

Fig. 18-36. Complete elimination of papillary hyperplasia must be accomplished surgically.

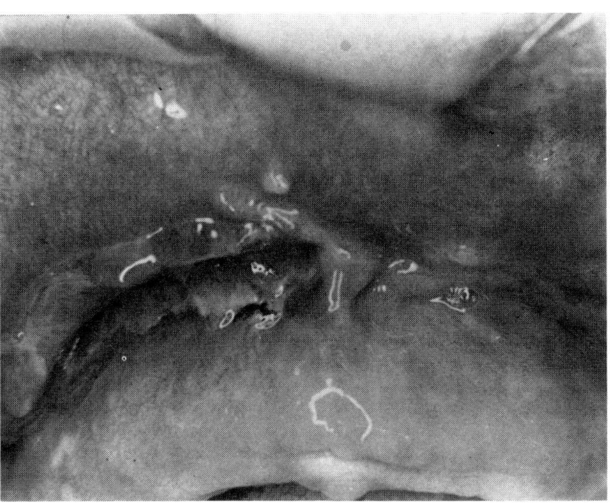

Fig. 18-37. An epulis fissuratum caused by irritation from overextended denture flange.

sorted to. As a rule, surgery should be avoided in these border tissues if possible because some degree of scar tissue formation will occur, thus complicating the problem of using the reflecting tissue to develop a border seal for the denture.

Tissue treatment material

Tissue treatment material is also referred to as tissue conditioner. It is a soft material that is applied temporarily to the tissue surface of a partial denture, either specially constructed for the purpose of supporting the material or to an already existing prosthesis that the patient is functioning with, in order to allow a more equal distribution of forces occurring against the denture and to permit the soft tissues to return to the normal architecture.

The material is nonirritating and nontoxic. It is soft elastic, so it does not undergo substantial permanent deformation. The softness and elasticity of most tissue conditioners last approximately 1 week, after which the material begins to harden and can itself become an irritant. To be effective in treating abused oral tissue, the conditioner must be changed every 4 or 5 days. It is to be hoped that materials with longer periods of clinical effectiveness will be introduced.

The tissue conditioner is usually supplied as a powder and a liquid (Fig. 18-38). The powder is acrylic polymer, usually ethyl methacrylate, and the liquid is usually a mixture of ethyl alcohol and an aromatic ester. The two combine to form a gel. The setting is a physical process; no chemical reaction is involved.

The mechanism of action of the material is a combination of distributing forces more evenly, obtaining more intimate soft tissue contact, and the physical act of massaging the tissue as the soft material compresses and relaxes during function. Through this action blood flow through the abused tissues is increased and edema and other by-products of the inflammatory process are removed at a faster rate.

Clinical procedures

If a new temporary partial denture is to be constructed solely to serve as a vehicle for the tissue conditioning material, the clinical procedures will be exactly the same as for constructing an interim or transitional partial denture. The laboratory procedures will vary slightly.

If an existing and serviceable prosthesis is available and if some relief space can be created or obtained on the tissue surface of the denture adjacent to the abused tissue, the prosthesis can be used as the vehicle to support the tissue treatment material. If the tissue surface of the partial denture is metallic, more difficulty will be encountered in using it as the vehicle since adequate relief cannot be obtained between the abused tissue and the metal and sufficient thickness of tissue conditioner must be present in order to be effective.

Laboratory procedures

After the casts have been mounted on an articulator and before any other laboratory procedures for the construction of the treatment partial denture are started, one thickness of baseplate wax is adapted to the cast over the area or areas of abused tissue (Fig. 18-39). This layer of wax will provide a space for the tissue treatment material that will be added after the partial denture is complete and the wax spacer removed.

The treatment partial denture can now be con-

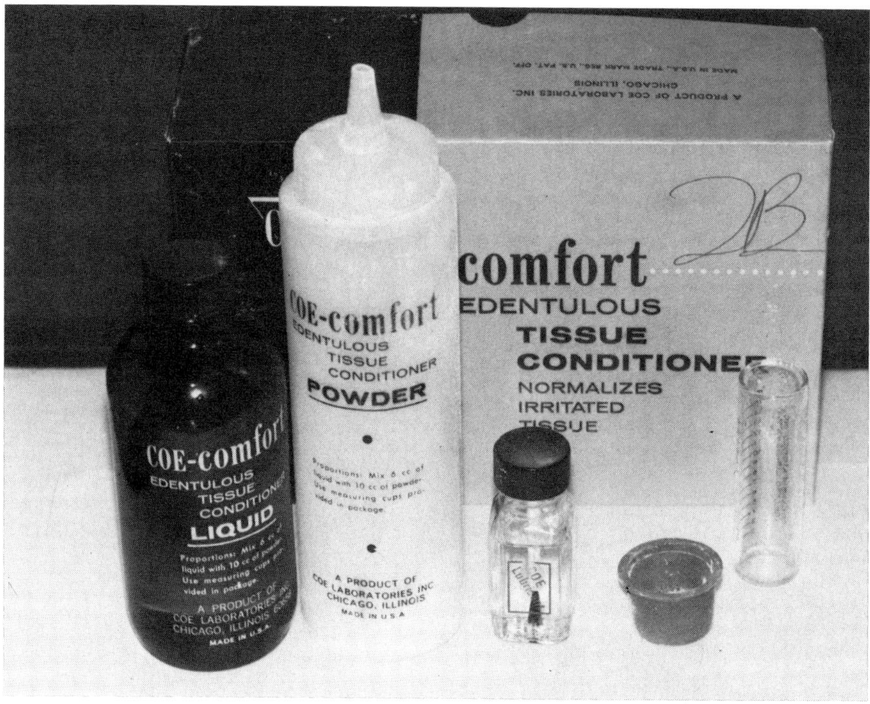

Fig. 18-38. Tissue-conditioning material is soft elastic plastic used to treat abused soft tissue.

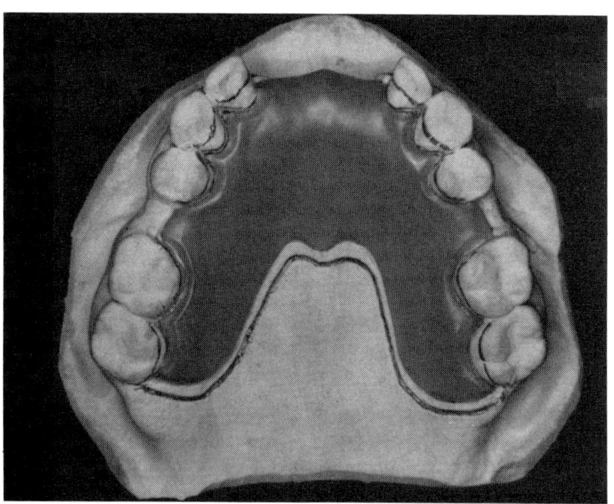

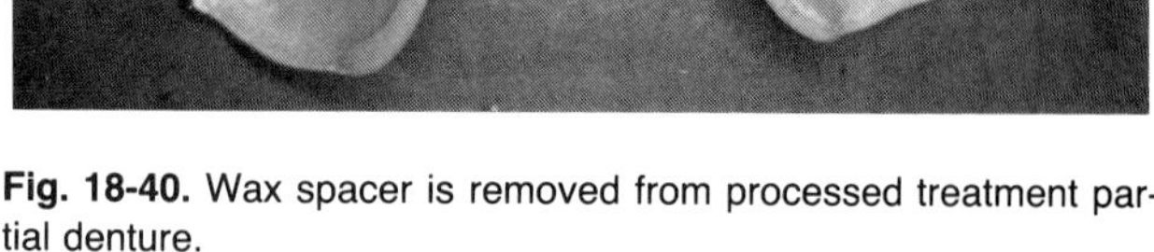

Fig. 18-39. Single layer of baseplate wax is adapted to cast over area of abused tissue. Wax acts as spacer for tissue-conditioning material.

Fig. 18-40. Wax spacer is removed from processed treatment partial denture.

structed following the same technique used for the interim partial denture.

The wax spacer is removed from the processed denture (Fig. 18-40), and the denture is finished and polished. The external surface of all temporary partial dentures must be brought to a high polish to prevent plaque and other debris from collecting on the surface.

Using the tissue conditioner

The treatment partial denture should be fitted to the mouth the same as any other temporary partial denture using pressure-indicating paste. The occlusion must be checked and refined following normal procedures. Then the tissue conditioner is applied as shown in Fig. 18-41.

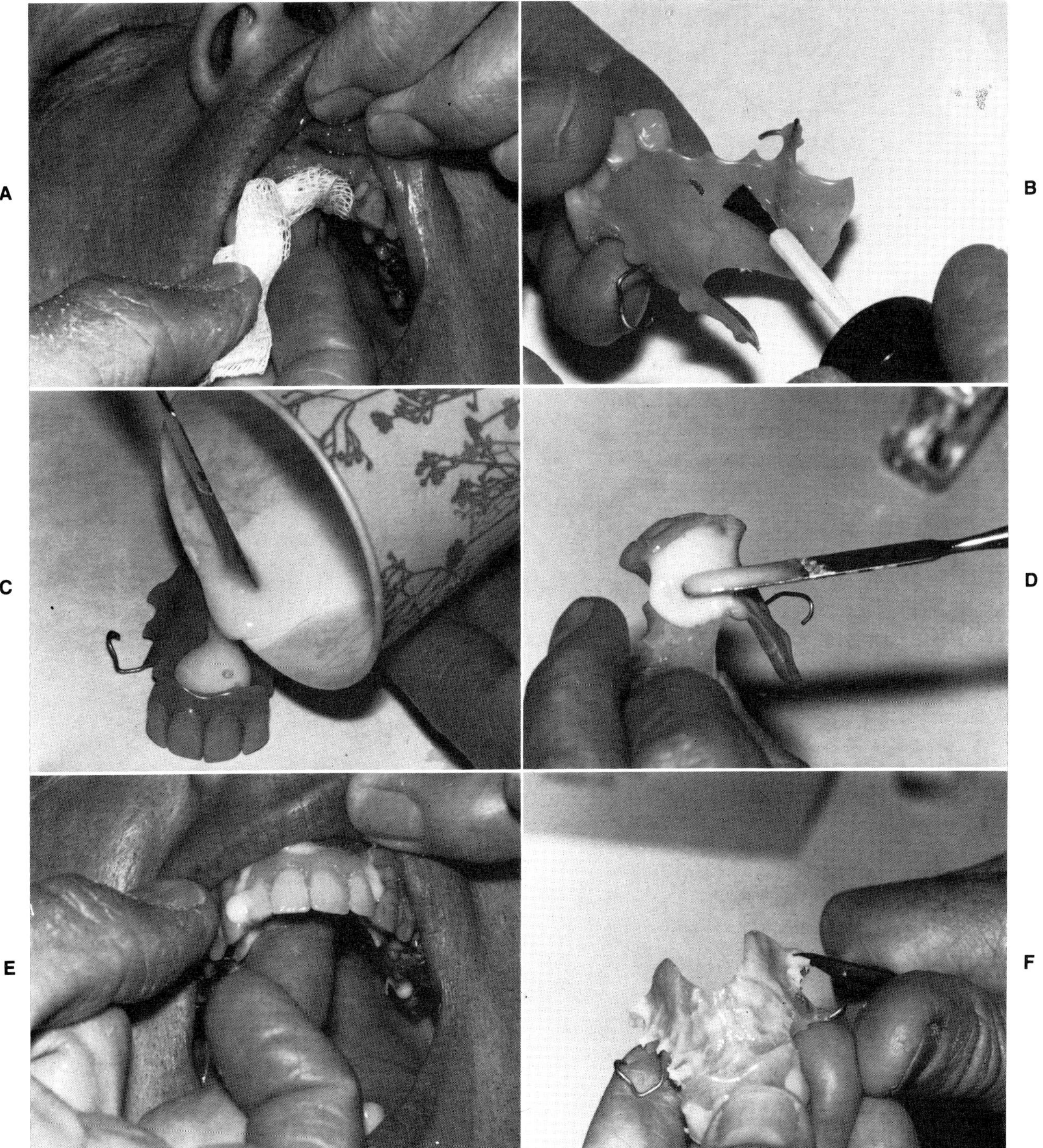

Fig. 18-41. A, Area of abused tissue is dried with gauze sponge, and arch is partially isolated with sponges. **B,** External surface of treatment denture is painted with separator. **C,** Tissue conditioner is mixed in disposable cup according to manufacturer's directions to consistency of heavy cream and flowed onto denture. **D,** Material is distributed evenly over surface of denture with cement spatula. Working time varies depending on manufacturer, but 1 minute is average. **E,** Denture is seated firmly in mouth. **F,** Excess material is trimmed with sharp blade.

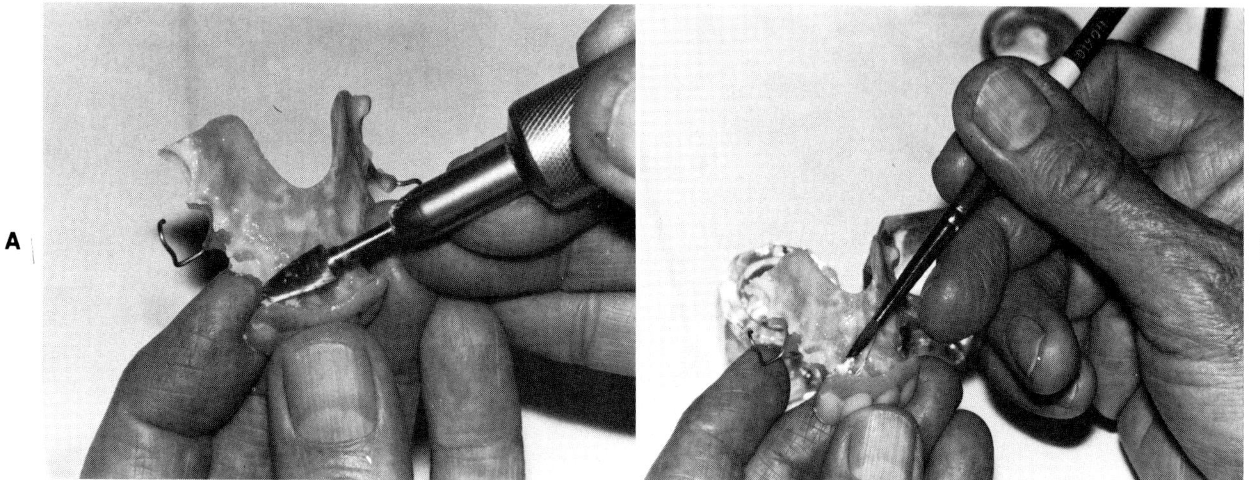

Fig. 18-42. A, Showthrough areas of hard denture base are removed with burs. **B,** New tissue conditioner is added to relieved areas.

The treatment partial denture with the tissue conditioning material in place is seated in the mouth under light pressure. The pressure should be maintained as the material flows. Border tissues should be manipulated to border mold the material. For a mandibular removable partial denture the tongue should be brought forward and into each cheek to define the lingual extension accurately. If posterior artificial teeth are present, the patient must close the teeth together while the material is still capable of flowing to align the artificial teeth properly with the opposing occlusion. Once the denture has been seated and aligned correctly, the patient should remain quiet for 4 to 5 minutes until the gel stage of the material has been reached. At that time the denture should be removed from the mouth and examined for completeness. If voids or bubbles are present, additions to the tissue conditioner may be made by the paint brush technique. The tip of a fine camel's hair brush is dipped in the liquid and touched to the powder. A small ball of material will collect on the brush tip and is transferred to the void area or to other defects.

If the denture base is exposed through the treatment material, these areas should be relieved and new material added (Fig. 18-42). The best way to relieve the denture base is by coating the surface of the treatment material with liquid soap and cutting away the exposed portion of the acrylic resin denture base with vulcanite burs. The liquid soap prevents the fragments of denture base that is being relieved from attaching to the surface of the conditioning material. The soap and grindings are washed from the denture, and additional material added by the brush technique. The denture must be reseated in the mouth while the material is still capable of flowing.

Before excess treatment material is trimmed away, the denture should be held under cool running water. Cooling the surface of the tissue conditioning material will make it easier to trim. Immediately after reaching the gel state the material is very sticky. The best method of trimming or removing excess treatment material is with a scalpel blade. The material should be trimmed to avoid leaving rough or irregular peripheral borders. There is no way to smooth or finish the margins except with a sharp knife or scissors.

The patient should be counselled in the home care of the treatment partial denture. The tissue conditioner should not be allowed to dry. For those short periods of time the denture is not in the mouth it must be submerged in water or cleansing solution. The partial denture should be worn full time except for cleaning after each meal.

Cleaning is best accomplished by holding the denture under cool running tap water or by brushing it gently with a soft brush.

Changing the vertical dimension of occlusion with treatment partial dentures

Altering a patient's existing vertical dimension of occlusion is discussed in Chapters 10 and 14. The reason for changing the vertical dimension will not be repeated. The warning, however, not to alter the vertical dimension without positive diagnostic findings will be repeated, along with the caution not to make changes in the vertical dimension of occlusion with permanent restorations until the patient has been subjected to a correction of the vertical dimension with temporary appliances for an extended period of time and has responded favorably.

When the vertical dimension of occlusion is altered

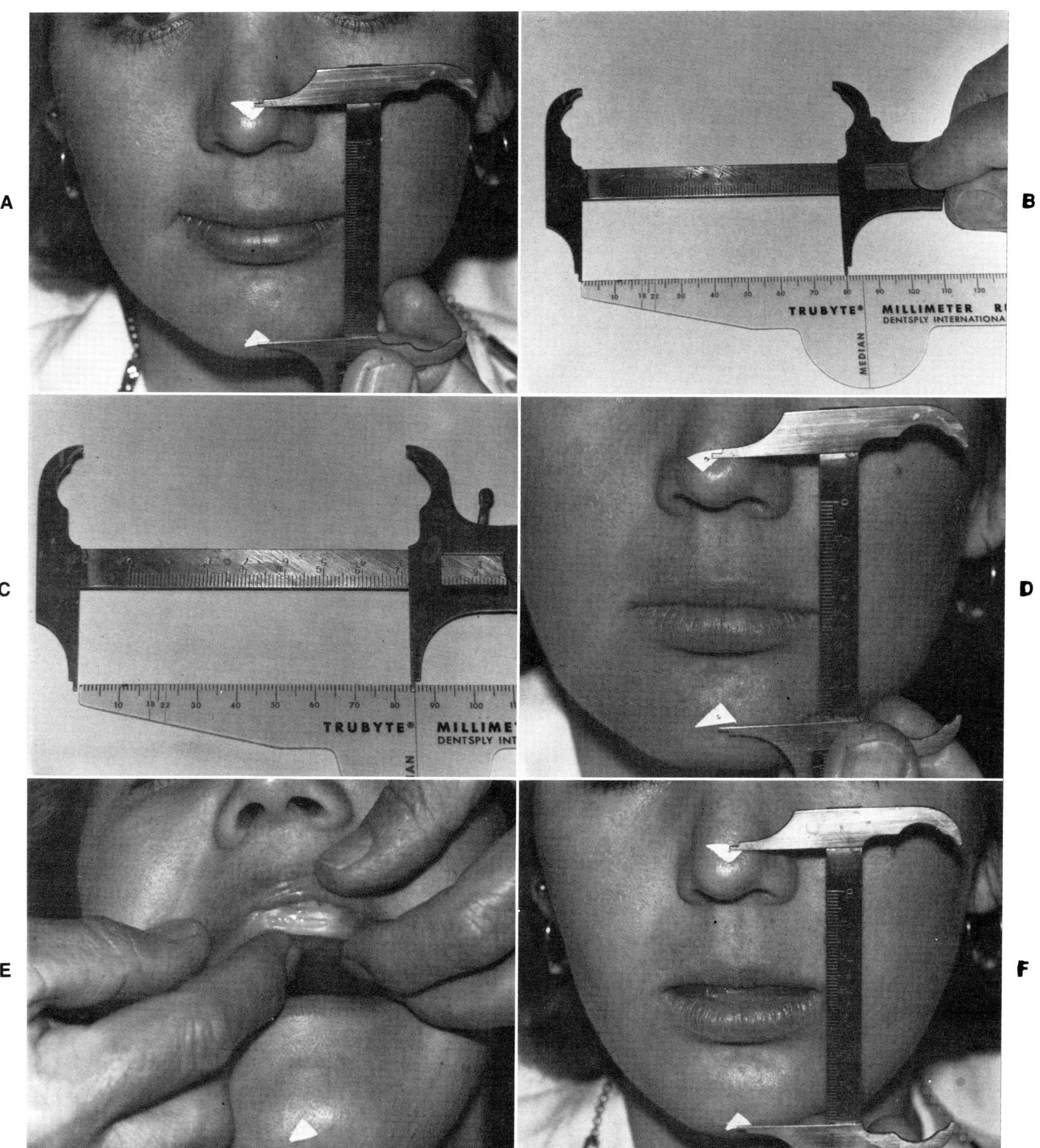

Fig. 18-43. A, Vertical dimension of occlusion is measured with teeth in contact. **B,** and **C,** Calipers are opened to proposed increased vertical dimension of occlusion. **D,** Increase in vertical dimension of occlusion is demonstrated by points on face. **E,** Several layers of baseplate wax are softened in 60° C (140° F) water bath and adapted over maxillary teeth. If patient is wearing removable partial denture, wax is adapted over prosthesis as well as natural teeth. Mandible is guided to terminal closure. **F,** Excess wax is removed after each trial closure. Wax is softened and trial closures repeated until all mandibular teeth contact record simultaneously at desired vertical dimension.

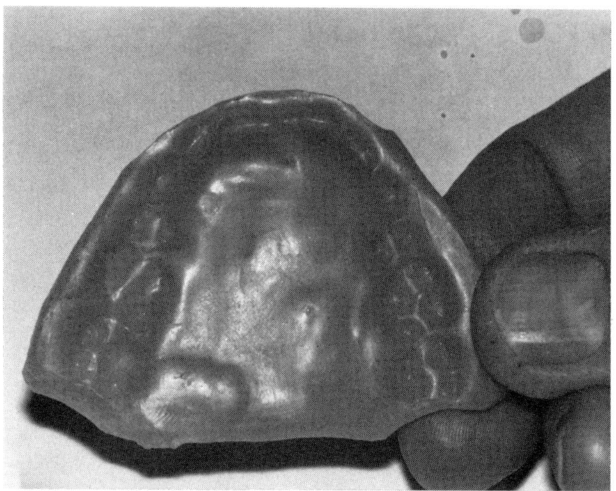

Fig. 18-44. Completed centric occlusion jaw relation record at new vertical dimension of occlusion.

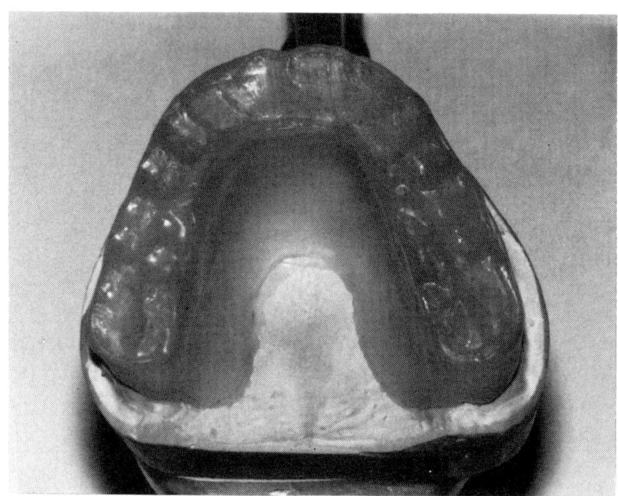

Fig. 18-45. Generated wax pathway is sealed to cast before processing. Excursions of mandibular teeth can be read in surface of wax.

with temporary appliances, all remaining teeth in both arches must be maintained in function against the appliance. The device is normally constructed to be worn over the maxillary teeth for convenience and to permit more freedom of tongue movement. All remaining mandibular teeth must contact the occluding surface of the prosthesis in centric relation and, if possible, in centric occlusion. This will prevent overeruption of teeth in the opposing arch that are not maintained in function. Covering all teeth in the supporting or maxillary arch will prevent individual teeth or small groups of teeth from being submerged because of extended overloading.

Clinical procedures

The maxillary cast for the patient whose vertical dimension of occlusion is to be increased temporarily is mounted on a semiadjustable articulator by using a face-bow transfer.

A centric jaw relation record is made at the proposed new vertical dimension of occlusion to mount the mandibular cast. (Figs. 18-43 and 18-44).

The lower teeth should contact the record in eccentric positions as well as in centric relation. To achieve this, the patient may be guided to produce a functionally generated path in the surface of the wax. This is accomplished by retruding the mandible to centric relation and guiding the patient with finger pressure to right and left lateral movements and straight protrusive excursions. The patient should start each movement at the centric relation position and terminate at the end of each excursive slide. The mouth should be opened at the end of the slide. Movement back to the centric relation position should not be attempted.

When the functionally generated path is complete, the wax pattern is removed from the teeth, taking care not to distort it. The wax pattern is seated on the maxillary cast, and the remainder of the appliance is waxed. The palatal extension should be in the form of a horseshoe major connector. The margins should be lightly beaded. The buccal or facial extension of the appliance should include the occlusal or incisal one third of the crowns of the teeth (Fig. 18-45). Retention for the appliance is provided by the close adaptation to the crowns of the teeth: clasps are rarely needed.

The functionally generated path technique will produce an accurate record, but it is difficult to maintain the desired degree of jaw opening. A technique that will produce an acceptable record may be accomplished more simply using a semiadjustable articulator.

The centric relation record at the increased vertical dimension of occlusion is accomplished on the patient as previously described. With this record the mandibular cast is mounted on the articulator.

The settings on the articulator are adjusted to the average readings. The horizontal condylar reading for the Hanau series articulators is set at 30 degrees, and the lateral condylar control is set at 15 degrees. The incisal guidance is set at 30 degrees also. See Chapter 14 for discussion of adjusting the Hanau articulator with a protrusive wax record. The wax eccentric record can now be generated on the articulator. The right and left lateral and protrusive pathways are repeated until the incisal guide pin remains in contact with the incisal guide

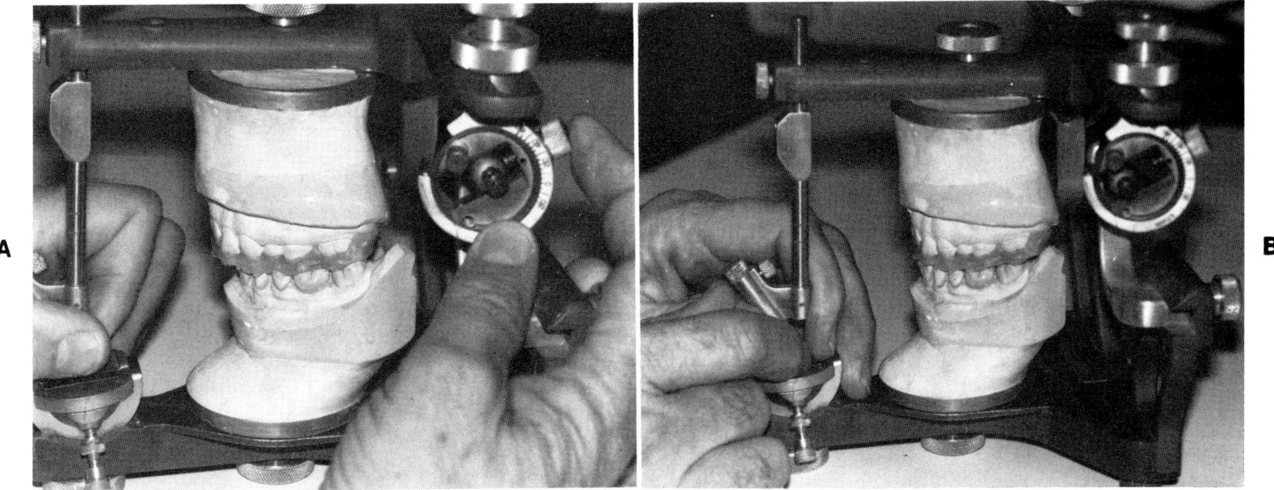

Fig. 18-46. A, Articulator is guided to right and left lateral excursions. **B,** Downward pressure on guide pin is maintained as articulator is moved into protrusive relationship.

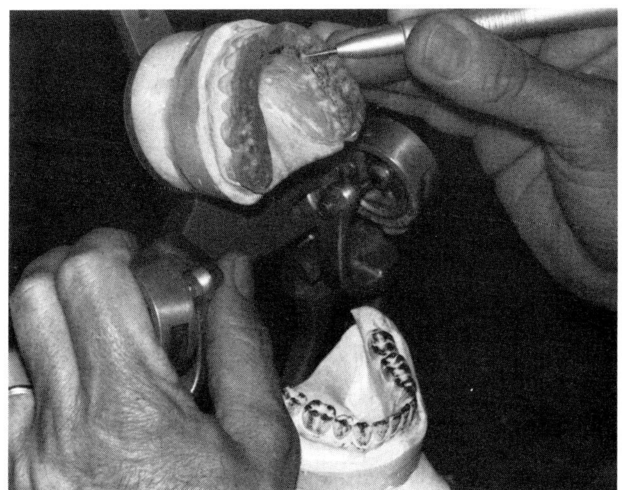

Fig. 18-47. Processing error is corrected on articulator before appliance is removed from cast.

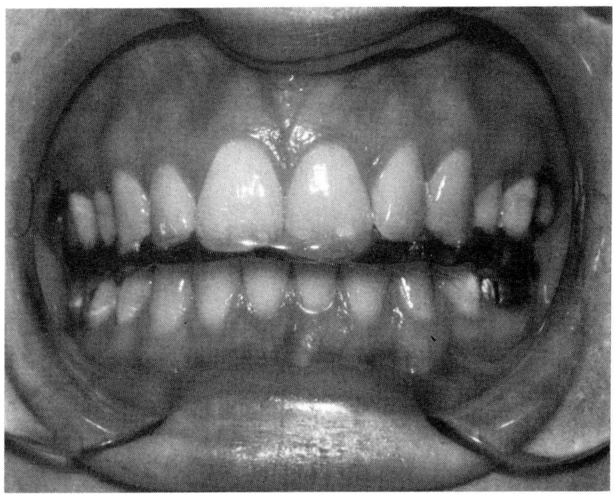

Fig. 18-48. Temporary appliance should be worn successfully for several months before permanent increase in vertical dimension of occlusion is attempted.

table throughout the excursions (Fig. 18-46). The presence of the guide pin ensures that the established vertical dimension of occlusion will not be altered.

Obviously the pathway generated by this technique will not be individualized for each patient. After the appliance is completed, it will be necessary to refine the occlusal contacts in the mouth. This can be accomplished using articulating ribbon or paper.

The completed wax pathway, still seated on the maxillary cast, is invested, packed, and processed (usually in clear acrylic resin). After processing, the cast is returned to the articulator to correct the processing error before the appliance is decast and polished (Fig. 18-47).

Patients receiving this type of treatment should be observed frequently following the insertion of the appliance. Construction of a permanent restoration at the new vertical dimension of occlusion should not be attempted until the patient has successfully worn the temporary appliance for at least several months (Fig. 18-48).

Surgical splints

The healing process of many surgical procedures performed in the oral cavity can be improved if the af-

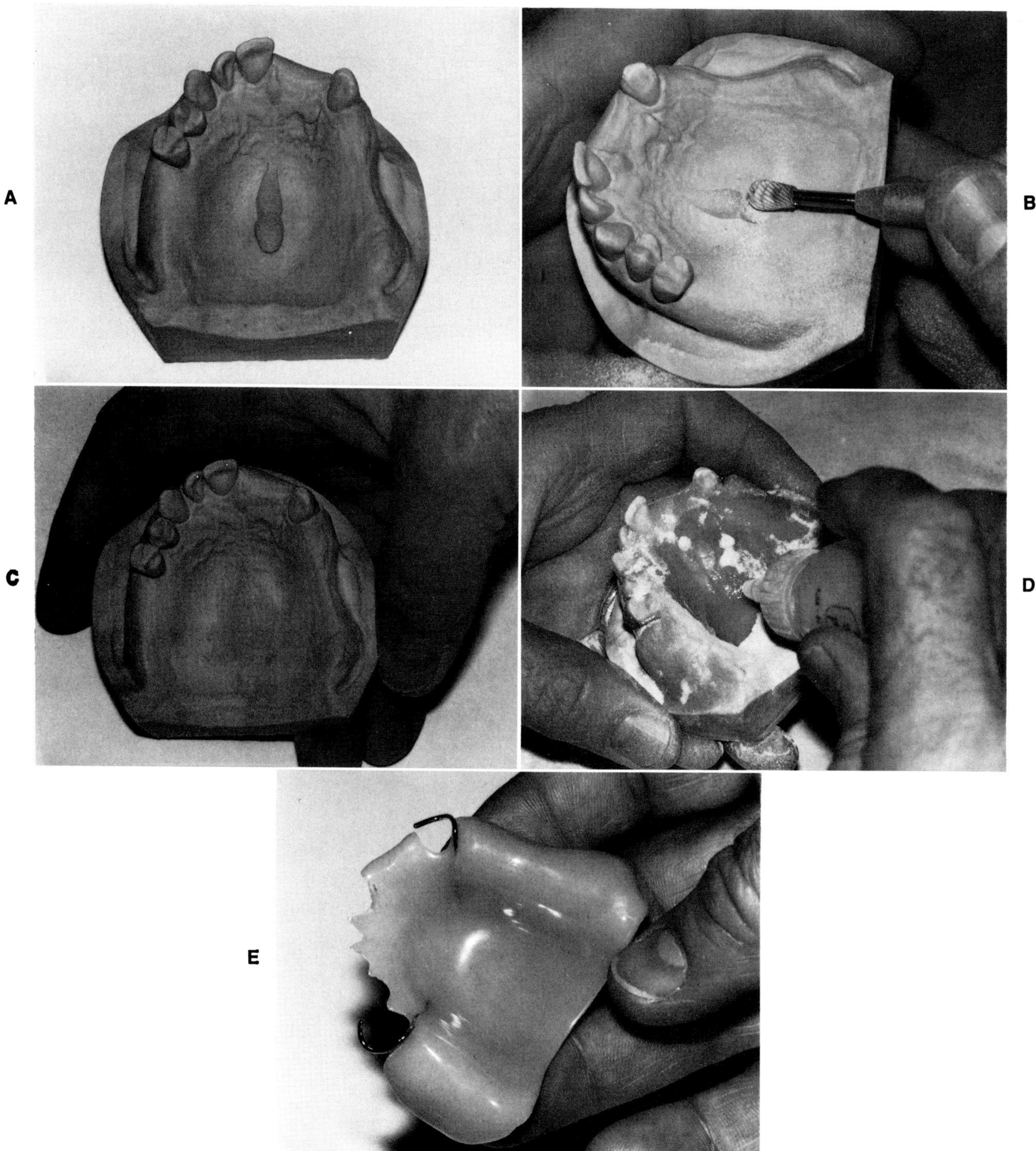

Fig. 18-49. A, Torus palatinus that must be surgically removed before permanent prosthesis can be constructed. **B,** Torus is removed from cast with acrylic bur. **C,** Site of torus is completely smoothed. **D,** Surgical splint is made using the sprinkle-on technique. Note wrought wire clasps that are used to retain splint. **E,** Completed splint should be highly polished in order to maintain surgical site as clean as possible.

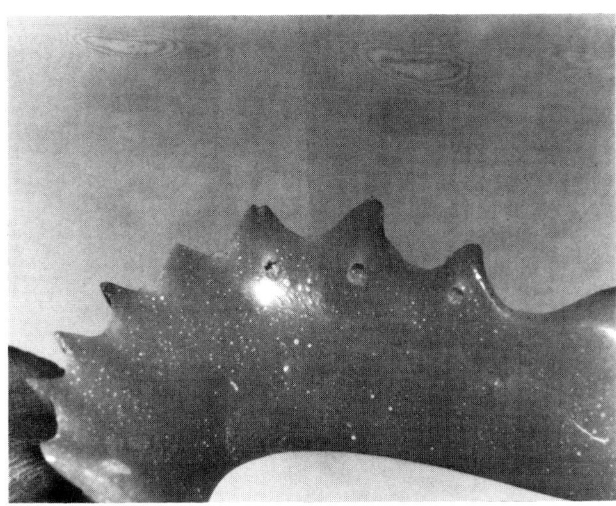

Fig. 18-50. Lingual splint to be used following mandibular tori removal has holes so that splint can be ligated to teeth with sutures passing through holes and around teeth.

fected tissues are supported or protected by a temporary surgical splint. The splint is constructed of autopolymerizing acrylic resin, usually by the sprinkle-on technique.

The surgical sites that most commonly lend themselves to support by a splint are palatal tissues and tissues on the lingual aspect of the mandibular ridge, the most common places for bony exostoses. Maxillary or mandibular tori can be removed and the site protected by the placement of an acrylic resin splint.

After the determination that surgical intervention is necessary, impressions in irreversible hydrocolloid can be made (Fig. 18-49). If the practitioner is not going to perform the surgery, consultation with the surgeon should be made to ascertain the desired contour of the area after the surgery is complete. The master cast should be scraped or cut to conform to the desired configuration. After the cast is reshaped, the splint is formed by the sprinkle-on method. Retention devices for the splint may be in the form of wrought wire clasps or, if more positive retention is desired, holes may be provided in the interproximal extension of the splint and the splint secured to the remaining teeth with sutures passing through the holes in the splint and through the interproximal spaces.

The splint may be lined with tissue-conditioning material for more intimate adaptation to the surgical site. This will help prevent saliva and other irritating material from collecting beneath the splint.

Palatal splints are especially helpful following surgery that includes reflection of a major portion of the palatal tissue. If the palate is not supported, hemorrhage between the bony hard palate and the soft tissue can grossly deform the tissue. In time the clot providing the deformation will resolve, but the patient will be subjected to a long period of discomfort.

Mucosa on the lingual aspect of the mandibular ridge is especially friable and sensitive. Protecting these tissues from the action of the tongue and from the effects of food being shunted over them will greatly decrease the postsurgical discomfort of the patient (Fig. 18-50).

Night guards and mouth protective devices

The purpose of a night guard is to protect the remaining teeth from self-inflicted damage during sleep. Actually, protective devices are designed and prescribed for patients to be worn at any time that oral habits are potentially damaging to the dentition.

The damaging habit is normally in the form of bruxism, unconscious grinding of the teeth during sleep or during periods of tension. The cause of bruxism is perhaps best left to texts dealing primarily with emotional responses of patients. The dental practitioner must recognize the condition and help the patient prevent unnecessary oral destruction until the underlying causes can be diagnosed and treated.

Night guards or occlusal protective guards may also be prescribed for patients with acute temporomandibular joint disturbances. These occlusal guides may be constructed of soft resilient resin or of hard acrylic resin.

The use of hard acrylic resin protective occlusal devices in the treatment of acute temporomandibular joint disturbances is based on the premise that the pain that the patient is feeling is caused by muscle spasms of the elevator muscles of the mandible. The spasms are produced as a result of the mandible being forced to deviate from its normal closing path because of the presence of deflective occlusal contacts. The interceptive contacts have usually been present for a long time but have been asymptomatic. Symptoms normally appear after or during a period when the patient is subjected to emotional distress. This is not to imply that all temporomandibular joint disturbances have a psychologic foundation, but a large percentage do.

The purpose of the hard acrylic resin occlusal guard is to break the cycle of the mandibular closing pathway that has set up the muscle spasms. The patient must be made to lose the sense or memory of the disruptive occlusal contacts that have triggered the painful syndrome.

Mouth guards are appliances that may be used by the dentulous patient or the partially edentulous patient to protect the remaining teeth and other oral structures from damage that can arise from physical contact in sports or other trauma-inducing incidents. These appliances not only protect the teeth and related structures from direct damage from blows but also protect the intracranial contents from the effects of trauma to the lower face by absorbing the effects of the trauma before it can be transmitted to the brain. Because of the necessity of absorbing the effects of trauma, the mouth guard is normally constructed of resilient resin.

There are many athletic mouth guards available for intraoral adaptation from drug stores or sports stores. These usually require softening in hot water and, while soft, fitted to the teeth. Obviously, the accuracy of fit is lacking in such home-prepared devices.

Clinical and laboratory procedures for hard acrylic resin occlusal guards

Accurate casts of both arches are made with irreversible hydrocolloid impressions. The maxillary cast is mounted on a semiadjustable articulator by using a face-bow transfer. The mandibular cast is mounted by using centric jaw relation records. Protrusive records are made to set the horizontal and lateral condylar guidances.

At the time of this clinical procedure the patient may be in considerable pain, and difficulty will normally be encountered in guiding the patient into the completely retruded position of centric relation. A convenient jaw position must be recorded with the understanding that, as acute symptoms subside following insertion of the guard, refinement in the occlusal contacts against the guard will be made.

Although it is possible to construct the occlusal guard of sprinkle-on resin, it is more accurate to develop the guard in baseplate wax and to invest and heat-process it.

The protective device is normally made to fit on the maxillary teeth and occlude with the mandibular teeth. Retention for the appliance is obtained from the close adaptation of the resin to the crowns of the teeth. The wax-up for the guard should cross the occlusal surfaces and contact the facial surfaces of the posterior teeth. It should cover the occlusal third of the facial surfaces. The palatal extension should be in the shape of a horseshoe major connector (Fig. 18-51).

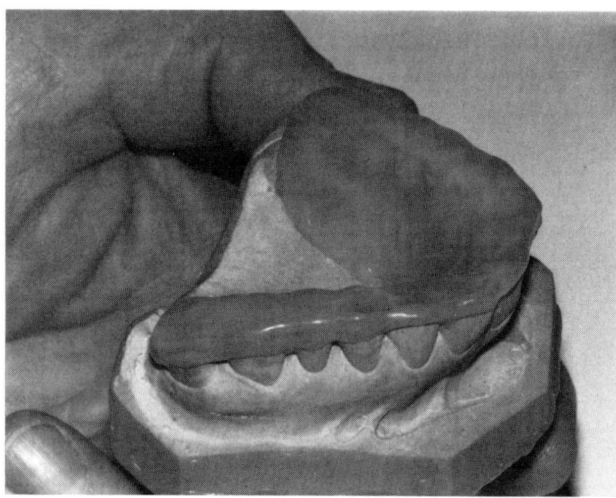

Fig. 18-51. Occlusal guard is retained by covering occlusal surfaces and one-third the facial surface of teeth.

The guard should be kept as thin as possible commensurate with maintaining adequate strength (Fig. 18-52). The thickness should rarely exceed 2 mm. After the baseplate wax has been shaped, the surface of the wax covering the occlusal and incisal surface of the teeth is uniformly softened. The articulator is closed to the point that will maintain a thickness of wax between 1 and 2 mm between opposing posterior teeth. Imprints of all occluding surfaces of the mandibular teeth must be evident. If any tooth is not in contact, wax should be pooled over the area and the articulator closed again until the imprint is clear. The depth of the cuspal or incisal imprints must not be excessive. Wax adjacent to the imprints should be removed so that the depth of the imprint does not exceed 2 mm.

The articulator is now closed and carried through protrusive and lateral movements so that the mandibular teeth will carve a path of movement in the wax (Fig. 18-53). This discursive movement of the articulator is continued until the multiple pathways being developed in the wax are smooth and clear. At this point the maxillary cast with the wax occlusal guard is invested, packed, and processed with clear heat-cured acrylic resin.

After the protective guard is recovered following the processing procedure, it is finished, polished, and prepared for delivery.

The guard is best and most accurately inserted with disclosing wax to locate areas of resin that are interfering with complete seating of the appliance (Fig. 18-54).

Once the guard is seated, articulating paper is used to obtain the best possible complete contact of the mandibular occlusal and incisal surfaces with the flat occlusal guard (Fig. 18-55).

The patient is dismissed with the instructions to wear the appliance full time for the next 24 hours except for cleaning the teeth and the guard and for eating. The patient should be placed on a completely soft diet so that tooth contacts with the guard out of the mouth will be avoided. In 24 hours relaxation of the muscle spasm will usually be evident. Mandibular repositioning will occur as muscle relaxation takes place. Adjustment of mandibular tooth contact with the guard must be reaccomplished as the mandible returns to its normal muscular position.

Acute symptoms of temporomandibular joint disturbances of this type can usually be controlled rapidly,

A B

C D

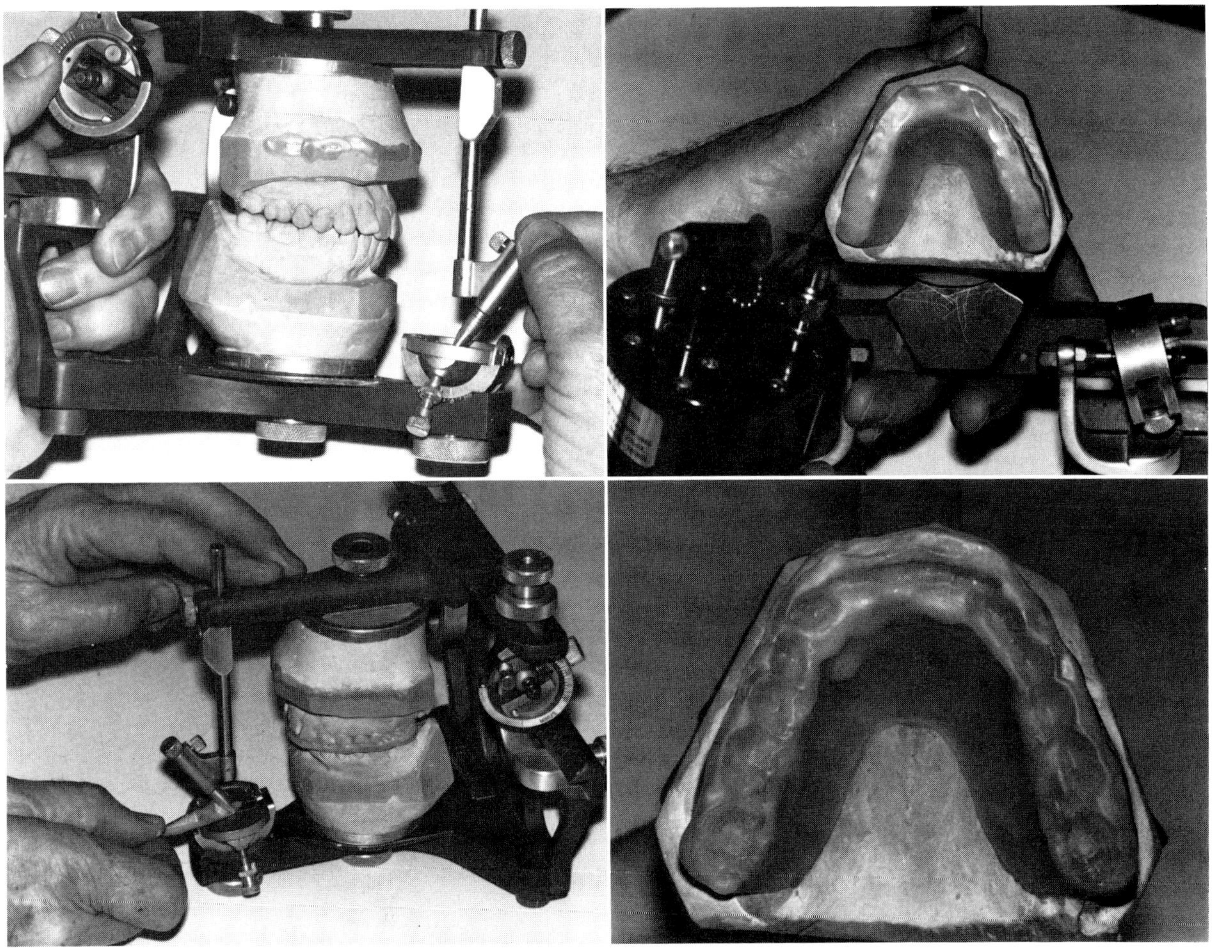

Fig. 18-52. A, Incisal guide pin is adjusted so that posterior teeth are separated between 1 and 2 mm. **B,** Baseplate wax is adapted over teeth and to proper outline form, horseshoe palatal design. Surface of wax is softened by flaming it. **C,** Articulator is closed until incisal pin contacts incisal table. **D,** Imprints of all teeth must be evident in wax.

A 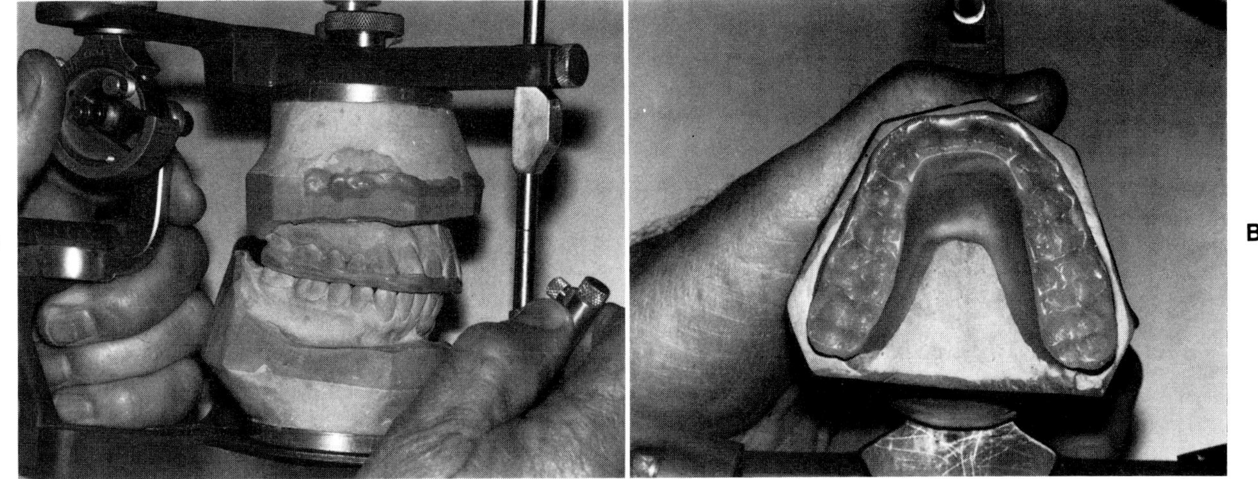 B

Fig. 18-53. A, Articulator is moved through all excursions as teeth contact wax and incisal guide pin stays in contact with guide table. **B,** Completed pathway showing tooth contact in all excursions. Thickness of occlusal guard must not exceed measurement of free-way space.

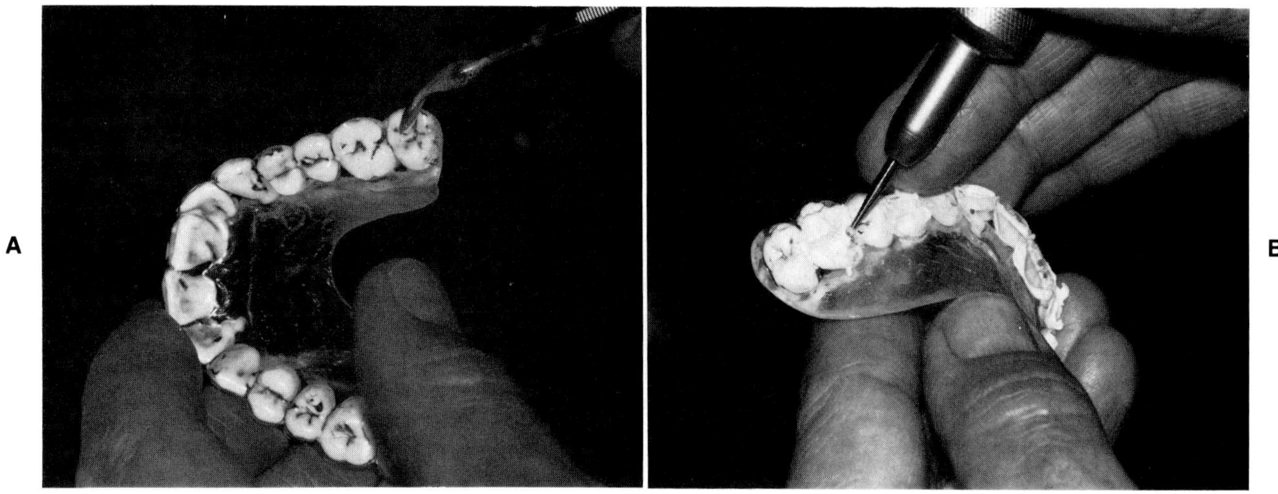

Fig. 18-54. A, Disclosing wax is flowed into tooth depressions of occlusal guard. **B,** Showthroughs of acrylic resin are relieved with small round bur to improve fit of guard to teeth.

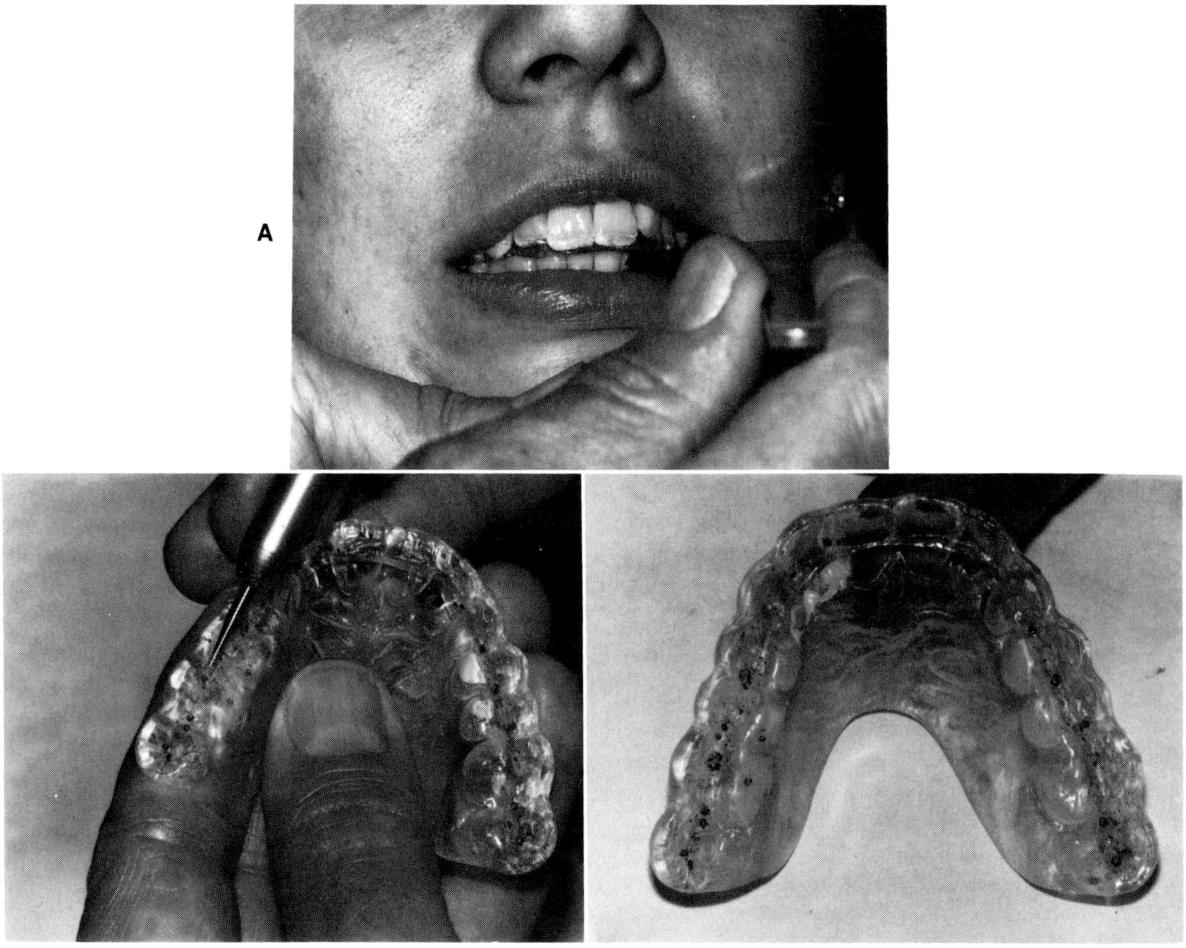

Fig. 18-55. A, Articulating paper is used in mouth to locate and correct premature occlusal contacts. **B,** Uniform occlusal contacts should be evident on surface of the guard. **C,** Final pattern of occlusal contacts.

but this should not mask the fact that a deep-seated and probably complicated problem still remains to be solved before the patient can be considered to be restored to health.

Clinical and laboratory procedures for soft resilient resin occlusal guards

The simplest method of preparing an accurate mouth guard is through the use of a vacuum machine. Several different makes are available on the commercial market. Some of the machines contain a heat source that softens the resin before the resin is adapted to a cast of the patient's maxillary arch.

The resilient material is supplied in 5- by 5-inch sheets. A thickness of the material of at least 1/8 inch should be used to provide sufficient resiliency to absorb the effects of trauma and protect the oral structures (Fig. 18-56).

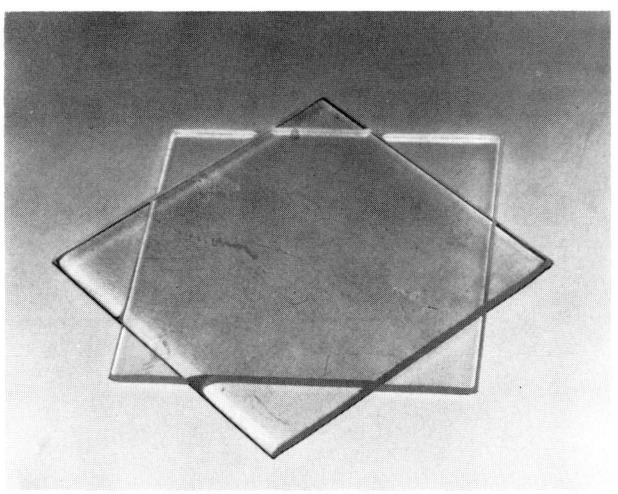

Fig. 18-56. Resilient mouth guard material is supplied in sheets 3 mm thick.

A

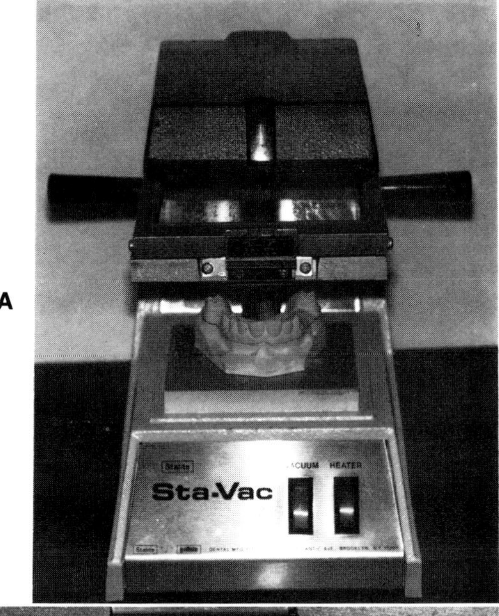

B

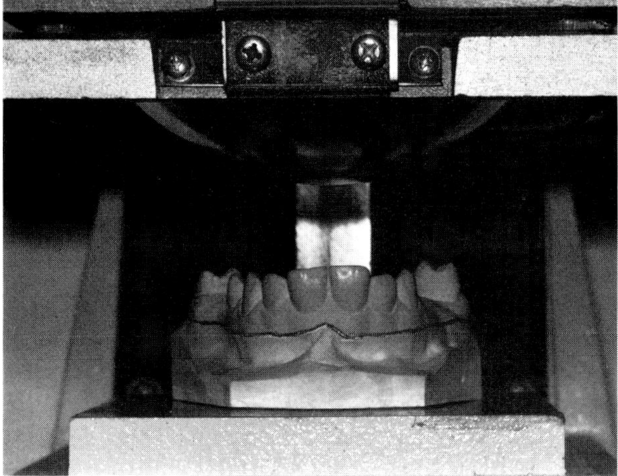

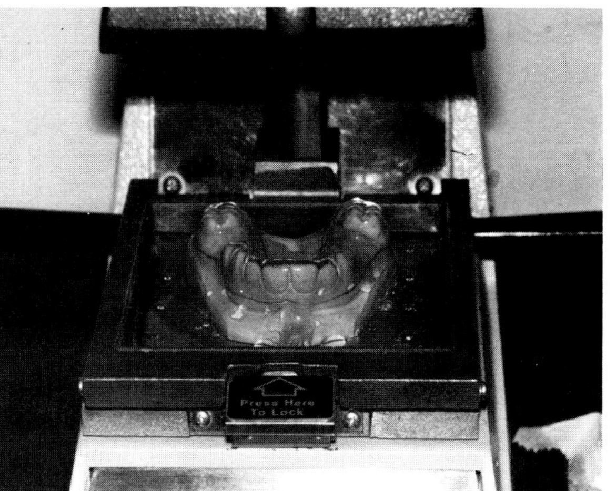

C

Fig. 18-57. A, Maxillary cast is positioned over vacuum intake as resilient material is held in heating unit above. **B,** As heat is absorbed, mouth guard material starts to slump. **C,** Upper member of machine is lowered so that guard material contacts cast, and vacuum is started.

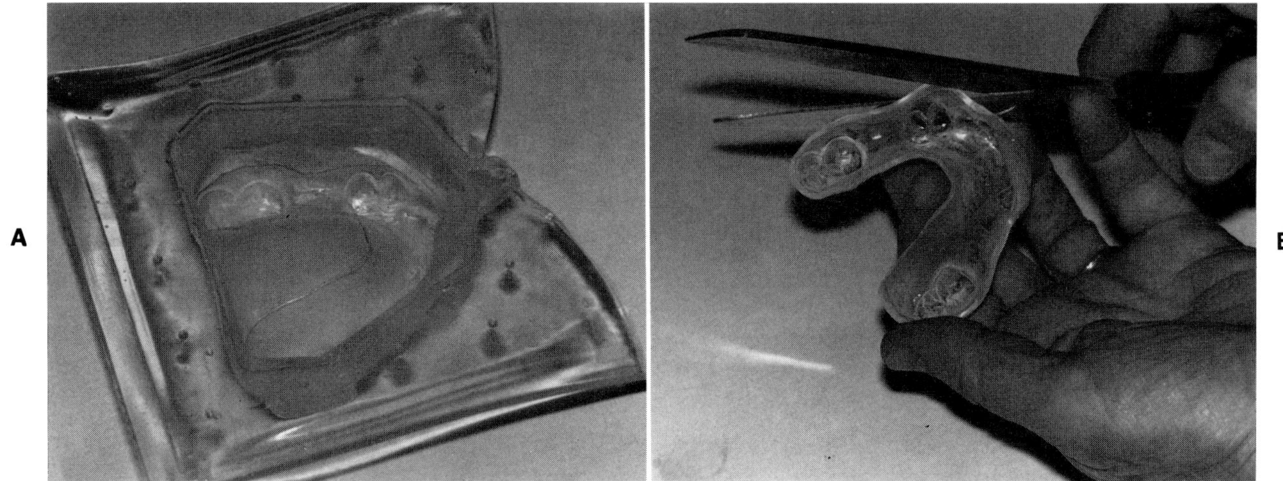

Fig. 18-58. A, Vacuum has pulled softened material into intimate contact with cast (cast removed). Outline of bead prepared in surface of cast can be easily read. **B,** Mouth guard is trimmed to outline form with scissors.

A maxillary cast made from an irreversible hydrocolloid impression is placed over the intake source of the vacuum machine (Fig. 18-57). The desired outline of the mouth guard should be drawn on the cast. Beading the outline with a small round excavator is helpful when trimming of the mouth guard is accomplished.

The outline should extend at least 5 mm onto the soft tissue facial to the teeth avoiding any impingement on frenum or muscle attachments. On the palate the outline should be in the form of a horseshoe with the margins at the junction of the horizontal and vertical slopes of the hard palate.

A sheet of material is attached to the heating source, which is positioned above the cast resting on the vacuum intake. If the electric heating device is not available, the material can be softened with a blow torch with a brush flame.

Once the material is softened as evidenced by the sagging of the center of the sheet, the resin is pulled down over the surface of the cast and the vacuum machine turned on. Air is pulled through the cast, producing an intimate adaptation of the resin to the surface of the cast. The edges of the sheet of resin form a peripheral seal around the cast so that a vacuum can be produced.

The resilient resin is teased off the cast and trimmed to the outline form indicated by the beading, which was transferred to the surface of the resin (Fig. 18-58). There are special burs available for use in trimming the resin. Regular burs used to trim hard resin will clog rapidly and are ineffective in cutting resilient resin.

Sharp edges of the mouth guard that are left after trimming with scissors may be rounded by flaming with an alcohol torch.

The mouth guard, when not in use, should be kept in water or preferably in a cleansing solution. The same solution used to cleanse complete dentures can be used safely.

IMMEDIATE PARTIAL DENTURES

Any of the previously discussed temporary partial dentures may be supplied as an immediate temporary partial denture. The term *immediate* describes a prosthesis that is inserted at the same appointment the tooth or teeth are extracted.

The advantages of such a service are obvious, particularly when anterior teeth are involved. The patient does not have to experience the embarrassment associated with missing anterior teeth. Although the vast majority of immediate partial dentures are constructed to replace missing anterior teeth, there are also advantages to replacing posterior teeth with an immediate prosthesis.

Replacing posterior teeth with the immediate partial denture protects the surgical site of the extraction from outside influence. Hemorrhage and swelling are controlled by the presence of the denture, and the postsurgical course is normally less troublesome to the patient. The denture also helps prevent migration of teeth adjacent to the edentulous area and overeruption of teeth opposing the missing teeth.

Permanent immediate partial dentures

If a decision is made to construct a definitive, or permanent, immediate partial denture (that is, using a cast metal framework), the decision must be made with knowledge that a try-in of the metal framework is difficult and that if the framework fails to seat at the time

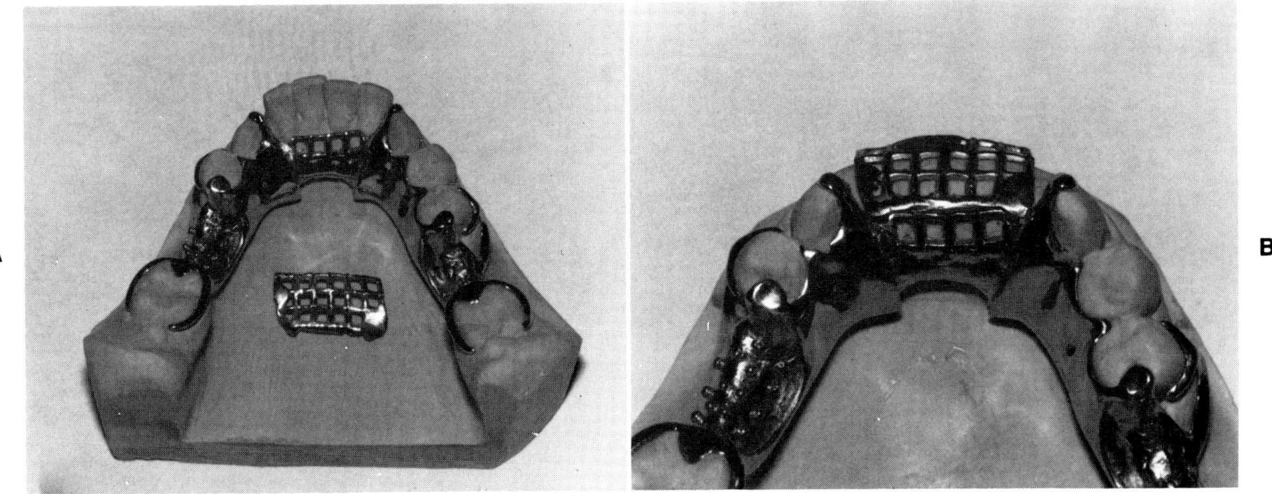

Fig. 18-59. A, Immediate permanent partial denture with acrylic resin retention minor connector separate. **B,** Teeth to be extracted and replaced are cut from cast and partial denture reassembled and soldered.

of insertion the patient will be left edentulous until reconstruction of the denture can be accomplished.

There are, however, techniques that will permit a try-in appointment. Construction of the framework is modified so that instead of the usual cast metal acrylic resin retention minor connectors, projections of wrought wire are cast to the framework to act as the retention minor connector for the denture base. These wires may be bent backward so as not to interfere with the teeth that will later be extracted during the framework try-in appointment. After the appointment the wires may be readjusted to the cast for positioning of the artificial teeth and waxing the denture base. Relining the denture base will be needed as healing and resorption of the edentulous areas take place.

A second technique is available for construction of a cast metal framework for an immediate partial denture of a more definitive type. This technique also permits the try-in of the framework before completing the prosthesis.

The master cast, properly relieved and blocked out, is duplicated in refractory material. The teeth that are to be extracted and replaced by the partial denture are cut from the duplicate refractory cast following the technique previously described.

The framework is waxed following an acceptable technique, but the acrylic resin retentive minor connector is not joined to the major connector. The acrylic resin connector should always be of the open latticework type, because relining after healing of the extraction sites will be required. The open latticework is the easiest type to reline or rebase.

The framework with the separate acrylic resin retention areas is invested and cast. The framework is now tried in and fitted to the abutment teeth. Some of the remaining teeth that are to be extracted and are adjacent to the abutment teeth may require slice preparations to permit the framework to be tried in. The slice preparations should be accomplished before making the final impression. The slice preparations also permit guiding planes to be developed on these abutment teeth.

Following the framework try-in appointment the teeth to be extracted are cut from the master cast in the same way that the teeth were cut from the refractory cast (Fig. 18-59). The framework is placed on the cast and the acrylic resin retention minor connectors placed in position. Space must be provided between the acrylic resin retention and the cast for the acrylic resin denture base. The minor connector is soldered to the framework using the electrosoldering machine (Fig. 18-60).

Temporary immediate partial dentures

The temporary immediate partial denture has the advantage that changes in the denture base or teeth can be made relatively easily as healing progresses or if there are patient objections to the appearance of the artificial teeth. In neither case, permanent or temporary, can the artificial teeth be tried in before the extraction.

The temporary partial denture can be used successfully over a long enough time to allow for complete healing before construction of the definitive prosthesis. Relining of the denture base will be necessary during the healing process. The reline may be done as a chairside procedure using mouth-curing resins (Fig. 18-61). This technique is not recommended as a form of long-

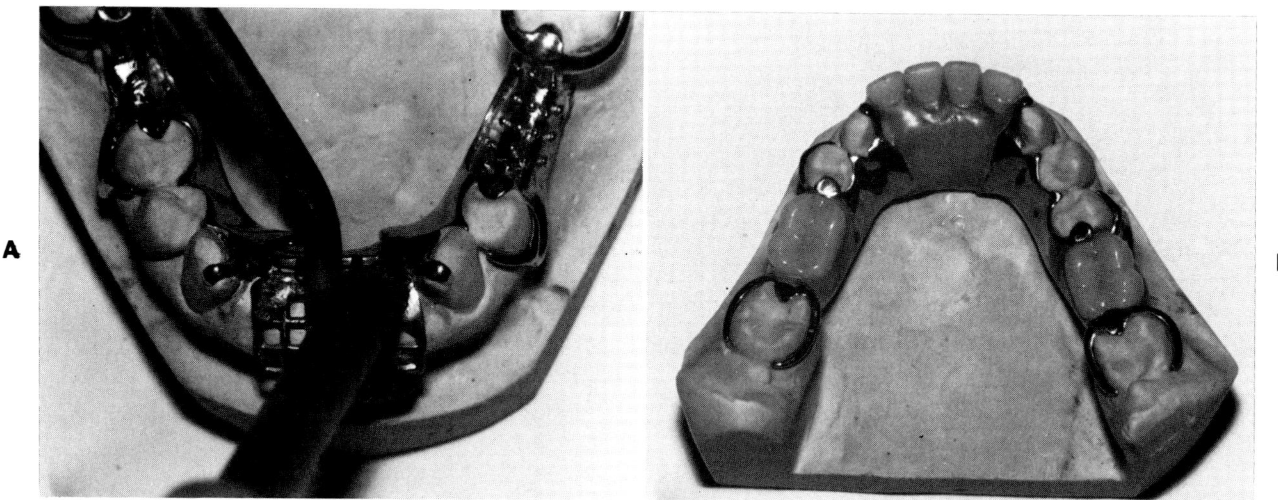

Fig. 18-60. **A,** Acrylic resin retention is soldered to framework. **B,** Denture teeth are set and denture base waxed to proper contour.

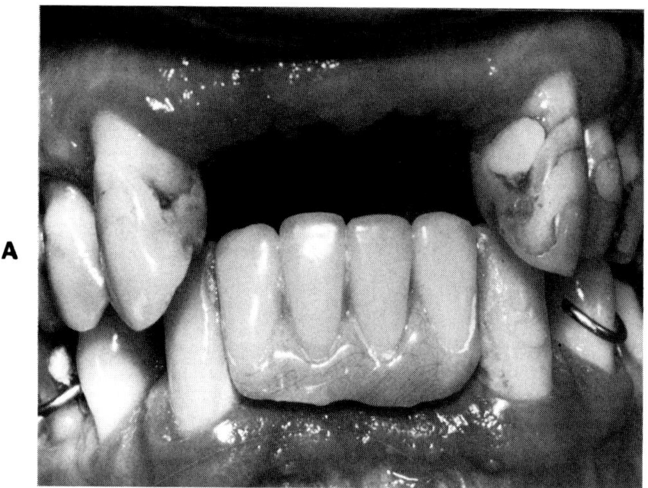

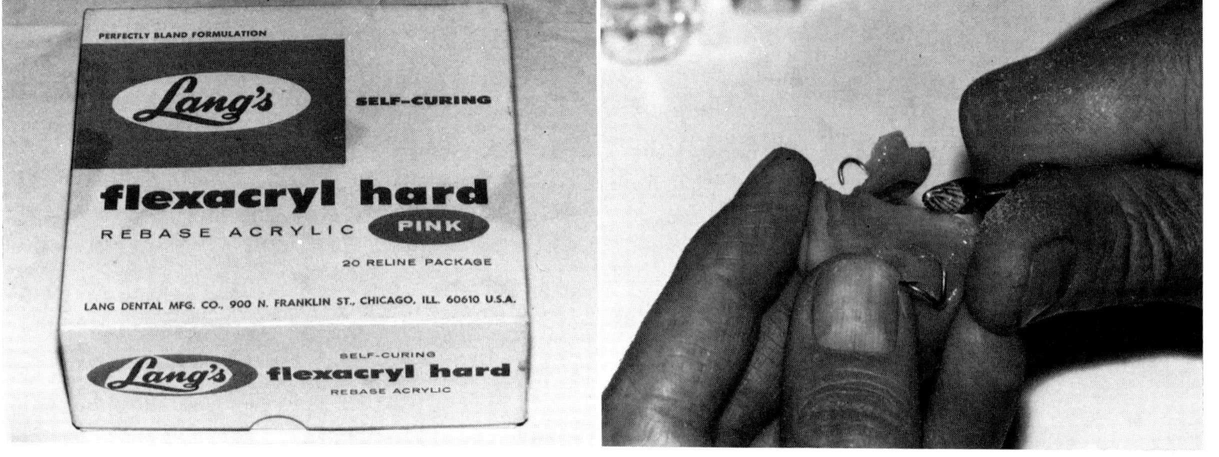

Fig. 18-61. **A,** Ridge resorption has occurred beneath temporary immediate partial denture base. **B,** Mouth-curing chairside reline material. Material is mixed, and flowed on denture base, and denture is seated in mouth. Material must be removed from mouth and trimmed before it becomes hard or it will lock into undercuts around teeth. **C,** Reline should not be considered permanent because material is porous.

term treatment because the mouth-cured resins tend to be porous and will absorb mouth fluids and become offensive if used for too long a time.

Whether the temporary or permanent approach is to be used to construct the immediate partial denture, the preparation of the master cast remains the same.

Clinical and laboratory procedures

If a permanent partial denture is to be made, final impressions are made after mouth preparation has been completed. Casts are poured in a minimum expansion dental stone. Jaw relation records may or may not be needed to mount the casts on an articulator so that the artificial teeth can be properly positioned.

After the casts have been mounted, the teeth to be replaced are removed from the cast (Fig. 18-62). They may be sectioned from the cast with a laboratory saw or can be cut free with a fissure bur in a straight handpiece. For either method care must be taken not to mar the proximal surfaces of teeth adjacent to those being removed or space available for the artificial teeth will be less in the mouth than it is on the cast.

The crown of the tooth should be removed cleanly and even with the gingival crevicular tissue first. Next the tooth socket should be formed into a slight concavity several millimeters deep at the center. Finally the surface of the cast facial to the socket should be scraped from a maximum depth of 1 mm at the edge of the socket downward along the root positon for a length of 4 to 5 mm. This step will help produce a closer adaptation of the inner surface of the denture base flange to the extraction site.

If a permanent partial denture is to be replacement, the cast should be blocked out and relieved as described in Chapter 11 and the framework constructed. After the framework is completed, it is repositioned on the master cast and the artificial teeth set.

If a temporary immediate partial denture is to be

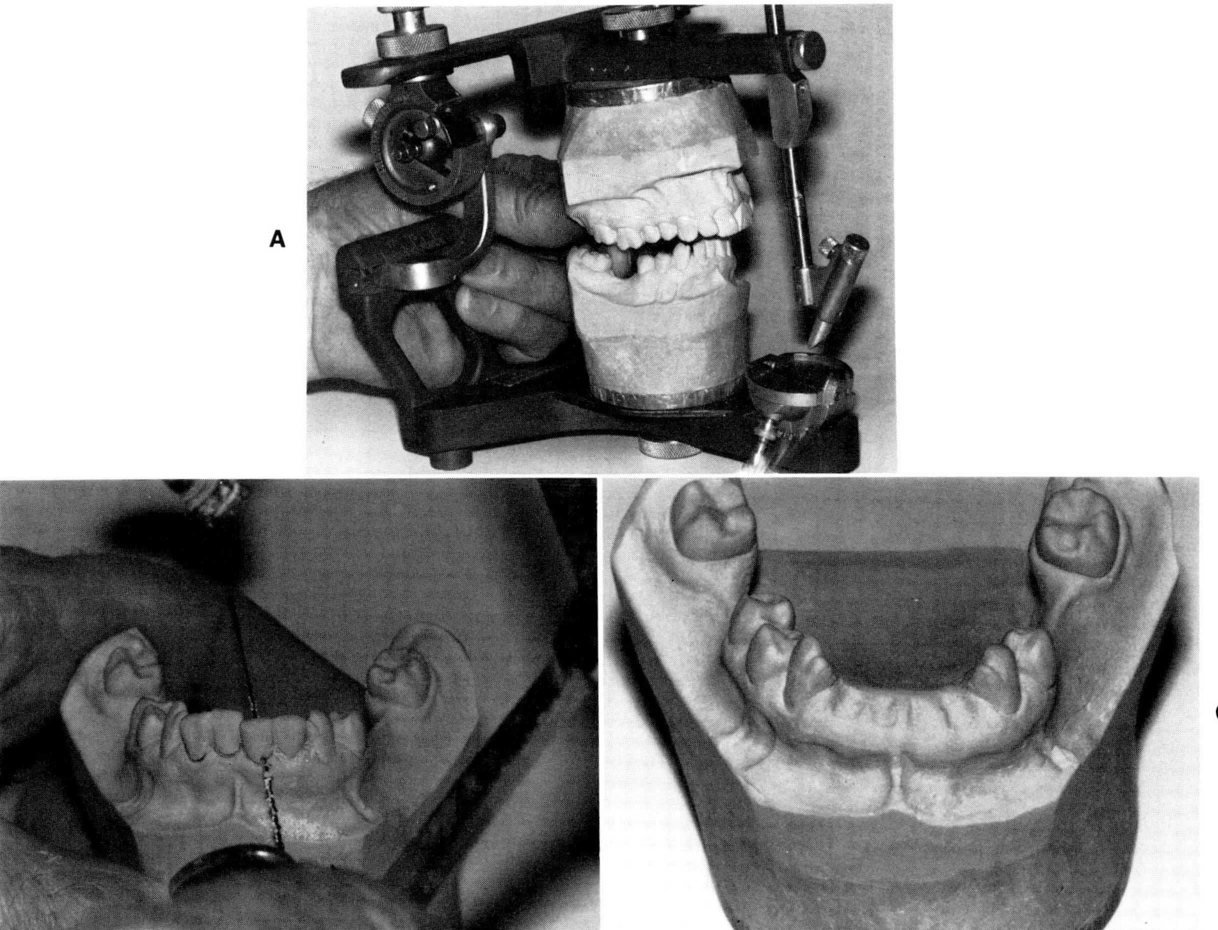

Fig. 18-62. A, Casts for immediate partial denture must be mounted on articulator. **B,** Teeth to be replaced are cut from cast. **C,** Slight concavity is prepared on ridge crest over tooth socket

constructed, the artificial teeth are selected and prepared as described in the construction of an interim partial denture.

Both the permanent and temporary immediate partial dentures are processed, finished, and polished as discussed previously.

Delivery of immediate partial denture

The teeth marked for extraction are removed with as little trauma to surrounding tissue as possible. The surgical site should be cleaned of areas of residual infection, redundant tissue, and detached bony fragments. Sutures may be placed if indicated.

To deliver a permanent immediate partial denture in the form least likely to produce postinsertion problems, disclosing wax should be used on the metallic portions of the denture contacting the teeth and on the denture bases to locate areas of the denture that are not fitting completely accurately (Fig. 18-63). In the presence of a bloody field these two procedures become much more difficult. Many patients, following surgery, are mentally not in the most receptive of moods for prolonged treatment. This is undoubtedly one of the greatest drawbacks in attempting to offer immediate permanent partial denture service. The occasion may demand too many compromises to arrive at a completely acceptable result. For this reason it is recommended that immediate patial denture treatment be offered as a temporary form of treatment to be followed in due process by treatment of a definitive nature.

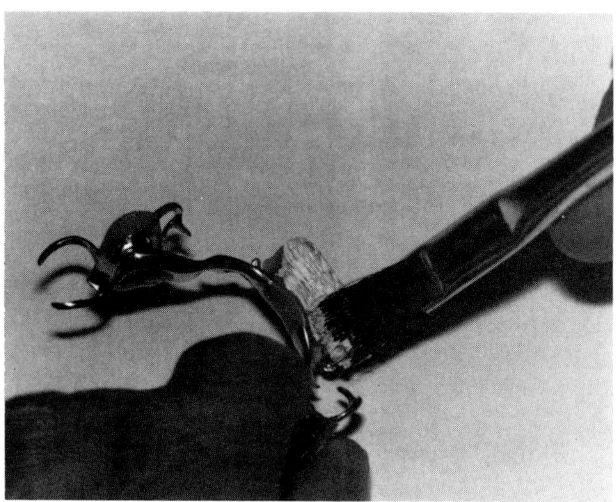

Fig. 18-63. Pressure-indicating paste is used on denture base at time of extraction to seat denture without excess pressure.

LENGTH OF APPOINTMENTS

The construction and insertion of most of these forms of temporary partial dentures and other removable appliances can normally be accomplished in two clinical appointments.

For the experienced practitioner the length of each appointment should not exceed 30 minutes. For the dental student each appointment should not be longer than 2 hours.

REFERENCE

De Van, M.M.: The transition from natural to artificial teeth, J. Prosthet. Dent. **11**:677-688, 1961.

BIBLIOGRAPHY

Bennett, C.G.: Transitional restorations for function and esthetics, J. Prosthet. Dent. **15**:867-872, 1965.

Blatterfein, L.: Role of the removable partial denture in the restoration of lost vertical dimension, N.Y. Univ. J. Dent. **10**:274-276, 1952.

Bolender, C.L., and others: Evaluation of treatment of inflammatory papillary hyperplasia of the palate, J. Prosthet. Dent. **15**:1013-1022, 1965.

Bruce, R.W., and Kobes, P.: Immediate removable partial dentures, J. Prosthet. Dent. **28**:36-42, 1972.

DeVan, M.M.: The additive partial denture: its principles and design (partial dentures), Northwest Dent. **35**:303-307, 1956.

Dreizin, S.: Nutritional changes in the oral cavity, J. Prosthet. Dent. **16**:1144-1150, 1966.

Ettinger, R.L.: The etiology of inflammatory papillary hyperplasia, J. Prosthet. Dent. **34**:254-259, 1975.

Frank, R.P.: Fabrication of temporary and treatment partial dentures, J. Prosthet. Dent. **30**:215-221, 1973.

Harvey, W.L.: A transitional prosthetic appliance, J. Prosthet. Den. **14**:60-70, 1964.

Lambson, G.O.: Papillary hyperplasia of the palate, J. Prosthet. Dent. **16**:636-645, 1966.

Reitz, P.V., and Weiner, M.G.: Fabrication of interim acrylic resin removable partial dentures with clasps, J. Prosthet. Dent. **40**:686-688, 1978.

Schopper, A.F.: Loss of vertical dimension: causes and effects: diagnosis and various recommended treatments, J. Prosthet. Dent. **9**:428-431, 1959.

Thomas, K.H.: Papillomatosis of the palate, Oral Surg. **5**:214-218, 1952.

Waldron C.A.: Oral leukoplakia, carcinoma, and the prosthodontist, J. Prosthet. Dent. **15**:367-376, 1965.

19 Complete denture opposing a removable partial denture

Many competent practitioners object to the use of a complete denture opposing either natural dentition or a prosthesis supported by natural dentition because of rapid and unequal destruction of the edentulous ridge (Fig. 19-1). However, most practitioners holding this belief are still reluctant to condemn healthy natural teeth. A compromise in treatment is generally followed.

INDICATIONS

The principal indication for the construction of a complete denture opposing a removable partial denture is a disparity in the jaw sizes or a gross malrelation of the jaws, usually a pronounced retrognathic relationship of the mandible to the maxilla. In these situations it is essential that every attempt be made to retain some teeth in the weaker of the two arches, normally the mandibular arch, but the maxillary arch when a prognathic jaw relationship is present (Figs. 19-2 and 19-3). A cleft or perforated palate that cannot be corrected surgically also necessitates retention of maxillary teeth even when the mandible has been made edentulous because the inability to obtain a peripheral seal makes the construction of a retentive complete denture an impossibility (Fig. 19-4). Other instances such as hemimaxillectomy also necessitate the retention of some teeth at all costs (Fig. 19-5). Such conditions are discussed in Chapter 23.

For patients with a relatively normal, or orthognathic, jaw relationship it is possible to deliver a complete maxillary denture opposing a mandibular partial denture with the expectation of acceptable results, but a complete mandibular denture opposing either natural maxillary dentition or a removable partial denture supported by natural teeth has little or no chance of success. The destruction of the mandibular edentulous ridge in the latter situation can be so rapid and complete as to render the patient a dental cripple. A mandibular complete denture without functioning posterior occlusion, for use as a esthetic replacement only, may be attempted, but chances for success are still poor. An endosseous implant to support a mandibular complete denture opposing a maxillary removable partial denture is also a hazardous procedure. The mandibular denture will be stabilized, but the concentration of forces passing through the implant posts to the substructure resting on the bone of the mandible can destroy the supporting bone.

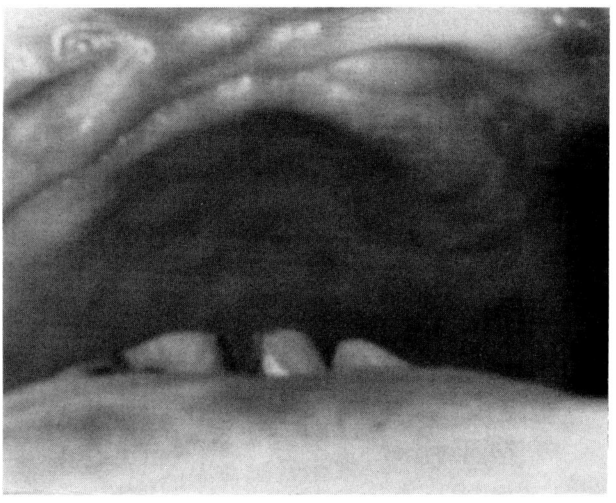

Fig. 19-1. Rapid destruction of edentulous ridge opposing natural dentition frequently occurs.

For these reasons the discussion in this chapter is limited to the construction of a maxillary complete denture opposing a mandibular partial denture.

If a Class III partial denture is to oppose a maxillary complete denture, an excellent technique is to complete the mandibular tooth-supported partial denture and establish or complete the occlusal plane before constructing the complete denture (Fig. 19-6). This technique should be followed only after a diagnostic mounting has shown the remaining natural teeth to be in favorable position in relation to the edentulous arch. Accepting malrelations of remaining mandibular teeth to either the correct buccolingual alignment or to the desired occlusal plane can do nothing but perpetuate the condition that contributed to the loss of the missing teeth originally.

This same approach to treatment planning may be used when fixed partial dentures are being constructed in one arch and a complete denture in the opposite arch

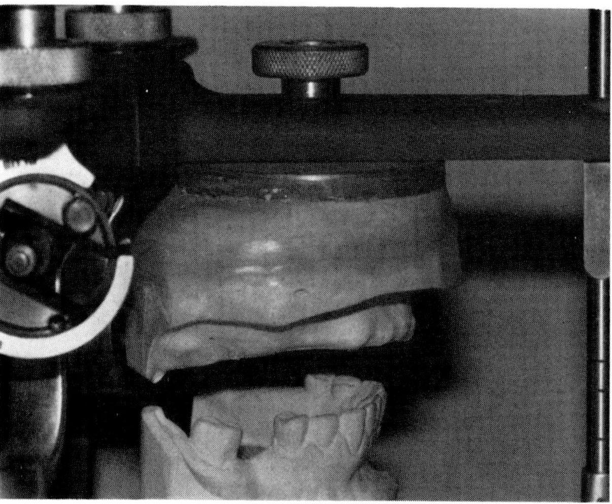

Fig. 19-2. Retrognathic jaw relationship. Mandible is weaker arch.

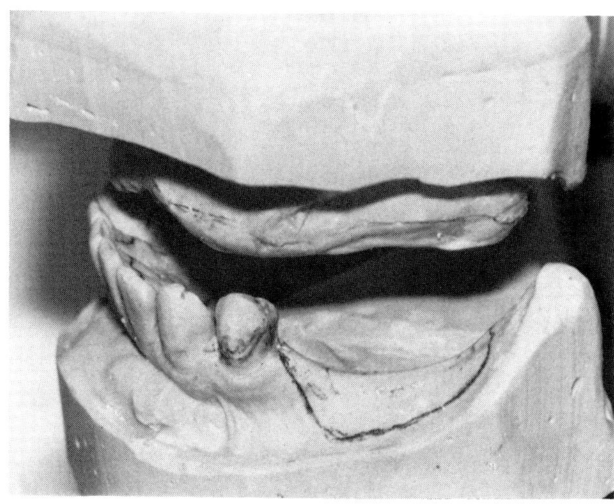

Fig. 19-3. Prognathic jaw relationship. Maxilla is weaker arch.

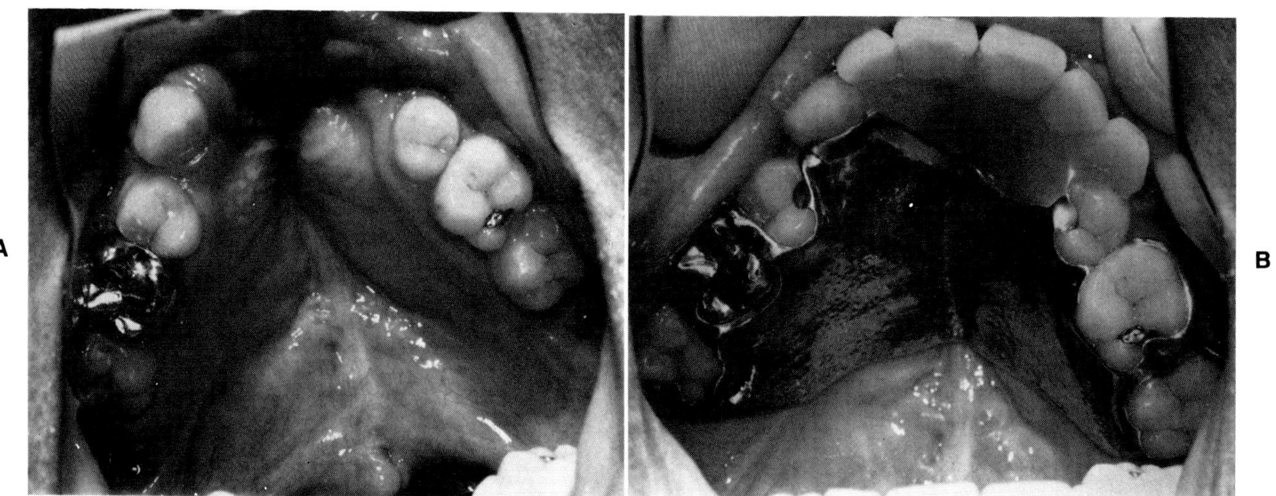

Fig. 19-4. Maxillary teeth must be retained when cleft or perforated palate is present. **A,** Partially edentulous arch. **B,** Same arch with removable partial denture in place.

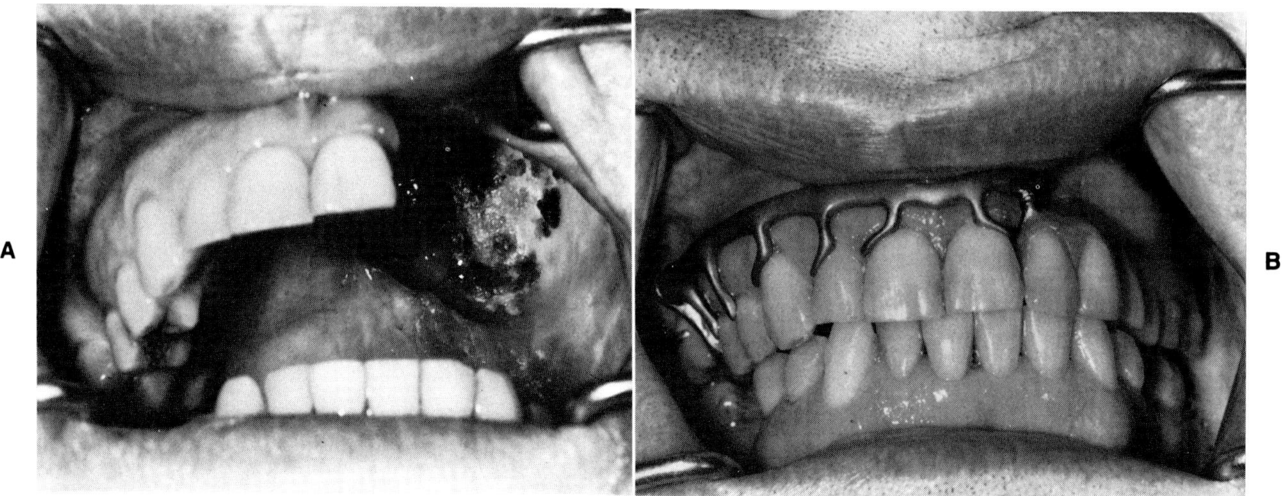

Fig. 19-5. Following extensive surgical procedures in either maxilla or mandible it is essential that some teeth be retained. **A,** Arch after surgery. **B,** Removable partial denture in place.

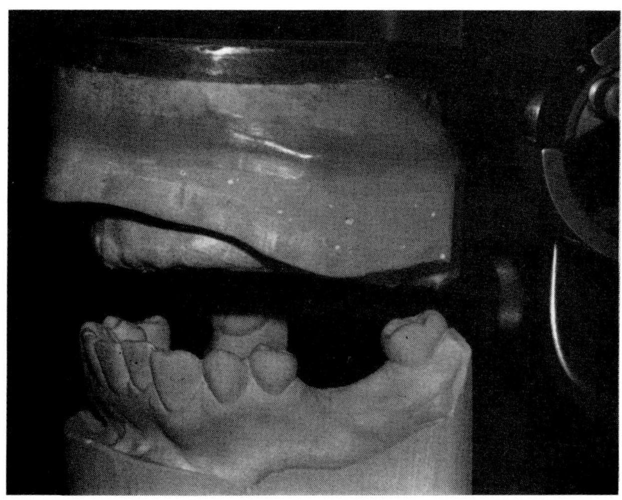

Fig. 19-6. When Class III partially edentulous arch opposes edentulous maxillary arch, mandibular removable partial prosthesis can be completed before maxillary denture is constructed.

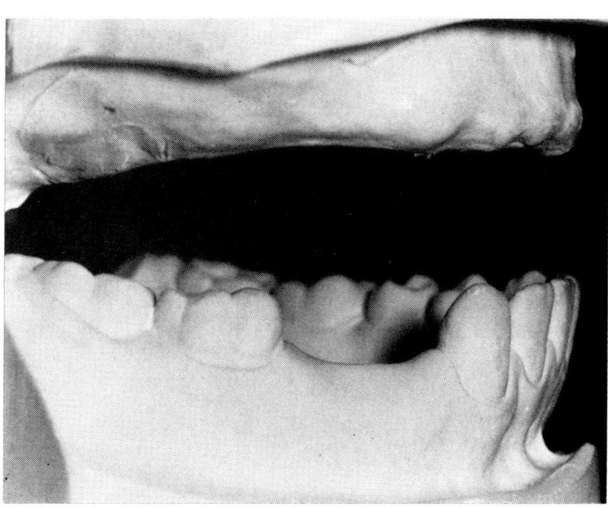

Fig. 19-7. Fixed partial dentures are completed to reestablish continuity of opposing arch before complete denture is constructed.

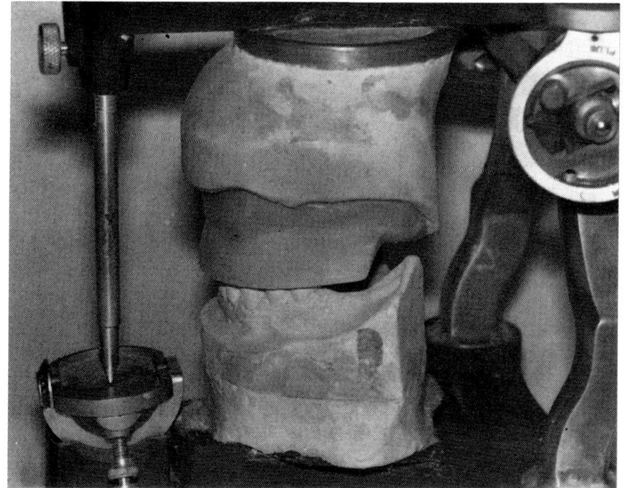

Fig. 19-8. Most favorable jaw relation for combination dentures is orthognathic relationship where complete maxillary denture opposes Class I mandibular partial denture.

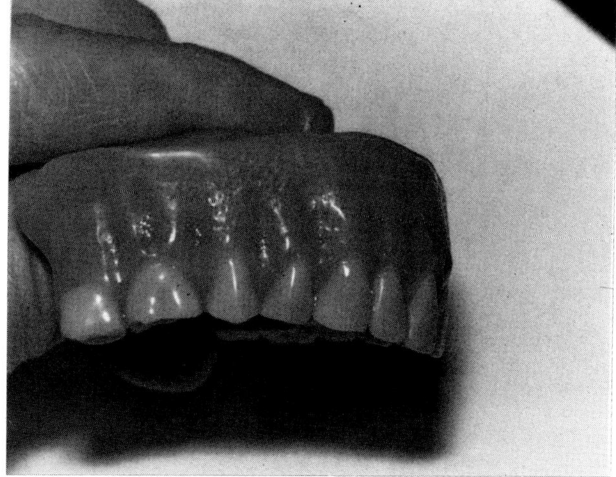

Fig. 19-9. Occlusal plane of preexisting complete denture that was constructed to occlude with natural teeth that have since been lost is often unacceptable. Reverse occlusal curve is demonstrated here.

(Fig. 19-7). The fixed partial denture should be completed first, and the occlusal plane, curve of Spee, and curve of Wilson established in harmony with the remaining natural teeth. When this has been accomplished, the complete denture can be made with occlusal harmony in all mandibular excursive movements.

MANDIBULAR DISTAL EXTENSION REMOVABLE PARTIAL DENTURE OPPOSING COMPLETE MAXILLARY DENTURE

The most frequently seen combination denture is a mandibular Class I or II partial denture opposing a maxillary complete denture (Fig. 19-8).

In unusual circumstances it might be possible to construct a mandibular partial denture to a preexisting clinically acceptable complete maxillary denture, but in most cases the occlusal plane and the tooth position in the maxillary denture will be less than ideal if the denture was constructed to oppose natural mandibular teeth that have since been extracted (Fig. 19-9). To obtain an acceptable result in the vast majority of cases, it will be necessary to construct new dentures and to develop the occlusal scheme simultaneously.

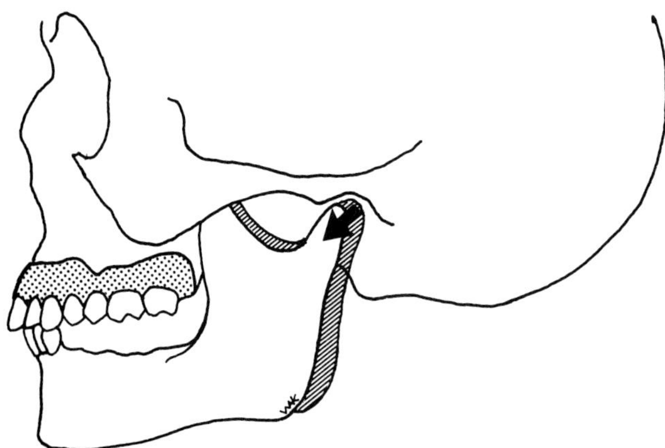

Fig. 19-10. When mandibular anterior teeth remain, patient will attempt to function in protrusive relationship to sense feeling of mastication.

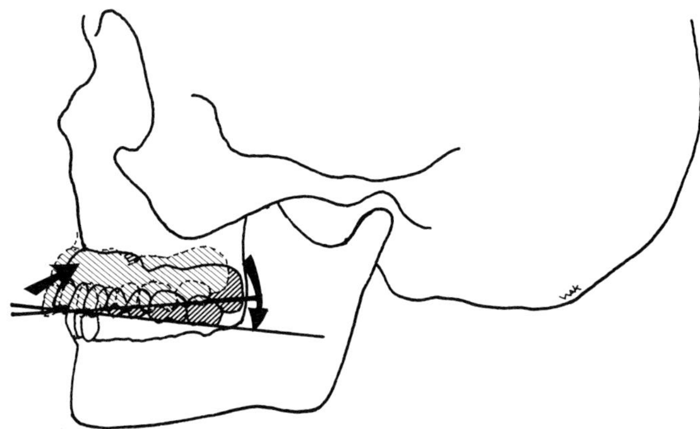

Fig. 19-11. As bone is resorbed from maxillary anterior ridge, denture will tip upward anteriorly and downward posteriorly.

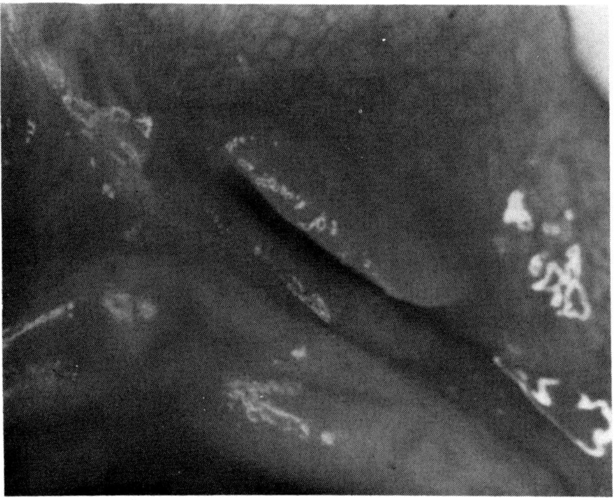

Fig. 19-12. Epulis fissuratum results from chronic irritation from overextended labial flange of denture.

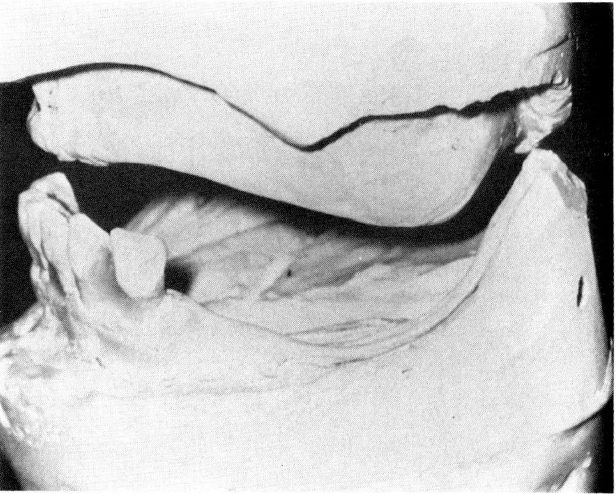

Fig. 19-13. Posterior downward tipping of maxillary denture produces overgrowth of fibrous tissue covering maxillary tuberosity.

Combination syndrome and associated changes

The destructive problems that may be encountered in constructing a mandibular distal extension partial denture against a complete maxillary denture have been called a combination syndrome by Kelly (1972). This combination syndrome consists of (1) loss of bone from the maxillary anterior edentulous ridge, (2) downgrowth of the maxillary tuberosities, (3) papillary hyperplasia of the tissues of the hard palate, (4) extrusion of the lower anterior teeth, and (5) loss of bone beneath the removable partial denture bases.

The combination syndrome usually has six associated changes: (1) loss of vertical dimension of occlusion, (2) occlusal plane discrepancy, (3) anterior spatial repositioning of the mandible, (4) development of epulis fissuratum, (5) poor adaptation of the prosthesis, and (6) periodontal changes.

These retrograde changes are probably triggered by the patient's functional habits. As long as any natural teeth remain in one arch, the patient will tend to function on these teeth regardless of their position because it is only through the masticatory sense nerve endings located in the periodontal ligament of the natural teeth that the patient can sense incising or mastication.

If the remaining natural teeth in the mandible are anterior teeth, as is usually the case, the majority of function will be taking place on the maxillary denture covering the anterior residual alveolar ridge (Fig. 19-10). This portion of the ridge is composed of cancellous bone and is subject to fairly rapid resorption if excessive force is placed against it. As ridge resorption occurs and progresses, the bony ridge is replaced by redundant soft tissue, initiating the combination syndrome and the associated changes.

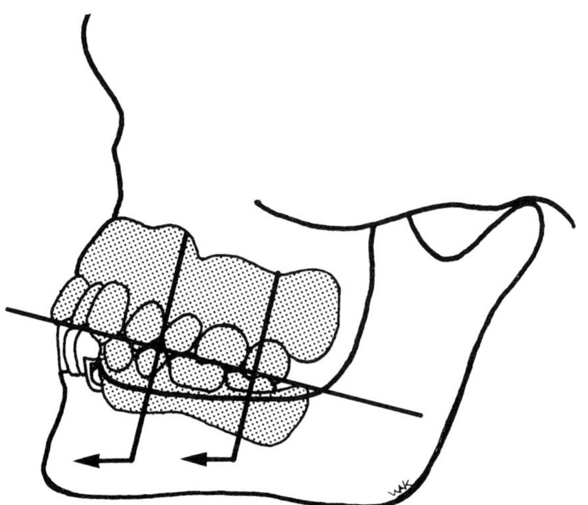

Fig. 19-14. As dentures settle as a result of ridge resorption, angulation of occlusal plane changes.

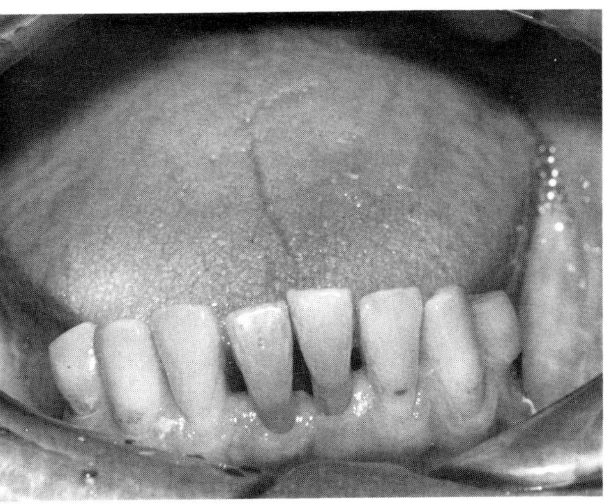

Fig. 19-15. As occlusal contact is lost between mandibular anterior teeth and complete denture, teeth may overerupt. Loosening and migration of these teeth are often seen.

As the resorptive changes occur in the maxillary anterior ridge, the vertical dimension of occlusion will begin to decrease as a result of settling of the maxillary anterior denture base. This in turn lowers the posterior occlusal plane. As the maxillary denture moves superiorly and anteriorly, the labial flange of the denture produces a low-grade irritation in the surrounding soft tissues, resulting in development of epulis fissuratum, and causes an associated overgrowth of fibrous tissue covering the maxillary tuberosities (Figs. 19-11 to 19-13). The change in the angulation of the occlusal plane may result in a protrusive or sliding contact of the mandibular teeth with the denture, which can contribute to the loss of support for the remaining natural teeth or precipitate periodontal changes.

As these changes progress, the retention and stability of the maxillary denture will decrease because of the changed shape and character of the supporting tissues. Papillary hyperplasia of the tissues of the hard palate, usually associated with poor oral hygiene, often results.

Resorption of bone under the denture base extensions of the mandibular removable partial denture with resultant settling of the partial denture occurs primarily because of the change in angulation of the occlusal plane (Fig. 19-14). Instead of occlusion occurring perpendicular to the residual ridge, it occurs at an angle that forces the mandible to assume a more anterior position.

The superior movement of the maxillary denture causes contact to be lost between the mandibular anterior teeth and the denture. To retain this contact, the mandibular teeth may overerupt, compounding the problem of periodontal support of these teeth (Fig. 19-15).

Another possibility is that the combination syndrome is triggered by the gradual resorption of bone beneath the mandibular distal extension bases. The inferior displacement of the mandibular partial denture is so gradual and slight that a patient may not seek professional help until many signs of the syndrome have appeared. The loss of posterior support in the mandible results in a decrease in posterior occlusal function and an increase in anterior occlusal function. The increased anterior load produces resorption of the maxillary anterior ridge, and the remaining steps in the syndrome follow in order.

Whatever the actual triggering mechanism, the probability of the syndrome must be recognized so its prevention can be included in the treatment process. Regular and frequent follow-up examinations, including no less than a remount procedure (See Chapter 16) at least once a year, are essential for patients with a complete denture opposing a removable partial denture. Too often the treatment offered is relining one or both prostheses, but unless changes in occlusal plane position, vertical dimension of occlusion, and mandibular position are recognized and corrected, relining will only perpetuate and magnify the destructive processes.

Clinical appointments

The sequence of appointments for patients requiring a complete maxillary denture opposing a mandibular Class I or II removable partial denture is important, because as little time as possible should elapse after final impressions are made of each arch until the prostheses are delivered to the patient.

The objectives of each appointment are listed, and clinical procedures are described for steps that are peculiar to the patient treatment of a complete denture opposing a removable partial denture. Those procedures that are involved in the planning, construction, and delivery of all removable partial dentures are discussed in other chapters of this book and can be referred to for greater detail. The clinical procedures required to accomplish the complete denture phase of treatment will also not be detailed here, but references to books on this subject are included at the close of the chapter.

Appointment 1—examination and preliminary impressions

If a combination denture is a distinct possibility, an in-depth diagnostic examination will be made to confirm or deny the feasibility of such treatment. Apparently healthy and strategically positioned teeth should not be removed until mounted diagnostic casts and other material can be used to show the patient the value of retaining these abutment teeth. The long-term importance of retaining teeth to preserve the remaining ridge should be stressed.

The examination should include history taking, digital and visual examination of the oral tissues, indicated radiographs, and the making of impressions of both arches in irreversible hydrocolloid. Complete diagnostic information is essential in arriving at the most reliable plan of treatment.

Appointment 2—diagnostic mounting and treatment plan

Before the second appointment baseplates must be constructed on the diagnostic casts (Fig. 19-16).

With the baseplates and occlusion rims constructed on the diagnostic casts, the centric jaw relation is established.

It is good practice to establish the tentative occlusal plane using the mandibular occlusion rim. The wax rim can be shaped so that it extends from the cusp tips of the remaining natural teeth (generally either one of the premolars or the canines) posteriorly to two-thirds the height of the pear-shaped pad (Fig. 19-17). It must be emphasized that this occlusal plane is tentative, only a point from which the actual plane will be determined.

Then, without permitting the opposing rims to contact, the dentist trims the maxillary rim to the proper anterior length and fullness to provide lip support (Fig. 19-18). Once the correct anterior rim length has been determined, the upper rim can be made parallel to the prosthetic plane, or the ala-tragus line (a plane originally proposed by Gysi running from the center of the tragus of the ear to the ala of the nose) (Fig. 19-19).

After the two occlusion rims have been shaped, they are removed from the mouth. The physiologic rest position of the mandible is determined from two marks, one on the tip of the nose and the other on the chin. The measurement of the physiologic rest position is reduced by 2 or 3 mm to arrive at the correct vertical dimension of occlusion with the proper amount of freeway space (Fig. 19-20).

The maxillary occlusion rim is now adjusted to the measurement of the vertical dimension of occlusion. At this stage the tentative mandibular occlusal plane is assumed correct. (It may be necessary to alter the position of the occlusal plane during the sixth appointment,

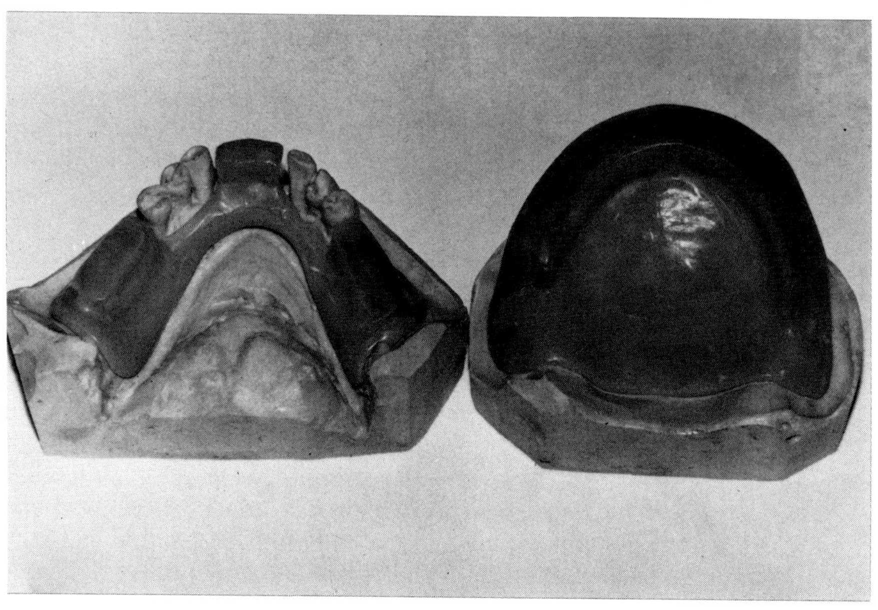

Fig. 19-16. Baseplates with wax occlusion rims are constructed for both arches.

after the diagnostic mounting has been completed and studied on the articulator.)

An important consideration in adjusting the length of the maxillary occlusion rim to meet the vertical dimension of occlusion is that the anterior length of the occlusion rim should be maintained if at all possible because the anterior length and fullness of the rim that have been established represent the position and length of the maxillary anterior teeth. To maintain this occlusal rim length, it is usually necessary to reduce the height of the lingual, or palatal, aspect of the anterior portion of the occlusion rim so that the lower anterior teeth may close sufficiently to reach the required vertical dimension of occlusion. This establishes the amount of vertical and horizontal overlap of the anterior teeth that will be required in the completed denture, which will be an important factor in the selection of the posterior occlusion (Fig. 19-21).

When the mandibular anterior teeth and the mandibular occlusion rim contact the maxillary occlusion rim simultaneously at the vertical dimension of occlusion, the centric jaw relation record can be made.

The correct vertical dimension of occlusion should be verified before the jaw relation is recorded. The simplest and most reliable method of verification is observation of the closest speaking space, the space between

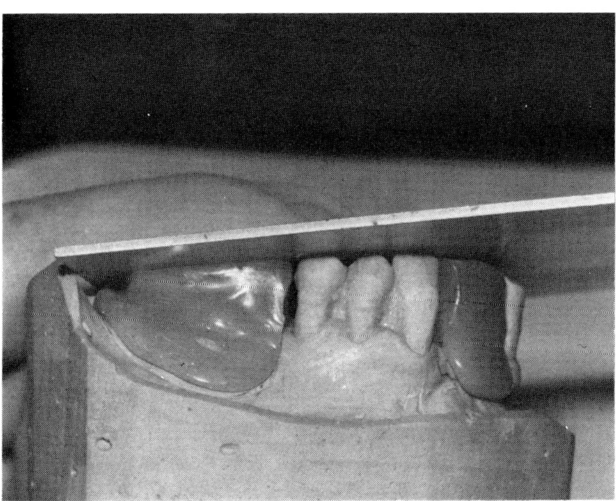

Fig. 19-17. The mandibular rim extends from cusp tips of remaining teeth posteriorly to two-thirds the height of pear-shaped pad.

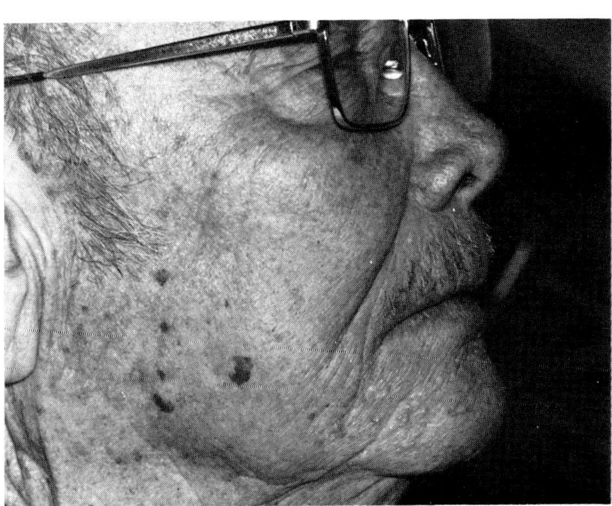

Fig. 19-18. Maxillary anterior rim is trimmed to proper length and lip support.

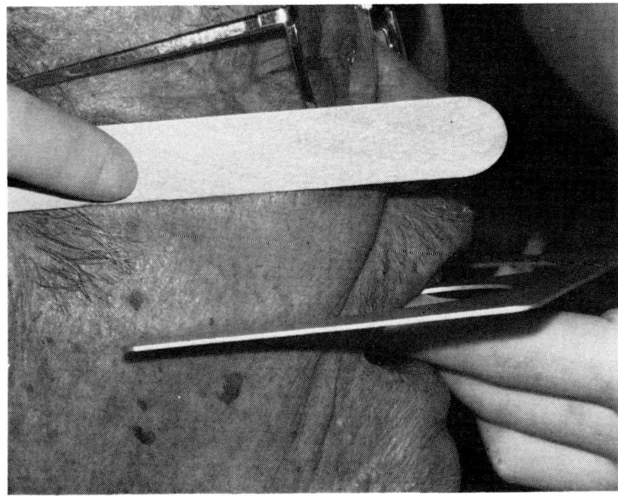

Fig. 19-19. Maxillary rim is adjusted so that it is parallel to ala-tragus line.

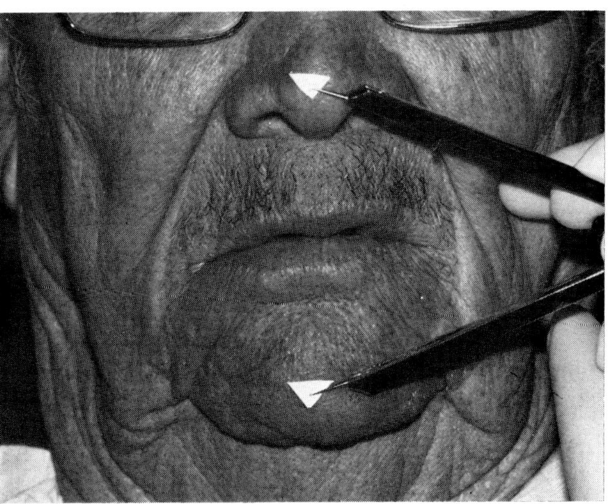

Fig. 19-20. Physiologic rest position is reduced by 2 or 3 mm to arrive at vertical dimension of occlusion.

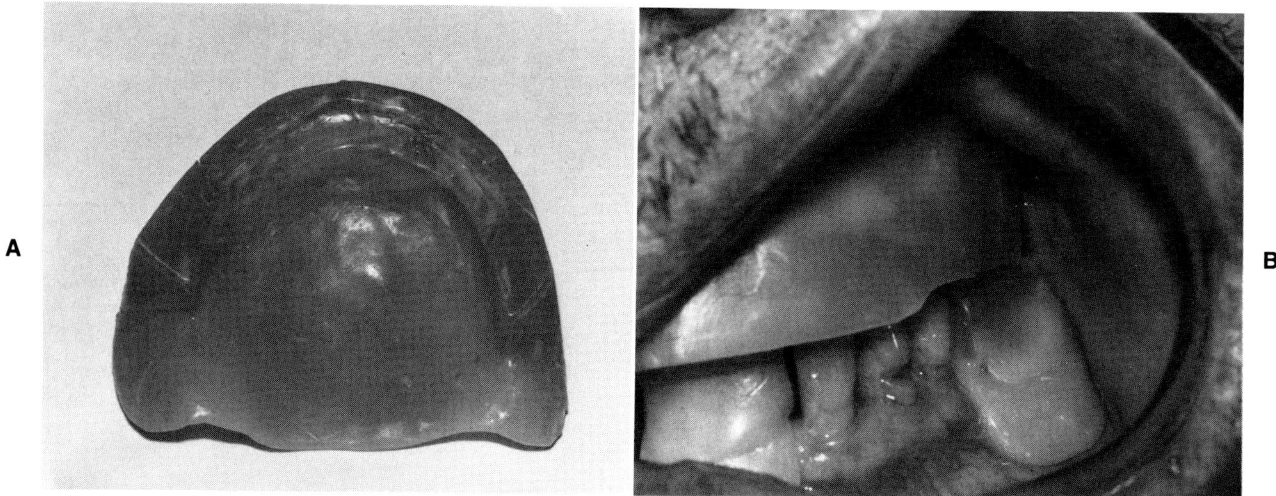

Fig. 19-21. A, Lingual portion of maxillary rim may have to be reduced in height to reach correct vertical dimension of occlusion without losing proper anterior length of rim. **B,** Reducing lingual portion of maxillary rim while maintaining anterior length establishes amount of horizontal and vertical overlap anterior teeth will eventually have.

the upper and lower anterior teeth during pronunciation of a sibilant, as described by Silverman. The closest speaking space should be approximately 1 mm. The patient is asked to count to ten, and the relationship of the mandibular teeth to the maxillary occlusion rim is observed. The closest relationship will occur as six and seven are spoken. Contact should not take place.

Recording the jaw relation. Several V-shaped notches are prepared in the surface of the mandibular occlusion rim. The notches should be at least 2 to 3 mm deep and 2 to 3 mm wide. A light coating of a lubricant, petrolatum, is placed over the surface of the occlusion rim.

The surface of the maxillary occlusion rim is prepared by drying with the air syringe. It is also helpful if a series of small holes are made in the surface of the wax with the pointed end of a No. 7 wax spatula. These holes will act as a retention device for the recording medium that will be added. The holes must not change the vertical dimension of occlusion.

A smooth mix of the zinc oxide–eugenol impression paste is made according to the manufacturer's directions. The mix is spread as an even coating 2 to 3 mm thick over the surface of the prepared maxillary occlusion rim (Fig. 19-22). The rim and baseplate are placed in the mouth, and the mandible is guided to its terminal hinge closure, centric jaw relation. Light contact between the mandibular teeth and rim and the maxillary rim must be maintained until the paste has set.

After the material has set, the mandible is teased open, still on the terminal hinge. The surface of the jaw relation record should be examined for clarity and for evidence of no excess pressure. Excess pressure would be shown by indentations of the mandibular teeth or occlusion rim into the maxillary rim. If the record is acceptable, it should be trimmed to expose only the occlusal surfaces of the mandibular rim with the notches and the incisal edges of the anterior teeth.

Completing the diagnostic mounting. The maxillary cast should be mounted on a semiadjustable articulator with a face-bow transfer to relate the cast to the condyles of the articulator. The use of a third point of reference for the face-bow transfer is helpful for correct positioning of the anterior teeth. (See Chapter 6.)

The mandibular cast is mounted on the articulator by using the centric jaw relation record. The casts are now related to each other and to the condyles of the articulator as the patient's jaws are related to each other. The casts can now be analyzed and a treatment plan formulated (Fig. 19-23).

Treatment planning. Following the second appointment, when all the diagnostic data have been gathered and the mounted diagnostic casts are available for study, the final treatment plan is formulated (Fig. 19-24).

Before any restorative work is begun, the mandibular diagnostic cast *must* be surveyed and designed. If teeth are to be extracted, they should be cut off the cast before the design is made.

Consideration should be given to all factors influencing the design of the framework as the treatment for the remaining teeth is planned.

Any required extractions or periodontal therapy should be scheduled as early as possible.

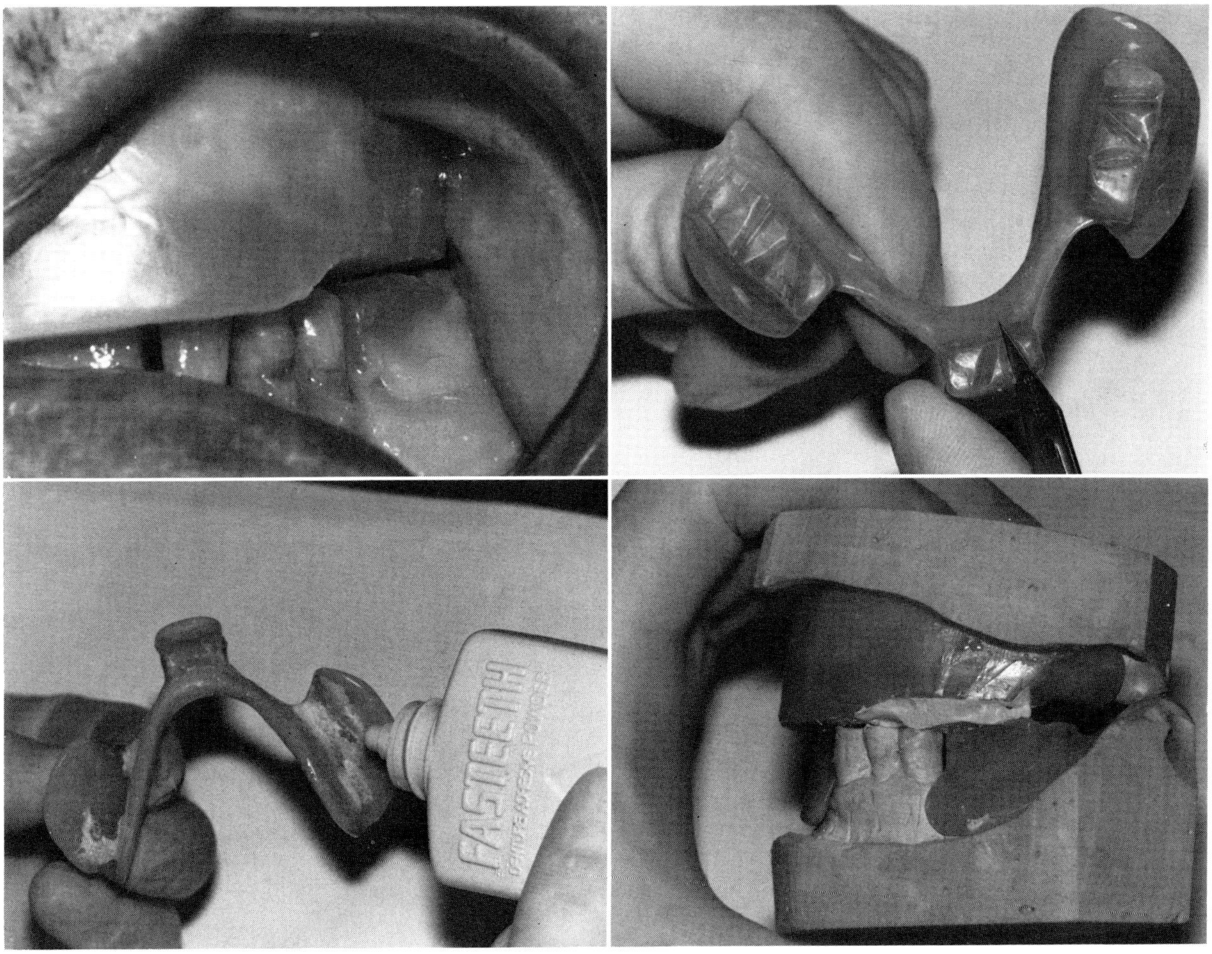

Fig. 19-22. A, Posterior section of occlusion rims do not contact at correct vertical dimension of occlusion. Small space should be present. Vertical dimension is maintained by anterior teeth contacting upper rim. **B,** Mandibular wax rim is notched. **C,** Denture adhesive may be used to stabilize either or both baseplates during recording procedure. **D,** Recording medium is placed on maxillary rim.

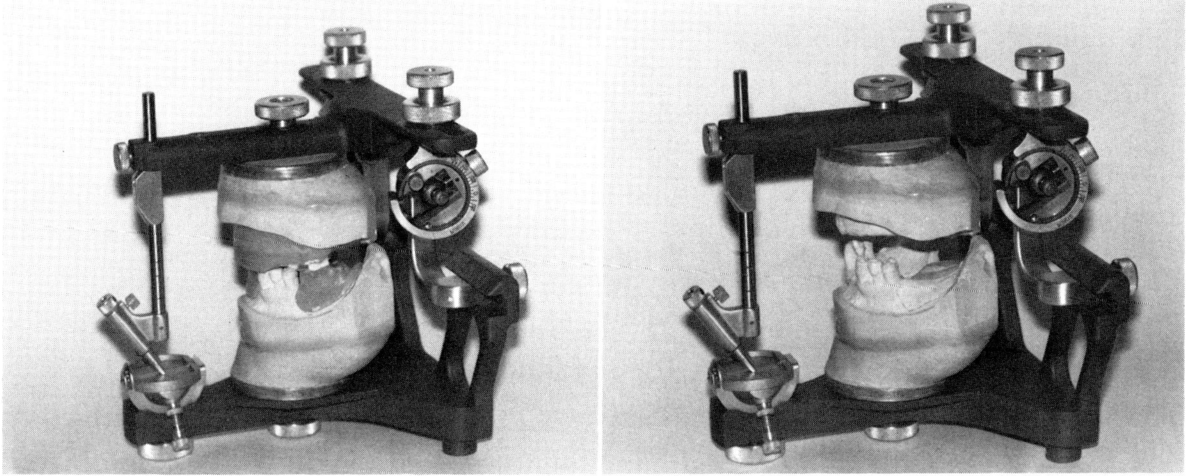

Fig. 19-23. Mounted casts can be analyzed and plan of treatment developed.

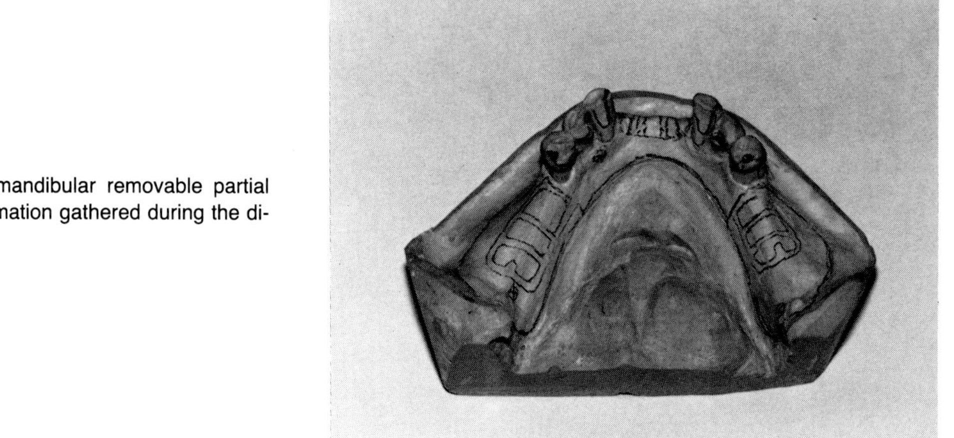

Fig. 19-24. Survey and design for mandibular removable partial denture are completed by using information gathered during the diagnostic phase.

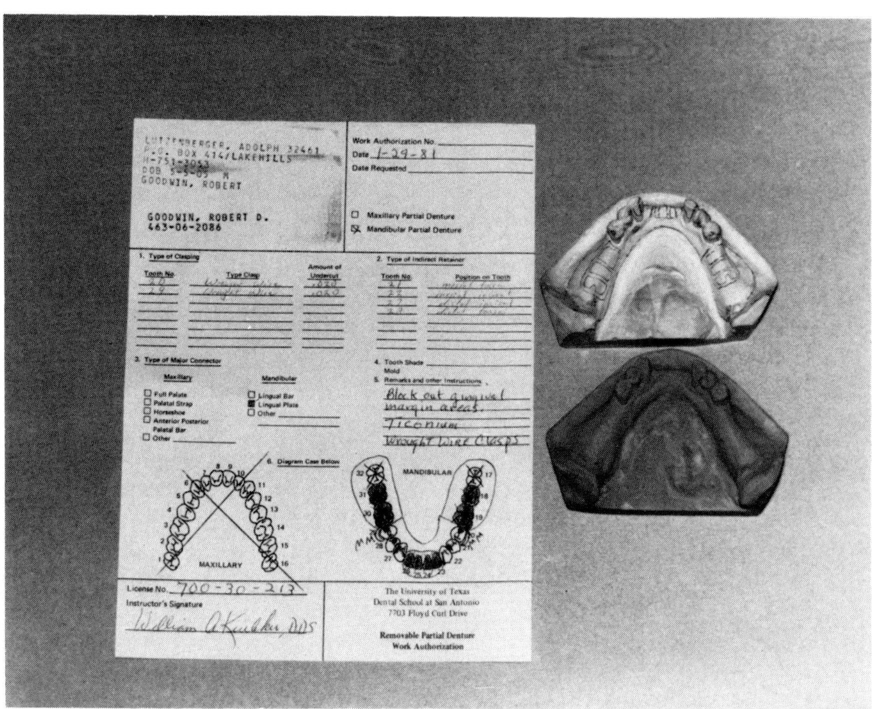

Fig. 19-25. Work authorization order, design cast, and master cast are forwarded to laboratory for construction of framework.

Appointment 3—mouth preparation and final impression for removable partial denture

This appointment is scheduled following completion of all preparatory work, including surgery, periodontal treatment, and restorative dentistry. The steps to be accomplished in this third appointment are (1) completion of mouth preparation on the remaining natural teeth, (2) making of final impressions with irreversible hydrocolloid, (3) pouring of the master cast in minimal expansion improved dental stone by using the two-pour technique, (4) trimming and inspecting the master cast, and (5) forwarding the master cast, design cast, and written work authorization order to the laboratory (Fig. 19-25).

Appointment 4—final maxillary impression

To conserve time, the final maxillary complete denture impression can be made while the laboratory is constructing the framework (Fig. 19-26).

A standard text on complete denture construction

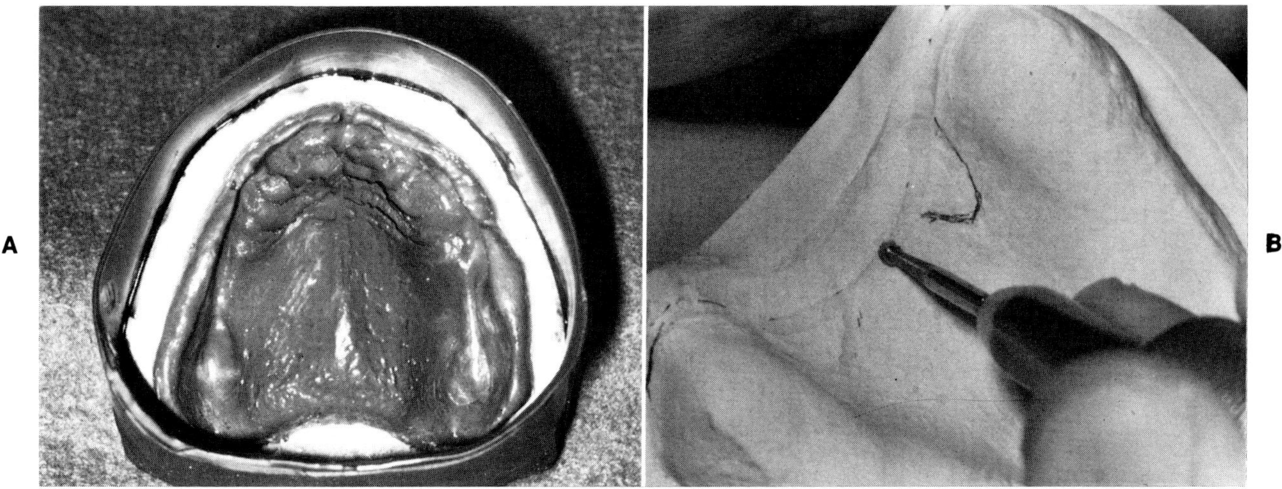

Fig. 19-26. A, Maxillary edentulous impression is made, boxed, and poured while framework is being constructed. B, Posterior palatal seal is prepared in master cast.

should be consulted for details on accomplishing an accurate impression. A number of techniques can yield acceptable results if attention is paid to details. The student should not fall prey to the idea that a special tray, a special material, or a short course will resolve problems caused primarily by lack of experience. Only diligent work, repetition, and time will overcome these problems.

Appointment 5—framework try-in and corrected cast impression

Before this appointment the framework received from the laboratory must be inspected and analyzed to make certain that the instructions to the laboratory were carried out and that the quality of construction is commensurate with good patient treatment.

The framework is tried in with disclosing wax. Minor discrepancies in the metal are eliminated and the fit of the framework to the teeth is refined (Fig. 19-27).

If time is available, a mandibular corrected cast impression is made with the material indicated for that patient, usually zinc oxide–eugenol paste or polysulfide rubber impression material (Fig. 19-28).

Appointment 6—jaw relation records and posterior tooth selection

Before this appointment an accurately fitting baseplate and occlusion rim should be constructed on the maxillary cast and baseplates should be attached to the framework made on the corrected mandibular master cast.

The mandibular occlusion rim is contoured so that its height is even with the remaining teeth and two-thirds that of the pear-shaped pad and so that it is centered over the edentulous ridge. Any necessary alterations in the height and position of the occlusal plane (realized following the diagnostic mounting procedure) should be made at this time.

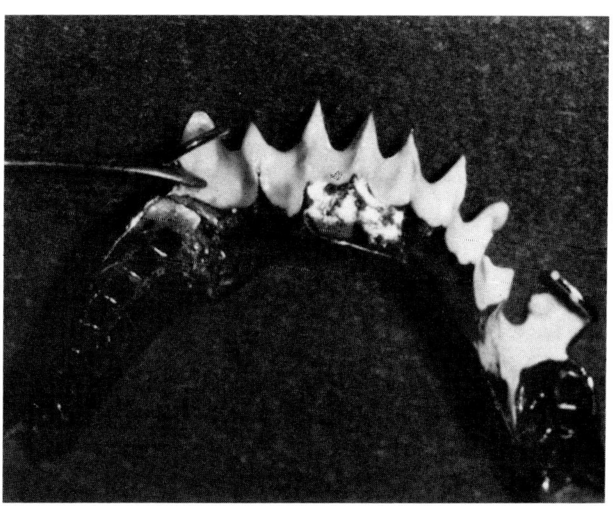

Fig. 19-27. Fit of framework is refined with disclosing wax.

After the labial surface of the maxillary rim has been contoured for lip support and lip length, the posterior height of the rim is reduced until the accepted vertical dimension is reached. It will usually be necessary to reduce the height of the lingual portion of the anterior occlusion rim to allow the lower anterior teeth to clear the previously established length of the upper rim. This technique and the reason for it are included in the discussion of the second clinical appointment for the combination dentures.

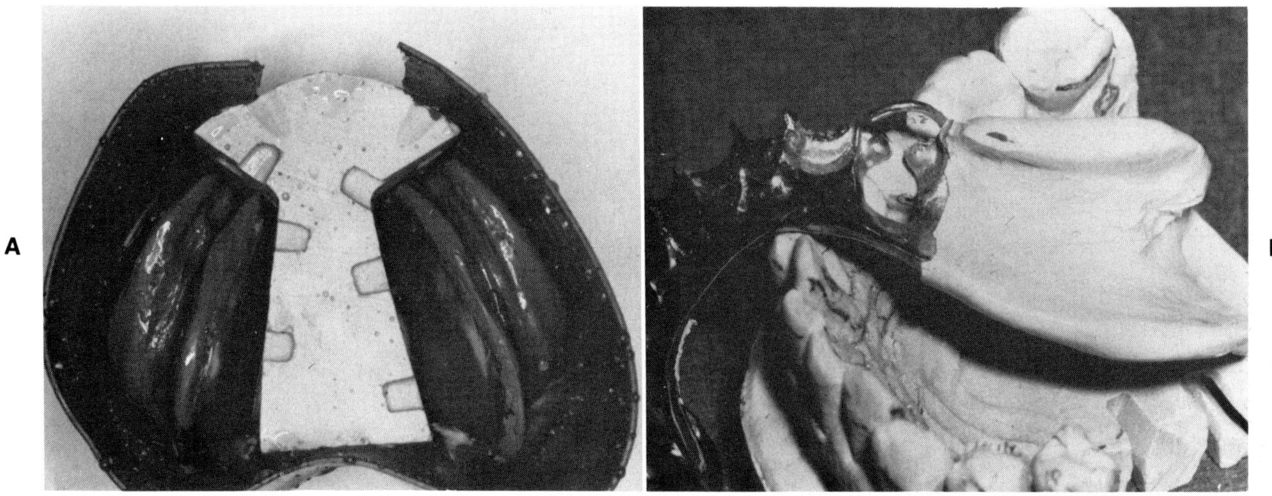

Fig. 19-28. Mandibular corrected cast impression may be made in polysulfide rubber impression material if edentulous ridge is undercut, **A,** or in zinc oxide–eugenol impression material, **B.**

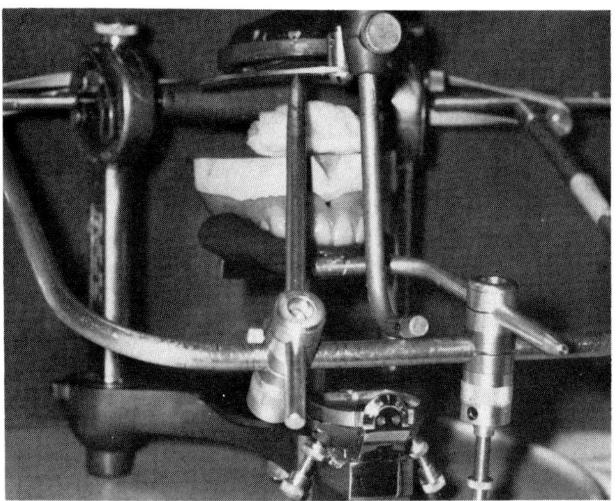

Fig. 19-29. Maxillary cast is mounted on articulator by using face-bow transfer if anatomic posterior denture teeth are planned.

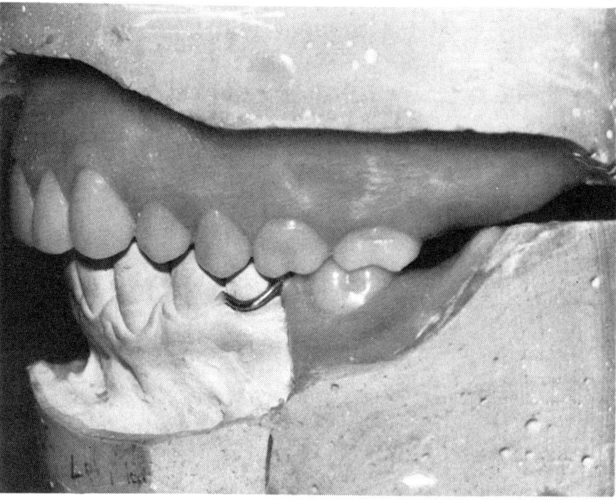

Fig. 19-30. Plastic posterior anatomic teeth are generally used in combination dentures. Note planned horizontal and vertical overlap of anterior teeth.

A face-bow fork is attached to the maxillary occlusion rim, and a face-bow transfer of the maxillary cast to the articulator is made if anatomic posterior teeth are to be used. If nonanatomic teeth are planned, the face-bow transfer is not necessary and the maxillary cast is arbitrarily mounted on the articulator (Fig. 19-29).

A centric jaw relation record is made to mount the mandibular cast to the maxillary cast on the articulator. If all the mandibular posterior teeth are missing, the recording medium may be placed on the lower rim and the upper rim indexed. If not enough lower teeth are missing to provide a long enough platform for a stable record, the recording medium may be placed over the surface of the entire maxillary rim and the lower rim indexed. This will include a record of the incisal edges of the anterior teeth as well as the indexed occlusion rim.

Posterior tooth selection. The shade of the remaining natural teeth must be taken, preferably in natural light. The shade of the replacement teeth must match as closely as possible that of remaining teeth.

The size of the artificial teeth to be used must be harmonious with the natural teeth. The bizygomatic width may be taken and the width of the maxillary cen-

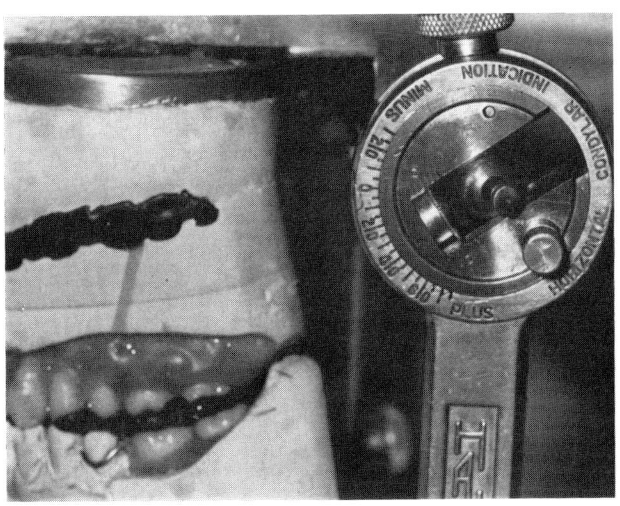

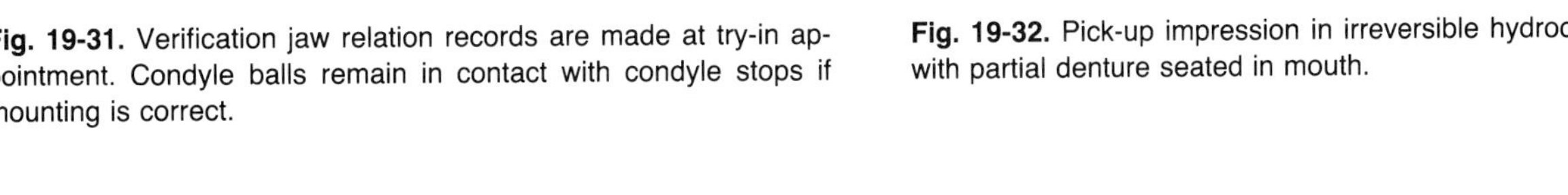

Fig. 19-31. Verification jaw relation records are made at try-in appointment. Condyle balls remain in contact with condyle stops if mounting is correct.

Fig. 19-32. Pick-up impression in irreversible hydrocolloid is made with partial denture seated in mouth.

tral incisors calculated, and this measurement used to begin tooth selection. A wider or narrower tooth may be substituted if the original measurement is not satisfactory.

Acrylic resin or plastic anatomic posterior teeth are used in most combination dentures (Fig. 19-30). The plastic teeth can best be adapted to the partial denture framework.

When all posterior teeth are replaced and adequate interridge distance is present, porcelain anatomic teeth can be used. They are considered to be more efficient than plastic, but more subject to breakage.

Occasionally when all posterior teeth are being replaced and when the vertical overlap of the anterior teeth is minimal, nonanatomic, or zero-degree, occlusion may be used. Care must be taken not to build in anterior interferences.

Perhaps the most ideal occlusal scheme can be developed by using opposing gold occlusal surfaces. (See Chapter 11.)

Appointment 7—esthetic try-in and jaw relation verification

By using phonetics, appearance, and measurements for free-way space, the vertical dimension of occlusion is checked. If it is incorrect, the posterior teeth of one denture are removed and replaced by a wax occlusion rim and the vertical dimension is increased or decreased as required.

If this corrective step is necessary, another appointment will be required to verify the jaw relation. If the vertical dimension of occlusion is acceptable, the next step is to verify the centric jaw relation (Fig. 19-31).

After the vertical dimension of occlusion and the centric jaw relation have been verified, the esthetic quality of the denture must be considered. The patient must be given the opportunity to observe the appearance of the dentures in as natural a setting as possible. Having a member of the family or a friend present to assure the patient of the favorable appearance of the dentures may do much to allay future problems. It is helpful, though not necessarily legally binding, if the patient signs an agreement as to the esthetic quality of the dentures.

Following this appointment the dentures are processed. Before decasting, the processing error must be corrected on the articulator.

Appointment 8—delivery of dentures

Pressure-indicating paste is painted on the tissue surface of the dentures and the dentures seated in the mouth. The areas of excessive pressure are corrected.

Remount casts for both dentures are constructed. For the maxillary complete denture the ridge area is blocked out with wet toweling or plasticene, and a cast is poured. The peripheries of the denture must be clearly defined in the cast.

With the partial denture seated in the mouth, a pick-up impression is made with irreversible hydrocolloids (Fig. 19-32). The partial denture must be seated in the impression when the remount cast is poured.

Undercuts in the denture base should be blocked out with baseplate wax or plasticene before the cast is poured.

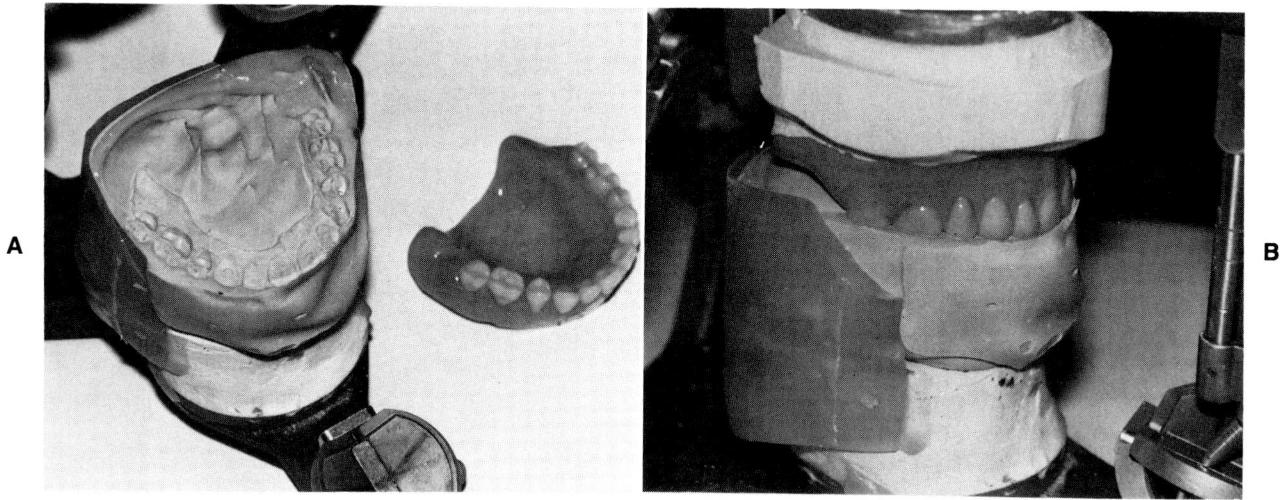

Fig. 19-33. If occlusal index was made from previous face-bow mounting, A, denture is seated in index and remounted on articulator, B. Otherwise, face-bow transfer is used to remount denture.

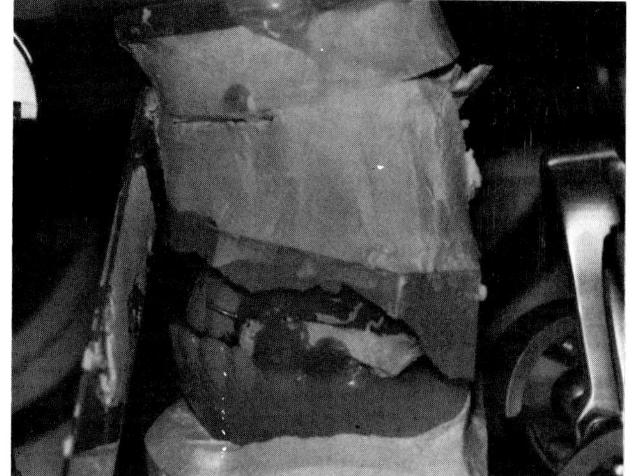

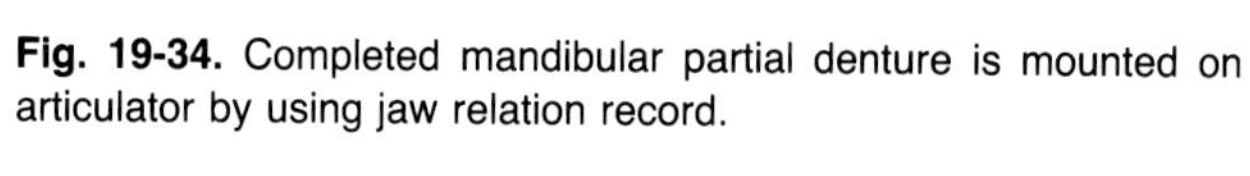

Fig. 19-34. Completed mandibular partial denture is mounted on articulator by using jaw relation record.

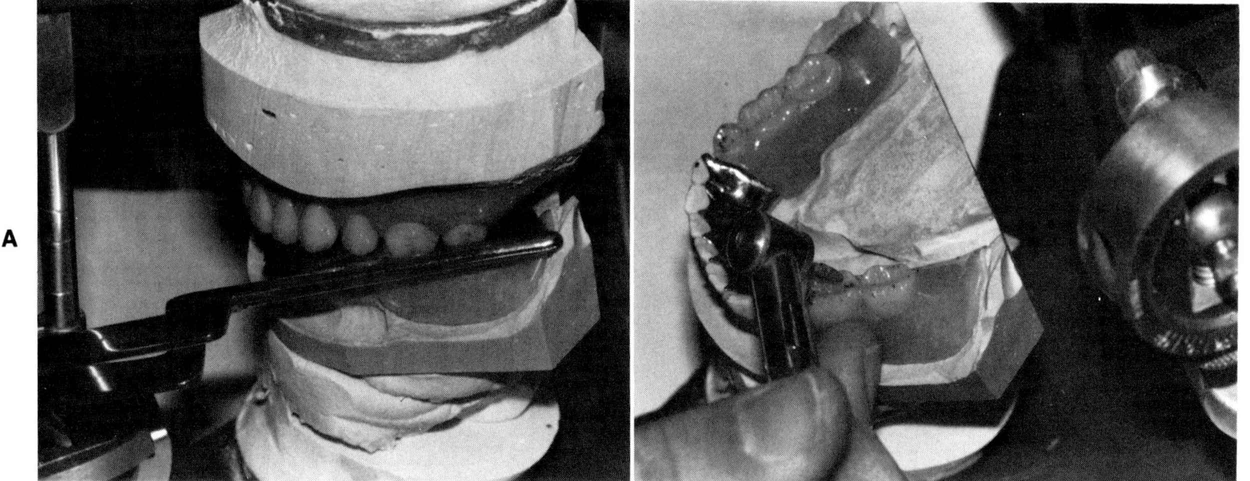

Fig. 19-35. A, Occlusal interferences are located by using articulating paper or ribbon held in a forceps. B, Corrections are made with mounted points.

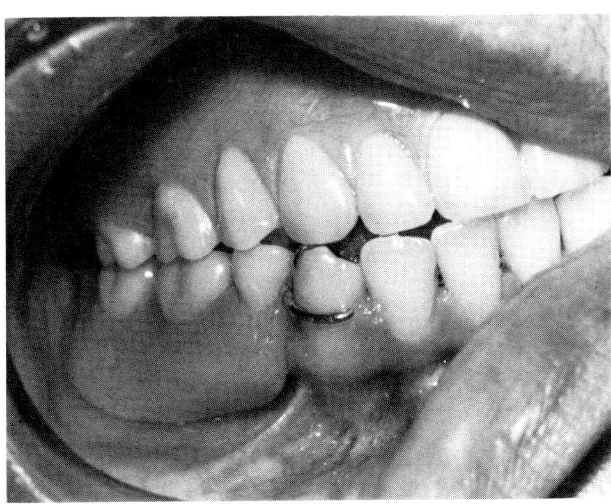

Fig. 19-36. Harmony in occlusion must be obtained before treatment can be considered successful.

The maxillary denture is mounted on the articulator by a face-bow transfer or by using an occlusal index that was made before the processed denture was removed from the cast and the articulator (Fig. 19-33).

A wax centric jaw relation record is made, and the mandibular partial denture and cast are mounted on the articulator (Fig. 19-34).

The mounting is verified by another centric jaw relation record. One must not proceed until the mounting is verified.

The occlusion is corrected and refined in both centric and eccentric positions (Figs. 19-35 and 19-36).

The patient should be instructed on home care of the prosthesis and oral hygiene.

The patient must be scheduled for a 24-hour observation appointment.

Appointment 9—postinsertion observation and adjustment

The patient's reaction to wearing the prosthesis is obtained.

The soft tissue and teeth are examined for evidence of abrasion, irritation, and excessive pressure. Any discrepancies are corrected.

Home care instructions are reinforced, and periodic maintenance and examination are arranged with the patient.

REFERENCES

Kelly, E.: Changes caused by a mandibular removable partial denture opposing a maxillary complete denture, J. Prosthet. Dent. **27**:140-150, 1972.

Silverman, M.M.: The Speaking Method in measuring vertical dimension, J. Prosthet. Dent. **3**:193-199, 1953.

BIBLIOGRAPHY

Oesterling, B.O.: Complete dentures opposite partial dentures: diagnostic factors, J. Am. Dent. Assoc. **63**:611-617, 1961.

Saunders, T.R., and others: The maxillary complete denture opposing the mandibular bilateral distal-extension partial denture: treatment considerations, J. Prosthet. Dent. **41**:124-128, 1979.

Spee, F.G.: The gliding path of the mandible along the skull, J. Am. Dent. Assoc. **100**:670-675, 1980, translated by Biedenbach, M.A., Hotz, M., and Hitchcock, H.P.

Tillman, E.J.: Removable partial upper and complete lower dentures, J. Prosthet. Dent. **11**:1098-1104, 1961.

Wilson, G.H.: A manual of dental prosthetics, Philadelphia, 1911, Lea and Febiger.

20 Other forms of the removable partial denture

For the most part this book describes the design, construction, and clinical appointments concerned with conventional extracoronal clasp–retained removable partial dentures. Temporary and immediate partial dentures are also discussed.

Other forms of removable partial dentures are available, and some are considered here. The basic rules of design and construction apply no matter what the reason for use.

GUIDE PLANE REMOVABLE PARTIAL DENTURES USED TO STABILIZE PERIODONTALLY WEAKENED TEETH

Indications

One important use for removable partial dentures and one that has been alluded to in the text is that of stabilizing teeth that have lost supporting bone. This form of removable partial denture differs from the normal concept of design and construction and yet still adheres to the basic design philosophy.

There have been many ways in which dental specialists and general practitioners have approached the problem of stabilizing weakened teeth. This lack of stability may have been brought about by natural destructive processes or as a result of therapy. The most definitive method of supporting these teeth is by the use of fixed periodontal prosthesis and, barring contraindications, their use should be considered the treatment plan of choice (Figs. 20-1 and 20-2). However, most people who have this problem of weakened teeth are in the fourth, fifth or sixth decade of life, and many have major medical problems that contraindicate the extensive treatment necessary for multiple fixed prostheses. Such patients and those whose dental prognosis is limited at best are of particular interest here.

Physiologically the periodontium permits a tooth to move in three different directions, vertically, mesiodistally, and buccolingually (Fig. 20-3). A number of investigators have shown that excessive lateral, or buccolingual, force is the most destructive of the directional forces. This is perhaps the principal reason why splinting with fixed prostheses is often not the answer to stabilizing weakened teeth. The fixed splint, unless it encircles nearly the entire arch, will provide increased resistance only to anteroposterior forces (Fig. 20-4). Little or no additional support is gained in a buccolingual direction. The removable partial denture, being anchored on both sides of the arch and joined together with a rigid major connector, can provide cross-arch stabilization to forces operating in a buccolingual direction (Fig. 20-5).

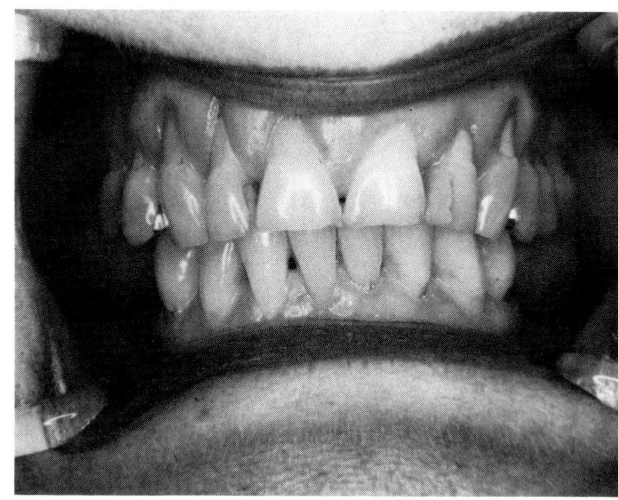

Fig. 20-1. Natural destructive processes occur when excessive forces are concentrated on few remaining teeth.

There have been many attempts to correlate the amount of tooth movement with periodontal health (Fig. 20-6). In all reported cases in which the splint-type guide plane removable partial denture (Fig. 20-7) has been worn, mobility of the teeth has remained the same or decreased. The basic concept in stabilizing weakened teeth is that the teeth must be held completely rigid. If any movement is allowed, an increase in mobility is to be expected.

Design

When the status of periodontally weakened teeth is evaluated, the following factors should be considered: (1) how the teeth can be protected from insult caused by continuous or intermittent movement, (2) how the

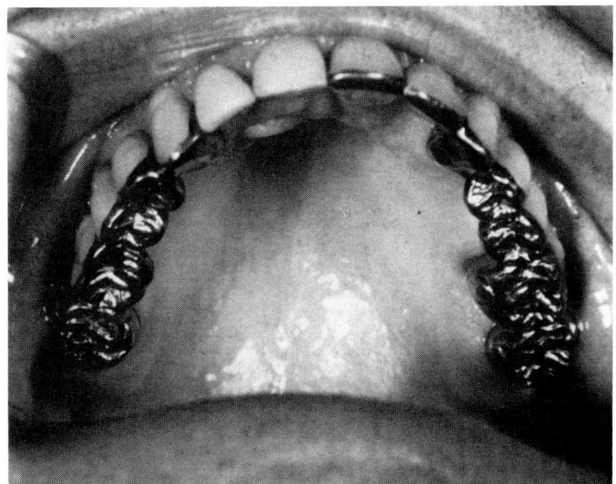

Fig. 20-2. Periodontally weakened teeth supported by fixed restorations.

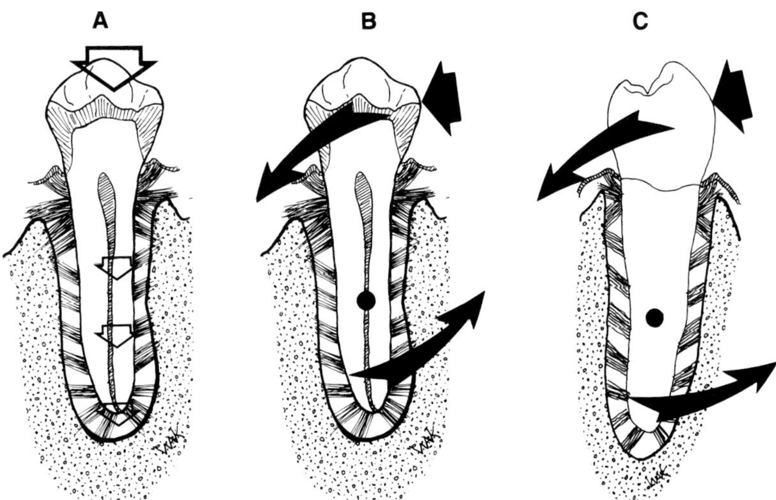

Fig. 20-3. Tooth may move vertically, **A,** mesiodistally, **B,** and buccolingually, **C.**

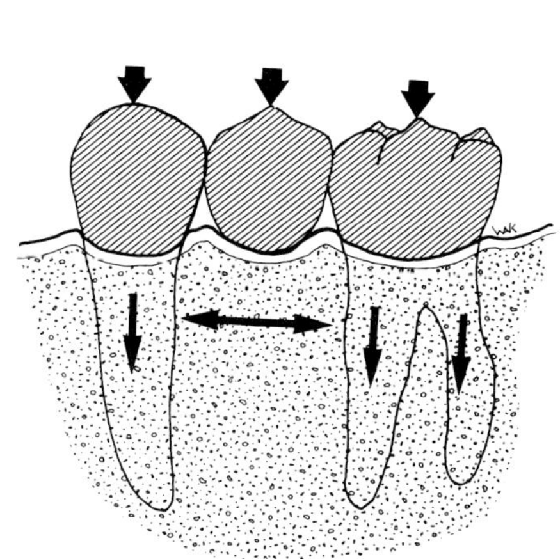

Fig. 20-4. Fixed partial denture or fixed splint provides stabilization in anteroposterior direction only (horizontal arrows).

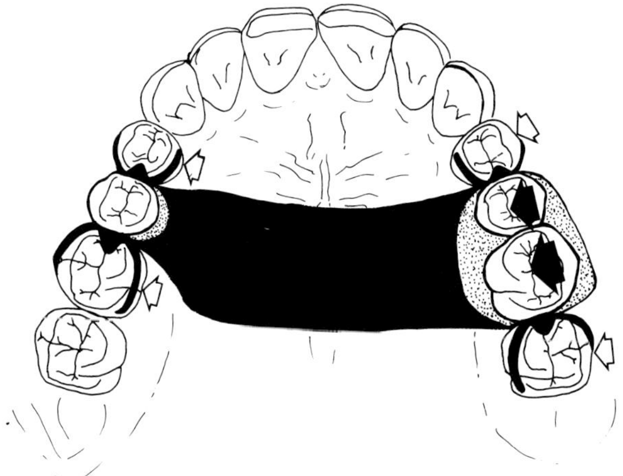

Fig. 20-5. Cross-arch stabilization is provided by removable partial denture. Occlusal forces (solid arrows) are resisted by abutment teeth on both sides of arch (open arrows) because of rigid major connector.

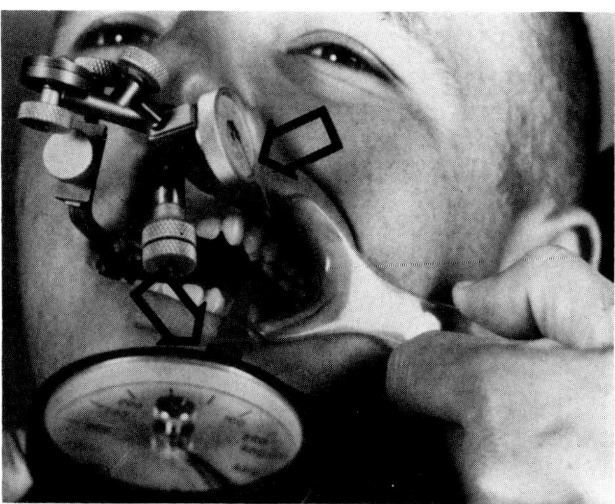

Fig. 20-6. Periodontometer (top arrow) and forcemeter (bottom arrow) are used to measure tooth mobility.

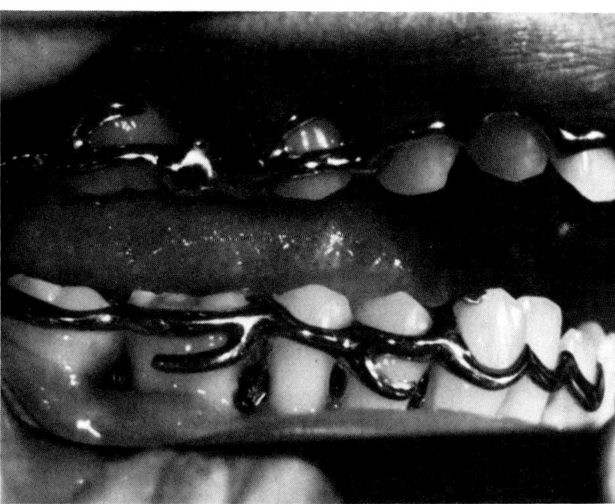

Fig. 20-7. Continuous loop removable splint rigidly supports weakened teeth.

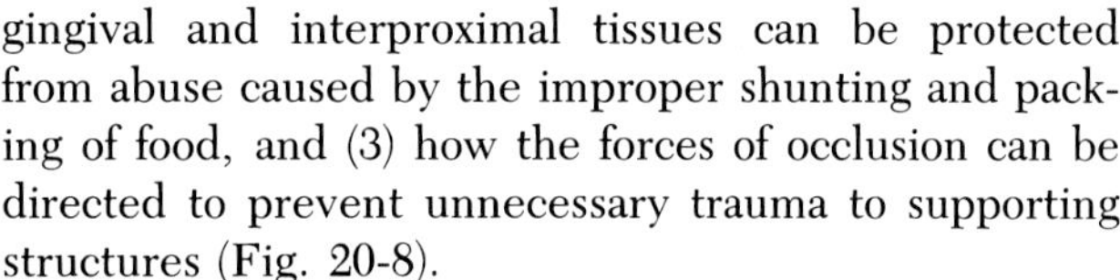

gingival and interproximal tissues can be protected from abuse caused by the improper shunting and packing of food, and (3) how the forces of occlusion can be directed to prevent unnecessary trauma to supporting structures (Fig. 20-8).

The partial denture design philosophy of broad stress distribution is the best method of obtaining the needed support for weakened teeth. The stress is distributed through the use of rigid major and minor connectors and multiple rests and clasps (Figs. 20-9 and 20-10). It must be remembered that not all clasps used will be retentive; many will be used only to prevent the tooth from being moved in a lateral, usually buccal, direction. Mouth preparation before the construction of the denture is extremely important. Periodontally weakened teeth must be supported rigidly not only when the prosthesis is in place, but also while the partial denture is being inserted and withdrawn.

It must be remembered that before a retentive clasp tip engages the largest bulge of a tooth, the reciprocating portion of that clasp, whether an arm, plate, or rest, should contact the opposite side of the tooth so that the retentive clasp tip will flex and not force the tooth to move (see Fig. 3-13). The framework should be completely passive as it lies in the mouth. Prevention of lateral pressures being distributed to supporting teeth, important in the design and construction of all removable partial dentures, becomes of critical importance in the treatment of weakened teeth because a large number of teeth, more than normal, will be contacted by the prosthesis, and multiple parallel guiding planes will be required. It may be difficult to prove that parallelism of these multiple surfaces has been achieved by mere visual inspection of the teeth. To make certain

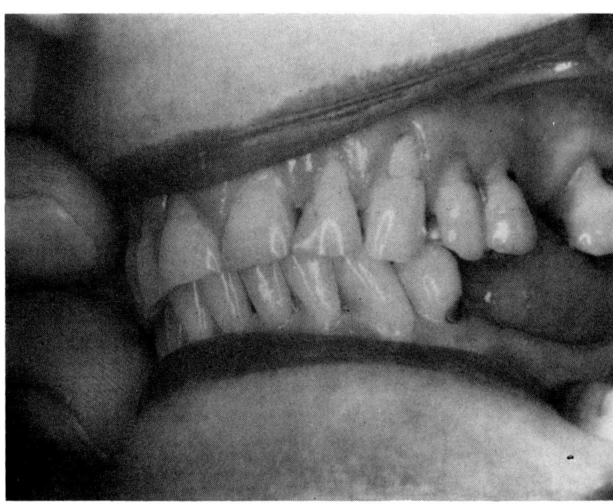

Fig. 20-8. Damage to supporting structure occurred because forces of occlusion were not distributed over wide enough area.

that the goal is being achieved or to locate surfaces that may need further correction, impressions of the arch should be made in irreversible hydrocolloid and casts poured in fast-setting artificial stone. Then these casts can be mounted on the surveyor and checked to be certain the guide planes are being developed at the proper positions. Corrections can be made at the same appointment by this technique. Although intraoral paralleling devices are available, with experience the techniques described can be accomplished effectively and accurately.

Polishing of all tooth surfaces that have been reshaped is imperative. Enamel surfaces may be highly polished with Carborundum-impregnated rubber

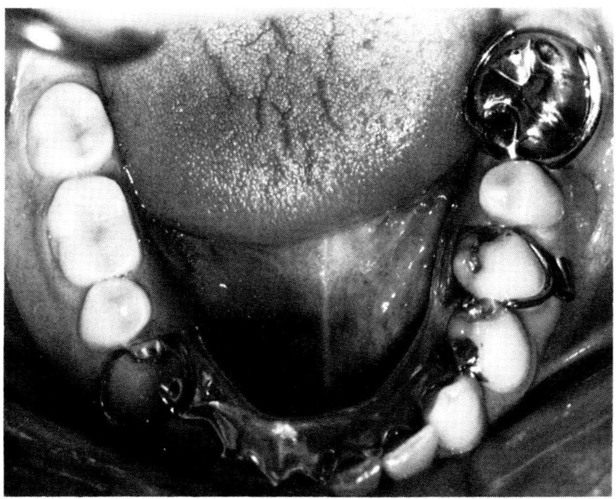

Fig. 20-9. Multiple rests and clasps are routinely designed to support periodontally weakened teeth.

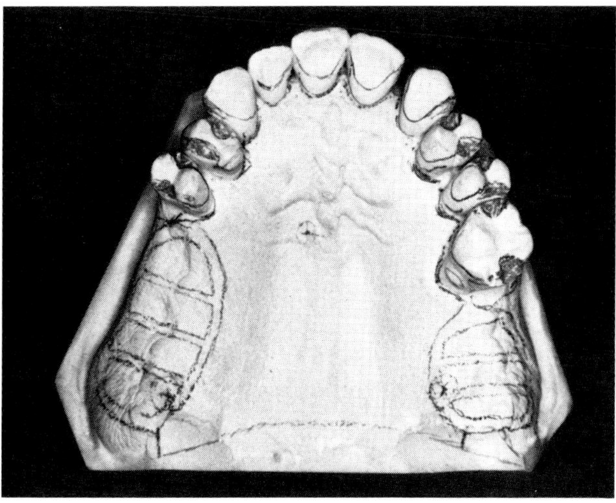

Fig. 20-10. Design for stabilizing removable partial denture follows philosophy of broad stress distribution.

wheels and points; pumice-incorporated wheels and points are not effective on enamel.

As mentioned previously, in those arches where bone loss is generalized and severe each posterior tooth should have support from both the buccal and lingual aspects. The support against movement in the buccal direction must come from buccal clasp arms. The use of multiple embrasure clasps, although not normally the most desirable form of clasping, is frequently necessary, particularly in arches where few, if any, teeth are missing. Removable splints may be made for arches with no missing teeth to provide support for the weakened teeth. Examples of this type of splint are depicted later in this chapter.

When multiple buccal clasp arms are designed, no more than two on each side of the arch should be retentive. The remainder should be rigid and designed to contact the tooth at or above the survey line (Fig. 20-11). Recontouring the buccal surfaces to lower the survey line toward the gingival attachment is extremely important to gain as much mechanical advantage against tipping forces as possible. It is also possible to gain a little esthetic value by keeping the clasps as low on the crown as possible.

If the patient under consideration for treatment is conscious of esthetics, the guide plane removable partial denture is not likely to prove satisfactory. A careful explanation should be offered to the patient that in order to maintain the natural teeth some display of metal will be necessary. Generally the only alternative to this form of treatment if the teeth have lost the majority of bony support is the complete denture, either conventional or overdenture. Esthetic qualities can be maintained or improved through the use of the complete

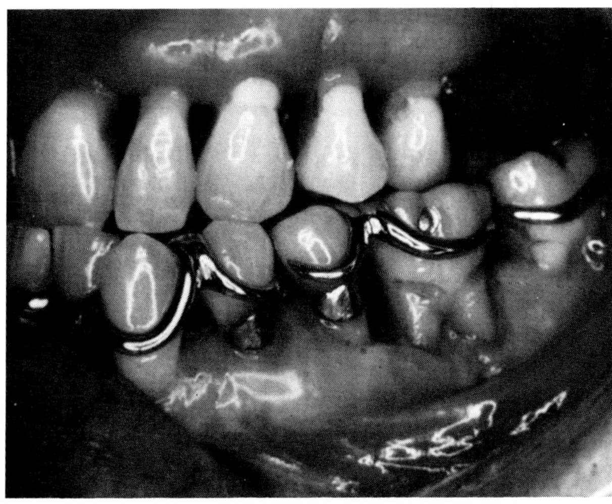

Fig. 20-11. There should never be more than two retentive buccal clasp arms on each side of arch. All other clasps must be positioned above height of contour.

denture, but the long-term prognosis for maintenance of the residual ridges is not favorable unless the overdenture concept is followed.

Role of lingual plate

Weakened anterior teeth usually will not require support from the facial surfaces. The muscular action of the lips during speech and eating is sufficient to prevent anterior migration except when tongue-thrusting habits are present or when bone loss is severe. A decision is often made to maintain mandibular anterior teeth as long as possible even when severe bone loss is present. It is possible under these conditions to prepare

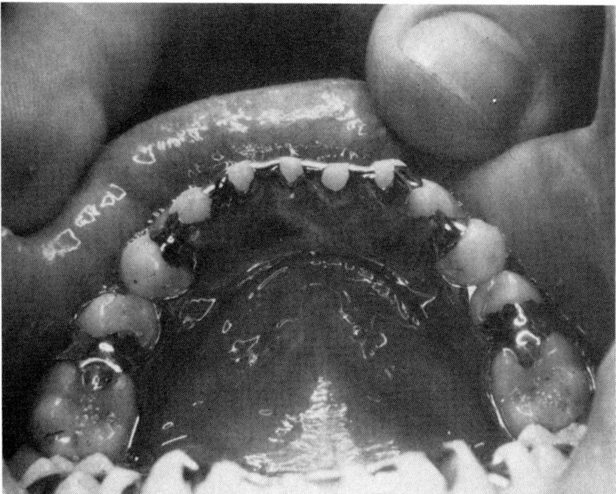

Fig. 20-12. Mesial and distal incisal rests may be used to stabilize weakened anterior teeth.

mesial and distal incisal rests on these teeth and to engage these rest seats with projections from the lingual plating (Fig. 20-12). This approach will hold these teeth extremely rigidly. (Another technique for supporting weakened anterior teeth is provided by the swing-lock partial denture, which is described later in the chapter.) The lingual plate serves as the major connector for the prosthesis and provides cross-arch stabilization as well as lingual support for the individual teeth (Fig. 20-13).

The role of the lingual plate is twofold: (1) To a major degree it contributes horizontal stability to a removable partial denture. (2) In the event that the removable partial denture is not used primarily to replace teeth but to act as a splint for the remaining natural teeth, it helps prevent the application of excessive lateral forces on the teeth.

The interproximal spaces for these weakened teeth will be larger than normal because of tissue recession around the necks of the teeth, so it is essential that the interproximal spaces lingual to the contact point be closed completely to prevent packing of food beneath the plate from an occlusal or incisal direction (Fig. 20-14). Several periodontal groups have shown that the lingual plate can perform this secondary function. When the interproximal extensions of the lingual plate are constructed properly, the design of the plate in these areas will be needle shaped and sharp (Fig. 20-15). From this pointed interproximal tip the plate should fall away to a razor-thin edge and just cover the cingulum of an anterior tooth or lie just occlusal to the largest convexity of a posterior tooth. The plate should fit the cingulum as accurately as an inlay fits its preparation. Food that passes over this portion of the lingual plate should be shunted away from the margin of the

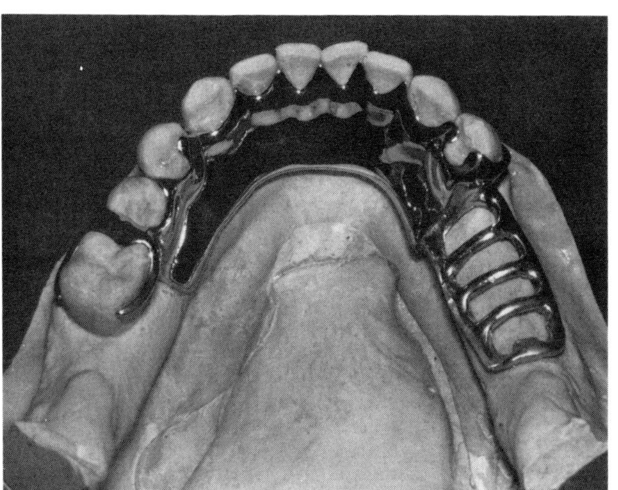

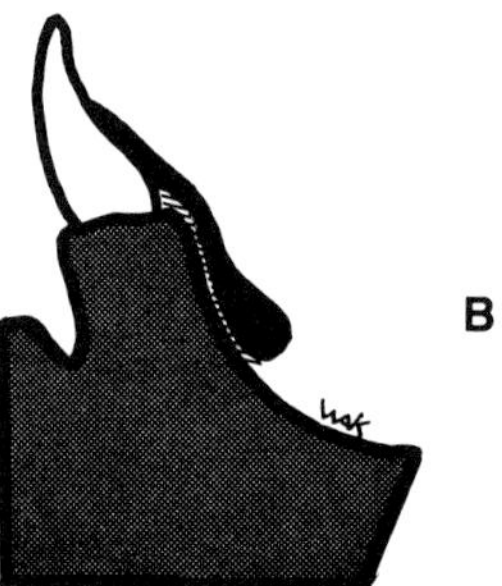

Fig. 20-13. A, Lingual plate provides cross-arch stabilization as well as support for individual teeth. B, Cross-sectional form of lingual plate major connector, consisting of half-pear shape at inferior border with thin metal plating extending onto teeth, provides excellent rigidity.

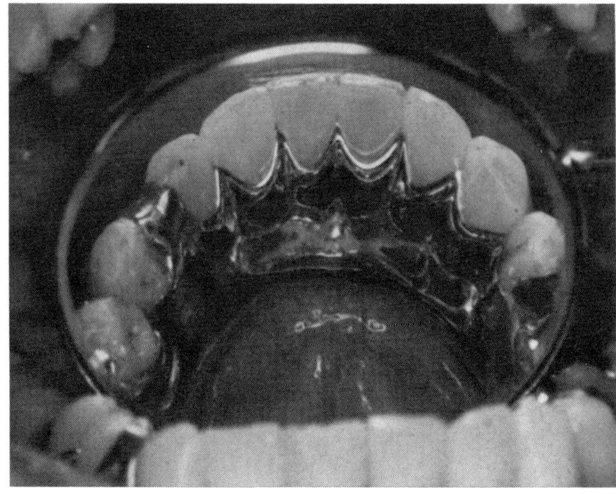

Fig. 20-14. Design of lingual plate must close interproximal spaces. Result is a scalloped appearance.

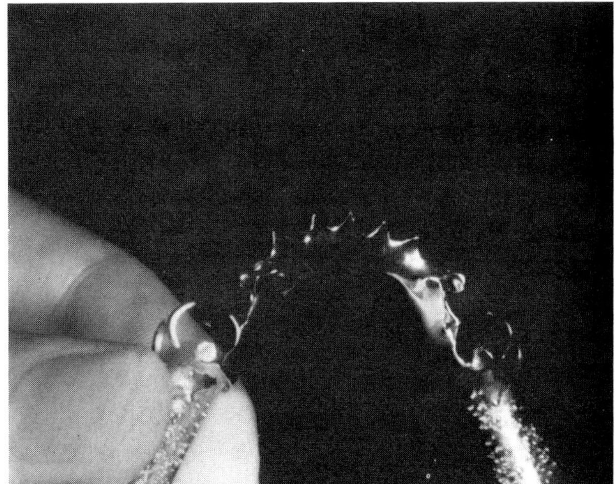

Fig. 20-15. Lingual plate in interproximal areas is needlelike with thin, sharp edges.

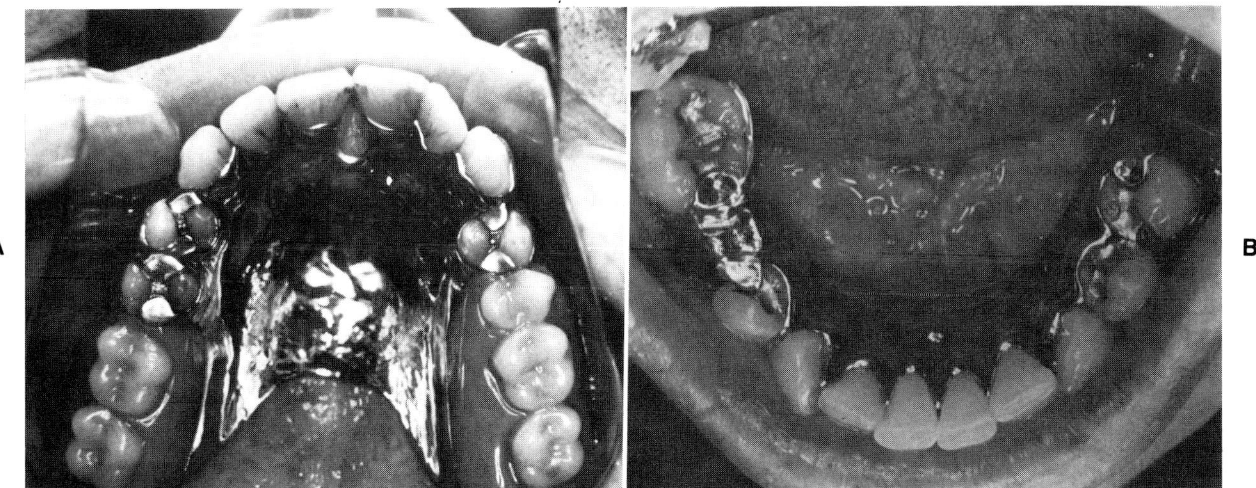

Fig. 20-16. Maxillary, **A,** and mandibular, **B,** removable partial dentures can stabilize periodontally weakened teeth.

major connector smoothly and completely. If the joint between the plate and the tooth is too thick, food and other debris will collect, increasing the difficulty of maintaining proper oral hygiene and contributing to the discomfort of the patient.

Fitting the framework

As for all removable partial dentures, it is imperative that the practitioner check the fit of the framework before completion. (This process is covered in detail in Chapter 12.)

Prognosis

The results of this form of treatment are encouraging. Clinical results have been consistently promising. Thus carefully planned, constructed, and fitted removable guide plane partial dentures can be effective in stabilizing weakened teeth (Fig. 20-16).

SWING-LOCK REMOVABLE PARTIAL DENTURES

In the swing-lock removable partial denture, first described by Dr. Joe J. Simmons in the *Texas Dental Journal* in February 1963, all or several of the remaining teeth are used to retain and stabilize the prosthesis against vertical displacement. The prosthesis consists of a hinged buccal or labial bar attached to a conventional major connector (Figs. 20-17 to 20-19). Retention and stabilization are provided by the bar.

The labial bar is generally designed with small vertical projection arms that contact the labial or buccal surfaces of the teeth gingival to the height of contour (Fig. 20-20). These vertical arms look like an I or T bar and provide both retention and stabilization for the prosthesis. The labial bar can also be designed with acrylic resin retention components (Fig. 20-21), in which case retention and stability are provided by an acrylic resin denture base attached to the labial bar. This design is

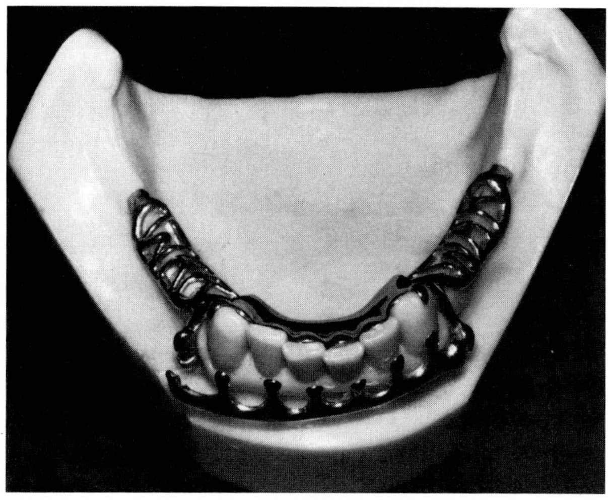

Fig. 20-17. Swing-lock removable partial denture framework with hinged labial bar.

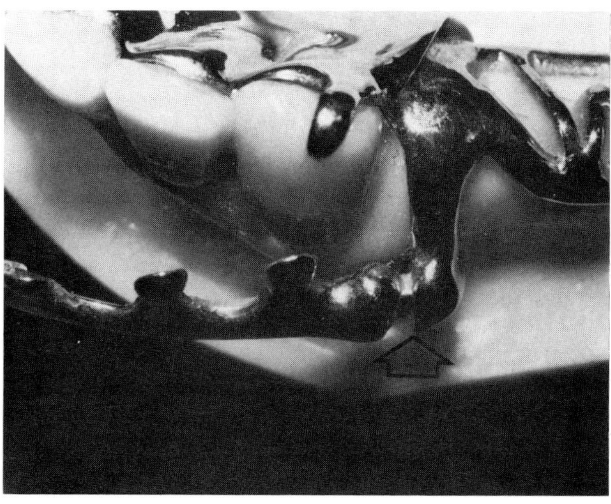

Fig. 20-18. Labial bar is attached to framework by hinge mechanism (arrow) that permits it to open and close like a gate.

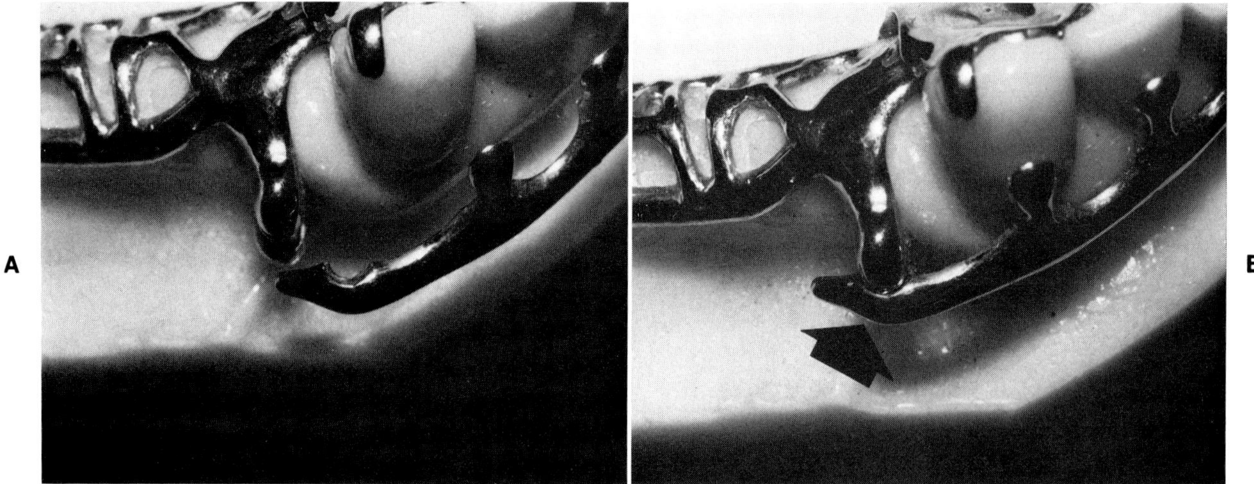

A B

Fig. 20-19. Locking mechanism in open **A**, and closed, **B**, positions.

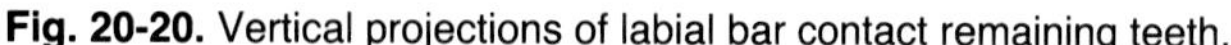

Fig. 20-20. Vertical projections of labial bar contact remaining teeth.

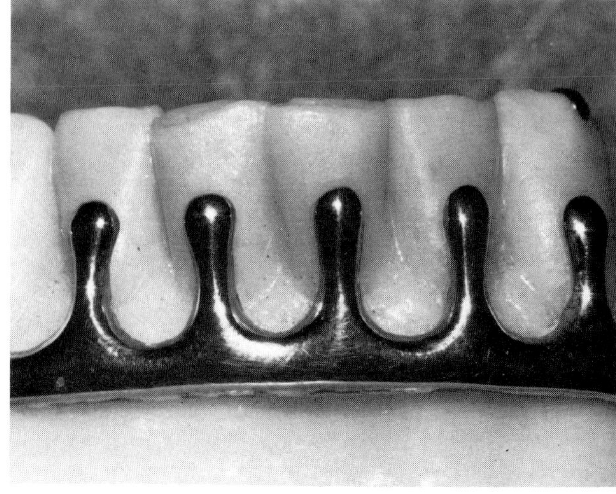

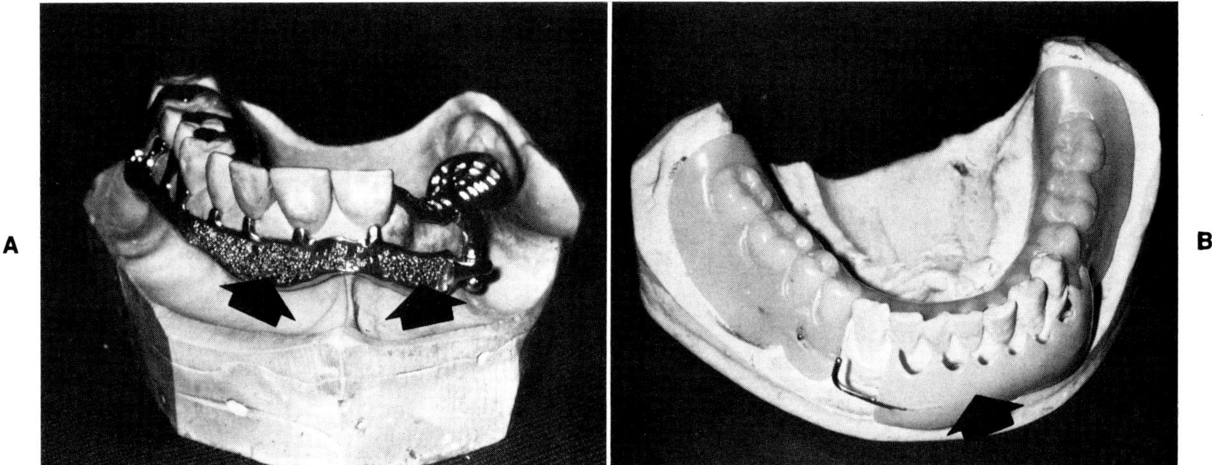

Fig. 20-21. **A,** Labial bar with bead retention (arrows) for attachment of acrylic resin gingival veneer. **B,** Acrylic resin and wire swing-lock prosthesis with labial gingival veneer (arrow). (Courtesy Dr. James Brudvik.)

used if the vertical projection bars would produce a poor esthetic result or if extensive loss of gingival tissue has occurred and a resin gingival veneer is needed to improve appearance.

Advantages

The primary advantage of the swing-lock concept of treatment is that it provides a relatively inexpensive method of using all or most of the remaining teeth for the retention and stabilization of a prosthesis. Alternatives to this type of treatment include (1) removal of the remaining teeth and (2) fixed splinting of the remaining teeth and construction of a conventional removable partial denture. The latter is relatively time consuming and expensive and presents problems if one of the splinted teeth fails. Loss of a splinted tooth could necessitate removal and reconstruction of a fixed splint, whereas a tooth can be removed and added to the major connector of a swing-lock prosthesis through a simple laboratory procedure.

Because the construction of a swing-lock removable partial denture is relatively simple and inexpensive, it can be used in situations for which more conventional types of treatment may appear hopeless.

Disadvantages

A swing-lock prosthesis can produce a relatively poor esthetic result for patients with short or extremely mobile lips. Obtaining perfect adaptation of a resin veneer is difficult because the path of insertion is dictated by the hinge movement of the labial bar.

The remaining teeth are grasped firmly by the prosthesis. A long distal extension base is likely to move toward the tissue under the forces of occlusion. This movement can tip the teeth grasped by the prosthesis (Fig. 20-22).

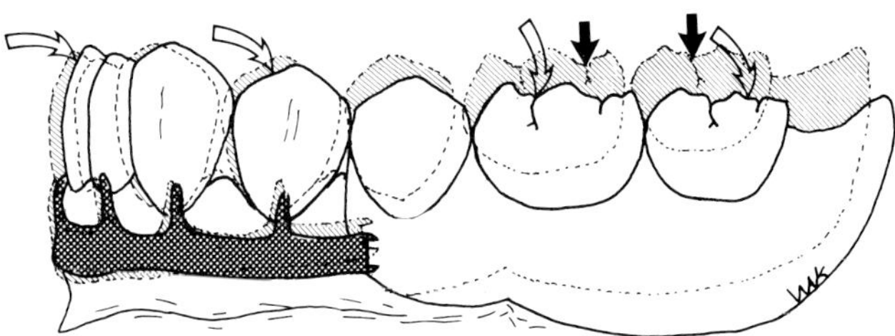

Fig. 20-22. Occlusal forces applied to swing-lock removable partial denture replacement teeth (solid arrows) can cause prosthesis to move toward tissue. Teeth contacted by prosthesis will tend to rotate distally.

Indications

There are a number of indications for use of the swing-lock design in the treatment of partially edentulous patients:

1. Too few remaining natural teeth for a removable partial denture of conventional design (Fig. 20-23)
2. Remaining teeth too mobile to serve as abutment teeth for conventional design (Fig. 20-24)
3. Position of remaining teeth not favorable for a conventional design (Fig. 20-25)
4. Retention and stabilization needed for maxillofacial prostheses such as obturators for postsurgical patients (Fig. 20-26) (see Chapter 23)
5. To retain a prosthesis for patients who have lost large segments of teeth and alveolar ridge through traumatic injury (Fig. 20-27)

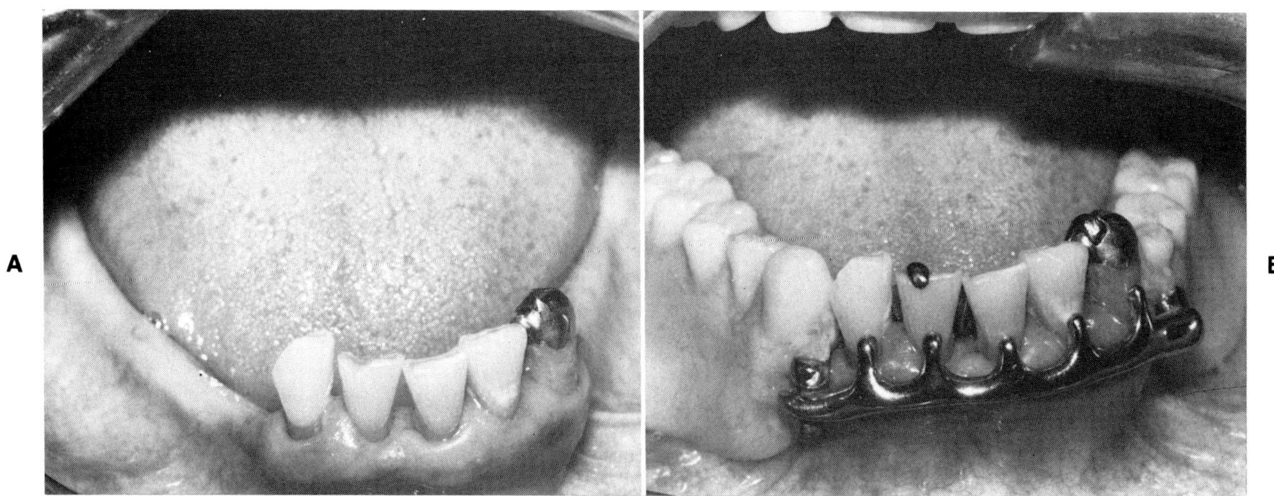

Fig. 20-23. A, Too few natural teeth remain to construct adequate conventional removable partial denture. **B,** Swing-lock partial denture in place.

Fig. 20-24. Remaining teeth exhibit mobility, contributing to poor prognosis for conventional removable partial denture.

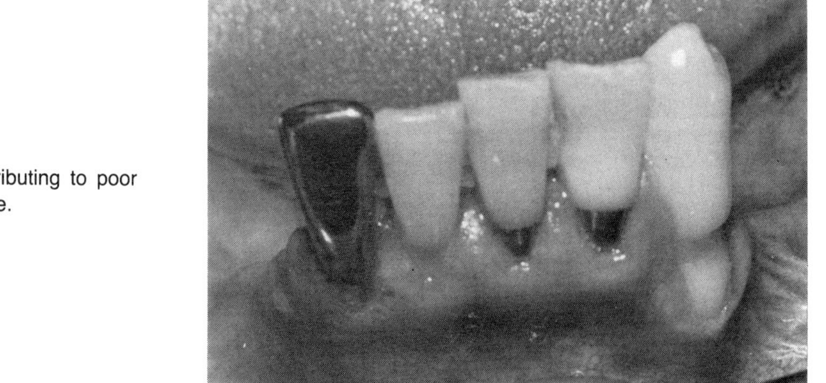

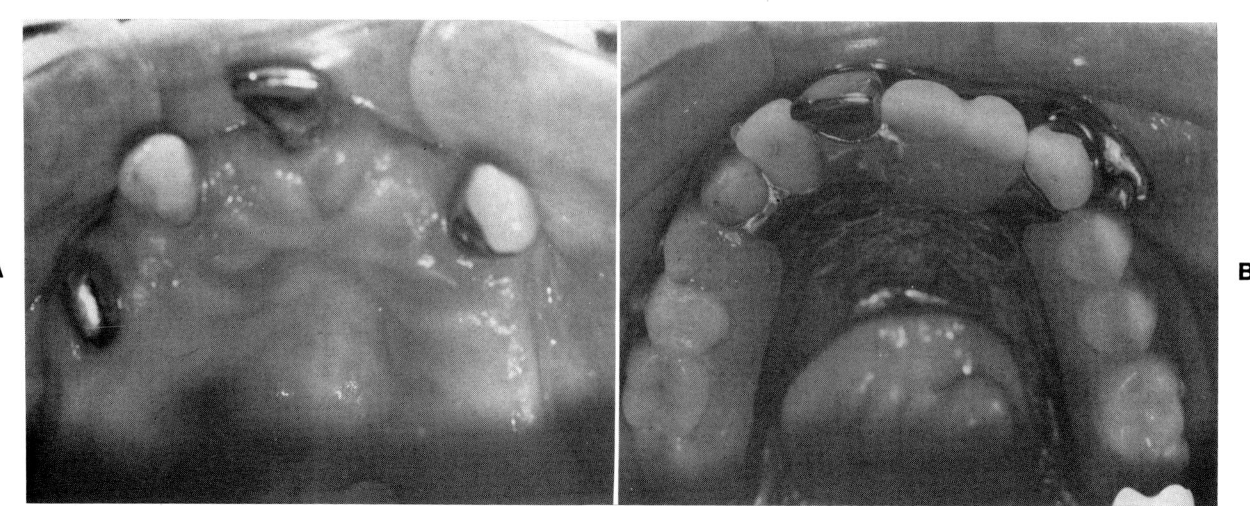

Fig. 20-25. A, Location of remaining teeth is unfavorable for design of conventional prosthesis. **B,** Swing-lock removable partial denture in place.

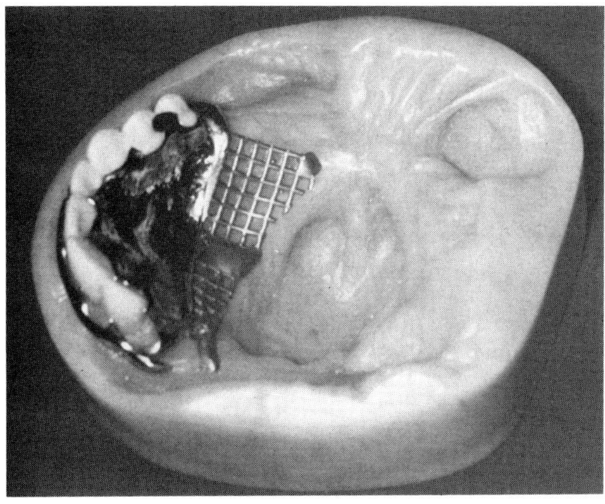

Fig. 20-26. All remaining teeth are used to support prosthesis for postsurgical patient.

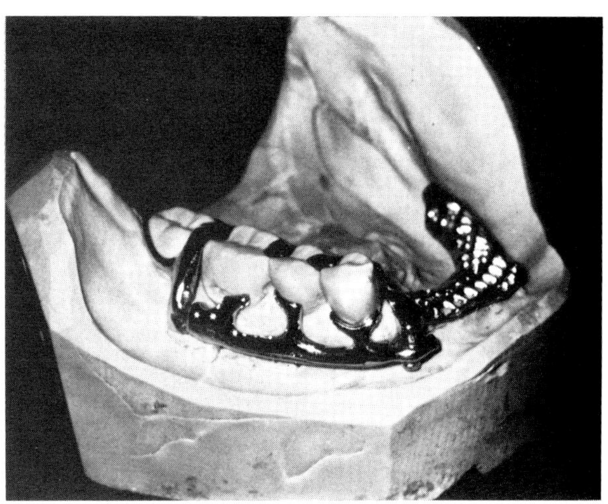

Fig. 20-27. Swing-lock denture framework for patient left with four posterior teeth on right side after automobile accident.

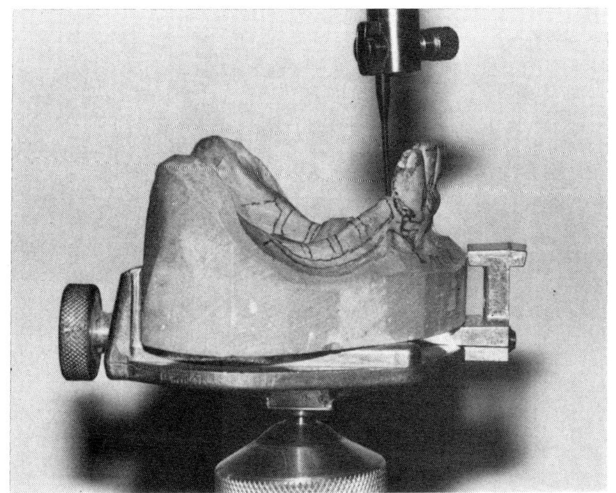

Fig. 20-28. Swing-lock prosthesis is designed with occlusal plane parallel with base of surveyor.

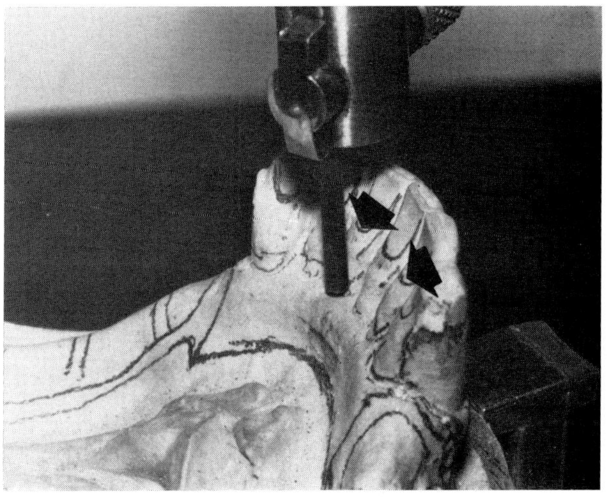

Fig. 20-29. Height of contour marked on all remaining teeth. Lingual plating must always extend above survey line (arrows).

Selection of metal for swing-lock framework

Chrome alloy is the material of choice for the metallic framework of a swing-lock removable partial denture. Gold is contraindicated because the hinge and lock mechanisms show noticeable wear in a relatively short time when gold is used and gold components must be made fairly bulky compared with chrome components to provide the necessary rigidity and strength.

Design

The path of insertion of a swing-lock prosthesis is from the lingual direction with the labial arm open. However, it is imperative that the cast be surveyed with the occlusal plane of the teeth parallel with the base of the surveyor (Fig. 20-28). Most forces applied to the prosthesis will be directed perpendicular to the occlusal plane. Survey lines are drawn on all the remaining teeth. Lingual plating is positioned above the survey line (Fig. 20-29). With the gate closed, the lingual plating and the rests in definite rest seats resist movement toward the tissue. The vertical projection extensions from the labial arm prevent occlusal movement (Fig. 20-30). All teeth contacted by the framework act collectively to prevent movement. Long distal extension bases can place tipping forces on all the teeth grasped by the prosthesis if the extension base moves toward the tissue.

The lingual plate major connector is usually the connector of choice for the mandibular arch (Fig. 20-31). A double lingual (Kennedy) bar can be used, but it has

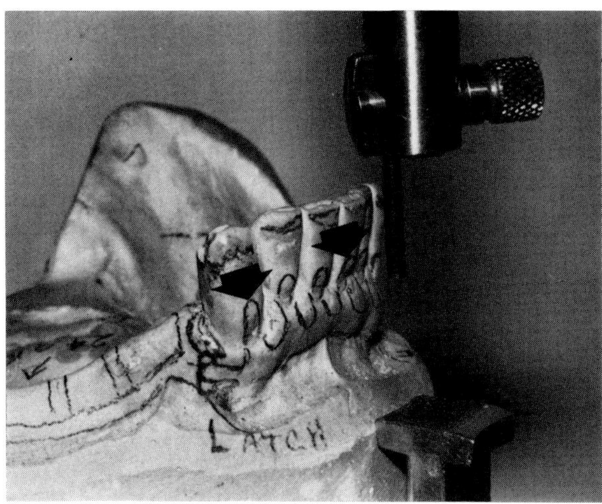

Fig. 20-30. Height of contour marked on labial surface of teeth. Vertical bar projections (arrows) must contact tooth below survey line to prevent occlusal movement of prosthesis.

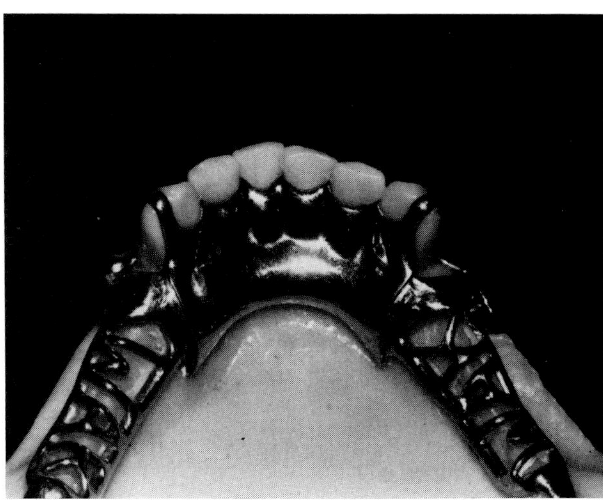

Fig. 20-31. Lingual plate is major connector of choice for mandibular swing-lock prosthesis.

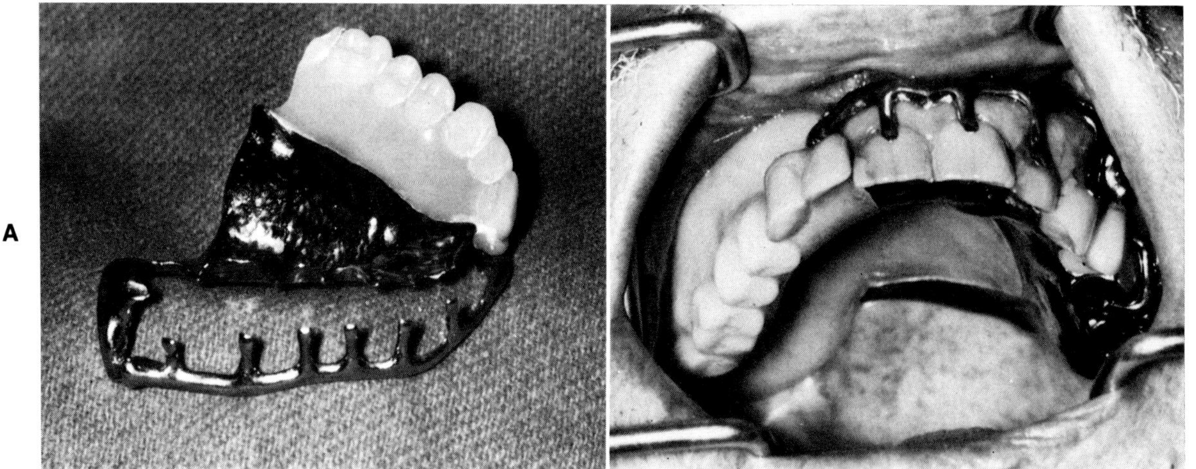

Fig. 20-32. Complete palate major connector provides most support for maxillary swing-lock removable partial denture. Connector may be constructed principally of metal, **A**, or it may be combination of resin and metal, **B**.

more disadvantages than advantages. The lingual plate major connector must be designed to provide rigidity and comfort. The active floor of the mouth is measured, and those measurements are transfered to the master cast to indicate the position of the inferior border of the major connector. The connector should be constructed with the same contour and size as a lingual bar, with lingual plating extending from the superior aspect of the bar to the correct position on the teeth. The lingual plating must be positioned above the survey line and is scalloped with extensions to the contact point areas of the teeth.

Major connectors for the maxillary arch should use as much of the palate as possible for support of the prosthesis. Full palatal coverage is generally indicated (Fig. 20-32). A closed horseshoe design can also be used if anatomic considerations or patient desires indicate the need for an opening in the palatal coverage. The remaining teeth are plated on the lingual surfaces, with the plating extending above the survey line.

The labial arm can be designed in two ways. The conventional design consists of a labial arm with I or T bar vertical projections that contact the labial or buccal surfaces of the teeth below the survey line (Fig. 20-33). An alternate approach is the use of acrylic resin retention loops on the labial arm and a processed resin ve-

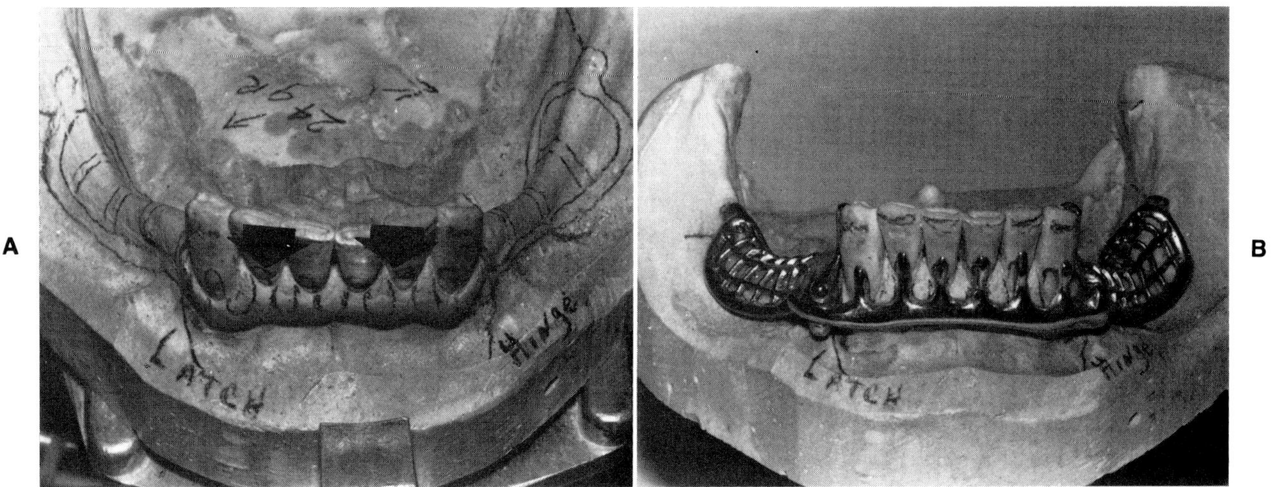

Fig. 20-33. **A,** Labial bar is designed with vertical projection bars contacting teeth below height of contour (arrows). **B,** Completed framework.

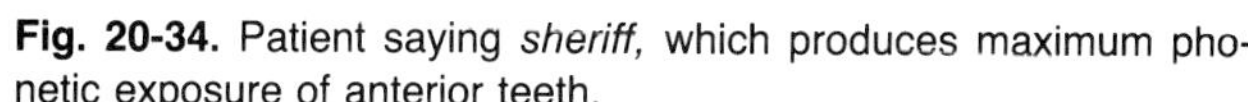

Fig. 20-34. Patient saying *sheriff,* which produces maximum phonetic exposure of anterior teeth.

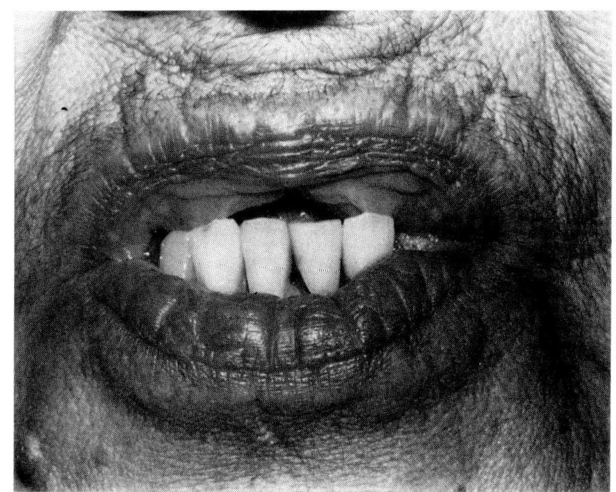

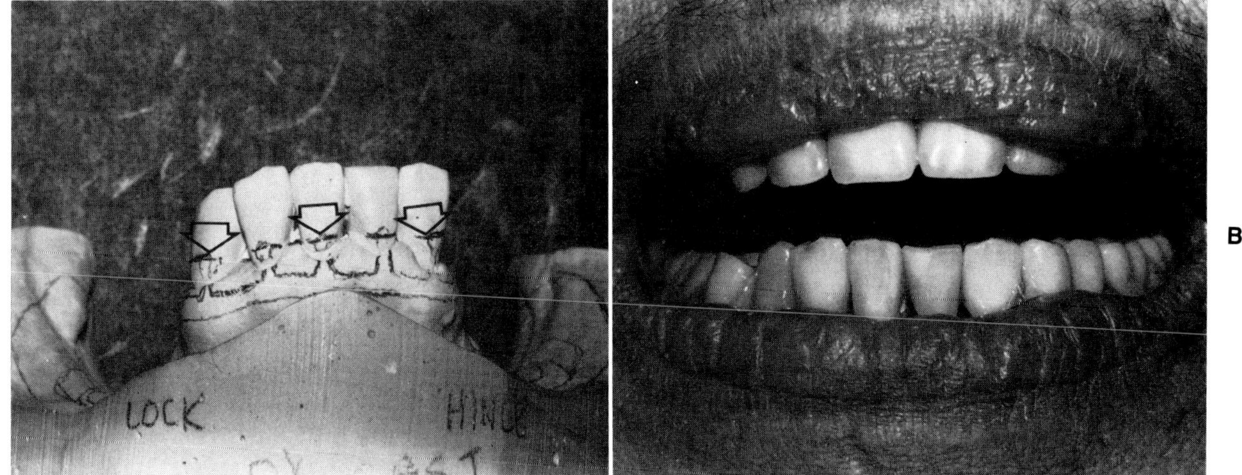

Fig. 20-35. **A,** Lines representing maximum phonetic exposure drawn on lower cast (arrows). Vertical projection arms designed to produce minimal display of metal. **B,** Vertical arms covered by lower lip.

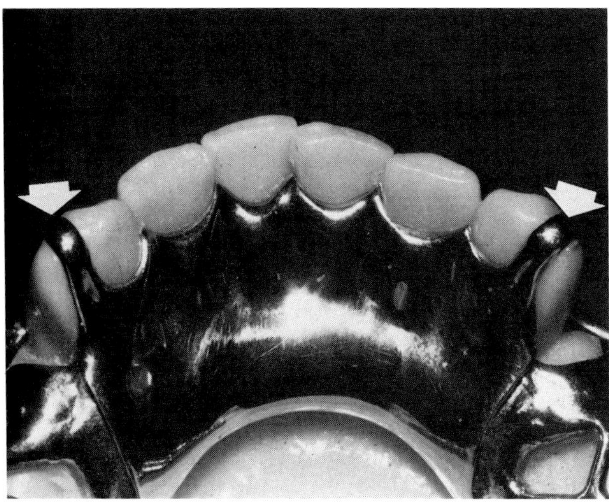

Fig. 20-36. Incisal rests placed on canines (arrows) to provide support and to prevent movement of prosthesis toward tissue.

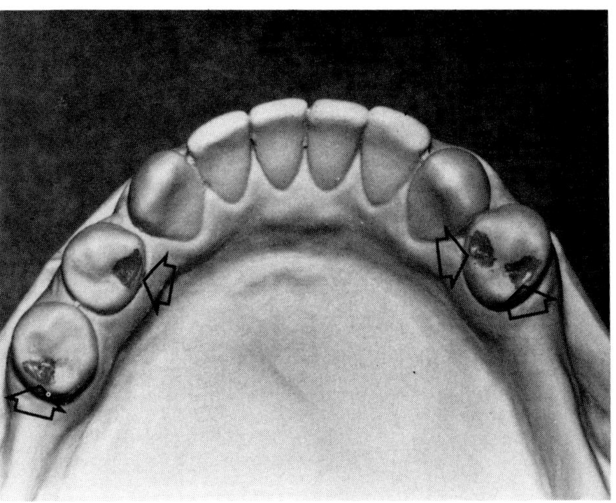

Fig. 20-37. Additional rests serve as indirect retainers.

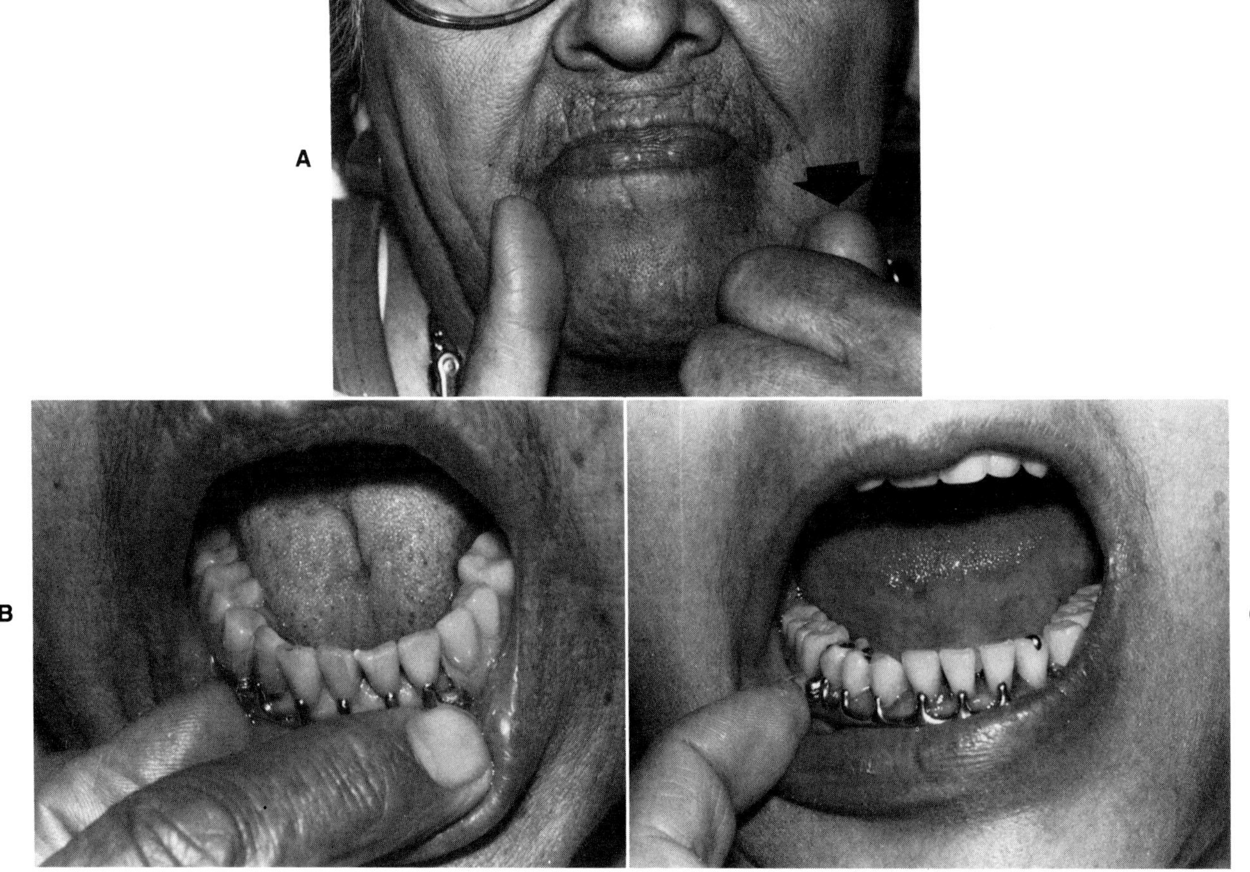

Fig. 20-38. Because patient has lost end of left thumb, **A,** (arrow), lock mechanism was placed for convenient opening with right thumb, **B. C,** Opening lock with forefinger is more convenient for this patient.

neer. This design is used if esthetics would be compromised by the show of metal or if a great loss of gingival tissue has occurred. The resin veneer design is usually used when the patient has mobile or short lips. The patient is asked to say words such as *sheriff* or *shepherd* to produce maximum movement of the lips and exposure of the teeth, and lines are drawn on the casts to indicate the position of maximum lip movement (Figs. 20-34 and 20-35). If metallic components would be visible and would be objectionable to the patient, the resin veneer is included in the design.

Although positioning of lingual plating above the survey line does prevent movement toward the tissue, well-designed rests in properly prepared rest seats ensure that the forces are directed along the long axis of the teeth. Rests are placed adjacent to edentulous areas (Fig. 20-36). If teeth are present distal to the first premolar, an additional rest is placed on the mesial occlusal surface of the first premolar or on the lingual or incisal surface of the canine (Fig. 20-37).

The location of the hinge and locking mechanisms is determined by the patient's ability to open the lock (Fig. 20-38). It is usually easier for a right-handed patient to open the locking mechanism if it is located on the right side of the prosthesis.

Impressions

Alginate (irreversible hydrocolloid) is the impression material of choice for the swing-lock denture. Most patients who require this type of treatment have gingival recession and large gingival embrasures. Rubber base impression material is too tough and will lock into undercut embrasure areas. Alginate, however, will tear and release without excessive application of force. It also possesses a sufficient degree of accuracy if it is handled properly.

The extension of the impression into the buccal and labial vestibular areas is critical. Frequently, a custom tray must be constructed to record these areas accurately. This is particularly true if the anterior teeth incline labially. Modeling plastic is used to border mold the vestibular areas of the tray to provide the proper extension. A custom tray must be constructed with sufficient relief to provide 5 to 6 mm of space for alginate around the remaining teeth. The tray should be prepared with several holes to help retain the alginate in the tray. If a stock tray is used, the edentulous areas should be corrected with modeling plastic. Alginate adhesive is painted in the tray and on its borders (Fig. 20-39).

Heavy-bodied alginate is used for making the impression. If this type of alginate is not available, less water should be used in mixing regular-bodied alginate. Good technique should be followed in making the impression, including isolating the mouth with gauze and finger placement of impression material around the teeth and into the vestibular areas. The impression is allowed to remain in the mouth for 2 minutes more than usual. This allows the alginate time to develop maximum strength. The impression is removed with a single snap, with the force applied along the long axes of the remaining teeth.

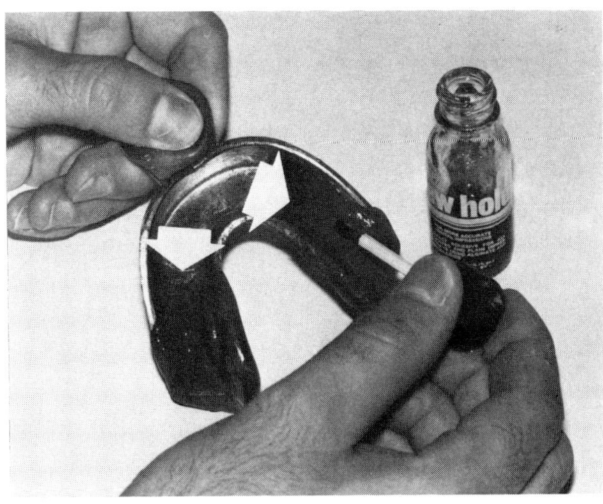

Fig. 20-39. Stock tray corrected with modeling plastic (arrows). Alginate adhesive painted on all internal and border areas of corrected tray.

The alginate will usually tear interproximally, particularly if open gingival embrasures are present. The torn surfaces are carefully approximated and luted in position with a small amount of sticky wax (Fig. 20-40). The interproximal contours are important because the framework will extend into these areas because of the lingual path of insertion. The impression is cleaned of saliva and is poured within 12 minutes with properly proportioned improved stone. A two-stage pour technique is used.

Fitting the framework

A critical procedure in the construction of a swing-lock prosthesis is the fitting of the framework to the teeth and to the opposing occlusion. Disclosing wax is added to all areas of the framework that contact the teeth with the exception of the labial arm, which is fitted later. The framework is then seated into position with the labial arm open. Closure of the labial arm should not be attempted until all other areas of the framework have been fitted. Pressure is applied to the framework in the direction of the path of insertion and in a vertical direction through pressure on the rests. The framework is removed and inspected under magnification for metallic showthrough areas. These areas

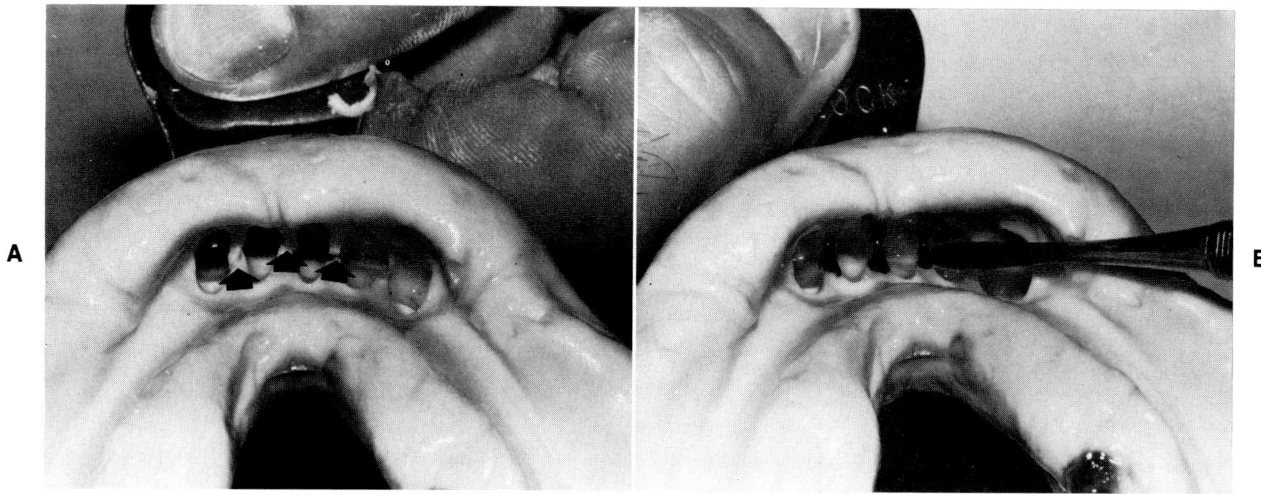

Fig. 20-40. A, Alginate impression material torn in gingival embrasure areas (arrows). B, Torn interproximal areas repositioned and luted with sticky wax.

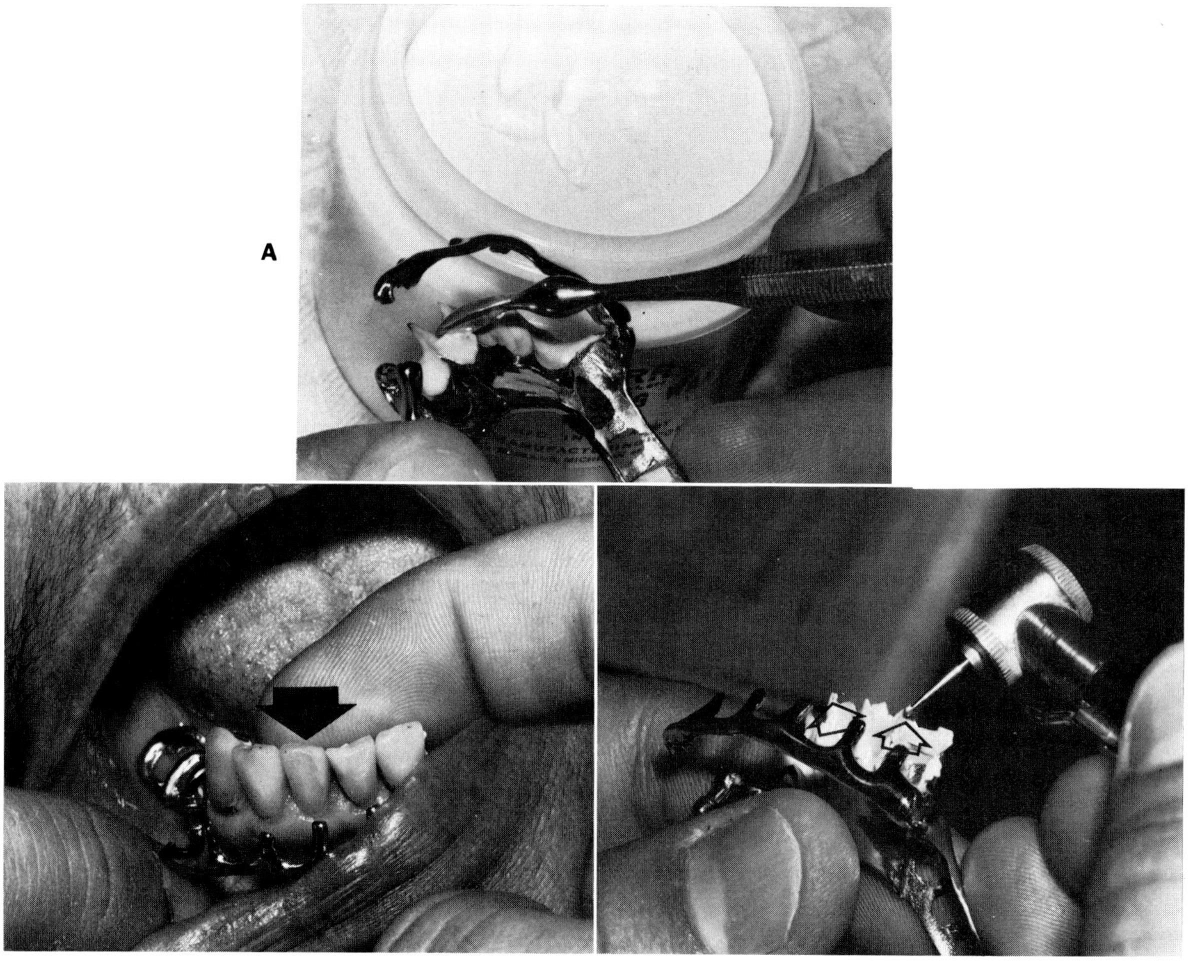

Fig. 20-41. A, Disclosing wax added to all areas of framework contacting teeth except labial arm. B, Framework seated and pressure applied to framework in labial direction (arrow). C, Metallic showthrough areas (arrows) removed with high-speed No. 2 round bur.

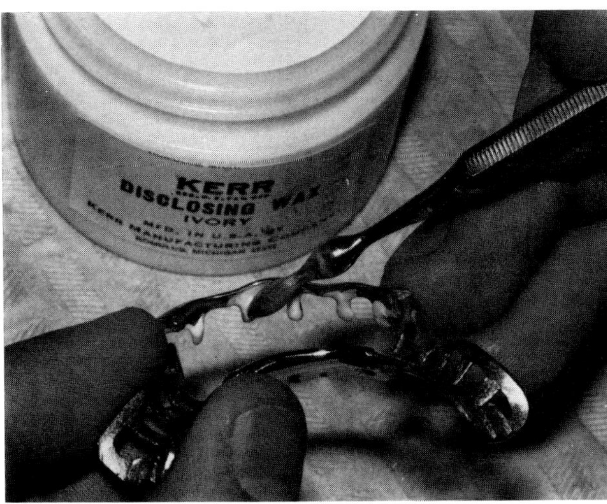

Fig. 20-42. Disclosing wax applied to vertical projections of labial arm.

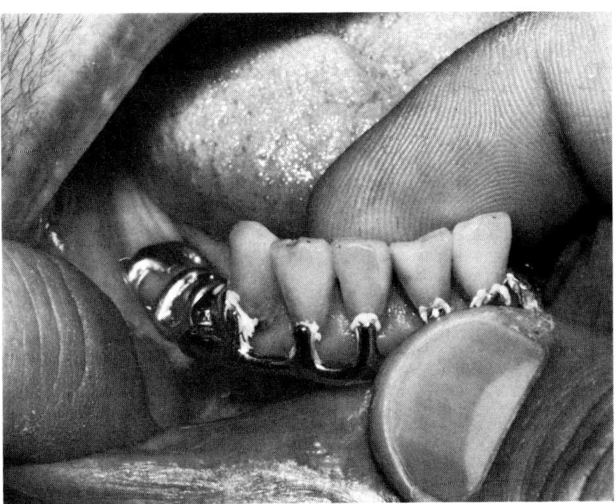

Fig. 20-43. Pressure to close arm applied first at hinge area, gradually progressing to lock.

are removed with a small round bur, and the procedure is repeated until the appearance of the wax indicates that the framework is completely seated (Fig. 20-41).

Disclosing wax is then applied to all areas of the labial arm that will contact teeth (Fig. 20-42). The framework is seated, and pressure is applied to the arm starting at the hinge area and progressing toward the lock (Fig. 20-43). If there appears to be resistance to total closure, the framework is removed, inspected, and those areas impeding closure are relieved (Fig. 20-44). This procedure is followed until the labial arm will close in the mouth with the same degree of force needed when the framework is on the cast. Care must always be exercised in closing the labial arm to avoid trapping and pinching the lip or cheek in the lock mechanism. Initially it may be necessary to use a blunt instrument to open the lock. After wearing the prosthesis for a short period, the patient will be able to open the locking mechanism with the thumbnail alone.

The occlusion must be checked and corrected to ensure that no part of the framework keeps the natural teeth apart.

Corrected cast procedure

All mandibular distal extension removable partial denture situations require the making of a corrected cast impression. Optimum support from the residual ridge is critical to the success of this type of treatment. Significant movement of the denture bases toward the tissue will quickly loosen the remaining teeth because the teeth are so firmly engaged by the framework.

Overdisplacement of tissue and overextension of denture base borders can also contribute to early failure to the prosthesis. Almost continuous force will be applied

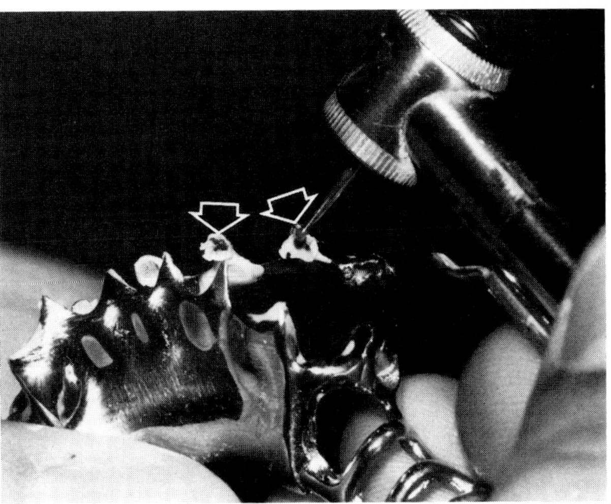

Fig. 20-44. Metallic showthroughs (arrows) are relieved.

to the remaining teeth if either of these conditions is present. Therefore the selection of the corrected cast impression material and care in border molding procedures are critical factors in this phase of treatment (Fig. 20-45).

Occlusion development

An occlusion should be developed that will minimize the lateral forces applied to the prosthesis. A "locked-in" occlusion with lateral interferences should be avoided.

Simultaneous occlusal contact between both the natural and artificial teeth at the patient's centric jaw relation is essential (Fig. 20-46). Premature contact of ar-

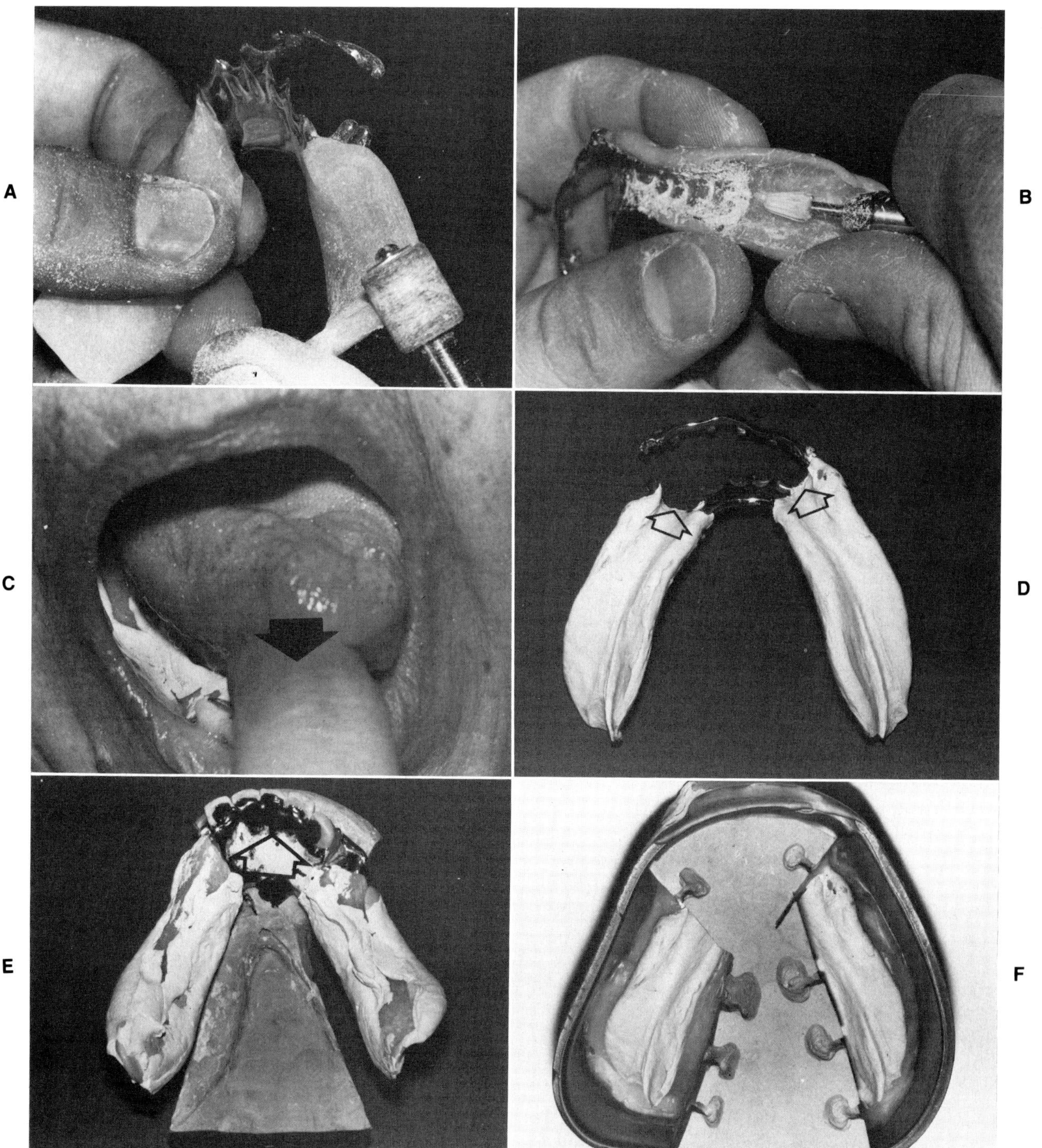

Fig. 20-45. A, Acrylic resin impression bases constructed on framework. **B,** After border molding is complete, internal surface of tray is relieved. **C,** Framework maintained in position by pressure applied to lingual aspect of major connector (arrow) in labial direction, closing gate. **D,** Corrected cast impression. Impression material on guiding planes (arrows) must be trimmed before framework is seated on cast. **E,** After ridge areas of cast are removed, impression is luted in position on cast with sticky wax (arrow). **F,** Impression beaded and boxed for pouring.

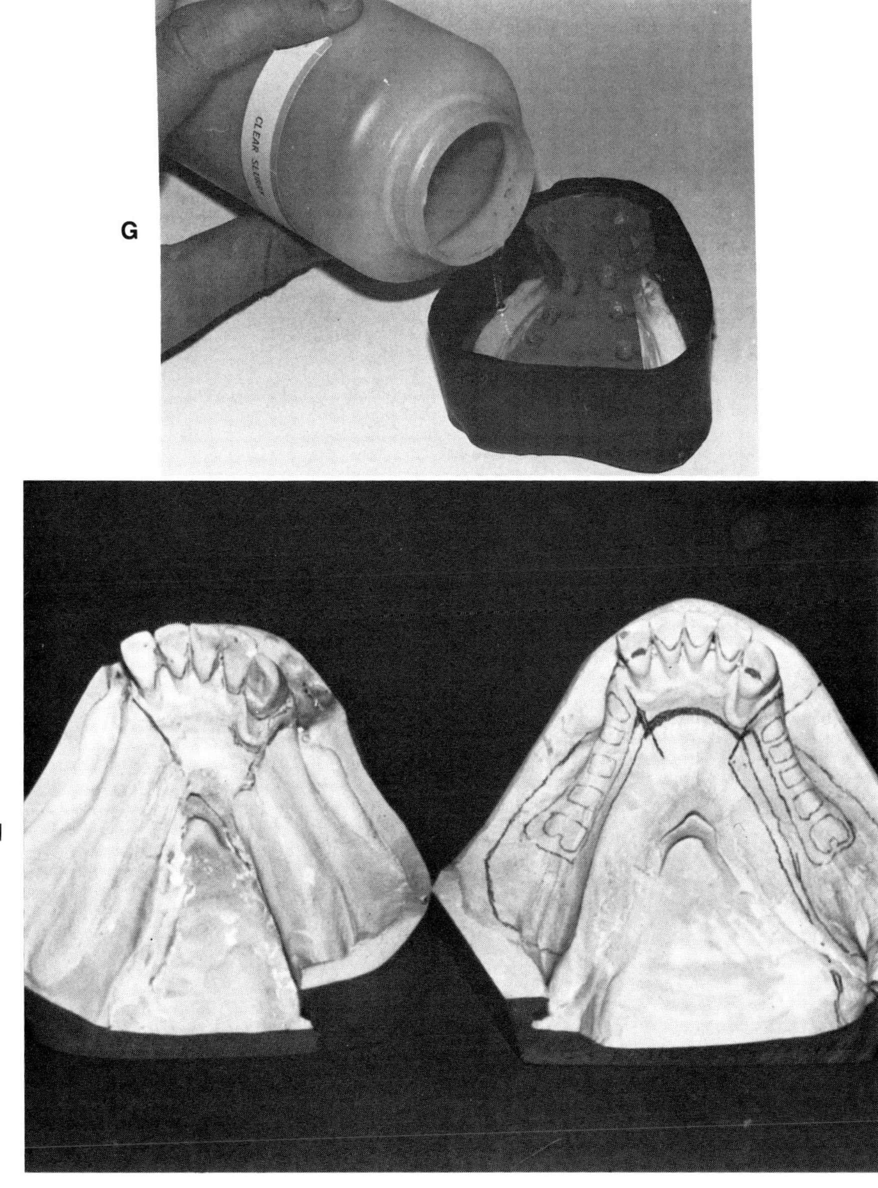

Fig. 20-45, cont'd. G, Clear slurry water poured into boxed impression to test seal. Original cast soaked for 5 minutes. **H,** Corrected cast, left; original, right.

A

B

C

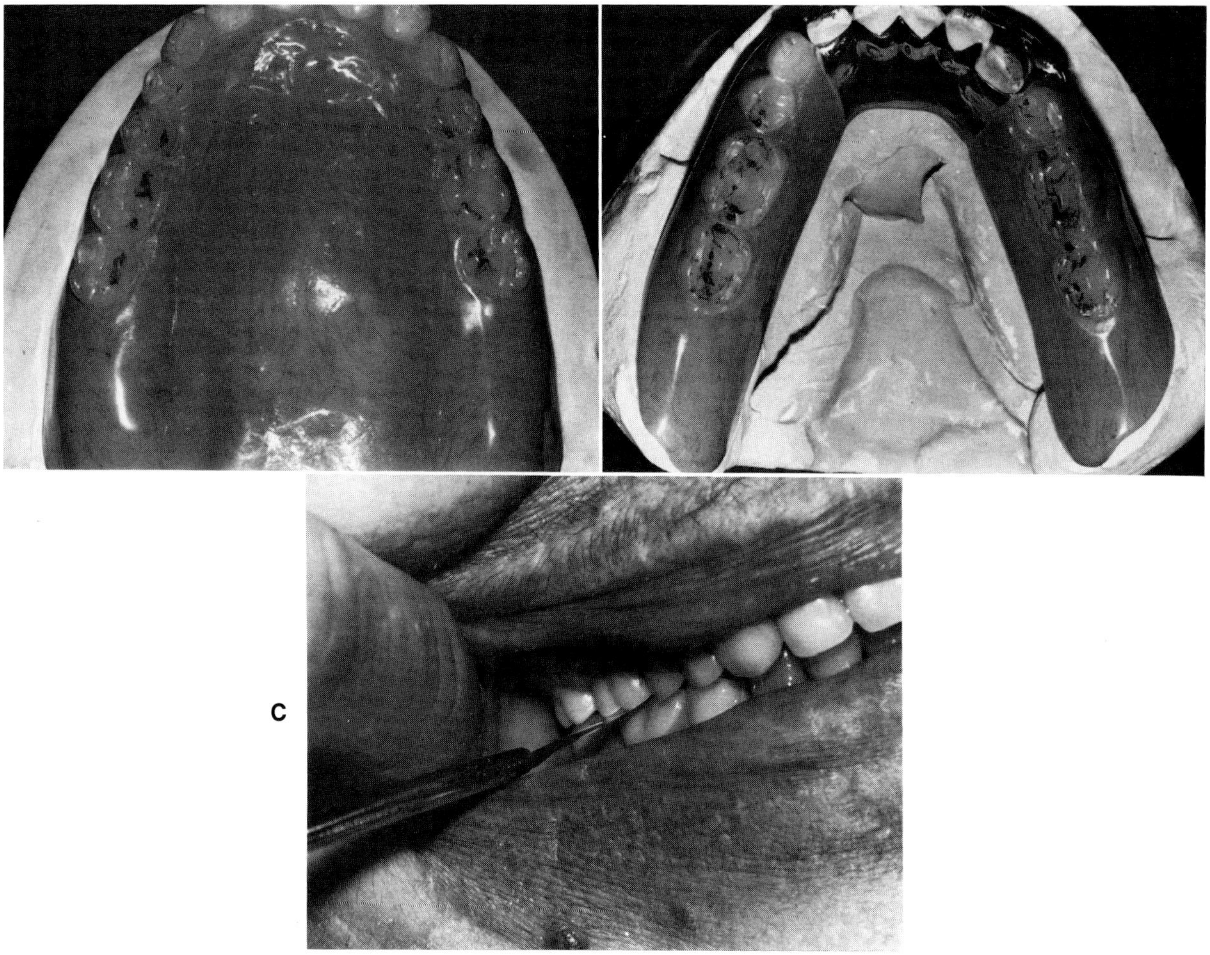

Fig. 20-46. A, Occlusal contact markings on maxillary denture are confined to lingual cusps. **B,** Mandibular contacts are in central groove area. **C,** Shim stock is used to verify equalized occlusal contacts.

tificial teeth on a distal extension base will hasten the loss of the remaining natural teeth.

Insertion of completed prosthesis

Pressure-indicator paste is used to locate pressure areas caused by the denture bases. The lingual path of insertion may cause insertion problems if the residual ridge is undercut on the buccal aspects. However, this is rarely a problem.

The occlusion is evaluated in centric and eccentric relations. Corrections are made if indicated.

If the swing-lock prosthesis is entirely tooth supported, the vertical struts of the labial arm can remain in intimate contact with the teeth for maximum retention. If long distal extension bases are involved or if the supporting tissues are easily displaced, maximum retention may be detrimental to the prognosis of the treatment. A two-prong pliers can be used to adjust the vertical projection arms slightly (Fig. 20-47). Reducing

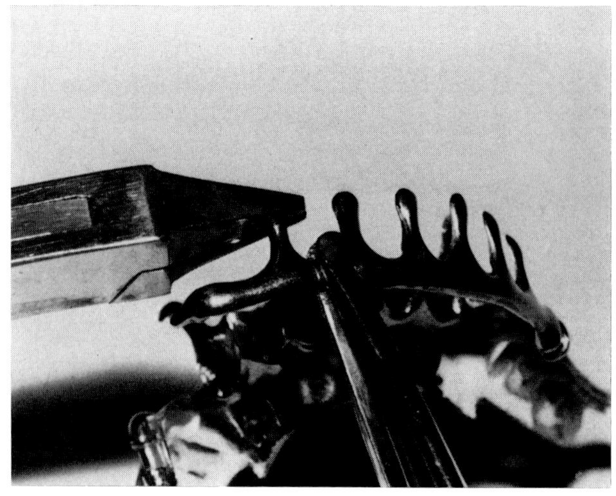

Fig. 20-47. Two-prong pliers may be used to adjust vertical projection arms.

retention by bending the arms slightly out of contact with the tooth will allow some movement of the denture bases toward the tissue without placing tipping forces on the remaining natural teeth.

Postinsertion care

Oral and prosthesis hygiene must be emphasized because the swing-lock denture's extensive tooth coverage complicates the maintenance of an adequate level of hygiene. Frequent observation and maintenance are essential to the success of the treatment.

Distal extension denture bases must be relined if any appreciable resorption of the residual ridges occurs. The impression of the denture base areas should be made with the labial arm locked to ensure that the framework is in its correct position. The impression must be made with the teeth out of occlusion.

Occasionally the lock mechanism will loosen after a time. It can be tightened by adjusting the labial bar. The bar is stabilized at both ends, and a finger is used to apply slight pressure against the bar in the direction away from the side that contacts the teeth (Fig. 20-48). This adjustment will usually necessitate slight adjustment of the vertical projection arms.

Teeth can be added to the swing-lock prosthesis as a relatively simple laboratory procedure. An alginate impression is made with the prosthesis in position and the labial arm unlocked. Usually the prosthesis will be retained in the impression. Undercuts in the denture base areas are blocked out, leaving only the borders exposed. A stone cast is poured. The labial arm will be enclosed by alginate, so special care should be taken in removing the impression from the cast. The safest procedure is to remove the tray from the impression material and cast and to peel the alginate away from the framework and cast. Retention can be soldered to the major connector and the replacement tooth attached with autopolymerizing acrylic resin.

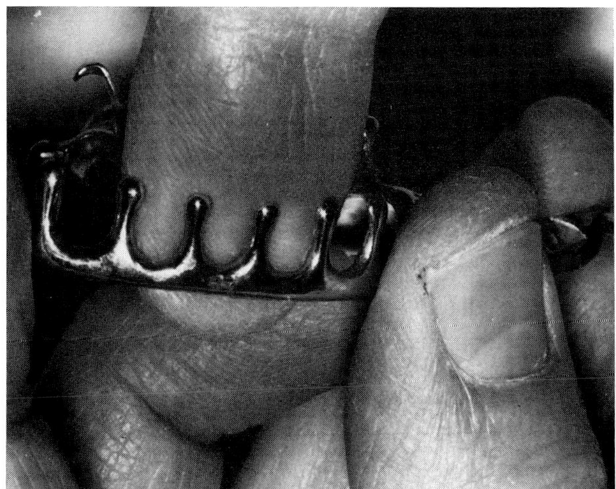

Fig. 20-48. Locking mechanism can be tightened by supporting ends of labial arm and gently applying pressure on lingual side of arm.

Prognosis

Clinical research has shown that teeth with unfavorable alveolar support can be retained for significant periods by the use of a well-constructed swing-lock prosthesis, provided the patient maintains an adequate level of oral hygiene.

Although some clinical steps vary slightly from those used in the construction of a conventional removable partial denture, they should not be too difficult for any dentist.

REMOVABLE PARTIAL OVERDENTURES

The overdenture concept has been used in complete denture treatment for several years with excellent results (Fig. 20-49). Increased patient comfort and preservation of the residual ridges are just two of the many advantages provided by this type of treatment.

Overdenture abutments can be as effective in providing support for removable partial dentures as for complete dentures. Strategically located abutment teeth can minimize or eliminate movement of a removable partial denture, thereby reducing the stress placed on the remaining teeth and the residual ridges (Fig. 20-50). These abutment teeth also help the prosthesis to withstand occlusal forces. Overdenture abutments can be used in the construction of a removable partial denture without any appreciable change in the procedures employed.

Indications

The indications for use of the overdenture concept in removable partial denture design are limited only by the imagination of the dentist and the requirements of the patient. However, most situations in which overdenture abutments are used to support removable partial dentures fall into one of the five general categories that follow.

Support for distal extension base

The distal extension removable partial denture has the greatest potential for applying harmful leverage-induced stresses to the abutment teeth. Every effort should be made to retain a posterior abutment tooth that can prevent movement of the distal extension base toward the tissue. Extruded molar teeth can frequently be treated with endodontic therapy and reduced in length to provide vertical support for the prosthesis

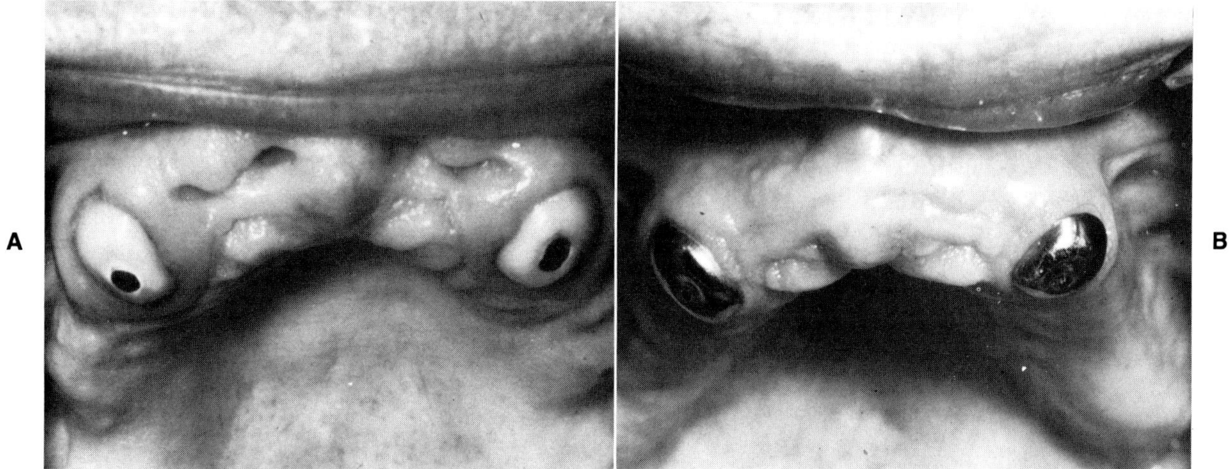

Fig. 20-49. Maxillary canines used to support overdentures. **A,** Polished dentin with amalgam restoration in pulp chamber. **B,** Gold copings on prepared canine teeth.

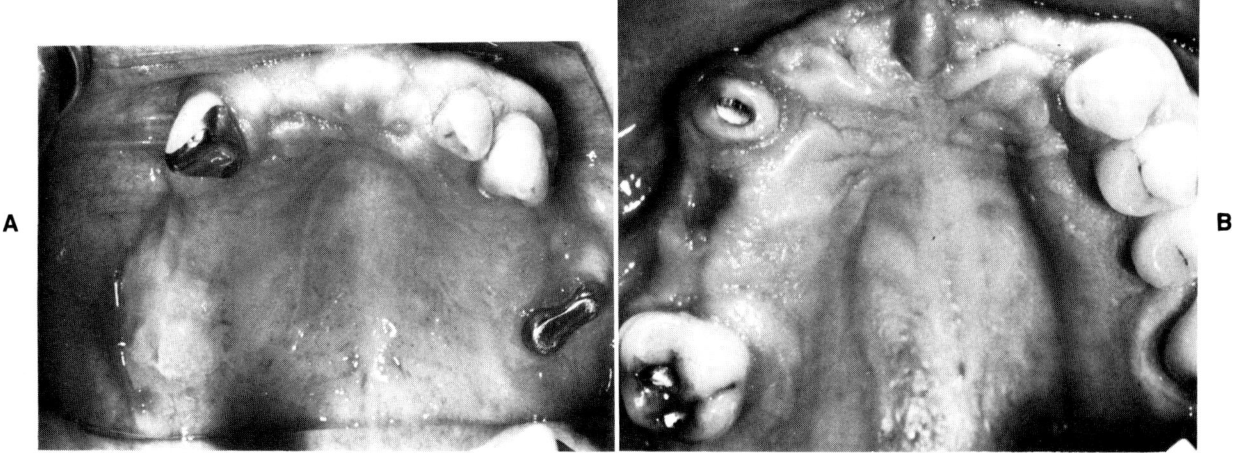

Fig. 20-50. A, Mesiobuccal and palatal root covered by coping to support removable partial overdenture. **B,** Unprotected canine supporting extensive anterior edentulous area.

(Fig. 20-51). In other situations endodontic treatment followed by hemisection will allow the use of a tooth with furcation involvement (Fig. 20-52).

Support for long-span anterior edentulous areas

Often overlooked but one of the most important indications for use of overdenture abutments is that of providing support for long anterior denture bases. Vertical overlap of the anterior teeth is usually essential in providing an adequate esthetic result. A great amount of lateral as well as tissueward force is applied to the anterior replacement teeth, causing movement of the prosthesis and resorption of the anterior ridge. This resorption compounds the problem and the replacement teeth for a new prosthesis will need to be set anterior to the ridge to provide adequate support of the lips. This vicious cycle leads to a poorer and poorer result. The retention of one or two anterior teeth can contribute greatly to avoiding these problems. Not only does the overdenture abutment provide support and limit movement of the prosthesis, but the presence of a healthy root in bone and under physiologic function discourages resorption of the alveolar bone in that area of the alveolar ridge (see Figs. 20-53 to 20-55).

Additional support for weak abutment tooth

A common diagnostic problem is present when a patient has lost considerable alveolar bone support

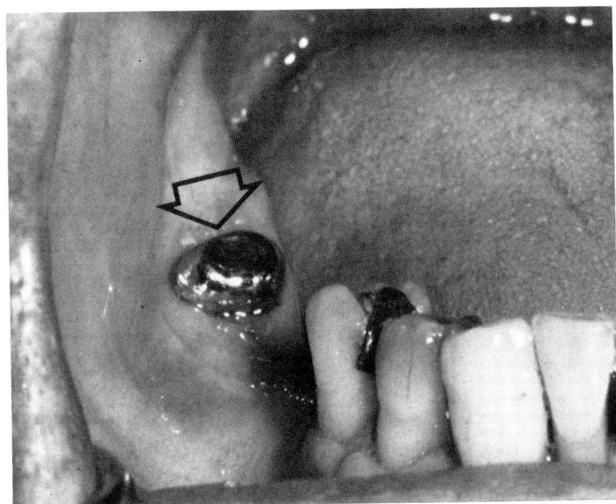

Fig. 20-51. Molar used as overdenture abutment (arrow) to provide support for distal extension denture base.

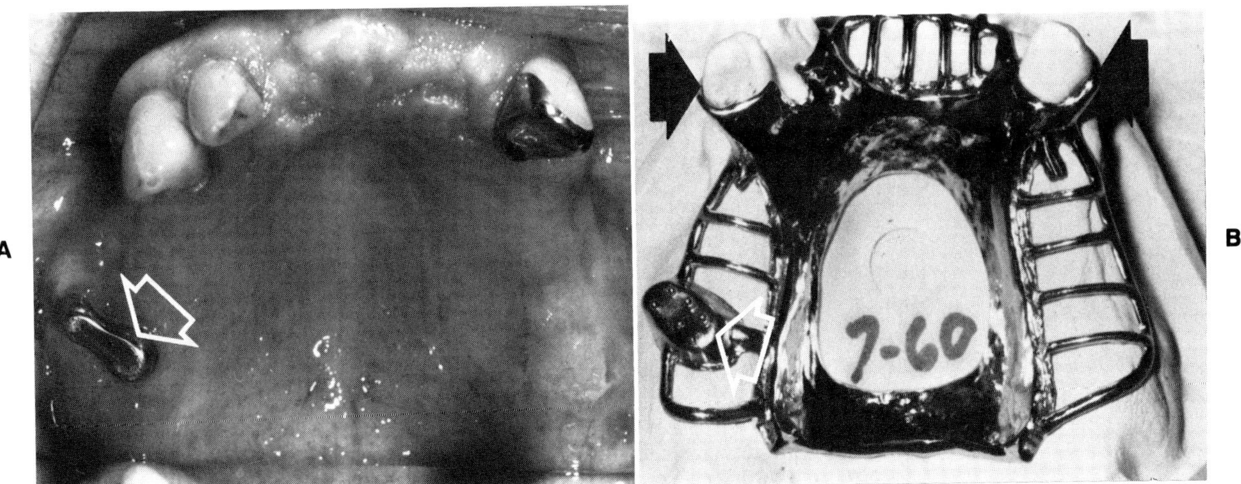

Fig. 20-52. A, This patient, in his late sixties, was reluctant to lose any more teeth. Bilateral distal extension removable partial denture with three remaining teeth does not have the best possible prognosis. Endodontic treatment and a hemisection on the maxillary right second molar were accomplished, and the tooth was used for posterior support. **B,** Although complete palatal coverage would have been the ideal in this situation, patient desires dictated use of closed horseshoe major connector. Wrought wire clasps (black arrows) were used on canines for retention. Metal-to-metal contact between framework and overdenture abutment was used (white arrow).

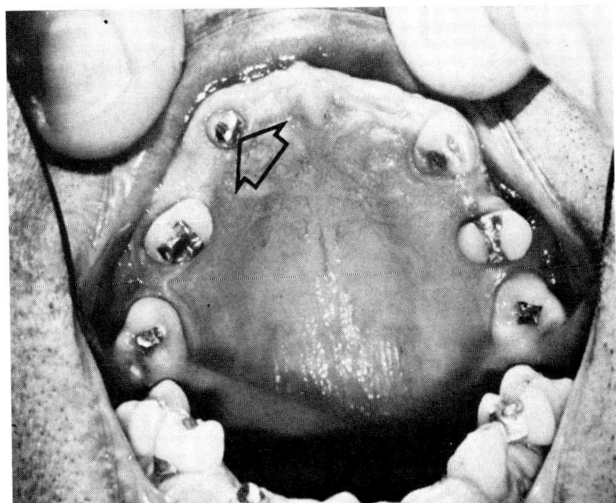

Fig. 20-53. Lateral incisor as overdenture abutment (arrow) for support of extensive anterior denture base.

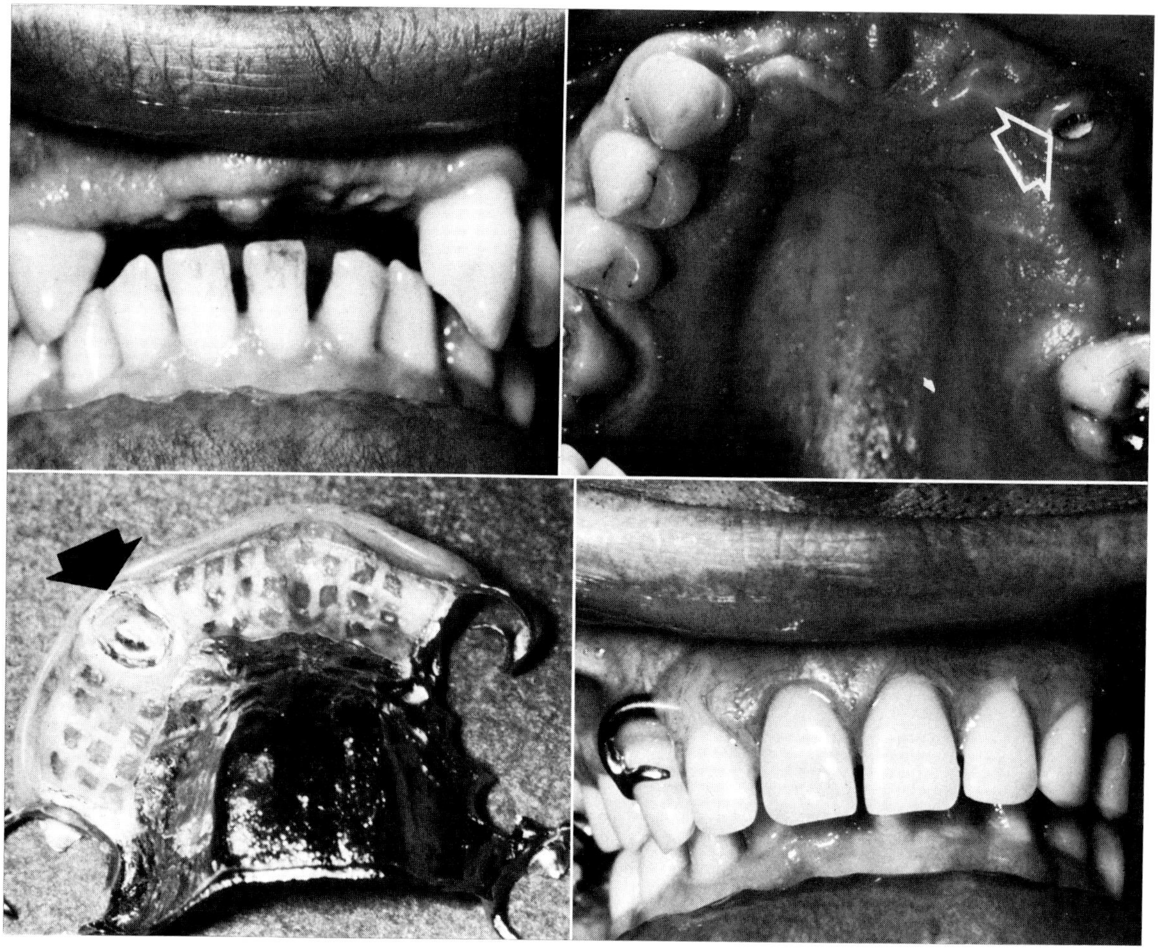

Fig. 20-54. A, This patient, in his late forties, had deep vertical overlap. Maxillary four incisor teeth and left first premolar had hopeless periodontal involvement. In addition, left canine had poor crown/root ratio and was mobile. Interim prosthesis was constructed, replacing four incisor teeth. **B,** Left canine became progressively more mobile, so was prepared as overdenture abutment (arrow) and added to interim prosthesis. **C,** Complete palatal coverage and overdenture abutment (arrow) used for support of prosthesis. **D,** Completed removable partial overdenture. Prosthesis was exceptionally stable and provided excellent result. This would probably not have been the case if overdenture abutment had not been used for support of anterior denture base.

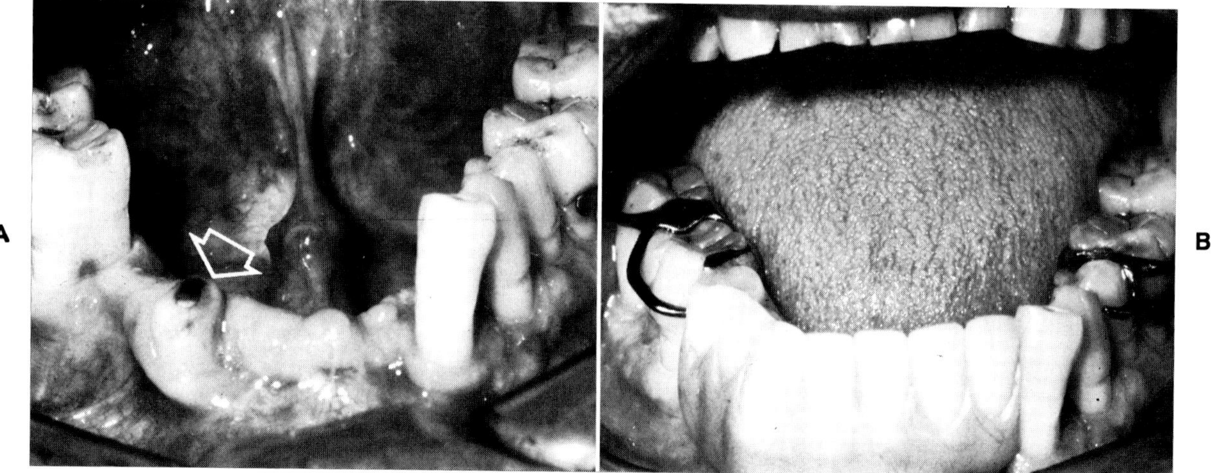

Fig. 20-55. A, Mandibular canine used as overdenture abutment (arrow). **B,** Completed prosthesis provided excellent support.

through periodontal disease. Usually several teeth are hopeless or have been lost, and no strong abutment teeth remain. Examples of this situation are shown in Figs. 20-56 and 20-57.

Support when few or weak teeth remain

The use of selected overdenture abutment teeth can sometimes allow the construction of a removable partial denture in situations that appear hopeless, such as those shown in Figs. 20-58 and 20-59.

Support for interim prosthesis

Occasionally a patient needs some type of prosthesis for esthetics or function but it is impossible to formulate a final treatment plan because the prognosis of some teeth remains in doubt. For instance, the patient's home maintenance procedures or the response to periodontal treatment may need to be evaluated before a final decision is made. A possible solution is illustrated in Fig. 20-60.

Diagnosis and treatment planning

Preparation of a diagnostic mounting and the survey and design of diagnostic casts are essential steps in developing a treatment plan. Decisions relative to the selection of teeth to be used as overdenture abutments as well as the types of restorations to be placed must be made with the ultimate design of the removable partial denture in mind.

Selection of overdenture abutment teeth

Criteria used for the selection of teeth to serve as overdenture abutments for removable partial dentures are similar to those used for complete dentures. The greatest differences are in the position of the selected teeth and in the concern for tissue undercuts.

Positional considerations

The selection of overdenture abutments is largely dependent on the position of the remaining teeth and the size of the edentulous areas. The selected tooth or teeth should be most beneficial in reducing stress to the abutment teeth and the residual ridge. The tooth adjacent to the abutment tooth may be selected if it is the best tooth available, but oral hygiene procedures are more difficult if an adjacent tooth is used.

The presence of a labial or buccal tissue undercut is not nearly as critical as for an overdenture abutment for a complete overdenture. It is not absolutely essential to get maximum extension of the borders of the prosthesis into the vestibule, because retention is provided by clasps and guiding planes. The borders of the remov-

Text continued on p. 616.

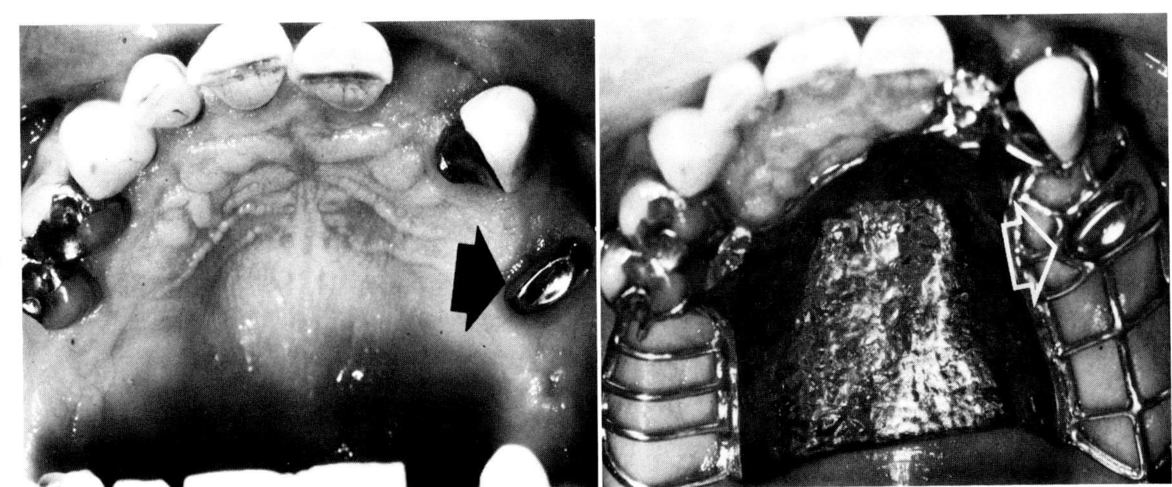

Fig. 20-56. A, This patient was in his late sixties. Maxillary left second premolar was mobile, and left canine had marginal crown/root ratio. Endodontic treatment was completed on second premolar, and tooth was prepared as overdenture abutment (arrow). **B,** Complete palatal coverage was used, with light wrought wire retention on canine. Acrylic resin retention minor connector was designed to avoid contact with overdenture abutment tooth (arrow). Fit of tissue surfaces and occlusion was perfected, and resin overlying overdenture abutment was relieved to eliminate contact with tooth. Hole was placed in denture base, and resin was prepared for butt joint. Tooth-colored autopolymerizing acrylic resin was placed in concavity. Patient was asked to close firmly on cotton roll placed on occlusal surfaces bilaterally to allow some tissue displacement before overdenture abutment came into contact with prosthesis. With prosthesis at rest, slight space is present between abutment tooth and denture base. This procedure will prevent movement of prosthesis with overdenture abutment acting as fulcrum point.

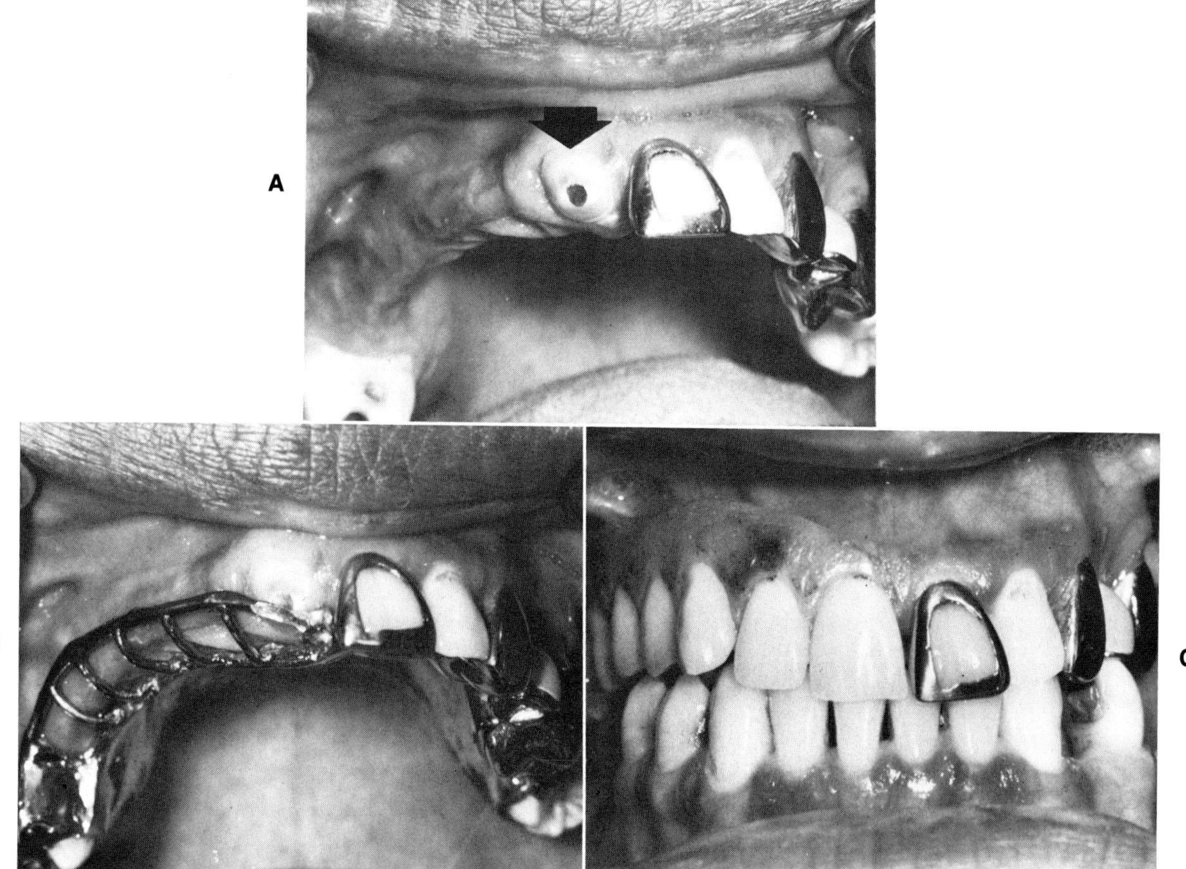

Fig. 20-57. Loss of teeth distal to central or lateral incisor teeth creates problems in construction of adequate prosthesis. Example is this man in his late forties. Maxillary right premolars and canine had been removed several years earlier, and prosthesis was constructed. Because of lateral forces and movement of prosthesis, right lateral incisor was lost shortly thereafter and was added to prosthesis. When patient came in for treatment, right central incisor was mobile, and considerable resorption of the residual ridge had occurred. **A,** Because removal of right central incisor would compound problem and hasten loss of remaining teeth, it was prepared as overdenture abutment (arrow). **B,** Complete palatal coverage and lingual plating were used to provide additional support and lateral stability. Acrylic resin retention was kept short of abutment tooth to allow replacement central incisor to be butted to ridge. Prosthesis was adapted to overdenture abutment tooth with autopolymerizing acrylic resin. Replacement teeth were placed, and selective grinding was accomplished to allow natural teeth to guide eccentric movements as much as possible. **C,** Prepared central incisor became firm, and prosthesis was stable and retentive.

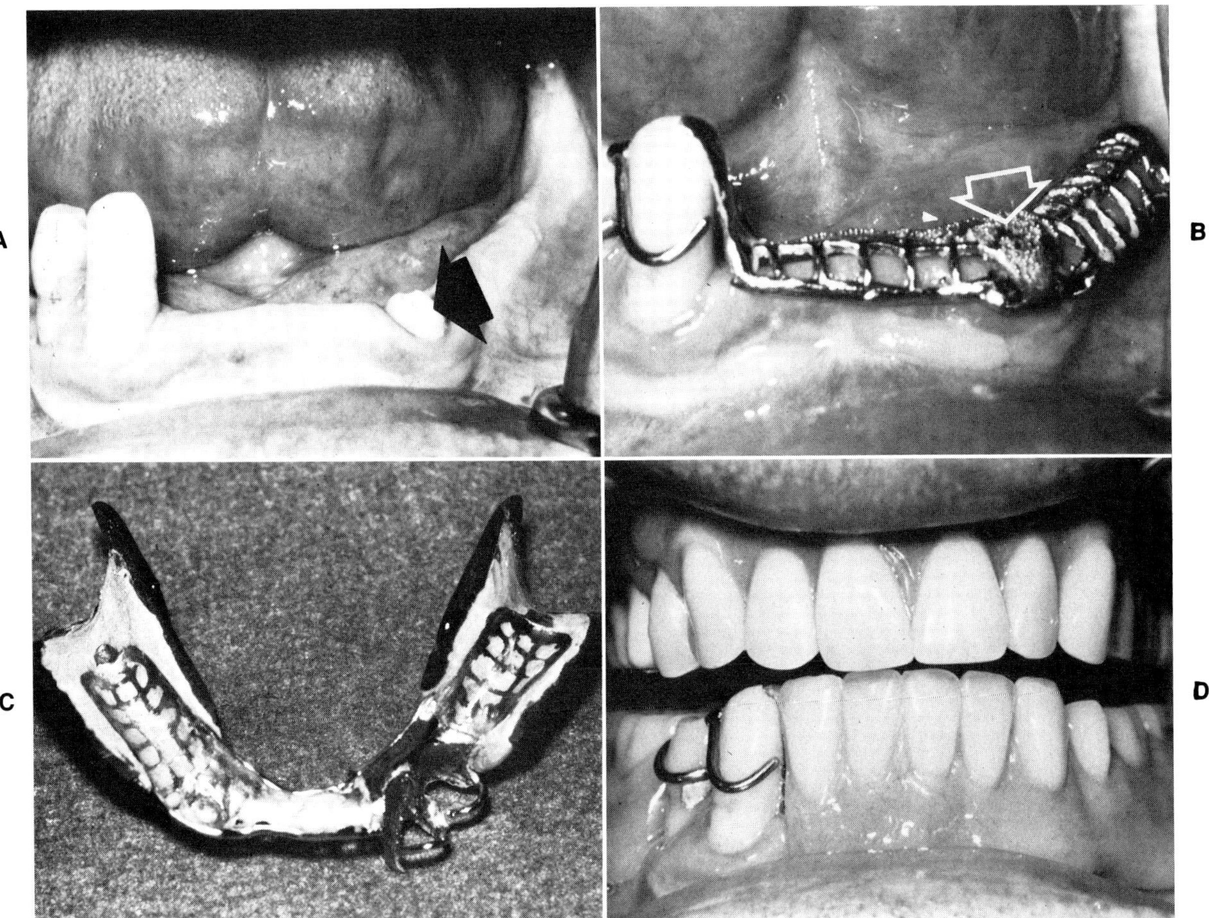

Fig. 20-58. This 50-year-old patient was completely edentulous in maxillary arch and had only three teeth remaining in mandibular arch. Right first premolar and canine were firm and had good crown/root ratios. Left canine had poor crown/root ratio and was mobile. All three remaining teeth had less than 2 mm of attached gingiva. Large tongue size and its retracted position suggested retention problems for complete denture. Left canine was treated with endodontic therapy and reduced in height to reduce mobility. Free gingival graft was used to create attached gingiva and to deepen labial vestibule. **A,** Left canine was prepared for overdenture coping (arrow). **B,** Prosthesis was designed with wrought wire clasps on right premolar and canine and metal-to-metal contact with overdenture abutment (arrow). **C,** Impression bases were border molded in preparation for making corrected cast impression to ensure adequate extension and fit of denture bases. **D,** Completed removable partial overdenture exhibits excellent retention and stability.

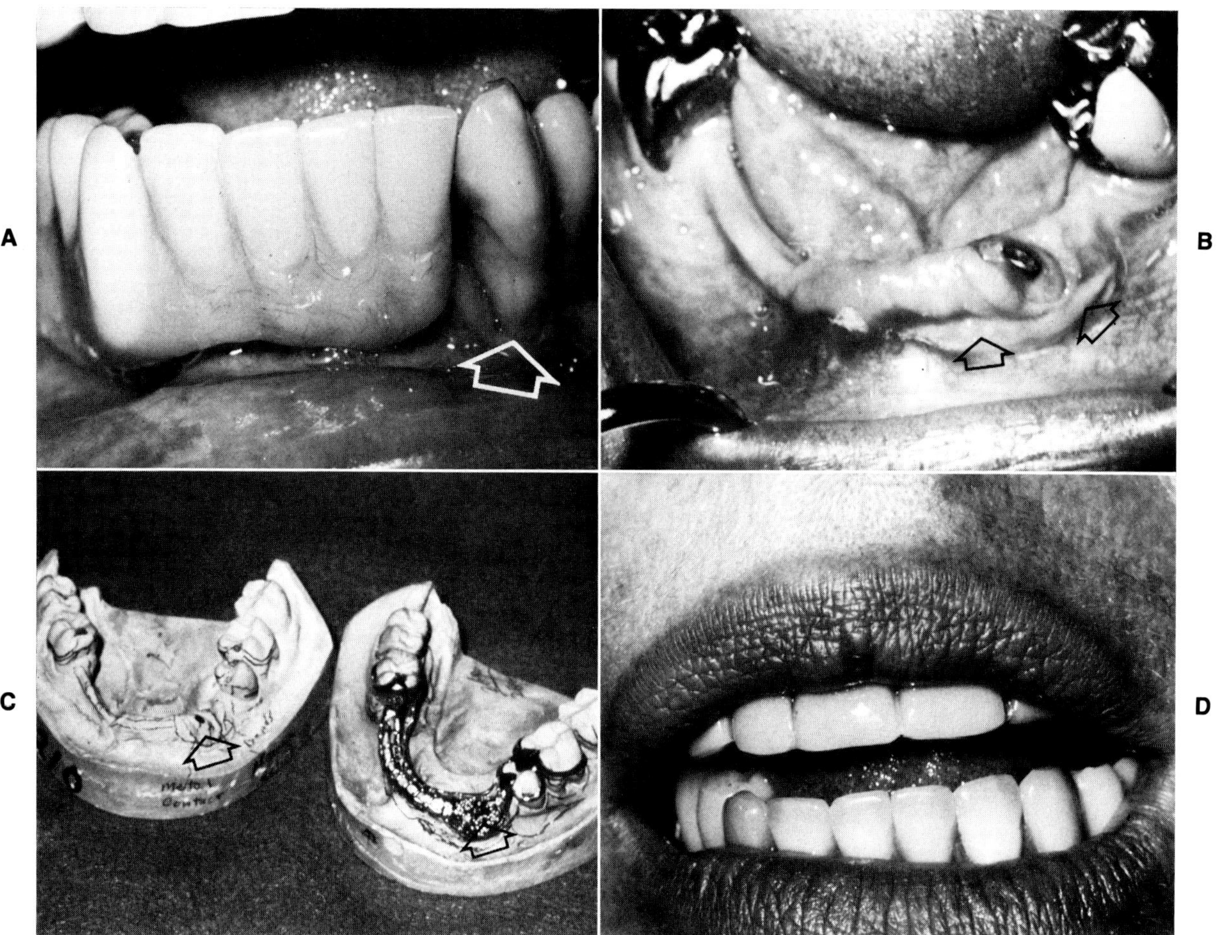

Fig. 20-59. This patient in her early forties had a molar-to-molar fixed partial denture in maxillary arch. Mandibular left first and second molars were splinted with gold crowns, as were second premolar and first molar on right side. Right canine had been removed several weeks earlier and had been added to removable partial denture. **A,** Left canine was mobile and did not have sufficient attached gingiva (arrow). All other mandibular teeth were missing. Loss of left canine would make successful construction and wear of mandibular removable partial denture extremely difficult. **B,** Endodontic treatment was completed on left canine, and tooth was prepared as overdenture abutment. (Note that canine was overprepared.) Replacement tooth was added to existing prosthesis, and **C,** a free gingival graft was placed to provide attached gingiva for canine. New framework using canine overdenture abutment (arrows) for support was constructed. Corrected cast impression was made to cover entire available residual ridge without interfering with function of surrounding structures. **D,** Completed prosthesis in place. Abutment tooth became firm and had adequate attached gingiva. Prosthesis was stable, and patient was pleased to be able to retain remaining teeth. It is doubtful that treatment would have been as successful without use of overdenture abutment.

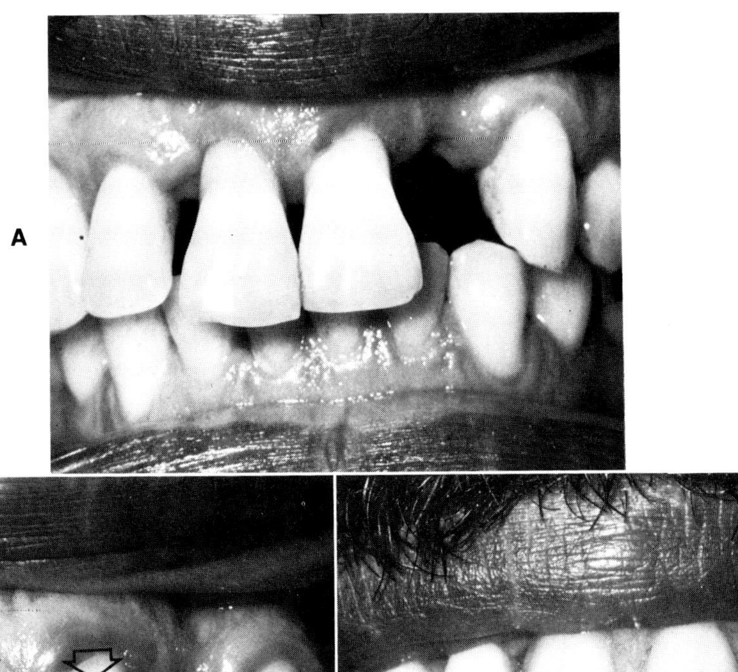

Fig. 20-60. This 51-year-old patient managed a small business and was concerned about his appearance. **A,** He exhibited moderate periodontal disease, and left lateral incisor had been removed 2 days earlier because of an acute periodontal abscess. Both central incisors had poor crown/root ratios but minimal pocket depth. Other areas of mouth exhibited deep pocket depth and gingival inflammation. Impressions were made for interim removable partial denture using central incisors as overdenture abutments. Shade was taken, and prosthesis was constructed in laboratory while endodontic treatment was being completed. **B,** Central incisors were prepared as overdenture abutments. Prosthesis was adapted to overdenture abutments with autopolymerizing acrylic resin. **C,** Patient was provided with prosthesis to fulfill his esthetic requirements while treatment planning and definitive periodontal and restorative procedures were being completed. Retained teeth provided support for prosthesis and helped prevent resorption of labial alveolar bone.

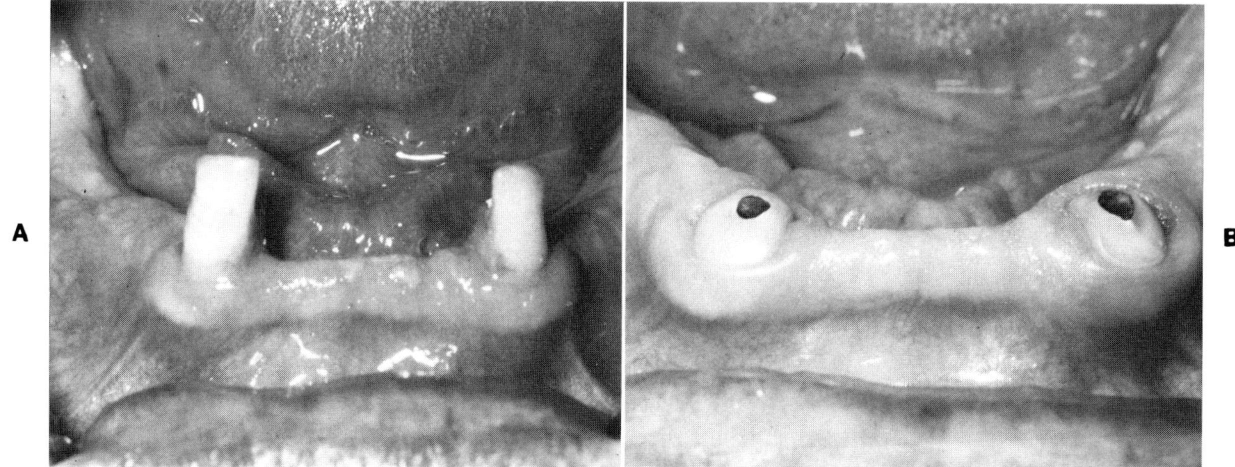

Fig. 20-61. A, Mandibular canines selected for support of overdenture. **B,** Teeth reduced to height of 2 to 3 mm above proximal gingival margin.

able partial denture base can be kept short to avoid the undercut, or the replacement tooth can be butted to the ridge.

Periodontal considerations

If the prospective overdenture abutment has periodontal problems, (1) excess pocket depth should be eliminated, (2) an ideal topography should be developed to allow the performance of meticulous oral hygiene procedures by the patient, and (3) sufficient (2 mm or more) attached gingiva must be present.

Mobility of the prospective abutment tooth is not extremely critical. The tooth will usually become firm after the clinical crown is reduced if the mobility is primarily caused by a poor crown/root ratio. Obviously the periodontium must be healthy or the abutment tooth will fail.

Endodontic considerations

Almost all overdenture abutment teeth require endodontic treatment so that the clinical crown can be reduced to an ideal length of 2 to 3 mm (Fig. 20-61). A rare exception is a tooth in which the pulp chamber is so extensively calcified that endodontic treatment is not necessary. When a tooth with a single root can be used as effectively as a multirooted tooth, economic factors favor selection of the single-rooted tooth.

Caries considerations

Obviously, rampant caries is a red flag when overdenture abutments are being considered. However, root caries is not uncommon when periodontal disease and treatment have exposed root surfaces and access for good oral hygiene has been difficult. A prospective abutment tooth in this situation would need to be rejected because of caries only if it were impossible to develop good margins for a coping. Use of the pulp chamber for retention allows the use of a coping in most instances even when caries destruction is extensive. Coping coverage of the overdenture abutment teeth is indicated if the size of the carious lesion or the presence of a restoration would leave the abutment tooth susceptible to fracture (Fig. 20-62). Generally the abutment tooth can be prepared, a restoration placed in the pulp chamber, and the abutment tooth used for support in its unprotected state (Fig. 20-63). The removable partial denture should be designed so that a coping can

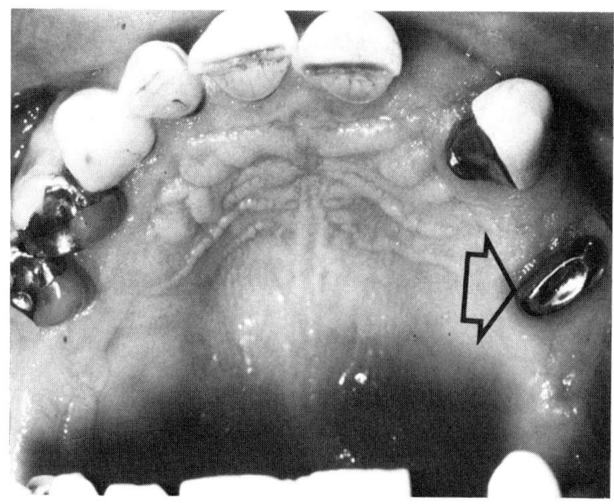

Fig. 20-62. Weakened overdenture abutment protected by gold coping (arrow).

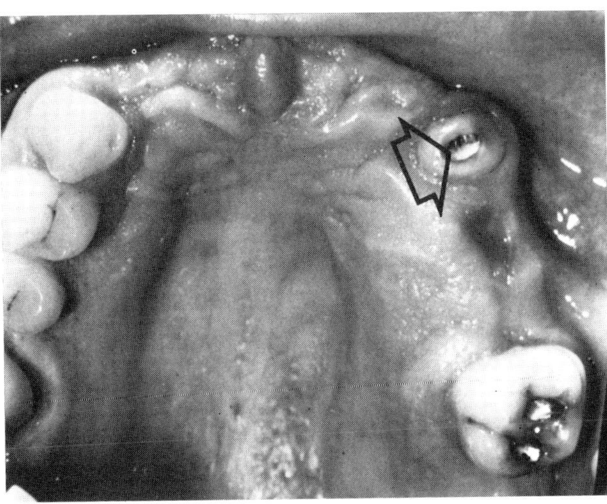

Fig. 20-63. Maxillary canine restored with amalgam restoration (arrow). Coping coverage not used.

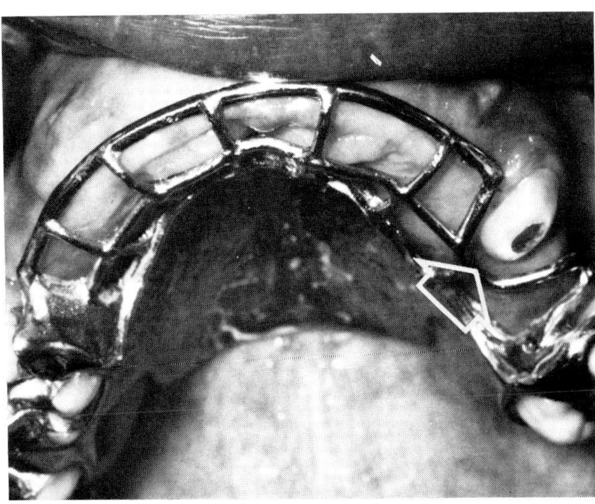

Fig. 20-64. Acrylic resin minor connector bypasses unprotected overdenture abutment tooth. Coping can be added later if needed.

be added to the abutment tooth later should this become necessary (Fig. 20-64).

Oral hygiene considerations

The success of the overdenture depends largely on the patient's ability to perform effective oral hygiene procedures. Any indication of inability to perform these procedures would contraindicate the overdenture.

Design

The design of a removable partial denture that uses overdenture abutments is essentially the same as for a conventional prosthesis. A few exceptions relative to selection of replacement teeth, choice of retentive clasps, and design of the denture base areas are necessary in some situations.

Acrylic resin teeth should always be used for replacement teeth over overdenture abutments because they are easier to modify and are less likely to fracture than porcelain teeth.

An example of the need for a possible change in clasp selection is a patient who is edentulous distal to the canine with the exception of a second premolar, which is to be used as an overdenture abutment. The premolar will help reduce the occlusal load on the residual ridge but may act as a fulcrum point if occlusal forces are applied distal to this abutment. Therefore the retentive clasp on the canine abutment should release easily. A light-gauge wrought wire clasp is probably the best choice in this situation (Fig. 20-65).

The prosthesis can be designed to contact the abutment tooth in one of three ways.

1. An attachment can be used that will provide retention for the prosthesis. Examples are studs such as the Rotherman,* Dalla Bona,* Gerber* GPC,* and Octolink* and other attachment systems such as the Zest Anchor* and the O-SO† attachment systems. In most instances adequate retention can be supplied by conventional abutment teeth, and the overdenture abutments are used only for vertical support.
2. The prosthesis can be designed to provide metal-to-tooth or metal-to-coping contact. This contact is accomplished through the use of a metal denture base or an acrylic resin minor connector that provides metal-to-tooth contact (Fig. 20-66). There are definite disadvantages to this approach: the prosthesis cannot be functionally fitted to the abutment tooth as easily as when the tooth is contacted by acrylic resin, and later placement or replacement of a coping is difficult if good contact between the tooth and the prosthesis is to be maintained.
3. The best and most commonly used approach is the development of resin-to-tooth contact (Fig. 20-67). The prosthesis is designed so that the acrylic resin retention minor connector does not cover or contact the abutment tooth. This allows the prosthesis to be functionally fitted under some occlusal force and to be modified if changes in the contour of the abutment tooth are required.

---

*APM Sterngold, 454 Peninseda Avenue, San Mateo, Calif. 94401.
†Scodenco, P.O. Box 35265, Tulsa, Okla. 74135.

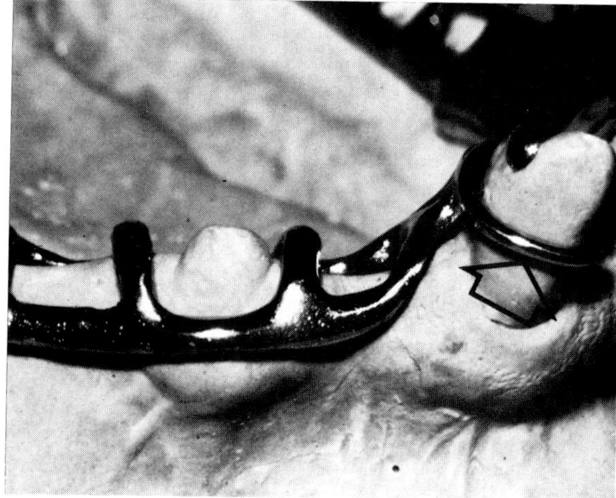

Fig. 20-65. Wrought wire clasp (arrow) used on canine to provide easy release should overdenture abutment become a fulcrum point.

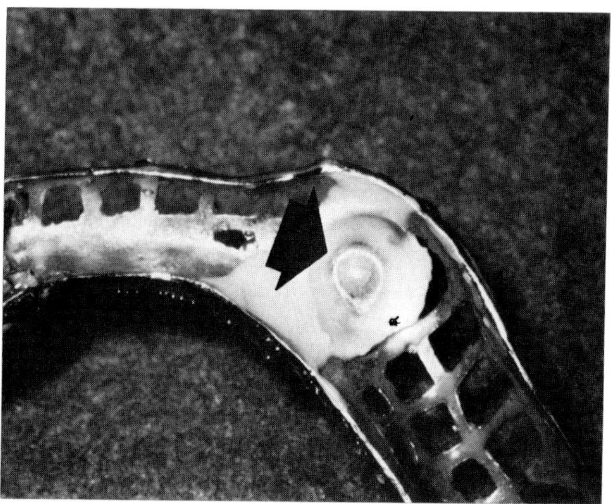

Fig. 20-66. Framework designed to provide metal contact with overdenture abutment (arrow). Disclosing wax is used to indicate undesirable contact areas.

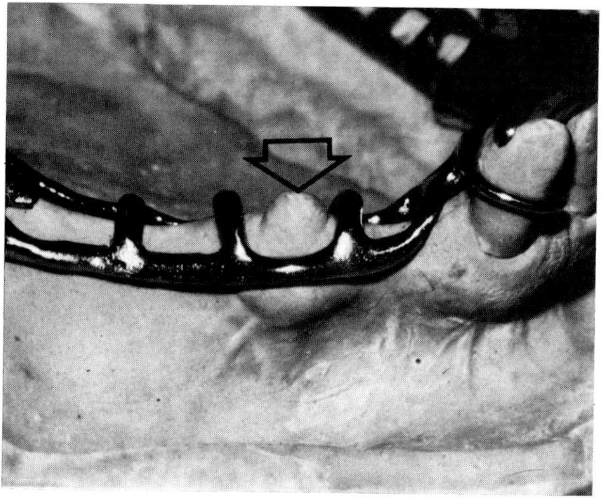

Fig. 20-67. Acrylic resin retention minor connector designed to bypass overdenture abutment (arrow), allowing resin-to-tooth contact by denture base.

Preparation of overdenture abutment

Adequate reduction of the abutment tooth is critical because a replacement tooth must be placed over the abutment tooth. Strength and esthetics are compromised by inadequate reduction (Fig. 20-68).

The preparation should extend 2 to 3 mm above the crest of the ridge (Fig. 20-69). The labial or buccal reduction is the most critical. Sufficient tooth reduction must be made to allow the placement of an artificial tooth in the same labiolingual position as the natural tooth. The taper of the preparation from the labiogingival margin to the center of the tooth must be 25 to 35 degrees. The proximal and lingual reductions are much less severe, with a 10- to 15-degree taper being adequate. The procedure is illustrated in Fig. 20-70.

Clinical procedures

Most of the clinical procedures are the same as for a conventional removable partial denture. Mouth preparation, impression making, and the fitting of the framework require no alterations in technique. The procedures for making a corrected cast impression are the same, even though an overdenture abutment is in the impression area. However, rubber base or silicone impression material should be used for the impression if there is a possibility that the abutment tooth is undercut.

Fitting the prosthesis to the abutment tooth

The best clinical results are obtained when the prosthesis is adapted to the abutment tooth at the time of insertion. A bur is used to remove all contact between the denture base and the overdenture abutment. Normal fitting procedures are accomplished, and the occlusion is perfected as for a conventional removable partial denture. The tissue surface of the acrylic resin base is prepared so that a butt joint will be formed when autopolymerizing resin is used to establish contact with the overdenture abutment. A small hole is placed through the acrylic resin base in the approximate center of the area occupied by the abutment. The hole should exit on the lingual side of the replacement tooth. Tooth-colored autopolymerizing acrylic resin is mixed, and a small amount is placed in the concavity occupied by the overdenture abutment tooth. The prosthesis is seated in the mouth while partial polymerization occurs. It is then removed and placed in warm water until polymer-

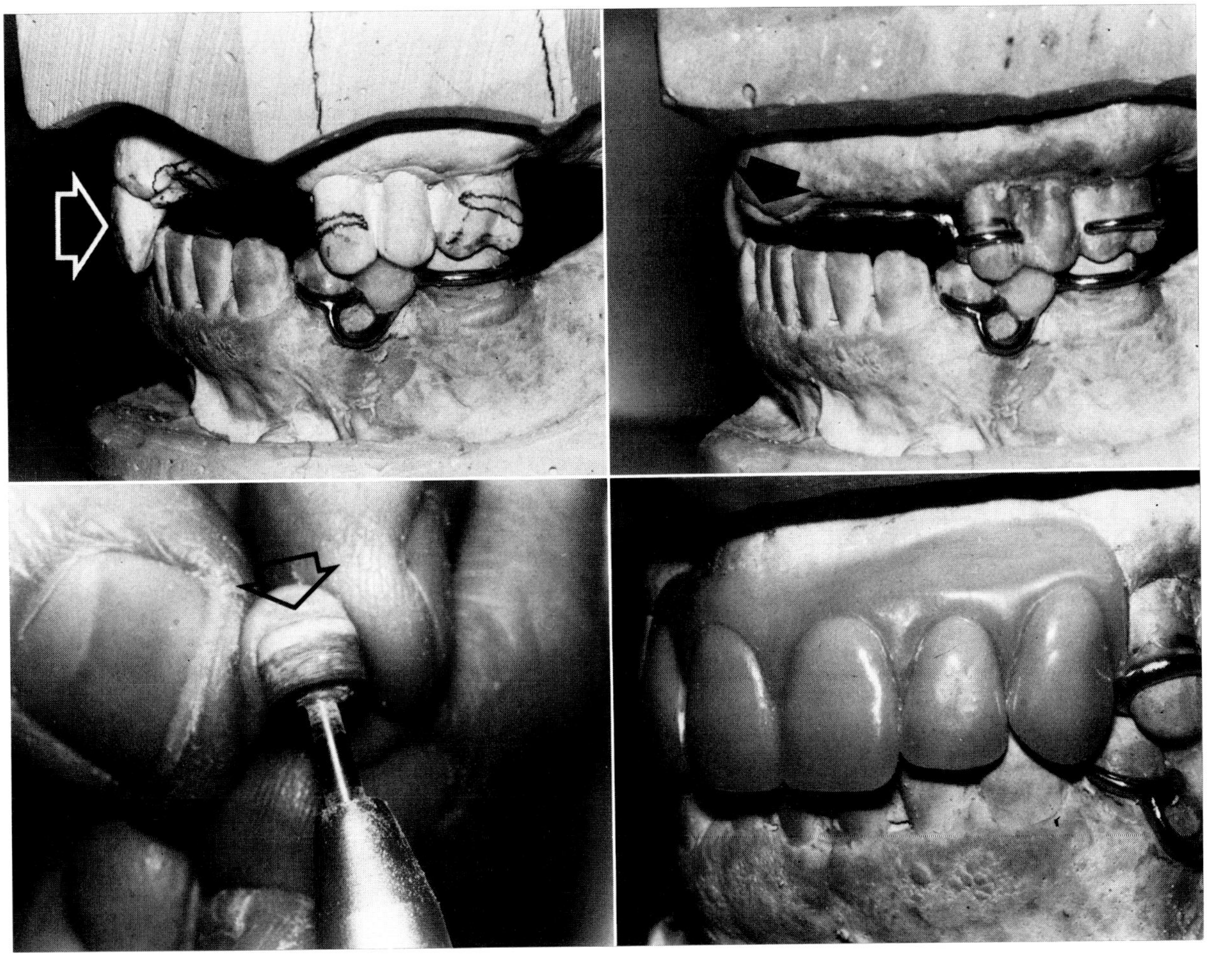

Fig. 20-68. Abutment tooth must be reduced sufficiently to allow esthetic placement of artificial tooth. **A,** Unprepared abutment tooth (arrow). **B,** Prepared tooth (arrow). **C,** Hollow grinding artificial tooth (arrow). **D,** Complete tooth arrangement.

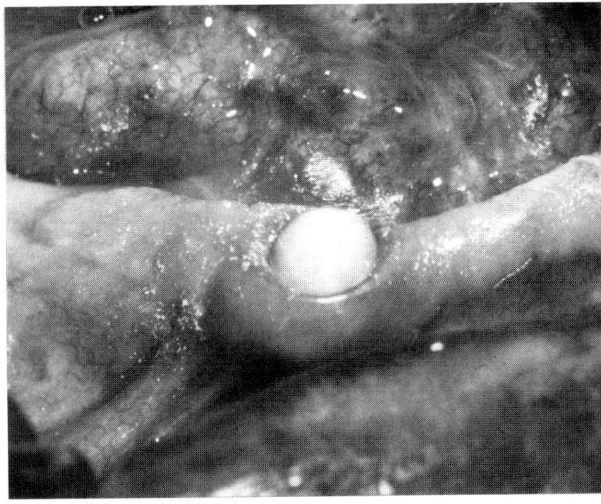

Fig. 20-69. Abutment reduced to 2 to 3 mm above proximal gingival margins.

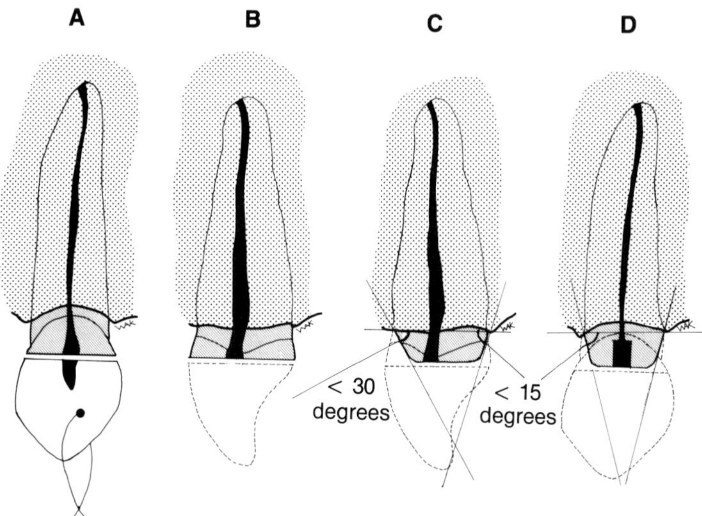

Fig. 20-70. A, Hole is prepared through clinical crown and dental floss threaded to secure crown when sectioned. **B,** Crown is sectioned 2 to 3 mm above proximal gingival margin. **C,** Labial aspect is tapered at approximately 30-degree angle to provide space for positioning of artificial tooth. **D,** Proximal and lingual surfaces are tapered approximately 15 degrees, and occlusal surface is rounded.

ization is complete. Any flash that goes beyond the butt joint preparation is removed with a bur. Resin is also removed in areas of contact with the free gingival margin. The resin that flowed through the hole in the base is finished flush with the polished surface (Fig. 20-71).

This technique allows the adaptation of the prosthesis to the overdenture abutment under varying degrees of occlusal force. If the edentulous area is small and the objective is a prosthesis that is entirely tooth borne, the patient simply closes into light centric occlusal contact. If the edentulous area is large and it is believed that some tissue displacement is desirable before contact with the overdenture abutment, the adaptation can be completed under some occlusal force. This can be accomplished by applying finger pressure or by having the patient close on a cotton roll placed over the replacement teeth.

Postinsertion care

The patient must be educated as to the importance of the overdenture abutments for the success of the prosthesis and as to the alternatives if the abutment tooth were lost. Ideally the patient will be motivated to perform the procedures necessary for maintaining good oral health.

Fluoride application to the prepared teeth helps prevent caries. The patient should be treated on the day of insertion and at subsequent recall appointments with a 2-minute application of 0.5% acidulated phosphate fluoride (APF) followed by a 2-minute application of 0.4% stannous fluoride ($SnF1_2$). The patient is also given a stable, water-free 0.4% $SnF1_2$ gel to be used on a daily basis after thorough cleaning of the prosthesis and the teeth. The gel can be used with a toothbrush to protect the remaining teeth as well as the abutment tooth. It should be placed in the concavity of the denture base that fits over the overdenture abutment tooth, and the prosthesis inserted in the mouth. The denture base acts as a carrying tray for the gel. The prosthesis is worn 4 to 5 minutes after which the patient can remove the prosthesis and expectorate, but not rinse.

Recall appointments at 3- to 4-month intervals should be used to evaluate plaque control and tissue response to the prosthesis. Continuous education and motivation are essential to the continued success of this treatment.

Prognosis

The chance for a successful prognosis is enhanced if the removable partial denture design is sound, if the fitting of the framework to the teeth and the bases to the tissue is accurate, and if the occlusion is of fine quality. However, no matter how meticulous, beautiful, and accurate the restorative procedures, the ultimate success depends on what the patient does.

These treatment procedures are within the capability of any dentist, because they vary little from routine clinical procedures used in treating the partially edentulous patient. Dental students have demonstrated their ability to master these procedures with relatively little difficulty.

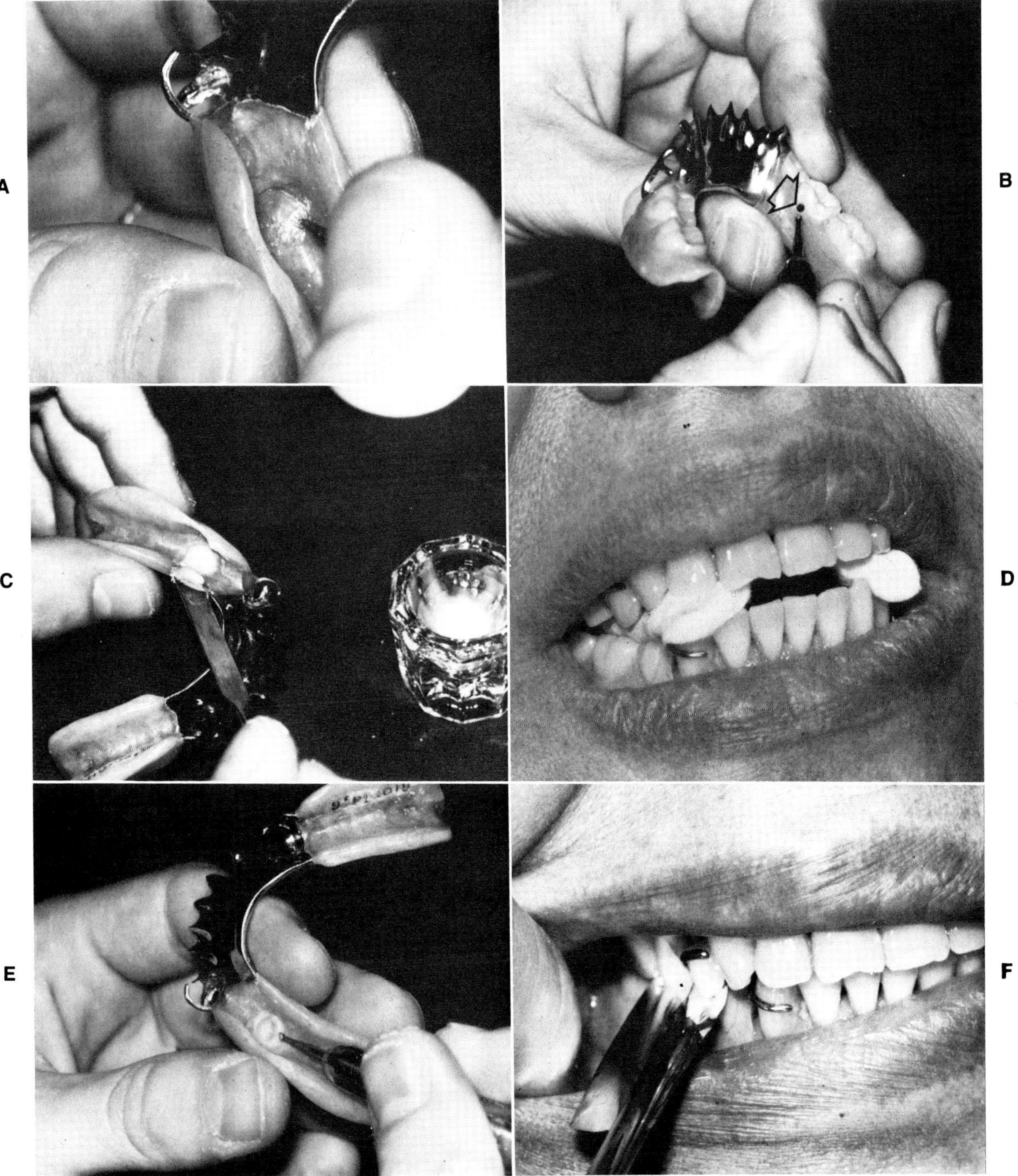

Fig. 20-71. Adapting denture base to overdenture abutment. **A,** Contact is removed between denture base and abutment tooth. Butt joint finish line is prepared. **B,** Escape hole is prepared (arrow). **C,** Tooth-colored autopolymerizing acrylic resin is placed in prepared concavity of denture base. **D,** Patient closes on cotton rolls. **E,** Acrylic resin flash is removed back to butt joint of finish line. **F,** Occlusion is carefully checked.

UNILATERAL REMOVABLE PARTIAL DENTURES

Several decades ago, before the advent of high-speed dental engines, many practitioners were reluctant to enter the laborious clinical sessions necessary to prepare several teeth for crowns to replace one or two missing teeth with a fixed partial denture. Frequently the practitioner and the patient shared a reluctance to prepare crowns on two uninvolved teeth to replace a single tooth. The prognosis for full coverage crown restorations was not favorable at that time.

To avoid this seemingly unnecessary tooth crown preparation, many practitioners resorted to removable prostheses to replace these single teeth or short-span edentulous spaces. If these spaces were unilateral, the removable partial dentures were designed to cover only the side of the arch with the missing teeth. This unilateral design concept was devised with the idea of contacting as little of the soft tissue and as few of the remaining teeth as possible. The practice of preventive dentistry and adequate home care instruction was not particularly in vogue at that time, so decay and gingival inflammation were constant problems.

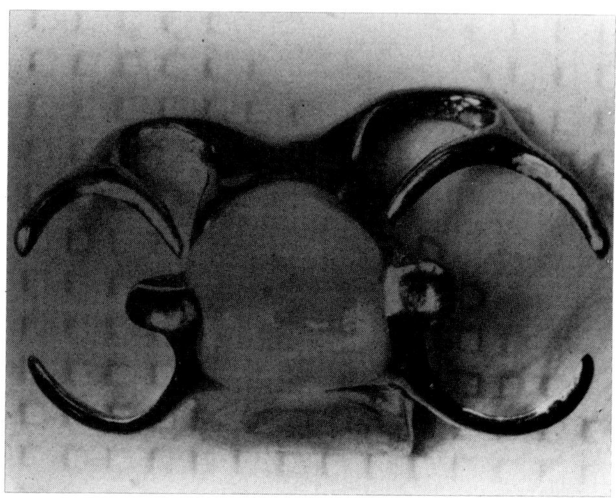

Fig. 20-72. Unilateral removable partial denture should be used with caution. It is potentially dangerous replacement.

Disadvantages

We do *not* advocate the use of the unilateral removable partial denture because it is potentially dangerous to the wearer (Fig. 20-72). Unless all dislodging forces can be totally controlled—which most of the time is difficult if not impossible—the chance of the denture becoming dislodged and aspirated is too great compared with what it can contribute to the overall health of the patient. It cannot be denied that many patients have worn unilateral partial dentures successfully for a number of years, but their use cannot be justified in light of the extremely serious potential consequence and the other currently available forms of treatment.

Limiting factors in selecting a unilateral partial denture for a treatment plan besides the obvious one just mentioned are mentioned in the following discussion.

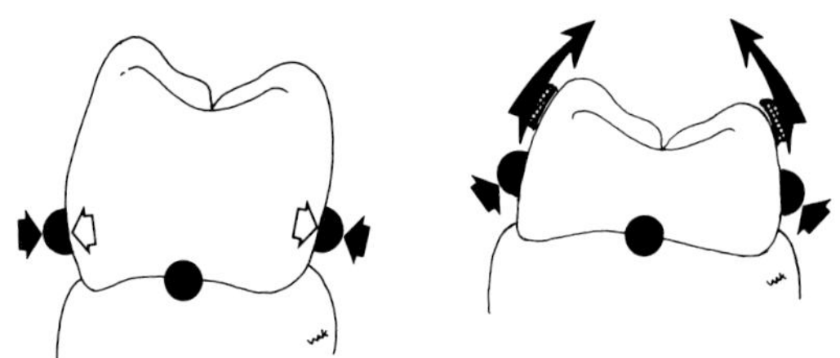

Fig. 20-73. For unilateral removable partial denture to be successful, clinical crown of abutment tooth must be long enough to resist rotational forces.

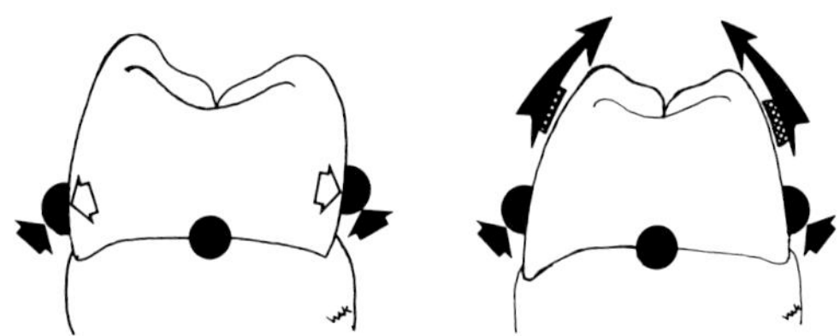

Fig. 20-74. The buccal and lingual surfaces of the abutment tooth must be parallel to resist tipping forces.

Design

The abutment teeth must have adequate clinical crown length (Fig. 20-73). A short crown will not offer sufficient resistance to rotational forces around an axis along the crest of the residual ridge. These rotational forces must be resisted or the partial denture will not be retained.

The buccal and lingual surfaces of the abutment teeth must be parallel or nearly parallel to each other in order to resist these tipping forces. If one or both surfaces are tapered or slanted occlusogingivally, little resistance to rotation in a direction away from the tapered surface will be encountered (Fig. 20-74).

Retentive undercuts should be available on both the buccal and lingual surfaces of each abutment tooth (Fig. 20-75). With this clasping configuration, complete resistance to rotational or dislodging forces should be present. With anything less than this, the partial denture could be dislodged during the chewing process.

The type of clasps used is not significant, because the prosthesis is tooth supported. The simplest type of clasp available to reach the retentive undercut and to meet the additional clasp requirements (for example,

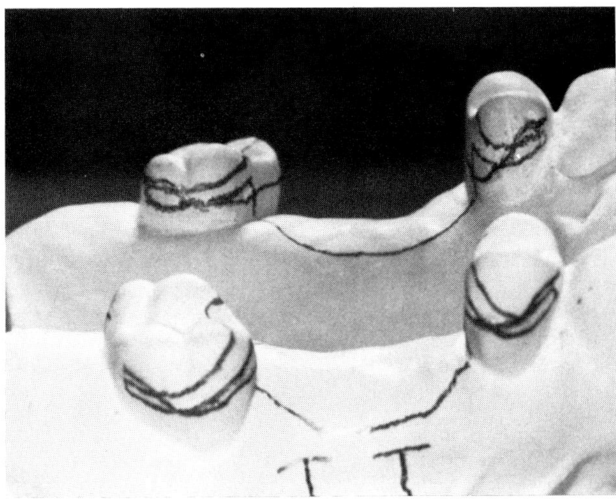

Fig. 20-75. Retentive undercuts must be available on both the buccal and lingual surfaces of abutment teeth.

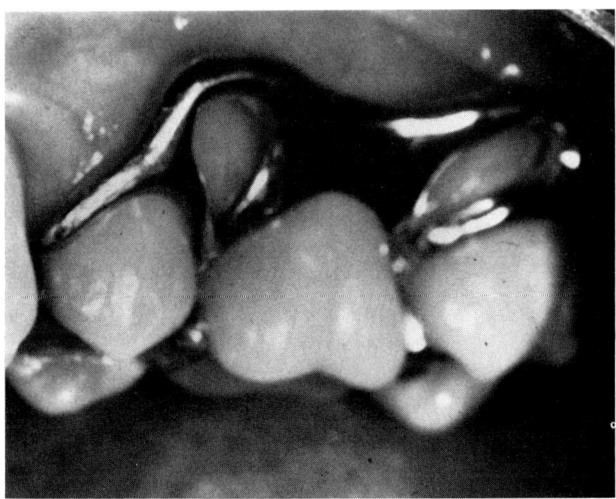

Fig. 20-76. Denture base contributes little to support of unilateral removable partial denture.

bracing, encirclement) should be selected. Occlusal rests must be designed at each end of the edentulous space to ensure total vertical support. If the prosthesis is not seated completely, greater problems will be faced in realizing passivity against rotational forces.

The artificial tooth replacement for the unilateral removable partial denture will normally be the tube tooth supported by a cast metal denture base. The edentulous ridge is not a contributing factor as far as support for the prosthesis is concerned, so extension of the denture base is not a factor.

The metal denture base can be made to fit the residual ridge more intimately if good impression techniques and good laboratory procedures are followed. This results in a more hygienic prosthesis, because food will not tend to collect under the denture base. The only support that may be derived from the denture base is some resistance to lateral and rotational forces. This resistance is limited; it should not be counted on to overcome a deficiency in support from the abutment teeth (Fig. 20-76).

The remainder of the procedure for using the unilateral partial denture in patient treatment is the same as for any conventional removable partial prosthesis. The cast framework must be fitted to the abutment teeth, and the final occlusion must be brought to a state of harmony with the remaining natural teeth.

Prognosis

Although unilateral removable partial dentures have been used successfully, we wish to reemphasize our objection to them because of the possibility of aspiration.

REFERENCE

Simmons, J.J.: Swinglock stabilization and retention, Texas Dent. J. 81:10-12, February 1963.

BIBLIOGRAPHY

Antos, E.W., Jr., and others: The swing-lock partial denture: an alternative approach to conventional removable partial denture service, J. Prosthet. Dent. **40**:257-262, 1978.

Beard, C.C., and Clayton, J.A.: Effects of occlusal splint therapy on TMJ dysfunction, J. Prosthet. Dent. **44**:324-335, 1980.

Brewer, A.A., and Morrow, R.M.: Overdentures, ed 2, St. Louis, 1980, The C.V. Mosby Co.

Firtell, D.N., and others: Root retention and removable partial denture design, J. Prosthet. Dent. **42**:131-134, 1979.

Fish, E.N.: Periodontal diseases: occlusal trauma and partial dentures, B. Dent. J. **95**:199-206, 1953.

Javed, N.S., and Dadmanesh, J.: Obturator design for hemimaxillectomy patients, J. Prosthet. Dent. **36**:77, 1976.

Jordan, L.G.: Treatment of advanced periodontal disease by prosthodontic procedures, J. Prosthet. Dent. **10**:908-911, 1960.

Lord, J.L. and Teel, S.: The overdenture, Dent. Clin. North Am. **13**:871, 1969.

Lord, J.L. and Teel, S.: The overdenture: patient selection, use of copings and follow-up evaluation, J. Prosthet. Dent. **32**:41-50, 1974.

McKinzie, J.S.: Mutual problems of the periodontist and prosthodontist, J. Prosthet. Dent. **5**:37-42, 1955.

Miller. P.A.: Complete dentures supported by natural teeth, J. Prosthet. Dent. **8**:924, 1958.

Morrow, R.M.: Handbook for immediate overdentures, St. Louis, 1979, The C.V. Mosby Co.

Muhlemann, H.R.: Periodontometry: a method of measuring tooth mobility, Oral Surg. **4**:1220, 1951.

Nevin, R.B.: Periodontal aspects of partial denture prosthesis, J. Prosthet. Dent. **5**:215-219, 1955.

Philips, W.L.: Impaction of dentures in the esophagus, J. Prosthet. Dent. **26**:222-224, 1971

Reitz, P.V., and others: An overdenture survey: second report, J. Prosthet. Dent. **43**:457-462, 1980.

Richard, G.E., and others: Hemisected molars for additional overdenture support, J. Prosthet. Dent. **38**:16-21, 1977.

Rudd, K.D., and O'Leary, T.J.: Stabilizing periodontally weakened teeth by using guide plane removable partial dentures, J. Prosthet. Dent. **16**:721-727, 1966.

Schooper, A.F.: Partial dentures and its relation to periodontics, J. Am. Dent. Assoc. **45**:415-421, 1952.

Schulte, J.K., and Smith, D.E.: Clinical evaluation of swinglock removable partial dentures. J. Prosthet. Dent. **44**:595-603, 1980.

Schuyler, C.H.: The partial denture as a means of stabilizing abutment teeth, J. Am. Dent. Assoc. **28**:1121-1125, 1941.

Seaman, F., and Shannon, I.L.: Fluoride treatment and microhardness of dentin, J. Prosthet. Dent. **41**:528-530, 1979.

Seeman, S.: A study of the relationship between periodontal disease and the wearing of partial dentures, Aust. Dent. J. **8**:206-208, 1963.

Simmons, J.J.: Swinglock clinical manual, Dallas, 1968, Ideal Development Company.

Sprigg, R.H.: Six year clinical evaluation of the Swing-lock removable partial denture, The Haus Turkheim memorial lecture, London, Spring 1970, The Anglo-Continental Dental Society.

Stewart, K.L., and Rudd K.D.: Stabilizing periodontally weakened teeth with removable partial dentures, J. Prosthet. Dent. **19**:475-482, 1968.

Strohaver, R.A., and Trovillion, H.M.: Removable partial overdentures, J. Prosthet. Dent. **35**:624-629, 1976.

Thayer, H.H., and Caputo, A.A.: Photoelastic stress analysis of overdenture attachments, J. Prosthet. Dent. **43**:611-617, 1980.

Toolson, L.B., and Smith, D.E.: A 2-year longitudinal study of overdenture patients: incidence and control of caries on overdenture abutments, J. Prosthet. Dent. **40**:486-491, 1978.

Trapozzano, V.R. and Winter, G.R.: Periodontal aspects of partial denture design, J. Prosthet. Dent. **2**:101-107, 1952.

21 Relining, rebasing, and repairing the removable partial denture

James S. Brudvik

Removable partial dentures require a level of maintenance that far exceeds that of the fixed restoration. Because removable partial denture wearers are encouraged to keep their dentures out of the mouth for a good part of the day, the potential exists for distortion and damage. The true removable partial denture—that is, one supported by edentulous ridges as well as abutment teeth—has a special need for relining or rebasing. When this distal extension denture loses soft tissue support and begins to rock around its fulcrum, in function it has the potential to damage the abutment teeth and gingival tissues.

Relining is the most basic of the partial denture maintenance techniques. It involves adding new denture base material to the existing resin to make up for the loss of tissue base contact caused by the resorption of the alveolar ridge. The addition can be done in the denture flask as part of a laboratory procedure or directly in the mouth using specially formulated resins. Both techniques have advantages but, because of the poor quality of resin that results from the mouth reline, that technique is normally reserved for temporary or transitional situations only.

Rebasing is completely a laboratory technique where the bulk of the denture base material along with the correcting impression material is removed and replaced by new resin. This approach results in a base of uniform quality but is technically complicated by the fact that the retentive meshwork is buried within the denture base and often without sufficient relief beneath the mesh to allow for adequate bulk of new resin.

When both the denture base and the denture teeth are involved in a maintenance or repair situation, the partial denture may need to be stripped of both teeth and denture base and reconstructed.

RELINING

In order to determine if a removable partial denture is in need of relining, some visual reference to the loss of supporting tissue must be established. Perhaps the easiest means of evaluating the space under the denture base is to place a thin mix of alginate (irreversible hydrocolloid) in the denture base area, seat the partial denture in the mouth and maintain its position until the alginate sets (Fig. 21-1). The denture can then be removed from the mouth, the amount of alginate present measured, and an informed clinical judgment made (Fig. 21-2). The alginate must be mixed with an increased water/power ratio to allow a minimum of tissue displacement. One scoop of alginate powder mixed with 2 measures of water will provide a usable mix. The alginate separates easily and cleanly from the denture after the evaluation is made.

It is also possible to evaluate the loss of support on distal extension partial dentures by applying a seating force on the extreme distal end of the denture base and watching an anterior indirect retainer lift off its rest preparation as the denture rotates around the fulcrum line (Fig. 21-3). The amount of space under the indirect retainer is an indicator of the amount of space to be found under the denture base. Some clinical judgment is essential here because the length of the distal extension base affects the amount of movement, as does the distance from the indirect retainer to the fulcrum line.

If two or more millimeters of alginate is present under the denture base or if the indirect retainer lifts two or more millimeters, the patient can be considered a candidate for a reline or rebase.

Impression technique

In order for a removable partial denture reline to be successful, the denture base must extend to cover the denture space. The impression material cannot be expected to extend the borders of the denture beyond the support of the denture base. If the existing denture is short of ideal coverage, a rebase should be used instead of a reline.

The resin denture base is prepared for the reline impression by removing a uniform amount of denture resin from the tissue side of the base as well as all undercut areas. This removal is often limited by the amount of resin under the retentive meshwork. The resin should be removed for two important reasons. First, space must be created so that there is no possibility that the semicontained impression material might displace soft tissue and distort the supporting struc-

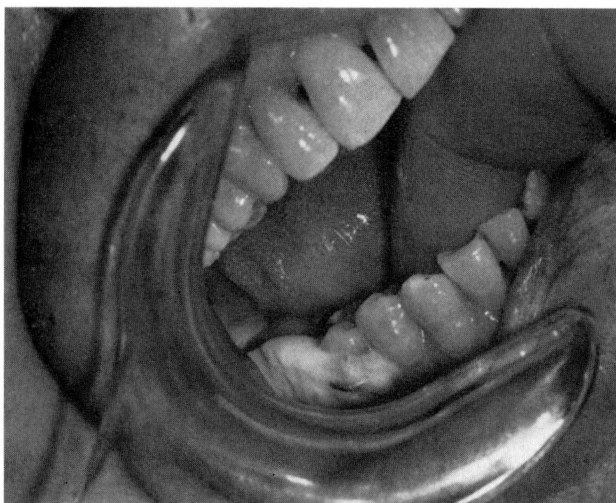

Fig. 21-1. Mandibular distal extension partial denture extension filled with thin mix of alginate and held with rests seated until alginate sets.

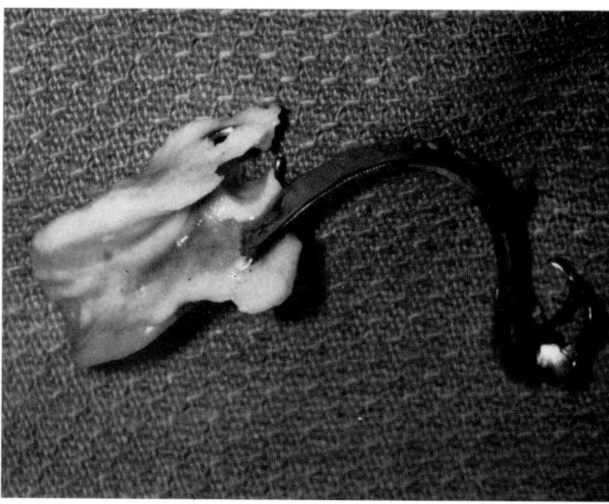

Fig. 21-2. Removable partial denture removed from mouth. Bulk of alginate on crest of ridge is good indication for need to reline.

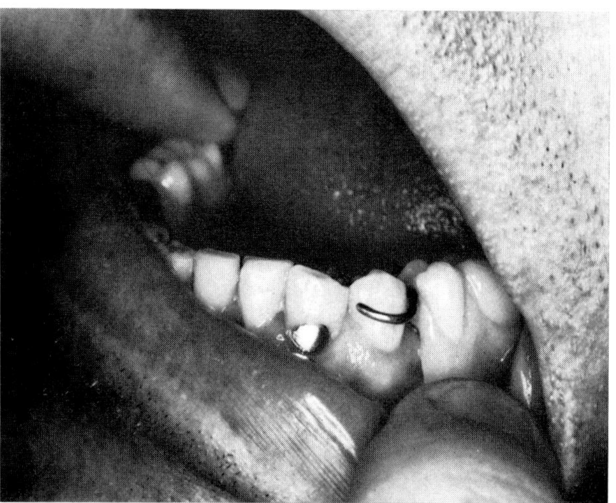

Fig. 21-3. Finger pressure applied to retromolar pad area of distal extension partial denture. Incisal rest on distal surface of left canine has rotated off tooth by more than a millimeter, indicating possible need for reline.

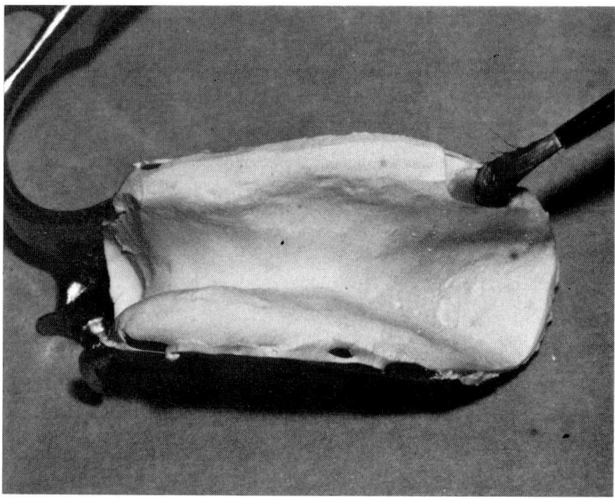

Fig. 21-4. Small artist's brush is used to add mouth temperature wax to correct impressions. When adding to rubber, silicone, or ether impression, thin layer of sticky wax applied to area with *very hot* spatula will greatly increase the adherence of wax. When wax is painted, it helps to have brush at temperature of wax (leave brush in wax pot for 30 seconds before painting).

tures, and second, the resin that has been in contact with the oral cavity must be removed so that the new resin will interface with material that is dense and uncontaminated.

The more displaceable tissue present in the denture base area, the greater the space required for the impression material. The choice of impression material itself also depends on the type of tissue to be impressed. Mobile tissue on the crest of the ridge is a good indication to use a free-flowing zinc oxide impression material. Polysulfide rubber, silicones, or mouth temperature wax can be used with confidence on the dense, firm edentulous ridge. Tissue-conditioning material can also be used as an impression material although it offers no particular advantage and can easily distort soft tissue.

The most critical step in the reline procedure is the maintenance of the tooth-framework relationship during the set of the impression material. Under *no* circumstances can the patient be allowed to bring his teeth into contact during the impression making. Rather, the dentist must hold the framework against the abutment teeth until the impression material is ready to be removed from the mouth. In this way soft tissue support will be in harmony with the tooth-framework relationship and is the only way that success in the reline procedure can be routinely accomplished.

When zinc oxide base impression materials are used, the clinician must remove any excess material that extrudes into tooth undercut areas or around active clasp arms. This is easily accomplished with an explorer or similar dental instrument in the hand that is not being used to maintain the tooth-framework relationship.

Small defects in the impression can usually be corrected with mouth temperature wax (Fig. 21-4). Thin extensions of impression material beyond the denture border should be removed as soon as the set impression is removed from the mouth. Rough edges created by the removal of extraneous material can be covered with a thin coat of mouth temperature wax and the completed reline impression reinserted in the mouth. At this time, an attempt to rock the framework around its fulcrum should be made to verify that the reline impression has indeed restored the desired support to the denture base.

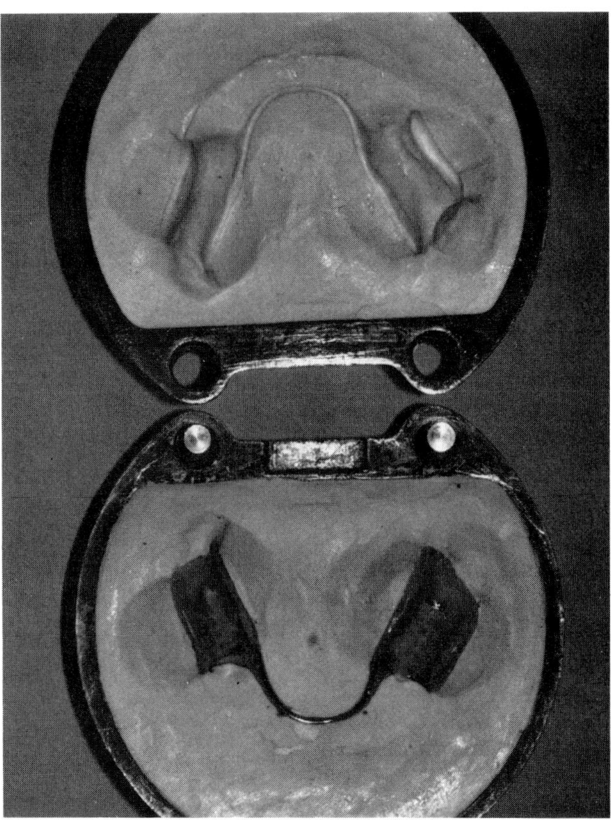

Fig. 21-5. Denture to be relined is found in one half of flask with stone replica of ridge tissues in other.

Laboratory technique

The completed partial denture reline impression is presented to the laboratory for processing.

The denture is first flasked in the conventional denture flask. As a routine partial denture is processed, the framework is included in the first half of the flasking by covering it and the stone teeth of the master cast with the investing plaster-stone mixture.

In the reline investing only the impression area remains with the first half of the flasking (Fig. 21-5). The entire partial denture is included in the second half of the flasking. This situation makes complete flask closure before processing *absolutely critical.* An error here will result in the entire partial denture being held up by the denture base. In conventional construction the failure to complete flask closure will result only in a prematurity on the denture teeth.

Depending on the instructions of the resin manufacturer, the partial denture can be flasked in dental stone. The flask can be warmed to facilitate the separation of zinc oxide base impression material or mouth temperature wax. Polysulfide rubber or silicones can be separated immediately after the flasking stone is set without the need for heat.

The denture base area is now completely cleared of impression material with an assortment of denture finishing burs. Separating material is applied to the cast in standard fashion. The resin is mixed to the manufacturer's directions and placed in the flask. Complete flask closure is essential.

The relined impression can also be mounted on a duplicating device. This device is commonly used for the reline procedure in complete dentures. Again, the entire partial denture must be in the top half of the mounting. The impression material is removed as in the flasked reline. Autopolymerizing denture resin is used with this device.

In either technique, once the resin is completely polymerized, the deflasking begins. This step is frought with the potential for damaging the partial denture. Clasp arms, in particular, are easily distorted from careless deflasking. The final deflasking should be done with a shell blaster to eliminate harming these metal components.

The now relined partial denture is shaped and polished in the same fashion as is done with initial processing.

Intraoral reline

There are commercially available autopolymerizing resins that are intended to be cured in the mouth. This type of reline is inferior to the laboratory reline, but there are indications for its use in temporary situations. The preparation of the denture base is the same as for the laboratory reline. The mouth-curing resin must be

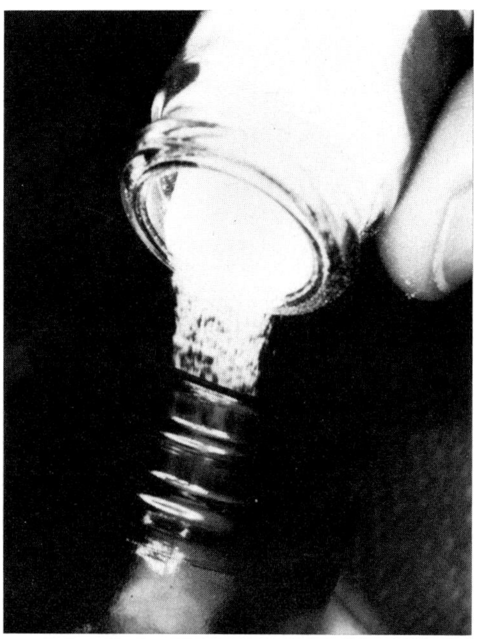

Fig. 21-6. Polymer sifted into monomer to reduce air entrapment.

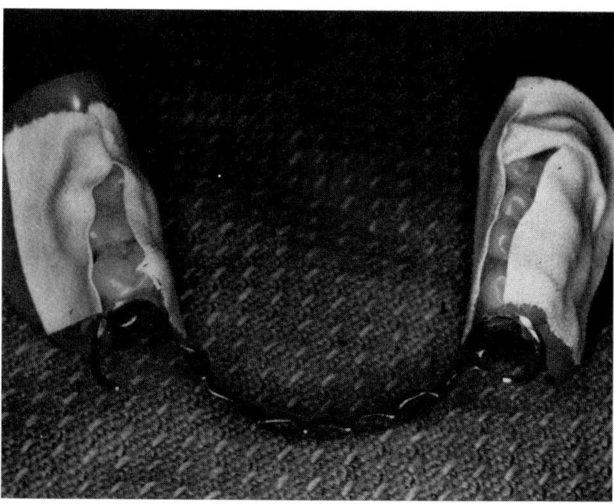

Fig. 21-7. External surface of partial denture prepared for intraoral reline.

mixed according to the manufacturer's directions, but special care must be taken to sift the polymer into the monomer without trapping air in the mixture (Fig. 21-6). Spatulation of the resin is not critical when the material is to be packed under pressure, but when the resin is used as both a relatively free-flowing impression as well as the final base, any air trapped in the mix will inevitably result in a porous resin base.

The denture base is prepared by covering the external surface with adhesive tape (Fig. 21-7). The tape prevents the resin from curing to the outer surface of the denture and the denture teeth. The inner surface is wetted with monomer and the prepared resin applied with a small spatula. Again, care must be taken not to trap air in the resin.

The partial denture is now placed in the mouth and held in proper relation by the clinician. At the time specified by the manufacturer, the denture is removed and any excess trimmed back to the original border with a sharp curved scissor (Fig. 21-8). The patient rinses the mouth with cold water to remove the taste of free monomer from the mix. The denture is then reseated while the resin is still plastic, and held in place until the directions indicate that the denture should be removed and placed in a pressure pot for final curing.

The resin used in this type of reline will completely polymerize in around 12 to 15 minutes from the start of the mix. When the resin is set, it can be finished in the conventional manner. It can be expected that the in-the-mouth reline will be porous and not color stable.

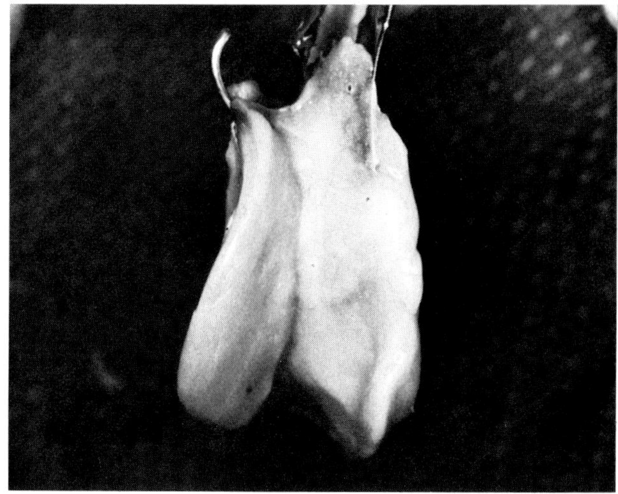

Fig. 21-8. Autopolymerizing resin is removed from mouth when suggested by manufacturer. Resin extending beyond internal finishing line must be removed when resin is still doughy.

Nevertheless, the procedure is quick and will return the partial denture to a stable relationship between the hard and soft tissue support.

REBASING

The rebasing procedure replaces the majority of the denture base and is indicated in situations where the denture borders do not extend to cover all the supporting soft tissue. It is often used when the denture has

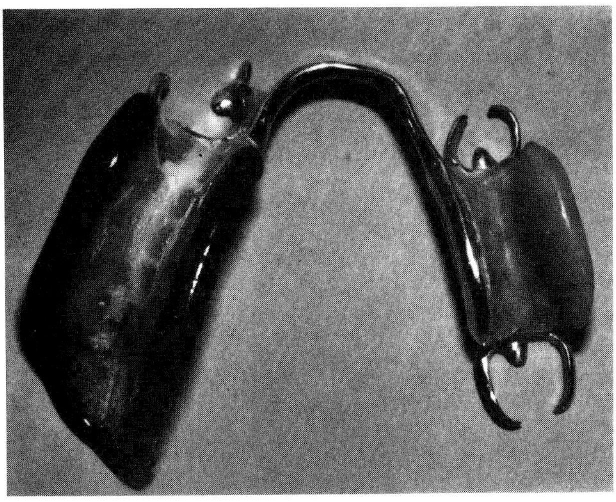

Fig. 21-9. Distal extension base has been relieved almost to meshwork and borders remolded in modeling compound.

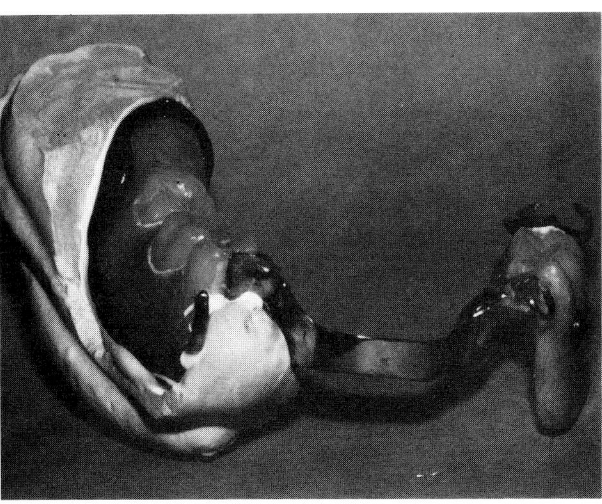

Fig. 21-10. Sectional cast poured against rebase impression. Cast should have sufficient undercuts on its base to lock it into first half of flasking stone.

been fractured in the denture base area or has become stained or discolored.

The denture resin is relieved as in the reline and shortened to allow room for a readaptation of the borders with modeling plastic. The modeling plastic is added in small increments and border molded in the same way a complete denture impression is extended to cover the entire denture base area (Fig. 21-9). When the border molding is complete, the base is covered with a suitable impression material and the final impression made with the framework positively related to the teeth.

It is best to pour a cast against the impression after it has been corrected for defects. The cast will only contact the soft tissue (edentulous ridge) area and not involve the framework at all (Fig. 21-10). On this cast the new peripheries can be blended into the polished surfaces of the denture base with the addition of small amounts of baseplate wax (Fig. 21-11). This procedure will give a nearly finished contour to the processed rebase and reduce finishing time.

The rebase impression is flasked in a conventional manner as described in the reline procedure. Again the entire partial denture will be held in the second half of the flask. Because wax and modeling plastic are involved in this impression, the flask should be subjected to a brief boilout procedure to soften these materials and ease separation of the flask. When the flask is opened and all traces if impression materials and wax removed, the remaining denture resin can be ground away to allow the majority of the finished rebase to be in new resin (Fig. 21-12). Obviously this resin removal must stop short of the denture teeth. Where anterior teeth are involved, the junction of the new resin and the existing denture base should be kept in an area that will not be visible when the patient smiles, because there will often be a faint line at this junction.

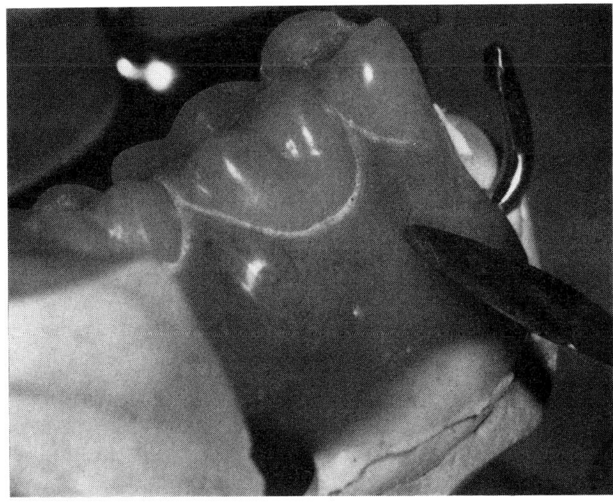

Fig. 21-11. Base contours reestablished with base plate wax before flasking.

The packing of the rebase in the flask is, as stated earlier, *absolutely critical.* Incomplete flask closure will

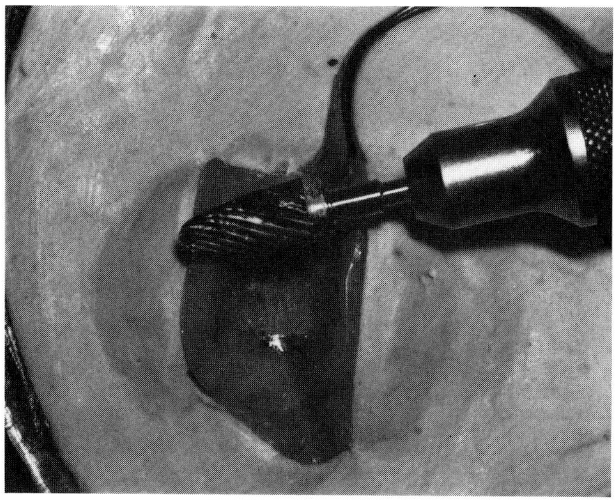

Fig. 21-12. Preparation for rebase requires that most of denture base be cut away to position just short of denture teeth.

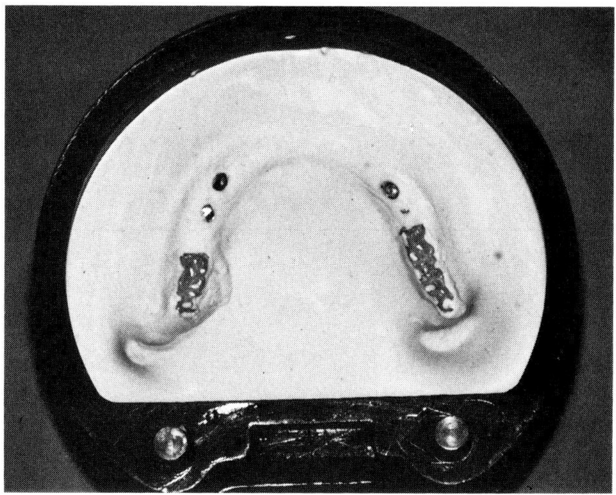

Fig. 21-13. First pour of second half of flasking carried just to occlusal surface of rests and denture teeth.

make the rebased partial denture unusable. Careful trial packing and attention to detail will eliminate these potential problems.

The recovery of the processed rebase or reline from the flask presents another possible problem area. Because the entire framework is enveloped in the second half of the flasking, the potential for damaging or distorting the frame, and especially the clasp arms, is great. Investing the second half in two stages can simplify this procedure. The first stage will consist of stone just covering the framework and up to the occlusal or incisal surfaces of the denture teeth (Fig. 21-13). When this is set, it is painted with separating medium and the flasking completed with a stone core. Recovery now consists of removing the stone core and carefully removing the thin stone covering with a laboratory knife or a pneumatic blade. This removal should be for bulk only and the final stone removal left to the shell blaster.

Attention to these details will greatly reduce deflasking and finishing time. The line of juncture of the new resin and the old is more an esthetic irritant than a structural flaw. Despite the utmost attention to detail it may still occur. Shaping the borders of the old resin to a 90-degree angle to the external surface greatly reduces the chances of having an observable line. When the new resin does not butt at right angles to the old, a flash of thin resin over the existing denture base resin will usually result in a prominent line. Where esthetics is not an issue, the junction should be rounded to reduce stress concentration and increase strength.

RECONSTRUCTING

If the denture base is destroyed or severely compromised and the framework still demonstrates a clinically acceptable fit, the partial denture can be reconstructed

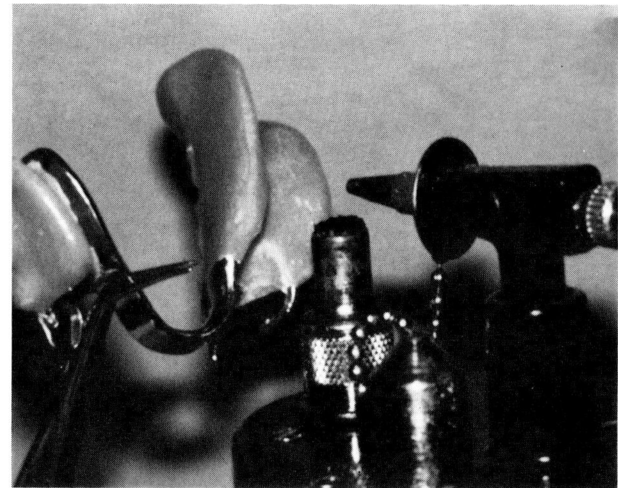

Fig. 21-14. Burning off unwanted denture flange before picking up casting from mouth to reconstruct denture.

by completely removing all resin and denture teeth. This is done by heating the resin from the tissue side while holding the framework in a cotton forceps or hemostat (Fig. 21-14). The resin will soften or even ignite and can then be pried from the retentive meshwork. The framework is then sandblasted to remove the residue from the resin and may be repolished in a normal manner.

The framework is then seated in the mouth and an alginate impression made over it (Fig. 21-15). The framework must be taken out of the mouth by the impression. If it remains in the mouth (separating from the alginate) the retentive clasp arms must be carefully adjusted to reduce the retention and the impression remade. The impression is poured in dental stone and

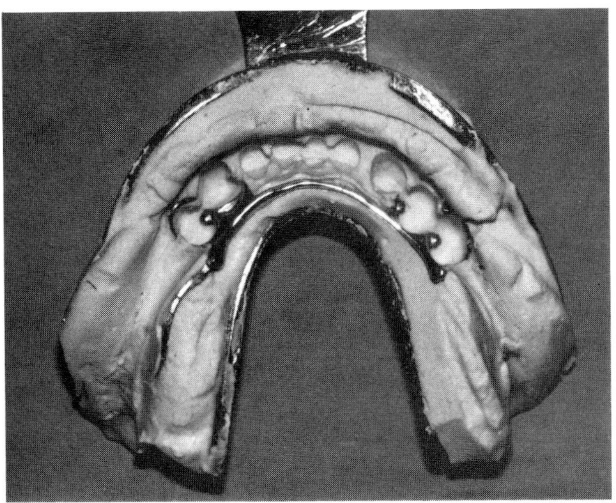

Fig. 21-15. Alginate impression picks up framework from mouth. Undersurface of occlusal rests are free of alginate, indicating that framework was fully seated during placing and setting of impression. Defects in edentulous areas will mandate altered cast impression.

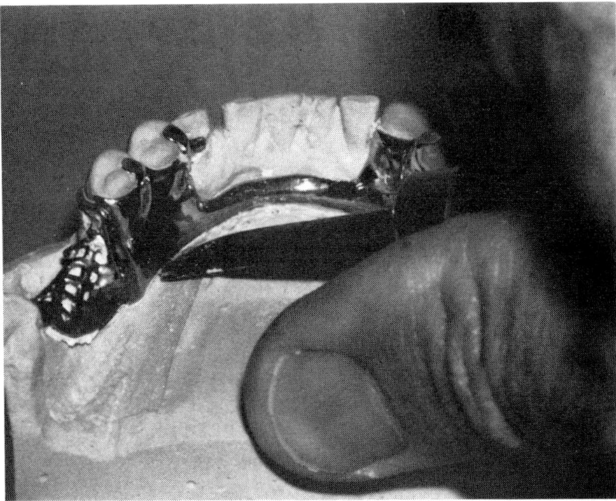

Fig. 21-16. Framework is gently pried from cast with care not to use clasp arms as purchase points.

allowed to completely set before any attempt to recover the cast is made.

After the impression is separated from the cast and the cast trimmed in the standard fashion, the framework is carefully separated from the stone cast by prying it along the inferior border of the major connector (Fig. 21-16). Force must not be applied to the retentive clasp arms. Obviously, distortion is possible in these areas. In some instances, some portions of the stone teeth will fracture during removal. This is not critical to success; the teeth can be attached to the cast with cyanoacrylate adhesive without influencing the final result. With the framework successfully removed from the cast, an analysis of the edentulous areas can be made. If an altered cast impression is indicated, a tray can be attached and the impression made in the conventional manner. If no further impression is indicated, the partial denture can be articulated and completed as if it were a routine construction.

In order to accurately record the tissues in the retentive meshwork area, impression material must be placed into the mesh with the finger or an incomplete impression is likely. There is no reason for the reconstructed partial denture not to be as successful as the original if routine insertion procedures and follow-up are done as indicated.

REPAIRS

Denture base and artificial teeth repairs

Impressions for denture base repairs

Occasions will arise where sections of the denture base have been fractured from the partial denture. If the section is available and can be accurately positioned

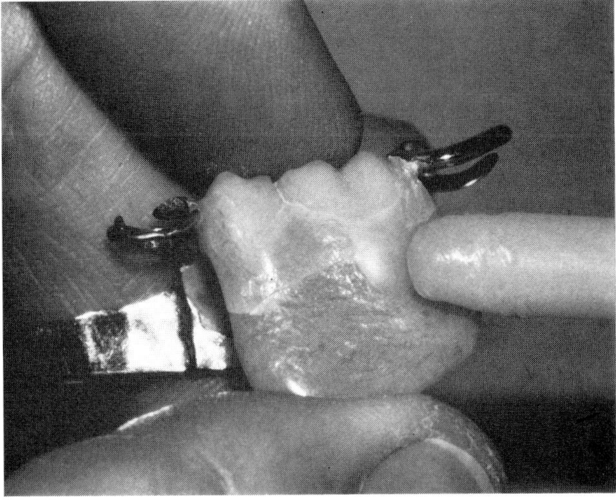

Fig. 21-17. Denture segments should be clean and dry before they are joined with sticky wax while held in precise relationship.

on the fracture site, the repair is a simple matter of luting the pieces together with sticky wax. Normally the clinician holds the sections together in the desired relationship while an assistant places small amounts of sticky wax along the fracture line (Fig. 21-17). Dental stone is poured against the tissue side of the denture base to preserve the relationship. When the stone has set, the denture is removed and cleansed of wax. The fracture line is opened and dovetailed (Fig. 21-18) and, after the cast is painted with a suitable separating material, the pieces of the denture are assembled and held in position with sticky wax or modeling plastic. Autopolymerizing resin can now be added to the prepared

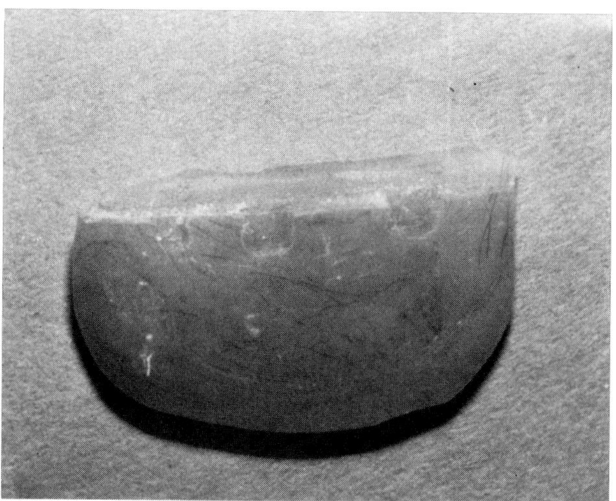

Fig. 21-18. Broken segment is offset and dovetailed on external surface to provide adequate space for quality resin repair.

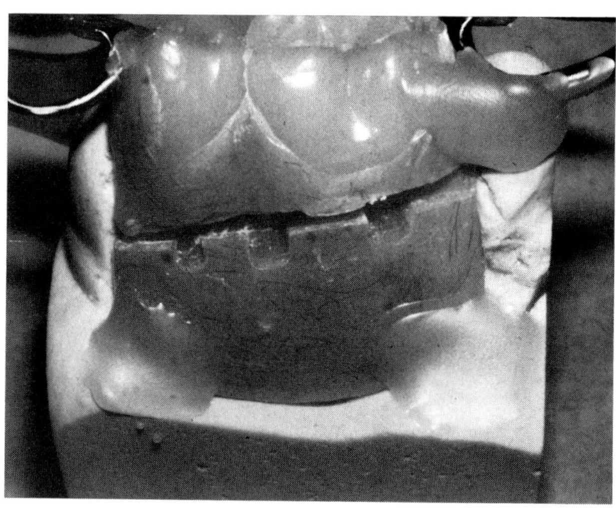

Fig. 21-19. Preparation of repair site is primarily at expense of flange to keep repair as far from denture teeth as possible.

fracture line by the salt-and-pepper method and the repair placed in a heated pressure pot to complete the curing cycle (Fig. 21-19).

If the broken segment(s) cannot be positively related, they should be discarded and the repair undertaken in the following manner (the same approach is indicated if the segments have been lost). If only a small segment is missing, it may be sufficient to simply adapt modeling plastic to the denture base and reconstruct that area in the mouth. The modeling plastic is added to the denture base with dry heat so that it will stick to the base. It is molded by hand to approximate the soft tissue contours, flamed, tempered in the water bath, and seated in the mouth. The plastic will need to be refined by scraping and reheating one or two times to achieve an impression that does not displace tissue. If the defect is large, it is advisable to first approximate the contour with modeling plastic and then reline both the plastic *and* the remainder of the denture base by molding a rebasing "wash" impression. The remainder of the repair is done as a rebase, as previously described.

Replacement of denture teeth

The replacement of a broken or missing denture tooth or teeth is a simple laboratory procedure requiring only that the clinician provide an accurate opposing cast and a jaw relation record. Often no actual record is necessary; only a marking of the opposing cast and the partial denture to indicate centric occlusion. If the partial denture is unstable against the opposing cast because of the loss of the denture teeth, then a positive centric occlusion record can be made by placing modeling plastic in the area of the missing teeth and making a recording. This record will always need to be refined by scraping off excess plastic, reheating, and remaking the closure. Modeling plastic is a wax and exhibits considerable shrinkage. Reheating only the surface and remaking the record can greatly reduce this shrinkage. Modeling plastic is preferred over other waxes because it is completely hard at room temperature.

If the repair is simply the replacement of a tooth with no fracture or loss of associated denture base, a tooth of the same mold and shade is selected and fitted into the existing space. Care should be taken to preserve the labial (or buccal) denture base with access gained by opening the lingual surface (Fig. 21-20). Resin teeth are almost universally used for repair because they are easily bound to the denture with the repair resin. The ridge lap area should be relieved to allow at least 2 mm of repair resin to bind the tooth to the base.

The replacement tooth should be luted to the adjacent denture teeth or framework with sticky wax in its desired position and the autopolymerizing resin added with a fine brush to control its placement (Fig. 21-21). The completed repair is best cured in a heated pressure pot. Careful addition of the repair resin will greatly reduce finishing time (Fig. 21-22). The completed repair is now articulated against the opposing cast and occlusal adjustments completed.

If a number of teeth are to be replaced or if associated denture base areas are missing, a mounting cast should be poured against the partial denture and that cast articulated with the opposing cast. The replacement teeth can now be positioned and the denture base relieved to accept them. Gingival contours are waxed in and the partial denture flasked and packed as de-

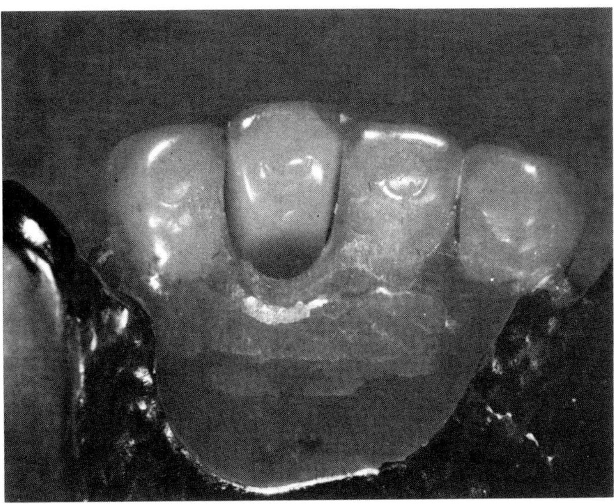

Fig. 21-20. Lingual surface prepared for replacement of single tooth. Adjacent resin and teeth have been relieved slightly to provide base of clean resin for repair.

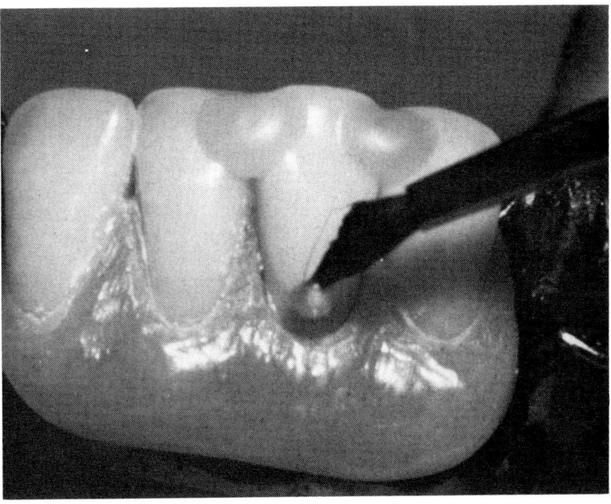

Fig. 21-21. Small amounts of freshly mixed repair resin are added to gingival repair space using small brush that has been contoured to sharp edge. With care at this point, little finishing will be needed.

scribed in the section on the rebase. This approach greatly reduces finishing time and results in a superior end result. The freehand placement of repair resin is difficult to control in extensive additions.

Adding teeth to denture following loss of natural teeth

The replacement of a natural tooth by adding a denture tooth to an existing partial denture requires both the recontouring of the denture base with impression material and an opposing cast with a centric occlusion record as described earlier. This type of repair is often complicated by the need to add clasps and rests or an extension of retentive meshwork or both.

The additional resin retention is easily accomplished by electrosoldering a loop of nonprecious clasp wire in the repair area. If only a single tooth is to be added adjacent to an existing resin denture base, no metal retention will be required.

A new retentive clasp arm can be adapted only if a cast of the remaining natural teeth has been made. This cast is obtained by making an alginate impression over the entire partial denture once the base has been redefined with modeling plastic in the area of the missing tooth. Because resorption of the extraction site will quickly occur, a precise impression is not now critical. The clasp arm is most commonly made of wrought wire and is attached to the resin of the denture base in the area of the added denture tooth. The replacement tooth or teeth are now added as previously described. When a number of teeth are added (as in the case of four mandibular incisors), the repair is really only transitional because the great soft tissue shrinkage and the difficulty of adding extensive resin retention do not make for a quality partial denture.

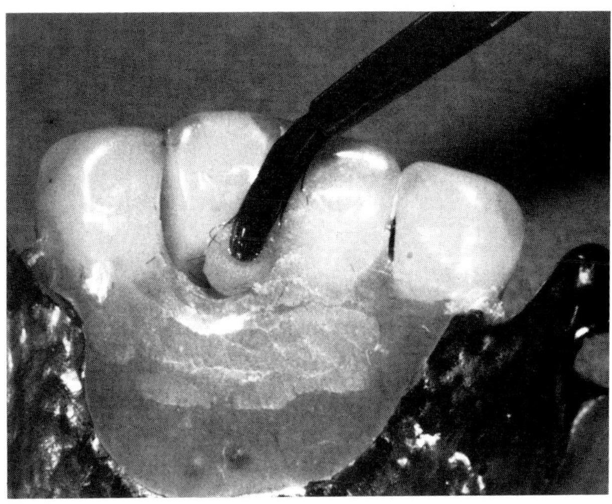

Fig. 21-22. Larger amounts of repair resin are carried by brush to lingual access area.

Design considerations. The addition of denture teeth can be made easier when the loss of the natural tooth is anticipated and the denture designed accordingly. For example, the addition of four mandibular incisors is much easier when a lingual plate has been used as the major connector as opposed to a lingual bar. Teeth with a questionable prognosis should be prepared for an occlusal rest and the casting designed to include that additional rest even if it would not normally be needed. This rest, in connection with the lingual plating, will make the addition of a clasp and denture tooth a simple procedure. The axial and facial surfaces of the once adjacent tooth (now the terminal abutment) should be recontoured for ideal clasping contour before the repair impression is made.

Metal repairs

Clasp addition

By far the most common metal repair for the removable partial denture is the addition of a retentive clasp arm. The clinical procedure for delivering this repair to the laboratory is the same if the reciprocal clasp is to be added. The partial denture must be picked up in the alginate impression so that the exact frame-to-tooth relationship is reproduced on the repair cast. Other retentive clasp arms may have to be adjusted slightly to reduce retention for this to occur. It is not necessary to pour the complete cast—only that area adjacent to the repair site is actually required for the clasp addition. The more teeth involved with the cast, the greater the difficulty in removing the frame without breaking the stone teeth.

The clinician must recover the cast in the office so that he may evaluate the abutment contour and prescribe the type and placement of the repair clasp. The

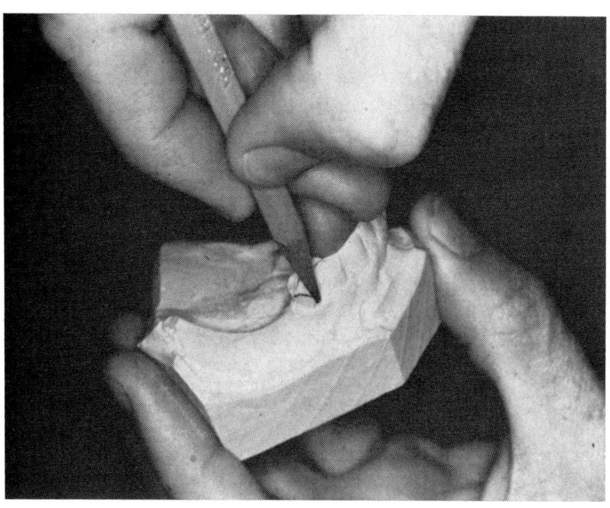

Fig. 21-23. Tooth contour and clasp placement for repair clasp is a clinical decision and should be part of work authorization to laboratory.

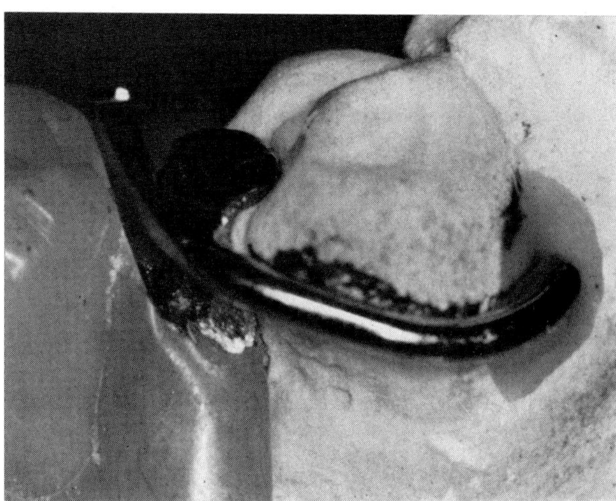

Fig. 21-24. Wrought repair clasp in place for electrosoldering to the rest–minor connector area.

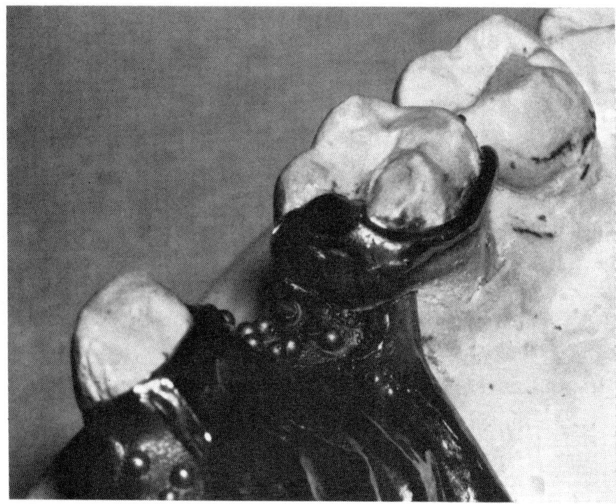

Fig. 21-25. This clasp addition illustrates proper position of soldering area, well into minor connector.

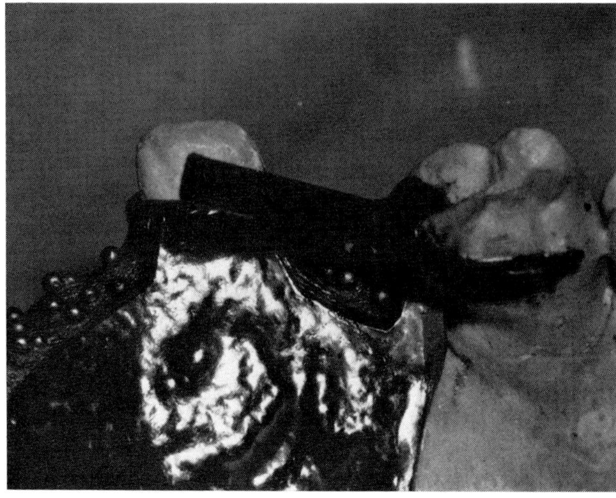

Fig. 21-26. Clasp addition waxed and sprued directly on repair cast. Small amount of investment suitable for alloy to be used can be painted on wax to strengthen repair segment before removing from cast.

design of the replacement clasp is drawn on the abutment tooth and the cast and denture submitted to the laboratory (Fig. 21-23).

The replacement clasp may be embedded in the resin of the denture base or electrosoldered to the framework itself (Fig. 21-24). When a resin attachment is used, the wire must be so contoured that resistance to dislodgement is inherent in the clasp form. Both infrabulge clasps and circumferential clasps are to be used in repair situations. They may be cast or wrought. The wrought clasp is normally chosen for repair situations because it is by far the easiest to construct. The use of cast clasps for repair situations requires the same procedures of blockout, duplication, waxing, and casting as did the original framework. When this is contemplated, the solder joint between the clasp and the framework must be placed well into the minor connector so that the joint is not involved in clasp flexure (Fig. 21-25). It is possible in certain situations for the laboratory to wax the replacement clasp directly on the stone tooth and carefully remove it for investment and casting (Fig. 21-26).

Electrosoldering with either precious or nonprecious solder is usually a simple procedure. Only when the solder joint is adjacent to the resin denture base is special care required so that an excessive amount of resin is not destroyed (Fig. 21-27).

The wrought clasp is adapted and soldered on the stone cast when this is desired. Half-round wires are available to be used as reciprocating (nonretentive) clasps. Round wire forms are almost universally prescribed for the retentive clasp arm.

Infrabulge clasps are normally easy to attach to the buccal resin denture base (Fig. 21-28). Circumferential clasps are usually best attached by bringing them transocclusally to the lingual surface of the denture base. The base is relieved but not perforated and the clasp added with autopolymerizing resin. Curing of the resin should take place in a heated pressure pot or, at a very minimum, in a closed container to claim the best results (Fig. 21-29).

The clinician should expect the clasp repair to be returned on the submitted cast with the clasp in contact with the stone tooth as designed.

Repair of major and minor connectors

It is clinically acceptable to section and solder major and minor connectors when the denture has been distorted and does not completely and passively seat on the abutment teeth.

The clinician will section the framework with a Carborundum "cut off" disk. The sections must now be seated in the mouth (Fig. 21-30). Ideally the sections will have an acceptable fit and the relationship can be captured in a plaster or resin index (Fig. 21-31). Should one or more of the pieces not fit satisfactorily, the denture must be remade.

The sectioned partial denture and the index are submitted to the laboratory where they are reassembled and a counter model of dental stone poured against the framework (Fig. 21-32). High heat platinum 0.001-inch foil is adapted to the counter model in the area of the disk cut only and the framework fluxed with fluoride-based flux (Fig. 21-33). Either precious metal solder or industrial brazing alloy can be used with the electrosoldering machine to complete the repair.

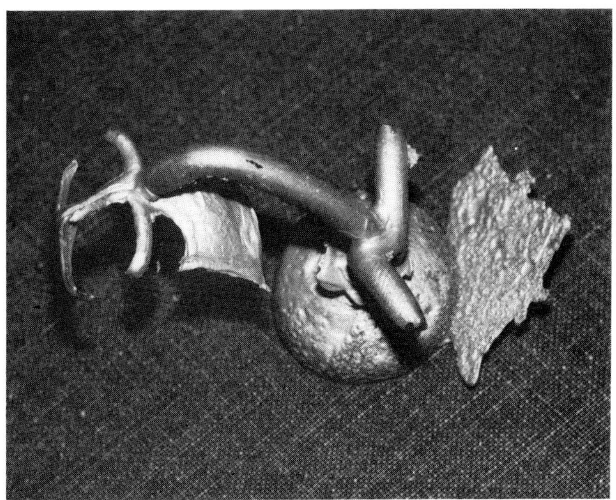

Fig. 21-27. Repair clasp (embrasure) is sprued and cast. Soldering will take place in major connector, well away from clasp.

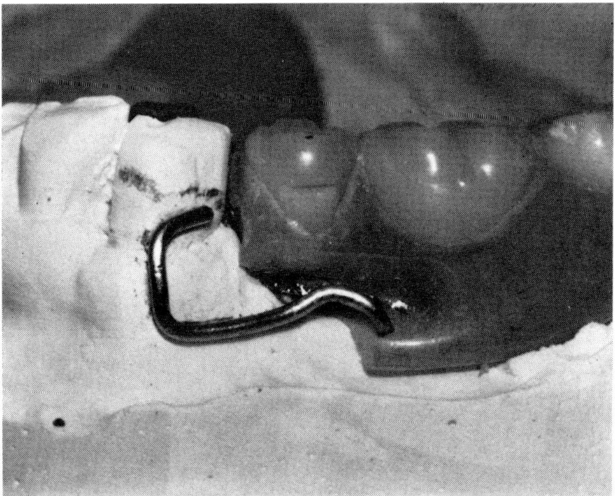

Fig. 21-28. Addition of wrought wire infrabulge repair clasp. Portion of wire that will be within repair resin is crimped so that it cannot rotate in resin. The Class V cavity in denture tooth is prepared to allow patient's fingernail to engage tooth rather than wire clasp during removal.

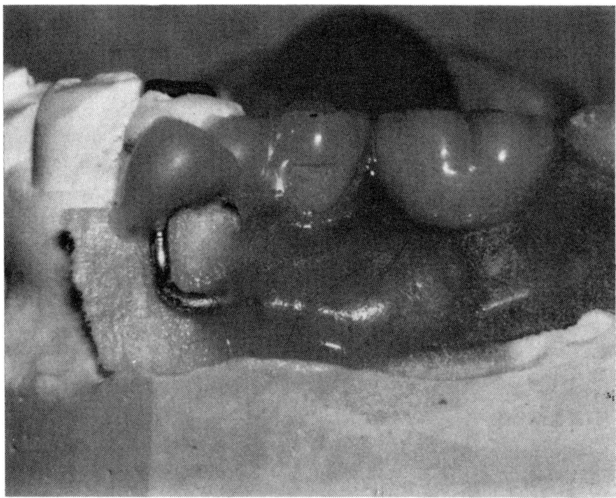

Fig. 21-29. With clasp tip waxed to stone tooth, repair resin is added and repair placed in pressure pot to complete processing.

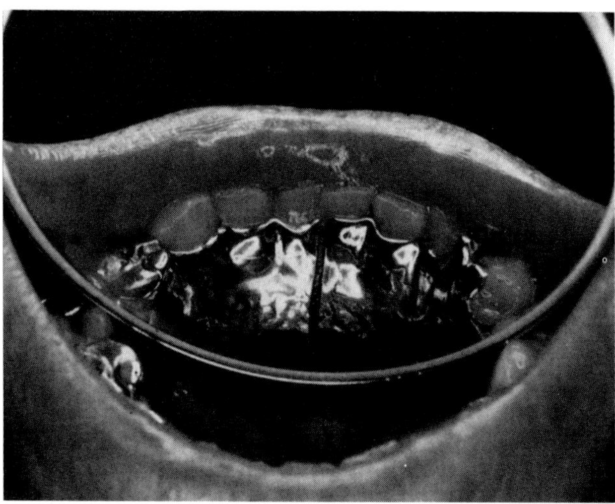

Fig. 21-30. Lingual plate major connector has been sectioned and seated in mouth. Sectioning cut should be as narrow as possible to decrease width of solder joint.

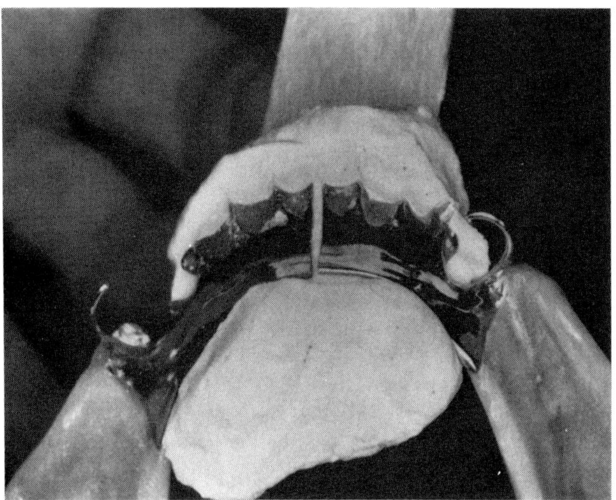

Fig. 21-31. Fast set plaster matrix carried to mouth on tongue blade makes accurate way of transferring repair relationship to laboratory.

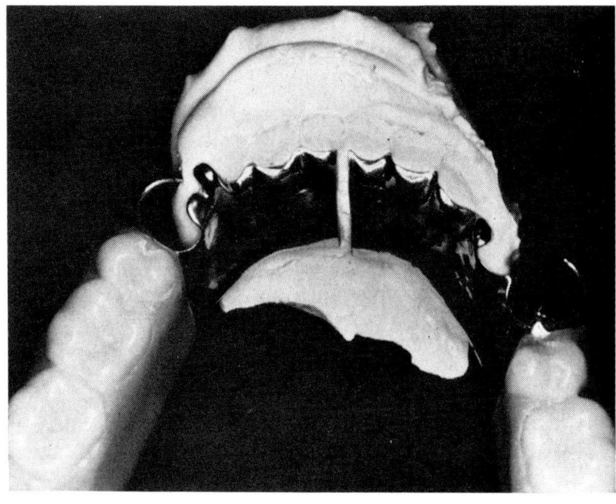

Fig. 21-32. Simple dental stone soldering cast for major connector repair. Cast is poured against plaster matrix and framework submitted by clinician.

Because the repair site may be many millimeters long, care must be taken not to stop the heating of the solder until the joint is complete. If the carbon tip of the soldering unit is removed from the joint before completion, oxidation can be expected to occur, which may make the addition of more soldering alloy difficult. A strip of solder a few millimeters longer than the joint should be used. If the joint is wider than a standard separating disk, a piece of nickel-chrome-cobalt wire can be adapted and placed in the joint before the soldering flux is added (Fig. 21-34). The presence of this wire will simplify soldering the wide joint.

The repaired major connector is finished and polished with the same materials and techniques as were used in the basic construction.

Individual tooth addition

When an individual tooth is to be added to an existing removable partial denture, the design of the existing major connector greatly influences the repair approach. When the lingual surface of the tooth to be replaced is covered with a major connector (lingual plate), the repair is limited to the soldering of a small wire loop to the denture (Fig. 21-35). The loop must be

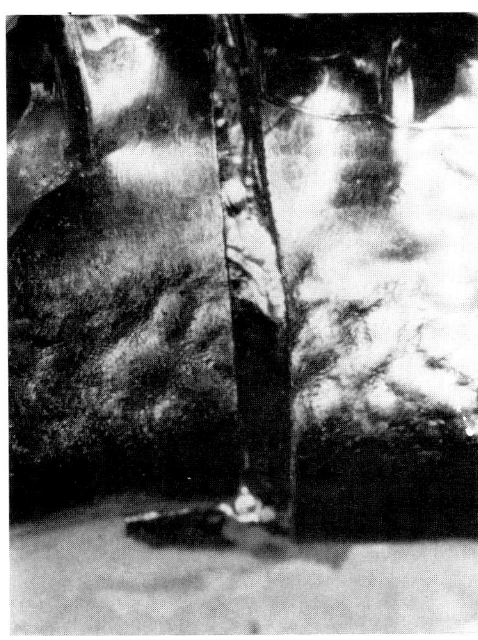

Fig. 21-33. Foil is extended slightly beyond actual repair boundary. With care, foil can be removed from solder joint and reused, because its high melting point keeps it from blending with solder.

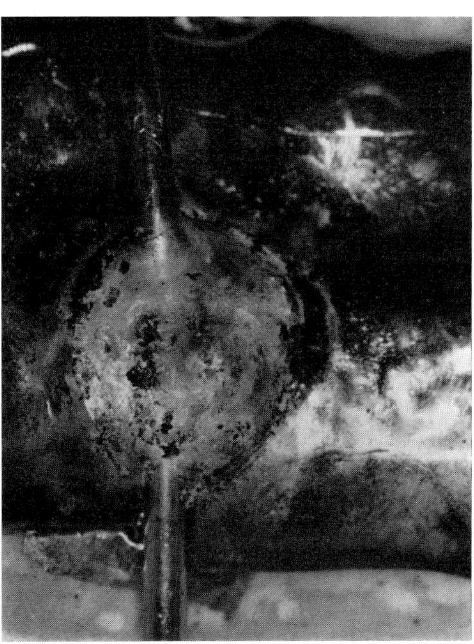

Fig. 21-34. Partially completed solder joint that shows position of wire used to fill wide joint. In actual practice, joint must be completed without interruption to keep joint from oxidizing and terminating flow of solder prematurely.

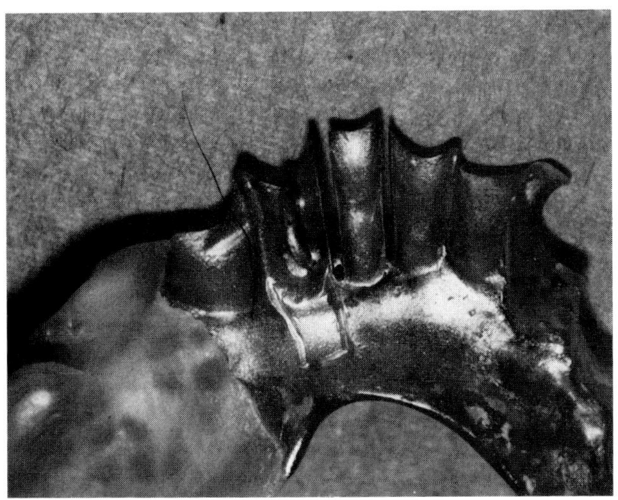

Fig. 21-35. Loop soldered to lingual plate for addition of single tooth. There is also finishing line present in the major connector, cut with an inverted cone stone, that will provide butt joint in repair resin and metal junction.

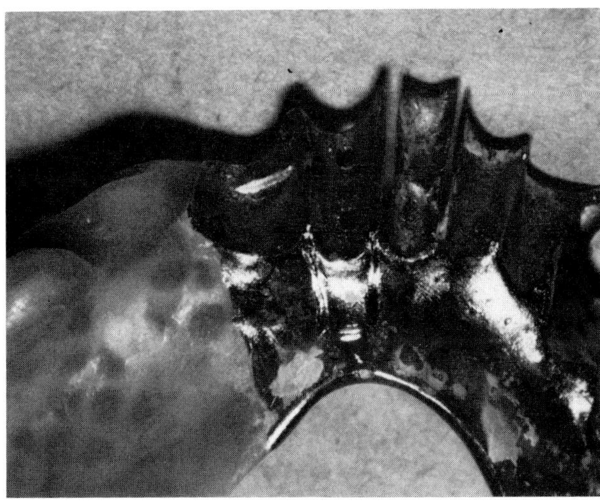

Fig. 21-36. Lingual plate perforated for placement of wire loop. Soldering takes place on outer surface where loop extends through holes.

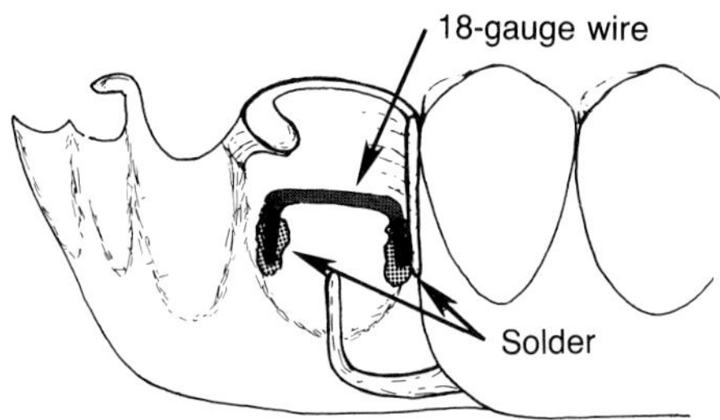

Fig. 21-37. Straight wires can be soldered between minor connectors in various areas in repair situations to provide retention for resin and denture teeth.

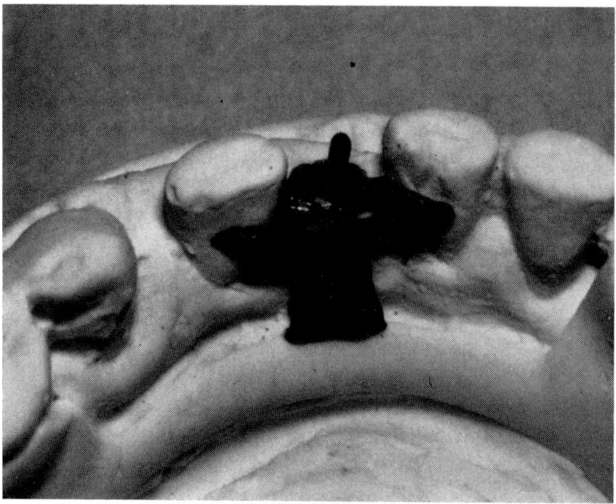

Fig. 21-38. A sectional refractory cast with an individual tooth replacement waxed. This repair addition will be soldered to lingual bar major connector.

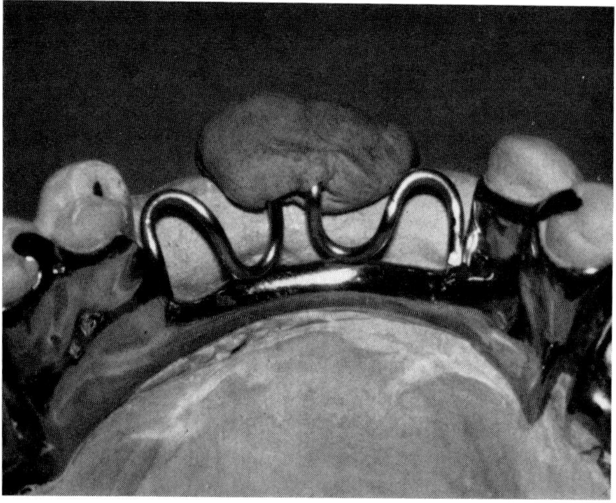

Fig. 21-39. Loop of 18-gauge nonprecious wire is held in position with clay in preparation for soldering retention for addition of a number of denture teeth.

placed so that it does not interfere with the positioning of the denture tooth (Fig. 21-36). An alternative to the loop is a straight piece of wire soldered at both ends to the interproximal area of the lingual plate (Fig. 21-37). The denture tooth, in either case, is first ground to an acceptable position in the arch with the denture removed from the repair cast (the cast is poured into an alginate impression of the jaw made with the denture in place as previously described). The lingual surface is then shaped to provide for the soldered retention and the repair completed with tooth-colored resin of the proper shade.

When the major connector does not involve the area of the tooth to be added, a major problem is encountered. Depending on the distance from the major connector to the repair tooth, a simple electrosoldered loop may not suffice. It may be necessary to duplicate the repair cast, with the denture in place, in refractory material and wax an addition to the major connector (Fig. 21-38). This wax form will be invested and cast with standard techniques. After fitting and finishing, the repair addition is electrosoldered as previously described. An internal finishing line must be available to create a butt joint between resin and metal. This line is created in the same way as in ordinary framework construction. Without an internal finishing line, the repair resin of either tooth or denture base will have no specific place to end, and the result will be a thin flash of uncontrolled resin that will percolate.

In every repair an attempt must be made to cut the finishing line in the major connector adjacent to the repair site. Ideally the connector will have sufficient bulk to allow at least 0.5 mm of finishing line depth. A No. 35 inverted cone carbide bur at high speed will provide a sharp line.

Denture base addition

The creation of retention for denture base addition is strictly a laboratory procedure, requiring only an accurate repair cast made with the existing partial denture in place. The area of the denture base addition must be fully extended and the desired outline of the additional denture base drawn on the cast. An opposing cast suitable for articulation is also required.

The laboratory will normally remove the existing denture base (if any) and adapt loops of at least 18 gauge wire for soldering to the framework (thinner wire will not be rigid enough) (Fig. 21-39). Section of standard retentive meshwork from scrap partial denture frameworks can also be used if their contour approximates the repair area (Fig. 21-40). Wire or cast sections are soldered using electrosoldering techniques previously described and are considered standard laboratory procedures. (Fig. 21-41).

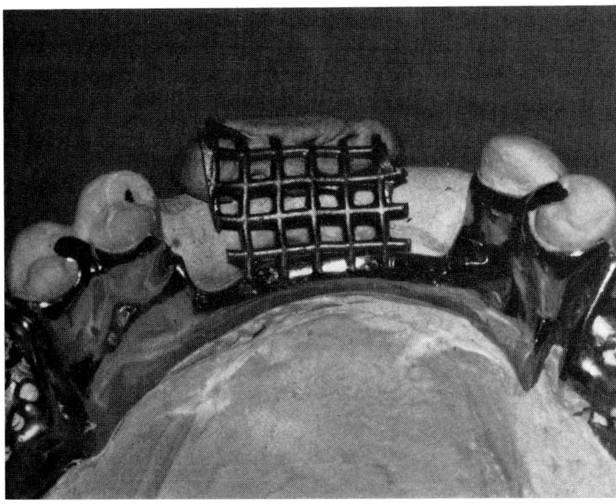

Fig. 21-40. Meshwork salvaged from another denture in place for soldering.

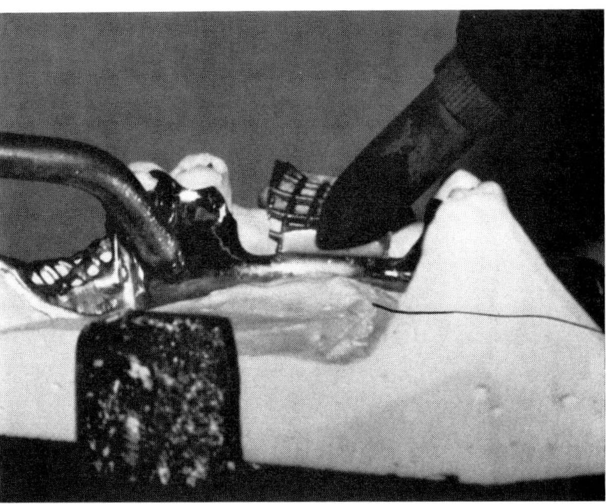

Fig. 21-41. Soldering tips in place for completing resin retention repair.

Again it is essential that the laboratory prepare an internal finishing line. Because an entire denture base is to be added, an external finishing line will also be required. The external line can be formed by building up an area on the major connector with solder just adjacent to the added retention (Fig. 21-42). This addition will require finishing with inverted cone stones or burs to provide a sharp finishing line. The denture base can now be waxed and the denture teeth positioned and processed in a routine manner.

CONSTRUCTING A CROWN UNDER EXISTING REMOVABLE PARTIAL DENTURE

Crown preparation

When an abutment tooth of an existing removable partial denture requires a cast restoration, a full veneer crown is almost always indicated. The preparation must conform to accepted resistance and retention forms and, in addition, have adequate tooth reduction to allow for rest seat preparation. There must also be sufficient reduction on the axial surfaces to allow a minimum of 1 mm of unveneered alloy between tooth and framework. When the crown is to be veneered with porcelain or resin, additional axial reduction is required to create 2.5 mm of space.

It is far easier to build a crown under an existing denture if veneering is not required. Every attempt should be made to use Type III gold unveneered. As a final check on tooth preparation, the denture must be seated in the mouth and the tooth-frame relation verified for adequate reduction (Fig. 21-43). If satisfactory, the tooth preparation can be polished and prepared for the impression procedure.

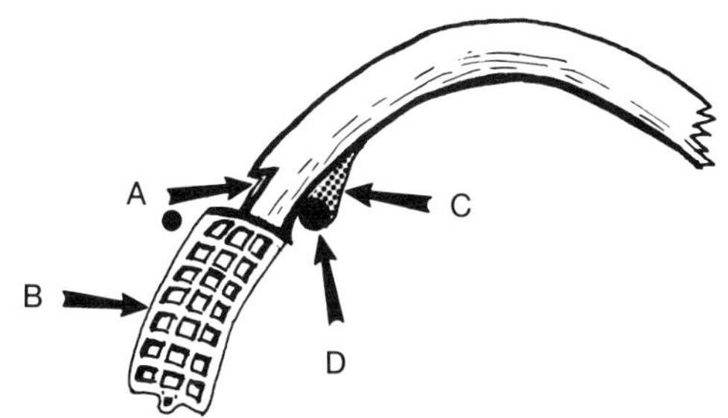

Fig. 21-42. This cross-sectional drawing illustrates relationship of meshwork and finishing lines in the addition repair. *A,* Internal finishing line cut into existing major connector. *B,* Retentive meshwork soldered to major connector. *C,* Solder joining wire, *D,* to major connector for additional thickness for creation of *external* finishing line. Metal along wire-casting junction will have to be sharpened with inverted cone stone to create final finishing line.

Impression with partial denture in place

As with most other partial denture repairs, a cast must be obtained from an impression made with the denture seated in the mouth. The denture must come off the teeth in the impression without any change in the tooth-frame relation. Impression materials that are strong when set are indicated for this type of impression (that is, polysulfide rubber or silicone in preference to reversible hydrocolloid).

A tray must be chosen that will fit over the partial denture with adequate clearance all around. Dentulous rim lock trays can be used in most situations. Because usually only one preparation is involved in this type of repair, there will be sufficient time to manipulate the

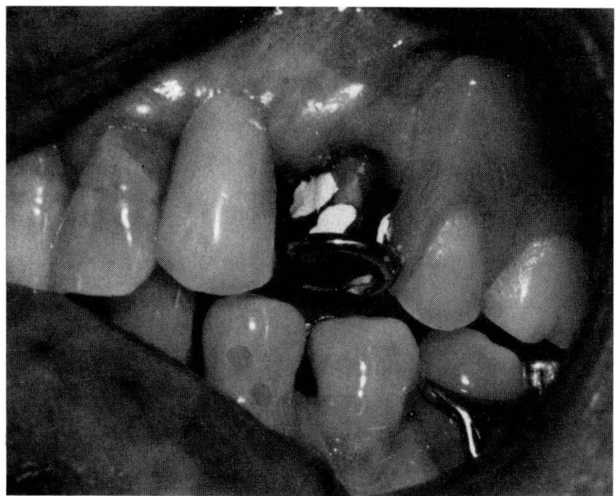

Fig. 21-43. Adequate space is apparent between prepared tooth and partial denture.

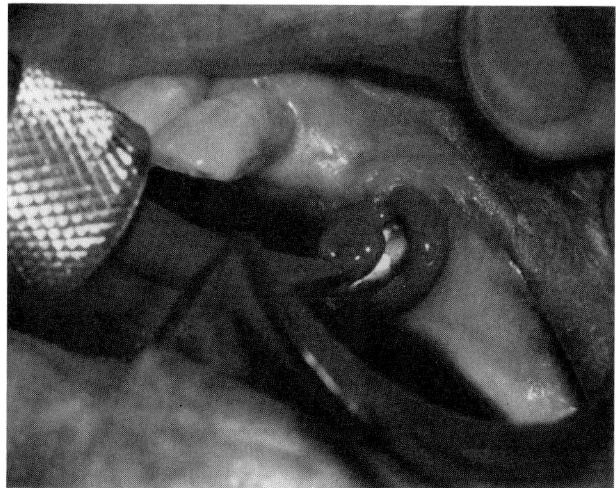

Fig. 21-44. Abutment tooth is covered with thin layer of impression material to include gingival sulcus.

stock tray to seat it properly to support the impression material without applying forces that might displace a distal extension denture base. If the base is displaced, the tooth-frame relationship will be changed and the resulting crown-frame relationship will be compromised.

The gingival tissues are retracted in the conventional manner and, at the appropriate time, the cord is removed and the injectable impression material placed into the gingival crevice and extended to cover the entire prepared tooth with a thin layer (1 to 2 mm) of impression material (Fig. 21-44). At this point the denture is seated in the mouth and the injection of impression material continued until the entire area of the prepared tooth and the adjacent parts of the denture are completely filled (Fig. 21-45). If the injection phase is done in excess, the tray need be considered primarily as a relating device to remove the partial denture from the mouth. This philosophy reduces the tendency to overseat the tray and greatly reduces the potential problems associated with movement of the denture. The tray material need only impress the occlusal surfaces of the remaining teeth. The denture will be locked into the impression by the rest and clasp(s) of the repair site.

A die pin is placed conventionally into the prepared tooth impression and the repair cast completed in a double pour (Fig. 21-46). The impression must be poured and recovered in the dental office so the clinician can verify the tooth-frame relationship as seen on the cast. If it does not duplicate the intraoral relationship, a compromising error has been made and the entire procedure must be redone. If the laboratory pours and separates the impression, there is no way the technician can verify the relationship, and no matter how well the crown is made, it may not relate to the framework when cemented.

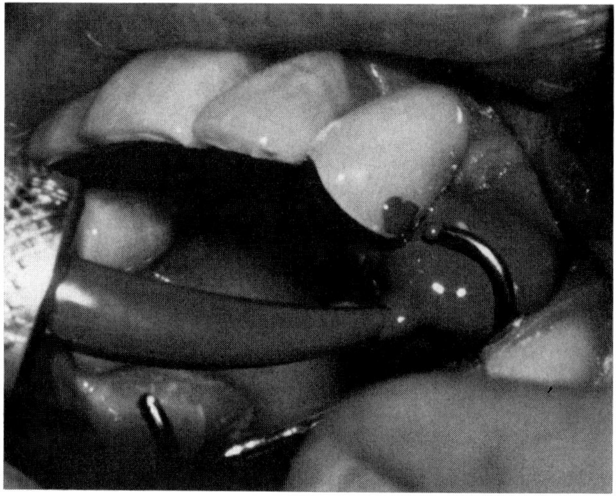

Fig. 21-45. With denture seated in mouth, additional syringe material is added to complete impression.

Perhaps of even greater significance is the responsibility of clinician to verify that the existing clasp or clasps are of good quality and of the form and material indicated for that particular situation. Any opportunity to improve the design of the partial denture by changing the clasping on the proposed crown should be taken. It is actually easier to contour the crown ideally and then add a new clasp, most commonly of wrought wire, as described elsewhere in this chapter (Fig. 21-47). If the clinical state of the denture justifies the cre-

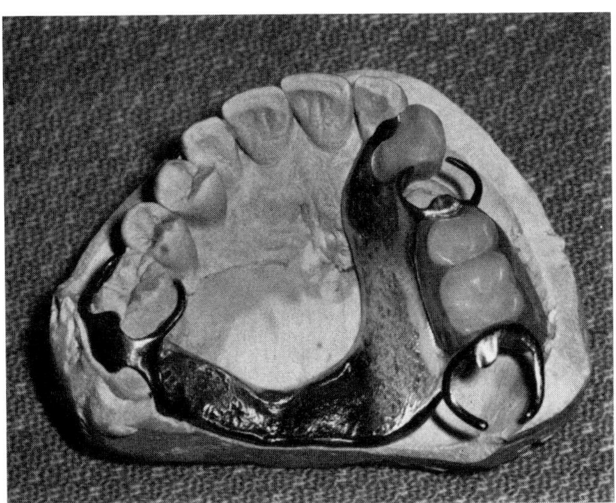

Fig. 21-46. Repair cast ready for laboratory. Impression was carefully blocked out with wax or clay in areas of clasp arms and minor connectors as well as the internal surface of denture base so that partial denture can easily be removed from cast and yet have positive seat against major connector.

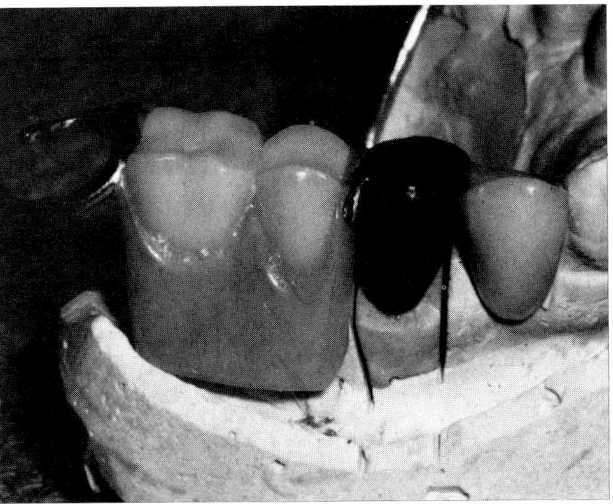

Fig. 21-47. Cast clasp has been removed from partial denture because it was not in ideal position. Repair clasp will be added to partial denture after completion of crown.

ation of a crown to fit the framework, the added cost of a clasp repair cannot be significant.

Whether the clasp is to be replaced or not, the technician articulates the casts and waxes a coping to include the margins. The coping and die are returned to the cast, the denture seated, and wax added to adapt the coping to the framework (Fig. 21-48). When the occlusal surface and the nonretentive axial surfaces are completed, wax is flowed onto the contact surface of the retentive clasp arm. At this point the framework is removed and sufficient wax added occlusally to the retentive area to provide the required height of contour and amount of undercut.

It is a clinical responsibility to prescribe the amount of undercut required. In most situations 0.010 inch to 0.015 inch will prove satisfactory for modern alloys. A dental surveyor is employed to verify the undercut placement. Again, the path of insertion is a clinical responsibility. It can normally be expected to be along the long axis of the abutment teeth.

There is a tendency to simply flow hot wax against the framework and accept the contour that results. Depending on the blockout involved in the construction phase, the waxed surfaces may give excessive crown-frame contact. This is potentially dangerous in mandibular distal extension situations where unacceptable forces may be placed on the abutment tooth if some freedom of movement is not created. The contour of the axial surface in these situations should be considered a clinical responsibility and be included on the work authorization order.

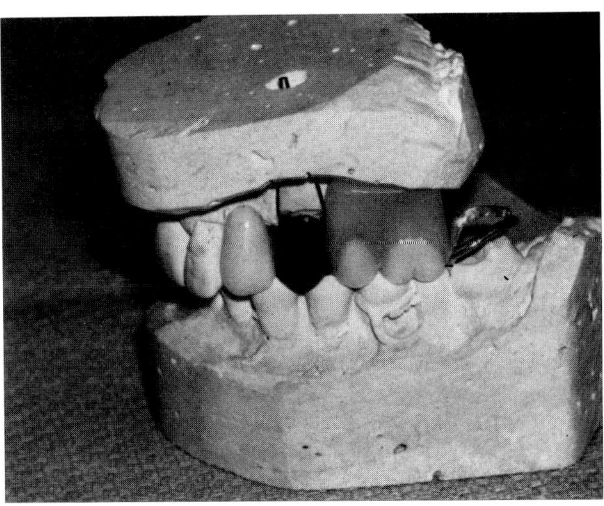

Fig. 21-48. Finished wax crown is in contact with rest and minor connector and in proper occlusion. It is ready to be veneered if necessary.

Veneering the repair crown

Veneering the crown adds greatly to construction time and is technique sensitive. Because porcelain must be built to excess, fired (with shrinkage) and shaped, the location of the prescribed retentive area becomes somewhat arbitrary.

The technique of choice when the crown must be veneered is to wax the crown as previously described, veneer the facial surface to accept porcelain, and remove the clasp arm that would lie on the porcelain (Fig. 21-49). The crown is cast and veneered to an ideal contour and, when stained and glazed, the crown is returned to the cast and a repair clasp of wrought wire in the de-

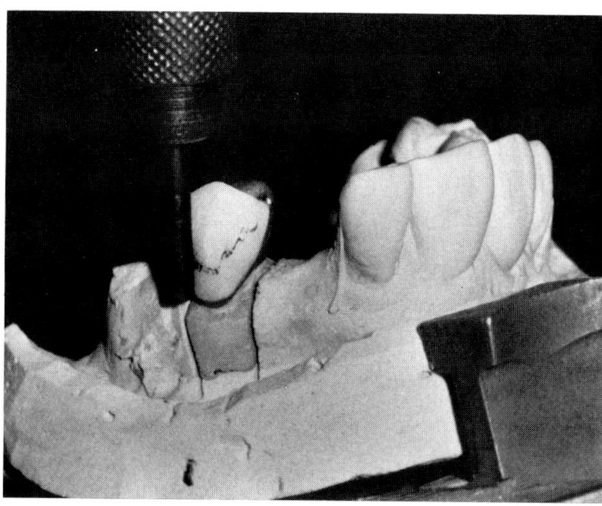

Fig. 21-49. Veneered repair crown is placed on dental surveyor to create ideal contours for replacement clasp. Building and contouring porcelain to existing clasp is difficult and usually results in an inferior repair addition.

sired form is added to the now ideal contour. In this way laboratory time in fitting the frame to the porcelain is eliminated and an ideal clasp-crown contour easily achieved. The repair clasp in this situation will be in harmony with the clinician's design philosophy.

CONCLUSION

Repair techniques, both clinical and laboratory, must be considered by dentists and technicians alike in their relationship to the entire mouth and not just as isolated additions or correction.

BIBLIOGRAPHY

Barrett, D.A., and Pilling, L.O.: The restoration of carious clasp-bearing teeth, J. Prosthet. Dent. **15**:309-311, 1965.

Bates, J.F.: Studies related to the fracture of partial dentures, Br. Dent. J. **120**:79-83, 1966.

Beckett, L.S.: Partial denture. The rebasing of tissue borne saddles: theory and practice, Aust. Dent. J. **16**:340-346, 1971.

Blatterfein, L.: Rebasing procedures for removable partial dentures, J. Prosthet. Dent. **8**:441-467, 1958.

Breithart, A.R.: Converting a tooth-supported denture to a distal extension removable partial denture, J. Prosthet. Dent. **18**:233, 1967.

Brudvik, J.S., and others: Repairs of metal parts removable partial dentures, J. Prosthet. Dent. **28**:205-208, 1972.

Ewing, J.E.: The construction of accurate full crown restorations for an existing clasp by using a direct metal pattern technique, J. Prosthet. Dent. **15**:889-899, 1965.

Goldberg, A.T., and Jones, R.D.: Constructing cast crowns to fit existing removable partial denture clasps, J. Prosthet. Dent. **36**:382-386, 1976.

Kelly, E.: Unbending the bent lingual bar, J. Prosthet. Dent. **25**:668-669, 1971.

Lewis, A.J.: Failure of removable partial denture casting during service, J. Prosthet. Dent. **39**:147-149, 1978.

McCartney, J.W.: Occlusal reconstruction and rebase procedure for distal extension removable partial dentures, J. Prosthet. Dent. **43**:695-698, 1980.

Reynolds, J.M.: Crown construction for abutments of existing removable partial dentures, J. Am. Dent. Assoc. **69**:423-426, 1964.

Scott, J., and Bates, J.F.: The relining of partial dentures involving precision attachments, J. Prosthet. Dent. **28**:325-333, 1972.

Stamps, J.T., and Tanquist, R.A.: Restoration of removable partial denture rest seats using dental amalgam, J. Prosthet. Dent. **41**:224, 1979.

Steffel, V.L.: Relining removable partial dentures for fit and function, J. Prosthet. Dent. **4**:496-509, 1954.

Teppo, K.W., and Smith, F.W.: A method of immediate clasp repair, J. Prosthet. Dent. **30**:77-80, 1975.

Warnick, M.E.: Cast crown restoration of a badly involved abutment to fit an existing removable partial denture, Dent. Clin. North Am. **14**:631-644, 1970.

Wilson, J.H.: Partial dentures—rebasing the saddle supported by the mucosa and alveolar bone, Dent. J. Aust. **24**:185-188, 1952.

Wilson, J.H.: Partial dentures—relining the saddle supported by the mucosa and alveolar bone, J. Prosthet. Dent. **3**:807-813, 1953.

22 Attachments for removable partial dentures

Merrill C. Mensor, Jr.

HISTORICAL BACKGROUND

The historical background on precision attachments is adequately covered by Raoul Boitel (1978). His review of the literature states that the primary development of attachments is an American innovation in removable partial denture construction dating from the turn of the century. He states that the European contributions have only had their impact on prosthodontics the last 30 years. The ingenuity of many attachment systems dazzles the mind of the uninitiated. The practicality, simplicity of assembly, and biomechanics of a few attachments have weathered the time and are representative subjects of this text. See Mensor (1980) for complete laboratory assembly procedures of representative attachments.

PRECISION ATTACHMENTS

Precision attachments as they relate to removable partial dentures have evolved as retainers or major connectors. The main purpose of the precision attachment is retention, stress direction, and concealment within the prosthesis. The attachment complex consists of a cast retainer, the attachment, and the partial denture.

The cast retainer is the primary unit designed to carry the attachment and may be single or multiple castings. Sometimes stability is enhanced by milled lingual retentive or bracing arms.

Attachments are machine fabricated or they may be constructed from resin patterns, ceramic cores, or as milled units. They may be precision or semiprecision. Some provide various degrees of resilience, whereas others are nonresilient.

In application, attachments are divided into four groups: intracoronal, extracoronal, combined (intra-extra coronal) and auxiliary as cross-arch units.

FRAMEWORK DESIGN

The framework design of the attachment-retained removable partial denture is dictated by the bearing area and the space closure (bounded or free end). The maxillary framework generally uses the skeletal support area of the palate, whereas the mandibular partial denture framework design is standard for all bilateral free-end partial dentures, and a modification of this design is used for unilateral applications.

Mandibular partial dentures

The elimination of clasps from the partial denture removes any orientation of the framework to the master cast unless lingual bracing-retentive arms have been milled into the design. As such, two temporary indirect retainers (minor connectors) are waxed up as part of the framework (Fig. 22-1) and provide a means of proper orientation for either picking up the attachments in the mouth or off the master cast. Failure to use these minor connectors will eliminate the orientation of the lingual bar to the relief area and cause lingual tissue impingement in the mouth. In the case of the resilient attachment, the lingual bar will dig into the lingual tissue and make the appliance useless.

The indirect retainer further allows the repositioning or resin pickup of the attachment, when necessary, before final delivery of the prosthesis. At that time the minor connectors are removed from the framework.

Relief for nonresilient partial dentures is developed on the master cast before duplication to provide for normal jaw flexion. This is in the order of 30-gauge wax relief with finish lines and saddle stops. Relief for resilient partial dentures must provide for both vertical and angular displacement; therefore the relief starts at 36-gauge occlusally and increases as a wedge to 20-gauge gingivally (Fig. 22-2). After duplication, the lingual bar is waxed with a definite egg contour toward the floor of the mouth (Fig. 22-3).

Maxillary partial dentures

The maxillary partial denture framework also requires temporary minor connectors for the orientation and testing of the framework, as well as the resin pickup of attachments in the mouth (Fig. 22-4). Under no circumstances should a horseshoe palate design be used, because maximum stability is achieved with broad palatal coverage of the skeletal support bone of the palate. Double beading will ensure a positive post dam palatal seal, but this should be done in concurrence with the dentist's digital palpation of the palate.

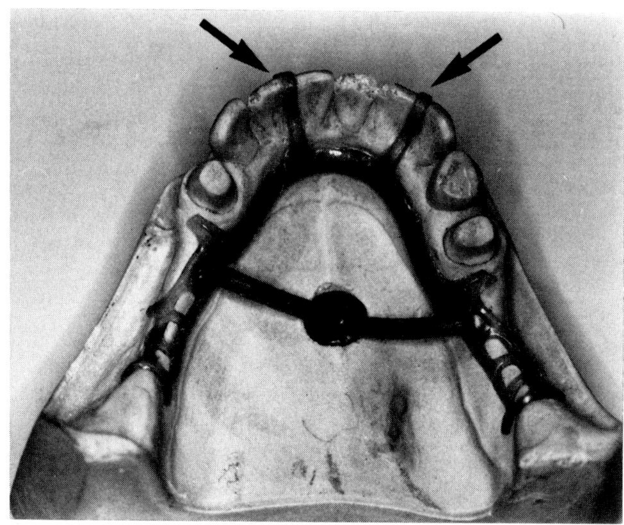

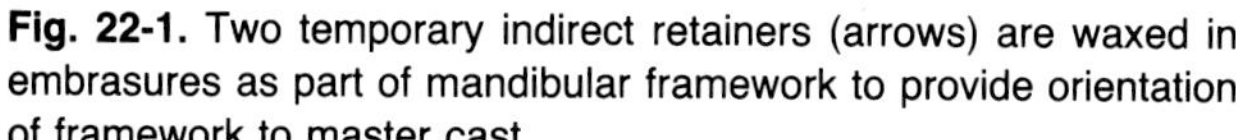

Fig. 22-1. Two temporary indirect retainers (arrows) are waxed in embrasures as part of mandibular framework to provide orientation of framework to master cast.

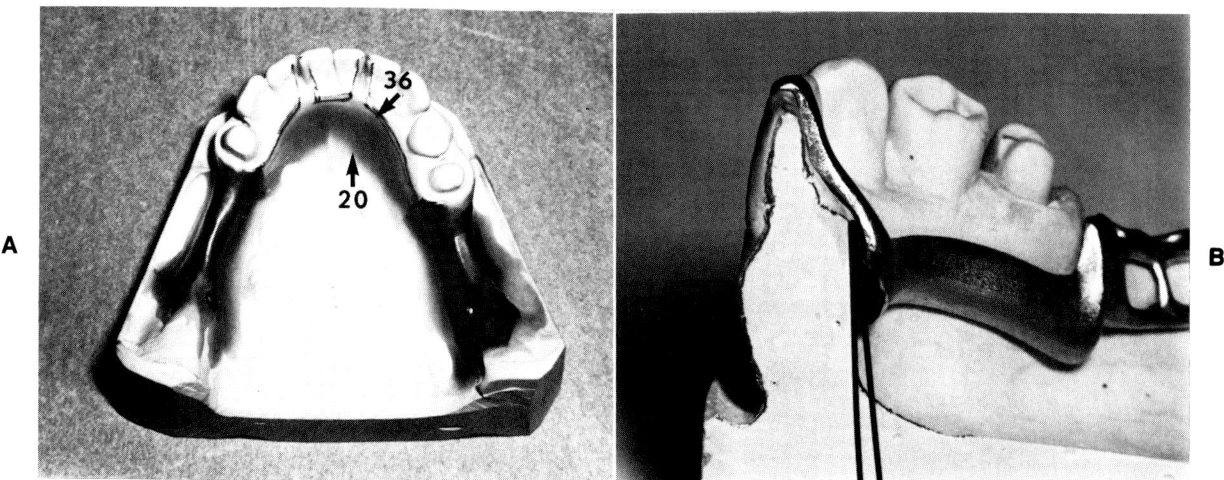

Fig. 22-2. A, For resilient mandibular partial denture one should wax out 36-gauge relief occlusally to 20-gauge relief gingivally and then duplicate in refractory investment. **B,** Relief (lines) provides space for vertical and angular displacement.

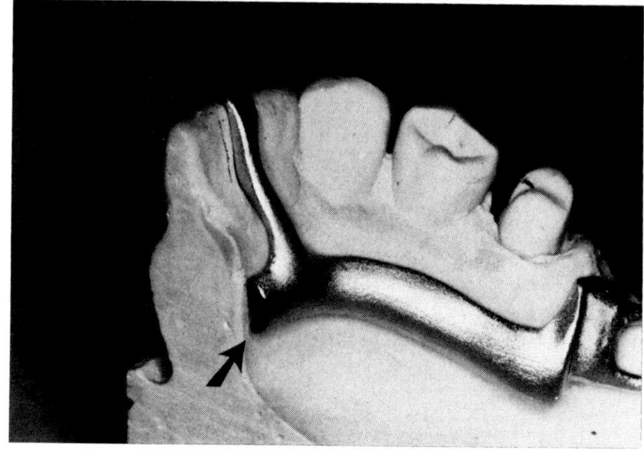

Fig. 22-3. Egg contour (arrow) on refractory cast prevents tissue impingement.

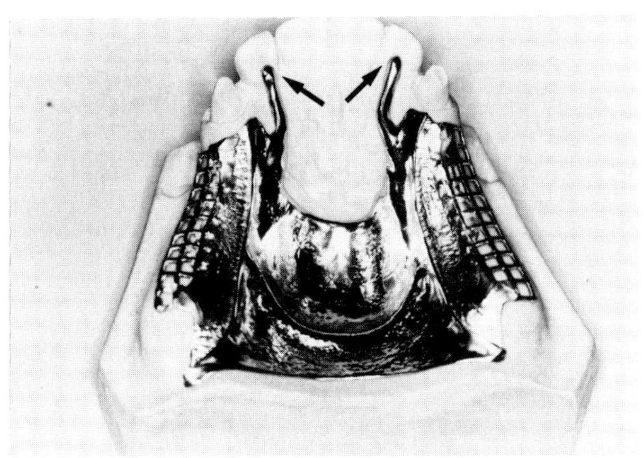

Fig. 22-4. Maxillary framework is waxed with two temporary indirect retainers either in embrasures or on cingula (arrows). This position can be determined from contact of opposing dentition.

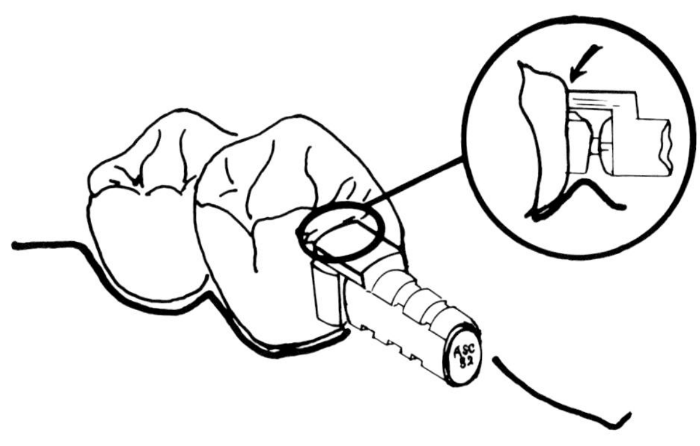

Fig. 22-5. ASC-52 attachments are spring-loaded universal joint stress directors. Miniature indirect retainer of an ASC-52 protect configuration (arrow) prevents lift (mandibular) or drop (maxillary) of saddle.

The bead is usually 2 mm in from the posterior border of the impression on the master cast and to the depth of a No. 2 round bur; the second bead, parallel to the first, is 2 mm further in. Palatal relief is provided over thin areas when indicated. A complete denture post dam may also be used.

INDICATIONS FOR ATTACHMENTS

Attachment usage must be considered separately for the maxillary and mandibular arches. Whereas the maxillary arch is basically rigid with broad palatal support, the mandible lacks broad support and is subject to the dynamics of multiflexion under functional loading.

Maxillary removable partial denture

Spring-loaded rigid and resilient attachments provide positive retention that is adjustable compared with pure frictional units that wear into a semiprecise attachment and require milled retentive arms for control.

Stress reduction is accomplished by a given path of insertion that does not jar the retainer tooth on insertion or removal, as do most retentive clasp systems. Esthetics is automatically provided by the concealment factor of the attachment removable partial denture. The increased cost factor of attachments must be weighed against the jarring and lack of esthetics of the clasp systems.

Mandibular removable partial denture

The above discussion applies to the mandibular partial denture with the additional consideration of the need for stress direction. Stress direction that provides universal joint action such as the ASC-52* (Fig. 22-5)

*Bell International, Inc., San Mateo, Calif. 94402.

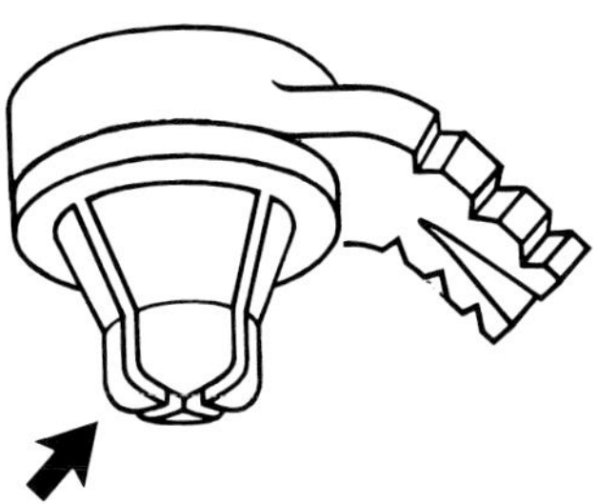

Fig. 22-6. CEKA With Wings is represented by extension of male housing. Male retention stud (arrow) is threaded into female. Designation of this CEKA is A-KS 694, 695, 696 Stress-Director.

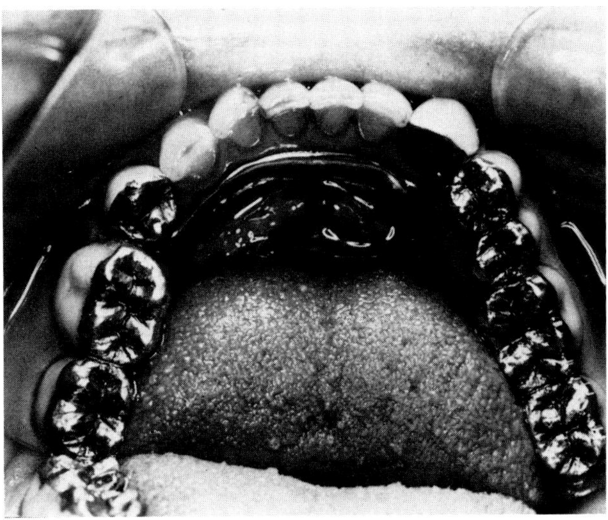

Fig. 22-7. Typical bilateral removable partial denture. Note single abutments carrying attachment-retained removable partial denture.

and the resilient CEKA* (Fig. 22-6) automatically reduces the requirement of double abutment retainer preparation required with a rigid system for a mandibular removable partial denture. The need for only two cast retainers significantly reduces the fabrication cost on a typical bilateral removable partial denture (Fig. 22-7).

The stress director requirements may be eliminated for the mandibular removable partial denture if it opposes a complete maxillary prosthesis or a full posterior free end maxillary partial denture. It may also be eliminated if only mandibular molars are replaced because in this situation the prosthesis is posterior to the major flexion area of the mandible whether the prosthesis opposes another prosthesis or complete dentition. A maxillary complete denture does provide some stress direction by the nature of its being soft tissue borne.

ATTACHMENT SELECTION

The following recommendations, taken from practice, will provide maximum retention with minimal torque to the abutment teeth and the underlying structures:

1. *Bounded edentulous areas:* rigid maxillary attachments; somewhat flexible mandibular attachments (use of P.D.,† M.S.,‡ or equivalent attachments).
2. *Free-end saddle design bilateral maxillary partial denture opposing fixed or bounded mandibular partial denture:* resilient or rigid attachments and wide palatal strap.
3. *Free-end saddle unilateral maxillary partial denture opposing fixed or bounded partial denture:* rigid or resilient attachments with cross-arch unit of same degree of movement and wide palatal strap.
4. *Free-end bilateral maxillary partial denture opposing free-end bilateral mandibular partial denture:* rigid maxillary attachments; stress-directed mandibular attachments.
5. *Free-end maxillary partial denture against same side free-end mandibular partial denture:* rigid maxillary attachments; resilient mandibular attachments.
6. *Free-end maxillary partial denture against opposite side free-end mandibular partial denture:* rigid maxillary attachments; resilient mandibular attachments.
7. *Rigid or bounded maxillary partial denture against free-end mandibular partial denture:* resilient unilateral or bilateral mandibular attachments.
8. *Complete maxillary denture against free-end mandibular partial denture:* rigid mandibular attachments. (Maxillary complete denture provides stress direction.)

*Jelenko, Armonk, N.Y. 10504.
†Dentalloy, Inc., Stanton, Calif. 90680
‡J.M. Ney Co., Bloomfield, Conn. 06002

The following is a list of attachments in order of use and preference:

1. *Rigid bounded attachments* (used with lingual retentive or bracing arms)
   Ancra*
   Ney†
   Stern-McCollum‡
   Stern .086, .096‡
2. *Rigid free-end maxillary attachments with bracing or retentive arms*
   Schatzmann‡
   CEKA§
   BIVAL||
3. *Resilient maxillary or mandibular attachments*
   ASC-52||
   Posterior protect (universal action; no torque)
   Anterior protect (universal action; no torque)
   CEKA§ (universal action; no torque)
   DALBO‡ (upper only unidirectional with torque)
4. *Cross-arch stabilizers*
   CEKA§ With Wings (rigid or resilient)
   A-KS (694, 695, 696) Stress-director
   (724, 725, 726) Rigid
   Snap-prox‡ Rigid
   ASC-52 Mini|| Protect or Regular
   Huser Hook‡ Resilient
   Roach*‡|| Resilient

CONTRAINDICATIONS

Attachment systems are contraindicated in the healthy mouth when the potential abutment teeth do not require restorations. Systems such as the Swing Lock or RPI partial denture serve adequately to provide support, but they have the negative factors of poor esthetics, potential decay of the abutment teeth, and increased torque potential especially on mandibular removable partial dentures. The lower cost factor of the clasp type removable partial denture along with the lower skill requirement is a definite plus for the patient requiring a predictable, utilitarian service.

Some attempt should be made to include the basic design of the attachment partial denture framework of the mandibular removable partial denture in the clasp frame so that it may be converted to an attachment-retained removable partial denture when abutment

*Degussa-ADER, Long Island City, N.Y. 11101.
†J.M. Ney Co., Bloomfield, Conn. 06002.
‡APM-Sterngold, Stamford, Conn. 06907.
§Jelenko, Armonk, N.Y. 10504
||Bell International, Inc. San Mateo, Calif. 94402

teeth require either cast retainers or stress reduction with one of the resilient attachments.

CLINICAL CONSIDERATIONS

First visit

Diagnostic casts

Clinical considerations follow a set procedure for all attachment-retained removable partial dentures. Diagnostic casts are mounted on an articulator with a jaw relation record. The space adjacent to the retainer is evaluated for occlusogingival clearance with an EM Gauge (Fig. 22-8, *A*) as it relates to an occluded set of casts. This measurement is then compared with the measurement listed for the various attachments on Card 1 or Card 2 of the EM Attachment Selector (Fig. 22-8, *B*). The attachment of choice is selected on the basis of the criteria presented in the discussion of attachment selection.

A

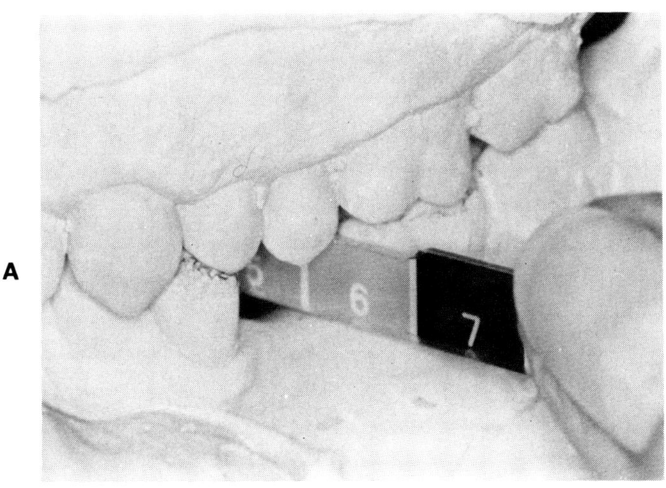

B

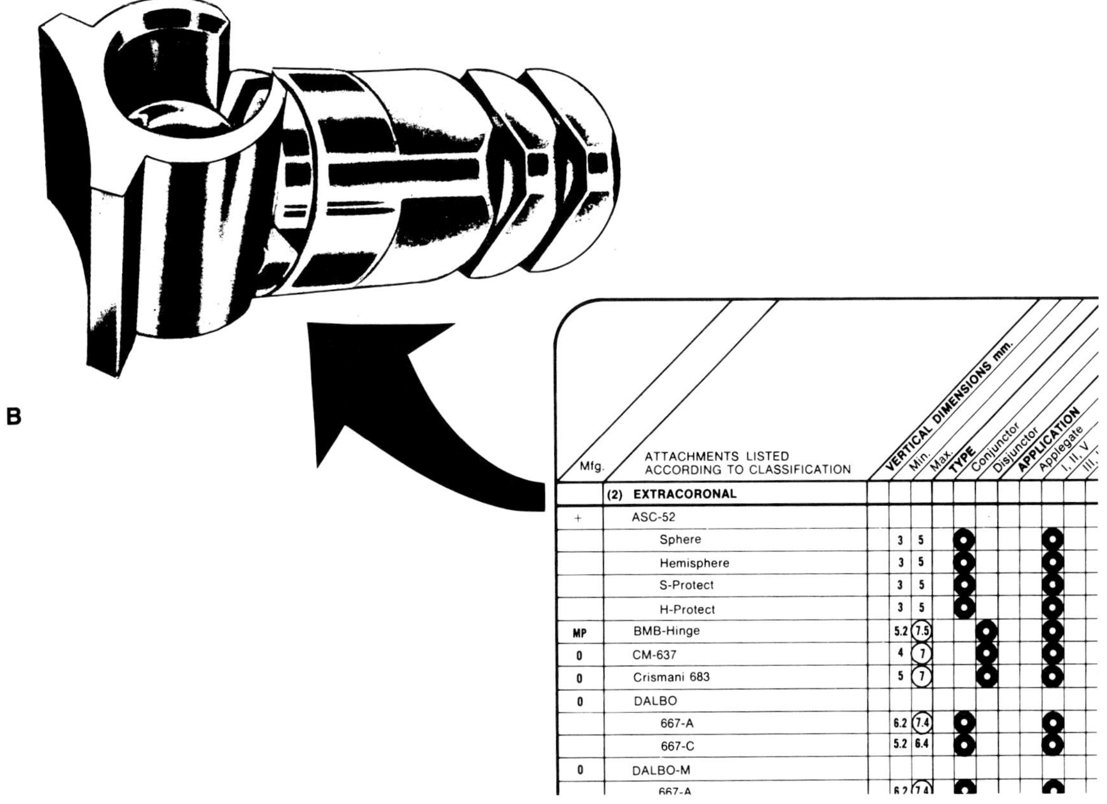

Fig. 22-8. A, EM gauge placed next to occluded abutment. Color-coded numeric readout is used with EM Attachment Selector, **B,** to choose attachments.

Instrumentation

The complexity of the restoration and the normality of the maxillomandibular relation of the patient determine the instrumentation required for assembly of the removable partial denture.

Generally, Arcon instrumentation (Fig. 22-9) with hinge axis location, interocclusal records, and mandibular movement recordings will reduce the probability of instrument error and the potential overload and malfunction of an attachment-retained removable partial denture.

Retainer preparation

Diagnostic preparations for rigid or resilient internal attachments are necessary. Overreduction of the abutments can diminish their strength with the possibility of pulpal involvement. Underreduction will result in overcontouring, potential for periodontal problems, and an occlusal overload.

CLINICAL PROCEDURES

A. Diagnostic casts
   1. Attachment selection
      a. EM gauge*
      b. EM Attachment Selector*
B. Maxillomandibular movement records
   1. Semiadjustable instruments
   2. Fully adjustable instruments
      a. Full recordings (stereograph)
      b. Simplex recording (with anterior couple)
C. Diagnostic retainer preparation
   1. Diagnostic preparation intracoronal
   2. Preparation with attachment as guide
      a. Box reduction
      b. Retainer preparation
      c. Accessory preparation
   3. Preparation to include lingual retentive or bracing arms
      a. Bracing arms
      b. Retentive arms
   4. Diagnostic preparation extracoronal
      a. Accessory retention grooves
   5. Splinting
      a. With attachments
      b. Attachments plus soldering
      c. Solder or multiple cast units

Second visit

Retainer preparation follows the diagnostic preparation determined from the first visit for internal attachments. Extracoronal attachment preparation does not require a diagnostic preparation. Both intracoronal and extracoronal retainers demand length and parallelism for retention, which can be enhanced with accessory retention grooves (Fig. 22-10). The gingival margin about the attachment should be at least 1 mm gingival to the attachment to protect the periodontium.

*Bell International, Inc., San Mateo, Calif. 94402.

Master impressions are made with full arch trays in the material of choice after gingitage, cord retraction, or electrosurgical reduction of the tissue about the preparation. The opposing cast is made with an irreversible hydrocolloid.

A kinematic face-bow transfer is recorded with three wax records for split cast verification of axis and centric relation.

Temporization should be customized either with Trim*-filled aluminum shells or plastic forms filled with Trim. It is essential that the temporary prostheses be well adapted not only to gingival fit but also to proximal and occlusal contact for stability during the fabrication period.

CLINICAL PROCEDURES

A. Prepare mouth as determined by diagnostic preparations
B. Master impressions
   1. Retraction or electrosurgery, or both
   2. Full arch impressions
      a. Relation cast
      b. Die cast
   3. Opposing cast alginate
   4. Maxillomandibular records
      a. Kinematic face-bow
      b. Three wax records
      c. Split cast verification
C. Temporization
   1. Aluminum shell filled with Trim* plus zinc oxide–eugenol
   2. Plastic forms filled with Trim* plus zinc oxide–eugenol
   3. Customized temporary prostheses from diagnostic casts

Laboratory work order

The laboratory work order should have instructions to compensate for final cement elevation of the castings and the removable partial denture, including the following instructions that relate to the type of attachment selected for the removable partial denture.

A. Retainer restorations only (balance of dentition not restored)
   1. Foil opposing teeth for wax-up.
   2. Place two 12-μm strips between casting and die, control centric stops.
   3. Return for try-in and occlusal control.
B. Retainer restoration, milled or resilient.
   1. Milled (automatically provides orientation for

*Harry J. Bosworth Co., Chicago, Il. 60605.

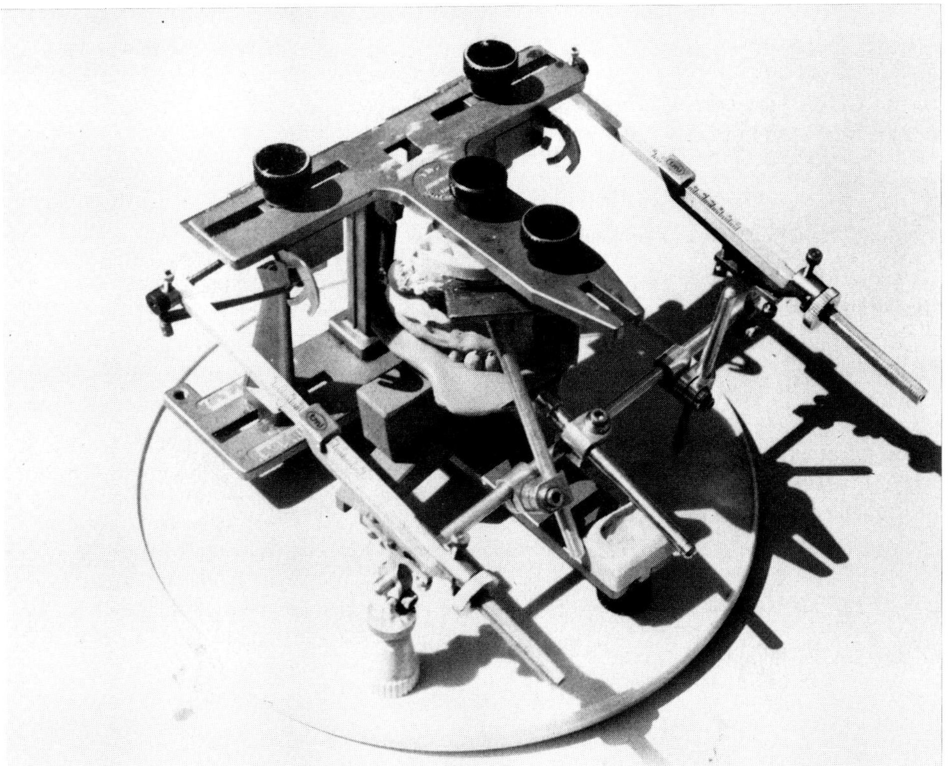

Fig. 22-9. Arcon instruments such as TMJ articulator (TMJ Instrument Co., Inc., Santa Ana, Calif. 92704) with TMJ kinematic face-bow attached provide computer programming for precise gnathologic techniques related to construction of removable partial dentures.

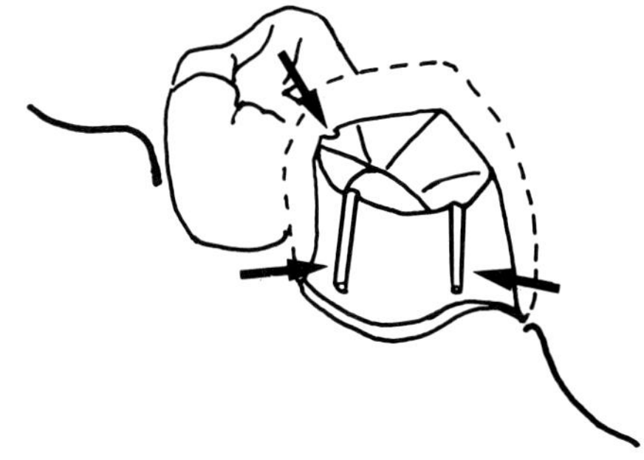

Fig. 22-10. Principal attachment retainer must have parallel retention grooves (arrows) to enhance retention and prevent rotation of cast retainer.

attachment and frame: return with base for altered cast following steps A 1 and 2).

2. Resilient (requires temporary indirect retainers for altered cast technique).

Third visit

Retainer control

The occlusal fit and function are controlled to compensate for final cement elevation either by temporizing the retainers with a mixture of Aquaphor, Pro-Tem cement, and powder of zinc oxy-phosphate cement or by placing two 12-μm Leader Tape* strips between the casting and the tooth for the elevation.

Removable partial denture casting control

The framework is positioned against the tooth retainer and the temporary indirect retainer to its seat. The cast base contact to the tissue is verified with PIP or an equivalent indicator. The attachment of choice is then set between the retainer and the framework with

*3M Co., St. Paul, Minn. 55101

Getz Minit Weld, and the partial saddle area is detailed for the final altered cast impression.

The altered cast impression should be boxed, poured, and mounted on the articulator before it is returned to the laboratory for completion.

CLINICAL PROCEDURES

A. Control retainer
   1. Fit of crown.
   2. Occlusal fit (elevate retainer crown and castings to compensate for final cement elevation).
      a. Protem cement,* Aquaphor,† and powder of zinc oxy-phosphate cement.
      b. Two strips of 12 mμ 3 M Leader Tape.

B. Partial denture casting
   1. Metal-to-tooth retainer and temporary indirect retainer.
   2. Base-to-tissue contact verified with PIP‡.
   3. Pick up attachment with Getz Minit Weld§.
   4. Detail for final altered cast impression.
   5. Return to articulator for boxing and pour altered cast.
   6. Return to laboratory for completion.

Fourth visit

Delivery of retainers and removable partial denture

Rigid system. The retainers are temporarily cemented following the technique described in the third visit. The partial denture is tested with PIP for tissue contact. It is then controlled for occlusal hold with 5-μm Mylar film, and any corrections are made at this time.

The retainers are now cleaned and prepared for final cementation. Following cementation, the removable partial denture is delivered without the attachment retention activated so that the patient can be instructed in the proper method of insertion and removal as well as maintenance of the appliance. The patient is dismissed with the activation of the attachments scheduled for the fifth visit.

Resilient system. The procedures for the resilient attachment system are the same as those for the rigid system, with the additional use of the temporary indirect retainers.

If the base and occlusion are correct and the attachment is out of phase, then the attachment section in the partial denture must be removed and repositioned with a resin pick-up using the temporary indirect retainers for orientation. If the base and attachments are correct and the occlusion is off, the occlusion must be corrected. If the base is off and the attachment and occlusion are correct, the partial denture must be rebased following the altered cast technique used in the third visit.

The attachments will be activated and the temporary indirect retainers will be removed at the fifth visit.

CLINICAL PROCEDURES: DELIVERY OF RETAINERS AND REMOVABLE PARTIAL DENTURES

A. Temporary cementation retainers (see third visit).

B. Use PIP on base; insert partial denture; test fit.

C. Use Mylar film for occlusion 12 μm, 5 μm.

D. If rigid, make corrections if necessary (milled lingual arm reference).

E. If resilient, make correction if necessary (temporary indirect retainer reference point).
   1. If base and vertical are correct but attachment is out of phase, reposition attachment.
      (1) Remove with heating rod.
      (2) Reposition with resin pick-up with indirect retainer as reference.
   2. If base correct but occlusion is off, correct occlusion.
   3. If base is off but attachment is correct, rebase (altered cast, remount, reprocess).

F. Cement retainers.

G. Deliver partial denture with attachment not activated and temporary indirect retainer present (resilient).

H. Instruct patient on insertion, removal, and maintenance.

I. Make appointment for control, activation, and removal of temporary indirect retainer (resilient).

Fifth visit

The rigid system removable partial denture is retested for fit of the base and occlusal holding as noted for the fourth visit, and the retention is activated. The resilient system is tested in the same way, the attachments are activated, and the temporary indirect retainers are removed (Fig. 22-11).

POSTINSERTION OBSERVATIONS

The occlusion of the partial denture is converted to cast metal 4 to 6 weeks after initial placement. The removable partial denture is remounted on the articulator with a new transfer cast, and the occlusion is refined by one of the acceptable techniques for fabricating the cast metal occlusion (Fig. 22-12).

The patient should have an initial 3-month recall appointment, after which appointments should be scheduled every 6 months for routine inspection and control or replacement of the spring retention units (Figs. 22-13 and 22-14).

---

*Profession Products Co., San Diego, Calif. 92101.

†Beiersdorf Inc., South Norwalk, Conn. 06854.

‡Mizzy, Inc., Clifton Forge, Va. 24422.

§Getz-Opotow, Elkgrove Village, Ill. 60007.

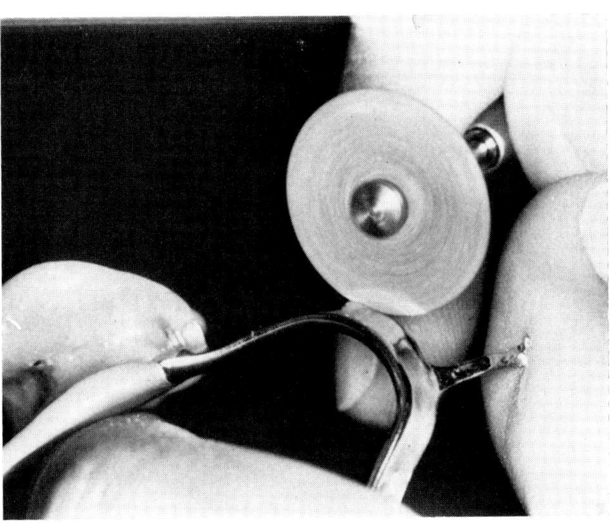

Fig. 22-11. Temporary indirect retainers are removed with disk, and occlusal surface of lingual bar is polished.

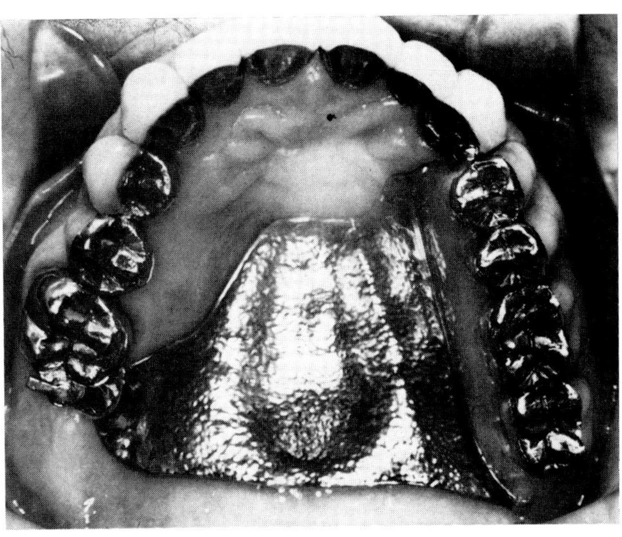

Fig. 22-12. Typical cast metal occlusion developed by drop wax correction of resin occlusion. Cast metal occlusal was cured onto denture base by using occlusal index.

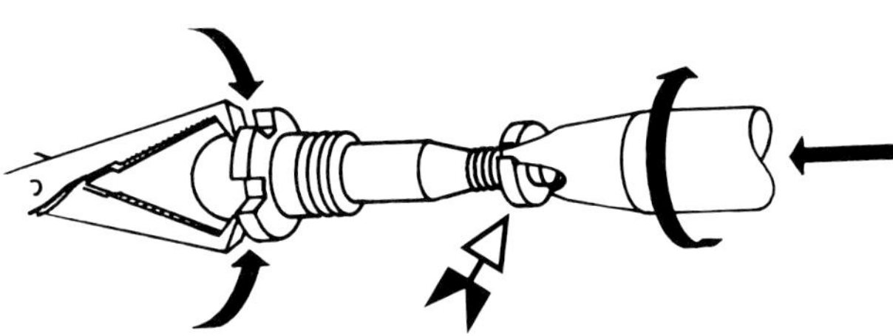

Fig. 22-13. Spring control for ASC-52 attachment is accomplished by holding dowel with rat-tooth plier while adjusting small collar (open arrow).

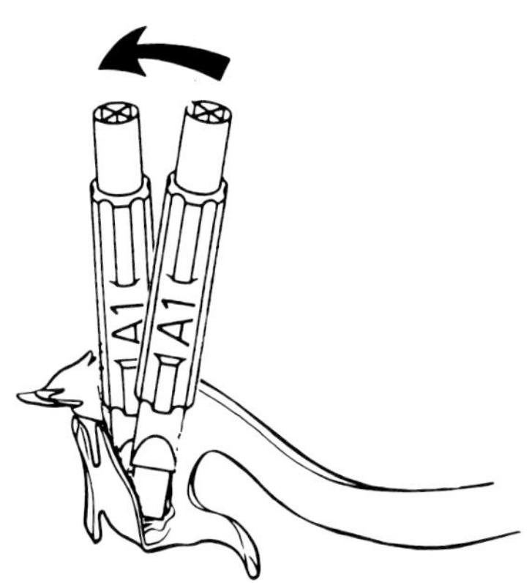

Fig. 22-14. The CEKA attachment is adjusted by inserting blade of CEKA A 1 tool into stud flange and working A 1 back and forth to increase retention.

AUXILIARY ATTACHMENTS (CROSS-ARCH STABILIZERS)

Auxiliary attachments are required for unilateral removable partial dentures. The CEKA With Wings is an ideal attachment to use as a cross-arch unit because its retention component is adjustable, interchangeable, and replaceable with little or no torque to the supporting retainer. It is available in either a rigid or resilient configuration (Figs 22-15 and 22-16). The rigid form is usually used because the elasticity of the palatal strap or lingual bar plus the normal flexion of the resilient attachment removable partial denture (mandibular) provides more than enough movement potential to allow full function of the attachment-retained removable partial denture.

The CEKA With Wings can be used with rigid or resilient CEKA or similar types such as the ASC-52. It can also be used with rigid systems of other designs. The supporting retainer should be full coverage or within the pontic of a fixed bridge.

Fabrication of CEKA

The resin pattern form of the CEKA (red for precious metals, blue for nonprecious metals) is aligned and waxed-up to be in harmony with the path of insertion of the corresponding attachment (Fig. 22-17).

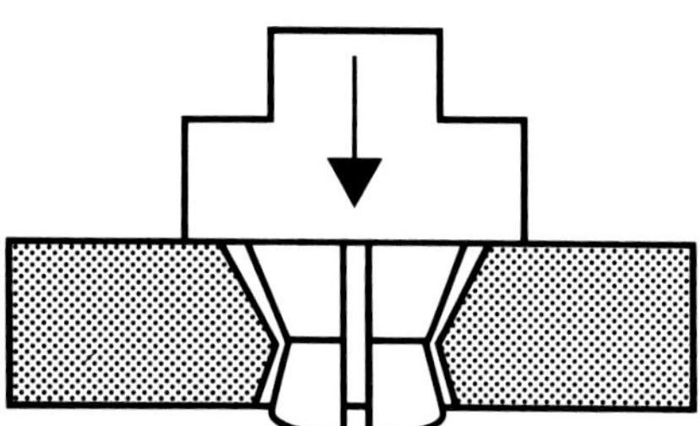

Fig. 22-15. Rigid CEKA attachments rest solidly against female component (shaded area).

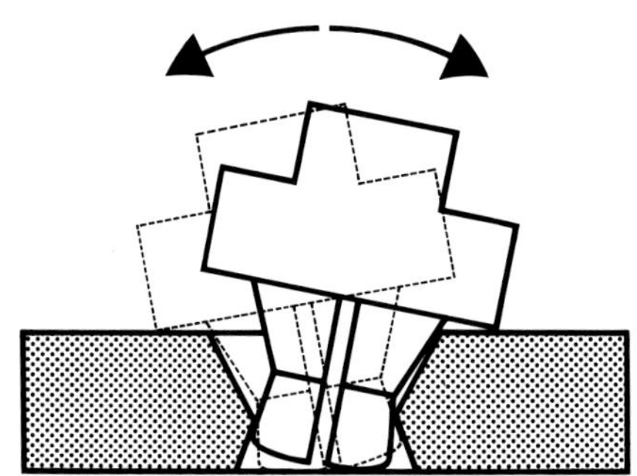

Fig. 22-16. Resilient CEKA attachments connect with female component (shaded area) but have vertical and universal joint function (arrows).

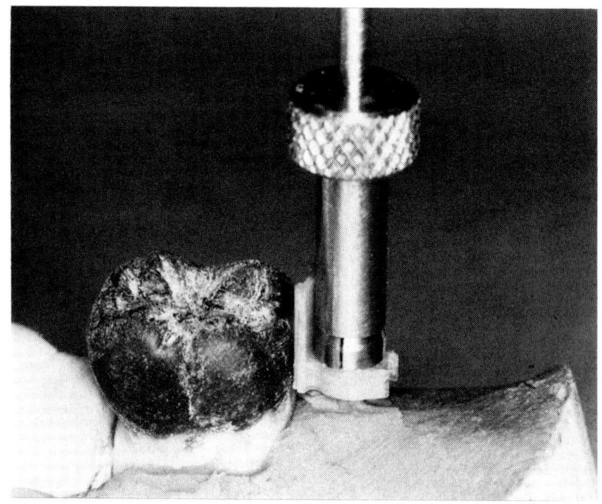

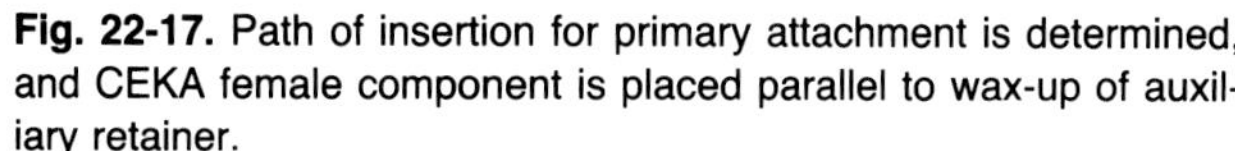

Fig. 22-17. Path of insertion for primary attachment is determined, and CEKA female component is placed parallel to wax-up of auxiliary retainer.

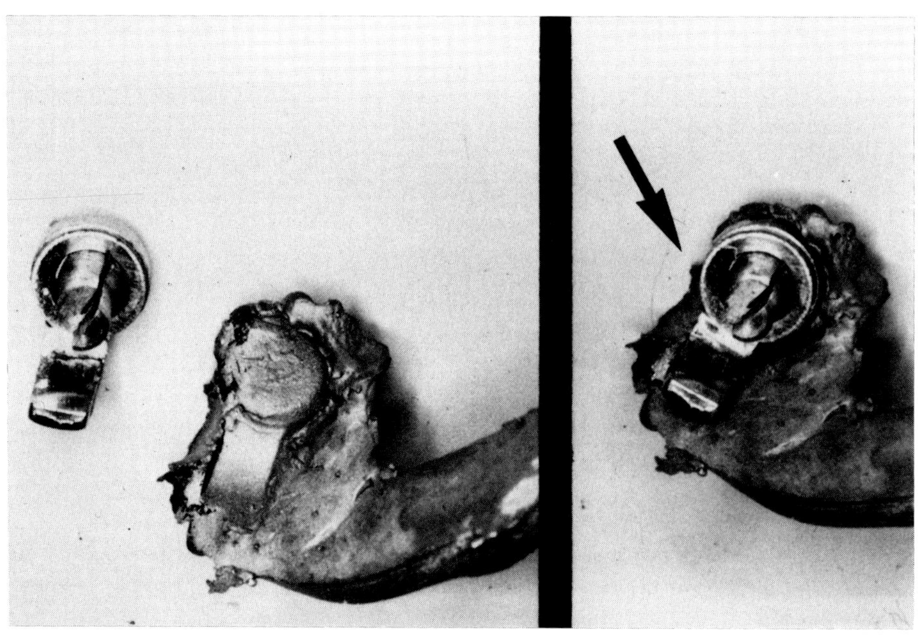

Fig. 22-18. Left, cast retainer with CEKA female component. Right, CEKA With Wings is adapted to conform with removable partial denture frame extension (arrow).

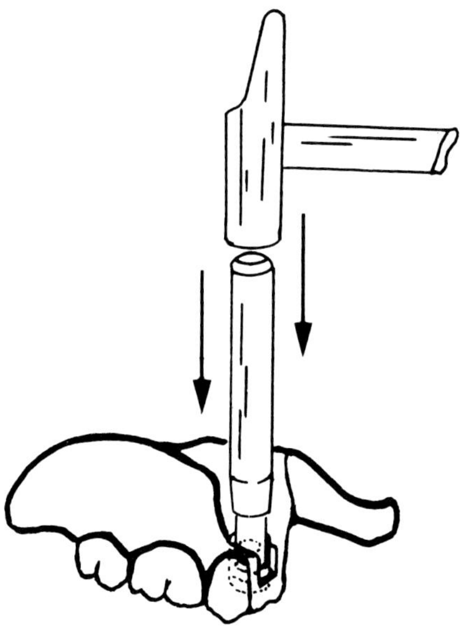

Fig. 22-19. CEKA male stud is riveted to place in female component with CEKA riveting tool H 6 a (resilient), H 6 b (solid).

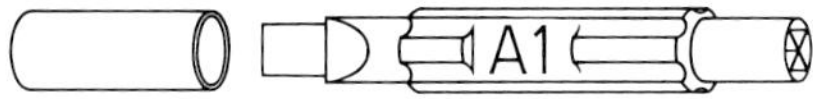

Fig. 22-20. CEKA attachment is activated with CEKA A 1 tool to provide positive retention.

The pattern is cast, and the wing section is fitted and bent to conform with the intended wax-up of the partial denture frame (Fig. 22-18).

The master cast is waxed for duplication to include the CEKA With Wings.

The cast framework is related to the CEKA and soldered or welded to the partial denture.

The CEKA male stud is placed into the female component and riveted to place (Fig. 22-19).

The CEKA male component is activated by using the activation tool (Fig. 22-20) with a back and forth action. The contralateral attachment is activated at the same time.

MAINTENANCE

Refer to the EM Attachment Selector and to the manufacturer's instructions for service recommendations. A detailed review is found in Mensor (1980).

SUMMARY

The attachment-retained removable partial denture presents a challenge in technical skill and understanding of the biomechanics of maxillomandibular function. The main functions of the attachment are retention, stress reduction, and concealment for esthetic purposes. The attachment-retained removable partial denture does attempt to return the patient to as near normal function and appearance as possible.

REFERENCES

Boitel, R.H.: Precision attachments: an overview. In Tylman, S.D., and Malone, W.F.: Tylman's theory and practice of fixed prosthodontics, ed. 7, St. Louis, 1978, The C.V. Mosby Co.

Mensor, M.C., Jr.: Precision removable partial dentures: attachments in fixed-removable prosthodontics. In Kornfeld, M.: Mouth rehabilitation: clinical and laboratory procedures, ed. 2, vol. 2, St. Louis, 1974, The C.V. Mosby Co.

Mensor, M.C., Jr.: Attachments in fixed prosthodontics. In Eissmann, H.F., and others: Dental laboratory procedures: fixed partial dentures, vol. 2, St. Louis, 1980, The C.V. Mosby Co.

23 Removable partial dentures in maxillofacial prosthetics

Stephen M. Parel

The partially edentulous maxillofacial patient may not fall within the parameters of conventional partial denture principles of treatment. The number and extent of contributing therapeutic factors for these patients can complicate the diagnosis and compromise the treatment. Without a complete understanding of these factors and their biologic or psychologic implications, any prosthodontic treatment may be subject to failure.

To understand more completely the application of removable partial dentures to maxillofacial prosthetics, it is helpful to consider the source of most of these defects. Removal of malignant or nonmalignant disease from the head and neck region accounts for the majority of jaw defects seen in a maxillofacial practice. Congenital deformities and trauma contribute to a lesser degree. Each of these patient categories will require a different approach to treatment, which will vary with the nature of the problem and adjunctive therapy required.

The cancer patient, for example, may need extensive preventive maintenance to provide resistance to rampant caries if ionizing radiation is used. Some may never be candidates for extractions, resulting in treatment plans necessarily including nonsalvageable teeth. The cleft palate patient may have such a poor psychologic self-image that home care and maintenance programs will be difficult or impossible to institute. This will in turn influence the choice of abutments and retainer design for maximum longevity. Past and proposed surgical reconstructive efforts for the trauma patient will also influence the timing and extent of partial denture intervention. Perhaps in no other area of prosthodontics do so many factors influence the ultimate goal of treatment, as so timelessly stated by M. M. DeVan (1952): "To perserve that which remains."

DEFECTS OF MAXILLA

Acquired defects

When the integrity of the maxilla or soft palate is compromised, a defect may be created that can cause significant functional and social problems. Speech will become nasal and often unintelligible if there is constant air escape into the nasopharynx or maxillary sinuses. Swallowing solids or liquids may be difficult and embarrassing, with nasal regurgitation the most common result.

The value of an obturating prosthesis is dramatically obvious in these cases, and is a most essential element in overall patient care (Rahn and Boucher, 1970). Hospital recovery time, for example, is significantly reduced when defect obturation is undertaken at the time of initial surgery (Nakamoto, 1971). Many patients with acquired defects of the maxilla and associated structures can be restored to 90% to 95% speech efficiency and quality with a carefully made obturator (Aramany, 1972; Kipfmueller and Lang, 1972; Subtelny and Koepp-Baker, 1961; Majid and others, 1974). The fact that most such acquired defects result from tumor removal makes a rapid recovery time and return to normal social activities even more essential.

Surgical obturators

It is obvious that the design of an obturating prosthesis must be carefully considered to reduce and distribute stress to the abutment teeth, because basal support tissue is sparse or totally absent (Zarb, 1967). These conditions, however, apply most frequently to the obturator for the completely healed defect, which is generally the second or third in a series of obturators these patients will receive. The first and possibly most important phase of treatment is the immediate, or surgical, obturator.

Preliminary planning is the key to the success of this treatment and a presurgical diagnostic impression is an absolute necessity (Rahn and others, 1979; Desjardins, 1977). This diagnostic cast and appropriate x-ray studies are presented to the surgeon in consultation before any surgery is undertaken. When the proposed extent of the resection is determined, the cast is returned to the laboratory for duplication and obturator construction (Fig. 23-1). There are often areas of uncertainty regarding tumor extension, and two or more obturators may have to be made to suit variations in the proposed final result.

The periodontal condition of the unaffected teeth is always a consideration in any obturating partial denture. The success of the surgical obturator, however,

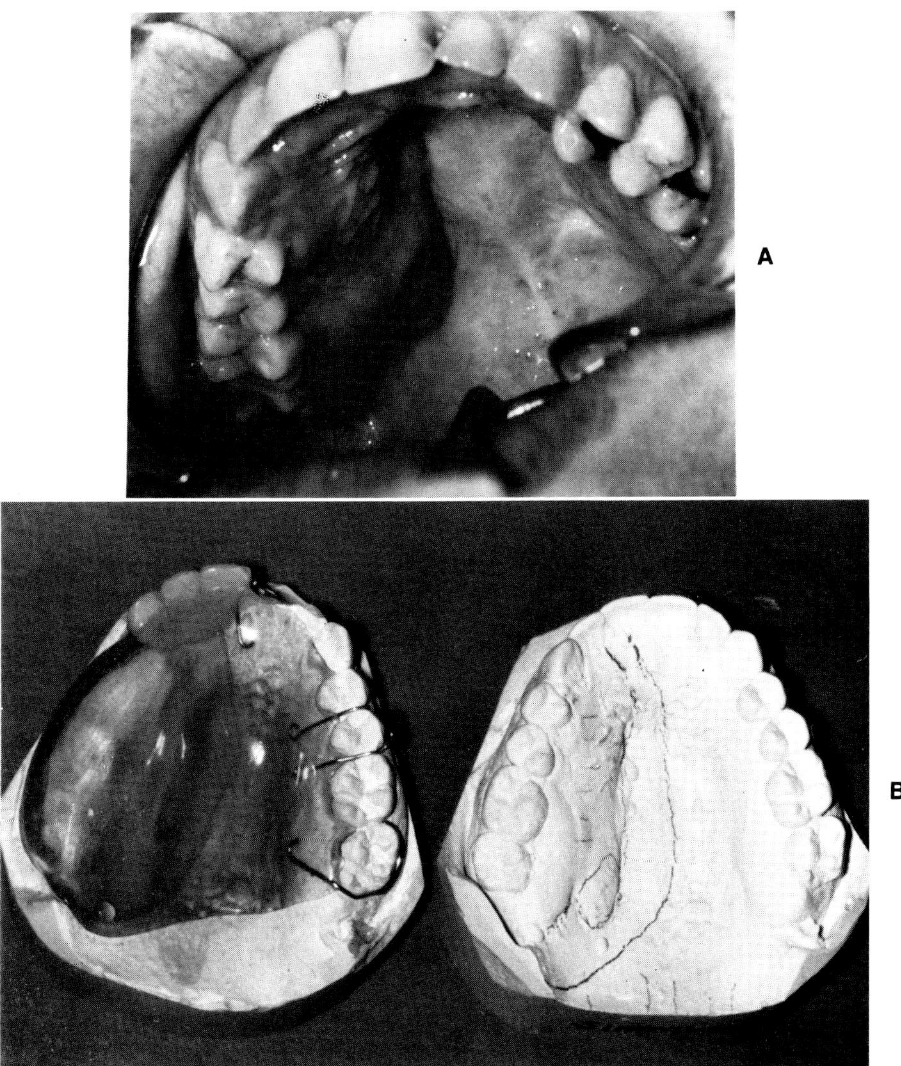

Fig. 23-1. A, Preoperative intraoral view showing palatal expansion from malignancy arising in maxillary sinus. **B,** Presurgical impression of defect and surrounding tissue with area of resection predicted by consultation with surgeon. Surgical obturator is made on duplicate cast using light wire retention.

may depend on periodontally involved teeth, which in any other circumstance would be candidates for immediate extraction.

The principal consideration in these cases is to gain as much stabilization as possible for the prosthesis during the initial healing period. This will improve the potential for adequate speech and function, but may include using prognostically poor teeth as abutments (Fig. 23-2). Light wrought wires will minimize the stresses induced by the cantilevered obturator and are relied on heavily with surgical obturators. Eliminating all posterior teeth and keeping the acrylic resin as thin as possible will reduce weight and further reduce stress to the abutments (Lang and Bruce, 1967). Anterior teeth may be successfully placed on a surgical prosthesis as an option, depending on the condition of the remaining dentition and the psychosocial needs of the patient (Fig. 23-3).

It is impossible to predict with accuracy the final defect size or location, so the obturating portion of the prosthesis will invariably need to be altered with a soft tissue–conditioning material in the operating suite (Fig. 23-4). The porous nature of these materials and the constantly changing defect dimensions will require the soft liner to be changed frequently during initial healing. This also allows supportive undercut areas of the defect to be used for reducing abutment stress.

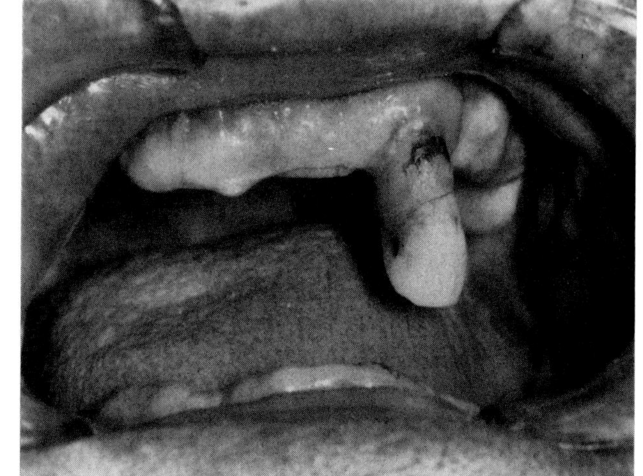

Fig. 23-2. Periodontally hopeless maxillary canine that will be called to support obturating maxillary prosthesis. These teeth are usually retained if at all possible to enhance support and stability.

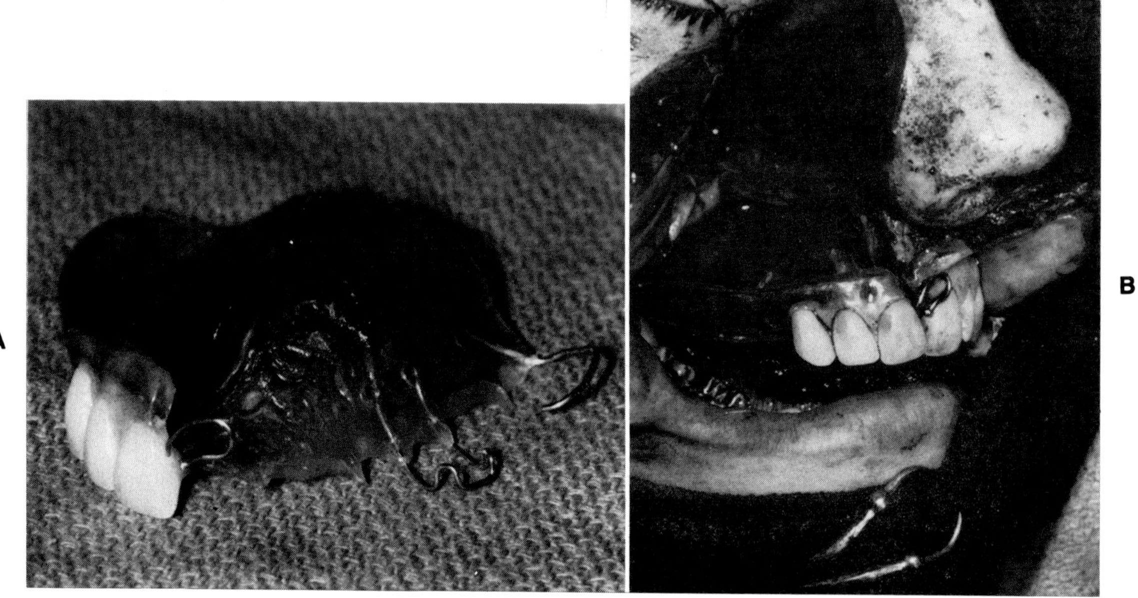

Fig. 23-3. A, Presurgically prepared maxillary obturator with anterior teeth. **B,** Obturator in place following Weber-Ferguson incision to expose tumor in maxillary sinus area.

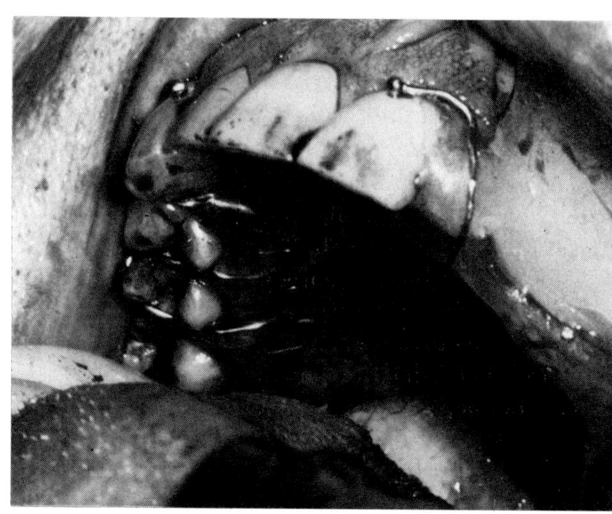

Fig. 23-4. Soft lining material adapted in operating room, which allows surgical obturator to effectively close defect area.

Interim obturator

When the defect has stabilized to the point that the continuous changes will be minimal, considerations for the treatment or short-term, obturator are begun (Stark, 1972). This is usually 2 to 4 weeks after the initial surgery. At this time the condition of abutments becomes a factor, because the interim prosthesis may have to serve for several months or an indefinite period. Patients with terminal disease, for example, may never progress past this stage. Those requiring radiation or extensive chemotherapy may depend on the interim prosthesis for extended periods as well.

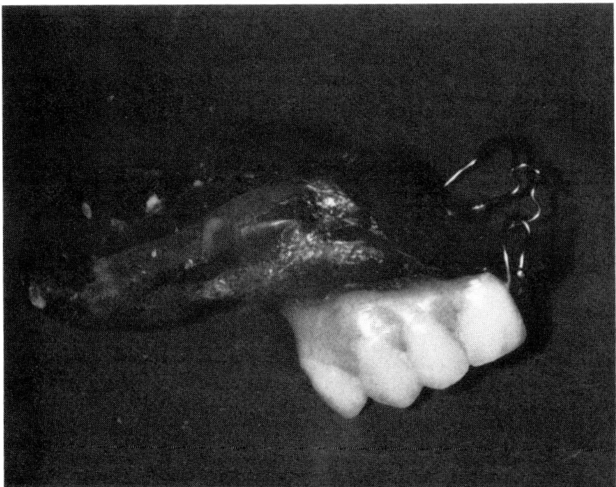

Fig. 23-5. Interim obturator with light wire clasping and additional anterior teeth for esthetic display only. This obturator will more accurately conform to margins of defect, because it is made shortly after surgery has been performed.

With the exception of the terminal patient, it is best to remove all hopeless teeth at this time and make appropriate plans for long-term retention of questionable teeth. This particularly is important for the patient scheduled to receive radiation therapy and is discussed in a subsequent section.

The interim obturator depends on light wire clasping (Fig. 23-5), but cast clasps may be used as an alternative. An acrylic resin base is still most practical for this prosthesis, and anterior teeth can usually be included with little complication (Fig. 23-6). Because the defect area will be recorded with reasonable accuracy in the impression, the need for soft relines is minimized or eliminated. This is a desirable feature of the interim prosthesis if long-term use is anticipated. Posterior occlusion should be avoided to reduce abutment stress and movement of the acrylic resin extension against healing tissues.

Definitive obturation

Individual patient responses to surgery and combined therapy (radiation, chemotherapy, and so on) will determine when the definitive obturator should be considered. This is when the condition and number of remaining teeth become most critical. All carious lesions should be restored and any hopeless teeth should be removed, or endodontically treated if extractions are contraindicated. A thorough periodontal evaluation of the remaining dentition should indicate which teeth may require splinting for maximum longevity and which teeth will be in most jeopardy when subjected to obturator-induced stresses. Only when all restorative, endodontic, and periodontal procedures are complete

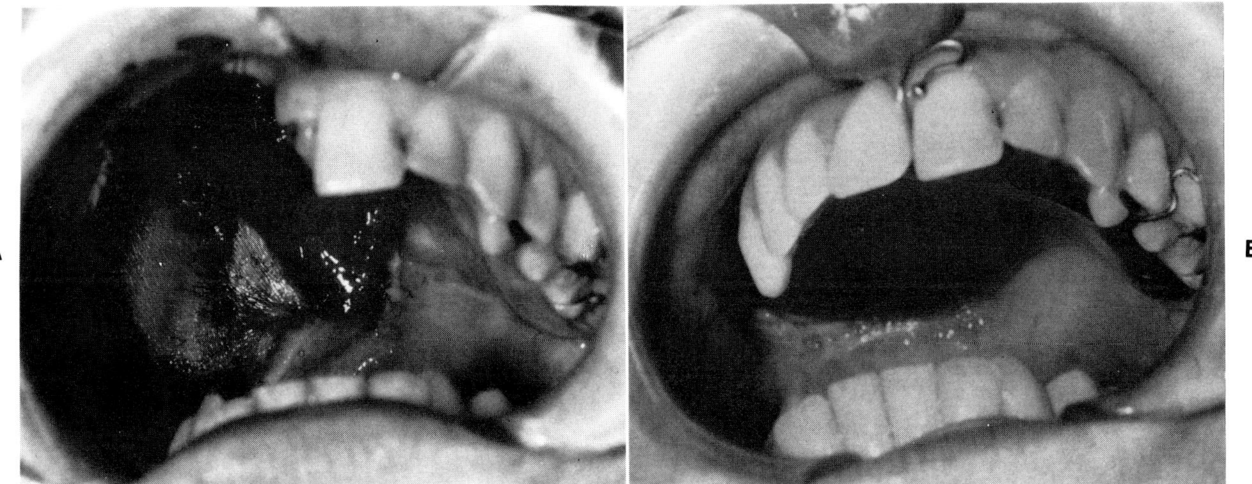

Fig. 23-6. A, Maxillary defect 10 days after surgery. Immature skin graft is visible, and granulation tissue is prevalent. **B,** Interim obturator in place following removal of surgical pack.

should the patient be considered for a definitive obturator prosthesis.

Philosophy of design. There is no unanimity of thought with regard to this type of obturator framework design, but three basic types of clasping can be applied to most cases: light steel or platinum gold paladium (PGP) wire soldered to a cast base; conventional infrabulge, circumferential, and cast variation clasps; and the hinged gate or swing-lock framework (Sprigg, 1977; Brown, 1970; Aramany, 1978; Simmons, 1963). Most clinicians are in agreement that there should be a retentive element as close to and as far from the defect as possible (Curtis and Beumer, 1979; Desjardins, 1978), but confusion remains as to the treatment of the individual abutments, particularly for the most common lateral resections.

Retention for an obturator should be designed to resist vertical and near vertical displacing forces. Some suggest using flexible wires only when relatively few teeth remain or a combination clasp assembly with one flexible retentive arm and a rigid bracing arm (Applegate and Nissle, 1951; Kelly, 1965).

Others feel that, because the obturator causes dramatically increased anteroposterior tooth movement in a lateral resection situation, splinting is of utmost importance (Feibiger and others, 1975). There is even some evidence that the swing-lock design should not be used at all unless splinting of the posterior teeth is first accomplished.

Cast clasps are probably the most universally used retention elements for obturators, yet there is still some disagreement as to whether lingual or buccal retention is appropriate. As the defect approaches the midline, the teeth farthest from the defect become more involved in resisting displacement, and the direction of displacement becomes more important. Lingual retentive arms on these teeth will serve to resist the downward displacement of the obturator extension and will disengage on occlusal or upward movement. Although disengagement is an asset, there is an accompanying reduction in retention resulting from the increase in rotation around the fulcrum line.

Because no cross-arch stabilization exists in these cases, there has been a suggestion that both lingual and buccal clasp arms be designed for "cross tooth" reciprocation and retention (Beumer and others, 1979). There has been some recent evidence that lingual retention, although superior initially, may not be advantageous through the complete range of displacing forces (Firtell and Grisius, 1980). The configuration of the normal lingual undercut allows for superior resistance in test situations, but the relatively quick loss of retention once the lingual clasp arm moves through a predicted range may be unfavorable as compared with the longer retentive period of the buccal arm through the same range.

Retentive elements on the most anterior abutments should be designed to release on vertical occlusal movement. The principal function of these retainers is to resist vertical downward forces of displacement and to a lesser degree, horizontal rotational movement. When this abutment is weak or has questionable defect side bone support, extra care must be taken with the choice and location of the retentive element, even to the point of designing a contingency clasp location in the framework if loss of this tooth seems eminent. A dual path of insertion has been suggested to use a weak anterior abutment for retention (King and Gay, 1979). This consists of establishing a divergent guide plane on the edentulous side of the tooth, which is engaged just before the framework is seated completely through a second path.

To completely understand the nature of forces placed on teeth by an obturator for a total lateral defect, an analysis of retention provided from the defect extension is necessary. If the resection and mouth opening allow, the obturator should cover as much of the lateral wall superiorly as possible (Zarb, 1967; Brown, 1970, Desjardins, 1978; Beumer, 1979; Brown, 1968). This will decrease the lever arm of displacing force to the teeth and provide an extremely valuable area of resistance to vertical displacement (Fig. 23-7). The scar band often produced at the skin graft–mucosa junction can create a horizontal shelf as well, which will enhance the resistance to vertical downward displacement (Fig. 23-8). There is no real purpose served in terms of resistance to vertical displacement by extending acrylic resin superiorly into the medial defect space past the junction of keratinized mucosa. In fact, the friable and sensitive nature of the respiratory mucosa in this area will usually not allow pressure or even intermittent contact.

If the soft palate is left intact and is relatively mobile, it is difficult to gain retention by actively engaging this margin. Since the soft palate margins change constantly during function, it is important to provide some inferior and superior posterior extension to the obturator to effect the maximum seal (Aramany and Myers, 1978). Only when the soft palate remnant is scarred and relatively immobile can resistance to vertical displacement be elicited in this area.

Several basic principles of partial denture design should be followed, regardless of philosophy adhered to in obturator construction (Frechette, 1956). There should be numerous and rounded rests that direct forces along the long axis of the teeth. Guide planes should be carefully planned for maximum bracing qualities and stability. Major connectors should be rigid and placed so impingement on soft tissues will be avoided.

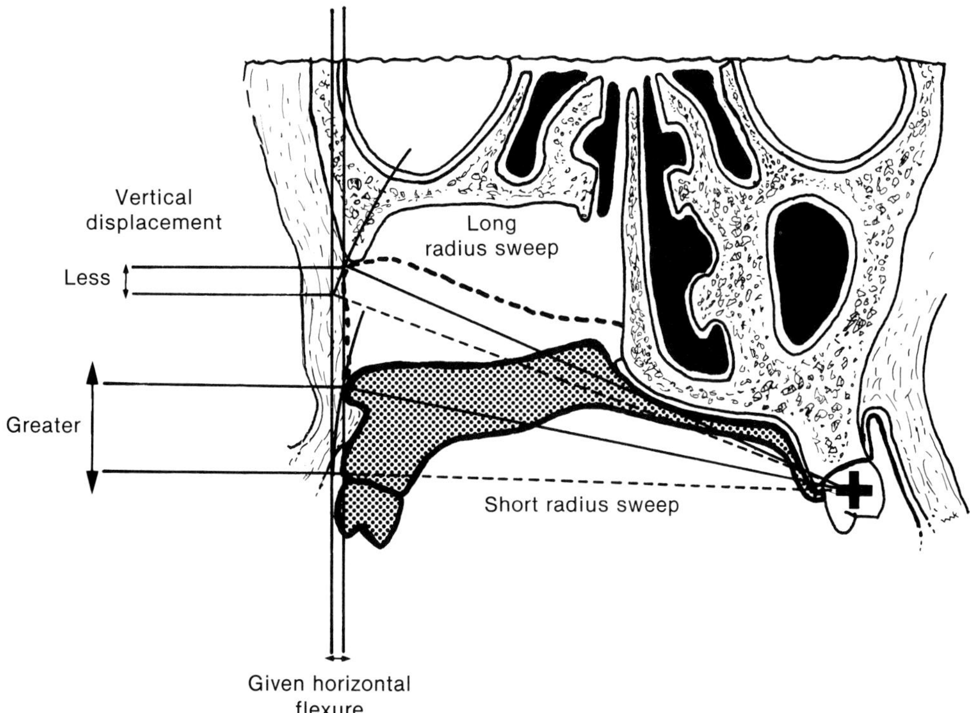

Fig. 23-7. Diagrammatic representation of decrease in vertical movement of obturator when flange is placed high, as opposed to being placed low into defect space. The longer the radius sweep from opposite abutment tooth, the less will be the vertical movement of obturator intraorally. It is therefore desirable to get maximum extension of the obturator bulb against lateral walls of maxillary cavity. (Redrawn from Brown, K. E.; Peripheral considerations to improving obturator retention, J. Prosthet. Dent. **20**:176, 1968).

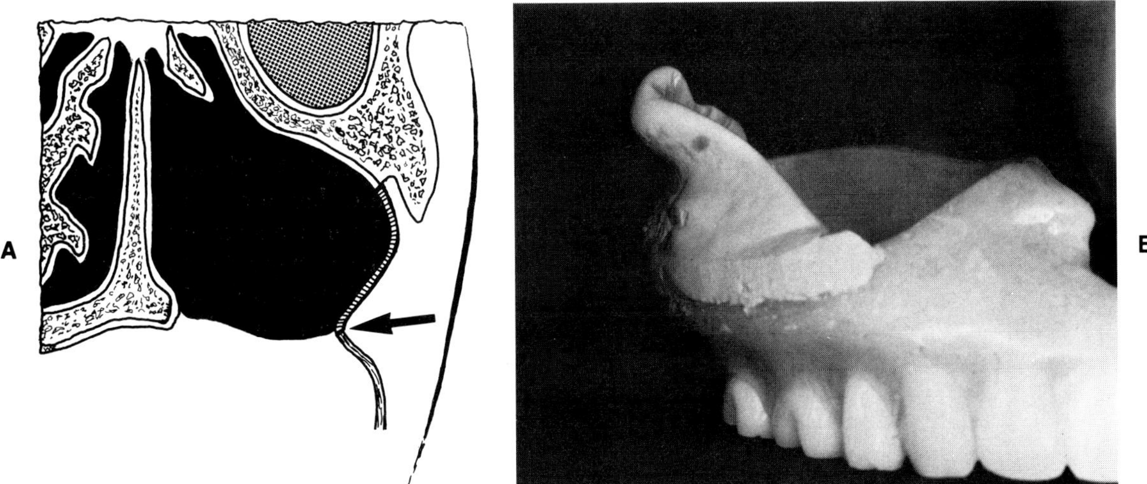

Fig. 23-8. A, Junction of oral mucosa and skin graft lining can provide excellent point of accessory retention for obturator bulb and should be used whenever possible. **B,** Lateral defect space traced in compound showing constriction of scar band and extension to lateral shelf created by tumor removal.

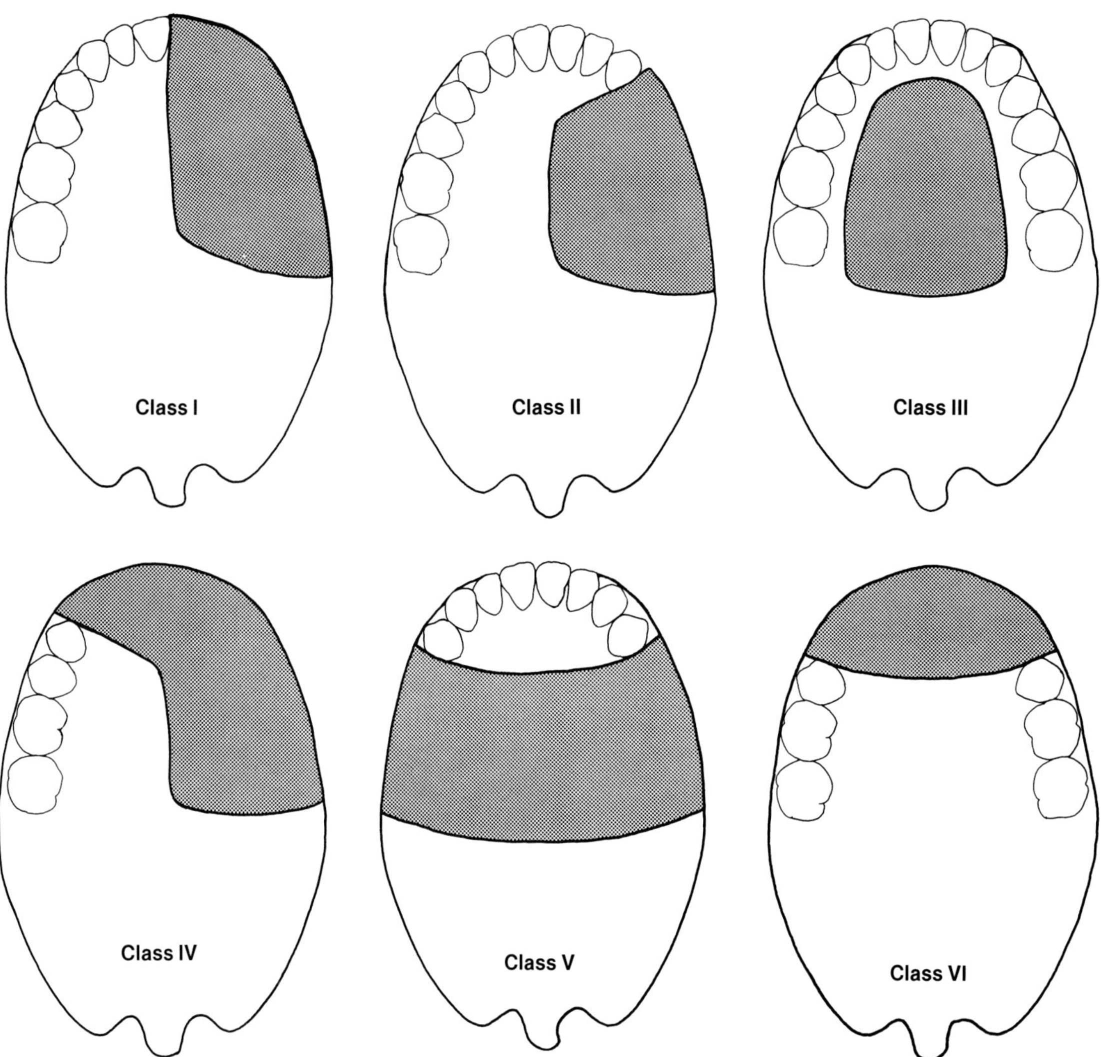

Fig. 23-9. Classification of maxillary defects as originally proposed by Aramany. (Redrawn from Aramany, M.A.; Basic principles of obturator design for partially edentulous patients, Part I, Classification. J. Prosthet. Dent. **40**:554, 1978.)

Retention—be it buccal, lingual, or both—should not exceed the limits of periodontal support. The clasp arms should be passive when not functionally stressed and provide only the minimal retention needed to resist displacement.

Design possibilities. Defects of the edentulous maxilla have been conveniently classified according to the defect location and its relation to the remaining teeth (Aramany, 1978). Classes I, II, and IV (the lateral defects with anterior margins approaching or crossing the midline) occur most frequently (Fig. 23-9). Although acquired defects of the soft palate do occur, they are considered in greater detail in the section on congenital defects of the maxilla.

Classes I, II, and IV. These defects are considered together because they are seen most often and share the same cantilever stress patterns. The most important factor to consider in these designs is the location of the fulcrum line in relation to remaining teeth. The triangle formed by the fulcrum and lines through the anterior and posterior teeth with the canine as an apex serves as a reference (Fig. 23-10). As this triangle flattens and diminishes in area, the stresses on the posterior teeth increase, leading to more difficult considerations of retention and stress distribution.

Of these three, the most favorable is the Class II defect because tripodal design can be integrated into the framework (Fig. 23-11). If the remaining anterior tooth

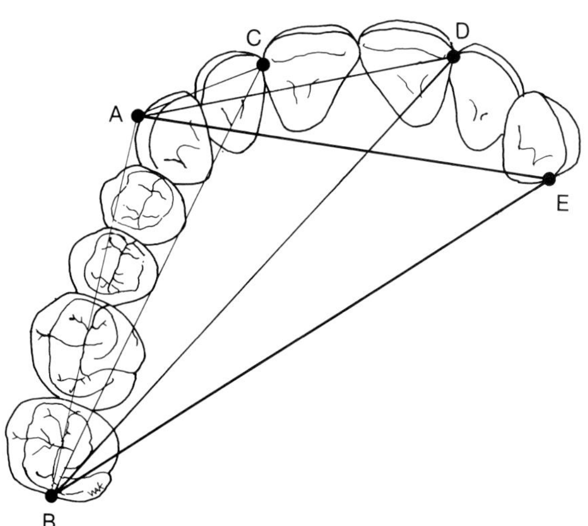

Fig. 23-10. As triangle formed between apex *(A)* and the distal abutment *(B)* or *(C, D, E)* narrows, rotational stress on nondefect side posterior abutments increases. This is caused by increase in lever action as the obturator portion of prosthesis grows larger.

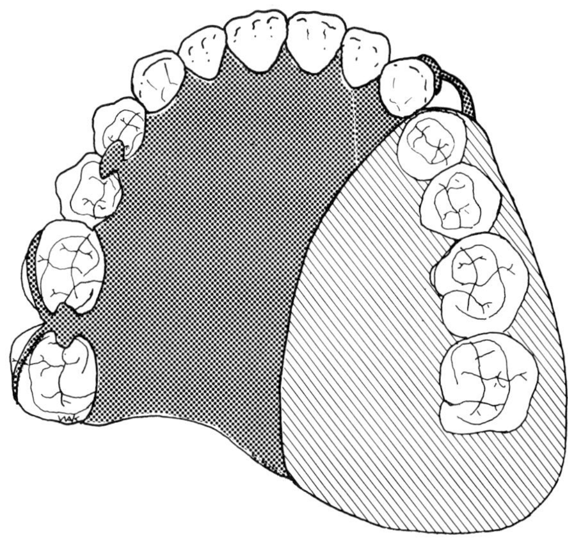

Fig. 23-11. Schematic drawing of potential design for Class II defect. Tripod design allows use of buccal retentive units on all abutment teeth.

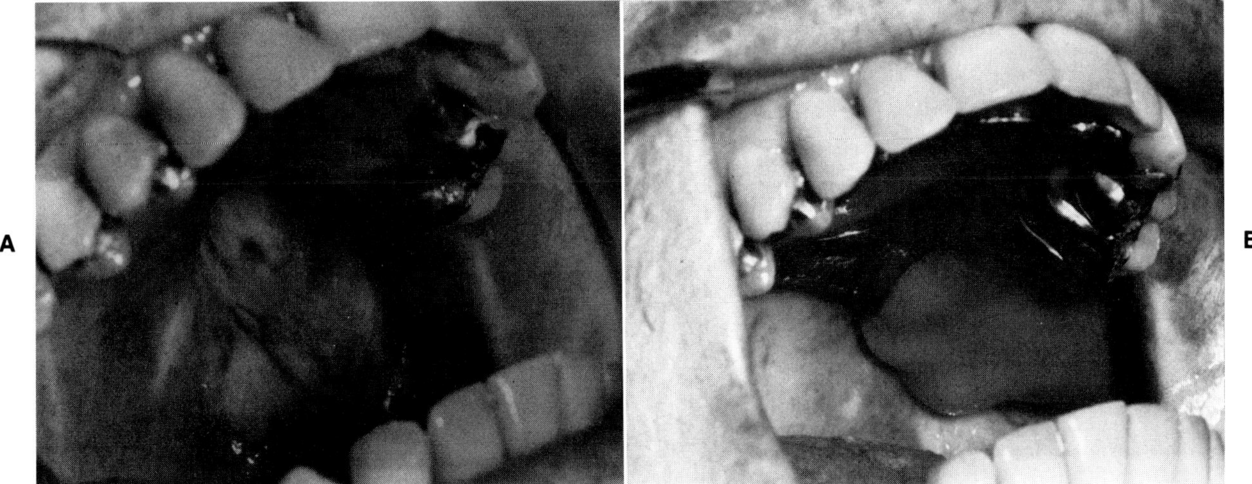

Fig. 23-12. A, Intraoral view of Class II defect. **B,** Obturator framework in place utilizing buccal retentive units on premolar and molar abutments bilaterally.

on the defect side is a canine, the prognosis for success is enhanced. The inclusion of posterior teeth on this side will aid further, but this is a relatively rare occurrence because eradication of disease from the maxillary sinus will usually involve both premolars. Generally conventional buccal retentive units can be used on the molars or second premolars. (Fig. 23-12).

The anterior abutment tooth must resist downward forces, and indirect retention should be distributed as evenly as possible. Cingulum rests are preferred over incisal rests on the anterior teeth. Care should be taken to avoid buccal retention in the canine–first premolar region of the unaffected side, because occlusal movement of the obturator could produce an extracting force on these teeth.

A hinged gate prosthesis for this defect would be unnecessarily cumbersome and may induce damaging stresses. Wrought wires are also unnecessary on the posterior teeth, but may help on the anterior abutment if tooth anatomy does not favor a cast clasp.

As the fulcrum line moves closer to the midline, the rotational forces become even more critical. At this point consideration to lingual retention on the molars becomes a more viable alternative.

The curvature of the remaining dentition will also be significant in planning retention for the Class I case because a broad arch will be more adaptable to tripodization and use of conventional buccal molar clasping (Fig. 23-13). In this case there will be a relatively long lever arm at right angles to the fulcrum line extending to the end of the obturator. Occlusal movement of the obturator at this point could cause a significant downward force on the first premolar and molars, which would necessitate eliminating any retentive elements on these

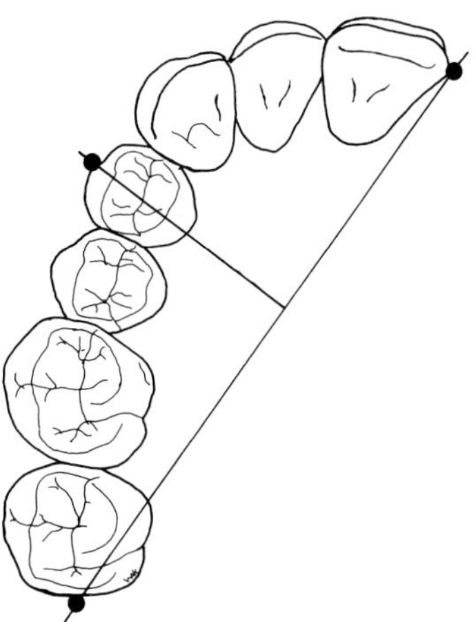

Fig. 23-13. Broad anterior dental arch allows for longer center fulcrum arm with possibility for tripodization and buccal molar clasping.

teeth. The narrow residual arch will most likely have a shorter obturator cantilever arm directed at the point of rotation on the molars, and may allow retentive elements to be placed in the canine region for additional resistance to displacement (Fig. 23-14).

The anterior clasping unit must be carefully considered, because central or lateral incisor root structure may not withstand the downward forces induced by obturator movement (Fig. 23-15). A substantial and well-designed guide plane will be important for adequate bracing. A flexible clasp arm that will disengage when occlusal forces direct the obturator upward will also promote longevity of this abutment (Fig. 23-16).

Class IV defects are difficult to obturate without subjecting the remaining teeth to potentially damaging forces. The case for diagonally reciprocating retention (lingual retention on the molars and buccal retention on the premolars) can be reasonably applied to the Class IV situation (Fig. 23-17). There is some justification for using only light wires in an acrylic resin base for definitive obturation if the remaining dentition is any less than optimal. Reducing the number of posterior occluding artificial teeth will further reduce the rotational tendencies of this prosthesis.

Class III. The Class III defect can be reasonably treated with nearly any combination of retentive elements, as long as the design does not exceed the limits of support offered by the remaining dentition (Fig. 23-18). It is usually unreasonable to expect any support from extensions into the defect space, although pro-

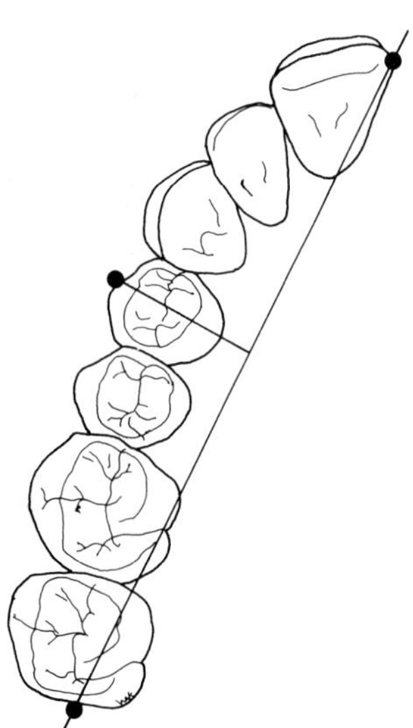

Fig. 23-14. Narrow residual arch decreases midline fulcrum distance and increases potential for rotational forces in axial plane. This will increase considerations for lingual clasping on molar abutment teeth.

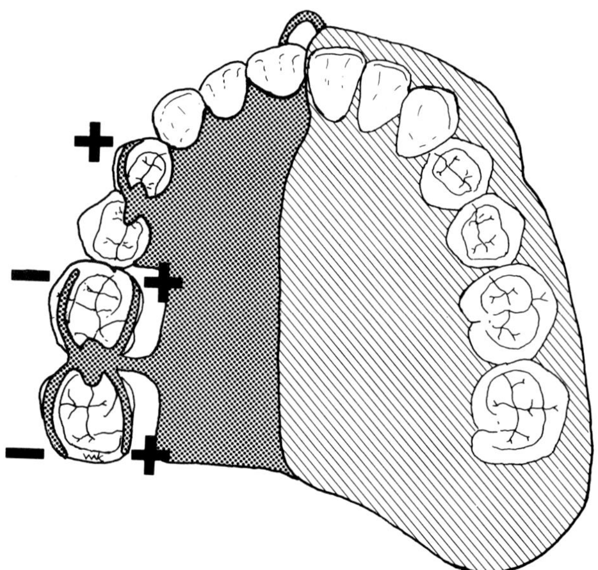

Fig. 23-15. Schematic drawing of potential design for Class I defect incorporating buccal clasping on premolar unit and lingual clasping on molar unit to reduce downward rotational movement produced by obturator extension.

cessed soft liner extensions above the lateral palatal shelves may be useful.

Class V. Although Class V defects occur infrequently, they can place tremendous stress on the remaining anterior teeth, particularly if the soft palatal remnant is not suitable for posterior support. Splinting the anterior teeth will offer additional resistance to the labial force exerted when the posterior extension drops. Occlusal forces on the obturator will also cause tremendous movement of the posterior abutments if the retainers are not designed to release in this situation (Fig. 23-19).

A sound argument can be made for the gate prosthesis, especially if the anterior teeth are adequately splinted (Fig. 23-20). This may more effectively distribute the gravitational forces inherent with such a large posterior extension (Javid and Dadmanesh, 1976; Simmons, 1963).

Class VI. The Class VI defect will usually be significantly smaller in area than the Class V defect making consideration of gravitational movement less important

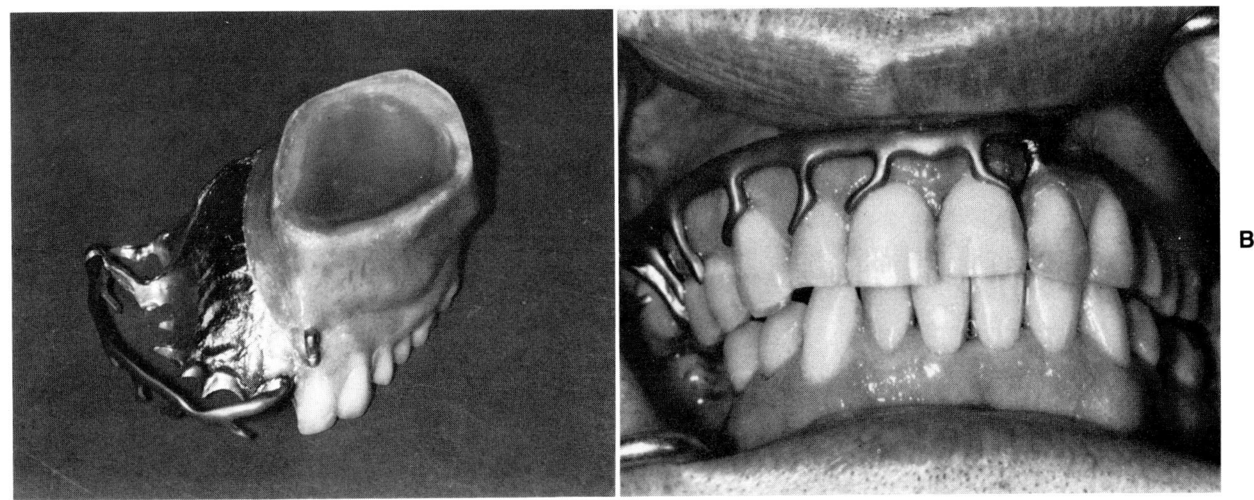

Fig. 23-16. A, Swing-lock partial denture design using long flexible hinging arm to engage anterior and posterior abutment teeth. **B,** Swing-lock partial design intraoral view using stress distribution to numerous abutment teeth.

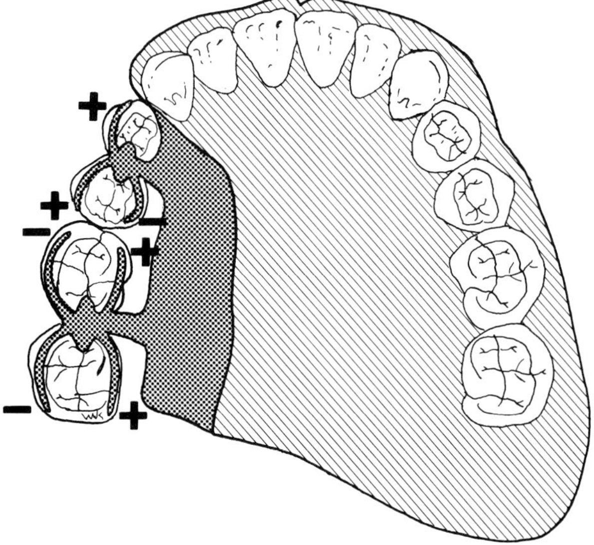

Fig. 23-17. Drawing of potential design for Class IV defect patient. Stresses to remaining dentition will be considerable in an obturator such as this, and care must be taken not to damage remaining dentition. Both buccal and lingual clasping elements are used.

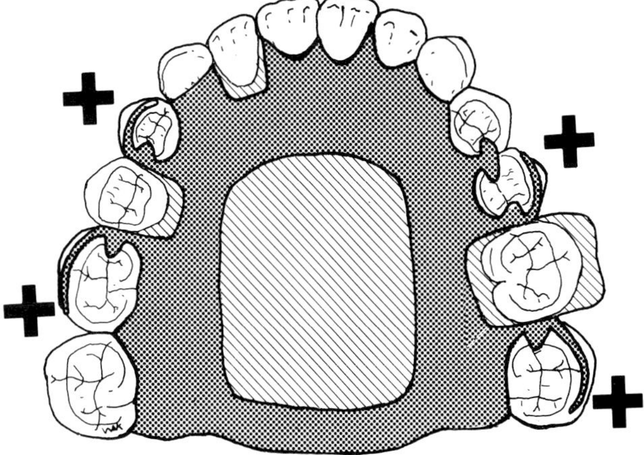

Fig. 23-18. Drawing of Class III defect. This is essentially a tooth-supported partial denture with central obturator extension. Conventional clasping elements can be used in pattern dictated by position and condition of remaining dentition.

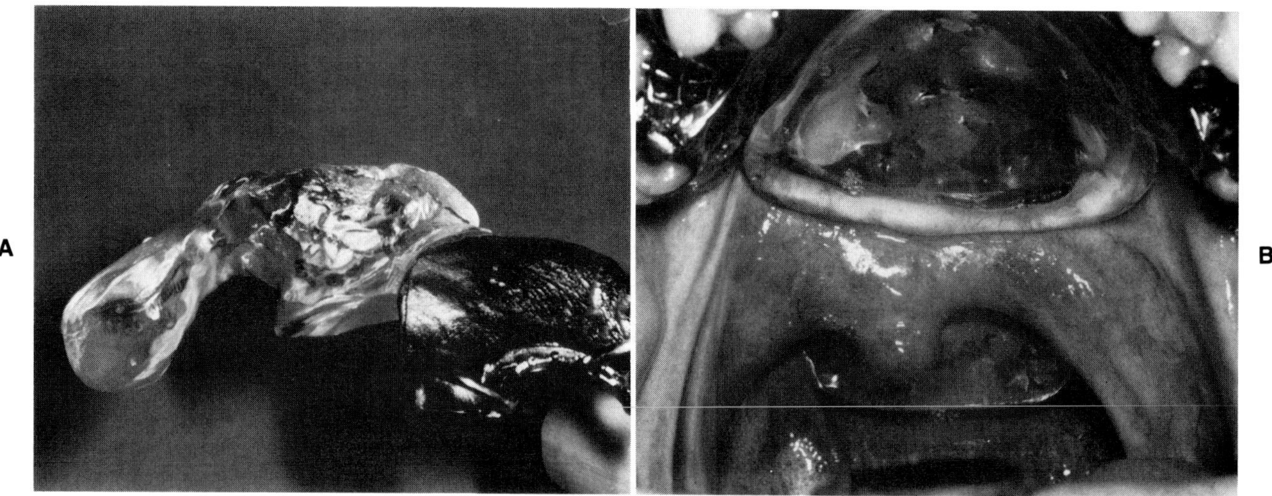

Fig. 23-19. A, Class V obturating partial denture with pharyngeal distal extension to compensate for lost palatal movement. **B,** Intraoral view showing obturating bulb extending beyond posterior abutments and into pharyngeal cavity.

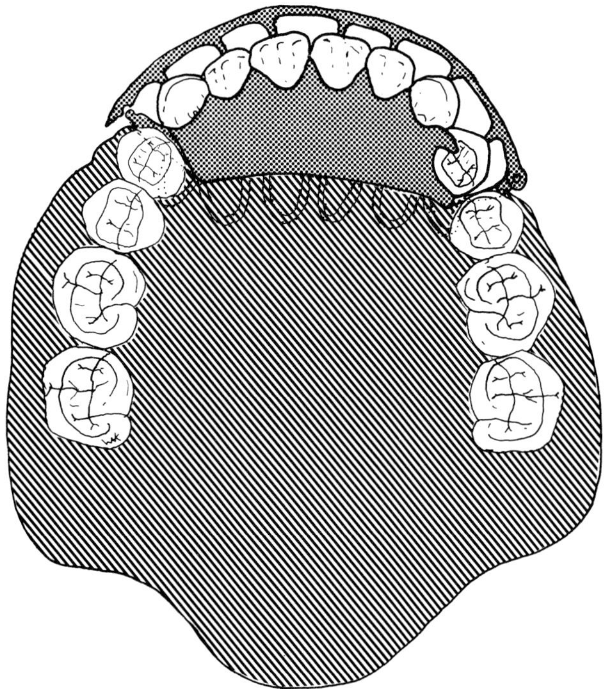

Fig. 23-20. Gate or swing-lock type prosthesis can distribute stresses to anterior abutment teeth and may provide favorable situation for support in Class V defect patient.

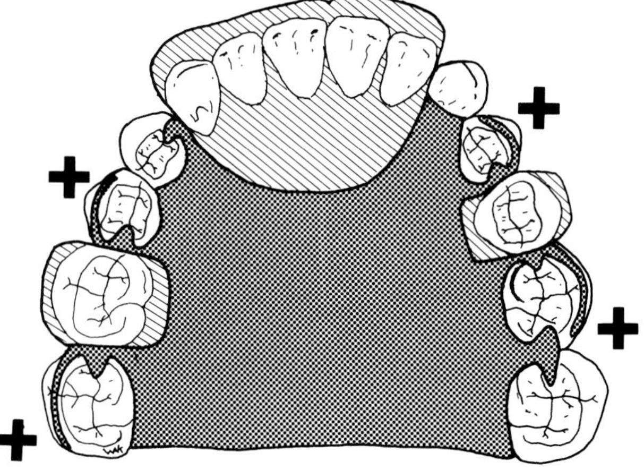

Fig. 23-21. Class VI defect will usually be less stressful to remaining anterior teeth and conventional clasping may be used to support this extension.

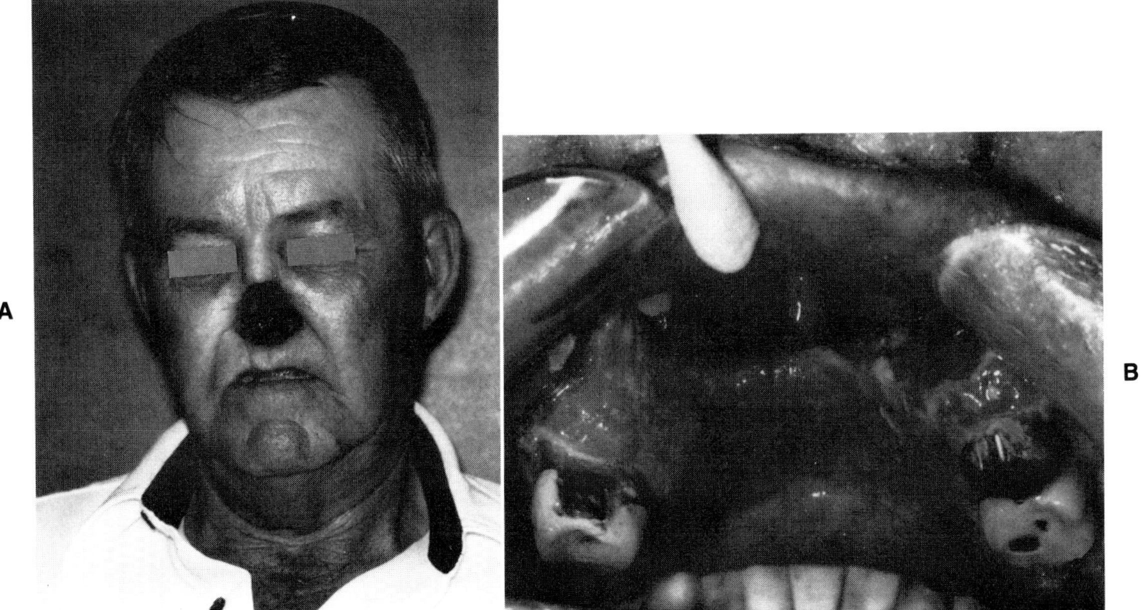

Fig. 23-22. A, Facial view of patient with intraoral/extraoral defect resulting from removal of squamous cell carcinoma. Upper lip is totally unsupported as result of surgical resection intraorally. (Partial denture made by Dr. E.N. Nichols.) **B,** Class VI defect created by surgical resection for removal of premaxillary malignancy.

Fig. 23-23. A, Double swing-lock partial denture with acrylic esthetic overlay engaging remaining dentition. **B,** Prosthetic nose magnetically attached to extension from obturator and nasal cavity. **C,** Completed facial and intraoral reconstruction with obturator supporting nasal prosthesis through magnetic retention. Upper lip is also supported by anterior teeth and obturator flange.

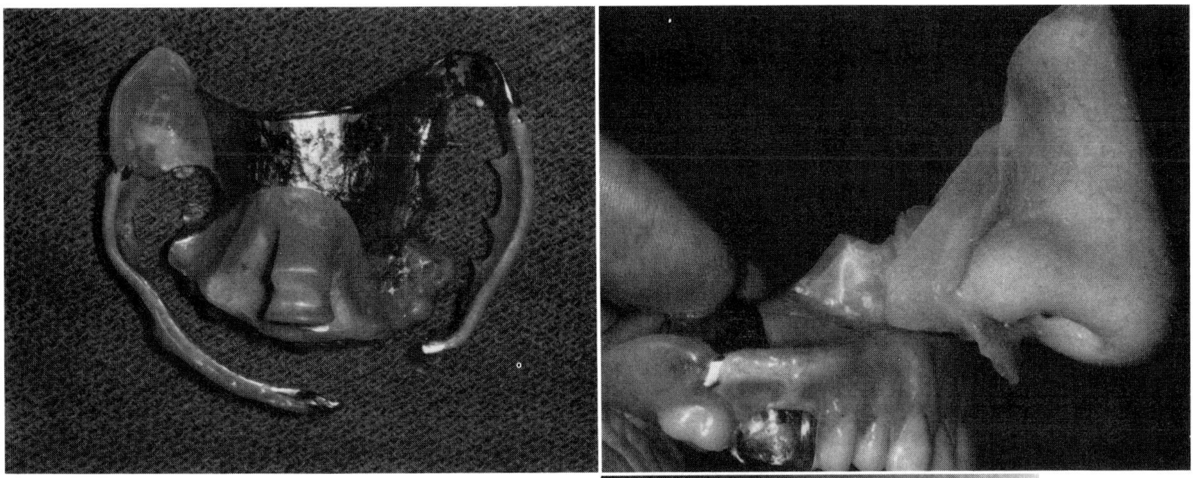

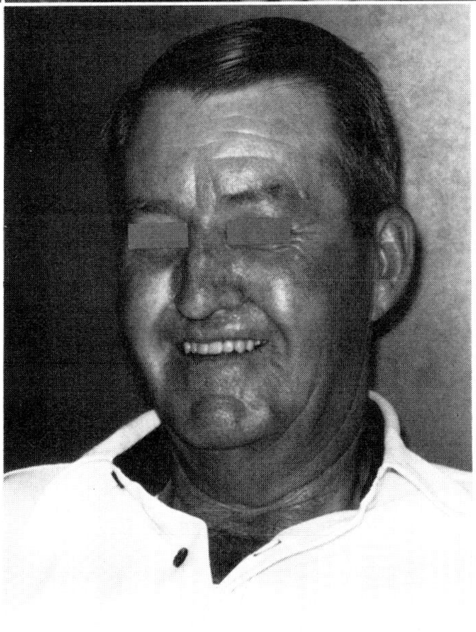

(Fig. 23-21). This prosthesis, however, may be called on to serve an entirely different function from the previously discussed obturators. A resection of this type can leave the upper lip totally unsupported, or missing altogether (Fig. 23-22). In the first instance, the acrylic resin extension will be designed to position and hold the lip in an esthetic position. If the lip is resected, the obturator may have to function to key or hold a facial prosthesis (Fig. 23-23). With the nose and lip intact, additional retention may be obtained with an obturator extension into the anterior base of the nasal sinus.

If the remaining teeth will tolerate full coverage, a cross-arch bar splint can be valuable in dissipating rotational stress to the anterior abutments. This will also allow a convenient accessory retention point to be incorporated into the finished prosthesis (Aramany, 1978; Adisman, 1962).

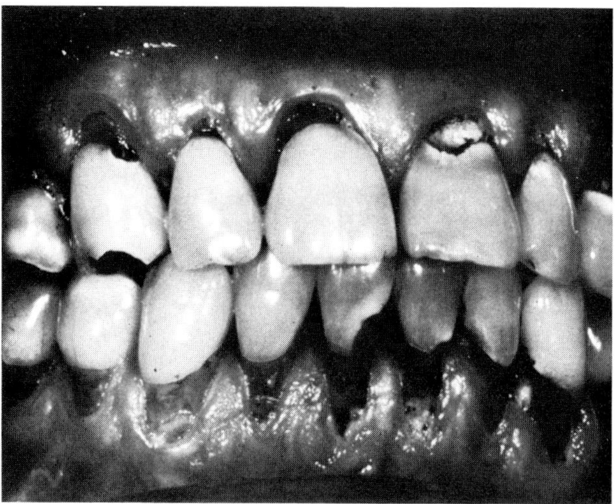

Fig. 23-24. Cervical and incisal carious activity typical of that precipitated by radiation to oral cavity and ensuing changes in salivary acidity.

Implications of ionizing radiation therapy

Any consideration of removable partial denture treatment for the patient with a head or neck malignancy must include an evaluation of the effects of radiation therapy. Whether administered before, after, or in lieu of surgery, the potential for damage to teeth and supporting structures is a critical factor in prosthetic reconstruction (Beumer and Curtis, 1979).

Radiation caries. There are two major complications from such ionizing radiation to the oral cavity and surrounding area. The first, and most easily treated, is the change in salivary flow and consistency during and following treatment. Although both the mucous and serous acini are affected, the serous components of the major salivary glands are most vulnerable to tumorcidal doses of ionizing radiation. The resultant loss of acinar function can be irreversible depending on the dose levels, and can cause dramatic changes in the inherent protective qualities of the normal saliva. The diminished flow, mucous nature, and increased acidity of the saliva create an environment where a rampant and unique type of cervical-incisal caries can occur (Fig. 23-24) (Del Regato, 1939; Beumer and Brady, 1978). This hard tissue breakdown is usually asymptomatic but can cause spontaneous amputation of nearly all remaining teeth if left untreated (Fig. 23-25).

There is an obvious need to control this activity if any tooth-tissue–borne prosthesis is to be considered. Fortunately, the conscientious and early application of top-

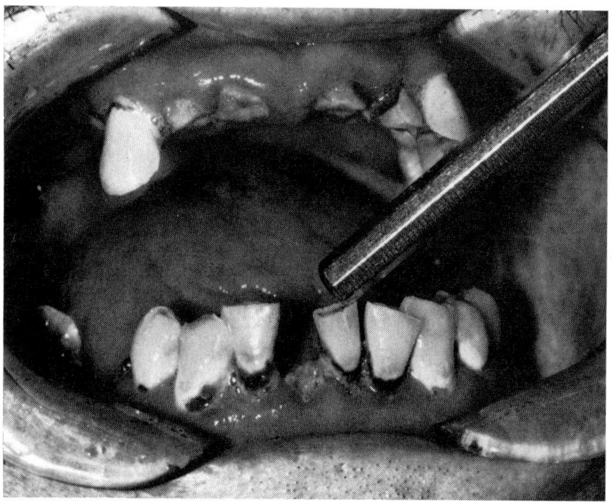

Fig. 23-25. Radiation caries developing to the point at which spontaneous amputation of dentition can occur. Lateral incisor is easily bent with mirror handle.

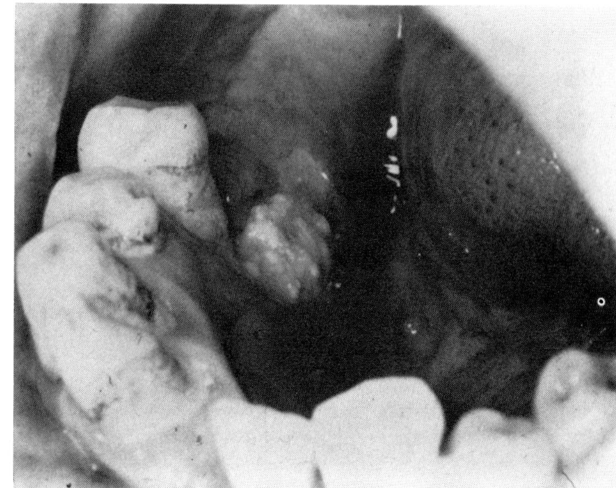

Fig. 23-26. Exposed lingual necrotic cortical bone caused by extraction of molar in irradiated field.

ical fluoride has proven extremely effective in dramatically reducing or eliminating radiation caries. A 1% sodium fluoride solution when applied daily in flexible carriers will protect the dentition to the extent that even minor existing lesions will be arrested. At this point, the dental restorations required to ensure competent abutments can be undertaken. Alloys can be placed without special precaution, leaving margins in self-cleansing areas where possible. Abutments requiring full coverage, however, should have subgingival margins, and partial coverage should be avoided. As long as this preventative measure stays in effect and follow-up is assured, the institution of fixed or removable restorations can be undertaken with relative security (Dreizen and others, 1977; Frank and others, 1965).

The near absence of saliva, however, may cause concern if the edentulous areas of support will be subjected to moderate prosthesis movement. The lubricating effect of normal saliva will be severely reduced, and tissue abrasion may become a problem. There are several saliva substitutes available, some with remineralizing components, that will alleviate this condition to some extent. The subjective evaluation of support tissue integrity and quality in each individual case will be the most important factor in predicting dry mouth patient response to a removable prosthesis.

Radiation necrosis

The second and most serious complication of radiation therapy is radiation-induced osteonecrosis (Fig. 23-26). This can occur anytime a break in epithelial continuity allows exposure of bone that has been or will be subjected to ionizing radiation. Although this can occur spontaneously, pretreatment extractions with inadequate healing time accounts for most cases of radiation necrosis. Posttreatment extractions of teeth in the fields of radiation most certainly pose the most risk for morbidity and should be avoided whenever possible. The use of a prosthesis on radiated mucosa may also induce a necrotic situation, particularly in the retromolar-lingual surface of the mandible where the mucosa is thin and vulnerable to penetration (Grant and Fletcher, 1966; Beumer and others, 1972). Osteonecrosis may occur in the maxilla, but is most commonly found in the mandible where treatment is most difficult and the sequlea are most serious (Fig. 23-27) (Bedwinek and others, 1976).

Fortunately, with early detection and conscientious conservative treatment, most cases of osteonecrosis can be resolved without surgery (Fig. 23-28) (Daly and Drane, 1972). Those that do not respond to conservative therapy can result in distressing deformities and the need for surgical intervention without evidence of malignant disease (Fig. 23-29). Such a result will most

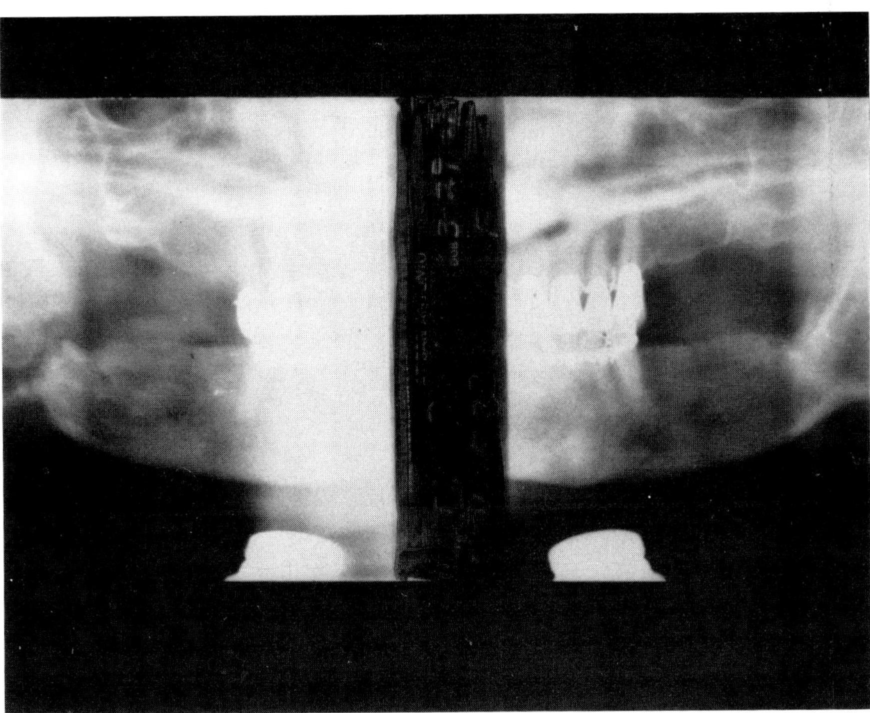

Fig. 23-27. Pathologic fracture at mandibular angle with bone necrosis evident radiographically. This occurred as result of extraction of tooth before radiation with inadequate healing time.

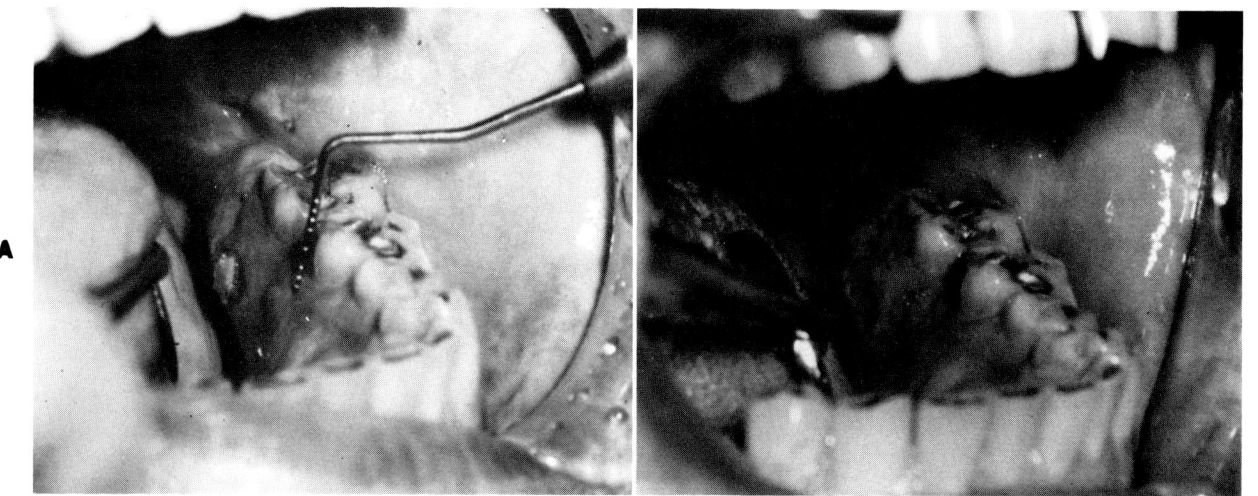

Fig. 23-28. **A,** Necrotic bone from lingual cortex of mandible. **B,** Granulation bed beneath exposed bone resulting from conservative treatment and fastidious hygiene.

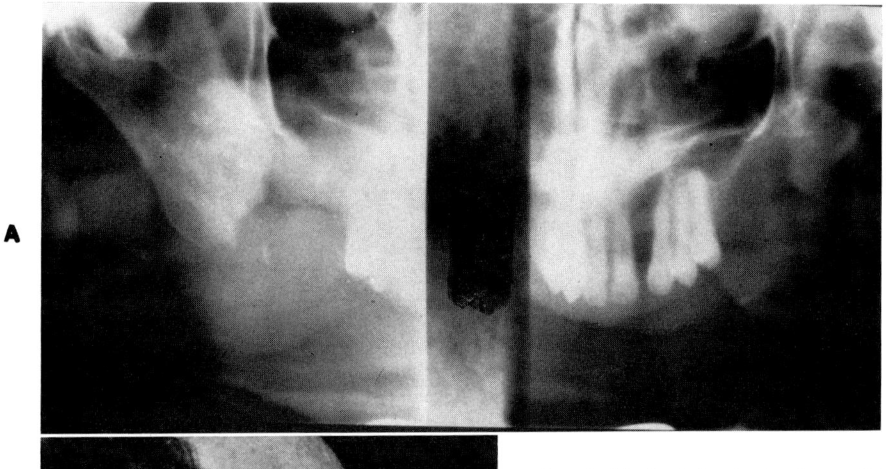

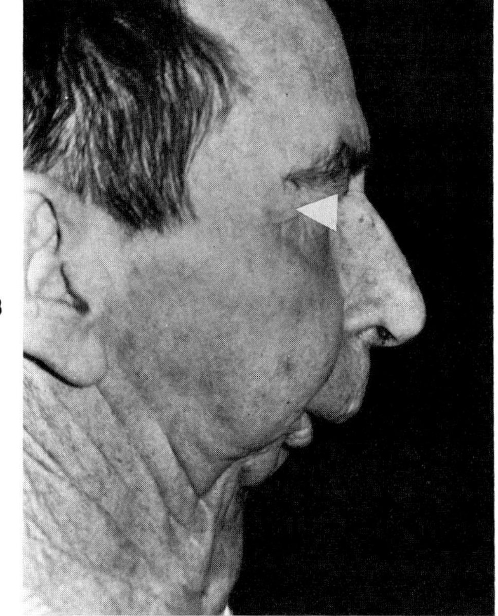

Fig. 23-29. **A,** Entire body of mandible lost from radionecrotic bone exposure intraorally. **B,** Profile of patient following surgery to remove necrotic bone from mandible. There was no recurrent tumor evident at time of surgical procedure.

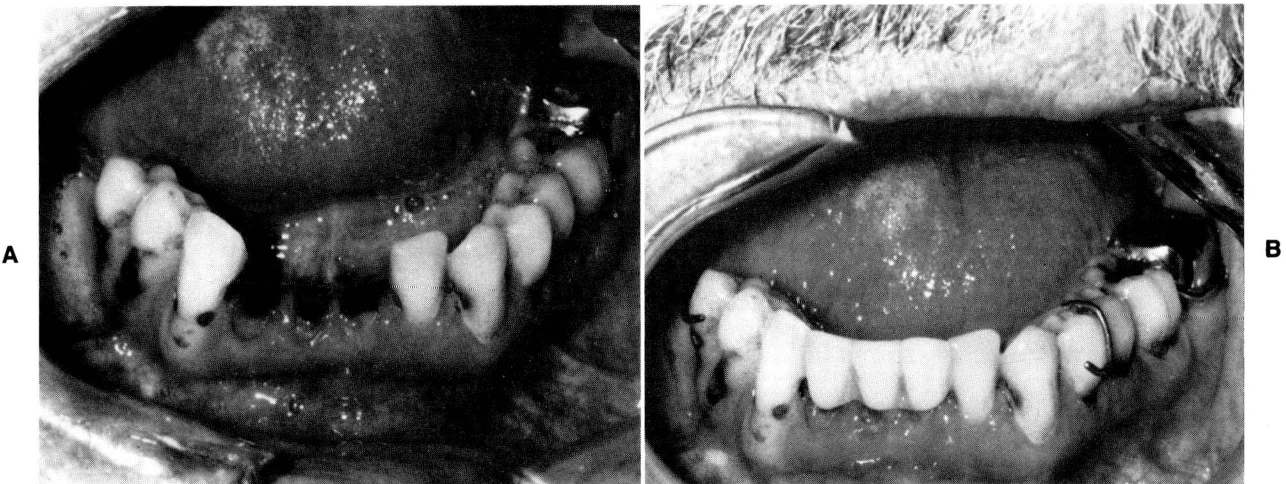

Fig. 23-30. **A,** Spontaneously amputated mandibular incisors as result of cervical radiation caries. No endodontic procedures were intitiated on these teeth. **B,** Light wire removable partial denture with pontics placed directly over residual root tips.

vividly demonstrate the importance of a coordinated approach to treatment planning between contributing services and the need for adequate patient education and follow-up care.

Should a tooth or teeth in a radiation field become unrestorable, there are several alternatives to forcep extractions that can be initiated. There has been some success with rubber band extractions of remaining tooth or root fragments. This involves using the conical shape of the root as a vehicle to slowly move a tensioned elastic band apically. This procedure, if done carefully, will allow granulation tissue to proceed into the extraction site behind the band until the entire root-bone surface has been covered. The tooth can then be removed without fear of exposing bone.

A less time-consuming approach is to amputate the tooth mechanically and institute endodontic procedures on the remaining root electively. The presence of such root fragments should not be an outright contraindication to denture or partial denture construction, as long as there is control over apical disease. Such sectioned teeth can, in fact, be used as partial overdenture abutments without complication (Fig. 23-30), if caries prevention for the remaining dentition is assured. Even the continuous erosion of a residual tooth fragment when prosthetically covered or left alone is preferred to the possible consequences of extraction (Fig. 23-31).

It is important to realize that a certain number of radiation patients will never be candidates for prosthetic rehabilitation. Even after the generally accepted waiting period of 6 months to a year (Daly and Drane, 1972; Krajicek, 1969), these patients will never return to complete epithelial health. Systemic complications (such as diabetes, chemotherapy) or topical abuse (smoking, alcohol intake) may further compromise support tissues to the point where risk factors make prosthetic implementation too hazardous.

Congenital defects

With presently available techniques and procedures, most congenital defects of the premaxilla, maxilla, and soft palate can be corrected surgically. Although this has changed the role of the prosthodontist in the care of patients with congenital defects over the past 2 decades, there are still important contributions to be made in the area of removable prosthodontics (Chierici, 1979).

Four basic descriptions of cleft palate configurations proposed by Veau in 1922 conveniently classify the basic palatal defects seen clinically (Fig. 23-32). The prosthesis made to correct these defects may serve to place tissue or fill a defect space and will have three parts (Fig. 23-33). The palatal portion is the framework and retentive elements that lie within the boundaries of the hard palate. The velar portion may help position the soft palate or may traverse the length of the soft palate area as a connecting extension. The pharyngeal section makes contact with the posterior and lateral pharyngeal wall, whether as an independent obturator or an integral part of the velar portion.

Palatal lift

Occasionally a patient will have a speech deficiency and a completely normal soft palate clinically, in which case a Class I submucous cleft may exist. In this instance there is incomplete muscle function in the mid-

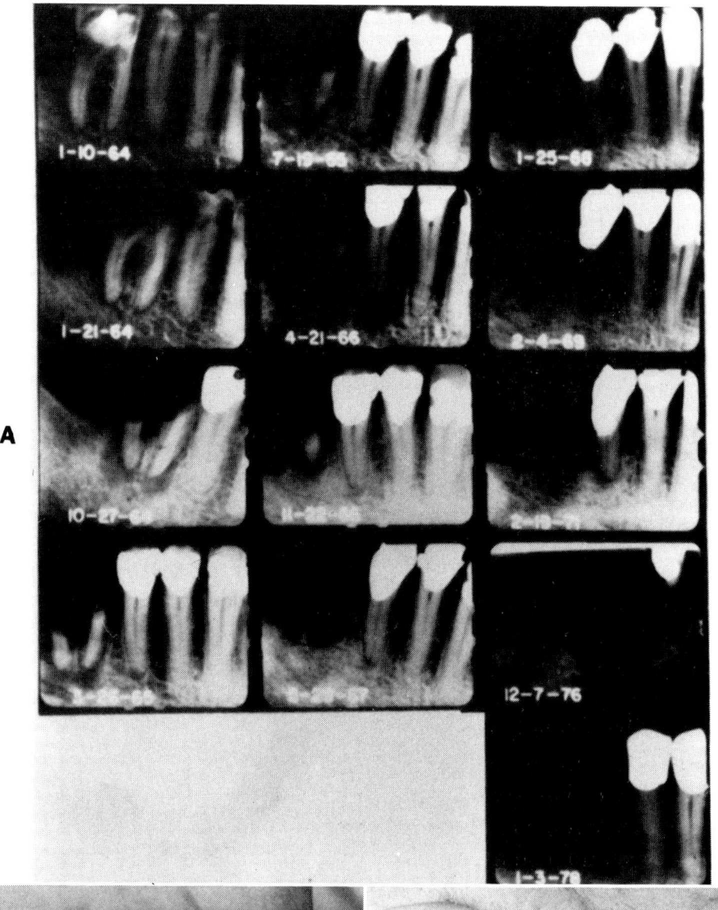

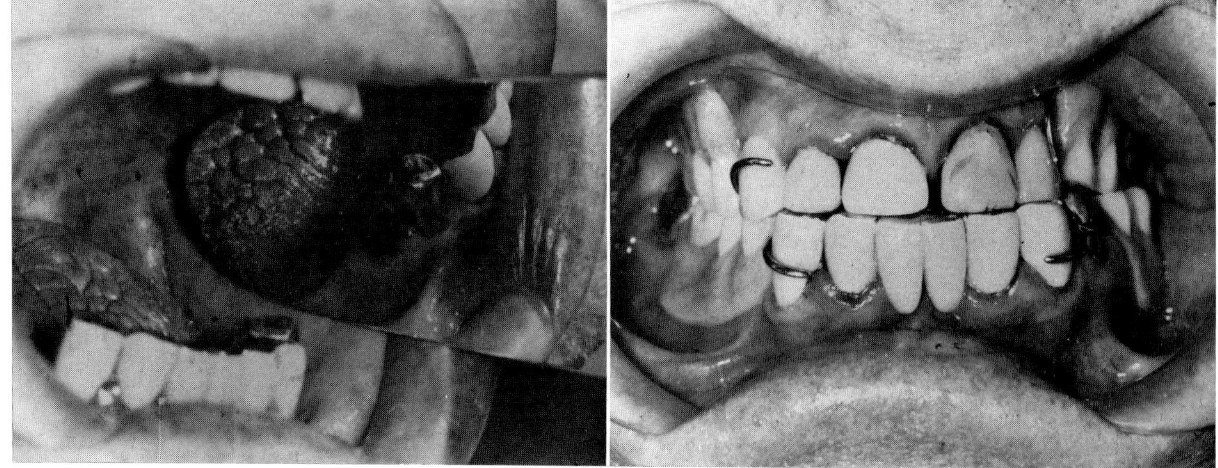

Fig. 23-31. A, Serial radiographs from 1964-1978 showing progression of radiation caries through one molar and premolar segment. No extractions were performed and residual tooth fragments exfoliated without exposing the mandibular bone, thus avoiding osteoradionecrosis. **B,** Remaining root tip in field of radiation that was left intact before reconstruction of removable partial denture. **C,** Removable partial dentures in place covering several residual root tips without complication. Fluoride therapy had been instituted at this time to limit carious activity to remaining dentition. (Partial dentures made by Dr. L.K. Sherrill.)

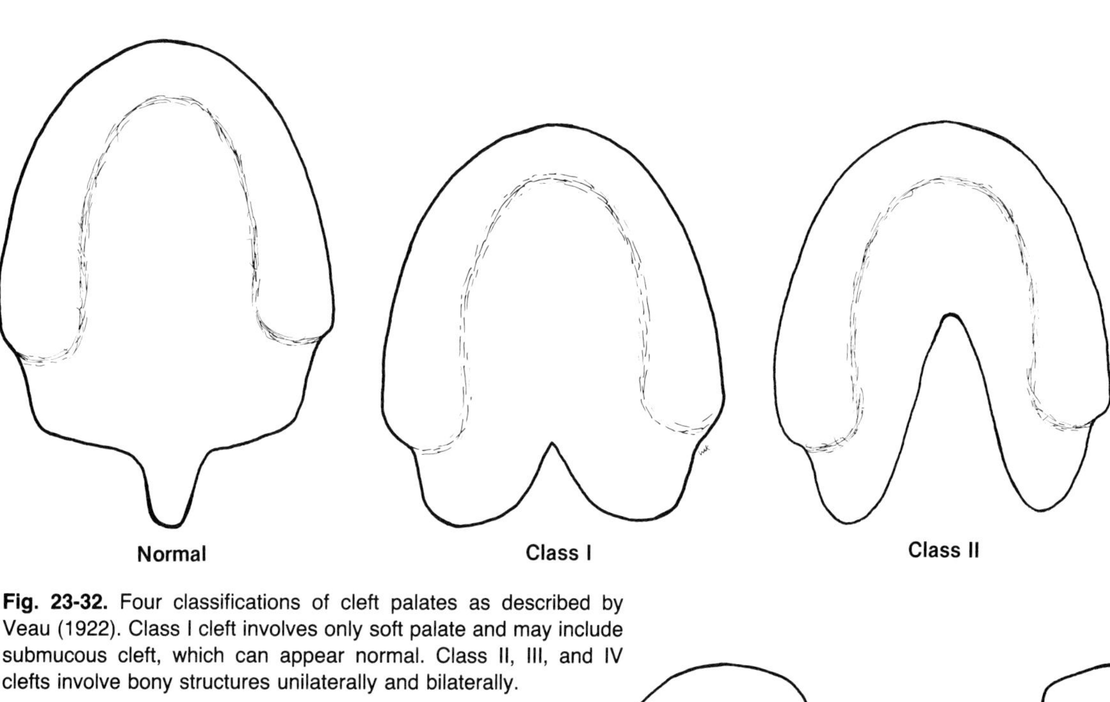

Class III

Class IV

Fig. 23-32. Four classifications of cleft palates as described by Veau (1922). Class I cleft involves only soft palate and may include submucous cleft, which can appear normal. Class II, III, and IV clefts involve bony structures unilaterally and bilaterally.

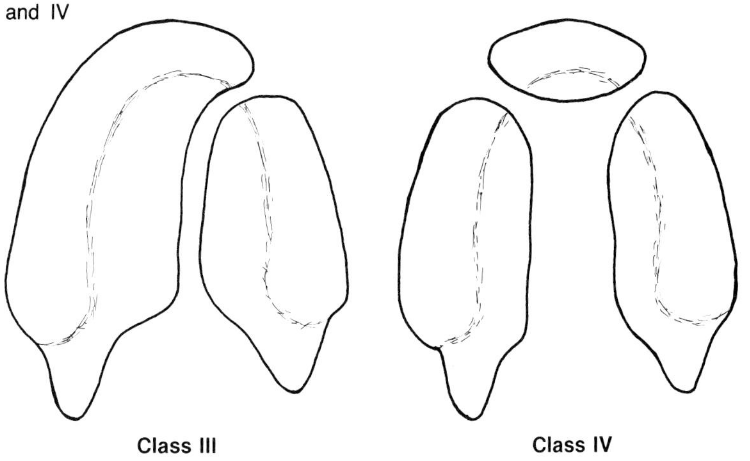

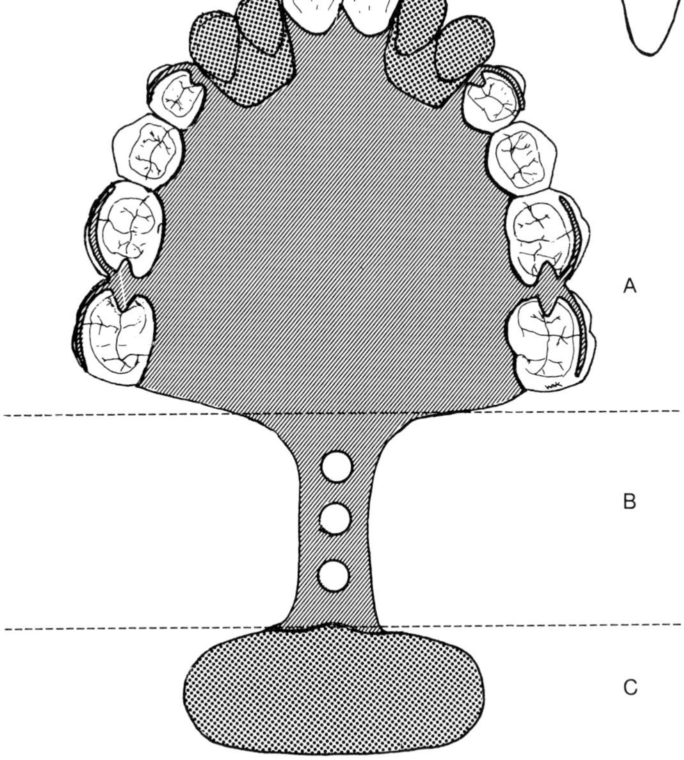

A

B

C

Fig. 23-33. Three basic parts of cleft palate prosthesis include palatal portion (*A*), the velar portion (*B*), which replaces the body of the soft palate, and the pharyngeal extension (*C*), which is the functional component providing contact with pharyngeal musculature.

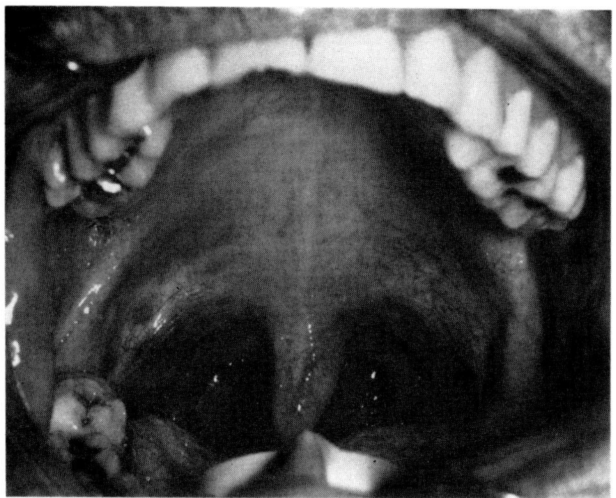

Fig. 23-34. Immobile soft palate as result of spinal cord injury, resulting in air escape through nose when speaking.

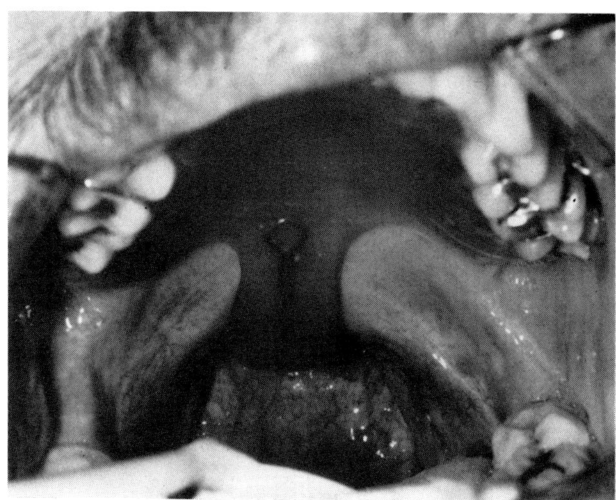

Fig. 23-35. Palatal lift prosthesis positioning nonfunctioning soft palate to more favorable location in relation to pharyngeal musculature.

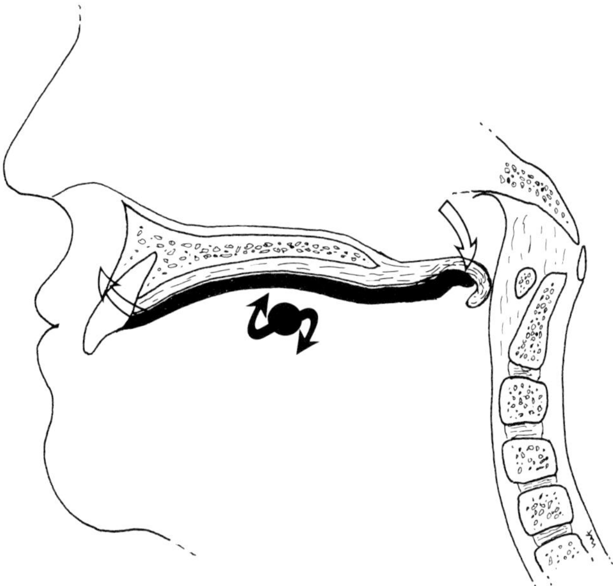

Fig. 23-36. Rotational forces of palatal lift type prosthesis will usually pivot around first molar area. This may require clasping into distal undercuts to resist downward force of soft palate against lift end of prosthesis.

line area, and the soft palate fails to make an adequate valve seal with the pharynx. Traumatic injuries or birth defects also result in a partial paralysis of an otherwise normal-appearing soft palate (Fig. 23-34).

When surgical procedures cannot provide adequate function for these patients, the prosthodontist may be called upon to provide a palatal lift prosthesis (Gibbons and Bloomer, 1958; Marshall and Jones, 1971). Whether or not there is cleft-related derangement of the dental arch in these cases, the framework must be designed to deal with substantial cantilever stresses. It may be advantageous to use wrought wire acrylic resin base prosthesis as a trial measure when attempting to position a soft palate to determine the amount of lift force necessary and the potential for successful treatment. In many cases, this prosthesis may be the only intervention necessary because the lifting action can stimulate enough pharyngeal activity to eventually eliminate the need for a palatal lift (Fig. 23-35).

There have been some preferences expressed to sequentially building up the velar portion, but present thinking favors positioning the soft palate at the desired level in one procedure. This will place a significant rotational force on the posterior abutments and place a vertical labial vector of force on the anterior teeth (Fig. 23-36). Adequate occlusal and cingulum rests are essential, and a labial bow may be beneficial in the acrylic resin base prosthesis. Splinting of the anterior teeth should be considered and molar clasping should be forgiving if long-term use is anticipated. Follow-up treatments should be assured and closely monitored.

Speech obturator

When the residual soft palate lacks sufficient length or is tissue deficient in the midline, a lift prosthesis will serve no purpose. In this instance the pharyngeal extension on the speech obturator can augment the soft palate and provide functional contact with the lateral and posterior pharyngeal musculature (Aran and Subtelny, 1959; Mazaheri, 1964; Sharry, 1962).

Most patients requiring such prosthetic pharyngeal augmentation can anticipate long-term use of their prosthesis. Fortunately, the velar and pharyngeal ex-

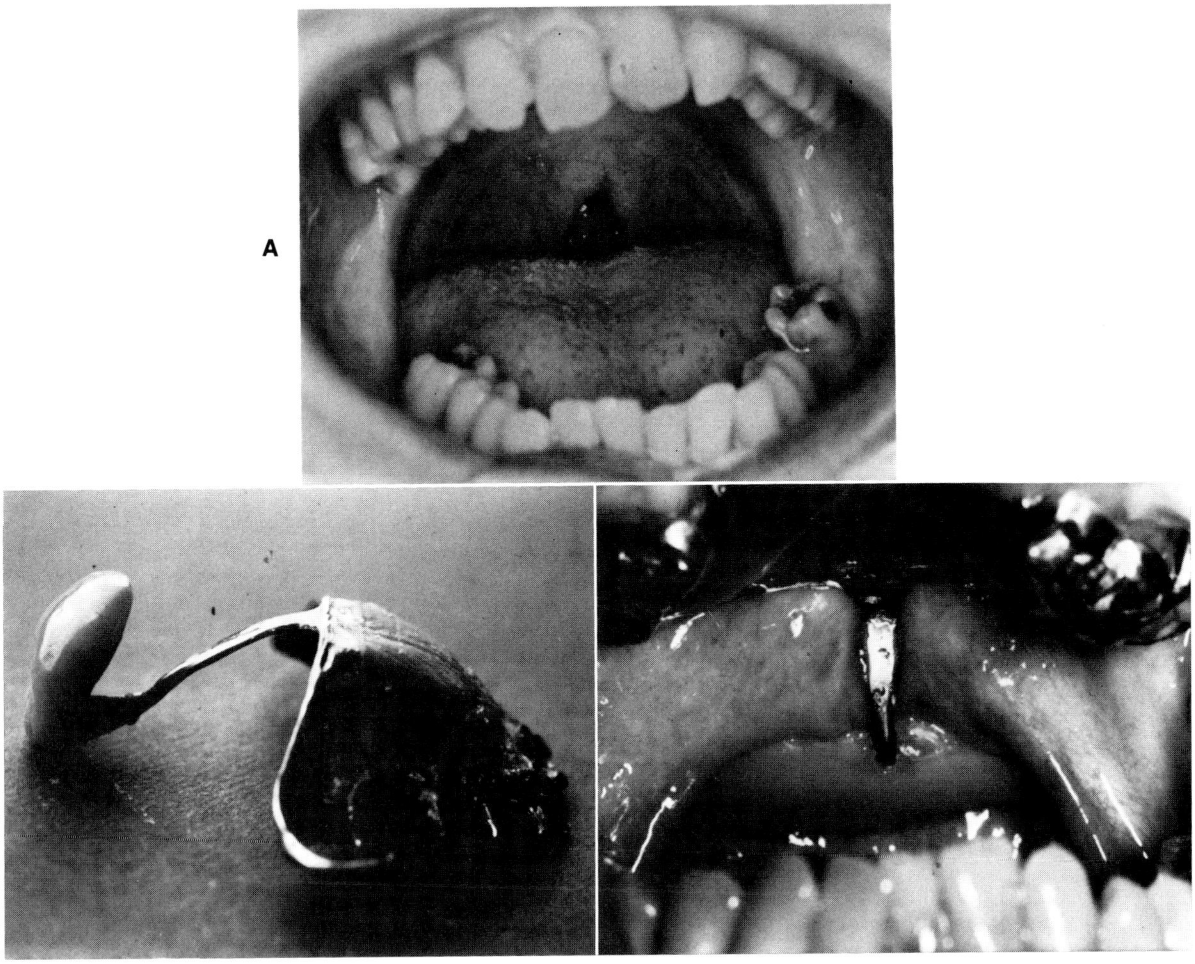

Fig. 23-37. A, Soft palate deficiency following insufficient surgical repair. Soft palate in this case is too short for lift prosthesis to be effective. **B,** Speech bulb appliance that will provide functional seal for residual soft palate against acrylic extension from partial denture. **C,** Intraoral view of large speech bulb in place with pharyngeal musculature relaxed.

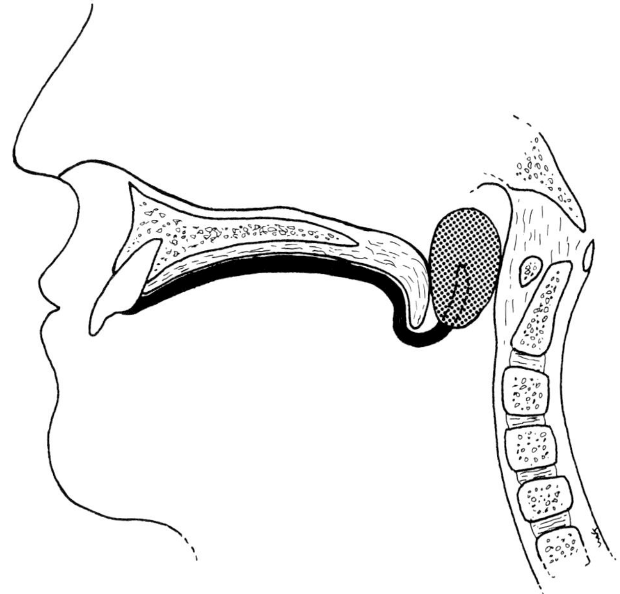

Fig. 23-38. Contact point of acrylic and soft tissue should be in region of palatal plane during function. This is region where normal musculature makes contact with pharyngeal wall.

tensions are not subjected to a constant displacing force as is the case with the palatal lift prosthesis. The acrylic resin extensions are functionally formed so that the soft tissues make intimate static contact but do not tend to displace the obturator (Fig. 23-37). This allows for greater freedom in design of the retentive elements and more advantageous use of conventional cast clasping (Fig. 23-38).

The framework should be designed to support the weight of the extension by distributing the stresses to the posterior abutments as evenly as possible (Fig. 23-39). The anterior force vector pattern is similar to that of the palatal lift, but generally of a lesser magnitude. The need for anterior splinting may be eliminated if adequate cingulum rests can be prepared.

DEFECTS OF MANDIBLE

When the continuity of the mandible is disrupted, a change in balance and symmetry will occur. Occlusal relationships are altered, and proprioceptive responses can be deranged to the point where both functional efficiency and appearance are severely compromised. Al-

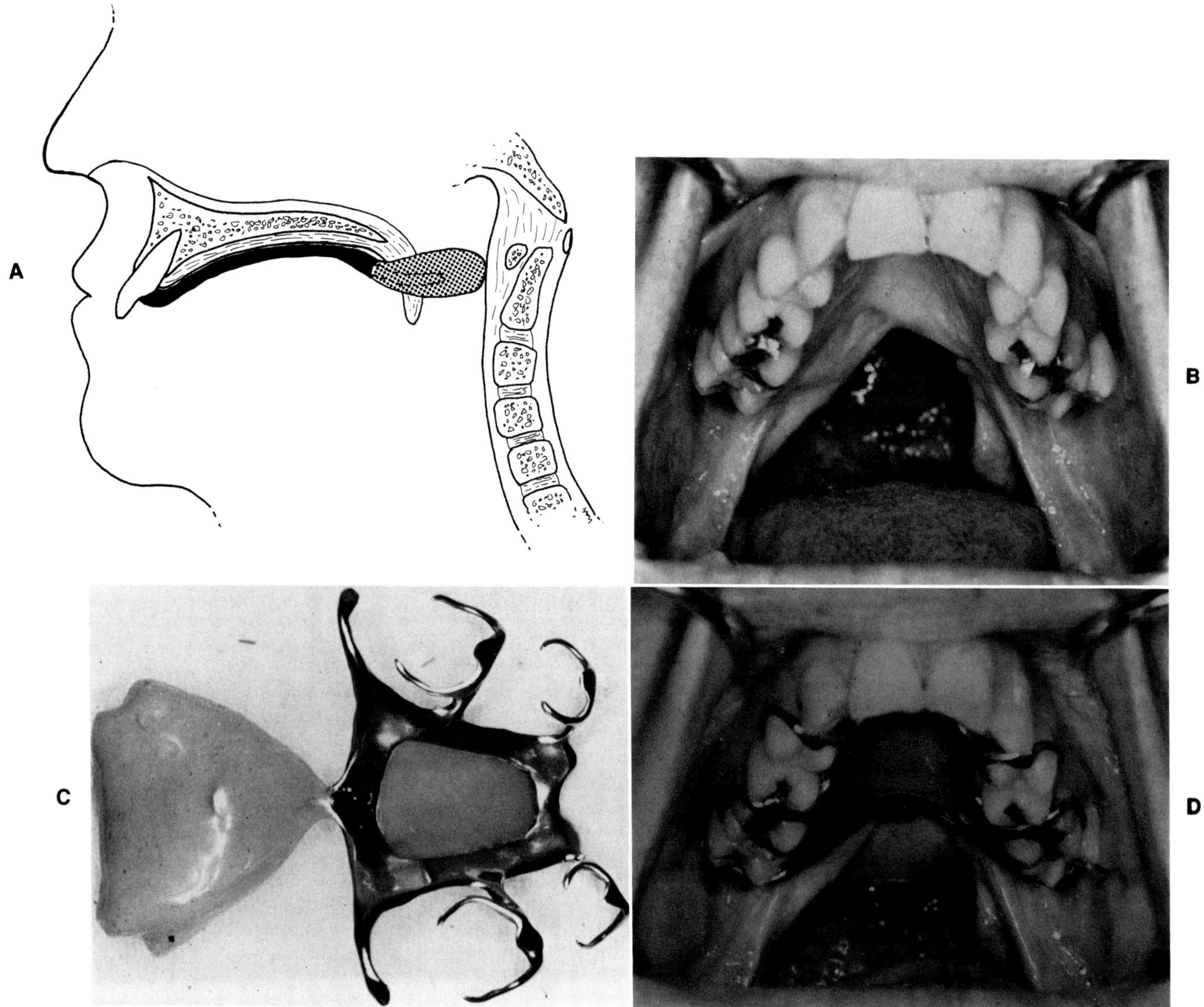

Fig. 23-39. A, Speech obturator prosthesis will generally traverse more linear path to pharyngeal wall and requires larger defect in soft palate. **B,** Intraoral view of large soft palatal defect that was not amenable to further surgical correction. **C,** Speech obturator appliance with velar and pharyngeal extension between tissue remnants of soft palate. **D,** Speech obturator in place showing draping effect of residual musculature around acrylic extensions of velar and pharyngeal portion.

though both the continuity and the discontinuity defects are debilitating, the discontinuity defects offer the most exaggerated compromise.

Discontinuity deviation

The most serious sequela of acquired mandibular discontinuity is deviation, which invariably occurs toward the operated side (Fig. 23-40). The severity and potential for correction of this misdirection will be largely determined by the nature of the initial disease process. Removal of benign tumors may result in little soft tissue deficit, and scarring should be minimal. These patients will be most amenable to physical and prosthetic correction of the midline discrepancy and are the best candidates for surgical reconstruction.

The removal of a mandibular maignancy, in contrast, usually requires adjacent soft tissue for closure, which may partially immobilize the tongue and restrict the dimensions of the oral cavity. The morbidity of this procedure is further increased if radiation therapy has been or will be used. This may require the intentional medial placement of the remaining mandible to avoid tension on the closure site and reduce the chance of subsequent fistula formation.

The dentulous mandibular discontinuity patient is at a tremendous advantage over their edentulous counterpart in the correction of deviation (Desjardins, 1978). Even a few teeth in poor condition may be adequate to allow the implementation of corrective measures that would otherwise be impossible.

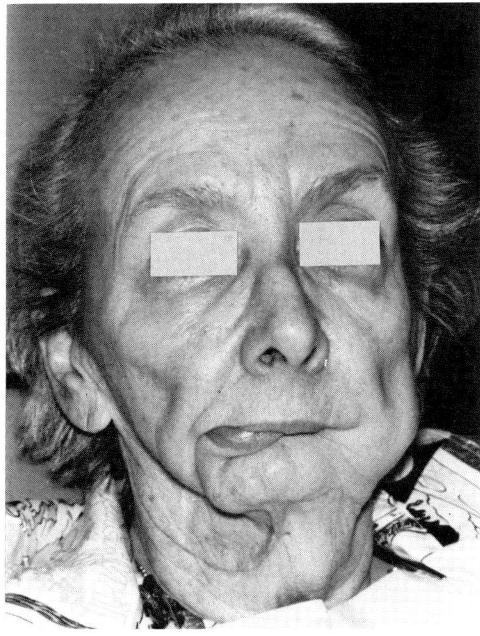

Fig. 23-40. Mandibular deviation produced by removal of large segment of mandibular body for treatment of malignant disease.

Treatment

There is some evidence that immediate postsurgical intermaxillary fixation is of benefit in preventing or minimizing deviation postoperatively (Adisman and Birnbach, 1966; Aramany and Myers, 1977; Desjardins, 1977). Maintaining this fixation for several weeks and reapplying elastic for several hours daily over an additional period preserve the proprioceptive occlusal relationships, and midline attainment is simplified.

There is disagreement as to whether immediate fixation is beneficial in all cases of mandibular resection, particularly with the patient who has undergone radiation therapy. Such fixation may in fact promote fistula formation and tissue breakdown when extensive resections require mandibular imbalance to obtain satisfactory closure.

Perhaps the most effective way to treat deviation is with early conscientious physical manipulation of the proximal fragment toward the unoperated side. This can be done as soon as healing will permit, usually within 2 weeks, and will be most effective in preventing scar contracture and breaking up muscle adhesions. In some cases, this physical therapy may be all that is required to attain an acceptable midline and occlusal relationship.

If the surgery has been extensive and combined with other modes of therapy, a deviation appliance may be necessary to maintain the desired mandibular position. The easiest and most practical such device consists of an acrylic resin ramp on the palatal incline of the nonaffected side (Fig. 23-41). This is a functionally generated platform that slopes occlusally away from the maxillary dentition and engages the remaining mandibular teeth as closure begins. The mandibular fragment is guided to a position of acceptable occlusion through the path of this ramp (Fig. 23-42). In most instances, such a guidance prosthesis is used as a training device and may be reduced in size or discarded if the patient develops a tendency toward a centric position naturally (Robinson and Rubright, 1964). Light wire embrasure or circumferential clasping will usually be adequate, with as many posterior teeth as possible used to counteract displacement. Because the ramp will lie within the confines of the hard palate, there is only a minimal tendency to develop damaging cantilever stresses to the support structures. Rarely is long-term use of a ramp prosthesis indicated, in which case a casting with conventional clasping can be considered.

Patients with consistent deviation and mechanically attainable midline position may require a flange prosthesis to consistently guide closure (Fig. 23-43). This prosthesis will be more permanent than the palatal ramp and will require careful consideration in clasp design. The mandibular flange portion of the prosthesis is

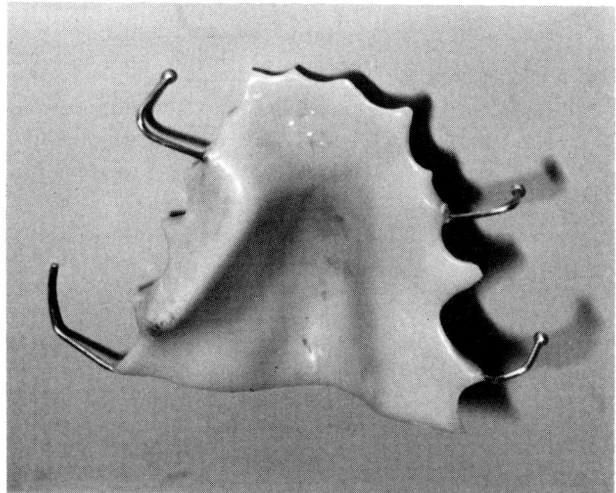

Fig. 23-41. Simple ramp-type deviation appliance that allows patient to reposition mandible by gliding down inclined plane provided.

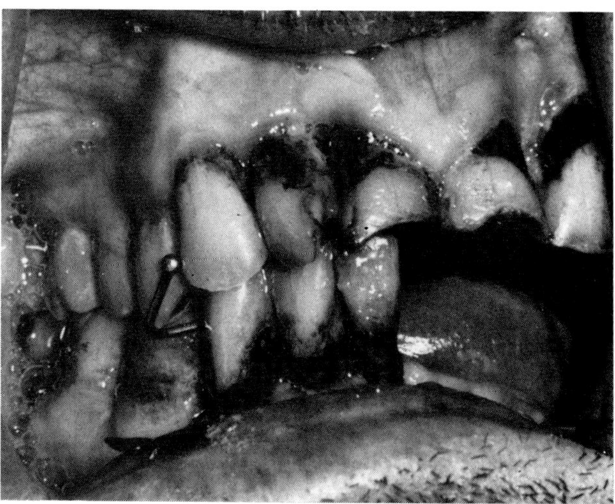

Fig. 23-42. Ramp appliance will allow relatively accurate midline positioning following creation of mandibular discontinuity defect if scarring is not too severe.

a flat cast or acrylic resin extension that will be long enough vertically to engage the buccal surface of the maxillary teeth on maximum functional opening (Fig. 23-44). A bracing bar or clasp surface is usually fabricated on the maxillary prosthesis to overlay the buccal enamel and contact the flange during the range of closure.

It is extremely important to consider the amount of cantilever stress that can be transferred to the mandibular dentition with a guiding flange prosthesis. The long vertical extension can create a lateral torque on the adjacent abutments and will induce a significant dislodging stress to the cross arch retainer when contact is made at maximal opening. There is no real way to avoid these stresses in designing the clasp elements, because prosthesis is useless without adequate retention. The retaining teeth should therefore be sound and not stressed beyond their physiologic limits.

Since the cast flange prosthesis may be used past the training period, emphasis must be placed on daily intermittent use. The prosthesis should never be worn at night, and never for prolonged periods during the day. Consistent follow-up with evaluation of mobility patterns and alveolar bone loss is mandatory. A permanently cemented cast overlay flange prosthesis can inflict significant hard and soft tissue destruction and should never be considered (Fig. 23-45).

The design of the definitive nonguiding prosthesis for the mandibulectomy patient will be based on the relation of the remaining teeth to the opposing occlusal surface. It is generally hazardous to expect the tissue overlying the defect space to support occlusal stresses without bone support. The choice of retention type and location is therefore not compromised by cantilever stresses such as those found in obturator partial denture design (Kratochvil, 1979). Following the principles of conventional partial denture construction, every attempt should be made to obtain cross-arch stabilization and full mucosal coverage over available support tissue.

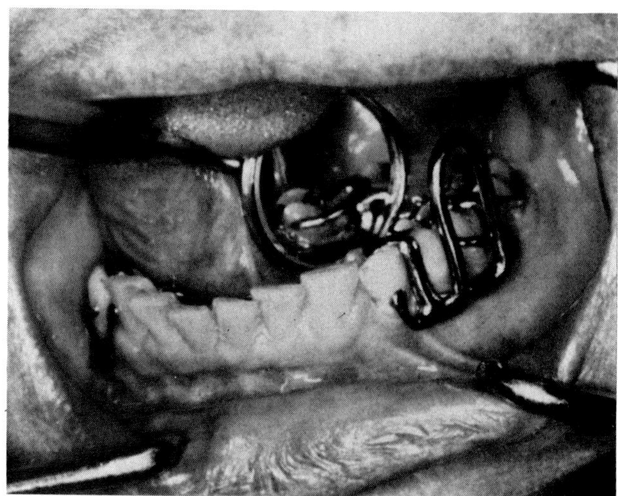

Fig. 23-43. Guiding planes attached to this removable partial denture framework can help correct mandibular deviation.

Some final considerations of mandibular discontinuity defects are necessary to obtain a complete understanding of the rehabilitative process. These patients will never attain the masticatory efficiency of the preoperative state because muscle inadequacy will not permit the same force of closure. It is also virtually impossible to develop consistent intercuspal contacts in a centric

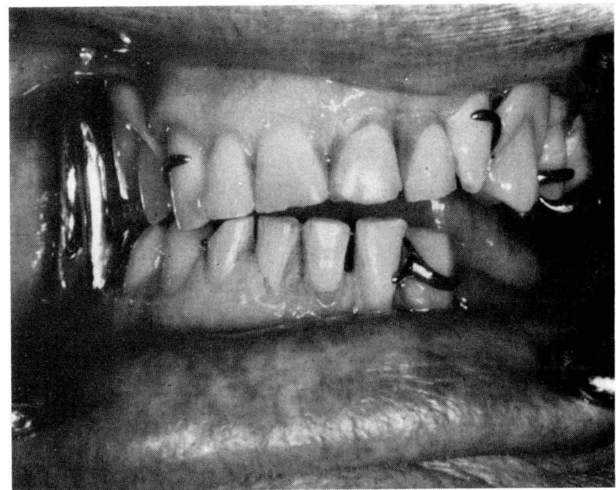

Fig. 23-44. Mandibular wire loop on flange prosthesis meets reciprocating plate attached to upper prosthesis to help obtain normal midline position. Stresses against this type of prosthesis can be severe because of extensive cantilevering, and such a prosthesis should be worn only intermittently.

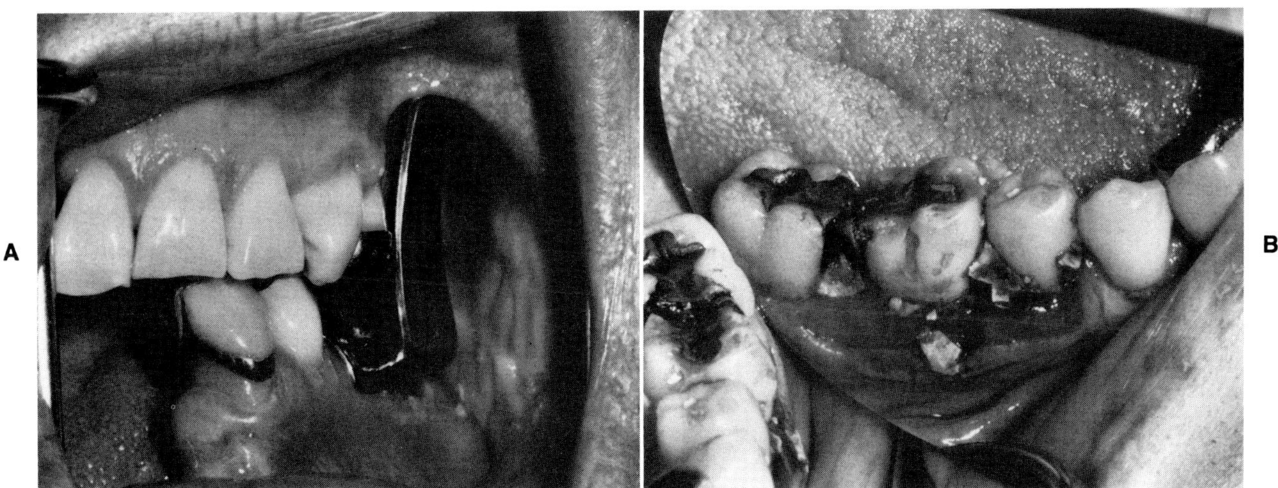

Fig. 23-45. A, Permanently cemented cast guide plane to control deviation of resected mandibular segment. **B,** Extensive periodontal destruction and severe tooth mobility resulting from use of this prosthesis over a 2-month period.

relation position if a complete lateral bone defect exists (Atkinson and Sheperd, 1969; Desjardins, 1977; Chalian and others, 1972). If the force of the muscles of mastication on the unaffected side is balanced by the suprahyoid group on the operated side, a lateral open bite and frontal rotation may occur even with optimal midline closure (Beumer and others, 1979). The tooth contacts made on initial intercuspation are generally not repeatable and will change as closure becomes more powerful, further exaggerating the apertognathia of the operated side dentition. No articulator can duplicate this occlusal pattern, and any definitive occlusal scheme will be a compromise. This is especially evident in patients with intractable deviation who require occlusal surfaces in bizarre positions (Fig. 23-46). This group will never approach a midline occlusion and represent a true test of prosthetic ingenuity and patient adaptability.

Continuity defects

Perhaps the most important consideration in planning the prosthetic reconstruction for patients with continuity defects is evaluation of the soft tissue support rather than remaining dentition. The most common continuity defects will involve a superior resection of alveolar or basal bone, leaving the inferior mandibular border intact. A similar situation may exist when bone grafts have been used to repair a discontinuity defect (Fig. 23-47).

When the soft tissue required for closure is compromised or brought from donor sites, there may never be

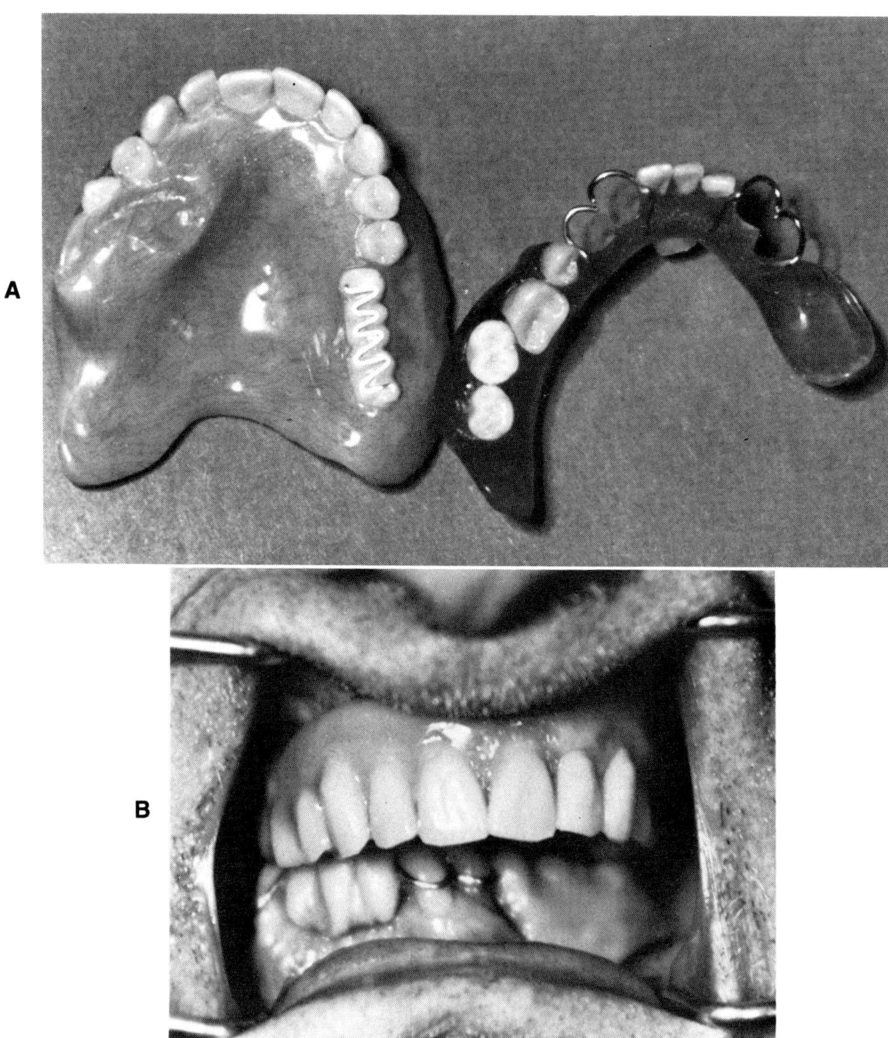

Fig. 23-46. A, Unusual occlusal patterns may result in prosthesis constructed for patient with uncontrollable deviation. **B,** Severe midline discrepancy dictated unusual occlusal positions and platforming, because this is only repeatable mandibular jaw position.

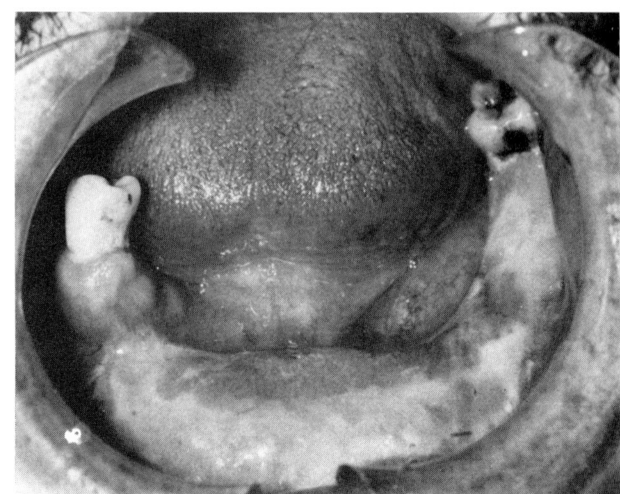

Fig. 23-47. Mandibular crestal bone defect with skin graft following removal of malignancy of anterior alveolar ridge. Inferior border remains intact, maintaining mandibular continuity.

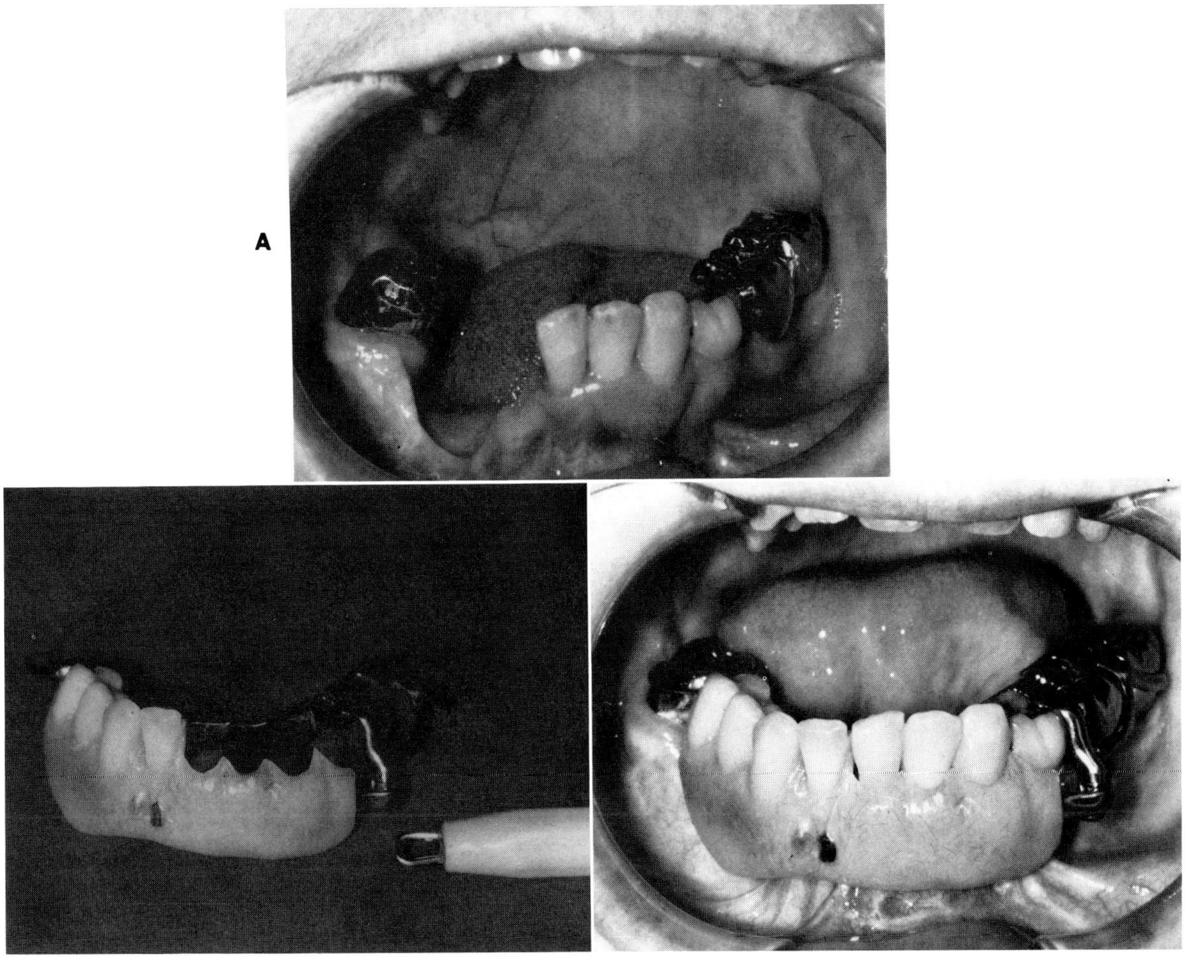

Fig. 23-48. A, Mandibular crestal defect resulting from severe alveolar ridge trauma. **B,** Swing-lock partial denture with esthetic overlay flange. This effectively splints remaining teeth and distributes stresses throughout lower arch. **C,** Completed prosthesis intraorally with acrylic flange extending into defect space.

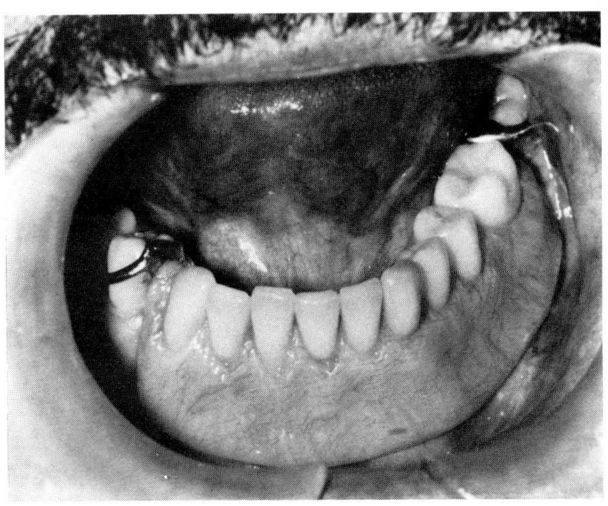

Fig. 23-49. Flexible clasping elements may be necessary when only a few teeth are called on to support prosthesis for large continuity defect.

any potential for prosthetic reconstruction, particularly if a significant part of the prosthesis is to be tissue borne.

With mucosal primary closure, however, the potential for skin grafting to create a suitable tissue-bearing surface exists. This is an important consideration in framework design because the vertical discrepancy in bone height can add to the length and angulation of the lever forces (Kratochvil, 1979; Kelly, 1950). Once an adequate tissue base has been established, consideration of the stress to the remaining dentition can be made. With sound abutments, retention can be designed to resist vertically dislodging movements using conventional clasping and multiple rests (Fig. 23-48). Retentive arms should disengage when occlusal force moves the denture base toward the tissue surface. Care must be taken not to overstress the abutments most distant from the defect because even normal tissue resiliency will produce significant movement if the lever arm past the fulcrum is long enough.

With questionable or terminal supporting teeth, the clasping can be designed to resist only lateral movement. This allows the prosthesis to be essentially tissue borne in a vertical direction. Flexible clasping may prolong the use of these abutments, allowing the construction of a relatively functional prosthesis in a situation that might otherwise be unrestorable (Fig. 23-49).

TRAUMATIC DEFECTS

Prosthetic restoration of traumatically induced oral defects differs from the treatment considerations for the previously discussed patients in several important ways. Although the size will vary, the defect location in the cancer patient is fairly predictable. This may not be true for the trauma patient, who has an endless variety of residual and missing or displaced tissue combinations. These patients are also in generally acceptable condition systemically, and may respond more favorably to surgical reconstruction without the complications surrounding most cancer treatment. In contrast to the patient with congenital defects, whose self-esteem may be low, the trauma patient is generally anxious to perform any task necessary to ensure an esthetically and functionally favorable result.

Unfortunately, the prosthodontist is often called on to restore structures that have been damaged to the point that even optimal surgical reconstruction leaves a less than ideal result. The treatment plan and execution may include compromise considerations unlike those found in any other area of prosthetic dentistry.

There is no real way to classify these situations, because their occurrance is so unpredictable. A review of several selected cases, therefore, will serve to emphasize the complications and hazards of dealing with traumatically damaged teeth and tissue.

Case one

This 24-year-old man suffered extensive midface damage from a self-inflicted gunshot wound (Fig. 23-50). Numerous plastic surgery procedures resulted in an acceptable facial reconstruction. Following intensive psychologic counseling, this patient sought definitive dental therapy.

The residual defect of the maxilla involved the entire premaxilla and left exposed maxillary sinus cavities bilaterally anterior to the second molars (Fig. 23-51). There was no vertical bone support anterior to the remaining teeth and no further surgical reconstructive procedures were planned. The remaining molars were sound but relatively mobile from constant occlusal trauma. Oral hygiene was poor.

Following a complete periodontal evaluation and subsequent period of home care therapy, this patient was evaluated for oral rehabilitation. As the patient's age and the importance of his remaining maxillary dentition were considered, it was felt that flexible wrought wire clasping would be most appropriate for gaining retention posteriorly. Some anterior support, however, was absolutely essential to ensure longevity for the molars. Extending the anterior superior acrylic resin into the horizontal shelf at the base of the nose provided adequate resistance to gravitational forces, and served to support an anterior artificial dentition (Fig. 23-52). Posterior teeth were considered but rejected for use in this prosthesis because of the lack of vertical resistance to the forces of mastication. In essence, the completed light-wire acrylic resin prosthesis was the definitive restoration for this particular case (Fig. 23-53).

Case two

A 21-year-old woman suffered extensive facial and oral damage from a close-range gunshot wound. The facial wounds were closed primarily with grafts, resulting in a commissure deficiency and relative microstomia. The lateral palatal deficiency was bordered by four intact teeth: a canine, one premolar, and two molars (Fig. 23-54). The canine was displaced laterally, but was relatively immobile. The labial and buccal sulcus areas had been grafted for increased depth on the edentulous side. At the request of the patient, no further oral reconstruction was performed, even though a commissurotomy procedure was indicated.

A transitional prosthesis was made 2 weeks after the sulcus procedure to maintain vestibular depth and provide much-needed anterior esthetic dentition. No attempt was made to provide a functional occluding surface at this time.

The cast framework used facial retention and multiple resting (Fig. 23-55). Lingual retention could have been used because the displacing forces were similar to those of an obturator. The anterior occlusion and tooth

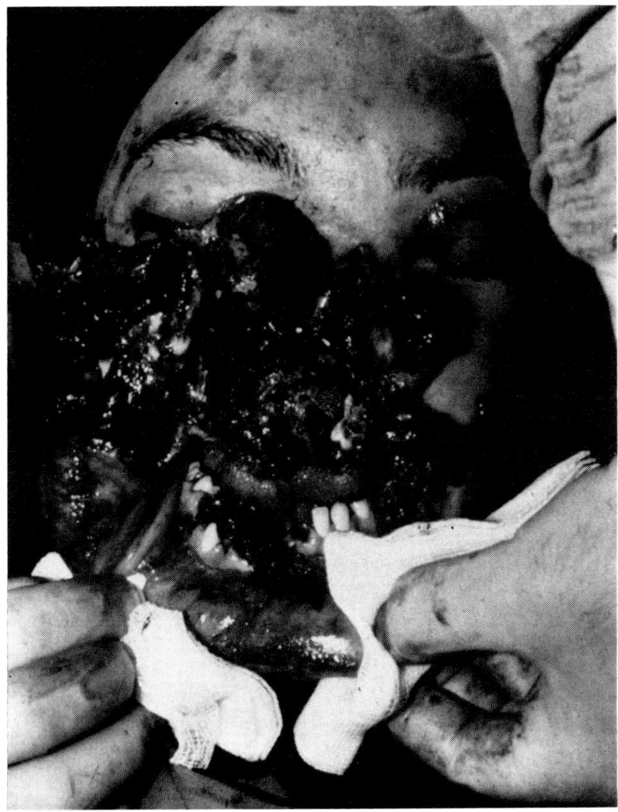

Fig. 23-50. Extensive midface trauma produced by shotgun blast.

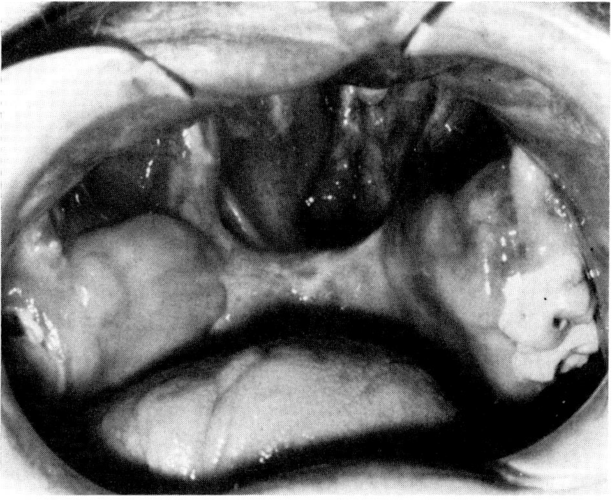

Fig. 23-51. Resulting maxillary defect from gunshot trauma depicted in Fig. 23-50. Only three molars remain to provide any support for intraoral prosthesis.

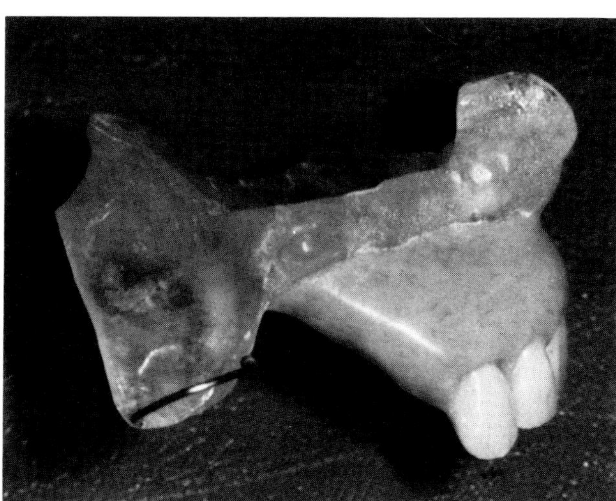

Fig. 23-52. Prosthesis provides esthetic display of anterior teeth only. No attempt was made to provide function past canines. Light wire clasping was used bilaterally to enhance long-term retention of abutment molars.

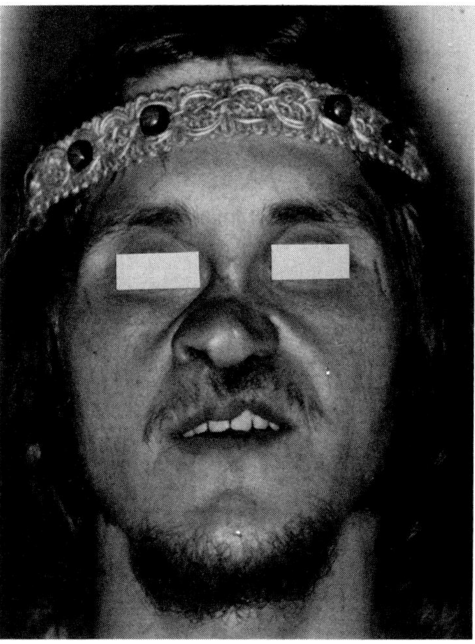

Fig. 23-53. Full face postoperative view of patient several years after initial trauma. Intraoral prosthesis provides some lip support and esthetic display of anterior teeth only.

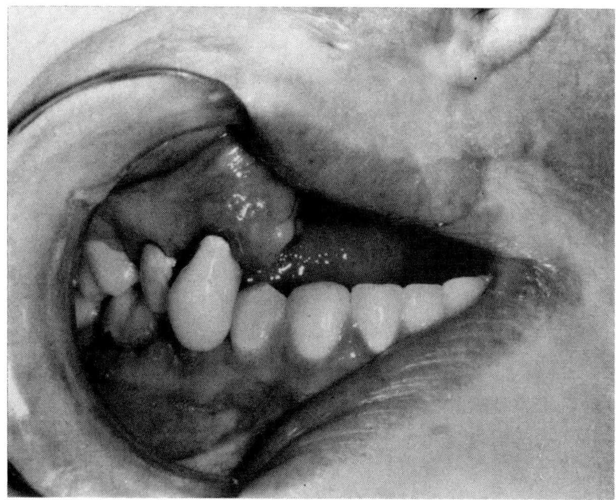

Fig. 23-54. Intact dentition following extensive midface trauma from gunshot wound. Premolar and molar teeth are in reasonable occlusion, but canine position indicates severe displacement.

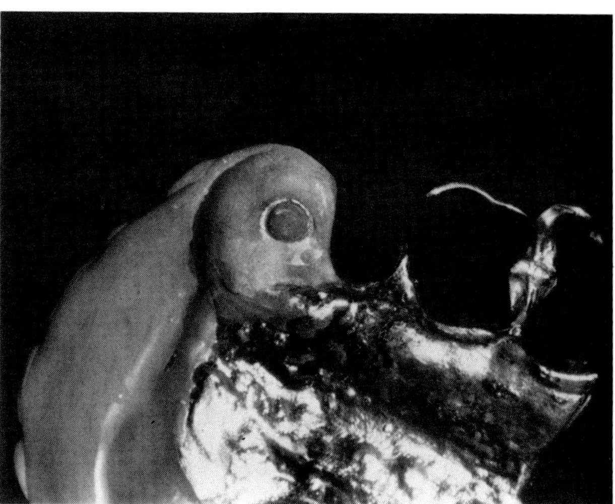

Fig. 23-55. Cast framework showing incorporated precision attachment beneath canine pontic.

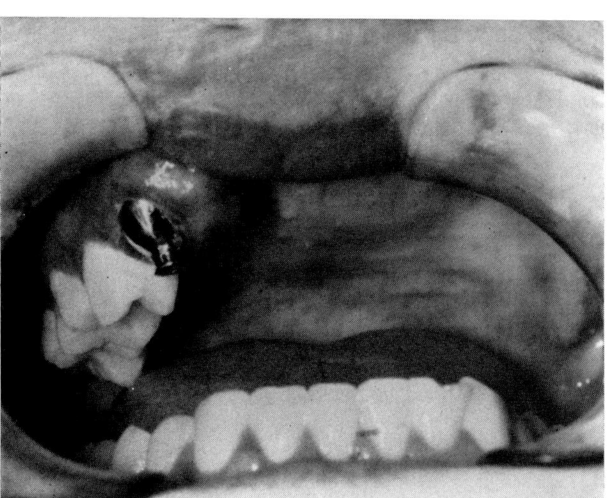

Fig. 23-56. Male portion of attachment was soldered to cast coping permanently cemented to endodontically treated canine.

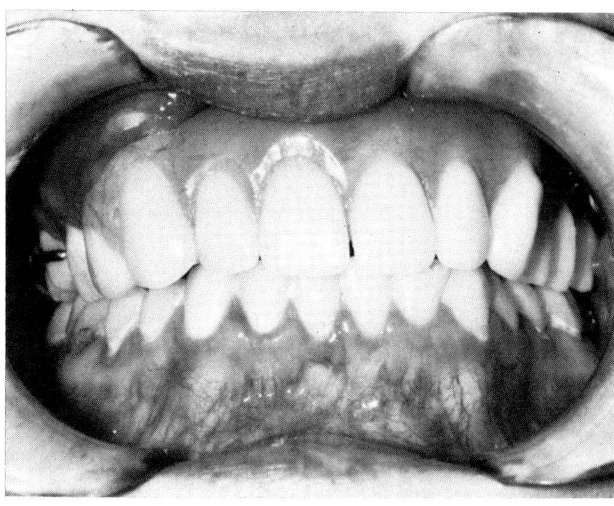

Fig. 23-57. Completed prosthesis is supported unilaterally by partial denture clasping elements and precision attachments beneath canine. This approach to treating anterior abutment was only way to ensure esthetic anterior tooth display without further surgical intervention to reposition displaced canine.

placement were compromised because of the canine position, which necessitated using this tooth as an overdenture abutment following endodontic intervention (Fig. 23-56). The posterior occlusion was functional only to the first molar area. Even with these less than ideal circumstances, the patient considered this a successful restoration (Fig. 23-57).

Case three

This 19-year-old man suffered extensive mid and lower face compression in an automobile accident. Following initial immobility and healing, several surgical procedures were necessary to reposition the maxilla and mandible in a relatively normal arch alignment.

The diagnostic cast mounting revealed an unusually broad maxilla and a relatively normal mandibular configuration. The lower soft tissue support was restricted and eventually increased with a vestibuloplasty procedure. The two lower molars were sound, but the anterior abutments were weak support teeth. The cast framework used both conventional molar clasping and a swing-lock anterior component to spread retentive forces evenly (Fig. 23-58). Several maxillary teeth were partially fractured during the accident and required full

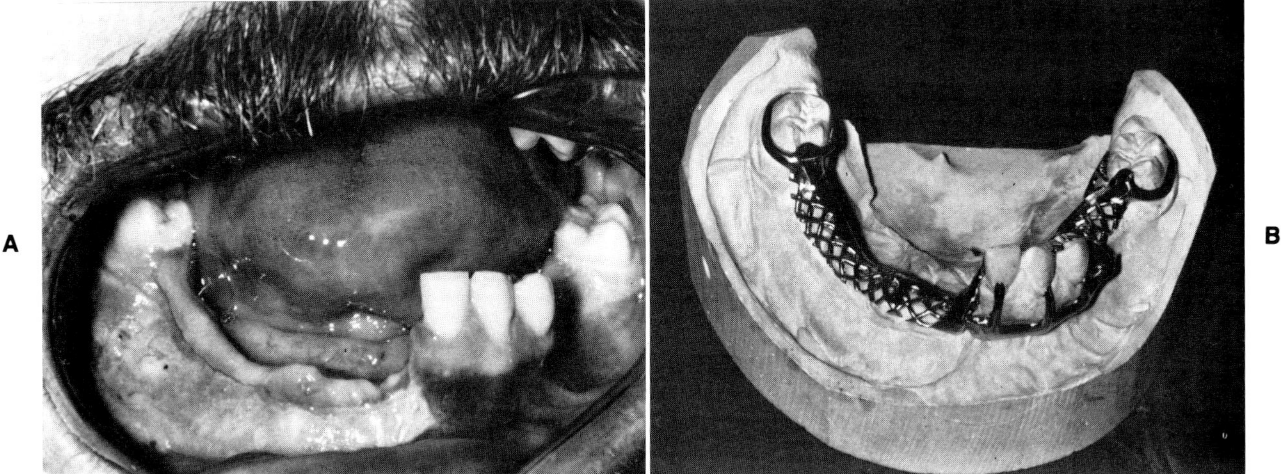

Fig. 23-58. A, Extensive oral trauma following automobile accident left several areas of missing teeth and alveolar bone. **B,** Partial denture framework for mandibular segment incorporates swing-lock anterior component with conventional clasping on remaining molars.

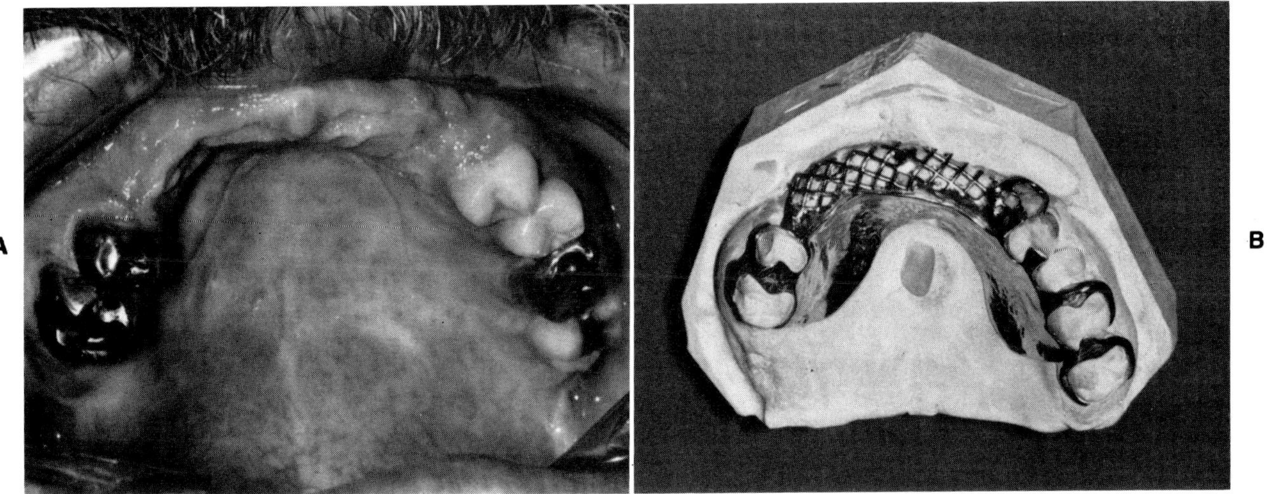

Fig. 23-59. A, Maxillary arch also shows signs of extensive tooth loss and bone destruction. There were numerous fractured and cracked cusps on some of remaining teeth, which required full coverage before construction of partial denture framework. **B,** Maxillary cast framework using conventional circumferential clasping on posterior abutments and I-bar anteriorly for esthetic purposes.

Fig. 23-60. Completed restoration intraorally showing acceptable but not ideal occlusion.

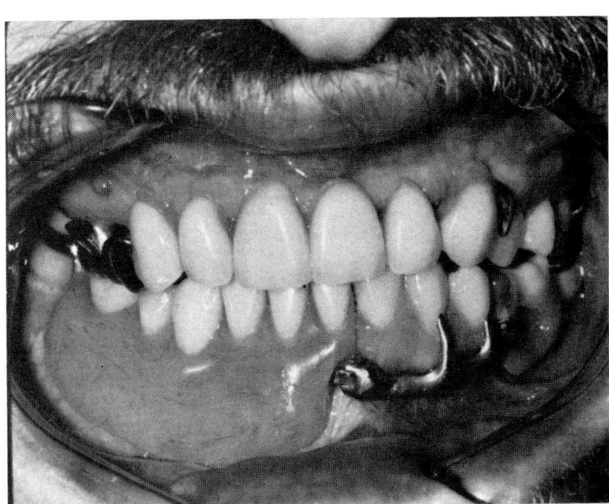

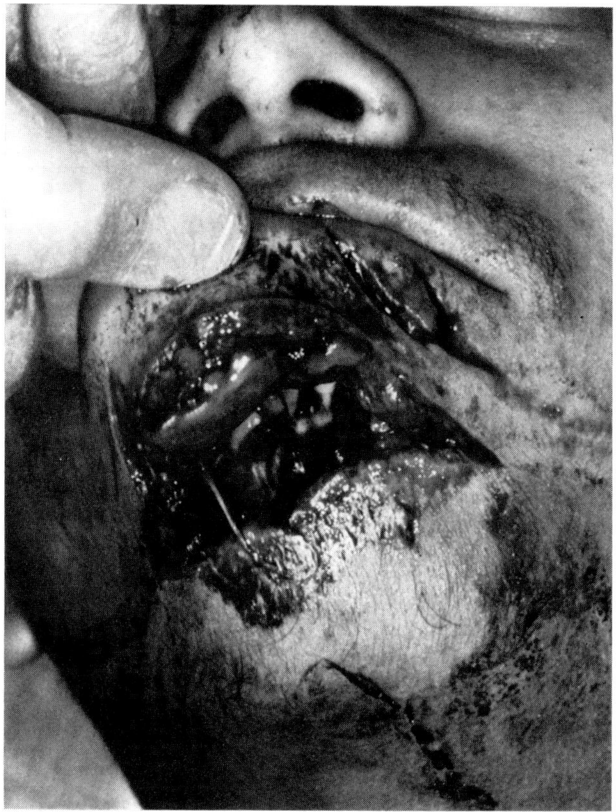

Fig. 23-61. Anterior facial lacerations and mandibular fracture following trauma from automobile accident.

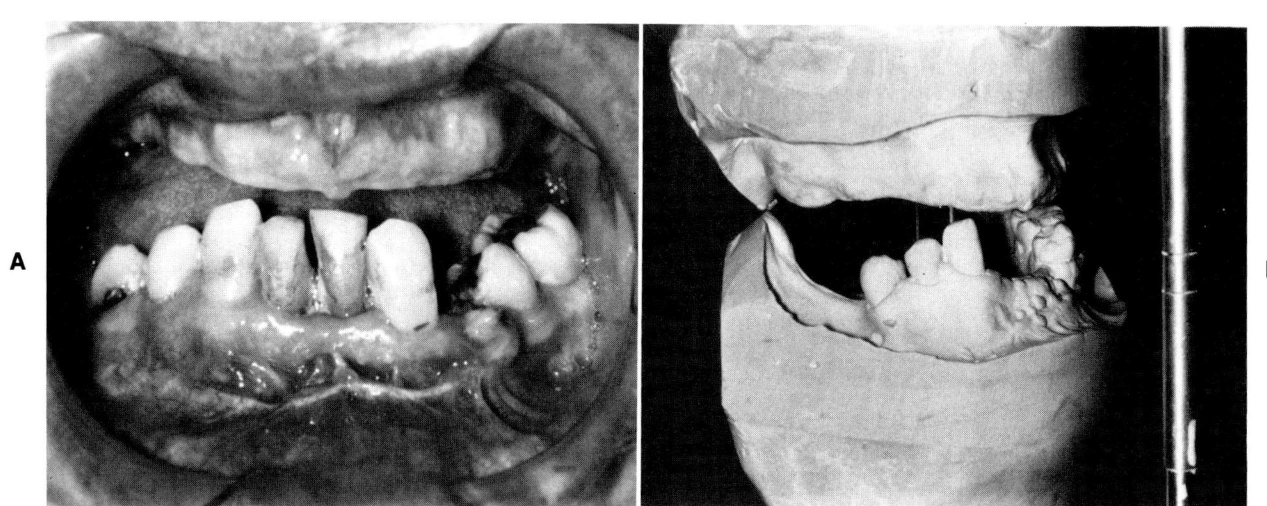

Fig. 23-62. A, Immediate postoperative occlusal interarch relationships showing significant arch discrepancy. **B,** Diagnostic mounting showing jaw relationship after removal of hopelessly damaged anterior teeth. Patient refused further surgery to correct arch relationship.

coverage and splinting. This was done only after careful evaluation for pulpal damage, which included long-term temporization and observation (Fig. 23-59 A, B)

Even though the final occlusal scheme was dictated by the abnormal ridge configurations, the resultant prosthesis served to successfully restore form and function to a severely disrupted oral cavity (Fig. 23-60).

Case four

This 51-year-old woman suffered extensive long bone damage and a severe mandibular fracture as a passenger in a motor vehicle accident (Fig. 23-61). The mandibular fractures were repaired primarily, but the badly comminuted bone fragments made restoration of an ideal occlusion difficult.

It became evident postoperatively that a significant discrepancy existed in the mandibular occlusal plane, which appeared to be amenable to surgical correction (Fig. 23-62). Unfortunately, the patient's psychologic state and overiding systemic disabilities made further surgery unfeasible. The most important considerations then became to retain as many usable teeth as possible while constructing a prosthesis that could function harmoniously with the maxillary dentition.

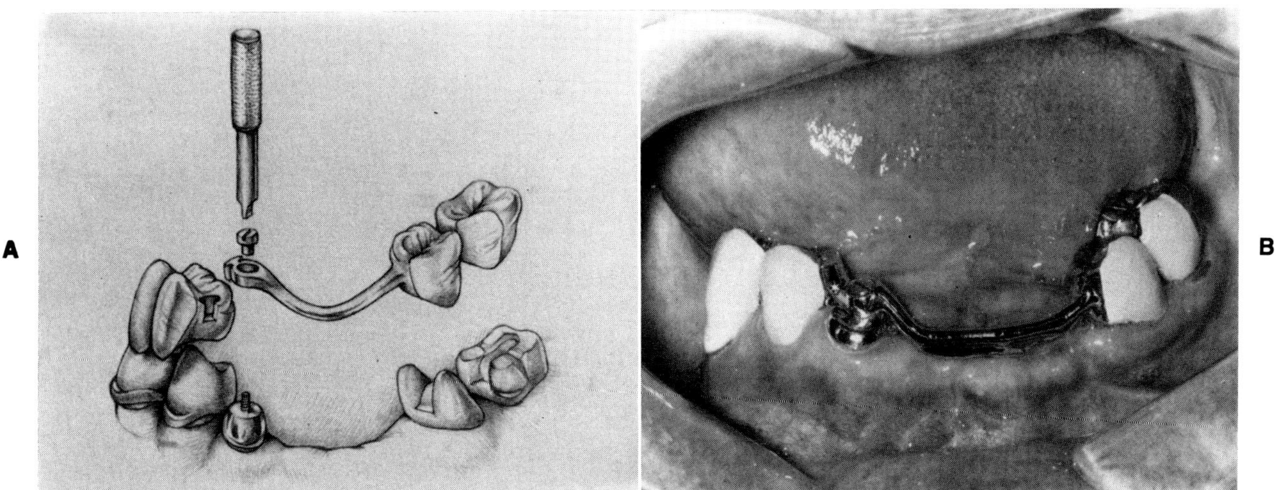

Fig. 23-63. A, Diagrammatic representation of fixed restorations required to overcome discrepancies in arch segment parallelism. **B,** Completed fixed restorations intraorally using a precision screw assembly on endodontically treated canine overdenture abutment and anterior clip-bar. Canine coping assembly is also interchangeable with other types of overdenture retention units as contingency factor in event other abutment teeth are lost.

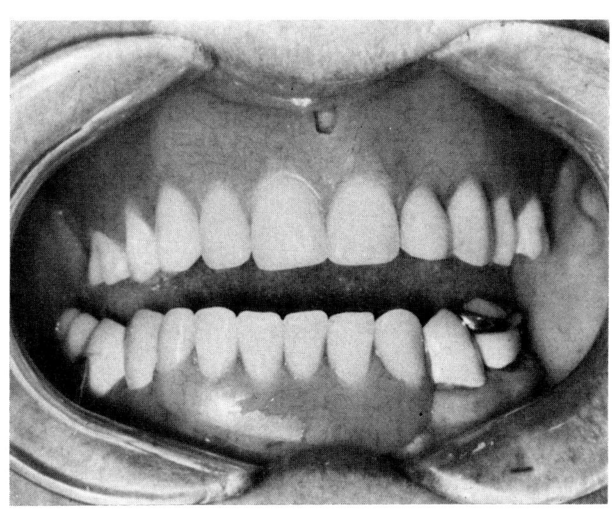

Fig. 23-64. Completed mandibular partial denture using conventional clasping posteriorly and embedded metal clip over bar splint for anterior retention.

The first procedure consisted of reducing the lower right canine to the point where the occlusal plane was no longer compromised. This required endodontic therapy and crown amputation. Cross-arch splinting was considered, but the divergence of the traumatized right and left dental segments eliminated a common path of insertion. A semiprecision key in the mesial surface of the right premolar allowed the fixed bar splint to seat through a dual path of insertion. Incorporating a precision screw assembly* over the canine abutment allowed full use of the substantial canine root support and minimized the potential for movement of the semiprecision key in the rest seat (Fig. 23-63). A clip assembly on the anterior bar provided retention to complement the conventional clasp elements on the posterior abutments (Fig. 23-64).

It is not uncommon for traumatized teeth to become symptomatic long after the initial trauma. This often requires planning for contingent situations in the construction of a removable or fixed partial denture. The screw on the canine coping in this case, for example, will accept several overdenture attachments. Such a consideration may be important if any of the remaining traumatized teeth ultimately fail as partial denture abutments.

SUMMARY

The variety and relationship of contributing diagnostic and treatment factors can make the completion of any removable partial denture for the patient with maxillofacial deformities a challenge. It is critical to have a thorough knowledge of the influence these factors may have on planning treatment and the hazards inherent to prosthetic intervention. Whether the ultimate prosthesis is a highly simplistic temporary treatment for the terminal patient, or a complex definitive restoration for the surgically compromised, this segment of our population can be most beneficially served by the efforts of the maxillofacial prosthodontist.

*Schubiger Screw, APM Sterngold, San Mateo, California.

REFERENCES

Adisman, I.K.: Removable partial dentures for jaw defects of the maxilla and mandible, Dent. Clin. North Am. **6**:849-70, 1962.

Adisman, I.K., and Birnbach, S.: Surgical prosthesis for reconstructive mandibular surgery, J. Prosthet. Dent. **16**:988, 1966.

Applegate, O.C., and Nissle, R.D.: Keeping the partial denture in harmony with biologic limitations, J. Am. Dent. Assoc. **43**:409-19, 1951.

Aramany, M.A.: Basic principles of obturator design for partially edentulous patients. Part I, Classification, J. Prosthet. Dent. **40**:554, 1978.

Aramany, M.A.: Basic principles of obturator design for partially edentulous patients. Part II, J. Prosthet. Dent. **40**:656, 1978.

Aramany, M.A., and Drane, J.B.: Effect of nasal extension sections on the voice quality of acquired cleft palate patients, J. Prosthet. Dent. **27**:144, 1972.

Aramany, M.A., and Myers, E.N.: Dental occlusion and arch relationship in segmental resection of the mandible. In Sisson, G.A., and Tardy, M.E., Plastic and reconstructive surgery of the face and neck, proceedings of the Second International Symposium, New York, 1977, Grune and Stratton.

Aramany, M.A., and Myers, E.N.: Prosthetic reconstruction following resection of the hard and soft palate. J. Prosthet. Dent. **40**:174, 1978.

Aran, A., and Subtelny, J.D.: Velopharyngeal function and cleft palate prosthesis, J. Prosthet. Dent. **9**:149, 1959.

Atkinson, H.F., and Sheperd, R.W.: Masticatory movements of patients after major oral surgery, J. Prosthet. Dent. **21**:175, 1969.

Bedwinek, J.M., and others: Osteoradionecrosis in patients treated with definitive radio therapy for squamous cell carcinomas of the oral cavity and naso and oropharynx, Radiology **119**:665, 1976.

Beumer, J., and Brady, F.: 1978 dental management of the irradiated patient, Int. J. Oral Surg. **7**:208, 1978.

Beumer, J., and Curtis, T.A.: Acquired defects of the mandible: etiology, treatment and rehabilitation. In Beumer, and others: Maxillofacial rehabilitation, St. Louis, 1979, The C.V. Mosby Co.

Beumer, J., and Curtis T.A., Radiation therapy of head and neck tumors: oral effects and dental manifestations. In Beumer, J., and others: Maxillofacial rehabilitation, St. Louis, 1979, The C.V. Mosby Co.

Beumer, J., and others: Hard and soft tissue necrosis following radiation therapy for oral cancer, J. Prosthet. Dent. **27**:640, 1972.

Beumer, J., and others: Radiation complications in edentulous patients, J. Prosthet. Dent. **36**:193, 1976.

Beumer, J., and others: Maxillofacial rehabilitation, prosthodontic and surgical considerations, St. Louis, 1979, The C.V. Mosby Co.

Brown, K.E.: Peripheral considerations to improving obturator retention, J. Prosthet. Dent. **20**:176, 1968.

Brown, K.E.: Clinical considerations improving obturator treatment, J. Prosthet. Dent. **24**:461, 1970.

Chalian, V.A., and others: Maxillofacial prosthetics: multidisciplinary practice, Baltimore, 1972, Williams and Wilkins Co.

Chierici, G., Cleft palate habilitation. In Beumer, J., and others: Maxillofacial rehabilitation, St. Louis, 1979, The C.V. Mosby Co.

Curtis, T.A., and Beumer, J.: Restoration of acquired hard palate defects: etiology, disability, and rehabilitation. In Maxillofacial rehabilitation, Beumer, J., and others: St. Louis, 1979, The C.V. Mosby Co.

Daly, T., and Drane, J.B.: Management of dental problems in irradiated patients, 1972, University of Texas Press.

Del Regato, B.O.A.: Dental lesions observed after roentgen therapy in cancer of the buccal cavity, pharynx, and larynx, Am. J. Roentgenol. Radium Ther., Nucl. Med. **42**:404, 1939.

DeVan, M.M.: The nature of the partial denture foundation: suggestions for its preservation, J. Prosthet. Dent. **2**:210, 1952.

Desjardins, R.P.: Early rehabilitative management of the mandibulectomy patient J. Prosthet. Dent. **38**:311, 1977.

Desjardins, R.P.: Obturator design for acquired maxillary defects, J. Prosthet. Dent. **39**:424-35, 1978.

Desjardins, R.P.: Occlusal considerations for the partial mandibulectomy patient J. Prosthet. Dent. **41**:308, 1979.

Desjardins, R.P., and Laney, W.R.: Prosthetic rehabilitation after cancer resection in the head and neck, Surg. Clin. North Am. **57**:809, 1977.

Dreizen, S., and others: Prevention of xerostomia related dental caries in irradiated cancer patients, J. Prosthet. Dent. **56**:99, 1977.

Feibiger, G.E., and others: Movement of abutments by removable partial denture frameworks with a hemimaxillectomy obturator J. Prosthet. Dent. **34**:555-61, 1975.

Firtell, D.M., and Grisius, R.J.: Retention of obturator-removable partial dentures: a comparison of buccal and lingual retention, J. Prosthet. Dent. **43**:212-17, 1980.

Frank, R.M., and others: Acquired dental defects and salivary gland lesions after irradiation for carcinoma, J. Am Dent. Assoc. **70**:868, 1965.

Frechette, A.R.: The influence of partial denture design on distributing of force to abutment teeth, J. Prosthet. Dent. **6**:195, 1956.

Gibbons, P., and Bloomer, H.: A supporting type prosthetic speech aid, J. Prosthet. Dent. **8**:362, 1958.

Grant, B.P., and Fletcher, G.H.: Analysis of complications following megevoltage therapy for squamous carcinoma of the tonsillar area, Am. J. Roentgenol., Radium Ther., Nucl. Med. **96**:28, 1966.

Javid, N.S., and Dadmanesh, J.: Obturator design for hemimaxillectomy patients, J. Prosthet. Dent. **36**:77-81, 1976.

Kelly, E.K.: Full and partial dentures after extensive bone grafts to the mandible, Dent. Digest **56**:159-64, 1950.

Kelly, E.K.: Partial denture design applicable to the maxillofacial patient, J. Prosthet. Dent. **15**:168-73, 1965.

King, G.E., and Gay W.D.: Application of various removable partial denture design concepts to a maxillary obturator prosthesis, J. Prosthet. Dent. **41**:316, 1979.

Kipfmueller, L.T., and Lang, B.R.: Pre-surgical maxillary prosthesis, an analysis of speech intelligibility, J. Prosthet. Dent. **28**:620-6, 1972.

Krajicek, D.D.: Oral radiation in prosthodontics, J. Am. Dent. Assoc. **78**:320, 1969.

Kratochvil, F.T.: Defects with mandibular continuity. In Beumer, J., and others: Maxillofacial rehabititation, St. Louis, 1979, The C.V. Mosby Co.

Kratochvil, F.T.: Lateral discontinuity defects, partial denture design. In Beumer, J., and others: Maxillofacial rehabilitation, St. Louis, 1979, The C.V. Mosby Co.

Lang, B.R., and Bruce, R.A.: Presurgical maxillary prosthesis, J. Prosthet. Dent. **17**:613, 1967.

Majid, A., and others: Speech intelligibility following prosthetic obturation of surgically acquired maxillary defects, J. Prosthet. Dent. **32**:87, 1974.

Marshall, R.C., and Jones, R.N.: Effects of a palatal left prosthesis upon the speech intelligibility of a dysarthyritic patient, J. Prosthet. Dent. **25**:327, 1971.

Mazaheri, M.: Prosthodontics in cleft palate treatment and research, J. Prosthet. Dent. **14**:1146, 1964.

Nakamoto, R.: Use of immediate obturators in maxillary resections, M.D. Anderson Hospital and Tumor Institute, Houston, Texas, Res. Rep. No. 20, 1971.

Rahn, A.O., and Boucher, C.J.: Maxillofacial prosthetics, principles and concepts, Philadelphia, 1970, W.B. Saunders Co.

Rahn, A.O., and others: Prosthodontic principles in surgical planning for maxillary and mandibular resection patients, J. Prosthet. Dent. **42**:429, 1979.

Robinson, J.E., and Rubright, W.C.: The use of a guide plane for maintaining the residual fragment in partial or hemimandibulectomy, J. Prosthet. Dent. **14**:922, 1964.

Sharry J.J.: Miscellaneous partial prosthodontics in complete denture prosthodontics, New York, 1962, McGraw-Hill Co.

Simmons, J.D.: Swing lock stabilization and retention, Tex. Dent. J. **81**:10, 1963.

Sprigg, R.H.: Prosthodontic treatment of unilateral defects, Presented at the 25th Annual Meeting of the American Academy of Maxillofacial Prosthetics, Orlando, Florida, 1977.

Stark, B.S.: Transitional prosthesis for dentulous hemimaxillectomy patients, J. Prosthet. Dent. **27**:73, 1972.

Subtelny, J.D., and Koepp-Baker, H.: Palatal function and cleft palate speech, J. Speech Hear. Disord. **26**:213, 1961.

Veau, V., and Ruppe, C.: Anatomie chirugicale de la division palatine, J. Chir. **20**:1, 1922.

Zarb, G.A.: The maxillary resection and its prosthetic replacement, J. Prosthet. Dent. **18**:268, 1967.

24 Removable partial dentures for the older adult

James S. Brudvik

The loss of teeth has always been associated with aging. In literature and art, references to this association abound. One might even suggest that we, as midtwentieth century Americans, accept as fact that, should we live long enough, we will become edentulous. In 1974 the National Center for Health Statistics reported that 40% of Americans over the age of 75 retain some or all of their natural teeth. The number of patients in this age group with *all* their teeth remaining and therefore *not* in need of prosthodontic therapy could be considered small based on dentistry's clinical perceptions.

As we look to the future, we can expect to find the partially edentulous group of older American growing as the years of therapy, based on caries prevention and oral hygiene care for periodontal tissues, manifest themselves. We can, therefore, expect an ever increasing percentage of our aging population to require removable partial dentures rather than complete dentures to restore their mouths esthetically and functionally.

GERONTOLOGY

The study of aging, and its effects, is called gerontology. It should be separated in our minds from geriatrics, which is an area of medicine dealing with disease in old age. Unfortunately, separating disease from aging is not a simple matter because chronic disease, in some form, is a part of all our lives and can be expected to increase as we age.

CHANGES THAT OCCUR WITH AGING

Social changes

The 1980 census indicated that 11% of Americans, or 23 million, are over 65 years of age. This percentage is predicted by many sources to increase to near 20% of our citizens by the turn of the century. There are more women than men in our elderly population (at age 85, there are 100 women for 48.5 men [U.S. Census, 1975]). Although our stereotype of the older dental patient may be that dear old lady in the local nursing home, it must be stressed that only a small proportion of the elderly are actually in an institution (5%). The fact is that the vast majority of older adults live with us in our community and can be expected to do so.

As people retire and move into their later years, they naturally have a loss of income that pension plans and social security benefits do not make up. They then face the distinct possibility that they may not be able to afford the cost of reconstructive dentistry and, therefore, allow their prosthodontic needs to go unfilled. At the present time, less than one third of older adults have any income besides Social Security. Anderson and others (1976) state that, among people over 65 who have incomes of less than $3000, only 16.5% visited a dentist in the preceeding 12 months. Since prosthodontic treatment is not covered under Medicare, and often limited under state-supported Medicaid, the potential for fee-for-service dentistry is not encouraging. It is quite possible, however, that as the percentage of the elderly in our voting population increases, we may see increased political pressure to adjust the social system to allow for funding of dental care.

Physiologic changes

The changes in this area that occur, as a result of age alone, are well documented. The elderly can be expected to suffer a loss in perception and in sensory response. Hearing, touch, smell, taste, and sight diminish with age. In fact, some of these sensory losses can occur early in life.

Fortunately, these changes are gradual, and compensatory mechanisms are strengthened as we age. Young dentists must be knowledgeable about these changes because they have not, as yet, begun to experience them themselves and may not, therefore, be fully aware just how they affect their dental treatment of the elderly.

A classic example might focus on the apparent inability of an elderly patient to adequately remove the plaque from abutment teeth *and* his removable partial denture. Before we lose all patience with him, we must remember that the loss of visual acuity, coupled with the equally discouraging reduction in psychomotor skill, may make the task of routine daily hygiene nearly impossible. Our ingenuity in developing alternative methods of care may make the difference between success and failure for our partial denture therapy.

The patient's ability to hear our instructions also

plays an important role in treatment. Presbycusis (progressive bilateral loss of the ability to hear tones in higher frequencies) is the most common deficiency in hearing in the elderly. Although hearing aids may make up some of this loss, by increasing the volume of the signal, this amplification also increases the backgrond noise and may only add to the frustration of trying to discriminate the sounds of our dental office and our requests.

Decreases in the acuity of taste and smell are not as clearly supported by clinical research as those in sight and hearing. In fact, definite controversy exists in these areas at the present time. It does appear that changes can be expected after 55 years of age, and if a change in taste is concomitant with the construction and delivery of removable partial dentures, it is easy to imagine the patient sayng, "I can't taste as well, now that I have these new partials."

There is good evidence to indicate that a number of medications, especially in the high doses that one may find in the chronically ill and aged patient, will alter taste sensations.

Psychomotor function is apt to be more related to health than sensory function is. Many of the chronic diseases of old age, especially arthritis, drastically alter the patient's ability to move and to control movement.

When we couple this impairment with the slower reaction times generally found in the older person, we can, again, see a need to alter our treatment approach to prosthodontic therapy.

Perception, memory and judgment, and the factors of cognition are also most apt to be related to health rather than to aging. Research on the brain and its effect on the aging process is literally just beginning. It is our perception, a reinforced stereotype, that old people become forgetful. We expect that they will forget our instructions, which may have, in fact, been presented in the worst possible way—that is, given quickly and briefly, with no feedback as to comprehension. We may have been interrupted several times in our discussion, and a series of background noises and events may have compounded the barriers to understanding.

When instructional material is presented in a structured manner in proper surroundings, there is no evidence to suggest that the retention of the elderly patient is any worse than that of the younger.

Normal and pathologic changes in the physiology of the elderly have no clear-cut separation. Even in the absence of disease, physiological functions begin to decline at 25 to 30 years of age and continue to do so until the biologic end. Aging appears to be best described as a reduction in the reserve capacity of the body. The aging process is seen first in those tissues that show the least growth in terms of cell division. The lens of the eye, cartilage, and the walls of arteries all show this reduction in cell multiplication.

Franks and Hedegard (1973) describe the changes in physical appearance, particularly the face, that have definite implications for the partial denture patient. A reduction in the amount of subcutaneous fat combined with the loss of elasticity of the skin results in the wrinkles of old age.

Habitual facial expression (repeated creasing of the skin in the same places) will eventually produce permanent lines that no amount of denture contour can erase. The elderly patients that expect their new dentures to eliminate the lines of age will certainly be disappointed and, unless informed of the biologic changes of ages, may condemn both denture and clinician.

Changes in the musculoskeletal system that concern us are primarily those of bone density that end in osteoporosis. It must be noted that the patterns of distribution of osteoporosis in the mandible do not depend on having teeth present. This condition is more apt to be seen in the elderly women patient and, although it does not contraindicate normal removable partial denture treatment, it does mandate more numerous follow-up appointments to ensure that potential loss of tissue-base contact does not go untreated.

Muscle weakness is also a consideration in the older adult. Muscle strength declines steadily from about the end of the second decade of life, and the muscles of mastication are no exception to this rule. Some of this loss is related to the actual reduction in the total number of muscle cells and the degeneration of motor end plates. Metabolic changes during muscle recovery from functional activities also lead to reduced strength. The older partial denture patient who complains of reduced capacity for extended mastication may require an explanation of these factors as an alternative to blaming the partial denture.

Joints, including the temporomandibular joint, undergo definite changes with age. Some are atrophic resulting from lack of function, decreased vascularity and, in the case of the jaw, a loss of elasticity of the articular disk. The great majority of problems are associated with the pathologic changes of arthritis.

Aging changes occur in all body systems, and current research activity in geriatrics has been greatly increased and stimulated by the National Institute on Aging since its inception in 1977.

Many of the stereotypes in the physiology of aging have been challenged, and new data are rapidly becoming available. Texts by Toga, Nandy, and Chauncey (1979), Franks and Hedegard (1973), among others, offer the student a comprehensive background in systemic, as well as oral, changes that develop with age.

Oral changes

Alveolar bone

As previously stated, bone becomes osteoporotic with age, a decrease in bone formation playing a larger role than any increase in osteoclastic activity. The bony changes are more apt to be endosteal than periosteal with the result that the body of the bone becomes more porous. It is widely held that osteoporotic bone is less resistant to trauma and disease because these two stimulate osteoclastic activity, exaggerating the already porous bone. One can assume, then, that osteoporosis will contribute to the development of periodontal disease (chronic) and perhaps alveolar ridge resorption as well. Animal studies indicate that anabolic steroids will alter the response of bone in osteoporosis. Since a good deal of research effort is now going into osteoporosis, both general and dental, one can hope to eventually have regimens of drug therapy to control this disease process.

Oral mucosa

The increases and decreases of keratinization with age are of particular importance in partial denture therapy, and a knowledge of these situations is essential to the clinician. Where keratinized tissue is normally present in the mouth, it tends to become more highly keratinized with a greater chance of edema and a flattening of the rete pegs. Where no keratinization is normal, the stratified squamous epithelium becomes thin and atrophic. With this in mind, careful attention to the quality of tissue adjacent to abutment teeth is essential to long-term success. Partial denture designs may have to be modified from the ideal to deal with the loss of attached keratinized gingiva in those patients who are not, for medical reasons, candidates for gingival grafting.

Salivary glands

Xerostomia, or dry mouth, is a *significant* factor in the response of both the hard and soft tissue of the mouth. It is commonly held that a decrease in salivary output (flow rate) is a inevitable result of age. Current research efforts indicate that in *nonmedicated* individuals there is *no* decrease in parotid fluid output related to age. It does appear, however, that there are changes in the chemical makeup and, therefore, the viscosity that do occur with age.

Certain pathologic conditions, coupled with the side effects of a number of medications commonly taken in old age, do create definite problems for the partial denture patient. Studies by Baum (1980) show a reduction of 25% in stimulated parotid saliva in the mouths of medicated, postmenopausal women. Reduced salivary output is an apparent serious factor in both dental decay and periodontal disease. In its most serious form (for example, after radiation therapy) patients often undergo complete destruction of exposed tooth surfaces unless aggressively managed with oral hygiene maintenance and fluoride application.

There are a variety of saliva substitutes available commercially. Perhaps the best known is the V.A. Oralube developed by Shannon in the Veterans' Administration. This solution, taken as prescribed, has been shown to give substantial relief to the mucositis and pain in the soft tissues as well as inducing rehardening of softened enamel surfaces.

An evaluation of the older denture patient's salivary output is an *essential* part of the diagnosis and prognosis for removable partial denture therapy.

Teeth

Color, position and inclination, contour, and the character of dentin and cementum change with age. These factors do contribute to our diagnosis and affect our treatment in the construction of removable partial dentures.

A slow, insidious mesial drift with wear at the contact areas of teeth appears to be a demonstrated, age-related manifestation. The crowded, crooked mandibular incisors commonly found in the older patient do often compromise our treatment, causing problems in the quality of fit of our major connectors. Esthetic replacement of missing anterior teeth requires an awareness of this condition and a commitment to building this age-related factor into our prostheses.

The change in hue of the teeth is also a major factor in the elderly denture patient. The patient's wish to regain a youthful appearance through the use of the lightest of available denture teeth runs counter to our knowledge that teeth do darken as they age, whether from years of staining or the progressive calcification of the underlying dentin. Simply the attrition of the incisal edges of anterior teeth with the corresponding loss of translucent enamel creates an illusion of a shade change.

Although attrition eventually exposes dentin and may initially result in tooth sensitivity, the calcification that begins at the exposed surface and progresses inwardly will eventually occlude the dentinal tubules. Although we may initially be concerned with preparing rest seats and guiding plane surfaces into dentin, experience indicates that in the older patient we do not expect to see decay occur in these areas, providing that the tooth structure has been adequately repolished and strict oral hygiene measures are enforced through annual recall.

In addition to the progressive calcification, the deposits of secondary dentin that occur with age also aid in our ability to create adequate rest preparations in abraded teeth with little fear of pulp exposure.

Age also results in the dentin of the root becoming

more transparent, although this does not create clinical problems. Cementum deposition, occurring in association with a healthy periodontium, appears to be continuous through life, but the phenomenon does not hold clinical significance for the partial denture patient.

Pulp

As age increases, the vascularity of the pulp decreases, as well as its nutrition and innervation. These factors may effect the patient's pain threshold. We are well aware of the deposition of secondary dentin, both the normal even deposition of dentin that is laid down in both crown and root and the localized dentin deposits that are irregular and reparative.

The incidence of mineralization of the pulp tissue usually increases with age, creating pulp stones, which may complicate necessary endodontic procedures.

Periodontium

Studies evaluating the periodontal ligament in cadaver material show a general decrease in the degree of cellularity in the area. The attachment is made up of fewer but thicker collagen bundles than in youth.

One would expect to find atherosclerotic changes in the small arteries and arterioles of the ligament because these vascular changes are common systemically in the elderly.

It is quite possible that these changes can lead to a level of relative ischemia in the periodontal ligament that in turn increases the susceptibility to periodontal disease because of decreased cellular nutrition and the reduction in the availability of natural defense mechanisms.

Currently there is much debate over gingival recession. Some authors believe it is inevitable; whereas others claim that in the absence of disease the normal attachment will remain at, or near, the cementoenamel junction throughout life.

The individual's response to plaque buildup appears to alter with age, becoming aggravated in the elderly who abstain from oral hygiene procedures.

The slower, delayed response of the periodontium to healthy stimulation coupled with the technical problems of oral hygiene, aggravated by failing eyesight and poor dexterity, places older partial denture patients in an almost impossible situation. They simply cannot be expected to maintain their mouths and prostheses plaque free and, therefore, they continue to contribute to their disease.

Systemic disease in older adults

Chronic disease and its management with drug therapy influence the treatment of the partially edentulous elderly patient. Although even a superficial evaluation of the myriad of chronic diseases affecting the geriatric patient is beyond the scope of this chapter, certain areas that show a special relation to partial denture therapy are reviewed.

Arteriosclerosis

Arteriosclerosis is a condition almost inevitably increasing with age and a common cause of cardiac arrhythmia. An affected heart is predisposed to develop arrythmias when irritated by epinephrine. Ischemic heart disease is identified with severe chest pains that often radiate to the arms. Occasionally in the elderly, this pain may be associated with the mandible and mandibular teeth. Transient cerebral ischemia is also often found in old age and can manifest as loss of vision in one eye, hemianesthesia, and hemiparesis. Since this problem can be brought on by drugs with hypotensive side effects, a careful history, coupled with consultation with physician and pharmacist, must be a element of treatment planning.

Hypertension

Since any dramatic rise or fall of blood pressure can lead to cerebrovascular accidents, those aspects of our partial denture therapy that might produce stress or pain must be analyzed. The evaluation of the elderly patient's blood pressure should certainly be mandatory at the initial stages of treatment because many older adults who are hypertensive are truly unaware of their condition.

In the chronic hypotensive patient, any sudden hypertension, which could be triggered by drug reaction, pain, or blood loss, can also be deadly, causing either myocardial or cerebral infarcts.

Postural hypotension

The elderly patient should never be subjected to a rapid change in posture as may occur by uprighting a dental chair too quickly. It is conceivable that an elderly hypotensive patient could collapse and fall if brought out of the dental chair quickly and without assistance. Unfortunately, many sedatives, antidepressants, and anti-hypertensive drugs commonly used by elderly patients have the ability to cause venous dilation and result in postural hypotension.

Emphysema

Reduced vital capacity, combined with any impediment to normal breathing, can result in a seriously compromised dental patient. Since asthma, bronchitis, and pneumonia can all be chronic in the elderly patient, and can be aggravated by drug therapy, especially narcotics, special precautions must be taken for these patients. Long sessions under a rubber dam and abnormal head position during mouth preparations and impressions must be carefully monitored and oxygen supplementation available. The anxiety brought on by an inability to breathe easily is a matter of real concern in the elderly.

Diabetes mellitus

As more diabetic patients survive to old age, thanks to modern treatment modalities, it is increasingly important to be aware of the severely compromised retardation of healing associated with this disease. Although the vast majority of diabetic patients will be controlled with insulin therapy, we can expect to see any trauma associated with our treatment to be magnified by complications in the repair process.

Pharmacology of older adults

The elderly patient population has far more need for medication than do younger patients. The older group uses *more than two times* the amount of drugs than the middle-aged population. We can expect that as the number of medications taken increases a similar increase in adverse drug reactions will occur. The dentist treating the older adult must also be aware of drug interaction as well. Current research indicates a far stronger relationship between medications and nutrition than previously imagined.

The complexities of drug usage in the elderly far exceed the dental clinician's opportunity to stay abreast of the situation; as a result, it is imperative that communication be established with the patient's physician. In addition, developing a pharmacist as a resource person for the interaction between the patient's current medications and those that we may wish to use in the course of our partial denture treatment will give the dentist additional confidence.

Since multiple diseases are to be expected in the elderly, it is not surprising to find that institutionalized elderly patients may be taking 10 to 12 different medications at the same time. Indeed, a large part of the nursing duties in nursing homes consists of drug monitoring.

There is more to drug therapy than simply prescribing medications and seeing that the patient takes them as directed. The four basic physiologic activities relative to drug use must be considered as they relate to the elderly.

Absorption

The ability of the elderly body to absorb a drug cannot be taken for granted. Since absorption is not consistent, correct dosage may be difficult to determine. Of particular importance are those drugs that are weakly acidic. Aspirin and barbiturates are less well absorbed because of decreased production of hydrochloric acid in the stomach.

Distribution

Since drugs are often stored in various body tissues after absorption, age-related changes in the storage tissues must be considered. Both fat and protein levels change with age. The fat proportion increases as body fluid and lean body mass decrease. Those drugs, such as phenobarbital and diazepam, that are fat soluble will be more apt to remain stored in fat and, as a result, the intensity of the action of the medication will decrease. The duration of the drugs action will be increased. Stored drugs are normally released into the blood in an orderly fashion. With so many factors involved, a variety of patient responses to drug distribution must be expected as the rule in the elderly patient.

Metabolism

Drugs are broken down to less toxic products as they are metabolized. In passing through the liver, as all absorbed drugs must, many are converted into water-soluble compounds so that they may be excreted via the kidney. Body changes that modify metabolism will leave drugs acting far beyond their planned time and result in toxic effects of accumulation. This is referred to as an increase in the half-life of the drug and is commonly seen in meperidine, barbituates, and tricyclic antidepressants, among other common medications for the elderly. Again careful monitoring is the only way to control toxicity, or its opposite, the lack of drug effectiveness.

Excretion

The elimination of the products of drug metabolism is equally important and definitely affected by the changes expected in aging. Since the kidneys are the major route for drug excretion, the decrease in the number of functioning glomerular tubules (up to 30%) in the elderly causes a decrease in the rate of excretion. This, in turn, allows an accumulation that may become toxic. Cardiac glycosides (digoxin), tetracycline, and sulfonamides represent this group of drugs.

The acid-base balance in the urine also plays an important role in the excretion of drugs. If a weakly acidic drug is given when the urine is strongly acidic, resorption in the tubules can occur, which will have the effect of giving a greater drug response than planned.

These physiologic considerations in the elderly may well be magnified by a variety of patient actions relative to their drug therapy. Ivey stresses four common problems when elderly patients are responsible for administering their own medications:

1. Failing eyesight makes for difficulty in reading labels.
2. Side effects may be forgotten or confused with symptoms of other conditions.

3. Carelessness in following the instructions relative to actually taking the medication.
4. Noncompliance with the drug regimen because of beliefs about medications (one study found that between 25% and 50% of outpatients completely failed to take their medication).

Among the medications apt to be prescribed during removable partial denture therapy, analgesics and sedatives deserve special mention. The elderly patient is more sensitive to drugs that act on the central nervous system. A progresssive age-related increase in relief of pain intensity with 10 mg morphine sulfate and 20 mg pentazocine has been reported.

Increased sensitivity to barbiturates may show a response that varies from restlessness to frank psychosis. There is a marked increase in the half-life of phenobarbital with clearance and distribution problems. The use of barbiturates is probably not worth the risk.

Among the principles written for prescribing for older adults, the following have special interest for the dentist:

1. Obtain a careful drug history from the patient's record (for those in institutions), or from the physician if dental medications are planned.
2. Titrate the dosage based on patient response.
3. Use smaller doses for the elderly.
4. Remember that drugs and combinations of drugs can cause illness.

Of those known to be responsible for the majority of adverse drug reactions, only aspirin is apt to be prescribed by a dentist relative to partial denture treatment in the older adult. It is effective to have an elderly patient monitored professionally, on a daily basis, during a postoperative period when aspirin is being given.

The dentist with older adult patients has an obligation to gain further knowledge in the pharmacologic aspects of medical treatment and to rely on physician and pharmacist in consultation for drug therapy in the elderly.

Nutrition changes

Oral health cannot be separated from general health where poor nutrition is involved. The elderly, for a variety of reasons, often have some form of malnutrition, often subclinical. The causes are usually related to economics but access to purchase food for the homebound may also be involved. Even when nutritional meals are provided, normal digestion and absorption may be greatly altered by disease, drug therapy, or both.

Inability to completely masticate food particles may play a important role in the enjoyment of eating, but it is unlikely that this is of great significance in the use of food. A number of studies have indicated that the volume of food an elderly individual consumes can be directly related to the ability to masticate comfortably and efficiently. Since many of the chronically ill, aged patients do not maintain their weight, the role of the nutritionist or dietician in institutional care is often greatly concerned with devising diets to keep the patient at a planned daily caloric intake, in addition to supervising levels of vitamins and minerals.

In as far as partial denture therapy can make mastication more comfortable and effective, we can contribute to the nutritional health of the patient. On the other hand, the elderly patient who continues to wear ill-fitting partial dentures may actually benefit by removing the dentures and switching to a softer diet. Relines, repairs, clasp adjusting, and the rebuilding of worn occlusal surfaces can often restore the effectiveness of a removable partial denture and may well be more practical than constructing new dentures for the older adult.

Nutrition and dental tissues

Fortunately, tooth structure is formed at the beginning of life and remains unaffected by the nutritional problems of old age. Soft tissues of the mouth and, in particular, those associated with the support of a denture base are affected by the general level of health as they respond to the stresses of partial denture wear. The following nutrition-related responses are of concern to us in the evaluation of soft tissue strength.

Fluid intake. Water (and its life-giving force) is really the keystone of health. It makes up roughly two thirds of body weight and is essential for normal function of *every* body process. In elderly patients we often find an easily disturbed water balance. A reduced fluid intake by the elderly is one way of combating the problem of frequent constant pressure to urinate. The dehydration that results not only leads to reduced cardiac output but to a dry mucosa as well.

Protein metabolism. The Food and Nutrition Board of the National Academy of Science formulates the Recommended Daily Dietary Allowances. For adults over 51 years, they give a protein allowance of 56 g for men and 46 g for women. The diets of many of the elderly are deficient in protein resulting in a potential for degeneration of connective tissue. Animal experiments have shown changes in gingival and periodontal tissues from this degeneration.

Fatty acids. Essential fatty acids are necessary to maintain good blood circulation. Some studies have shown that the rate of absorption of fat is slowed in the elderly and that lipemia may result. We would be wise to recommend to our patients that they spread out their fat intake to cover all three basic meals for the day to keep a steady absorption rate.

Minerals and vitamins. Although these elements are essential for the various chemical processes of the body, it is rare to find an actual intake deficiency in the modern diet. There may well be problems associated with absorption, metabolism, and excretion related to vitamins and minerals, which would affect the elderly patient, but a determination of these relationships is outside the realm of dental practice. Fortunately, research in trace element analysis has greatly expanded the ability of medicine to diagnose imbalance in these areas. In most major medical centers, specific analysis and counseling are currently available. It is likely that imbalances in mineral elements play a role in the development of chronic diseases.

Calcium and vitamin C are of special interest for the partial denture patient. Calcium, along with phosphorus and fluorine, plays a definite role in the maintenance of the bony tissues. Calcium, at a daily level of 1000 mg/day (preferably in the diet), is considered a minimum level for patients with osteoporosis and a good maintenance level for any elderly person.

Vitamin C, in large doses, is still controversial. Some clinicians have reported success with a regimen of 4 g/day for a month followed by 2 g/day for chronic soft tissue soreness under dentures.

Drugs and nutrition. Drug therapy, as stated earlier, is a major item in the management of acute and chronic disease in the elderly. Various drugs may greatly decrease absorption, usage, and excretion of nutrients and, as a result, render inadequate what appear to be the recommended nutritional levels. In addition, drug therapy often reduces appetite, which in turn exaggerates the effect of the drug on the patient's nutritional balance.

A nutritional analysis should be an integral part of the diagnosis and treatment planning phase of partial denture therapy. Although this may not always be practical in routine situations, elderly patients with constant soft tissue problems should be referred for nutritional analysis and, if indicated, supportive therapy.

CLINICAL CONSIDERATIONS

In every aspect of removable partial denture therapy, there are special considerations that should be made for the older patient. Although they will not all be a part of every patient's treatment, they should be considered an essential check list as treatment progresses.

Impressions

Rebound of soft tissues

Denture base tissues will be deformed by the wearing of existing partial dentures. When final impressions are made of tissue at rest, it will be necessary to keep the old dentures out of the mouth for some period of time before the impressions are made. The elderly patient will require *far* more time for tissue rebound than the younger patient. Even in a healthy, older mouth, 24 hours of tissue rest should be the minimum.

Protection of lips

Older tissues can be expected to be both dry and friable. The distension of the lips during impression procedures often results in cracked lips with hemorrhage. A liberal application of petroleum jelly is an essential preventive measure.

Tray selection and modification

As tissues age, they lose their elasticity. Trays may have to be modified (made smaller) to even get them in the mouth. Some compromise in the preliminary impression may be made, trying to capture minimum tissue coverage and then constructing "dainty" custom trays for final impressions.

Maintenance of airway

Even a partial obstruction of the elderly patient's airway during actual impression making may lead to panic, especially among those patients who do not fully understand what is happening. Allow the patient to assume the most comfortable body and head position for him even if this puts the clinician in an abnormal position. Use a minimum of impression material. Make a few practice runs with the tray so that the patient is fully aware of the sequence. Stay with the patients during the set of the material to constantly reassure them and to be available to remove excess material that might pass to the posterior of the mouth.

Stabilization of loose teeth

Since many patients can be expected to have some teeth that lack bony support, there is some risk of extracting them in the impression or, at a minimum, causing the patient discomfort during removal of the impression. These teeth can be temporarily splinted to adjacent teeth by placing any of the zinc oxide type of jaw registration materials interproximally. If placed on dry tooth surfaces, these materials will provide a temporary bond and can later be removed with ease.

Preparation of abutment teeth

Although dentin can be exposed with little fear of sensitivity or subsequent decay in the elderly patient, *special* attention must always be given to the potential for cervical caries. It is not unusual to have spontaneous horizontal crown fracture from unnoticed root decay. The reasons for the marked increase in cervical decay in the elderly are varied. Any change in salivary output is certainly suspect.

This type of decay can proceed so rapidly that teeth can be lost between annual recall visits, particularly if the elderly patient's hygiene procedures fail dramatically for any reason.

Every attempt to keep the margins of restorations, especially crowns, away from the gingival tissues must be made. When they are exposed, they are more easily reached during oral hygiene procedures and more easily examined for evidence of cervical decay.

Partial denture design

Simplicity should be the key to the design of the denture for the elderly patient. Precision attachments requiring coordination to insert and remove are not indicated. Retention should be minimal because it is not unusual to find the elderly patient unable to remove an overly retentive partial denture, especially as eye-hand coordination decreases in advanced age. When possible, Class V–like cavities should be cut into denture teeth, preferably first premolars, to provide purchase points for removal of the denture so that the patient will not put undesirable leverage on buccal retention clasp arms.

Jaw relation records and occlusion

Although interocclusal records for complete dentures are often difficult to make for the elderly because of their lack of muscle control and habitual patterns, those records for removable partial dentures should not be much different than for younger patients. *Special care* must be taken to not be aggressive in attempting to retrude the mandible. Even with an explanation, many older adults resent the dentist pushing on their jaw because they feel severe pain with what the dentist thinks is hardly any force at all. Better results can be obtained by slowly and repeatedly explaining and demonstrating on the dentist's own mandible just what is expected and then letting the patients retrude the mandible by themselves with only the lightest guidance.

Occlusal schemes should be simple without excessive contact or steep cusp guidance. Monoplane posterior teeth in the mandibular denture with 20-degree teeth in the maxillary denture will provide limited point contact and reduce frictional resistance to smooth nonmasticatory eccentric movements. Bilateral simultaneous contact in the second premolar–first molar area is to be desired, with anterior teeth and second molars out of contact when a mandibular removable partial denture opposes a maxillary complete denture.

Insertion of partial denture

With the routine partial denture patient, resin denture borders can be extended to the absolute limits of the denture-bearing area knowing that little damage can occur beyond minor soreness if the denture is actually overextended. With the older patient, concern over retarded healing of denture border trauma suggests a denture base that is *slightly* underextended. Previous denture experience is most likely to have been with bases giving less than ideal coverage, and a new denture with much greater base coverage is often objectionable to the patient.

Final denture borders and the internal surfaces of the denture bases must be carefully examined under good illumination to remove any sharp contours that might traumatize the tissues.

The elderly denture patient should *always* be seen 24 hours after insertion to eliminate the cause of any tissue trauma before ulceration can begin. The patient must be instructed to remove the partial denture if the mouth becomes sore and above all *not* to wear the denture during the first night. The combination of a lower pain response and delayed healing of soft tissue can quickly create a situation where the denture must be completely removed until complete healing occurs and the insertion procedures begun again. The nursing staff for the institutional patient must be alerted to examine the mouth of the chronically ill, compromised patient, who may not be aware of the trauma caused by the new denture.

Transitional partial denture

There will be many instances in the treatment of the partially edentulous older patient where the dentist will be tempted to give up on the remaining teeth and construct complete dentures, immediate or overdenture. The complete dentures may be well made in every way but the patient unable to adapt to them. Especially in the chronically ill and aged patient with few teeth remaining, every effort should be made to postpone to the end the extraction of the last tooth. Even in the presence of severe mobility, consideration should be given to maintain the tooth unless the patient is in pain, or if x-ray evaluation shows periapical disease. Often the aged patient will not adapt to complete dentures, particularly the lower, and will be unable to keep the lower denture in position in the mouth. Constructing a transitional denture so that teeth can be added to as teeth are lost can help the patient slowly adapt to the denture while there are still teeth remaining to provide support and stability against horizontal movement.

For the transitional denture to be successful, it must have all the features of the complete denture it may indeed become. Controversy exists whether to use wire occlusal and incisal rests in the transitional denture. It would seem that when a stable tooth with good bone support exists, it should help distribute vertical load. Mobile teeth with poor prognoses are best left without rests or locking denture contours that would luxate the tooth. The resin surfaces adjacent to the teeth should be highly polished with rubber points and pumice to remove roughness that would tend to hold plaque and debris.

The borders of the transitional partial denture should be those of a complete denture when possible. It may be possible to have a complete periphery with holes for the natural teeth if only a few remain. Where there are more remaining teeth adjacent to one another, the denture base will most likely *not* extend to the vestibule buccal to them.

The occlusal scheme should be that of a complete denture.

Remaining natural teeth that have extruded beyond the desired occlusal plane should be recontoured to reduce the disturbance in the plane. This reduction is usually possible without causing sensitivity because of the aging changes in the dentin and the pulp heights.

It is not intended that the transitional partial denture be overly retentive through the use of clasp arms. Wire clasp arms placed at the height of contour on selected teeth will give a great measure of lateral support without exerting undue torquing forces in function. Wire I-bar clasps are particularly effective in the transitional denture.

As the patient adapts to the transitional denture and becomes able to manage it in mastication, weak teeth can be extracted and easily replaced with denture teeth and flange contours when necessary.

It should be the deliberate effort of every dentist working with the older partially edentulous patient to see that the patient does not become totally edentulous in old age. Quality removable partial dentures, designed and constructed with the knowledge of the considerations and compromises in the elderly patient, coupled with the last resort of the transitional partial denture, can achieve this desirable goal.

REFERENCES

Anderson, R., and others: Two decades of health services, Cambridge, 1976, Ballinger Pub. Co.

Baum, B.J.: Research on oral physiology and aging. Chicago, Nov. 19-20, 1980, Symposium, American Dental Association Conference, The oral health care needs of the elderly.

Franks, A.S., and Hedegard, B.: Geriatric dentistry, Philadelphia, 1973, J.B. Lippincott Co.

Ivey, M.: Medication use in the elderly. In Carnavali, D.L., and others, editors: Nursing management for the elderly, Philadelphia, 1979, J.B. Lippincott Co.

Toga, C.J., Nandy, K., and Chauncey, H.: Geriatric dentistry: clinical application of selected biomedical and psychological topics. Lexington, Mass. 1979, D.C. Heath & Co.

BIBLIOGRAPHY

Behnke, J.A., and others: The biology of aging, New York, 1978, Plenum Press.

Hickey, T.: Health and aging, Monterey, Calif. 1980, Brooks/Cole Pub. Co.

Kiyak, H.A., and Brudvik, J.: Syllabus on geriatric dentistry, Seattle, 1981, University of Washington School of Dentistry.

Kutscher, A., and Goldberg, I.: Oral care of the aging and dying patient, Springfield, Ill, 1973, Charles C Thomas.

Langer, A.: Oral signs of aging and their clinical significance, Geriatrics **31**:63-69, 1976.

Massler, M.: Geriatric dentistry: root caries in the elderly, J. Prosthet. Dent. **44**:147-149, 1980.

Vestal, R.: Drug use in the elderly: a review of problems and special considerations, Drugs **16**:358-382, 1978

Index

B

D

Q

R

S

U

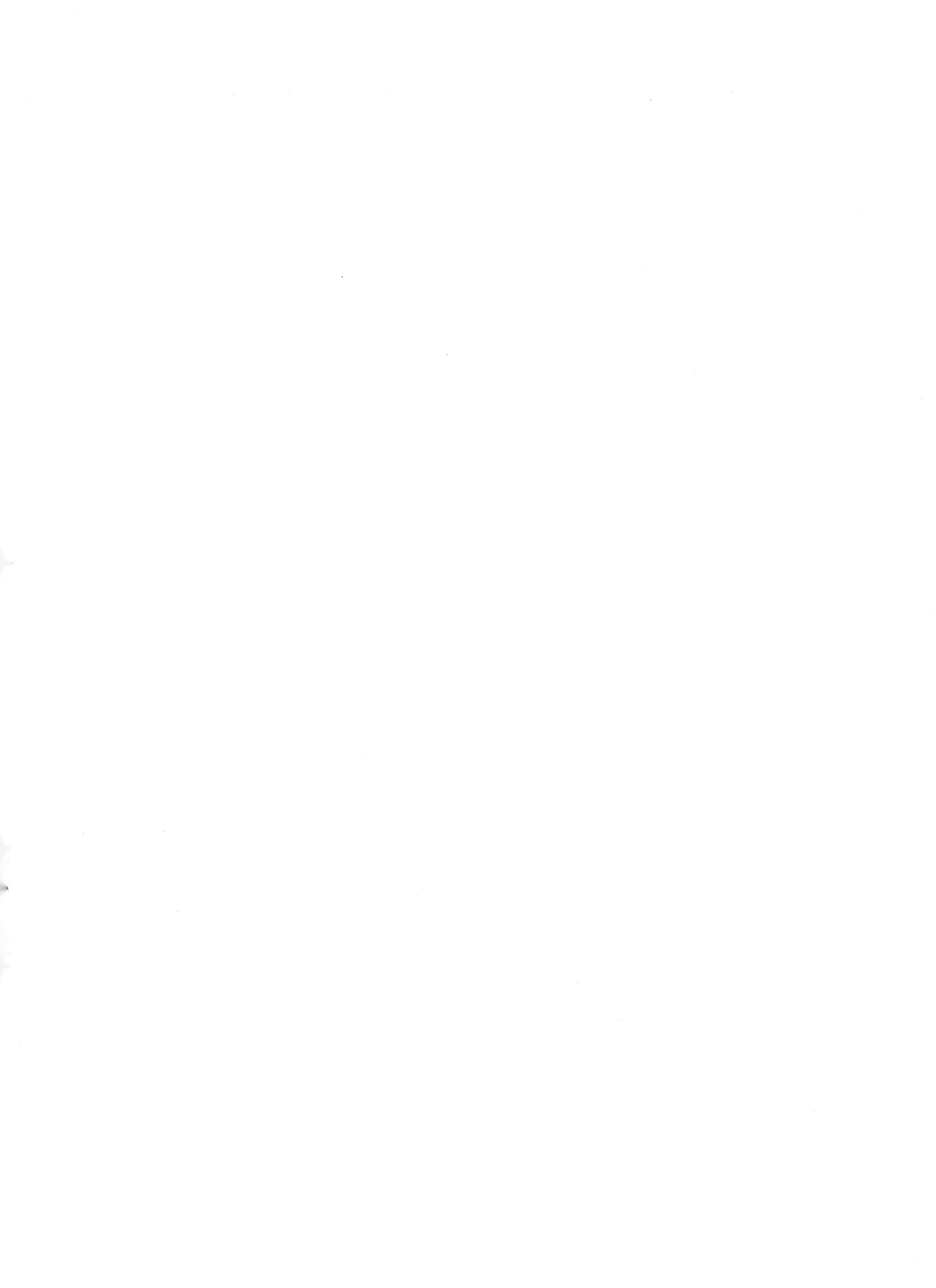